CONTENTS

Color Pill Atlas follows page xvi

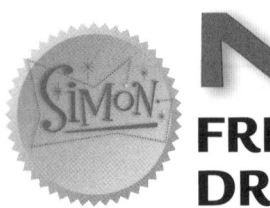

NEW!
FREE INTERNET DRUG UPDATES!

Your purchase of this book entitles you to receive our free online drug updates on SIMON. To help you keep pace with the constant changes in pharmacology, W.B. Saunders Company provides periodic drug information updates on our SIMON web site.

sign on at:

http://www.wbsaunders.com/SIMON/SaundersNDH

to be assured of receiving the most up-to-the-minute drug information including*:

information:

✔ *New drug entries*

✔ Brief *updates on other recently approved drugs*

✔ Names and brief descriptions of *new over-the-counter drugs*

✔ Drug alerts, including information about *drugs taken off the market*, significant *new uses, contraindications, dosage changes, and more...*

Visit our SIMON web site at
http://www.wbsaunders.com/SIMON/SaundersNDH today
to access this important information!

---

* Not every update will include each of these items. Information released by the FDA and other developments will determine the contents of each update.

SAUNDERS NURSING DRUG HANDBOOK 2003

BARBARA B. HODGSON, RN, OCN

Cancer Institute
St. Joseph's Hospital
Tampa, Florida

ROBERT J. KIZIOR, BS, RPh

Education Coordinator
Department of Pharmacy
Alexian Brothers Medical Center
Elk Grove Village, Illinois

SAUNDERS

An Imprint of Elsevier Science

Philadelphia / London / New York / St. Louis / Sydney / Toronto

SAUNDERS
An Imprint of Elsevier Science

The Curtis Center
Independence Square West
Philadelphia, Pennsylvania 19106

Saunders Nursing Drug Handbook 2003   **ISBN 0-7216-9565-5**
**Copyright 2003, 2002, 2001, 2000, 1999, 1998, 1997, 1996, 1995, 1994, 1993,
    Elsevier Science (USA). All rights reserved.**

Notice

Pharmacology is an ever-changing field. Standard safety precautions must be
followed, but as new research and clinical experience broaden our knowledge, changes in treatment and drug therapy become necessary or appropriate. Readers are advised to check the most current product information provided by the manufacturer of each drug to be administered to verify the
recommended dose, the method and duration of administration, and contraindication. It is the responsibility of the treating physician, relying on experience and knowledge of the patient, to determine dosages and the best treatment for each individual patient. Neither the Publisher nor the author assume
any liability for any injury and/or damage to persons or property arising from
this publication.

THE PUBLISHER

Vice President and Publishing Director, Nursing: Sally Schrefer
Editor: Robin Carter
Developmental Editor: Gina Hopf
Editorial Assistant: Jamie Randall

SH/RDC

ISSN 1098-8661

Printed in the United States of America.

Last digit is the print number: 9   8   7   6   5   4   3   2   1

To my daughter, Lauren, a true friend, for her unconditional love
To my son-in-law, Jim, always available to help, to talk
To my daughter, Kathryn, always supportive, always encouraging
And to my son, Keith, who is a source of great pride to us all.

Barbara Hodgson

To all health care professionals, who in the expectation of little glory or material reward dedicated themselves to the art and science of healing.

Robert Kizior

AUTHOR BIOGRAPHIES

BARBARA HODGSON

Born and raised in Michigan, Barbara was married and raising a young family in Chicago when she decided to fulfill a lifelong dream and become a nurse. After graduation, she started her own business as author and publisher of **Medcards, The Total Medication Reference Guide,** the first of its kind. These drug cards were designed to assist nursing students in understanding drug information to give knowledgeable care to their patients.

In 1981, she met co-author Robert (Bob) Kizior, who was teaching a pharmacology class. After class, Barbara approached him and asked if he would be interested in working on **Medcards** with her. He agreed, and together they became so successful that a few years later Barbara was able to fulfill another dream and move to Florida.

By 1987, Barbara was approached by W.B. Saunders and asked to author the **Saunders Nursing Drug Handbook.** Since then, Barbara and Bob have worked together on this handbook and on two more drug resources, the **Saunders Electronic Nursing Drug Cards** and the **Saunders Drug Handbook for Health Professions.**

Barbara specializes in oncology at the Cancer Institute, St. Joseph's Hospital, in Tampa, Florida. Barbara's daughter Lauren and her husband, Jim, are emergency nurses. Her daughter Kathryn is a research biologist. Her son, Keith, is a student and plans to become an emergency nurse.

Barbara's favorite interests are spending time with her very busy, tight-knit family and when she has a rare moment, getting her hands full of dirt working in her garden.

ROBERT (BOB) KIZIOR

Bob graduated from the University of Illinois School of Pharmacy and is licensed to practice in the state of Illinois. He has worked as a hospital pharmacist for thirty-two years at Alexian Brothers Medical Center in Elk Grove Village, Illinois—a suburb of Chicago. Bob is the Clinical Education Coordinator for the Department of Pharmacy where he participates in educational programs for pharmacists, nurses, physicians, and patients. He plays a major role in conducting Drug Utilization Reviews and is co-chair of the Medication Safety Subcommittee that is focused on identifying and preventing medication errors within the medical center. His hospital experience is diverse and includes participation in clinical pharmacy initiatives on inpatient units and in the surgical pharmacy satellite. Bob is a former adjunct faculty member at William Rainey Harper Community College in Palatine, Illinois. It was there that Bob first met Barbara and commenced their long-standing professional association.

An avid fan of Big Ten college athletics, Bob also has eclectic tastes in music that range from classical, big band, rock 'n roll, and jazz to country and western. Bob spends much of his free time reviewing the professional literature to stay current on new drug information. He and his wife, Marcia, and their two Labrador retrievers—Caty and Zak—enjoy escape weekends at their year-round lake house in central Wisconsin.

CONSULTANT REVIEWERS

Katherine B. Barbee, MSN, ANP,
  F-NP-C
Kaiser Permanente
Washington, District of Columbia

Marla J. DeJong, RN, MS, CCRN,
  CEN, Capt.
Wilford Hall Medical Center
Lackland Air Force Base, Texas

Diane M. Ford, RN, MS, CCRN
Andrews University
Berrien Springs, Michigan

Denise D. Hopkins, PharmD
Clinical Instructor of Pharmacy
  Practice
College of Pharmacy
University of Arkansas
Little Rock, Arkansas

Barbara D. Horton, RN, MS
Arnot Ogden Medical Center
  School of Nursing
Elmira, New York

Mary Beth Jenkins, RN, CCRN,
  CAPA
Elliott One Day Surgery Center
Manchester, New Hampshire

Kelly W. Jones, PharmD, BCPS
Associate Professor of Family
  Medicine
McLeod Family Medicine Center
McLeod Regional Medical Center
Florence, South Carolina

Linda Laskowski-Jones, MS, RN,
  CS, CCRN, CEN
Christiana Care Health Systems
Newark, Delaware

Denise Macklin, BSN, RNC, CRNI
President, Professional Learning
  Systems, Inc.
Marietta, Georgia

Judith L. Myers, MSN, RN
Health Sciences Center
St. Louis University School of
  Nursing
St. Louis, Missouri

Kimberly R. Pugh, MSEd, RN, BS
Nurse Consultant
Baltimore, Maryland

Regina T. Schiavello, BSN, RNC
Wills Eye Hospital
Philadelphia, Pennsylvania

Gregory M. Susla, PharmD, FCCM
National Institutes of Health
Bethesda, Maryland

STUDENT REVIEWER PANEL

Elizabeth Bartol
York College of Pennsylvania
York, Pennsylvania

Victoria Bird
Lincoln University
Jefferson City, Missouri

Amy Blaum
Southeastern Louisiana University
Baton Rouge, Louisiana

Misty ReNea Cheesman
University of Missouri
Sinclair School of Nursing
Columbia, Missouri

Susanna Cooke
College of St. Benedict
St. Joseph, Montana

Lisa Edmondson
York College
York, Pennsylvania

Wendy A. Foster, BS
University of Texas Health Science
    Center
San Antonio, Texas

Jacquie Frieke
Westmoreland County
    Community College
Youngwood, Pennsylvania

Juliet Fundora
Southeastern Louisiana University
Baton Rouge, Louisiana

Rachel A. Gerken
University of Missouri
Sinclair School of Nursing
Columbia, Missouri

Shayne M. Gray, RN, BSN
Intensive Care Nurse
The University of Arkansas for
    Medical Sciences Hospital
Little Rock, Arkansas
Former Nursing Student
College of Nursing
University of Arkansas for Medical
    Sciences
Little Rock, Arkansas

Jill Hall, RN
Pediatric Intensive Care Unit
Miller Children's Hospital
Long Beach, California
Former Nursing Student
Golden West College
Huntington Beach, California

Stelena N. Harrison
Seattle University
Seattle, Washington

Suzanne Heroux
Arizona State University West
Glendale, Arizona

Elizabeth Hoogmoed, RN, BSN
Valley Hospital
Ridgewood, New Jersey
Former Nursing Student
William Patterson University
Wayne, New Jersey

Akara Ingram
University of Missouri
Sinclair School of Nursing
Columbia, Missouri

Tammy F. Jones
Lexington Community College
Lexington, Kentucky

PREFACE

Nurses face many challenges in today's environment, not the least of which is familiarity with the large number of medications available. New medications are being introduced, and new applications, dosage forms, and different routes of administration for existing medications are increasing at a rapid rate. This voluminous amount of drug information must be integrated into the patient care environment quickly.

Saunders Nursing Drug Handbook 2003 is designed as an easy-to-use source of current drug information needed by the busy nurse. What separates this book from others is that it guides the nurse through patient care to better practice, and to better care.

This handbook contains:

1. **A fully updated and expanded IV Compatibility chart.** This handy trifold chart is bound into the handbook to prevent accidental loss.

2. **The Classifications section.** Presents the action and uses for some of the most common clinical and pharmacotherapeutic classes. Three *new* classes have been added in this edition—ACE inhibitors II, antimigraine (triptans), and proton pump inhibitors. Unique to this handbook, each class provides an at-a-glance table that compares all the generic drugs within the classification according to product availability, dosages, side effects, and other characteristics. Its green full-page color tab ensures you can't miss it!

3. **An attractive four-color atlas of medications.** Contains photographs of more than 100 of the most commonly used oral medications. The medications, both brand and generic, are shown in their different dosage forms. Just look for the blue full-page color tab to help you identify those medications presented to you sans prescription bottle or order! A 🖋 appears in the individual drug entries when there is a corresponding illustration in the atlas.

4. **An alphabetical listing of drug and herbal entries by generic name.** Green letter thumb tabs help you page through this section quickly. *New* to this edition, are full entries for 19 of the most commonly used herbs, each indicated with a green leaf 🌿. To make scanning pages easier each new entry begins with a shaded box containing the generic name, pronunciation, trade names, fixed-combinations, and classifications.

5. **A comprehensive reference section.** The reference section is updated, expanded, and contains one *new* appendix—Drugs of Abuse. The herbal therapies appendix has been expanded to include more than 40 entries. Other appendixes include vital information on poison

antidotes, calculation of doses, controlled drugs, FDA pregnancy categories, normal laboratory values, signs and symptoms of electrolyte imbalance, and techniques of medication administration.

6. **The New Drug Supplement.** We endeavor to include all of our drug entries in the A–Z portion of the handbook, but when the FDA releases a drug late in the season we include its monograph here to provide you with all the most current information. Each New Drug Supplement entry includes the class, action, use, routes, dosages, and side effects of the generic drug.

7. **The indexes.** *New* to this edition is a Therapeutic Treatment index, which allows the nurse to locate drugs appropriate for a broad range of clinical indications. Look for the full-page black tab to locate this resource. The general index is at the back of the book on light green pages. Undoubtedly the most comprehensive tool to help you navigate the handbook, the general index is organized by showing generic drug names in **bold,** trade names in regular type, classifications in *italics,* and the page number of the main drug entry listed first and in **bold.**

8. **A mini CD.** Saunders Nursing Drug Handbook 2003 has a Windows-compatible mini CD-ROM packaged in the back of the book. The software features 60 preformatted drug cards for commonly used medications. Users can print these portable drug cards in full color or black and white.

A DETAILED GUIDE TO THE SAUNDERS NURSING DRUG HANDBOOK

An intensive review by Consultant Reviewers and the Student Reviewer Panel helped us to revise the **Saunders Nursing Drug Handbook** so that it is most useful in educational and clinical practice. The main objective of the handbook is to provide essential drug information in a user friendly format. The bulk of the handbook contains an alphabetical listing of drug entries by generic name.

To maintain the portability of this handbook and meet the challenge of keeping content current we have also included additional information for some medications on a SIMON Internet site. SIMON also includes drug alerts (e.g., medications removed from the market) and drug updates (e.g., new drugs, updates on existing entries). Information is periodically added, allowing the nurse to keep abreast of current drug information. The drug entries with SIMON enhancement are indicated with a ✳ next to the generic drug name.

You'll also notice that some entries for infrequently used medications are condensed to reflect only the absolutely essential points the nurse should know when called upon to administer them. These abbreviated entries always include the generic name, pronunciation, brand names, classification, action, uses, precautions, interactions, availability, indications/routes/dosage, side effects, adverse reactions/toxic effects, and nursing implications. IV drug entries also include administration/handling, IV incompatibilities, and IV compatibilities information.

New to this edition is our treatment of IV information. A *new* IV Compatibilities heading for drugs administered by direct IV push, via Y-site, or via IV piggyback appears in every IV drug entry. We also incorporated the IV Incompatibilities heading ⊘. The drugs listed in this section are not compatible with the generic drug when administered direct by IV push, via Y-site, or via IV piggyback. We have highlighted the intravenous drug information with a special heading icon ⚕ and have broken it down by IV Storage, IV Reconstitution, and Rate of IV Administration. To aid in the care of volume-restricted patients, selected drug entries include a maximum concentration heading.

We revised the order of entries to follow the logical thought process that the nurse undergoes whenever a drug is ordered for a patient:

- What is the drug?
- How is the drug classified?
- What does the drug do?
- What is the drug used for?
- Under what conditions should you *not* use the drug?
- How do you administer the drug?
- How do you store the drug?
- What is the dose of the drug?
- What should you monitor the patient for once he or she has received the drug?
- What do you assess the patient for?
- What interventions should you perform?
- What should you teach the patient?

The following are included within the drug entries:

Generic Name, Pronunciation, Trade Names. Each entry begins with the generic name and pronunciation followed by the U.S. and Canadian trade names. Exclusively Canadian trade names are followed by a black maple leaf. Trade names that were most prescribed in the year 2000 are underlined in this section.

Do Not Confuse With. Drug names that sound similar to the generic and/or brand names are listed under this heading to help you avoid potential medication errors.

Fixed-Combination Drugs. Where appropriate, fixed-combinations, or drugs made up of two or more generic medications, are listed with the generic drug.

▶ **Pharmacotherapeutic and Clinical Classification Names.** Each full entry includes both the pharmacotherapeutic and clinical classifications for the generic drug. When available, the page number of the classification description in the front of the book is provided in this section as well.

Action/*Therapeutic Effect*. This section describes how the drug is predicted to behave, with the expected therapeutic effect given in *italics*.

Pharmacokinetics. This section includes the absorption, distribution, metabolism, excretion, and half-life of the medication. *New* to this edition are protein-binding percentages and information on the dialysis of each medication.

Uses/*Unlabeled*. The listing of uses for each drug includes both the FDA uses and unlabeled uses, which appear in *italics*.

Precautions. This heading incorporates a discussion on when the generic drug is contraindicated or should be used with caution. The cautions warn the nurse of specific situations in which a drug should be closely monitored. ▷ **Lifespan Considerations** includes the pregnancy category and lactation data as well as age-specific information concerning children and the elderly.

Interactions. This heading enumerates drug, food, and herbal interactions with the generic drug. As the number of medications a patient receives increases, awareness of drug interactions becomes more important. *New* to this edition is information on therapeutic and toxic blood levels in addition to the altered lab values that show what effects the drug may have on lab results.

Product Availability. Each drug monograph gives the form and availability of the drug and indicates whether the drug is obtainable by prescription (Rx) or over the counter (OTC).

Administration/Handling. Instructions for administration are given for each route of administration (e.g., PO, IM, rectal). Special handling such as refrigeration is also included where applicable. **IV administration** 𝕄 is broken down by storage (including how long the medication is stable once reconstituted), reconstitution, and rate of administration (how fast the IV should be given).

IV Compatibilities. *New* to this edition we've paired compatibilites with **IV Incompatibilities** ⊘ to give the nurse the most comprehensive compatibility information possible when administering medications by direct IV push, via a Y-site, or via IV piggyback.

Indications/Routes/Dosage. This edition we've expanded information on pediatric dosing in this section. Each full entry provides specific dosing guidelines for adults, the elderly, children, and patients with renal and/or hepatic impairment. Dosages are clearly indicated for each approved indication and route.

Side Effects. Side effects are defined as those responses that are usually predictable with the drug, are *not* life-threatening, and may or may not require discontinuation of the drug. Unique to this handbook, side effects are grouped by frequency and occurrence percentages so the nurse can focus on patient care without wading through myriad signs and symptoms of side effects.

Adverse Reactions/Toxic Effects. Adverse reactions and toxic effects are very serious and often life-threatening, undesirable responses that require prompt intervention from a health care provider.

Nursing Implications. Nursing implications are organized as care is organized. That is:

- What needs to be assessed or done before the first dose is administered? (Baseline Assessment)
- What interventions and evaluations are needed during drug therapy? (Intervention/Evaluation)
- What explicit teaching is needed for the patient and family? (Patient/Family Teaching)

Saunders Nursing Drug Handbook is an easy-to-use source of current drug information for nurses, students, and other health care providers. It is our hope that this handbook will help you provide quality care to your patients.

We welcome any comments you may have that would help us to improve future editions of the handbook. Please contact us via the publisher at *www.wbsaunders.com/SIMON/SaundersNDH.*

Barbara B. Hodgson, RN, OCN
Robert J. Kizior, BS, RPh

Acetaminophen/Codeine

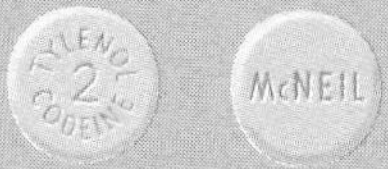

*Tylenol with Codeine
300/15mg: McNeil*

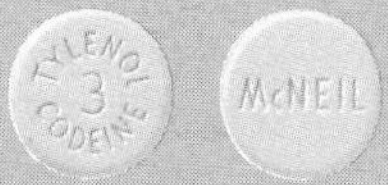

*Vicodin
500/5mg: Knoll*

*Tylenol with Codeine
300/30mg: McNeil*

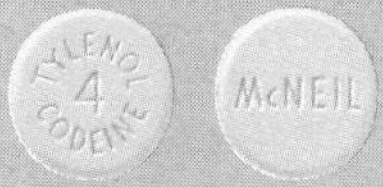

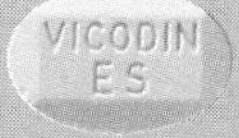

*Vicodin ES
750/7.5mg: Knoll*

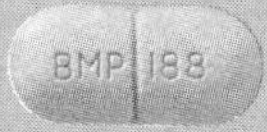

*Tylenol with Codeine
300/60mg: McNeil*

*Anexsia
650/7.5mg: Monarch*

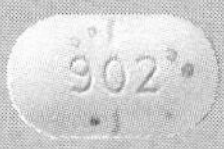

Acetaminophen/ Hydrocodone

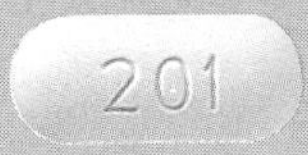

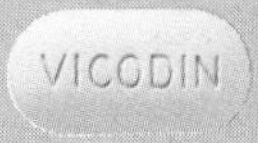

*Lorcet Plus
650/7.5mg: Forest*

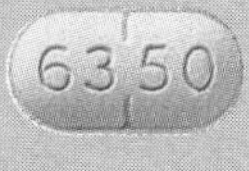

*Lortab
500/5mg: Whitby*

*Lorcet
650/10mg: Forest*

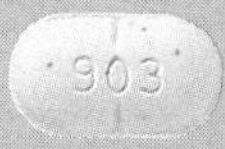

*Lortab
500/7.5mg: Whitby*

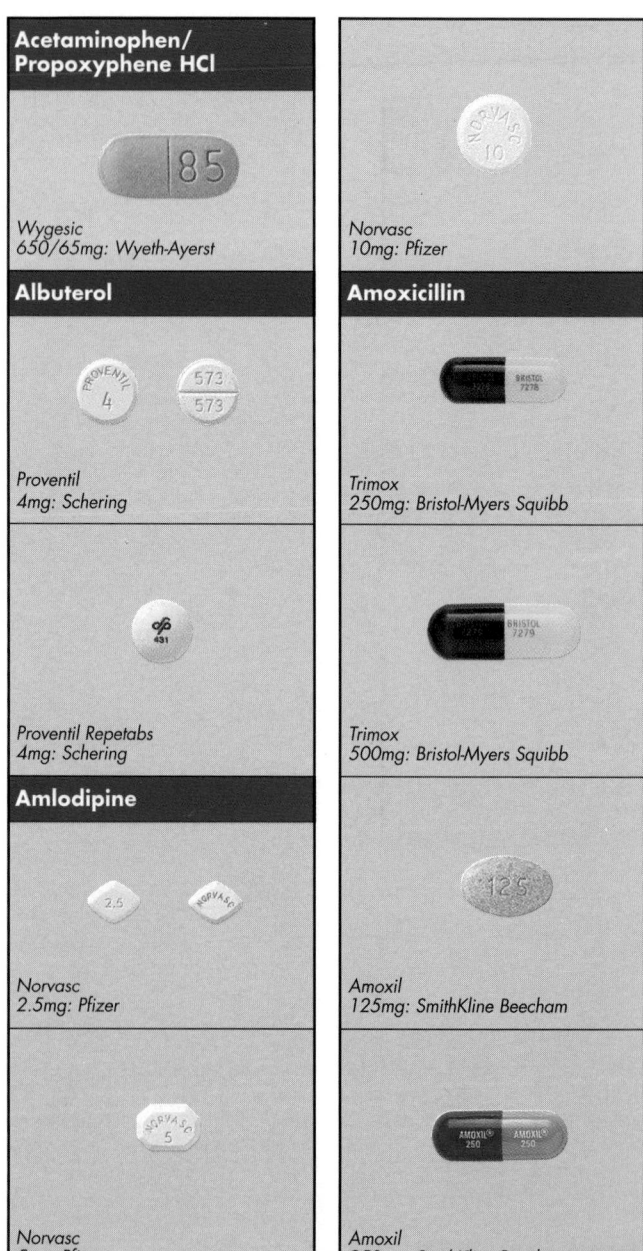

Acetaminophen/ Propoxyphene HCl

*Wygesic
650/65mg: Wyeth-Ayerst*

Albuterol

*Proventil
4mg: Schering*

*Proventil Repetabs
4mg: Schering*

Amlodipine

*Norvasc
2.5mg: Pfizer*

*Norvasc
5mg: Pfizer*

*Norvasc
10mg: Pfizer*

Amoxicillin

*Trimox
250mg: Bristol-Myers Squibb*

*Trimox
500mg: Bristol-Myers Squibb*

*Amoxil
125mg: SmithKline Beecham*

*Amoxil
250mg: SmithKline Beecham*

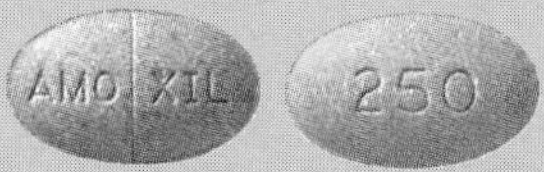

Amoxil
250mg: SmithKline Beecham

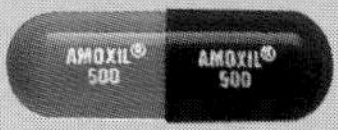

Amoxil
500mg: SmithKline Beecham

Amoxicillin/Clavulanate

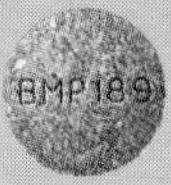

Augmentin
125/31.25mg: SmithKline Beecham

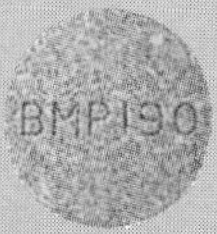

Augmentin
250/62.5mg: SmithKline Beecham

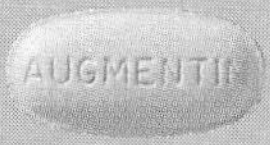

Augmentin
250/125mg: SmithKline Beecham

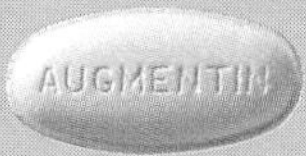

Augmentin
500/125mg: SmithKline Beecham

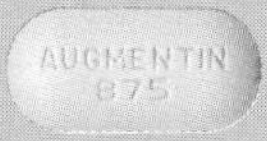

Augmentin
875/125mg: SmithKline Beecham

Azithromycin

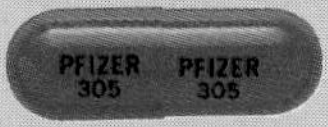

Zithromax
250mg: Pfizer

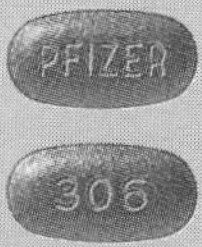

Zithromax
250mg: Pfizer

Cephalexin

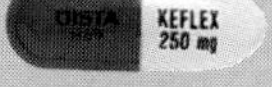

Keflex
250mg: Dista

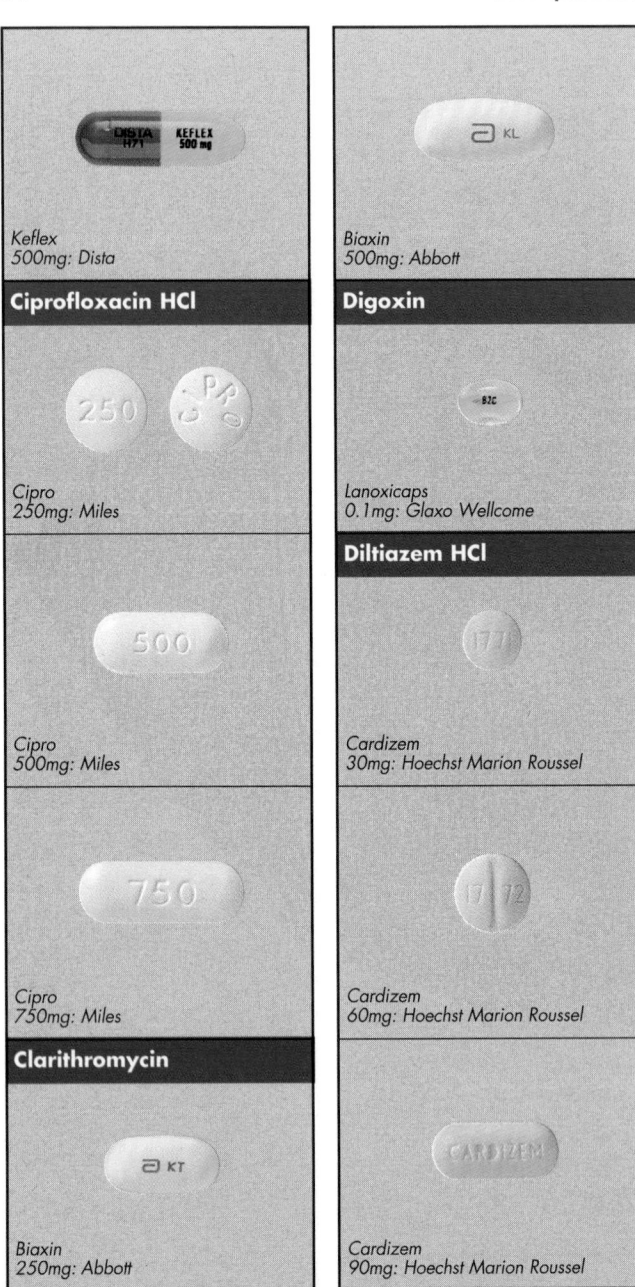

Keflex
500mg: Dista

Ciprofloxacin HCl

Cipro
250mg: Miles

Cipro
500mg: Miles

Cipro
750mg: Miles

Clarithromycin

Biaxin
250mg: Abbott

Biaxin
500mg: Abbott

Digoxin

Lanoxicaps
0.1mg: Glaxo Wellcome

Diltiazem HCl

Cardizem
30mg: Hoechst Marion Roussel

Cardizem
60mg: Hoechst Marion Roussel

Cardizem
90mg: Hoechst Marion Roussel

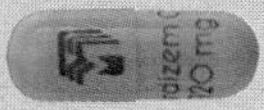

Cardizem CD
120mg: Hoechst Marion Roussel

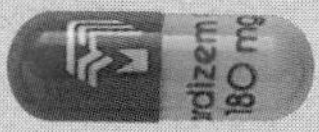

Cardizem CD
180mg: Hoechst Marion Roussel

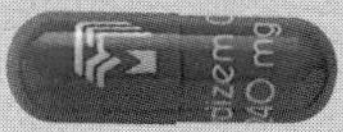

Cardizem CD
240mg: Hoechst Marion Roussel

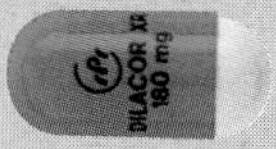

Dilacor XR
180mg: Rhone-Poulenc Rorer

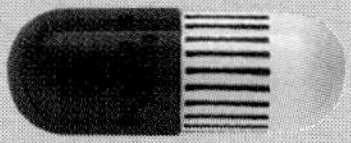

Dilacor XR
240mg: Rhone-Poulenc Rorer

Enalapril

Vasotec
2.5mg: Merck

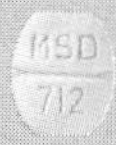

Vasotec
5mg: Merck

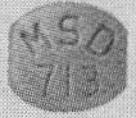

Vasotec
10mg: Merck

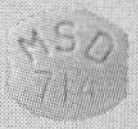

Vasotec
20mg: Merck

Estrogens, Conjugated

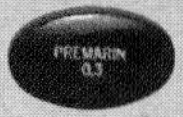

Premarin
0.3mg: Wyeth-Ayerst

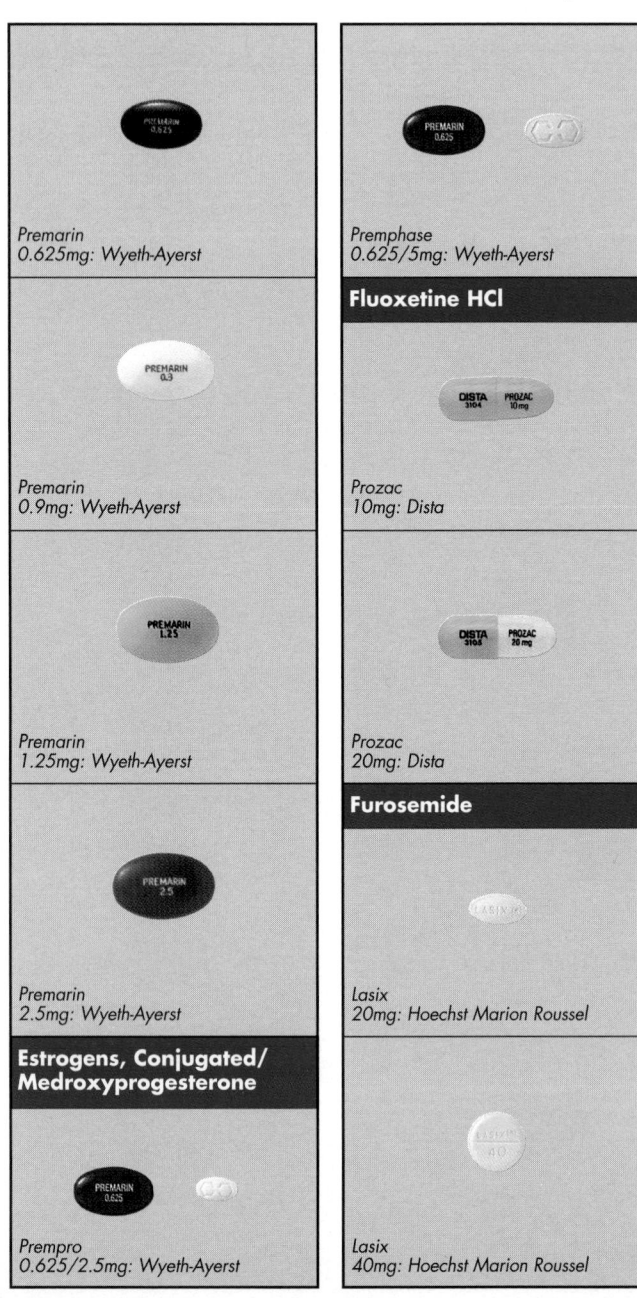

Premarin
0.625mg: Wyeth-Ayerst

Premarin
0.9mg: Wyeth-Ayerst

Premarin
1.25mg: Wyeth-Ayerst

Premarin
2.5mg: Wyeth-Ayerst

**Estrogens, Conjugated/
Medroxyprogesterone**

Prempro
0.625/2.5mg: Wyeth-Ayerst

Premphase
0.625/5mg: Wyeth-Ayerst

Fluoxetine HCl

Prozac
10mg: Dista

Prozac
20mg: Dista

Furosemide

Lasix
20mg: Hoechst Marion Roussel

Lasix
40mg: Hoechst Marion Roussel

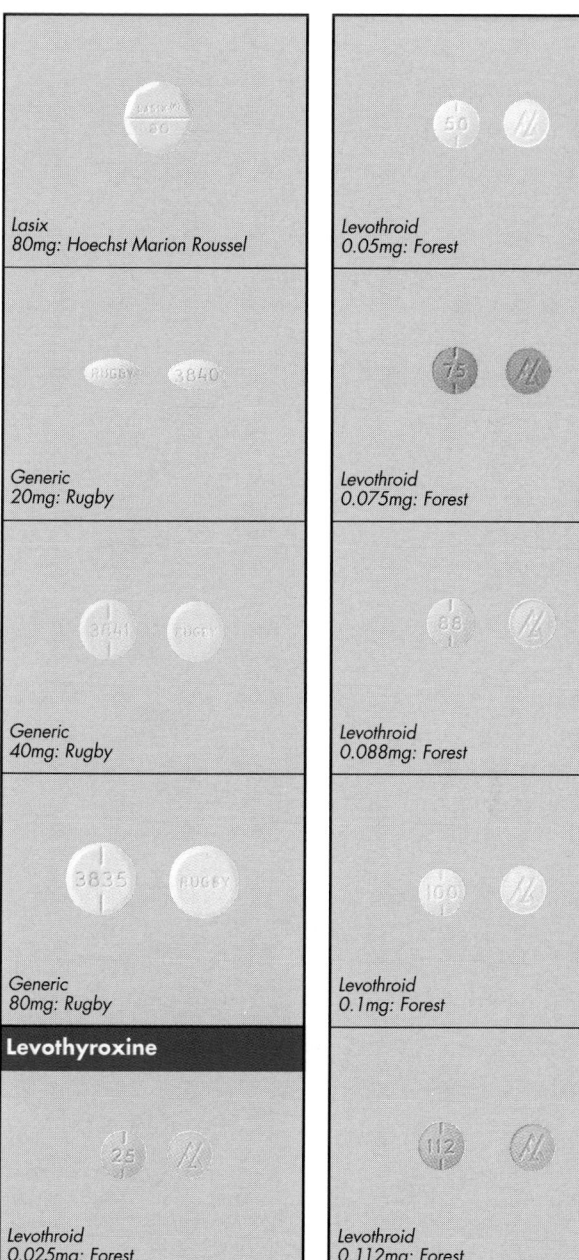

Lasix
80mg: Hoechst Marion Roussel

Levothroid
0.05mg: Forest

Generic
20mg: Rugby

Levothroid
0.075mg: Forest

Generic
40mg: Rugby

Levothroid
0.088mg: Forest

Generic
80mg: Rugby

Levothroid
0.1mg: Forest

Levothyroxine

Levothroid
0.025mg: Forest

Levothroid
0.112mg: Forest

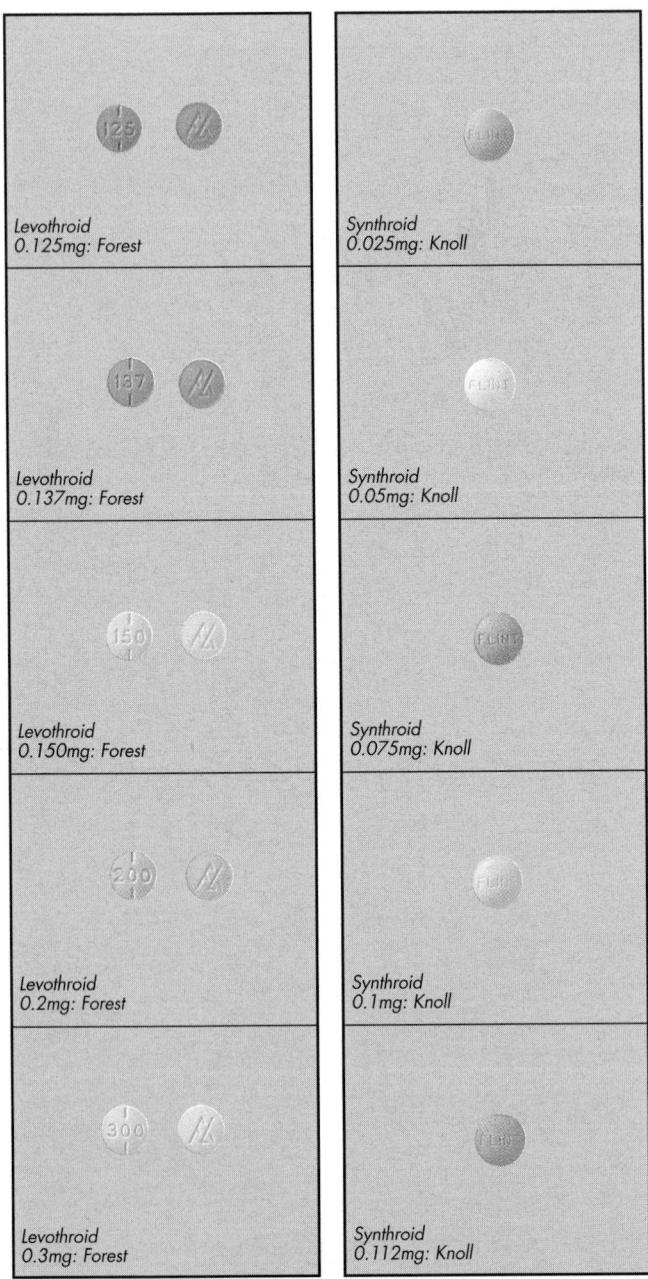

Levothroid
0.125mg: Forest

Synthroid
0.025mg: Knoll

Levothroid
0.137mg: Forest

Synthroid
0.05mg: Knoll

Levothroid
0.150mg: Forest

Synthroid
0.075mg: Knoll

Levothroid
0.2mg: Forest

Synthroid
0.1mg: Knoll

Levothroid
0.3mg: Forest

Synthroid
0.112mg: Knoll

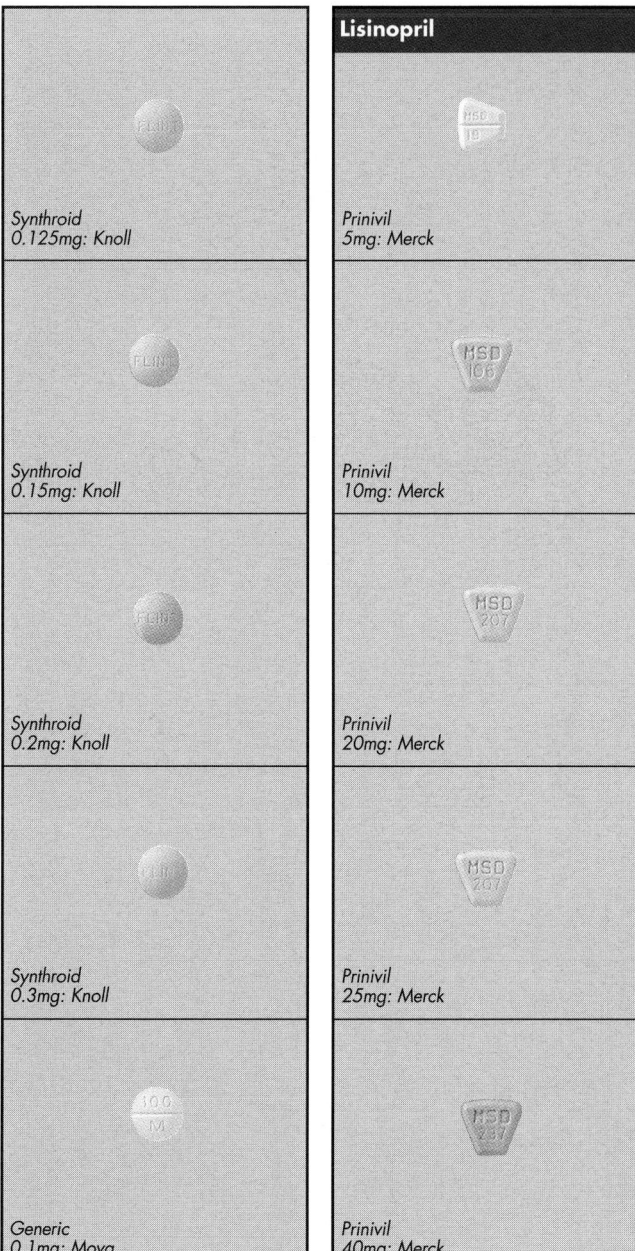

Lisinopril

Synthroid
0.125mg: Knoll

Prinivil
5mg: Merck

Synthroid
0.15mg: Knoll

Prinivil
10mg: Merck

Synthroid
0.2mg: Knoll

Prinivil
20mg: Merck

Synthroid
0.3mg: Knoll

Prinivil
25mg: Merck

Generic
0.1mg: Mova

Prinivil
40mg: Merck

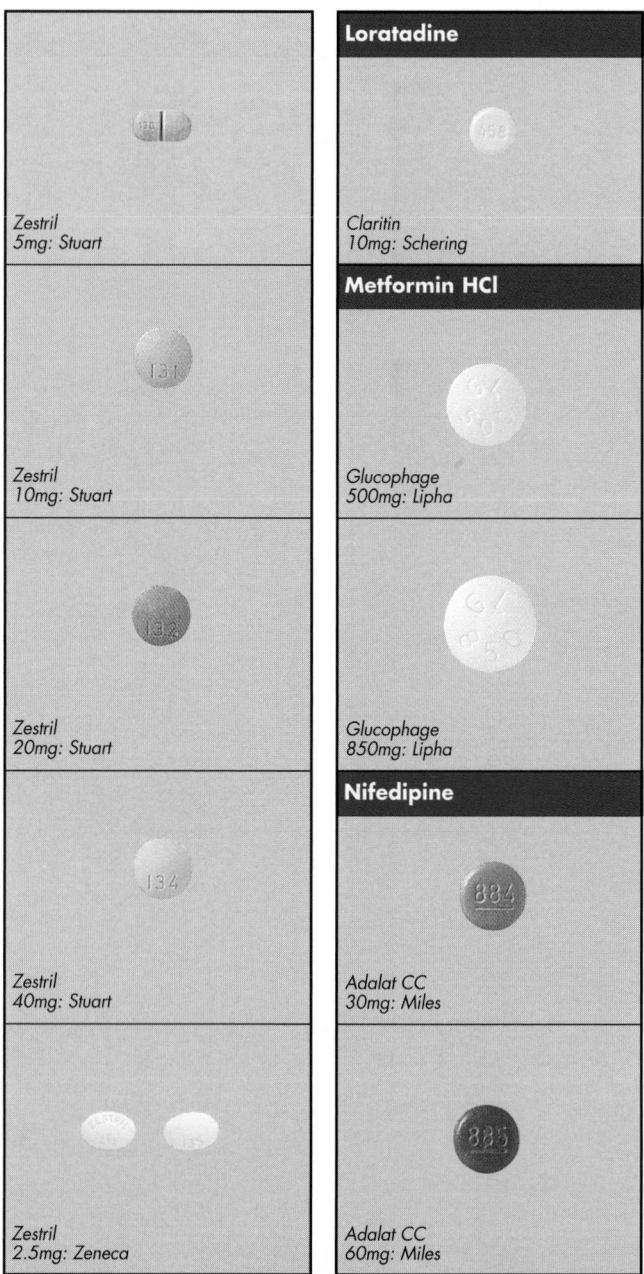

Zestril
5mg: Stuart

Zestril
10mg: Stuart

Zestril
20mg: Stuart

Zestril
40mg: Stuart

Zestril
2.5mg: Zeneca

Loratadine

Claritin
10mg: Schering

Metformin HCl

Glucophage
500mg: Lipha

Glucophage
850mg: Lipha

Nifedipine

Adalat CC
30mg: Miles

Adalat CC
60mg: Miles

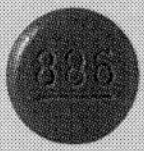

Adalat CC
90mg: Miles

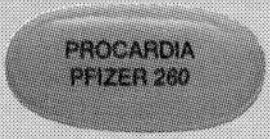

Procardia
10mg: Pfizer

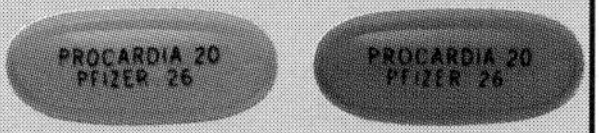

Procardia
20mg: Pfizer

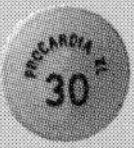

Procardia XL
30mg: Pfizer

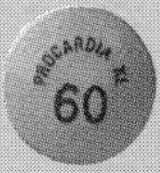

Procardia XL
60mg: Pfizer

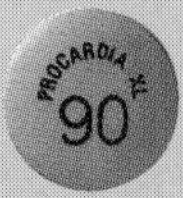

Procardia XL
90mg: Pfizer

Omeprazole

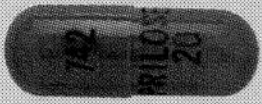

Prilosec
20mg: Merck

Paroxetine HCl

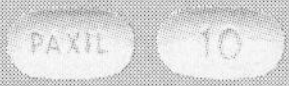

Paxil
10mg: SmithKline Beecham

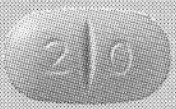

Paxil
20mg: SmithKline Beecham

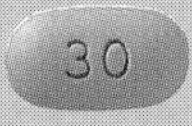

Paxil
30mg: SmithKline Beecham

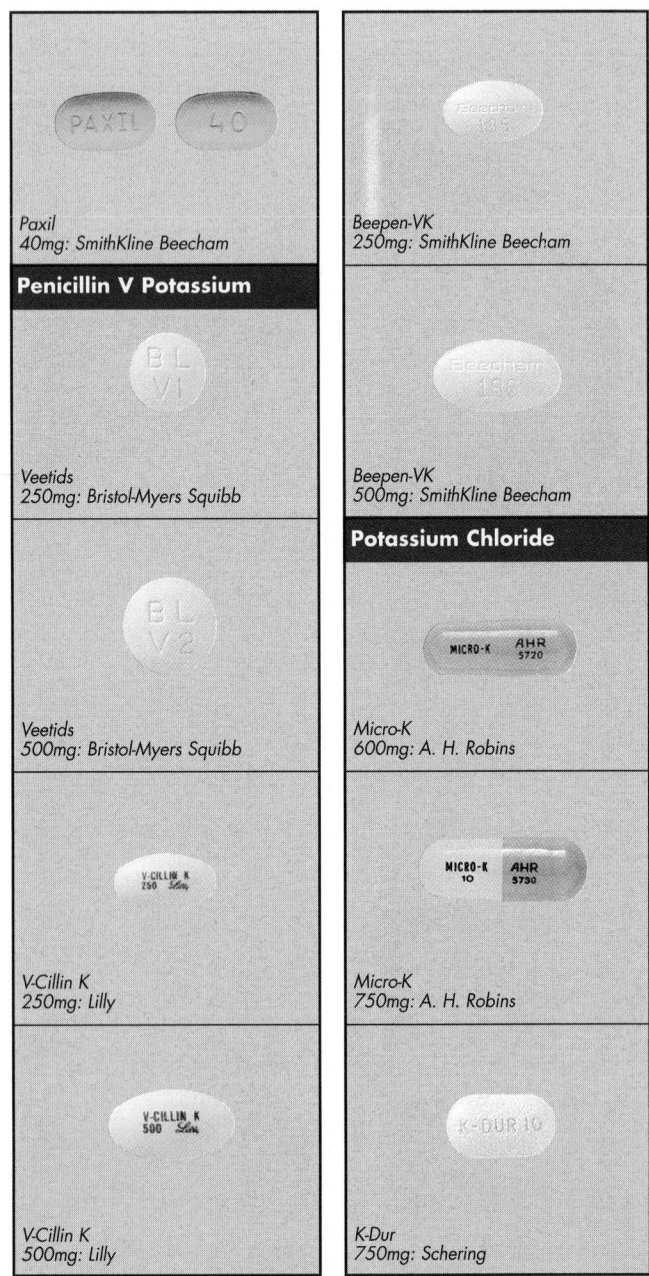

Paxil
40mg: SmithKline Beecham

Penicillin V Potassium

Veetids
250mg: Bristol-Myers Squibb

Veetids
500mg: Bristol-Myers Squibb

V-Cillin K
250mg: Lilly

V-Cillin K
500mg: Lilly

Beepen-VK
250mg: SmithKline Beecham

Beepen-VK
500mg: SmithKline Beecham

Potassium Chloride

Micro-K
600mg: A. H. Robins

Micro-K
750mg: A. H. Robins

K-Dur
750mg: Schering

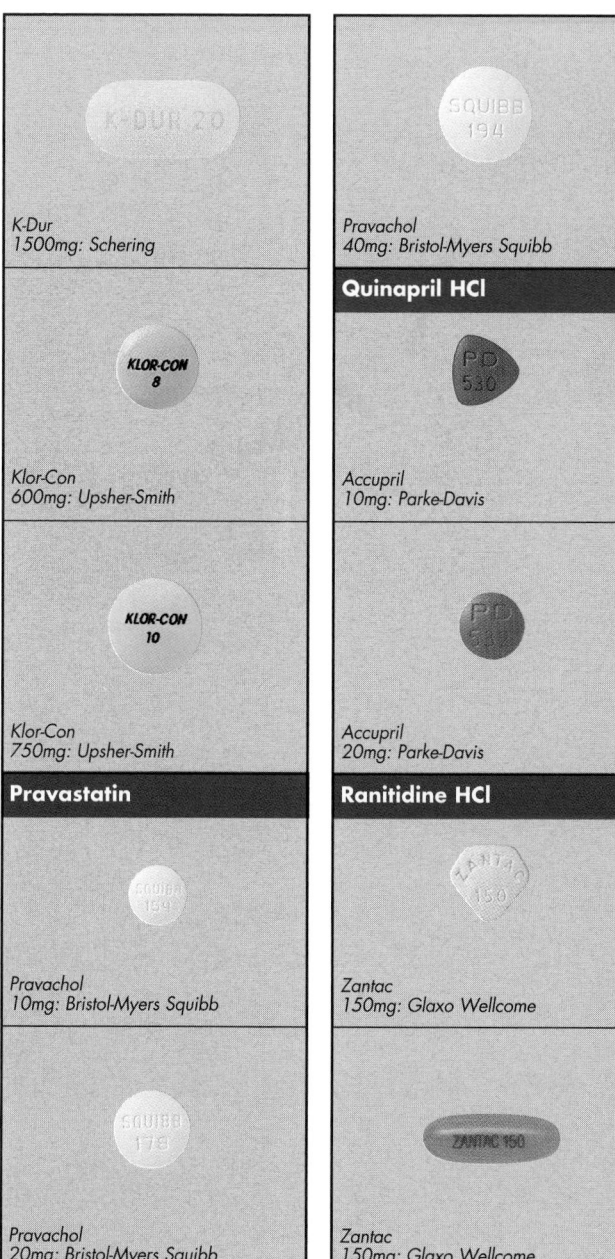

K-Dur
1500mg: Schering

Pravachol
40mg: Bristol-Myers Squibb

Quinapril HCl

Klor-Con
600mg: Upsher-Smith

Accupril
10mg: Parke-Davis

Klor-Con
750mg: Upsher-Smith

Accupril
20mg: Parke-Davis

Pravastatin

Ranitidine HCl

Pravachol
10mg: Bristol-Myers Squibb

Zantac
150mg: Glaxo Wellcome

Pravachol
20mg: Bristol-Myers Squibb

Zantac
150mg: Glaxo Wellcome

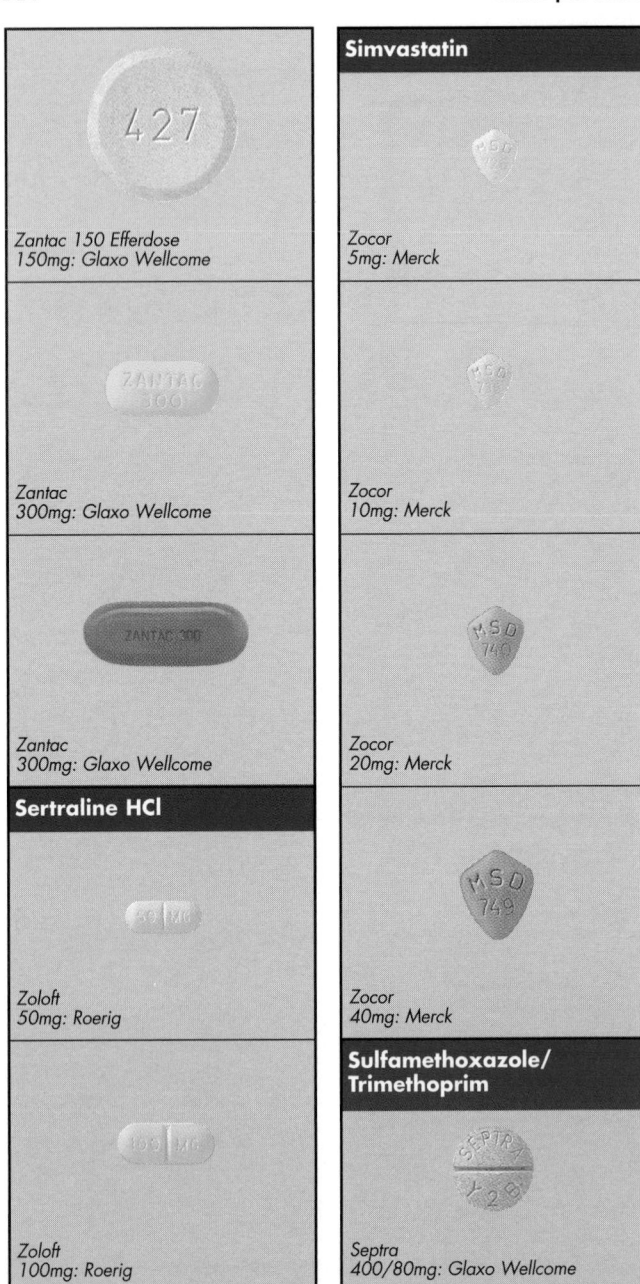

Zantac 150 Efferdose
150mg: Glaxo Wellcome

Zantac
300mg: Glaxo Wellcome

Zantac
300mg: Glaxo Wellcome

Sertraline HCl

Zoloft
50mg: Roerig

Zoloft
100mg: Roerig

Simvastatin

Zocor
5mg: Merck

Zocor
10mg: Merck

Zocor
20mg: Merck

Zocor
40mg: Merck

**Sulfamethoxazole/
Trimethoprim**

Septra
400/80mg: Glaxo Wellcome

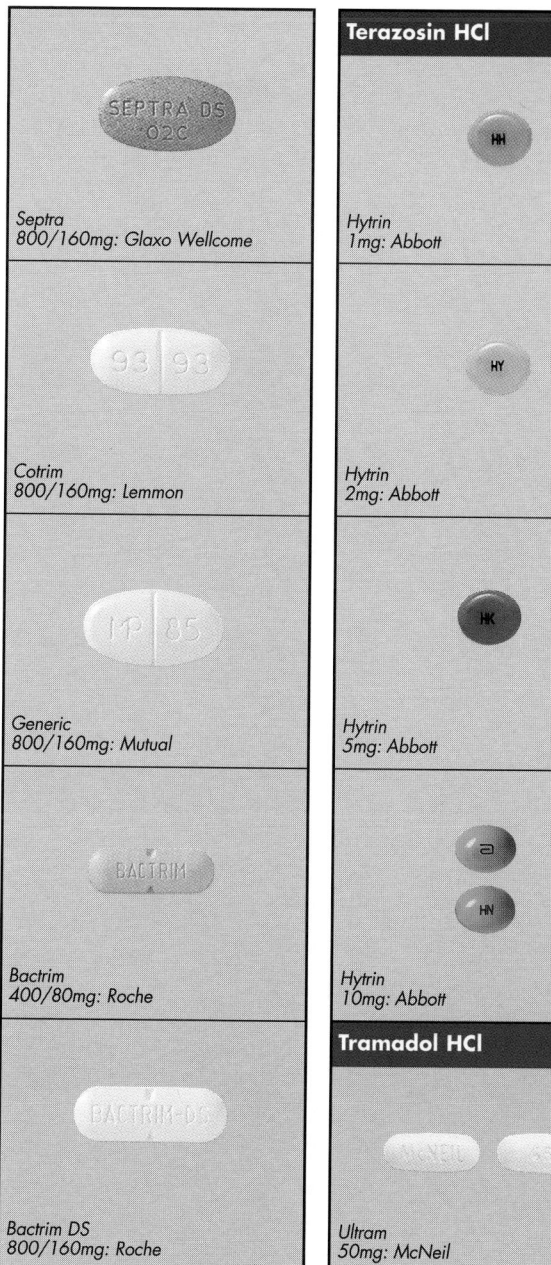

Septra
800/160mg: Glaxo Wellcome

Cotrim
800/160mg: Lemmon

Generic
800/160mg: Mutual

Bactrim
400/80mg: Roche

Bactrim DS
800/160mg: Roche

Terazosin HCl

Hytrin
1mg: Abbott

Hytrin
2mg: Abbott

Hytrin
5mg: Abbott

Hytrin
10mg: Abbott

Tramadol HCl

Ultram
50mg: McNeil

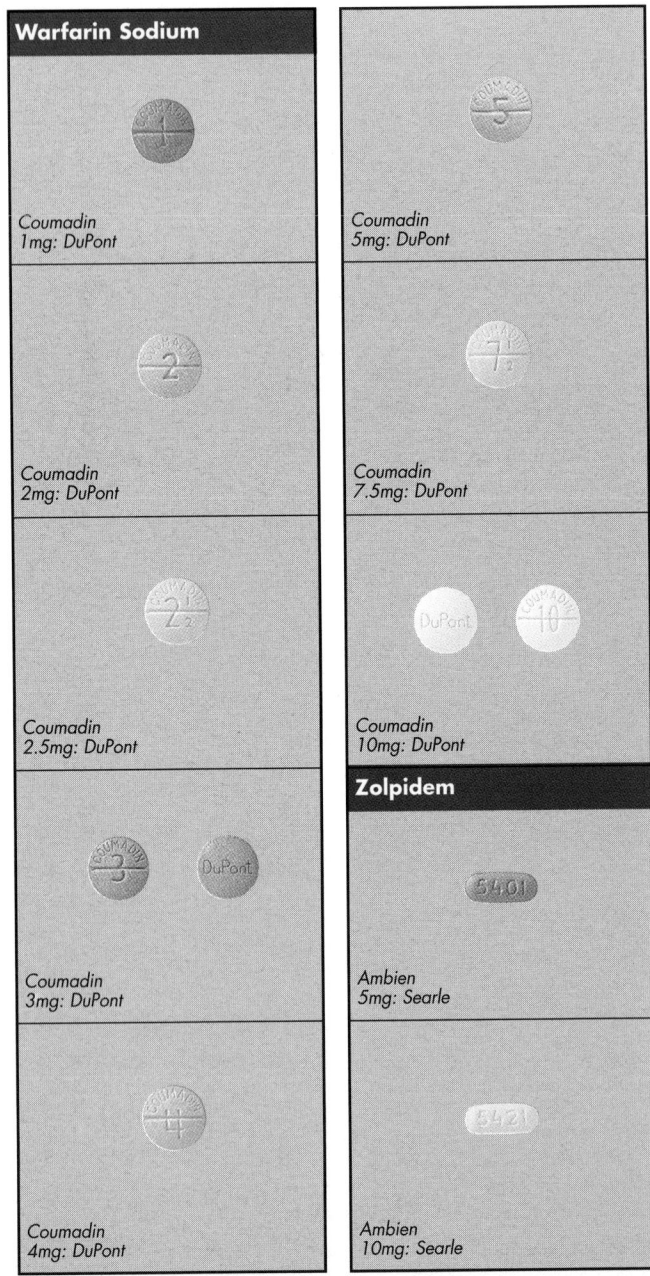

Warfarin Sodium

Coumadin
1mg: DuPont

Coumadin
2mg: DuPont

Coumadin
2.5mg: DuPont

Coumadin
3mg: DuPont

Coumadin
4mg: DuPont

Coumadin
5mg: DuPont

Coumadin
7.5mg: DuPont

Coumadin
10mg: DuPont

Zolpidem

Ambien
5mg: Searle

Ambien
10mg: Searle

ACKNOWLEDGMENTS

I offer a special heartfelt thank you to my co-author, Bob Kizior, for his continuing, superb work. Without Bob's effort in this major endeavor, this book would not have reached the par excellence it has achieved. We are indebted to Robin Carter, our nursing editor, for her consistent encouragement, and to Gina Hopf, our developmental editor, who kept such a close eye on this project, assisting our walk through the maze to final production. I thank my siblings, Milt, Bruce, Jane, Rich, Vance, and Greg, who have encouraged me through the years; Jim Witmer for all his knowledgeable input, motivation, and support; and Andrew Ross, who enlightens my family so dearly.

Barbara Hodgson

ILLUSTRATION CREDITS

Behrman RE (ed.): *Nelson Textbook of Pediatrics,* 15th ed. Philadelphia: WB Saunders Company, 1996.

Boothby WM, Sandiford RBL: *Boston Med Surg J* 185:337, 1921.

Kee JL, Hayes ER (eds.): *Pharmacology: A Nursing Process Approach,* 3rd ed. Philadelphia: WB Saunders Company, 2000.

Lehne RA: *Pharmacology for Nursing Care,* 4th ed. Philadelphia: WB Saunders Company, 2000.

Mosby's GenRx, 11 th ed. St. Louis: Mosby, 2001.

CONTENTS

Color Pill Atlas follows page xvi

Drug Classification Contents

Anesthetics: General

USES

IV anesthetic agents are used to induce general anesthesia. The general anesthetic state consists of unconsciousness, amnesia, analgesia, immobility, and attenuation of autonomic responses to noxious stimuli.

Volatile inhalation agents produce all the components of the anesthetic state but are administered through the lungs via an anesthesia machine. Agents for use include desflurane, sevoflurane, isoflu-

rane, enflurane, and halothane. They are used in practice to maintain general anesthesia.

ACTION

IV anesthetic agents: Most agents produce CNS depression by action on the GABA receptor complex. GABA is the primary inhibitory neurotransmitter in the CNS. Ketamine produces dissociation between the thalamus and the limbic system.

Volatile inhalation agents: Not fully understood, but may disrupt neuronal transmission throughout the CNS. These agents may either block excitatory or enhance inhibitory transmission through axons or synapses.

ANESTHESICS: GENERAL

Name	Availability	Uses	Dosage Range	Side Effects
Etomidate (Amidate)	**I:** 2 mg/ml	IV induction	0.2–0.6 mg/kg	Myoclonus, pain on injection, nausea, vomiting, respiratory depression
Ketamine (p. 628) (Ketalar)	**I:** 10 mg/ml, 50 mg/ml, 100 mg/ml	Analgesia, sedation, IV induction	1–4.5 mg/kg	Delirium, euphoria, nausea, vomiting
Methohexital (p. 720) (Brevital)	**Powder for injection:** 500 mg	IV induction, sedation	50–120 mg	Cardiovascular depression, myoclonus, nausea, vomiting, respiratory depression

Midazolam (p. 743) (Versed)	I: 1 mg/ml, 5 mg/ml	Anxiolytic, amnesic, sedation	1–5 mg titrated slowly	Respiratory depression
Propofol (p. 936) (Diprivan)	I: 10 mg/ml	Sedation, IV induction maintenance	0.5 mg/kg, 2–2.5 mg/kg, 100–200 mcg/kg/min	Cardiovascular depression, delirium, euphoria, pain on injection, respiratory depression
Thiopental (p. 1075) (Pentothal)	**Powder for injection:** 2.5% (25 mg/ml)	IV induction	Titrate vs. pt response. **Average:** 50–75 mg	Cardiovascular depression, nausea, vomiting, respiratory depression

I: injection.

Anesthetics: Local

USES

Local/regional anesthesia is selective for the surgical site. Epidural, spinal (intrathecal), IV regional, peripheral nerve block, topical or local infiltration can be selected. Local anesthetics prevent the initiation of electrical impulses necessary for spinal and peripheral nerve conduction.

ACTION

Most local anesthetics fall into one of two groups: esters or amides. Both provide anesthesia and analgesia by reversibly binding to and blocking sodium (Na) channels. This slows the rate of depolarization of the nerve action potential, and propagation of the electrical impulses needed for nerve conduction is prevented.

Anesthetics: Local *(continued)*

ANESTHETICS: LOCAL

Name	Uses	Maximum Recommended Dosage (mg)	Onset/Duration	Side Effects
Esters				
Chloroprocaine (p. 229) (Nesacaine)	Local infiltrate Nerve block Spinal	600–800	Fast/Short	Excitation (e.g., convulsions) followed by depression (drowsiness to unconsciousness), bradycardia, heart block, decreased contractile force, hypotension, hypersensitivity reaction
Procaine (p. 926) (Novocaine)	Local infiltrate Nerve block Spinal	400–500	Fast/Short	Same as above
Tetracaine (p. 1070)	Topical Spinal	100 (topical)	Slow/Long	Same as above
Amides				
Bupivacaine (p. 146) (Marcaine, Sensorcaine)	Local infiltrate Nerve block Epidural Spinal	175	Moderate/Long	Same as above
Etidocaine (Duranest)	Local infiltrate Nerve block Epidural	300	Fast/Long	Same as above

Levobupivacaine (p. 656) (Chirocaine)	Nerve block Epidural	—	Moderate/Long	Same as above
Lidocaine (p. 662)	Local infiltrate Nerve block Spinal Epidural Topical IV regional	300	Fast/Moderate	Same as above
Mepivacaine (p. 707) (Carbocaine, Polocaine)	Local infiltrate Nerve block Epidural	300	Moderate/Moderate	Same as above
Ropivacaine (Naropin)	Local infiltrate Nerve block Epidural Spinal	200	Moderate/Long	Same as above

Note: Most side effects are manifestations of excessive plasma concentrations.

Fast: <1 hr; Long: 3–12 hrs; Moderate: 1–3 hrs.

Angiotensin-converting enzyme (ACE) inhibitors

USES

Treatment of hypertension (HTN), adjunctive therapy for congestive heart failure (CHF).

ACTION

ACE inhibitors act primarily through suppression of the renin-angiotensin-aldosterone system. Produce a reduction in peripheral arterial resistance, an increase in cardiac output, and little or no change in heart rate.

Angiotensin-converting enzyme (ACE) inhibitors *[continued]*

ACE INHIBITORS

Name	Availability	Uses	Dosage Range (mg/day)	Side Effects
Benazepril (p. 111) (Lotensin)	**T:** 5 mg, 10 mg, 20 mg, 40 mg	HTN	**HTN:** 5–80 mg	Headaches, dizziness, fatigue, cough
Captopril (p. 165) (Capoten)	**T:** 12.5 mg, 25 mg, 50 mg, 100 mg	HTN CHF	**HTN:** 50–450 mg **CHF:** 12.5–450 mg	Insomnia, headaches, dizziness, fatigue, GI complaints, cough, rash
Enalapril (p. 395) (Vasotec)	**T:** 2.5 mg, 5 mg, 10 mg, 20 mg **IV:** 1.25 mg/ml	HTN CHF	**HTN:** 10–40 mg **(IV:** 1.25 mg q6h) **CHF:** 5–20 mg	Chest pain, hypotension, headaches, fatigue, dizziness
Fosinopril (p. 496) (Monopril)	**T:** 10 mg, 20 mg, 40 mg	HTN CHF	**HTN:** 10–80 mg **CHF:** 20–40 mg	Hypotension, nausea, vomiting, cough
Lisinopril (p. 668) (Prinivil, Zestril)	**T:** 2.5 mg, 5 mg, 10 mg, 20 mg, 40 mg	HTN CHF	**HTN:** 10–40 mg **CHF:** 5–20 mg	Chest pain, hypotension, headaches, dizziness, fatigue, diarrhea
Moexipril (p. 760) (Univasc)	**T:** 7.5 mg, 15 mg	HTN	**HTN:** 7.5–30 mg	Dizziness, fatigue, diarrhea, cough
Perindopril (p. 879) (Aceon)	**T:** 2 mg, 4 mg, 6 mg	HTN	**HTN:** 4–16 mg	Hypotension, dizziness, fatigue, syncope, cough
Quinapril (p. 954) (Accupril)	**T:** 5 mg, 10 mg, 20 mg, 40 mg	HTN CHF	**HTN:** 10–80 mg **CHF:** 10–40 mg	Chest pain, hypotension, headaches, dizziness, fatigue, diarrhea, nausea, vomiting, cough
Ramipril (p. 963) (Altace)	**C:** 1.25 mg, 2.5 mg, 5 mg, 10 mg	HTN CHF	**HTN:** 2.5–20 mg **CHF:** 1.25–10 mg	Hypotension, headaches, dizziness, cough
Trandolapril (p. 1112) (Mavik)	**T:** 1 mg, 2 mg, 4 mg	HTN CHF	**HTN:** 1–4 mg **CHF:** 1–4 mg	Dizziness, dyspepsia, cough, asthenia, syncope, myalgia

C: capsules; **CHF:** congestive heart failure; **HTN:** hypertension; **IV:** intravenous; **T:** tablets.

Angiotensin II Receptor Antagonists

USES

Treatment of hypertension (HTN) alone or in combination with other antihypertensives.

ACTION

Angiotensin II receptor antagonists (AIIRA) block vasoconstrictor and aldosterone-secreting effects on angiotensin II by selectively blocking the binding of angiotensin II to AT_1 receptors in vascular smooth muscle and adrenal gland, causing vasodilation and decrease in aldosterone effects.

ANGIOTENSIN II RECEPTOR ANTAGONISTS

Name	Availability	Uses	Dosage Range (mg/day)	Side Effects
Candesartan (p. 161) (Atacand)	**T:** 4 mg, 8 mg, 16 mg, 32 mg	HTN	2–32 mg	Headaches, upper respiratory tract infections, pain, dizziness
Eprosartan (p. 409) (Teveten)	**T:** 400 mg, 600 mg	HTN	400–800 mg	Headaches, upper respiratory tract infections, myalgia
Irbesartan (p. 608) (Avapro)	**T:** 75 mg, 150 mg, 300 mg	HTN	75–300 mg	Headaches, upper respiratory tract infections
Losartan (p. 683) (Cozaar	**T:** 25 mg, 50 mg, 100 mg	HTN	25–100 mg	Dizziness, headaches, upper respiratory tract infections, diarrhea, fatigue, cough
Telmisartan (p. 1053) (Micardis)	**T:** 40 mg, 80 mg	HTN	20–80 mg	Upper respiratory tract infections, dizziness, back pain, sinusitis, diarrhea
Valsartan (p. 1143) (Diovan)	**T:** 80 mg, 160 mg	HTN	80–320 mg	Dizziness, headaches, upper respiratory tract infections, diarrhea, fatigue

HTN: hypertension; **T:** tablets.

Antacids

USES

Relief of symptoms associated with hyperacidity (e.g., heartburn, acid indigestion, sour stomach), hyperacidity associated with gastric/duodenal ulcers, treatment of pathological gastric hypersecretion associated with Zollinger-Ellison syndrome, symptomatic treatment of gastroesophageal reflux disease (GERD), prevention and treatment of upper GI stress-induced ulceration and bleeding (especially in ICU).

Aluminum carbonate and hydroxide in conjunction with a low-phosphate diet to reduce elevated phosphate in pts with renal insufficiency. Calcium for calcium deficiency, magnesium for magnesium deficiency.

ACTION

Act primarily in the stomach to neutralize gastric acid (increase pH). Antacids do not have a direct effect on acid output. The ability to increase pH depends on the dose, dosage form used, presence or absence of food in the stomach, and acid neutralizing capacity (ANC). ANC is the number of mEq of hydrochloric acid that can be neutralized by a particular weight or volume of antacid.

Reduce elevated phosphate by binding with phosphate in the intestine to form an insoluble complex, which is then eliminated.

ANTACIDS

Antacid	Brand Names	Availability	Dosage Range	Side Effects
Aluminum				
Carbonate (p. 37)	Basaljel	**T, C:** 608 mg **S:** 400 mg/5 ml	2 **T** or **C** or 10 ml **S** up to 12 times/day	Chalky taste, mild constipation, stomach cramps *Long-term use:* Neurotoxicity in dialysis pts, hypercalcemia, osteoporosis *Large doses:* Fecal impaction, swelling of feet/legs

| Hydroxide (p. 37) | Amphojel, AluTab, Dialume | **T:** 300 mg, 500 mg, 600 mg
C: 500 mg | 500–1500 mg 3–6 times/day | Same as above |

Calcium

| Carbonate (p. 157) | Tums, Maalox, Antacid | **T (chewable):** 500 mg, 750 mg, 1,000 mg | 500–1,500 mg as needed | Chalky taste
Large doses: Fecal impaction, swelling of feet/legs, metabolic alkalosis
Long-term use: Difficult/painful urination |

Magnesium

| Hydroxide (p. 689) | Milk of Magnesia | **T (chewable):** 311 mg
L: 400 mg/5 ml, 800 mg/5 ml | **T:** 622–1,244 mg up to 4 times/day
L: 2.5–7.5 ml up to 4 times/day | Chalky taste, diarrhea, laxative effect, electrolyte imbalance (dizziness, irregular heartbeat, fatigue) |
| Oxide (p. 689) | Mag-Ox 400, Maox 420 | **T:** 400, 420, 500 mg | 400–800 mg/day | Same as above |

C: capsules; **L:** liquid; **S:** suspension; **T:** tablets.

Antianxiety

USES

Treatment of anxiety. Additionally, some benzodiazepines are used as hypnotics, anticonvulsants to prevent delirium tremens during alcohol withdrawal and as adjunctive therapy for relaxation of skeletal muscle spasms. Midazolam, a short-acting benzodiazepine, is used for preoperative sedation and relief of anxiety for short diagnostic endoscopic procedures (see individual monograph for midazolam).

Antianxiety [continued]

ACTION

Benzodiazepines are the largest and most frequently prescribed group of antianxiety agents. The exact mechanism is unknown but may increase the inhibiting effect of gamma-aminobutyric acid (GABA), which inhibits nerve impulse transmission by binding to specific benzodiazepine receptors in various areas of the central nervous system (CNS).

ANTIANXIETY

Name	Availability	Uses	Dosage Range (mg/day)	Side Effects
Alprazolam (p. 31) (Xanax)	**T:** 0.25 mg, 0.5 mg, 1 mg, 2 mg **S:** 0.5 mg/5 ml, 1 mg/ml	Anxiety, panic disorder	0.75–10 mg	Drowsiness, weakness or fatigue, ataxia, slurred speech, confusion, lack of coordination, impaired memory, paradoxical agitation, dizziness, nausea
Chlordiazepoxide (p. 227) (Librium, Libritabs)	**C:** 5 mg, 10 mg, 25 mg **T:** 10 mg, 25 mg **I:** 100 mg	Anxiety, alcohol withdrawal	5–300 mg	Same as above
Clonazepam (p. 260) (Klonopin)	**T:** 0.5 mg, 1 mg, 2 mg	Anticonvulsant, panic disorder	1–6 mg	Same as above
Clorazepate (p. 265) (Tranxene)	**C:** 3.75 mg, 7.5 mg, 15 mg **SD:** 11.25 mg, 22.5 mg	Anxiety, alcohol withdrawal, anticonvulsant	7.5–90 mg	Same as above

Diazepam (p. 334) (Valium)	**T:** 2.5 mg, 5 mg, 10 mg **S:** 5 mg/5 ml, 5 mg/ml **I:** 5 mg/ml	Anxiety, alcohol withdrawal, anticonvulsant, muscle relaxant	2–40 mg	Same as above
Lorazepam (p. 681) (Ativan)	**T:** 0.5 mg, 1 mg, 2 mg **S:** 2 mg/ml **I:** 2 mg/ml, 4 mg/ml	Anxiety	0.5–10 mg	Same as above
Oxazepam (p. 844) (Serax)	**C:** 10 mg, 15 mg, 30 mg **T:** 15 mg	Anxiety, alcohol withdrawal	30–120 mg	Same as above

C: capsules; **I:** injection; **S:** solution; **SD:** single dose; **T:** tablets.

Antiarrhythmics

USES

Prevention and treatment of cardiac arrhythmias, such as premature ventricular contractions, ventricular tachycardia, premature atrial contractions, paroxysmal atrial tachycardia, atrial fibrillation and flutter.

ACTION

The antiarrhythmics are divided into four classes based on their effects on certain ion channels and/or receptors located on the myocardial cell membrane. Class I is further divided into three subclasses (1A, 1B, 1C) based on electrophysiologic effects.

Class I: Block cardiac sodium channels and slow conduction velocity, prolonging refractoriness and decreasing automaticity of sodium-dependent tissue.

Class IA: Block sodium and potassium channels.

Class IB: Shorten the repolarization phase.

Class IC: No effect on repolarization phase, but slow conduction velocity.

Class II: Slow the sinus and atrioventricular (AV) nodal conduction.

Class III: Block cardiac potassium channels, prolonging the repolarization phase of electrical cells.

Class IV: Inhibit the influx calcium through its channels, causing slower conduction through the sinus and AV nodes

Antiarrhythmics [continued]

ANTIARRHYTHMICS

Name	Availability	Uses	Dosage Range	Side Effects
Class IA				
Disopyramide (p. 362) (Norpace SR, Norpace CR)	**C:** 100 mg, 150 mg **C (ER):** 100 mg, 150 mg	AF, WPW, PSVT, PVCs, VT	400–800 mg/day	Dry mouth, blurred vision, urinary retention, CHF, proarrhythmia
Procainamide (p. 923) (Pronestyl, Pronestyl SR, Procan SR)	**T:** 250 mg, 375 mg, 500 mg **C:** 250 mg, 375 mg, 500 mg **T (SR):** 250 mg, 500 mg, 750 mg, 1,000 mg **I:** 100 mg/ml, 500 mg/ml	AF, WPW, PVCs, VT	**A (PO):** 250–500 mg q3h **(ER):** 250–750 mg q6h	Hypotension, fever, agranulocytosis, SLE, headaches, proarrhythmia
Quinidine (p. 956) (Quinidex, Quinaglute)	**T:** 200 mg, 300 mg **T (ER):** 300 mg, 324 mg **I:** 80 mg/ml	AF, WPW, PVCs, VT	**A:** 200–600 mg q2–4h **(ER):** 300–600 mg q8h	Diarrhea, hypotension, nausea, vomiting, cinchonism, fever, thrombocytopenia, proarrhythmia
Class 1B				
Lidocaine (p. 662) (Xylocaine)	**I:** 300 mg for IM **IV Infusion:** 2 mg/ml, 4 mg/ml	PVCs, VT, VF	**IV:** 50–100 mg bolus, then 1–4 mg/min infusion	Drowsiness, agitation, muscle twitching, seizures, paresthesias, proarrhythmia
Mexiletine (p. 742) (Mexitil)	**C:** 150 mg, 200 mg, 250 mg	PVCs, VT, VF	**A:** 600–1,200 mg/day	Drowsiness, agitation, muscle twitching seizures, paresthesias, proarrhythmia, nausea, vomiting
Tocainide (p. 1096) (Tonocard)	**T:** 400 mg, 600 mg	PVCs, VT, VF	**A:** 1,200–1,800 mg/day	Drowsiness, agitation, muscle twitching seizures, paresthesias, proarrhythmia, nausea, vomiting, diarrhea, agranulocytosis

Class 1C

Flecainide (p. 461) (Tambocor)	T: 50 mg, 100 mg, 150 mg	AF, PSVT, ventricular arrhythmias (life-threatening)	Dizziness, tremors, lightheadedness, flushing, blurred vision, metallic taste, proarrhythmia
Propafenone (p. 935) (Rythmol)	T: 150 mg, 225 mg, 300 mg	PAF, WPW, ventricular arrhythmias (life-threatening)	Dizziness, blurred vision, taste disturbances, nausea, asthma worsening, proarrhythmia
Moricizine (p. 764) (Ethmozine)	T: 200 mg, 250 mg, 300 mg	Life-threatening ventricular arrhythmias	Nausea, dizziness, perioral numbness, euphoria

Class II (Beta Blockers)

Acebutolol (p. 5) (Sectral)	C: 200 mg, 400 mg	AF, A flutter, PSVT, PVCs	Bradycardia, hypotension
Esmolol (p. 418) (Brevibloc)	I: 10 mg/ml, 250 mg/ml	AF, A flutter, PSVT, PVCs	Same as above
Propranolol (p. 940) (Inderal)	T: 10 mg, 20 mg	AF, A flutter, PSVT, PVCs	A: 10–30 mg 3–4 times/day	Same as above

Class III

Amiodarone (p. 50) (Cordarone, Pacerone)	T: 200 mg, 400 mg I: 50 mg/ml	AF, PAF, PSVT, life-threatening ventricular arrhythmias	A (PO): 800–1,600 mg/day for 1–3 wks, then 600–800 mg/day. (IV): 150 mg bolus, then IV infusion	Blurred vision, photophobia, constipation, ataxia, proarrhythmia

(continued)

ANTIARRYTHMICS *(continued)*

Name	Availability	Uses	Dosage Range	Side Effects
Class III *(continued)*				
Sotalol (p. 1025) (Betapace)	**T:** 80 mg, 120 mg, 160 mg, 240 mg	AF, PAF, PSVT, life-threatening ventricular arrhythmias	**A:** 160–640 mg/day	Fatigue, dizziness, dyspnea, bradycardia, proarrhythmia
Ibutilide (p. 569) (Corvert)	**I:** 0.1 mg/ml	AF, A flutter	**A (>60 kg):** 1 mg over 10 min **(<60 kg):** 0.01 mg/kg over 10 min	torsades de pointes
Dofetilide (p. 371) (Tikosyn)	**C:** 125 mcg, 250 mcg, 500 mcg	AF, A flutter	**A:** Individualized	Same as above
Class IV (Calcium Channel Blockers)				
Verapamil (p. 1151) (Isoptin)	**I:** 5 mg/2 ml	AF, A flutter, PSVT	**A (IV):** 5–10 mg	Hypotension, bradycardia, dizziness, headaches, constipation
Diltiazem (p. 351) (Cardizem)	**I:** 25 mg/ml vials, **Infusion:** 1 mg/ml	AF, A flutter, PSVT	**A (IV):** 20–25 mg bolus, then infusion of 5–15 mg/hr	Same as above

A: adults; **AF:** atrial fibrillation; **A flutter:** atrial flutter; **C:** capsules; **CR:** controlled-release; **ER:** extended-release; **I:** injection; **PAF:** paroxysmal atrial fibrillation; **PSVT:** paroxysmal supraventricular tachycardia; **PVCs:** premature ventricular contractions; **SR:** sustained-release; **T:** tablets; **VF:** ventricular fibrillation; **VT:** ventricular tachycardia; **WPW:** Wolff-Parkinson-White syndrome.

Antibiotics

USES

Treatment of wide range of gram-positive or gram-negative bacterial infections; suppression of intestinal flora before surgery; control of acne; prophylactically to prevent rheumatic fever; prophylactically in high-risk situations (e.g., some surgical procedures or medical states) to prevent bacterial infection.

ACTION

Antibiotics (antimicrobial agents) are natural or synthetic compounds that have the ability to kill or suppress the growth of micro-organisms. One means of classifying antibiotics is by their antimicrobial spectrum. Narrow-spectrum agents are effective against few micro-organisms (e.g., aminoglycosides are effective against gram-negative aerobes), whereas broad-spectrum agents are effective against a wide variety of micro-organisms (e.g., fluoroquinolones are effective against gram-positive cocci and gram-negative bacilli).

Antimicrobial agents may also be classified based on their mechanism of action.

• Agents that inhibit cell wall synthesis or activate enzymes that disrupt cell wall, causing a weakening in the cell wall, cell lysis, and death. Include penicillins, cephalosporins, vancomycin, and imidazole antifungal agents.

• Agents that act directly on cell wall, affecting permeability of cell membranes, causing leakage of intracellular substances. Include antifungal agents amphotericin and nystatin, polymyxin, and colistin.

• Agents that bind to ribosomal subunits, altering protein synthesis and eventually causing cell death. Include aminoglycosides.

• Agents that affect bacterial ribosome function, altering protein synthesis and causing slow microbial growth. Do not cause cell death. Include chloramphenicol, clindamycin, erythromycin, tetracyclines.

• Agents that inhibit nucleic acid metabolism by binding to nucleic acid or interacting with enzymes necessary for nucleic acid synthesis. Inhibit DNA or RNA synthesis. Include rifampin, metronidazole, quinolones (e.g., ciprofloxacin).

• Agents that inhibit specific metabolic steps necessary for micro-organisms, causing a decrease in essential cell components or synthesis of nonfunctional analogues of normal metabolites. Include trimethoprim and sulfonamides.

• Agents that inhibit viral DNA synthesis by binding to viral enzymes necessary for DNA synthesis, preventing viral replication. Include acyclovir, vidarabine.

Antibiotics [continued]

SELECTION OF ANTIMICROBIAL AGENTS

The goal of therapy is to produce a favorable therapeutic result by achieving antimicrobial action at the site of infection sufficient to inhibit the growth of the microorganism. The agent selected should be the most active against the most likely infecting organism, least likely to cause toxicity or allergic reaction. Factors to consider in selection of an antimicrobial agent include:

- Sensitivity pattern of the infecting microorganism.
- Location and severity of infection (may determine route of administration).
- Pt's ability to eliminate the drug (status of renal and liver functions).
- Pt's defense mechanisms (includes both cellular and humoral immunity).
- Pt's age, whether pregnant, genetic factors, allergies, CNS disorder, pre-existing medical problems.

CATEGORIZATION OF ORGANISMS BY GRAM STAINING:

Gram-positive Cocci	Gram-negative Cocci	Gram-positive Bacilli	Gram-negative Bacilli
Aerobic	**Aerobic**	**Aerobic**	**Aerobic**
Staphylococcus aureus	*Neisseria gonorrhoeae*	*Listeria monocytogenes*	*E. coli*
Staphylococcus epidermidis	*Neisseria meningitidis*	*Bacillus antrocis*	*Klebsiella pneumoniae*
Streptococcus pyogenes	*Moraxella catarrhalis*	*Corynebacterium diphtheriae*	*Proteus mirabilis*
Streptococcus pneumoniae		**Anaerobic**	*Serratia marcescens*
Viridans streptococci		*Clostridium difficile*	*Pseudomonas aeruginosa*
Enterococcus faecalis		*Clostridium perfringens*	*Enterobacter spp.*
Enterococcus faecium		*Clostridium tetani*	*Haemophilus influenzae*
Anaerobic		*Actinomyces spp.*	*Legionella pneumophila*
Peptostreptococcus spp.			**Anaerobic**
Peptococcus spp.			*Bacteroides fragilis*
			Fusobacterium spp.

Antibiotic: Aminoglycosides

USES

Treatment of serious infections when other, less toxic agents are not effective, are contraindicated, or require adjunctive therapy (e.g., with penicillins or cephalosporins). Used primarily in the treatment of infections caused by gram-negative micro-organisms, such as those caused by *Proteus, Klebsiella, Pseudomonas,*

Escherichia coli, Serratia, and *Enterobacter.* Inactive against most gram-positive micro-organisms. Not well absorbed systemically from GI tract (must be administered parenterally for systemic infections). Oral agents are given to suppress intestinal bacteria.

ACTION

Bactericidal. Transported across bacterial cell membrane; irreversibly binds to specific receptor proteins of bacterial ribosomes. Interfere with protein synthesis, preventing cell reproduction and eventually causing cell death.

ANTIBIOTIC: AMINOGLYCOSIDES

Name	Availability	Dosage Range	Side Effects
Amikacin (p. 42) (Amikin)	I: 250 mg/ml, 50 mg/ml	**A:** 15 mg/kg/day **C:** 15 mg/kg/day	Nephrotoxicity, neurotoxicity, ototoxicity (both auditory and vestibular), hypersensitivity (skin itching, redness, rash, swelling)
Gentamicin (p. 516) (Garamycin)	I: 40 mg/ml, 10 mg/ml	**A:** 3–5 mg/kg/day **C:** 6–7.5 mg/kg/day	Same as amikacin
Neomycin (p. 797)	T: 500 mg	**A:** 1 g for 3 doses as preop	Nausea, vomiting, diarrhea
Netilimicin (p. 802) (Netromycin)	I: 100 mg/ml	**A:** 3–6.5 mg/kg/day **C:** 5.5–8 mg/kg/day	Same as amikacin
Streptomycin (p. 1036)	I: 1 g	**A:** 15 mg/kg/day **C:** 20–40 mg/kg/day **Maximum:** 1 g	Same as amikacin Peripheral neuritis (numbness), optic neuritis (any vision loss)

(continued)

CLASSIFICATIONS

ANTIBIOTIC: AMINOGLYCOSIDES (continued)

Name	Availability	Dosage Range	Side Effects
Tobramycin (p. 1093) (Nebcin)	**I:** 40 mg/ml, 10 mg/ml	**A:** 3–5 mg/kg/day **C:** 6–7.5 mg/kg/day	Same as amikacin

A: adults; **C:** capsules; **C:** (dosage); children; **I:** injection; **T:** tablets.

Antibiotic: Cephalosporins

USES

Broad-spectrum antibiotics, which, like penicillins, may be used in a number of diseases, including respiratory diseases, skin and soft tissue infection, bone/joint infections, genitourinary infections, prophylactically in some surgical procedures.

First-generation cephalosporins have good activity against gram-positive organisms and moderate activity against gram-negative organisms, including *Escherichia coli, Klebsiella pneumoniae, Proteus mirabilis.*

Second-generation cephalosporins have increased activity against gram-negative organisms.

Third-generation cephalosporins are less active against gram-positive organisms but more active against the Enterobacteriaceae with some activity against *Pseudomonas aeruginosa.*

Fourth-generation cephalosporins have good activity against gram-positive organisms (e.g., *Staphylococcus aureus*) and gram-negative organisms (e.g., *Pseudomonas aeruginosa*).

ACTION

Cephalosporins inhibit cell wall synthesis or activate enzymes that disrupt cell wall, causing a weakening in the cell wall, cell lysis, and cell death. May be bacteriostatic or bactericidal. Most effective against rapidly dividing cells.

ANTIBIOTIC: CEPHALOSPORINS

Name	Availability	Dosage Range	Side Effects
First-Generation			
Cefadroxil (p. 183) (Duricef)	**C:** 500 mg **T:** 1 g **S:** 125 mg/5 ml, 250 mg/5 ml, 500 mg/5 ml	**A:** 1–2 g/day **C:** 30 mg/kg/day	Abdominal or stomach cramps/pain, fever, nausea, vomiting, diarrhea, headaches, oral/vaginal candidiasis
Cefazolin (p. 185) (Ancef, Kefzol)	**I:** 500 mg, 1 g, 2 g	**A:** 0.75–6 g/day **C:** 25–100 mg/kg/day	Same as above
Cephalexin (p. 217) (Keftab)	**C:** 250 mg, 500 mg **T:** 250 mg, 500 mg, 1 g	**A:** 1–4 g/day **C:** 25–100 mg/kg/day	Same as above
Second-Generation			
Cefaclor (p. 181) (Ceclor)	**C:** 250 mg, 500 mg **T (ER):** 375 mg, 500 mg **S:** 125 mg/5 ml, 187 mg/5 ml, 250 mg /5 ml, 375 mg/5 ml	**A:** 250–500 mg q8h **C:** 20–40 mg/kg/day	Same as cefadroxil May have serum sickness like reaction
Cefmetazole (p. 193) (Zefazone)	**I:** 1 g, 2 g	**A:** 4–8 g/day	Same as cefadroxil
Cefotetan (p. 197) (Cefotan)	**I:** 1 g, 2 g	**A:** 1–6 g/day	Same as cefadroxil May cause unusual bleeding/bruising
Cefoxitin (p. 199) (Mefoxin)	**I:** 1 g, 2 g	**A:** 3–12 g/day	Same as cefadroxil

(continued)

ANTIBIOTIC: CEPHALOSPORINS *(continued)*

Name	Availability	Dosage Range	Side Effects
Second-Generation *(continued)*			
Cefpodoxime (p. 202) (Vantin)	**T:** 100 mg, 200 mg **S:** 50 mg/5 ml, 100 mg/5 ml	**A:** 200–800 mg/day **C:** 10 mg/kg/day	Same as cefadroxil
Cefprozil (p. 203) (Cefzil)	**T:** 250 mg, 500 mg **S:** 125 mg/5 ml, 250 mg/5 ml	**A:** 0.5–1 g/day **C:** 30 mg/kg/day	Same as above
Cefuroxime (p. 213) (Ceftin, Kefurox, Zinacef)	**T:** 125 mg, 250 mg, 500 mg **S:** 125 mg/5 ml, 250 mg/5 ml **I:** 750 mg, 1.5 g	**A (PO):** 0.25–1 g/day; **(IM/IV):** 2.25–9 g/day **C (PO):** 250–500 mg/day; **(IM/IV):** 50–100 mg/kg/day	Same as above
Loracarbef (p. 678) (Lorabid)	**C:** 200 mg, 400 mg **S:** 100 mg/5 ml, 200 mg/5 ml	**A:** 200–800 mg/day **C:** 15–30 mg/kg/day	Same as above
Third-Generation			
Cefdinir (p. 187) (Omnicef)	**C:** 300 mg **S:** 125 mg/5 ml	**A:** 600 mg/day **C:** 14 mg/kg/day	Same as above
Cefditoren (p. 189) (Spectracef)	**T:** 200 mg	**A:** 400–800 mg/day	Same as above
Cefixime (p. 192) (Suprax)	**T:** 200 mg, 400 mg **S:** 100 mg/5 ml	**A:** 400 mg/day **C:** 8 mg/kg/day	Same as above
Cefotaxime (p. 195) (Claforan)	**I:** 500 mg, 1 g, 2 g	**A:** 2–12 g/day **C:** 100–200 mg/kg/day	Same as above

Ceftazidime (p. 205) (Fortaz, Tazicef, Tazidime)	I: 500 mg, 1 g, 2 g	A: 0.5–6 g/day C: 90–150 mg/kg/day	Same as above
Ceftibuten (p. 207) (Cedax)	C: 400 mg S: 90 mg/5 ml, 180 mg/5 ml	A: 400 mg/day C: 9 mg/kg/day	Same as above
Ceftizoxime (p. 209) (Cefizox)	I: 500 mg, 1 g, 2 g	A: 1–12 g/day C: 150–200 mg/kg/day	Same as above
Ceftriaxone (p. 211) (Rocephin)	I: 250 mg, 500 mg, 1 g, 2 g	A: 1–4 g/day C: 50–100 mg/kg/day	Same as above

Fourth-Generation

| Cefepime (p. 190) (Maxipime) | I: 500 mg, 1 g, 2 g | A: 1–6 g/day | Same as above |

A: adults; **C:** capsules; **C** (dosage); children; **I:** injection; **S:** suspension; **T:** tablets.

Antibiotic: Fluoroquinolones

USES

Fluoroquinolones act against a wide range of gram-negative and gram-positive organisms. They are used primarily in the treatment of lower respiratory infections, skin/skin structure infections, UTIs, and sexually transmitted diseases.

ACTION

Bactericidal. Inhibit DNA gyrase in susceptible micro-organisms, interfering with bacterial DNA replication and repair.

Antibiotic: Fluoroquinolones *(continued)*

ANTIBIOTIC: FLUOROQUINOLONES

Name	Availability	Dosage Range	Side Effects
Ciprofloxacin (p. 243) (Cipro)	**T:** 250 mg, 500 mg, 750 mg **S:** 5 g/100 ml **I:** 200 mg, 400 mg	**A (PO):** 250–750 mg q12h **(IV):** 200–400 mg q12h	Dizziness, headaches, nervousness, drowsiness, insomnia, abdominal pain, nausea, diarrhea, vomiting
Enoxacin (p. 397) (Penetrex)	**T:** 200 mg, 400 mg	**A:** 200–400 mg q12h	Same as above
Gatifloxacin (p. 509) (Tequin)	**T:** 200 mg, 400 mg **I:** 200 mg, 400 mg	**A:** 200–400 mg q12h	Same as above
Levofloxacin (p. 656) (Levaquin)	**T:** 250 mg, 500 mg, 750 mg **I:** 250 mg, 500 mg, 750 mg	**A (PO/IV):** 250–750 mg/day as single dose	Same as above
Lomefloxacin (p. 672) (Maxiquin)	**T:** 400 mg	**A:** 400 mg/day	Same as above
Moxifloxacin (p. 767) (Avalox)	**T:** 400 mg **I:** 400 mg	**A:** 400 mg/day	Same as above
Norfloxacin (p. 823) (Noroxin)	**T:** 400 mg	**A:** 400 mg q12h	Same as above
Ofloxacin (p. 831) (Floxin)	**T:** 200 mg, 300 mg, 400 mg **I:** 200 mg, 400 mg	**A (PO/IV):** 200–400 mg q12h	Same as above
Sparfloxacin (p. 1027) (Zagam)	**T:** 200 mg	**A:** 400 mg once, then 200 mg/day	Same as above

A: adults; **I:** injection; **S:** suspension; **T:** tablets.

Antibiotic: Macrolides

USES

Macrolides act primarily against gram-positive micro-organisms and gram-negative cocci. Azithromycin and clarithromycin appear to be more potent than erythromycin. Macrolides are used in the treatment of pharyngitis/tonsillitis, sinusitis, chronic bronchitis, pneumonia, uncomplicated skin/skin structure infections.

ACTION

Bacteriostatic or bactericidal. Reversibly bind to the P site of the 50S ribosomal subunit of susceptible organisms, inhibiting RNA-dependent protein synthesis.

ANTIBIOTIC: MACROLIDES

Name	Availability	Dosage Range	Side Effects
Azithromycin (p. 98) (Zithromax)	T: 250 mg, 600 mg S: 100 mg/5 ml, 200 mg/5 ml, 1 g packet I: 500 mg	A (PO): 500 mg once, then 250 mg days 2–5 (IV): 500 mg/day C (PO): 10 mg/kg once, then 5 mg/kg/day on days 2–5	PO: Nausea, diarrhea, vomiting, abdominal pain IV: Pain, redness, swelling at injection site
Clarithromycin (p. 253) (Biaxin)	T: 250 mg, 500 mg T (XL): 500 mg S: 125 mg/5 ml	A: 250–500 mg q12h C: 7.5 mg/kg q12h	Headaches, loss of taste, nausea, vomiting, diarrhea, abdominal pain/discomfort
Dirithromycin (p. 360) (Dynabec)	T: 250 mg	A, C (>12 yrs): 500 mg/day as a single daily dose	Dizziness, nausea, vomiting, diarrhea, abdominal pain, headaches, weakness

(continued)

CLASSIFICATIONS

ANTIBIOTIC: MACROLIDES *(continued)*

Name	Availability	Dosage Range	Side Effects
Erythromycin (p. 415) (E-Mycin, Erytab, PCE, Eryc, EES, Eryped, Erythrocin)	**T:** 200 mg, 250 mg, 333 mg, 400 mg, 500 mg **C:** 250 mg **S:** 125 mg/5 ml, 200 mg/5 ml, 250 mg/5 ml, 400 mg/5 ml, 100 mg/2.5 ml	**A (PO):** 250–500 mg q6h **C (PO):** 30–50 mg/kg/day **A, C (IV):** 15–20 mg/kg/day **Maximum:** 4 g/day	**PO:** Nausea, vomiting, diarrhea, abdominal pain **IV:** Inflammation, phlebitis at injection site

A: adults; **C:** capsules; **C** (dosage): children; **I:** injection; **S:** suspension; **T:** tablets; **XL:** long acting.

Antibiotic: Penicillins

USES

Penicillins may be used to treat a large number of infections, including pneumonia and other respiratory diseases, urinary tract infections, septicemia, meningitis, intra-abdominal infections, gonorrhea and syphilis, bone/joint infection. Penicillins are classified based on an antimicrobial spectrum:

Natural penicillins are very active against gram-positive cocci but ineffective against most strains of *Staphylococcus aureus* (inactivated by enzyme penicillinase). *Penicillinase-resistant penicillins* are effective against penicillinase-producing *Staphylococcus aureus* but are less effective against gram-positive cocci than the natural penicillins.

Broad-spectrum penicillins are effective against gram-positive cocci and some gram-negative bacteria (e.g., *Hemophilus influenzae, Escherichia coli, Proteus mirabilis*). *Extended-spectrum penicillins* are effective against *Pseudomonas aeruginosa, Enterobacter, Proteus* species, *Klebsiella,* and some other gram-negative microorganisms.

ACTION

Penicillins inhibit cell wall synthesis or activate enzymes, which disrupt bacterial cell wall, causing a weakening in the cell wall, cell lysis, and cell death. May be bacteriostatic or bactericidal. Most effective against bacteria undergoing active growth and division.

ANTIBIOTIC: PENICILLINS

Name	Availability	Dosage Range	Side Effects
Natural			
Penicillin G benzathine (p. 867) (Bicillin)	**I:** 600,000 units, 1.2 million units, 2.4 million units	**A:** 1.2 million units/day **C:** 0.3–1.2 million units/day	Mild diarrhea, nausea, vomiting, headaches, sore mouth/tongue, vaginal itching/discharge, allergic reaction (including anaphylaxis, skin rash, hives, itching)
Penicillin G potassium (p. 867) (Pfizerpen)	**I:** 1, 2, 3, 5 million unit vials	**A:** 2–24 million units/day **C:** 100–250,000 units/kg/day	Same as above
Penicillin G procaine (p. 867) (Crystacillin)	**I:** 600,000 units, 1.2 million units, 2.4 million units	**A, C:** 0.6–1.2 million units/day	Same as above
Penicillin V (p. 870) (Pen-Vee K, V-Cillin-K)	**T:** 250 mg, 500 mg **S:** 125 mg/5 ml, 250 mg/5 ml	**A:** 0.5–2 g/day **C:** 25–50 mg/kg/day	Same as above

(continued)

ANTIBIOTIC: PENICILLINS *(continued)*

Name	Availability	Dosage Range	Side Effects
Penicillinase-Resistant			
Cloxacillin (p. 268) (Tegopen)	**C:** 250 mg, 500 mg **S:** 125 mg/5 ml	**A:** 1–2 g/day **C:** 50–100 mg/kg/day	Same as penicillin G benzathine
Dicloxacillin (p. 340) (Dynapen, Pathocil)	**C:** 125 mg, 250 mg, 500 mg **S:** 62.5 mg/5 ml	**A:** 1–2 g/day **C:** 12.5–25 mg/kg/day	Same as above Increase risk of liver toxicity
Nafcillin (p. 778) (Nafcil, Unipen)	**C:** 250 mg **I:** 500 mg, 1 g, 2 g	**A (PO):** 1–6 g/day. **(IV):** 2–6 g/day **C (PO):** 25–50 mg/kg/day. **(IV):** 50 mg/kg/day	Same as penicillin G benzathine
Oxacillin (p. 843) (Bactocill)	**C:** 250 mg, 500 mg **S:** 250 mg/5 ml **I:** 250 mg, 500 mg, 1 g, 2 g	**A (PO/IV):** 2–6 g/day **C (PO/IV):** 50–100 mg/kg/day	Same as above
Broad-Spectrum			
Amoxicillin (p. 56) (Amoxil, Polymox, Trimox)	**T:** 125 mg, 250 mg, 500 mg, 875 mg **C:** 250 mg, 500 mg **S:** 50 mg/ml, 125 mg/5 ml, 250 mg/5 ml	**A:** 0.75–1.5 g/day **C:** 20–40 mg/kg/day	Same as above
Amoxicillin/clavulanate (p. 58) (Augmentin)	**T:** 250 mg, 500 mg, 875 mg **T (chewable):** 125 mg, 200 mg, 250 mg, 400 mg **S:** 125 mg/5 ml, 200 mg/5 ml, 250 mg/5 ml, 400 mg/5 ml	**A:** 0.75–1.5 g/day **C:** 20–40 mg/kg/day	Same as above

Ampicillin (p. 63) (Omnipen, Polycillin, Principen)	**C:** 250 mg, 500 mg **S:** 125 mg/5 ml, 250 mg/5 ml **I:** 125 mg, 250 mg, 500 mg, 1 g, 2 g	**A:** 1–12 g/day **C:** 50–200 mg/kg/day	Same as above
Ampicillin/sulbactam (p. 65) (Unasyn)	**I:** 1.5 g, 3 g	**A:** 6–12 g/day	Same as above
Bacampicillin (p. 102) (Spectrobid)	**T:** 400 mg	**A:** 800–1,600 mg/day **C:** 25–50 mg/kg/day	Same as above
Extended-Spectrum		
Carbenicillin (p. 169) (Geocillin)	**T:** 382 mg	**A:** 382–764 mg 4 times/day	Same as above
Piperacillin/tazobactam (p. 898) (Zosyn)	**I:** 2.25 g, 3.375 g, 4.5 g	**A:** 2.25–4.5 g q6–8h	Same as above
Ticarcillin/clavulanate (p. 1082) (Timentin)	**I:** 3.1 g	**A:** 3.1 g q4–6h	Same as above

A: adults; **C:** (dose): children; **I:** injection; **S:** suspension; **T:** tablets.

Anticoagulants/Antiplatelets/Thrombolytics

USES

Treatment and prevention of venous thromboembolism, acute myocardial infarction, acute cerebral embolism; reduce risk of acute myocardial infarction, total mortality in pts with unstable angina; occlusion of saphenous grafts following open heart surgery; embolism in select pts with atrial fibrillation, prosthetic heart valves, valvular heart disease, cardiomyopathy. Heparin also used for acute/chronic consumption coagulopathies (disseminated intravascular coagulation).

ACTION

Anticoagulants: Inhibit blood coagulation by preventing the formation of new clots and extension of existing ones. *Do not dissolve formed clots.* Anticoagulants are subdivided into two common classes: *Heparin:* Indirectly interferes with blood coagulation by blocking the conversion of prothrombin to thrombin and fibrinogen to fibrin. *Coumarin:* Acts indirectly to prevent synthesis in the liver of vitamin K-dependent clotting factors.

Antiplatelets: Interfere with platelet aggregation. Effects are irreversible for life of platelet. Medications in this group act by different mechanisms and are used in combinations to provide desired effect.

Thrombolytics: Act directly or indirectly on fibrinolytic system to dissolve clots (converting plasminogen to plasmin, an enzyme that digests fibrin clot).

ANTICOAGULANTS/ANTIPLATELETS/THROMBOLYTICS

Name	Availability	Uses	Dosage Range	Side Effects
Anticoagulants				
Dalteparin (p. 304) (Fragmin)	**I:** 2,500 IU, 5,000 IU	DVT prophylaxis, unstable angina	**DVT:** 2,500–5,000 IU/day **Angina:** 120 IU/kg q12h	Hematoma at injection site, bleeding
Danaparoid (p. 305) (Organan)	**I:** 750 units	DVT prophylaxis	750 units q12h	Pain at injection site, bleeding

Enoxaparin (p. 397) (Lovenox)	I: 30 mg, 40 mg, 60 mg, 80 mg, 100 mg	DVT treatment/prophylaxis, DVT, unstable angina	**DVT prophylaxis:** 40 mg/day or 30 mg q12h **DVT, angina:** 1 mg/kg q12h	Same as dalteparin
Heparin (p. 543)	I: 5,000 units, 10, 000 units, 20,000 units **Infusion**	DVT prophylaxis, thrombosis, embolism, coagulopathies	**DVT prophylaxis:** 5,000 units q8–12h **DVT, embolism:** IV bolus, then IV infusion of 20,000–40,000 units/day	Bleeding
Tinzaparin (p. 1088) (Innohep)	I: 20,000 IU/ml	DVT treatment	175 IU/kg once daily	Same as danaparoid
Warfarin (p. 1168) (Coumadin)	T: 1 mg, 2 mg, 2.5 mg, 3 mg, 4 mg, 5 mg, 6 mg, 7.5 mg, 10 mg	Thromboembolic complications with AF, PE, DVT	Initially, 5–10 mg, then 2–10 mg/day	Same as heparin

Antiplatelets

Abciximab (p. 2) (ReoPro)	I: 2 m/ml	ACS	IV bolus of 0.25 mg/kg, then 10 mcg/min	Bleeding, hypotension
Anagrelide (p. 69) (Agrylin)	C: 0.5 mg, 1 mg	Thrombocythemia	2–10 mg/day	Abdominal pain, weakness, dizziness, shortness of breath
Aspirin (p. 83)	T: 80 mg, 160 mg, 325 mg	Atherosclerotic events	81–325 mg/day	GI irritation
Clopidogrel (p. 264) (Plavix)	T: 75 mg	Atherosclerotic events	75 mg/day	Pain, dizziness, heartburn, headaches, flulike symptoms
Dipyridamole (p. 360) (Persantine)	T: 25 mg, 50 mg, 75 mg	Thromboembolic complications	75–100 mg 4 times/day	Abdominal discomfort, diarrhea, dizziness, headaches

(continued)

ANTICOAGULANTS/ANTIPLATELETS/THROMBOLYTICS *(continued)*

Name	Availability	Uses	Dosage Range	Side Effects
Antiplatelets				
Eptifibatide (p. 411) (Integrilin)	**I:** 0.75 mg/ml, 2 mg/ml	ACS	IV bolus of 180 mcg/kg, then 2 mcg/kg/min	Same as abciximab
Ticlopidine (p. 1084) (Ticlid)	**T:** 250 mg	Stroke	250 mg 2 times/day	Skin rash, abdominal pain, diarrhea, nausea, indigestion
Tirofiban (p. 1090) (Aggrastat)	**I:** 50 mcg/ml, 250 mcg/ml	ACS	IV bolus of 0.4 mcg/kg/min, then 0.1 mcg/kg/min	Same as abciximab
Thrombolytics				
Alteplase (p. 35) (Activase)	**I:** 50 mg, 100 mg	AMI, acute ischemic stroke, PE	**IV:** 100 mg over 3 hrs (PE over 2 hrs)	Same as abciximab
Anistreplase (p. 71) (Eminase)	**I:** 30 units	AMI	**IV:** 30 units over 2–5 min	Same as above
Reteplase (p. 969) (Retavase)	**I:** 10 units	AMI	**IV:** 10 units q30min 2 times	Same as above
Streptokinase (p. 1033)	**I:** 250,000 units, 500,000 units, 1.5 million units	AMI, PE, arterial thrombus	**AMI:** 1.5 million units over 60 min **PE, arterial thrombus:** 250,000 unit bolus, then 100,000 units/hr	Same as above
Tenectaplase (p. 1057) (TNKase)	**I:** 50 mg	AMI	Based on pt weight. **Maximum:** 50 mg	Same as above

ACS: acute coronary syndrome; AF: atrial fibrillation; AMI: acute myocardial infarction; C: capsules; DVT: deep vein thrombosis; I: injection; IU: international units; PE: pulmonary embolism; T: tablets.

Anticonvulsants

USES

Anticonvulsants are used to treat seizures. Seizures can be divided into two broad categories: partial seizures and generalized seizures. Partial seizures begin focally in the cerebral cortex undergoing limited spread. Simple partial seizures do not involve loss of consciousness, but may evolve secondarily into generalized seizures. Complex partial seizures involve impairment of consciousness.

Generalized seizures may be convulsive or nonconvulsive and usually produce immediate loss of consciousness.

ACTION

Anticonvulsants can prevent or reduce excessive discharge of neurons with seizure foci or decrease the spread of excitation from seizure foci to normal neurons. The exact mechanism is unknown but may be due to: (1) suppressing sodium influx, (2) suppressing calcium influx, or (3) increasing the action of GABA, which inhibits neurotransmitters throughout the brain.

ANTICONVULSANTS

Name	Availability	Uses	Dosage Range	Side Effects
Barbiturates				
Phenobarbital (p. 881)	**T:** 30 mg, 60 mg, 100 mg **I:** 65 mg, 130 mg	Tonic-clonic, partial; status epilepticus	**A (PO):** 100–300 mg/day **(IM/IV):** 200–600 mg **C (PO):** 3–5 mg/kg/day **(IM/IV):** 100–400 mg	CNS depression, sedation, paradoxical excitement and hyperactivity, rash
Primidone (p. 920) (Mysoline)	**T:** 50 mg, 250 mg **S:** 250 mg/5 ml	Complex, partial, akinetic, tonic-clonic	**A:** 750–2,000 mg/day **C:** 10–25 mg/kg/day	CNS depression, sedation, paradoxical excitement and hyperactivity, rash, dizziness, ataxia

(continued)

ANTICONVULSANTS *(continued)*

Name	Availability	Uses	Dosage Range	Side Effects
Benzodizepines				
Clonazepam (p. 260) (Klonopin)	**T:** 0.5 mg, 1 mg, 2 mg	Petit mal, akinetic, myoclonic, absence seizure	**A:** 1.5–20 mg/day	CNS depression, sedation, ataxia, confusion, depression
Diazepam (p. 334) (Valium)	**T:** 2 mg, 5 mg, 10 mg **I:** 5 mg/ml **R:** 2.5 mg, 5 mg, 10 mg, 20 mg	Adjunctive therapy status epilepticus	**A (PO):** 4–40 mg/day **(IM/IV):** 5–30 mg **C (PO):** 3–10 mg/day **(IM/IV):** 1–10 mg	CNS depression, sedation, confusion, depression, respiratory suppression
Hydantoins				
Fosphenytoin (p. 497) (Cerebyx)	**I:** 50 mg PE/ml	Status epilepticus, seizures occurring during neurosurgery	**A:** 15–20 mg PE/kg bolus, then 4–6 mg PE/kg/day maintenance	Burning, itching, paresthesia nystagmus, ataxia
Phenytoin (p. 889) (Dilantin)	**C:** 100 mg **T (chewable):** 50 mg **S:** 125 mg/5 ml **I:** 50 mg/ml	Tonic-clonic psychomotor seizures	**A (PO):** 300–600 mg/day **IV:** 150–250 mg **C (PO):** 4–8 mg/kg/day **IV:** 10–15 mg/kg	Nystagmus, ataxia, hypertrichosis, gingival hyperplasia, rash, osteomalacia, lyphadenopathy
Miscellaneous				
Carbamazepine (p. 167) (Tegretol)	**S:** 100 mg/5 ml **T (chewable):** 100 mg **T:** 200 mg **T (ER):** 100 mg, 200 mg, 400 mg **C (ER):** 200 mg, 300 mg	Complex partial, tonic-clonic, mixed seizures, trigeminal neuralgia	**A:** 800–1,200 mg/day **C:** 400–800 mg/day	Dizziness, diplopia, leukopenia

Gabapentin (p. 502) (Neurontin)	**C:** 100 mg, 300 mg, 400 mg	Partial seizures with and without secondary generalization	**A:** 900–1,800 mg/day	CNS depression, fatigue, somnolence, dizziness, ataxia
Lamotrigine (p. 642) (Lamictal)	**T:** 25 mg, 100 mg, 150 mg, 200 mg	Partial seizures	**A:** 100–500 mg/day	Dizziness, ataxia, somnolence, diplopia, nausea, rash
Oxcarbazepine (p. 846) (Trileptal)	**T:** 150 mg, 300 mg, 600 mg	Partial seizures	**A:** 900–1,800 mg/day	Drowsiness, dizziness, blurred vision
Tiagabine (p. 1081) (Gabitril)	**T:** 4 mg, 12 mg, 16 mg, 20 mg	Partial seizures	**A:** Initially, 4 mg up to 56 mg **C:** Initially, 4 mg up to 32 mg	Dizziness, asthenia, nervousness, tremors, abdominal pain
Topiramate (p. 1103) (Topamax)	**T:** 25 mg, 100 mg, 200 mg	Partial seizures	**A:** 25–400 mg/day **C:** 1–9 mg/kg/day	Difficulty concentrating, speech problems, fatigue
Valproic acid (p. 1140) (Depakene, Depakote)	**C:** 250 mg **S:** 250 mg/5 ml **Sprinkles:** 125 mg **T:** 125 mg, 250 mg, 500 mg **T (ER):** 500 mg **I:** 100 mg/ml	Complex partial seizures, absence seizures	**A, C:** 15–60 mg/kg/day	Nausea, vomiting, tremors, thyrombocytopenia, hair loss, liver dysfunction
Zonisamide (p. 1186) (Zonegran)	**C:** 100 mg	Partial seizures	**A:** 500 mg/day	Somnolence, dizziness, anorexia, headaches, nausea

A: adults; **C:** capsules; **C** (dosage): children; **ER:** extended-release; **I:** injection; **R:** rectal; **S:** suspension; **T:** tablets.

Antidepressants

USES

Used primarily for the treatment of depression. Imipramine is also used for childhood enuresis. Clomipramine is used only for obsessive-compulsive disorder (OCD). Monoamine oxidase (MAO) inhibitors are rarely used as initial therapy except for pts unresponsive to other therapy or when other therapy is contraindicated.

ACTION

Antidepressants are classified as tricyclic, MAO inhibitors, or second-generation antidepressants (futher subdivided into selective serotonin reuptake inhibitors [SSRIs] and atypical antidepressants). Depression may be due to reduced funcitoning of monoamine neurotransmitters (e.g., norepinephrine, serotonin [5-HT], dopamine) in the CNS (decreased amount and/or decreased effects at the receptor sites).

Antidepressants block metabolism, increase amount/effects of monoamine neurotransmitters and act at receptor sites (change responsiveness/sensitivities of both pre- and postsynaptic receptor sites).

ANTIDEPRESSANTS

Name	Availability	Uses	Dosage Range (mg/day)	Side Effects
Tricyclics				
Amitriptyline (p. 52) (Elavil, Endep)	**T:** 10 mg, 25 mg, 59 mg, 75 mg, 100 mg, 150 mg	Depression	40–300 mg	Drowsiness, blurred vision, constipation, confusion, postural hypotension, conduction defects, weight gain, seizure tendency
Clomipramine (p. 259) (Anafranil)	**C:** 25 mg, 50 mg, 75 mg	OCD	25–250 mg	Same as above
Desipramine (p. 320) (Norpramin, Pertofrane)	**T:** 10 mg, 25 mg, 50 mg, 75 mg, 100 mg, 150 mg	Depression	25–100 mg	Same as above

Doxepin (p. 381) (Sinequan)	**C:** 10 mg, 25 mg, 50 mg, 75 mg, 100 mg, 150 mg **OC:** 10 mg/ml	Depression	25–300 mg	Same as above
Imipramine (p. 579) (Janimine, Tofranil)	**T:** 10 mg, 25 mg, 50 mg **C:** 75 mg, 100 mg, 125 mg, 150 mg	Depression, enuresis	30–300 mg	Same as above
Nortriptyline (p. 825) (Aventyl, Pamelor)	**C:** 10 mg, 25 mg, 50 mg, 75 mg **S:** 10 mg/5 ml	Depression	25–100 mg	Same as above
Protriptyline (p. 945) (Vivactil)	**T:** 5 mg, 10 mg	Depression	15–60 mg	Same as above

Monoamine Oxidase Inhibitors

Phenelzine (p. 880) (Nardil)	**T:** 15 mg	Depression	15–90 mg	Sedation, hypertensive crisis, weight gain, orthostatic hypotension
Tranylcypromine (p. 1114) (Parnate)	**T:** 10 mg	Depression	30–60 mg	Same as above

Selective Serotonin Reuptake Inhibitors

Citalopram (p. 248) (Celexa)	**T:** 20 mg, 40 mg **S:** 10 mg/5 ml	Depression	25–60 mg	Insomnia or sedation, nausea, agitation, headaches
Fluoxetine (p. 475) (Prozac)	**C:** 10 mg, 20 mg, 40 mg **T:** 10 mg **S:** 20 mg/5 ml	Depression, OCD, bulimia	10–80 mg	Same as above
Fluvoxamine (p. 488) (Luvox)	**T:** 25 mg, 50 mg, 100 mg	OCD	100–300 mg	Same as above

(continued)

ANTIDEPRESSANTS *(continued)*

Selective Serotonin Reuptake Inhibitors *(continued)*

Paroxetine (p. 860) (Paxil)	**T:** 10 mg, 20 mg, 30 mg, 40 mg **S:** 10 mg/5 ml	Depression, OCD, panic attack, social anxiety disorder	20–50 mg	Same as citalopram
Sertraline (p. 1007) (Zoloft)	**T:** 25 mg, 50 mg, 100 mg **S:** 20 mg/ml	Depression, OCD, panic attack	50–200 mg	Same as above

Atypical

Bupropion (p. 146) (Wellbutrin)	**T:** 75 mg, 100 mg **SR:** 100 mg, 150 mg	Depression	150–450 mg	Insomnia, irritability, seizures
Mirtazepine (p. 753) (Remeron)	**T:** 15 mg, 30 mg, 45 mg	Depression	15–45 mg	Sedation, dry mouth, weight gain, agranulocytosis, liver toxicity
Nefazodone (p. 794) (Serzone)	**T:** 50 mg, 100 mg, 150 mg, 200 mg, 250 mg	Depression	200–600 mg	Sedation, orthostatic hypotension, nausea
Trazodone (p. 1117) (Desyrel)	**T:** 50 mg, 100 mg, 150 mg, 300 mg	Depression	50–600 mg	Sedation, orthostatic hypotension, priopism
Venlafaxine (p. 1149) (Effexor)	**T:** 25 mg, 37.5 mg, 50 mg, 75 mg, 100 mg **T (ER):** 37.5 mg, 75 mg, 150 mg	Depression, anxiety	75–375 mg	Increased blood pressure, agitation, sedation, insomnia, nausea

C: capsules; **ER:** extended-release; **OC:** oral concentrate; **OCD:** obsessive compulsive disorder; **S:** suspension; **SR:** sustained-release; **T:** tablets.

Antidiabetics

USES

Insulin: Treatment of insulin-dependent diabetes (type 1) and noninsulin-dependent diabetes (type 2). Also used in acute situations such as ketoacidosis, severe infections, major surgery in otherwise noninsulin-dependent diabetics. Administered to pts receiving parenteral nutrition. Drug of choice during pregnancy

Sulfonylureas: Control hyperglycemia in type 2 diabetes not controlled by weight and diet alone. Chlorpropamide also used in adjunctive treatment of neurogenic diabetes insipidus.

Alpha-glucosidase inhibitors: Adjunct to diet to lower blood glucose in pts with type 2 diabetes mellitus whose hyperglycemia cannot be managed by diet alone.

Biguanides: Adjunct to diet to lower blood glucose in pts with type 2 diabetes mellitus whose hyperglycemia cannot be managed by diet alone.

Thiazolinediones: Adjunct in pts with type 2 diabetes currently on insulin therapy.

ACTION

Insulin: A hormone synthesized and secreted by beta cells of Langerhans' islet in the pancreas. Controls storage and utilization of glucose, amino acids, and fatty acids by activated transport systems/enzymes. Inhibits breakdown of glycogen, fat, protein. Insulin lowers blood glucose by inhibiting glycogenolysis and gluconeogenesis in liver; stimulates glucose uptake by muscle, adipose tissue. Activity of insulin is initiated by binding to cell surface receptors.

Sulfonylureas: Stimulate release of insulin from beta cells; increase sensitivity of insulin to peripheral tissue. Endogenous insulin must be present for oral hypoglycemics to be effective.

Alpha-glucosidase inhibitors: Work locally in small intestine, slowing carbohydrate breakdown and glucose absorption.

Biguanides: Decrease hepatic glucose output; enhance peripheral glucose uptake.

Thiazolinediones: Decrease insulin resistance.

Antidiabetics *(continued)*

ANTIDIABETICS

INSULIN

Name	Onset [hrs]	Peak [hrs]	Duration [hrs]	Side Effects
Rapid Acting				
Lispro (p. 590) (Humalog)	1/4	1/2–1½	4–5	Hypoglycemia, weight gain, lipodystrophy, local skin reactions
Insulin aspart (p. 590) (NovoLog)	5–10 min	1–3	3–5	Same as above
Regular (p. 590) (Humulin R, Novolin R)	1/2–1	2–4	5–7	Same as above
Intermediate Acting				
Lente (p. 590) (Humulin L, Novolin L)	1–3	6–14	24	Same as above
NPH (p. 590) (Humulin N, Novolin N)	1–2	6–14	24	Same as above
Long Acting				
Glargine (p. 590) (Lantus)	—	—	24	Same as above
Ultralente (p. 590) (Humulin U)	6	18–24	36	Same as above

ORAL AGENTS

Name	Availability	Dosage Range	Side Effects
Sulfonylureas			
Acetohexamide (p. 10) (Dymelor)	**T:** 250 mg, 500 mg	0.25–1.5 g/day	Hypoglycemia, weight gain
Chlorpropamide (p. 230) (Diabinese)	**T:** 100 mg, 250 mg	100–500 mg/day	Same as above
Glimepiride (p. 523) (Amaryl)	**T:** 1 mg, 2 mg, 4 mg	1–8 mg/day	Same as above
Glipizide (p. 524) (Glucotrol)	**T:** 5 mg, 10 mg **T (ER):** 5 mg	**T:** 2.5–40 mg/day **ER:** 5–20 mg/day	Same as above
Glyburide (p. 529) (Diabeta, Micronase)	**T:** 1.25 mg, 2.5 mg, 5 mg **PT:** 1.5 mg, 3 mg	**T:** 1.25–20 mg/day **PT:** 1–12 mg/day	Same as above
Tolazamide (p. 1097) (Tolinase)	**T:** 100 mg, 250 mg, 500 mg	0.2–1 g/day	Same as above
Tolbutamide (p. 1099) (Orinase)	**T:** 250 mg, 500 mg	0.5–3 g/day	Same as above
Alpha Glucosidase Inhibitors			
Acarbose (p. 4) (Precose)	**T:** 25 mg, 50 mg, 100 mg	75–300 mg/day	GI flatulence, diarrhea
Miglitol (p. 747) (Glyset)	**T:** 25 mg, 50 mg, 100 mg	75–300 mg/day	Same as above

(continued)

ANTIDIABETICS *(continued)*

ORAL AGENTS *(continued)*

Name	Availability	Dosage Range	Side Effects
Biguanides			
Metformin (p. 714) (Glucophage)	**T:** 500 mg, 850 mg **XR:** 500 mg	**T:** 0.5–2.5 g/day **XR:** 1,500–2,000 mg/day	Cramping, diarrhea, lactic acidoses (rare)
Meglitinides			
Nateglinide (p. 400) (Starlix)	**T:** 60 mg, 120 mg	60–120 mg 3 times/day	Hypoglycemia, weight gain
Repaglinide (p. 967) (Prandin)	**T:** 0.5 mg, 1 mg, 2 mg	0.5–1 mg with each meal (**maximum:** 16 mg/day)	Same as above
Thiazolidinediones			
Pioglitazone (p. 897) (Actos)	**T:** 15 mg, 30 mg, 45 mg	15–45 mg/day	Mild anemia, mild to moderate edema, weight gain
Rosiglitazone (p. 994) (Avandia)	**T:** 2 mg, 4 mg, 8 mg	4–8 mg/day	Same as above

XR: extended-release; **PT:** prestab; **T:** tablets.

Antidiarrheals

USES

Acute diarrhea, chronic diarrhea of inflammatory bowel disease, reduction of fluid from ileostomies.

ACTION

Systemic agents: Act at smooth muscle receptors (enteric), disrupting peristaltic movements, decreasing GI motility, increasing transit time of intestinal contents.

Local agents: Adsorb toxic substances and fluids to large surface areas of particles in the preparation. Some of these agents coat and protect irritated intestinal walls. May have local anti-inflammatory action.

ANTIDIARRHEALS

Name	Availability	Type	Dosage Range
Bismuth subsalicylate (p. 127) (Pepto-Bismol)	**T:** 262 mg **C:** 262 mg **L:** 130 mg/15 ml, 262 mg/ 15 ml, 524 mg/15 ml	Local	**A:** 2 T or 30 ml **C (9–12 yrs):** 1 T or 15 ml **C (6–9 yrs):** 2/3 T or 10 ml **C (3–6 yrs):** 1/3 T or 5 ml
Diphenoxylate (with atropine) (p. 358) (Lomotil)	**T:** 2.5 mg **L:** 2.5 mg/5 ml	Systemic	**A:** 5 mg 4 times/day **C:** 0.3–0.4 mg/kg/day in 4 divided doses (**L**)
Kaolin (with pectin) (p. 626) (Kaopectate)	Suspension	Local	**A:** 60–120 ml after each bowel movement **C (6–12 yrs):** 30–60 ml **C (3–6 yrs):** 15–30 ml
Loperamide (p. 675) (Imodium)	**C:** 2 mg **T:** 2 mg **L:** 1 mg/5 ml, 1 mg/ml	Systemic	**A:** Initially, 4 mg; 16 mg/day maximum **C (8–12 yrs):** 2 mg 3 times/day **(5–8 yrs):** 2 mg 2 times/day **(2–5 yrs):** 1 mg 3 times/day (**L**)

A: adults; **C:** capsules; **C** (dosage); children; **L:** liquid; **T:** tablets.

Antifungals: Topical

USES

Treatment of tinea infections, cutaneous candidiasis (moniliasis) due to *Candida albicans*.

ACTION

Exact mechanism unknown. May deplete essential intracellular components by inhibiting transport of potassium, other ions into cells; alter membrane permeability, resulting in loss of potassium, other cellular components.

ANTIFUNGALS: TOPICAL

Name	Availability	Dosage Range	Side Effects
Butenafine (Mentax)	**C:** 1%	2 times/day	Burning, stinging, itching, contact dermatitis, erythema
Ciclopirox (p. 238) (Loprox)	**C:** 1% **L:** 1%	2 times/day	Irritation, pruritus, redness
Clioquinol (Vioform)	**C:** 3% **O:** 3%	2–3 times/day	Irritation, stinging, swelling
Clotrimazole (p. 266) (Lotrimin, Mycelex)	**C:** 1% **L:** 1% **S:** 1%	2 times/day	Erythema, stinging, blistering, edema, itching
Econazole (Spectazole)	**C:** 1%	1–2 times/day	Burning, stinging, irritation, erythema
Ketoconazole (p. 630) (Nizoral)	**C:** 2%	1–2 times/day	Irritation, itching, stinging
Miconazole (p. 742) (Micatin, Monistat)	**C:** 2% **P:** 2%	2 times/day	Irritation, burning, allergic contact dermatitis

Nystatin (p. 826) (Mycostatin, Nilstat)	C: 100,000 g O: 100,000 g P: 100,000 g	2–3 times/day	Irritation
Oxiconazole (p. 847) (Oxistat)	C: 1 % L: 1%	1–2 times/day	Pruritus, burning, stinging, irritation, pain, tingling
Terbinafine (p. 1063) (Lamisil)	C: 1% G: 10 mg	1–2 times/day	Irritation, burning, itching, dryness
Tolnaftate (p. 1102) (Tinactin)	C: 1% G: 1% S: 1%	2 times/day	Mild irritation
Triacetin (Fungoid)	C: 1% S: 1%	3 times/day	Irritation
Undecylenic acid (Desenex, Cruex, Caldesene)	C, O, P	As needed	None significant

C: cream, **G:** gel; **L:** lotion; **O:** ointment; **P:** powder; **S:** solution.

Antiglaucoma Agents

USES

Reduction of elevated IOP in pts with open-angle glaucoma and ocular hypertension.

ACTION

Medications that decrease intraocular pressure (IOP) by increasing outflow of aqueous humor:

- *Miotics (direct acting):* cholinergic agents or miotics stimulate ciliary muscles, leading to increases in contraction of the iris sphincter muscle.

Antiglaucoma Agents *(continued)*

ACTION *(cont.)*

• *Miotics (indirect acting):* Primarily inhibit cholinesterase, allowing accumulation of acetylcholine, prolonging parasympathetic activity.

• *Sympathomimetics:* Increase both the rate of fluid flow out of the eye and decrease the rate of aqueous humor production.

Medications that decrease IOP by decreasing aqueous humor production:

• *Alpha-2 agonists:* Activate receptors in ciliary body, inhibiting aqueous secretion and increasing ureoscleral aqueous outflow.

• *Beta blockers:* Reduce production of aqueous humor.

• *Carbonic anhydrase inhibitors:* Reduce fluid flow into the eye by inhibiting enzyme carbonic anhydrase.

• *Prostaglandins:* Increase outflow of aqueous fluid through uveoscleral route.

ANTIGLAUCOMA AGENTS

Name	Availability	Dosage Range	Side Effects
Miotics			
Carbachol (p. 167) (Isopto Carbachol)	**S:** 0.75%, 1.5%, 2.25%, 3%	1 drop 2 times/day	Ciliary or accommodative spasm, blurred vision, reduced night vision, sweating, increased salivation, urinary frequency, nausea, diarrhea
Pilocarpine (p. 895) (Isopto Carpine)	**S:** 0.25%, 0.5%, 1%, 2%, 3%, 4%, 5%, 6%, 8%, 10%	1–2 drops 3–4 times/day	Same as above
Echothiophate (p. 391) (Phospholine Iodide)	**S:** 0.03%, 0.06% 0.125%, 0.25%	1 drop 2 times/day	Headaches, accommodative spasm, sweating, vomiting, nausea, diarrhea, tachycardia
Physostigmine (p. 893) (Eserine)	**O:** 0.25%	Apply up to 3 times/day	Blurred vision, eye pain

Sympathomimetics

Epinephrine (p. 401) (Epifrin, epinal)	**S:** 0.5%, 1%, 2%	1 drop 1–2 times/day	Mydriasis, blurred vision, tachycardia, hypertension, tremors, headaches, anxiety
Dipivefrin (p. 360) (Propine)	**S:** 0.1%	1 drop q12h	Ocular congestion, burning, stinging

Alpha Agonists

Apraclonidine (p. 74) (Iopidine)	**S:** 0.5%	1–2 drops 3 times/day	Ocular allergic-like reactions, hypersensitivity reaction, change in visual activity, lethargy
Brimonidine (p. 140) (Alphagan)	**S:** 0.2%	1–2 drops 2–3 times/day	Ocular allergy, headaches, drowsiness, fatigue

Prostaglandins

Latanoprost (p. 645) (Xalantan)	**S:** 0.005%	1 drop daily in evening	Burning, stinging, iris pigmentation
Bimatoprost (p. 126) (Lumigan)	**S:** 0.03%	1 drop daily in evening	Ocular hyperemia, eylash growth, pruritus
Travoprost (p. 1117) (Travatan)	**S:** 0.004%	1 drop daily in evening	Ocular pyeremia, eye discomfort, foreign body sensation, pain, pruritis

Beta Blockers

Betaxolol (p. 120) (Betoptic)	**Suspension:** 0.25% **S:** 0.5%	1–2 drops 1–2 times/day	Transient irritation, burning, tearing, blurred vision
Carteolol (p. 177) (Ocupress)	**S:** 1%	1 drop 2 times/day	Mild, transient ocular stinging, burning, discomfort

(continued)

ANTIGLAUCOMA AGENTS *(continued)*

Name	Availability	Dosage Range	Side effects
Beta Blockers *(continued)*			
Levobunolol (p. 656) (Betagan)	**S:** 0.25%, 0.5%	1 drop 1–2 times/day	Local discomfort, conjunctivitis, brow ache, tearing, blurred vision, headaches, anxiety
Metipranolol (p. 732) (Optipranolol)	**S:** 0.3%	1 drop 2 times/day	Transient irritation, burning, stinging, blurred vision
Timolol (p. 1085) (Timoptic)	**S:** 0.25%, 0.5% **G:** 0.25%, 0.5%	**S:** 1 drop 2 times/day **G:** 1 drop daily	Same as above
Carbonic Anhydrase Inhibitors			
Acetazolamide (p. 9) (Diamox)	**T:** 125 mg, 250 mg **C:** 500 mg	0.25–1 g/day	Diarrhea, loss of appetite, metallic taste, nausea, tingling in hands/fingers
Brinzolamide (Azopt)	**Suspension:** 1%	1 drop 3 times/day	Blurred vision, bitter taste
Dorzolamide (p. 379) (Trusopt)	**S:** 2%	1 drop 2–3 times/day	Burning, stinging, blurred vision, bitter taste

C: capsules, **G:** gel; **O:** ointment; **S:** solution; **T:** tablets.

Antihistamines

USES

Symptomatic relief of upper respiratory allergic disorders. Allergic reactions associated with other drugs respond to antihistamines, as do blood transfusion reactions. Used as a second-choice drug in treatment of angioneurotic edema. Effective in treatment of acute urticaria and other dermatologic conditions. May also be used for preop sedation, Parkinson's disease, and motion sickness.

ACTION

Antihistamines (H_1 antagonists) inhibit vasoconstrictor effects and vasodilator effects on endothelial cells of histamine. They block increased capillary permeability, formation of edema/wheal caused by histamine. Many antihistamines can bind to receptors in CNS, causing primarily depression (decreased alertness, slowed reaction times, somnolence) but also stimulation (restlessness, nervousness, inability to sleep). Some may counter motion sickness.

ANTIHISTAMINES

Name	Availability	Dosage Range	Side Effects
Chlorpheniramine (p. 231) (Chlor-Trimeton)	**T:** 4 mg **T (chewable):** 2 mg **T (SR):** 8 mg, 12 mg **S:** 2 mg/5 ml	**A:** 2–4 mg q4–6h or **SR:** 8–12 mg q12–24h **C:** 0.35 mg/kg/day	Dry mouth, urinary retention, blurred vision
Brompheniramine (p. 142) (Dimetane)	**T:** 4 mg **T (SR):** 4 mg, 6 mg **S:** 2 mg/5 ml	**A:** 4–8 mg q4–6h or **SR:** 8–12 mg q12–24h **C:** 0.5 mg/kg/day	Same as chlorpheniramine
Dexchlorpheniramine (Polaramine)	**T:** 2 mg **S:** 2 mg/5 ml	**A:** 2 mg q4–6h **C:** 0.5–1 mg q4–6h	Same as chlorpheniramine

(continued)

ANTIHISTAMINES *(continued)*

Name	Availability	Dosage Range	Side Effects
Diphenhydramine (p. 356) (Benadryl)	**T:** 25 mg, 50 mg **C:** 25 mg, 50 mg **L:** 6.25 mg/5 ml, 12.5 mg/5 ml	**A:** 25–50 mg q6–8h **C (6–11 yrs):** 12.5–25 mg q4–6h **(2–5 yrs):** 6.25 mg q4–6h	Dry mouth, urinary retention, blurred vision, sedation, dizziness, paradoxical excitement
Clemastine (p. 254) (Tavist)	**T:** 1.34 mg, 2.68 mg **S:** 0.67 mg/5 ml	**A:** 1.34–2.68 mg q8–12h **C (6–12 yrs):** 0.67–1.34 mg q8–12h	Same as diphenhydramine
Promethazine (p. 932) (Phenergan)	**T:** 12.5 mg, 25 mg, 50 mg **S:** 6.25 mg/5 ml, 25 mg/5 ml	**A:** 25 mg at at bedtime or 12.5 mg q8h **C:** 0.5 mg/kg at bedtime or 0.1 mg/kg q6–8h	Same as diphenhydramine
Cyproheptadine (Periactin)	**T:** 4 mg **S:** 2 mg/5 ml	**A:** 4 mg q8h **C:** 0.25 mg/kg/day	Same as diphenhydramine
Azatadine (Optimine)	**T:** 1 mg	**A:** 1–2 mg q12h **C:** 0.05 mg/kg/day	Same as diphenhydramine
Hydroxyzine (p. 563) (Atarax, Vistaril)	**T:** 10 mg, 25 mg, 50 mg, 100 mg **C:** 25 mg, 50 mg , 100 mg **S:** 10 mg/5 ml, 25 mg/5 ml	**A:** 25 mg q6–8h **C:** 2 mg/kg/day	Same as diphenhydramine
Cetirizine (p. 219) (Zyrtec)	**T:** 5 mg, 10 mg **S:** 5 mg/5 ml	**A:** 5–10 mg/day **C (6–12 yrs):** 5–10 mg/day **(2–5 yrs):** 2.5–5 mg/day	Minimal CNS and anticholinergic side effects
Fexofenadine (p. 455) (Allegra)	**T:** 30 mg, 60 mg, 180 mg	**A:** 60 mg q12h or 180 mg/day **C (6–11 yrs):** 30 mg q12h	Same as cetirizine
Loratidine (p. 680) (Claritin)	**T:** 10 mg **S:** 1 mg/ml	**A:** 10 mg/day **C (6–12 yrs):** 10 mg/day	Same as cetirizine

A: adults; **C:** capsules, **C** (dosage) children; **L:** liquid; **S:** syrup; **SR:** sustained-release; **T:** tablets.

Antihyperlipidemics

USES

Cholesterol management.

ACTION

Bile acid sequestrants: Bind bile acids in the intestine; prevent active transport and reabsorption and enhance bile acid excretion. Depletion of hepatic bile acids results in the increased conversion of cholesterol to bile acids.

HMG-CoA reductase inhibitors (statins): Inhibit HMG-CoA reductase, the last regulated step in the synthesis of cholesterol. Cholesterol synthesis in the liver is reduced.

Niacin (nicotinic acid): Reduces hepatic synthesis of triglycerides and secretion of VLDL by inhibiting the mobilization of free fatty acids from peripheral tissues.

Fibric acid: Increases the oxidation of fatty acids in the liver, resulting in reduced secretion of triglyceride-rich lipoproteins and increases lipoprotein lipase activity and fatty acid uptake.

ANTIHYPERLIPIDEMICS

Name	Availability	Primary Effect	Dosage Range (per day)	Side Effects
Bile Acid Sequestrants				
Cholestyramine (p. 235) (Questran, Prevalite)	**P:** 4 g	Decreases LDL	4–8 g	GI complaints, reduced absorption of other drugs
Cholestipol (Colestid)	**T:** 1 g **G:** 5 g	Decreases LDL	**T:** 2–16 g **G:** 5–30 g	Same as cholestyramine
Colesevelam (p. 272) (Welchol)	**T:** 625 mg	Decreases LDL	4–6 T	Same as cholestyramine

(continued)

ANTIHYPERLIPIDEMICS *(continued)*

Name	Availability	Primary Effect	Dosage Range (per day)	Side Effects
HMG-CoA Reductase Inhibitors (Statins)				
Atorvastatin (p. 88) (Lipitor)	**T:** 10 mg, 20 mg, 40 mg. 80 mg	Decreases LDL, TG Increases HDL	10–80 mg	Headaches, dizziness, nausea, vomiting, diarrhea, myalgia, increased LFTs, rhabdomyolysis
Fluvastatin (p. 487) (Lescol)	**C:** 20 mg, 40 mg **T (ER):** 80 mg	Decreases LDL, TG Increases HDL	20–80 mg	Same as above
Lovastatin (p. 685) (Mevacor)	**T:** 10 mg, 20 mg, 40 mg	Decreases LDL, TG Increases HDL	10–80 mg	Same as above
Pravastatin (p. 912) (Pravachol)	**T:** 10 mg, 20 mg, 40 mg	Decreases LDL, TG Increases HDL	10–40 mg	Same as above
Simvastatin (p. 1014) (Zocor)	**T:** 5 mg, 10 mg, 20 mg, 40 mg, 80 mg	Decreases LDL, TG Increases HDL	5–80 mg	Same as above
Niacin				
Nicotinic acid (p. 803) *Crystalline* (Niacor)	**T:** 500 mg	Decreases LDL, TG Increases HDL	Up to 6 g	Flushing, liver toxicity, increased glucose, GI complaints, gout
Nicotinic acid (p. 803) *Long-acting* (Niaspan)	**T(ER):** 500 mg, 750 mg, 1,000 mg	Decreases LDL, TG Increases HDL	Up to 2,000 mg	Same as above
Fibric Acid				
Clofibrate (p. 259) (Atromid-S)	**C:** 500 mg	Decreases TG	2 g	GI complaints, increased risk of gallstones
Gemfibrozil (p. 512) (Lopid)	**T:** 600 mg	Decreases TG	1,200 mg	Dyspepsia, abdominal pain, diarrhea, nausea, vomiting, fatigue
Fenofibrate (p. 445) (Tricor)	**C:** 67 mg, 134 mg, 200 mg	Decreases TG	67–200 mg	Diarrhea, nausea, constipation, abdominal pain, back pain, headaches

C: capsules; **G:** granules; **HDL:** high-density lipoprotein; **LDL:** low-density lipoprotein; **LFTs:** liver function tests; **P:** powder; **T:** tablets; **T (ER):** tablets – extended-release; **TG:** triglycerides.

Antihypertensives

USES

Treatment of mild to severe hypertension.

ACTION

Many groups of medications are used in the treatment of hypertension. In addition to the alpha-adrenergic central agonists, peripheral antagonists, and vasodilators listed below, refer to the classifications of diuretics, beta-adrenergic blockers, calcium channel blockers, and ACE inhibitors or to individual drug monographs.

Alpha agonists (central action): Stimulate alpha$_2$-adrenergic receptors in the cardiovascular centers of the CNS, reducing sympathetic outflow and producing an antihypertensive effect.

Alpha antagonists (peripheral action): Block alpha$_1$-adrenergic receptors in arterioles and veins, inhibiting vasoconstriction and decreasing peripheral vascular resistance, causing a fall in B/P.

Vasodilators: Directly relax arteriolar smooth muscle, decreasing vascular resistance. Exact mechanism unknown.

ANTIHYPERTENSIVES

Alpha Agonists: Central Action

Name	Availability	Dosage Range	Side Effects
Clonidine (p. 262) (Catapres)	**T:** 0.1 mg, 0.2 mg, 0.3 mg **P:** 0.1 mg/hr, 0.2 mg/hr, 0.3 mg/hr	**PO:** 0.2–0.8 mg/day **Topical:** 0.1–0.6 mg/wk	Sedation, dry mouth, constipation, sexual dysfunction, bradycardia
Guanabenz (p. 540) (Wytensin)	**T:** 4 mg, 8 mg	**PO:** 8–32 mg/day	Same as above
Guanfacine (p. 540) (Tenex)	**T:** 1 mg, 2 mg	**PO:** 1–3 mg/day	Same as above

(continued)

ANTIHYPERTENSIVES *(continued)*

Name	Availability	Dosage Range	Side Effects
Alpha Agonists: Central Action *(continued)*			
Methyldopa (p. 724) (Aldomet)	**T:** 125 mg, 250 mg, 500 mg	**PO:** 0.5–3 g/day	Same as above Forgetfulness, depression, nasal stuffiness
Alpha Agonists: Peripheral Action			
Doxazosin (p. 380) (Cardura)	**T:** 1 mg, 2 mg, 4 mg, 8 mg	**PO:** 2–16 mg/day	Dizziness, vertigo, headaches
Prazosin (p. 915) (Minipress)	**C:** 1 mg, 2 mg, 5 mg	**PO:** 6–20 mg/day	Dizziness, lightheadedness, headaches, drowsiness
Terazosin (p. 1062) (Hytrin)	**C:** 1 mg, 2 mg, 5 mg, 10 mg	**PO:** 1–20 mg/day	Dizziness, headaches, asthenia
Vasodilators			
Hydralazine (p. 548) (Apresoline)	**T:** 10 mg, 25 mg, 50 mg, 100 mg	**PO:** 40–300 mg/day	Anorexia, nausea, diarrhea, vomiting, headaches, palpitations
Minoxidil (p. 751) (Loniten)	**T:** 2.5 mg, 10 mg	**PO:** 10–40 mg/day	Fast/irregular heartbeat, hypertrichosis, swelling of feet/legs

C: capsules; **P:** patch; **T:** tablets.

Antimigraine (triptans)

USES

Treatment of migraine headaches with or without aura in adults 18 yrs or older.

ACTION

Triptans are selective agonists of the serotonin (5-HT) receptor that inhibit neuropeptide release and vasodilation, causing vasoconstriction.

TRIPTANS

Name	Availability	Dosage Range	Contraindications	Side Effects
Almotriptan (p. 29) (Axert)	**T:** 6.25 mg, 12.5 mg	6.25–12.5 mg; may repeat in >2 hrs	Ischemic heart disease, angina pectoris, arrhythmias, previous myocardial infarction, uncontrolled hypertension	Drowsiness, dizziness, fatigue, hot flashes, chest tightness, tingling in extremities, nausea, vomiting
Frovatriptan (p. 499) (Frova)	**T:** 2.5 mg	2.5 mg; may repeat in >2 hrs; no more than 3 **T**/day	Same as above	Same as above
Naratriptan (p. 790) (Amerge)	**T:** 1 mg, 2.5 mg	2.5 mg; may repeat once >4 hrs	Same as above	Same as above
Rizatriptan (p. 990) (Maxalt, Maxalt MLT)	**T:** 5 mg, 10 mg **DT:** 5 mg, 10 mg	5 or 10 mg; may repeat in >2 hrs	Same as above	Same as above

(continued)

TRIPTANS

Name	Availability	Dosage Range	Contraindications	Side Effects
Sumatriptan (p. 1044) (Imitrex)	**T:** 25 mg, 50 mg **NS:** 5 mg, 20 mg **I:** 6 mg	**PO:** 25–100 mg; may repeat q2h **NS:** 5–20 mg; may repeat in >2 hrs **SubQ:** 6 mg; may repeat in >1 hr	Ischemic heart disease, angina pectoris, arrhythmias, previous myocardial infarction, uncontrolled hypertension	Drowsiness, dizziness, fatigue, hot flashes, chest tightness, tingling in extremities, nausea, vomiting
Zolmitriptan (p. 1183) (Zomig)	**T:** 2.5 mg, 5 mg **DT:** 2.5 mg, 5 mg	2.5–5 mg; may repeat in >2 hrs	Same as above	Same as above

DT: disintegrating tablets; **I:** injection; **NS:** nasal spray; **T:** tablets.

Antipsychotics

USES

Antipsychotics are primarily used in managing psychotic illness (esp. in pts with increased psychomotor activity). They are also used to treat the manic phase of bipolar disorder, behavioral problems in children, nausea and vomiting, intractable hiccups, anxiety and agitation, as adjunct in treatment of tetanus, and to potentiate effects of narcotics.

ACTION

Effects of these agents occur at all levels of the CNS. Antipsychotic mechanism unknown, but may antagonize dopamine action as a neurotransmitter in basal ganglia and limbic system. Antipsychotics may block postsynaptic dopamine receptors, inhibit dopamine release, increase dopamine turnover.

These medications can be divided into the phenothiazines and nonphenothiazines (miscellaneous). In addition to their use in symptomatic treatment of psychiatric illness, some have antiemetic, antinausea, antihistamine, anticholinergic, and/or sedative effects.

ANTIPSYCHOTICS

Name	Availability	Dosage	Relative Side Effects Profile				
			EPS	Anticholinergic	Sedation	Hypotension
Chlorpromazine (p. 231) (Thorazine)	**T:** 10 mg, 25 mg, 50 mg, 100 mg, 200 mg **SR:** 30 mg, 75 mg, 100 mg **OC:** 30 mg/ml, 100 mg/ml	50–2,000 mg/day	Moderate	Moderate	High	High
Clozapine (p. 268) (Clozaril)	**T:** 25 mg, 100 mg	75–900 mg/day	Rare	High	High	High
Fluphenazine (p. 478) (Prolixin)	**T:** 1 mg, 2.5 mg, 5 mg, 10 mg **I:** 25 mg/ml **OC:** 5 mg/ml	**PO:** 2–40 mg/day **I:** 12.5–75 mg q2wks	High	Low	Low	Low
Haloperidol (p. 540) (Haldol)	**T:** 0.5 mg, 1 mg, 2 mg, 5 mg, 10 mg, 20 mg **I:** 5 mg/ml **OC:** 2 mg/ml	2–40 mg/day	High	Low	Low	Low
Loxapine (p. 686) (Loxitane)	**C:** 5 mg, 10 mg, 25 mg, 50 mg **OC:** 25 mg/ml **I:** 50 mg/ml	20–250 mg/day	High	Low	Moderate	Moderate
Mesoridazine (p. 712) (Serentil)	**T:** 10 mg, 25 mg, 50 mg, 100 mg **I:** 25 mg/ml **OC:** 25 mg/ml	100–400 mg/day	Low	High	High	High
Olanzapine (p. 833) (Zyprexa, Zydis)	**T:** 2.5 mg, 5 mg, 7.5 mg, 10 mg, 15 mg, 20 mg **DT:** 5 mg, 10 mg	10–20 mg/day	Low	Low	Moderate	Low

(continued)

ANTIPSYCHOTICS *(continued)*

Name	Availability	Dosage	Relative Side Effects Profile				
			EPS	Anticholinergic	Sedation	Hypotension
Quetiapine (p. 952) (Seroquel)	**T:** 25 mg, 100 mg, 200 mg, 300 mg	100–800 mg/day	Rare	Low	Moderate	Moderate
Risperidone (p. 982) (Risperdal)	**T:** 0.25 mg, 0.5 mg, 1 mg, 2 mg, 3 mg, 4 mg **OC:** 1 mg/ml	2–6 mg/day	Low	Low	Low	Moderate
Thioridazine (p. 1076) (Mellaril)	**T:** 10 mg, 15 mg, 25 mg, 50 mg, 100 mg, 150 mg, 200 mg **OC:** 30 mg/ml, 100 mg/ml	50–800 mg/day	Low	High	High	High
Thiothixene (p. 1079) (Navane)	**C:** 1 mg, 2 mg, 5 mg	5–60 mg/day	High	Low	Low	Low
Trifluoperazine (p. 1127) (Stelazine)	**T:** 1 mg, 2 mg, 5 mg, 10 mg **I:** 5 mg/ml **OC:** 2 mg/ml	5–80 mg/day	High	Low	Low	Low
Ziprasidone (p. 1180) (Geodon)	**C:** 20 mg, 40 mg, 60 mg, 80 mg	40–160 mg/day	Low	Low	Low to moderate	Low to moderate

C: capsules; **DT:** disintegrating tablets; **I:** injection; **OC:** oral concentrate; **SR:** sustained-release; **T:** tablets.

Antivirals

USES

Treatment of HIV infection. Treatment of CMV retinitis in pts with AIDS, acute herpes zoster (shingles), genital herpes (recurrent), mucosal and cutaneous herpes simplex virus, chicken pox, and influenza A viral illness.

ACTION

Effective antivirals must inhibit virus-specific nucleic acid/protein synthesis. Possible mechanisms of action of antivirals used for non-HIV infection may include interfering with viral DNA synthesis and viral replication, inactivation of viral DNA polymerases, incorporation and termination of the growing viral DNA chain, prevention of release of viral nucleic acid into the host cell, or interference with viral penetration into cells.

ANTIVIRALS

Name	Availability	Uses	Side Effects
Abacavir (p. 1) (Ziagen)	**T:** 300 mg **OS:** 20 mg/ml	HIV infection	Nausea, vomiting, loss of appetite, diarrhea, headaches, fatigue
Acyclovir (p. 12) (Zovirax)	**T:** 400 mg, 800 mg **C:** 200 mg **I:** 50 mg/ml	Mucosal/cutaneous HSV-1 and HSV-2, varicella zoster (shingles), genital herpes, herpes simplex, encephalitis, chicken pox	Malaise, anorexia, nausea, vomiting, lightheadedness
Amantadine (p. 38) (Symmetrel)	**C:** 100 mg **S:** 50 mg/5 ml	Influenza A	Anxiety, dizziness, lightheadedness, headaches, nausea, loss of appetite
Amprenavir (p. 67) (Agenerase)	**C:** 50 mg, 150 mg **OS:** 15 mg/ml	HIV infection	Hyperglycemia, rash, abdominal pain, nausea, vomiting, diarrhea
Cidofovir (p. 238) (Vistide)	**I:** 75 mg/ml	CMV retinitis	Decreased urination, fever, chills, diarrhea, nausea, vomiting, headaches, loss of appetite

(continued)

ANTIVIRALS *(continued)*

Name	Availability	Uses	Side Effects
Delavirdine (p. 316) (Rescroptor)	**T:** 100 mg, 200 mg	HIV infection	Diarrhea, fatigue, rash, headaches, nausea
Didanosine (p. 342) (Videx)	**T:** 25 mg, 50 mg, 100 mg, 150 mg, 200 mg **C:** 125 mg, 200 mg **Powder for suspension:** 100 mg, 167 mg, 250 mg	HIV infection	Peripheral neuropathy, anxiety, headaches, rash, nausea, diarrhea, dry mouth
Efavirenz (p. 392) (Sustiva)	**C:** 50 mg, 100 mg, 200 mg	HIV infection	Diarrhea, dizziness, headaches, insomnia, nausea, vomiting, drowsiness
Famciclovir (p. 440) (Famvir)	**T:** 125 mg, 250 mg, 500 mg	Herpes zoster, genital herpes	Headaches
Foscarnet (p. 493) (Foscavir)	**I:** 24 mg/ml	CMV retinitis, HSV infections	Decreased urination, abdominal pain, nausea, vomiting, dizziness, fatigue, headaches
Ganciclovir (p. 505) (Cytovene)	**C:** 250 mg, 500 mg **I:** 500 mg	CMV retinitis, CMV disease	Sore throat, fever, unusual bleeding/bruising
Indinavir (p. 584) (Crixivan)	**C:** 200 mg, 400 mg	HIV infection	Blood in urine, weakness, nausea, vomiting, diarrhea, headaches, insomnia, altered taste
Lamivudine (p. 640) (Epivir)	**T:** 100 mg, 150 mg **OS:** 5 mg/ml, 10 mg/ml	HIV infection	Nausea, vomiting, stomach pain, tingling, numbness
Lopinavir/irtonavir (p. 677) (Kaletra)	**C:** 133/33 mg **OS:** 80/20 mg	HIV infection	Diarrhea, nausea
Nelfinavir (p. 796) (Viracept)	**T:** 250 mg **Powder:** 50 mg/g	HIV infection	Diarrhea
Nevirapine (p. 802) (Viramune)	**T:** 200 mg	HIV infection	Chills, fever, sore throat, rash, abdominal pain, nausea, diarrhea, headaches

Oseltamivir (p. 842) (Tamiflu)	**C:** 75 mg **S:** 12 mg/ml	Influenza	Diarrhea, nausea, vomiting
Ribavirin (p. 974) (Virazole)	**Aerosol:** 6 g	Lowers respiratory infections in infants, children due to respiratory syncytial virus (RSV)	Anemia
Ritonavir (p. 985) (Norvir)	**C:** 100 mg **OS:** 80 mg/ml	HIV infection	Weakness, diarrhea, nausea, decreased appetite, vomiting, altered taste
Saquinavir (p. 999) (Invirase)	**C:** 200 mg	HIV infection	Weakness, diarrhea, nausea, mouth ulcers, abdominal pain
Stavudine (p. 1030) (Zerit)	**C:** 15 mg, 20 mg, 30 mg, 40 mg **OS:** 1 mg/ml	HIV infection	Numbness in hands/feet, decreased appetite, chills, fever, rash
Tenofovir (p. 1061) (Viread)	**T:** 300 mg	HIV infection	Diarrhea, nausea, pharyngitis, headaches
Valacyclovir (p. 1136) (Valtrex)	**T:** 500 mg	Herpes zoster, genital herpes	Headaches, nausea
Valganciclovir (p. 1139) (Valcyte)	**T:** 450 mg	CMV retinitis	Anemia, abdominal pain, diarrhea, headaches, nausea, vomiting, numbness in hands/feet
Zalcitabine (p. 1173) (Hivid)	**T:** 0.375 mg, 0.75 mg	HIV infection	Numbness in arms, feet, legs, joint pain, rash, nausea, vomiting
Zanamivir (p. 1175) (Relenza)	**Inhalation:** 5 mg	Influenza	Cough, diarrhea, dizziness, headaches, nausea, vomiting
Zidovudine (p. 1177) (Retrovir)	**T:** 300 mg **C:** 100 mg **S:** 50 mg/5 ml	HIV infection	Unusual tiredness, fever, chills, headaches, nausea, muscle pain

C: capsules; **I:** injection; **OS:** oral solution; **S:** syrup; **T:** tablets.

Beta-Adrenergic Blockers

USES

Management of hypertension, angina pectoris, arrhythmias, hypertrophic subaortic stenosis, migraine headaches, myocardial infarction (prevention), glaucoma.

ACTION

Beta-adrenergic blockers competitively block beta$_1$-adrenergic receptors, located primarily in myocardium, and beta$_2$-adrenergic receptors, located primarily in bronchial and vascular smooth muscle. By occupying beta-receptor sites, these agents prevent naturally occurring or administered epinephrine/norepinephrine from exerting their effects. The results are basically opposite to those of sympathetic stimulation.

Effects of beta$_1$-blockade include slowing heart rate, decreasing cardiac output and contractility; effects of beta$_2$-blockade include bronchoconstriction, increased airway resistance in pts with asthma or COPD. Beta blockers can affect cardiac rhythm/automaticity (decrease sinus rate, SA, AV conduction; increase refractory period in AV node). Decrease systolic and diastolic B/P; exact mechanism unknown, but may block peripheral receptors, decrease sympathetic outflow from CNS, or decrease renin release from kidney. All beta blockers mask tachycardia that occurs with hypoglycemia. When applied to the eye, reduce intraocular pressure and aqueous production.

BETA-ADRENERGIC BLOCKERS

Name	Availability	Selectivity	Dosage Range	Side Effects
Acebutolol (p. 5) (Sectral)	**C:** 200 mg, 400 mg	Beta$_1$	200–1,200 mg/day	Lightheadedness, fatigue, weakness, decreased sexual ability, trouble sleeping
Atenolol (p. 86) (Tenormin)	**T:** 25 mg, 50 mg, 100 mg	Beta$_1$	50–100 mg/day	Same as above
Betaxolol (p. 120) (Kerlone)	**T:** 10 mg, 20 mg	Beta$_1$	10–20 mg/day	Same as above

Bisoprolol (p. 128) (Zebeta)	**T:** 5 mg, 10 mg	Beta$_1$	2.5–20 mg/day	Same as above
Carteolol (p. 177) (Cartrol)	**T:** 2.5 mg, 5 mg	Beta$_1$, beta$_2$	2.5–10 mg/day	Same as above
Carvedilol (p. 177) (Coreg)	**T:** 3.125 mg, 6.25 mg, 12.5 mg, 25 mg	Beta$_1$, beta$_2$, alpha$_1$	12.5–50 mg/day	Same as above
Esmolol (p. 418) (Brevibloc)	**I:** 10 mg/ml, 250 mcg/ml	Beta$_1$	50–200 mcg/kg/min	Same as above
Metoprolol (p. 736) (Lopressor)	**T:** 50 mg, 100 mg/ml **I:** 1 mg/ml	Beta$_1$	50–450 mg/day	Same as above
Nadolol (p. 775) (Corgard)	**T:** 20 mg, 40 mg, 80 mg, 120 mg, 160 mg	Beta$_1$, beta$_2$	40–320 mg/day	Same as above
Penbutolol (p. 864) (Levatol)	**T:** 20 mg	Beta$_1$, beta$_2$	10–40 mg/day	Same as above
Pindolol (p. 897) (Visken)	**T:** 5 mg, 10 mg	Beta$_1$, beta$_2$	10–60 mg/day	Same as above
Propranolol (p. 940) (Inderal)	**T:** 10 mg, 20 mg, 40 mg, 60 mg, 80 mg, 90 mg, **C(SR):** 60 mg, 80 mg, 120 mg, 160 mg **S:** 4 mg/ml, 8 mg/ml **I:** 1 mg/ml	Beta$_1$, beta$_2$	80–320 mg/day	
Sotalol (p. 1025) (Betapace)	**T:** 80 mg, 120 mg, 160 mg, 240 mg	Beta$_1$, beta$_2$	160–640 mg/day	Same as above
Timolol (p. 1085) (Blocacren)	**T:** 5 mg, 10 mg, 20 mg	Beta$_1$, beta$_2$	10–60 mg/day	Same as above

C: capsules; **I:** injection; **S:** solution; **SR:** sustained-release; **T:** tablets.

Bronchodilators

USES

Relief of bronchospasm occurring during anesthesia and in bronchial asthma, bronchitis, emphysema.

ACTION

Inhaled corticosteroids: Exact mechanism unknown. May act as anti-inflammatories, decrease mucus secretion.

Beta₂-adrenergic agonists: Stimulate beta receptors in lung, relax bronchial smooth muscle, increase vital capacity, decrease airway resistance.

Anticholinergics: Inhibit cholinergic receptors on bronchial smooth muscle (block acetylcholine action).

Leukotriene modifiers: Decrease effect of leukotrienes, which increase migration of eosinophils, producing mucus/edema of airway wall, causing brochoconstriction.

Methylxanthines: Directly relax smooth muscle of bronchial airway, pulmonary blood vessels (relieve bronchospasm, increase vital capacity). Increase cyclic 3,5-adenosine monophosphate.

BRONCHODILATORS

Name	Availability	Dosage Range	Side Effects
Beta Agonists			
Albuterol (p. 22) (Proventil, Ventolin, Ventolin Rotacaps, Volmax, AccuNeb)	T: 2 mg, 4 mg T (SR): 4 mg, 8 mg S: 2 mg/5 ml MDI (Neb): 0.5%, 2.5 mg/3 ml, 1.25 mg/3 ml, 0.63 mg/3 ml	A, C (MDI): 2 puffs q4-6h as needed A, C (Rotacaps): 1-2 caps q4-6h as needed A (Neb): 2.5 mg q4-6h as needed C (Neb): 0.1-0.15 mg/kg q4-6h as needed A [T(SR)]: 4-8 mg q12h C [T(SR)]: 4 mg q12h	Tremors, tachycardia, palpitations, hypokalemia

Bitolterol (p. 130) (Tornalate)	MDI (Neb): 0.2%	A, C (MDI): 2 puffs q4–6h as needed A (Neb): 1.5–3.5 mg 2–4 times/day as needed C (Neb): 1.5 mg 2–4 times/day as needed	Same as above
Formoterol (p. 491) (Foradil)	C: 12 mcg		Same as above
Isoetharine (p. 614)	Neb: 1%		Same as above
Levalbuterol (p. 653) (Xopenex)	Neb: 0.63 mg/3 ml, 1.25 mg/3 ml	A: 0.63 mg q6–8h as needed	Same as above
Metaproterenol (p. 713) (Alupent, Metaprel)	MDI (Neb): 5% S: 10 mg/5 ml T: 10 mg, 20 mg		Same as above
Pirbuterol (Maxair)	MDI	A, C: 2 puffs q4–6h as needed	Same as above
Salmeterol (p. 996) (Serevent)	MDI C: 50 mcg	A (MDI): 2 puffs q12h C: 1–2 puffs q12h A, C (C): 1 inhalation q12h	Same as above
Terbutaline (p. 1064) (Brethine, Bricanyl)	MDI T: 2.5 mg, 5 mg		Same as above

Inhaled Anti-Inflammatory Agents

| Beclomethasone (p. 109) (Beclovent, Vanceroil, QVAR) | MDI | 1–2 inhalations 2–4 times/day | Oropharyngeal candidiasis, dysphonia, hoarseness, cough |
| Budesonide (p. 142) (Pulmicort) | MDI
Neb | MDI (A): 1–4 inhalations 2 times/day
C (>6 yrs): 1–2 inhalations 2 times/day | Same as above |

(continued)

BRONCHODILATORS *(continued)*

Inhaled Anti-Inflammatory Agents *(continued)*

Name	Availability	Dosage Range	Side Effects
Cromolyn (p. 285) (Intal)	MDI Neb	**MDI: C (>5 yrs):** 2 inhalations up to 4 times/day **Neb: C (>2 yrs):** 20 mg 4 times/day	Cough, urticaria, bronchospasm
Flunisolide (p. 470) (AeroBid)	MDI	**A:** 2–4 inhalations 2 times/day **C (6–15 yrs):** 1–2 inhalations 2 times/day	Same as beclomethasone
Fluticasone (p. 484) (Flovent)	MDI Rotadisk	**MDI: A, C (>12yrs):** 2 inhalations 2 times/day **Rotadisk: A, C (>4 yrs):** 1 inhalations 2 times/day	Same as beclomethasone
Nedocromil (p. 793) (Tilade)	MDI	**A, C (>6 yrs):** 2 inhalations 4 times/day	Unpleasant taste, headaches, nausea
Triamcinolone (p. 1121) (Azmacort)	MDI	**A:** 2 inhalations 3–4 times/day or 4–8 inhalations 2 times/day **C:** 1–2 inhalations 3–4 times/day or 2–6 inhalations 2 times/day	Same as beclomethasone

Leukotriene Modifiers

Name	Availability	Dosage Range	Side Effects
Montelukast (p. 762) (Singulair)	T: 4 mg, 5 mg, 10 mg	**A:** 10 mg/day **C (6–14 yrs):** 5 mg/day **C (2–5 yrs):** 4 mg/day	Dyspepsia, increased liver function tests
Zafirlukast (p. 1171) (Accolate)	T: 10 mg, 20 mg	**A, C (>12 yrs):** 20 mg 2 times/day **C (5–11 yrs):** 10 mg 2 times/day	Same as above
Zileuton (p. 1179) (Zyflo)	T: 600 mg	**A:** 600 mg 4 times/day	Same as above

A: adults; **C:** capsules; **C** (dosage): children; **MDI:** metered dose inhaler; **Neb:** nebulization; **S:** syrup; **T:** tablets; **T (SR):** tablets, sustained-release.

Calcium Channel Blockers

USES

Treatment of essential hypertension, treatment and prophylaxis of angina pectoris (including vasospastic, chronic stable, unstable), prevention/control of supraventricular tachyarrhythmias, prevention of neurologic damage due to subarachnoid hemorrhage.

ACTION

Calcium channel blockers inhibit the flow of extracellular Ca^{+2} ions across cell membranes of cardiac cells, vascular tissue. They relax arterial smooth muscle, depress the rate of sinus node pacemaker, slow AV conduction, decrease heart rate, produce negative inotropic effect (rarely seen clinically due to reflex response). Calcium channel blockers decrease coronary vascular resistance, increase coronary blood flow, reduce myocardial oxygen demand. Degree of action varies with individual agent.

CALCIUM CHANNEL BLOCKERS

Name	Availability	Dosage Range	Side Effects
Amlodipine (p. 55) (Norvasc)	**T:** 2.5 mg, 5 mg, 10 mg	2.5–10 mg/day	Abdominal pain, flushing, headaches
Bepridil (p. 115) (Vascor)	**T:** 200 mg, 300 mg, 400 mg	200–400 mg/day	Diarrhea, dizziness, nausea
Diltiazem (p. 351) (Cardizem)	**T:** 30 mg, 60 mg, 90 mg **T (SR):** 120 mg, 180 mg, 240 mg **C (SR):** 60 mg, 90 mg, 120 mg, 180 mg, 240 mg, 300 mg, 360 mg **I:** 5 mg/ml	**PO:** 120–360 mg/day **I:** 20–25 mg IV bolus, then 5–15 mg/hr infusion	Dizziness, drowsiness
Felodipine (p. 444) (Plendil)	**T:** 2.5 mg, 5 mg, 10 mg	5–10 mg/day	Peripheral edema, headaches

(continued)

CALCIUM CHANNEL BLOCKERS *(continued)*

Name	Availability	Dosage Range	Side Effects
Isradipine (p. 623) (DynaCirc)	**T:** 5 mg, 10 mg **C:** 2.5 mg, 5 mg	5–20 mg/day	Headaches
Nicardipine (p. 805) (Cardene)	**C:** 20 mg, 30 mg **C (ER):** 30 mg, 45 mg, 60 mg **I:** 2.5 mg/ml	**PO:** 60–120 mg/day	Flushing, feeling of warmth
Nifedipine (p. 809) (Adalat, Procardia)	**C:** 10 mg, 20 mg **T (ER):** 30 mg, 60 mg, 90 mg	30–120 mg/day	Peripheral edema, dizziness, flushed face, headaches, nausea
Nimodipine (p. 812) (Nimotop)	**C:** 30 mg	60 mg q4h for 21 days	Nausea
Verapamil (p. 1151) (Calan, Isoptin)	**T:** 40 mg, 80 mg, 120 mg **T (SR):** 120 mg, 180 mg, 240 mg	120–480 mg/day	Constipation, nausea

C: capsules; **ER:** extended-release; **I:** injection; **SR:** sustained-release; **T:** tablets.

Cancer Chemotherapeutic Agents

USES

Treatment of a wide variety of cancers; may be palliative or curative. Treatment of choice in hematologic cancers. Frequently used as adjunctive therapy, e.g., with surgery or irradiation; most effective when tumor mass has been removed or reduced by radiation. Often used in combinations to increase therapeutic results; decrease toxic effects. Certain agents may be used in non-malignant conditions; polycythemia vera, psoriasis, rheumatoid arthritis, or immuno-suppression in organ transplantation (used only in select cases that are severe and unresponsive to other forms of therapy). Refer to individual monographs.

ACTION

Most antineoplastics inhibit cell replication by interfering with supply of nutrients or genetic components of the cell (DNA or RNA). Some antineoplastics, referred to as cell cycle-specific (CCS), are particularly effective during a specific phase of cell reproduction (e.g., antimetabolites and plant alkaloids). Other antineoplastics, referred to as cell cycle-nonspecific, act independently of a specific phase of cell division (e.g., alkylating agents and antibiotics). Some hormones are also classified as antineoplastics. Although not cytotoxic, they act to depress cancer growth by altering the hormone environment. In addition, there are a number of miscellaneous agents acting through different mechanisms.

CANCER CHEMOTHERAPEUTIC AGENTS

Name	Availability	Side Effects
Aldesleukin (p. 602) (Proleukin)	**I:** 22 million units **Powder**	Hypotension, sinus, tachycardia, nausea, vomiting, diarrhea, renal impairment, anemia, rash, fatigue, agitation, pulmonary congestion, dyspnea, fever, chills, oliguria, weight gain, dizziness
Alemtuzumab (p. 22) (Campath)	**I:** 30 mg/3 ml	Rigors, fever, fatigue, hypotension, neutropenia, anemia, sepsis, dyspnea, bronchitis, pneumonia, urticaria
Alitretinoin (p. 26) (Panretin)	**Gel:** 0.1%	Burning, pain, edema, dermatitis, rash, skin disorders
Altretamine (p. 37) (Hexalen)	**C:** 50 mg	Nausea, vomiting, myelosuppression, peripheral neuropathy, altered mood, ataxia, dizziness, nervousness, vertigo
Aminoglutethimide (Cytadren)	**T:** 250 mg	Orthostatic hypotension, hypothyroidism, vomiting, anorexia, rash, drowsiness, headaches, fever, myalgia
Anastrozole (p. 70) (Arimidex)	**T:** 1 mg	Peripheral edema, chest pain, nausea, vomiting, diarrhea, constipation, abdominal pain, anorexia, pharyngitis, vaginal hemorrhage, anemia, leukopenia, rash, weight gain, sweating, increased appetite, pain, headaches, dizziness, depression, paresthesias, hot flashes, increased cough, dry mouth, asthenia, dyspnea, phlebitis

(continued)

CANCER CHEMOTHERAPEUTIC AGENTS *(continued)*

Name	Availability	Side Effects
Arsenic trioxide (p. 77) (Trisenox)	I: 10 mg/ml	AV block, GI hemorrhage, hypertension, hypoglycemia, hypokalemia, hypomagnesemia, neutropenia, oliguria, prolonged QT interval, seizures, sepsis, thrombocytopenia
Asparaginase (p. 81) (Elspar)	I: 10,000 units	Anorexia, nausea, vomiting, liver toxicity, pancreatitis, nephrotoxicity, clotting factor abnormalities, malaise, confusion, lethargy, EEG changes, respiratory distress, fever, hyperglycemia, depression, stomatitis, allergic reactions, drowsiness
BCG (p. 107) (Tice BCG, Theracys)	I: 50 mg, 81 mg	Nausea, vomiting, anorexia, diarrhea, dysuria, hematuria, cystitis, urinary urgency, anemia, malaise, fever, chills
Bexarotene (p. 123) (Targretin)	C: 75 mg Gel: 1%	Anemia, dermatitis, fever, hypercholesterolemia, infection, leukopenia, peripheral edema
Bicalutamide (p. 125) (Casodex)	T: 50 mg	Gynecomastia, hot flashes, breast pain, nausea, diarrhea, constipation, nocturia, impotence, pain, muscle pain, asthenia, abdominal pain
Bleomycin (p. 134) (Blenoxane)	I: 15 units, 30 units	Nausea, vomiting, anorexia, stomatitis, hyperpigmentation, nail changes, alopecia, pruritus, hyperkeratosis, urticaria, pneumonitis progression to fibrosis, decreased weight, rash
Busulfan (p. 149) (Myleran)	T: 2 mg	Nausea, vomiting, hyperuricemia, myelosuppression, skin hyperpigmentation, alopecia, anorexia, decreased weight, diarrhea, stomatitis
Capecitabine (p. 163) (Xeloda)	T: 150 mg, 300 mg	Nausea, vomiting, diarrhea, stomatitis, bone marrow depression, hand-and-foot syndrome, dermatitis, fatigue, anorexia
Carboplatin (p. 171) (Paraplatin)	I: 50 mg, 150 mg, 450 mg	Nausea, vomiting, nephrotoxicity, bone marrow suppression, alopecia, peripheral neuropathy, hypersensitivity, ototoxicity, asthenia, diarrhea, constipation
Carmustine (p. 175) (BCNU)	I: 100 mg	Anorexia, nausea, vomiting, bone marrow depression, pulmonary fibrosis, pain at injection site, diarrhea, skin discoloration.
Chlorambucil (p. 224) (Leukeran)	T: 2 mg	Bone marrow suppression, dermatitis, nausea, vomiting, liver toxicity, anorexia, diarrhea, abdominal discomfort, rash

Cisplatin (p. 246) (Platinol)	**I:** 50 mg, 100 mg	Nausea, vomiting, nephrotoxicity, bone marrow depression, neuropathies, ototoxicity, anaphylactic-like reactions, hyperuricemia, hypomagnesemia, hypophosphatemia, hypokalemia, hypocalcemia, pain at injection site
Cladribine (p. 251) (Leustatin)	**I:** 1 mg/ml	Nausea, vomiting, diarrhea, bone marrow depression, chills, fatigue, rash, fever, headaches, anorexia, diaphoresis
Cyclophosphamide (p. 290) (Cytoxan)	**I:** 100 mg, 200 mg, 500 mg, 1 g, 2 g **T:** 25 mg, 50 mg	Nausea, vomiting, hemorrhagic cystitis, bone marrow depression, alopecia, interstitial pulmonary fibrosis, amenorrhea, azoospermia, diarrhea, darkening skin/fingernails, headaches, diaphoresis
Cytarabine (p. 296) (Cytosar, ARA-C)	**I:** 100 mg, 500 mg, 1 g, 2 g	Anorexia, nausea, vomiting, stomatitis, esophagitis, diarrhea, bone marrow depression, alopecia, rash, fever, neuropathies, abdominal pain
Dacarbazine (p. 299) (DTIC)	**I:** 200 mg	Nausea, vomiting, anorexia, liver necrosis, bone marrow depression, alopecia, rash, facial flushing, photosensitivity, flulike syndrome, confusion, blurred vision
Dactinomycin (p. 302) (Cosmegen)	**I:** 0.5 mg vial	Nausea, vomiting, stomatitis, esophagitis, pharyngitis, GI ulceration, proctitis, diarrhea, bone marrow depression, alopecia, erythema, acne, skin eruptions, hypocalcemia, fever, fatigue, myalgia, anorexia
Daunorubicin (p. 312) (Cerubidine)	**I:** 20 mg	CHF, nausea, vomiting, stomatitis, mucositis, diarrhea, red urine, bone marrow depression, alopecia, fever, chills, abdominal pain
Daunorubicin (p. 312) (DaunoXome)	**I:** 50 mg	Nausea, diarrhea, abdominal pain, anorexia, vomiting, stomatitis, myelosuppression, rigors, back pain, headaches, neuropathy, depression, dyspnea, fatigue, fever, cough, allergic reactions, sweating
Denileukin (p. 318) (Ontak)	**I:** 300 mcg/2 ml	Hypersensitivity reaction, back pain, dyspnea, rash, chest pain, tachycardia, asthenia, flulike syndrome, chills, nausea, vomiting, infection
Docetaxel (p. 367) (Taxotere)	**I:** 20 mg, 80 mg	Hypotension, nausea, vomiting, diarrhea, mucositis, bone marrow suppression, rash, paresthesia, hypersensitivity, fluid retention, alopecia, asthenia, stomatitis, fever

(continued)

CANCER CHEMOTHERAPEUTIC AGENTS *(continued)*

Name	Availability	Side Effects
Doxorubicin (p. 383) (Adriamycin)	**I:** 10 mg, 20 mg, 50 mg, 75 mg, 150 mg, 200 mg	Cardiotoxicity, including CHF; arrhythmias, nausea, vomiting, stomatitis, esophagitis, GI ulceration, diarrhea, anorexia, red urine, bone marrow depression, alopecia, hyperpigmentation of nail beds and skin, local inflammation at injection site, rash, fever, chills, urticaria, lacrimation, conjunctivitis
Doxorubicin (p. 383) (Doxil)	**I:** 20 mg, 50 mg	Neutropenia, palmoplantar erythrodysesthesia syndrome, cardiomyopathy, CHF
Epirubicin (p. 404) (Ellence)	**I:** 2 mg/ml	Anemia, leukopenia, neutropenia, infection, mucositis
Estramustine (p. 425) (Emcyst)	**C:** 140 mg	Increased risk of thrombosis, gynecomastia, nausea, vomiting, diarrhea, thrombocytopenia, peripheral edema
Etoposide (p. 435) (VePesid)	**I:** 20 mg/ml **C:** 50 mg	Nausea, vomiting, anorexia, bone marrow depression, alopecia, diarrhea, somnolence, peripheral neuropathies
Exemestane (p. 437) (Aromasin)	**T:** 25 mg	Dyspnea, edema, hypertension, mental depression
Floxuridine (p. 461) (FUDR)	**I:** 500 mg vial	Aphthous, stomatitis, enteritis
Fludarabine (p. 464) (Fludara)	**I:** 50 mg	Nausea, diarrhea, stomatitis, bleeding, anemia, bone marrow depression, skin rash, weakness, confusion, visual disturbances, peripheral neuropathy, coma, pneumonia, peripheral edema, anorexia
Fluorouracil (p. 473)	**I:** 50 mg/ml **Cream:** 1%, 5% **Solution:** 1%, 2%, 5%	Nausea, vomiting, stomatitis, GI ulceration, diarrhea, anorexia, bone marrow depression, alopecia, skin hyperpigmentation, nail changes, headaches, drowsiness, blurred vision, fever
Flutamide (p. 483) (Eulexin)	**C:** 125 mg	Hot flashes, nausea, vomiting, diarrhea, hepatitis, impotence, decreased libido, rash, anorexia

Gemcitabine (p. 510) (Gemzar)	I: 200 mg, 1 g	Increased LFTs, nausea, vomiting, diarrhea, stomatitis, hematuria, myelosuppression, rash, mild paresthesias, dyspnea, fever, edema, flulike symptoms, constipation
Gemtuzumab (p. 514) (Mylotarg)	I: 5 mg/20 ml	Anemia, hematuria, liver toxicity, pneumonia, herpes simplex, nausea, vomiting, dyspnea, headaches, hypotension, hypoxia, mucositis, myelosuppression, peripheral edema, tachycardia, thrombocytopenia
Goserelin (p. 535) (Zoladex)	I: 3.6 mg, 10.8 mg	Hot flashes, sexual dysfunction, decreased erections, gynecomastia, breast swelling, lethargy, pain, lower urinary tract symptoms, headaches, nausea, depression, sweating
Hydroxyurea (p. 562) (Hydrea)	C: 500 mg	Anorexia, nausea, vomiting, stomatitis, diarrhea, constipation, bone marrow depression, fever, chills, malaise
Idarubicin (p. 571) (Idamycin)	I: 5 mg, 10 mg, 20 mg	CHF, arrhythmias, nausea, vomiting, stomatitis, bone marrow depression, alopecia, rash, urticaria, hyperuricemia, abdominal pain, diarrhea, esophagitis, anorexia
Ifosfamide (p. 573) (Ifex)	I: 1 g, 3 g	Nausea, vomiting, hemorrhagic cystitis, bone marrow depression, alopecia, lethargy, somnolence, confusion, hallucinations, hematuria
Imatinib (p. 575) (Gleevec)	C: 100 mg	Nausea, fluid retention, hemorrhage, musculoskeletal pain, arthralgia, weight gain, pyrexia, abdominal pain, dyspnea, pneumonia
Interferon alfa 2A (p. 593) (Roferon A)	I: 3 million units, 6 million units, 9 million units, 18 million units	Anorexia, nausea, diarrhea, bone marrow depression, pruritus, myalgia, dizziness, headaches, paresthesias, numbness, fatigue, fever, chills, dyspnea, flulike symptoms, vomiting, coughing, altered taste
Interferon alfa 2B (p. 594) (Intron A)	I: 3 million units, 5 million units, 10 million units, 18 million units, 25 million units, 50 million units	Mild hypotension, hypertension, tachycardia with high fever, nausea, diarrhea, altered taste, weight loss, thrombocytopenia, bone marrow depression, rash, pruritus, myalgia, arthralgia associated with flulike syndromes
Irinotecan (p. 609) (Camptosar)	I: 40 mg, 100 mg	Diarrhea, nausea, vomiting, abdominal cramping, anorexia, stomatitis, increased SGOT, severe myelosuppression, alopecia, sweating, rash, decreased weight, dehydration, increased alkaline phosphatase, headaches, insomnia, dizziness, dyspnea, cough, asthenia, rhinitis, fever, pain, back pain, chills

(continued)

CANCER CHEMOTHERAPEUTIC AGENTS *(continued)*

Name	Availability	Side Effects
Letrozole (p. 648) (Femara)	**T:** 2.5 mg	Hypertension, nausea, vomiting, constipation, diarrhea, abdominal pain, anorexia, rash, pruritus, musculoskeletal pain, back pain, arm and leg pain, arthralgia, fatigue, headaches, dyspnea, coughing, hot flashes
Leuprolide (p. 651) (Lupron)	**I:** 3.75 mg, 5 mg, 7.5 mg, 11.25 mg, 15 mg, 22.5 mg, 30 mg	Hot flashes, gynecomastia, nausea, vomiting, constipation, anorexia, dizziness, headaches, insomnia, paresthesis, bone pain
Lomustine (p. 674) (CeeNu)	**C:** 10 mg, 40 mg, 100 mg	Anorexia, nausea, vomiting, stomatitis, liver toxicity, nephrotoxicity, bone marrow depression, alopecia, confuson, slurred speech
Mechlorethamine (p. 696) (Mustargen)	**I:** 10 mg/ml	Severe nausea and vomiting, metallic taste, diarrhea, bone marrow depression, alopecia, phlebitis, vertigo, tinnitus, hyperuricemia, infertility, azoospermia, anorexia, headaches, drowsiness, fever
Megestrol (p. 699) (Megace)	**T:** 20 mg, 40 mg **Suspension:** 40 mg/ml	Deep vein thrombosis, Cushing-like syndrome, alopecia, carpal tunnel syndrome, weight gain, nausea
Melphalan (p. 702) (Alkeran)	**T:** 2 mg	Anorexia, nausea, vomiting, bone marrow depression, diarrhea, stomatitis
Mercaptopurine (p. 707) (Purinethol)	**T:** 50 mg	Anorexia, nausea, vomiting, stomatitis, liver toxicity, bone marrow depression, hyperuricemia, diarrhea, rash
Methotrexate (p. 720)	**T:** 2.5 mg, 5 mg, 7.5 mg, 10 mg, 15 mg **I:** 5 mg, 50 mg, 100 mg, 200 mg, 250 mg	Nausea, vomiting, stomatitis, GI ulceration, diarrhea, liver toxicity, renal failure, cystitis, bone marrow suppression, alopecia, urticaria, acne, photosensitivity, interstitial pneumonitis, fever, malaise, chills, anorexia
Mitomycin-C (p. 755) (Mutamycin)	**I:** 20 mg, 40 mg	Anorexia, nausea, vomiting, stomatitis, diarrhea, renal toxicity, bone marrow depression, alopecia, pruritus, fever, hemolytic uremic syndrome, weakness

Mitotane (p. 757) (Lysodren)	**T:** 500 mg	Anorexia, nausea, vomiting, diarrhea, skin rashes, depression, lethargy, somnolence, dizziness, adrenal insufficiency, blurred vision, decreased hearing
Mitoxantrone (p. 757) (Novantrone)	**I:** 20 mg, 25 mg, 30 mg	CHF, tachycardia, EKG changes, chest pain, nausea, vomiting, stomatitis, mucositis, myelosuppression, rash, alopecia, urine color change to bluish green, phlebitis, diarrhea, cough, headaches, fever
Nilutamide (p. 811) (Nilandron)	**T:** 50 mg	Hypertension, angina, hot flashes, nausea, anorexia, increased liver enzymes, dizziness, dyspnea, visual disturbances, impaired adaptation to dark, constipation, loss of libido
Paclitaxel (p. 853) (Taxol)	**I:** 30 mg, 100 mg	Hypertension, bradycardia, EKG changes, nausea, vomiting, diarrhea, mucositis, bone marrow depression, alopecia, peripheral neuropathies, hypersensitivity reaction, arthralgia, myalgia
Pegaspargase (Oncaspar)	**I:** 750 IU/ml	Hypotension, anorexia, nausea, vomiting, liver toxicity, pancreatitis, depression of clotting factors, malaise, confusion, lethargy, EEG changes, respiratory distress, hypersensitivity reaction, fever, hyperglycemia, stomatitis
Pentostatin (p. 874) (Nipent)	**I:** 10 mg	Nausea, vomiting, liver disorder, elevated LFTs, leukopenia, anemia, thrombocytopenia, rash, fever, upper respiratory infection, fatigue, hematuria, headaches, myalgia, arthralgia, diarrhea, anorexia
Plicamycin (p. 902) (Mithracin)	**I:** 2.5 mg	Anorexia, nausea, vomiting stomatitis, diarrhea, clotting factor disorders, facial flushing, mental depression, confusion, fever, hypocalcemia, hypophosphatemia, hypokalemia, headaches, dizziness, rash
Procarbazine (p. 926) (Matulane)	**C:** 50 mg	Nausea, vomiting, stomatitis, diarrhea, constipation, bone marrow depression, pruritus, hyperpigmentation, alopecia, myalgia, paresthesias, confusion, lethargy, mental depression, fever, liver toxicity, arthralgia, respiratory disorders
Rituximab (p. 987) (Rituxan)	**I:** 100 mg, 500 mg	Hypotension, arrhythmias, peripheral edema, nausea, vomiting, abdominal pain, leukopenia, thrombocytopenia, neutropenia, rash, pruritis, urticaria, angiooedema, myalgia, headaches, dizziness, throat irritation, rhinitis, bronchospasm, hypersensitivity reaction

(continued)

CANCER CHEMOTHERAPEUTIC AGENTS (continued)

Name	Availability	Side Effects
Streptozocin (p. 1036) (Zanosar)	**I:** 1 g	May lead to insulin-dependent diabetes, nausea, vomiting, nephrotoxicity, renal tubular acidosis, bone marrow depression, lethargy, diarrhea, confusion, depression
Tamoxifen (p. 1049) (Nolvadex)	**T:** 10 mg, 20 mg	Skin rash, nausea, vomiting, anorexia, menstrual irregularities, hot flashes, pruritus, vaginal discharge or bleeding, bone marrow depression, headaches, tumor or bone pain, ophthalmic changes, weight gain, confusion
Temozolamide (p. 1055) (Temodar)	**C:** 5 mg, 20 mg, 100 mg, 250 mg	Amnesia, fever, infection, leukopenia, neutropenia, peripheral edema, seizures, thrombocytopenia
Teniposide (p. 1059) (Vumon)	**I:** 50 mg/5 ml	Hypotension with rapid infusion, diarrhea, nausea, vomiting, mucositis, bone marrow depression, alopecia, anemia, rash, hypersensitivity reaction
Thioguanine (p. 1075)	**T:** 40 mg	Anorexia, stomatitis, bone marrow depression, hyperuricemia, nausea, vomiting, diarrhea
Thiotepa (p. 1077) (Thioplex)	**I:** 15 mg	Anorexia, nausea, vomiting, mucositis, bone marrow depression, amenorrhea, reduced spermatogenesis, fever, hypersensitivity reactions, pain at injection site, headaches, dizziness, alopecia
Topotecan (p. 1105) (Hycamtin)	**I:** 4 mg	Nausea, vomiting, diarrhea, constipation, abdominal pain, stomatitis, anorexia, neutropenia, leukopenia, thrombocytopenia, anemia, alopecia, headaches, dyspnea, paresthesia
Toremifene (p. 1107) (Fareston)	**T:** 60 mg	Elevated LFTs, nausea, vomiting, constipation, skin discoloration, dermatitis, dizziness, hot flashes, sweating, vaginal discharge, vaginal bleeding, ocular changes, cataracts, anxiety
Trastuzumab (p. 1115) (Herceptin)	**I:** 440 mg	CHF, S3 gallup, nausea, vomiting, diarrhea, abdominal pain, anorexia, rash, peripheral edema, back pain, bone pain, asthenia, headaches, insomnia, dizziness, cough, dyspnea, rhinitis, pharyngitis
Tretinoin (p. 1119) (Vesanoid)	**C:** 10 mg	Flushing, nausea, vomiting, diarrhea, constipation, dyspepsia, mucositis, leukocytosis, dry skin/mucus membranes, rash, itching, alopecia, dizziness, anxiety, insomnia, headaches, depression, confusion, intracranial hypertension, agitation, dyspnea, shivering, fever, visual changes, earaches, hearing loss, bone pain, myalgia, arthralgia

Valrubicin (p. 1143) (Valstar)	**I:** 200 mg/5 ml	Dysuria, hematuria, urinary frequency/incontinence, red color in urine, urinary urgency
Vinblastine (p. 1155) (Velban)	**I:** 10 mg	Nausea, vomiting, stomatitis, constipation, bone marrow depression, alopecia, peripheral neuropathy, loss of deep tendon reflexes, paresthesias, diarrhea
Vincristine (p. 1157) (Oncovin)	**I:** 1 mg, 2 mg, 3 mg	Nausea, vomiting, stomatitis, constipation, pharyngitis, polyuria, bone marrow depression, alopecia, numbness, paresthesias, peripheral neuropathy, loss of deep tendon reflexes, headaches, abdominal pain
Vinorelbine (p. 1159) (Navelbine)	**I:** 10 mg, 50 mg	Elevated LFTs, nausea, vomiting, constipation, ileus, anorexia, stomatitis, bone marrow suppression, alopecia, vein discoloration, venous pain, phlebitis, interstitial pulmonary changes, asthenia, fatigue, diarrhea, peripheral neuropathy, loss of deep tendon reflexes

C: capsules; **I:** injection; **T:** tablets.

Cardiac Glycosides (Inotropic Agents)

USES

CHF, atrial fibrillation, atrial flutter, paroxysmal atrial tachycardia, treatment of cardiogenic shock with pulmonary edema.

ACTION

Direct action on myocardium causes increased force of contraction, resulting in increased stroke volume and cardiac output. Depression of SA node, decreased conduction time through AV node, and decreased electrical impulses due to vagal stimulation slow heart rate. Improved myocardial contractility is probably due to improved transport of calcium, sodium, and potassium ions across cell membranes.

Cardiac Glycosides (Inotropic Agents) (continued)

CARDIAC GLYCOSIDES (INOTROPIC AGENTS)

Name	Availability	Dosage Range	Side Effects
Digoxin (p. 348) (Lanoxin)	C: 0.05 mg, 0.1 mg, 0.2 mg T: 0.125 mg, 0.25 mg E: 0.05 mg/ml I: 0.1 mg/ml, 0.25 mg/ml	PO/IV: 0.125–0.375 mg/day	Arrhythmias, blurred vision, confusion, hallucinations, nausea, vomiting, diarrhea, abdominal pain
Inamrinone	I: 5 mg/ml	IV: 0.75 mg/kg bolus, then 5–10 mcg/kg/min infusion	Arrhythmias, hypotension
Milrinone (p. 748) (Primacor)	I: 1 mg/ml	IV: 50 mcg/kg bolus, then 0.375–0.75 mcg/kg/min infusion	Arrhythmias, hypotension, headaches

C: capsules; E: elixir; I: injection; T: tablets.

Cholinergic Agonists/Anticholinesterase

USES

Paralytic ileus and atony of urinary bladder. Myasthenia gravis (weakness, marked fatigue of skeletal muscle). Terminates, reverses effects of neuromuscular blocking agents.

ACTION

Cholinergic Agonists: Referred to as muscarinics or parasympathetics and consist of two basic drug groups: choline esters and cholinomimetic alkaloids. Primary action mimics actions of acetylcholine at postganglionic parasympathetic nerves. Primary properties include the following: *Cardiovascular system:* Vasodilation, decreased cardiac rate, decreased conduction in SA, AV nodes, decreased force of myocardial contraction. *Gastrointestinal:* Increased tone, motility of GI smooth muscle, increased secretory activity of GI tract. *Urinary tract:* Increased contraction of detrusor muscle of urinary bladder, resulting in micturition. *Eye:* Miosis, contraction of ciliary muscle. *Anticholinesterase (anti-ChE)* also known as cholinesterase inhibitors: Inactivates cholinesterase, which prevents acetylcholine breakdown, causing acetylcholine to accumulate at cholinergic receptor sites. These agents can be considered indirect-acting cholinergic agonists. Primary properties include action of cholinergic agonists just noted. *Skeletal neuromuscular junction:* Effects are dose dependent. At therapeutic doses, increases force of skeletal muscle contraction; at toxic doses, reduces muscle strength.

CHOLINERGIC AGONISTS/ANTICHOLINESTERASE

Name	Availability	Uses	Dosage Range	Side Effects
Bethanechol (p. 122) (Urecholine)	**T:** 5 mg, 10 mg, 25 mg, 50 mg **I:** 5 mg/ml	Nonobstructive urinary retention	**PO:** 10–50 mg 3–4 times/day **SubQ:** 2.5–5 mg 3–4 times/day	Increased urinary frequency, salivation, belching, nausea, dizziness
Edrophonium (Tensilon)	**I:** 10 mg/ml	Diagnosis of myasthenia gravis reverses tubocurarine	**IV:** 10 mg over 30 seconds up to 40 mg	Bradycardia, nausea, vomiting, diarrhea, urinary frequency
Neostigmine (p. 799) (Prostigmin)	**T:** 15 mg **I:** 0.25 mg/ml, 0.5 mg/ml, 1 mg/ml	Symptomatic control of myasthenia gravis, neuromuscular blocker	**PO:** 15–365 mg/day **SubQ, IM:** 0.5 mg **IV:** 0.5–2 mg	Diarrhea, increased sweating, nausea, vomiting, stomach cramps
Pyridostigmine (p. 949) (Mestinon)	**T:** 60 mg **T (ER):** 180 mg **S:** 60 mg/5 ml **I:** 5 mg/ml	Treats myasthenia gravis, reverses tubocurarine	**PO:** 60–1,500 mg/day **IM:** 0.5–1.5 mg/kg **IV:** 0.1–0.25 mg/kg	Diarrhea, increased sweating, nausea, vomiting, stomach cramps

I: injection; **S:** suspension; **T:** tablets.

Corticosteroids

USES

Replacement therapy in adrenal insufficiency, including Addison's disease. Symptomatic treatment of multiorgan disease/conditions. Rheumatoid and osteo arthritis, severe psoriasis, ulcerative colitis, lupus erythematosus, anaphylactic shock, status asthmaticus, organ transplant.

ACTION

Suppress migration of polymorphonuclear leukocytes (PML) and reverse increased capillary permeability by their anti-inflammatory effect. Suppress immune system by decreasing activity of lymphatic system.

CORTICOSTEROIDS

Name	Availability	Route of Administration	Side Effects
Beclomethasone (p. 109) **(Beclovent, Beconase,** **Vanceril, Vancenase)**	**Inhalation** **Nasal:** 42 mcg/spray, 84 mcg/spray	Inhalation, intranasal	**I:** Cough, dry mouth/throat, headaches, throat irritation **Nasal:** Headaches, sore throat, sores inside nose
Betamethasone (p. 118) **(Celestone, Diprosone)**	**I:** 4 mg/ml	IV, intralesional, intra-articular	Nausea, vomiting, increased appetite, weight gain, trouble sleeping
Budesonide (p. 142) **(Rhinocort, Pulmicort)**	**Nasal:** 32 mcg/spray	Intranasal	**Nasal:** Headaches, sore throat, sores inside nose
Cortisone (p. 280) **(Cortone)**	**T:** 5 mg, 10 mg, 25 mg	PO	Same as betamethasone

Dexamethasone (p. 324) (Decadron)	**T:** 0.5 mg, 1 mg, 4 mg, 6 mg **OS:** 0.5 mg/5 ml **I:** 4 mg/ml	PO, parenteral	Same as betamethasone
Fludrocortisone (p. 466) (Florinef)	**T:** 0.1 mg	PO	Same as betamethasone
Flunisolide (p. 470) (Aeirobid, Nasalide)	**Inhalation** **Nasal:** 25 mcg/spray	Inhalation, intranasal	Same as beclomethasone
Fluticasone (p. 484) (Flonase, Flovent)	**Inhalation:** 44 mcg, 110 mg/ 220 mcg **Nasal:** 50 mg, 100 mcg	Inhalation, intranasal	Same as beclomethasone
Hydrocortisone (p. 554) (Cortef, Solu-Cortef)	**T:** 5 mg, 10 mg, 25 mg **I:** 100 mg, 250 mg, 500 mg, 1 g	PO, parenteral	Same as betamethasone
Methylprednisolone (p. 728) (Solu Medrol)	**T:** 4 mg **I:** 40 mg, 125 mg, 500 mg, 1 g, 2 g	PO, parenteral	Same as betamethasone
Prednisolone (p. 916) (Prelone)	**T:** 5 mg **OS:** 5 mg/5 ml, 15 mg/5 ml	PO	Same as betamethasone
Prednisone (p. 918) (Deltasone)	**T:** 1 mg, 2.5 mg, 5 mg, 10 mg, 20 mg, 50 mg	PO	Same as betamethasone
Triamcinolone (p. 1121) (Azmacort, Kenalog)	**T:** 4 mg, 8 mg **Inhalation:** 100 mcg	PO, inhalation	Same as betamethasone **I:** Cough, dry mouth/throat, headaches, throat irritation

I: injection; **OS:** oral suspension; **T:** tablets.

Corticosteroids: Topical

USES

Provide relief of inflammation/pruritus associated with corticosteroid-responsive disorders: e.g., contact dermatitis, eczema, insect bite reactions, first- and second-degree localized burns/sunburn.

ACTION

Diffuse across cell membranes, form complexes with cytoplasm. Complexes stimulate protein synthesis of inhibitory enzymes responsible for anti-inflammatory effects (e.g., inhibit edema, erythema, pruritus, capillary dilation, phagocytic activity).

Topical corticosteroids can be classified based on potency.

Low potency: Modest anti-inflammatory effect, safest for chronic application, facial and intertriginous application, with occlusion, for infants/young children.

Medium potency: For moderate inflammatory conditions (e.g., chronic eczematous dermatoses). May use for facial and intertriginous application for only limited time.

High potency: For more severe inflammatory conditions (e.g., lichen simplex chronicus, psoriasis). May use for facial and intertriginous application for short time only. Used in areas of thickened skin due to chronic conditions.

Very high potency: Alternative to systemic therapy for local effect (e.g., chronic lesions caused by psoriasis). Increased risk of skin atrophy. Used for short periods on small areas. Avoid occlusive dressings.

CORTICOSTEROIDS: TOPICAL

Name	Availability	Potency	Side Effects
Alclometasone (p. 22) (Aclovate)	**C, O:** 0.05%	Low	Burning, stinging, irritation, itching, rash
Amcinonide (p. 40) (Cyclocort)	**C, O, L:** 0.1%	High	Same as above

Betamethasone dipropionate (p. 118) (Diprosone)	**C, O, G, L:** 0.05%	High	Same as above
Betamethasone valerate (p. 118) (Valisone)	**C:** 0.01%, 0.05%, 0.1% **O:** 0.1% **L:** 0.1%	High	Same as above
Clobetasol (p. 259) (Temovate)	**C, O:** 0.05%	High	Same as above
Desonide (p. 324) (Tridesilon)	**C, O, L:** 0.05%	Low	Same as above
Desoximetasone (p. 324) (Topicort)	**C:** 0.25%, 0.5% **O:** 0.25% **G:** 0.05%	High	Same as above
Dexamethasone (p. 324) (Decadron)	**C:** 0.1%	Medium	Same as above
Flucinonide (p. 472) (Lidex)	**C, O, G:** 0.05%	High	Same as above
Fluocinolone (p. 472) (Synalar)	**C:** 0.01%, 0.025%, 0.2% **O:** 0.025%	High	Same as above
Flurandrenolide (Cordran)	**C, O, L:** 0.025%, 0.05%	Medium	Same as above
Fluticasone (p. 484) (Cutivate)	**C:** 0.05% **O:** 0.005%	Medium	Same as above
Halobetasol (p. 540) (Ultravate)	**C, O:** 0.05%	High	Same as above

(continued)

CORTICOSTEROIDS: TOPICAL (continued)

Name	Availability	Potency	Side Effects
Hydrocortisone (p. 554) (Cort-Dome, Hytone)	**C, O:** 0.5%, 1%, 2.5%	Medium	Same as above
Mometasone (p. 762) (Elocon)	**C, O, L:** 0.1%	Medium	Same as above
Prednicarbate (p. 916) (Dermatop)	**C:** 0.1%	—	Same as above
Triamcinolone (p. 1121) (Aristocort, Kenalog)	**C, O, L:** 0.025%, 0.1%, 0.5%	Medium	Same as above

C: cream; **G:** gel; **L:** lotion; **O:** ointment.

Diuretics

USES

Thiazides: Management of edema resulting from a number of causes (e.g., CHF, hepatic cirrhosis); hypertension either alone or in combination with other antihypertensives.

Loop: Management of edema associated with CHF, cirrhosis of liver, and renal disease. Furosemide used in treatment of hypertension alone or in combination with other antihypertensives.

Potassium-sparing: Adjunctive treatment with thiazides, loop diuretics in treatment of CHF and hypertension.

C L A S S I F I C A T I O N S

ACTION

Diuretics act to increase the excretion of water/sodium and other electrolytes via the kidneys. Exact mechanism of antihypertensive effect unknown; may be due to reduced plasma volume or decreased peripheral vascular resistance. Subclassifications of diuretics are based on their mechanism and site of action.

Thiazides: Act at the cortical diluting segment of nephron, block reabsorption of Na, Cl, and water; promote excretion of Na, Cl, K, and water.

Loop: Act primarily at the thick ascending limb of Henle's loop to inhibit Na, Cl, and water absorption.

Potassium-sparing: Spironolactone blocks aldosterone action on distal nephron (causes K retention, Na excretion). Triamterene, amiloride act on distal nephron, decreasing Na reuptake, reducing K secretion.

DIURETICS

Name	Availability	Dosage Range	Side Effects
Thiazides			
Chlorothiazide (p. 231) (Diuril)	**T:** 250 mg, 500 mg **S:** 250 mg/5 ml **I:** 500 mg	5–20 mg/day	Confusion, fatigue, muscle cramps, upset stomach
Chlorthalidone (p. 233) (Hygroton)	**T:** 15 mg, 25 mg, 50 mg, 100 mg	25–200 mg/day	Same as above
Hydrochlorothiazide (p. 550) (Hydrodiuril)	**T:** 25 mg, 50 mg, 100 mg **C:** 12.5 mg **Solution:** 50 mg/15 ml	25–100 mg/day	Same as above
Indapamide (p. 583) (Lozol)	**T:** 1.25 mg, 2.5 mg	2.5–5 mg/day	Same as above

(continued)

DIURETICS *(continued)*

Thiazides *(continued)*

Name	Availability	Dosage Range	Side Effects
Metolazone (p. 734) (Diulo, Zaroxolyn)	**T:** 2.5 mg, 5 mg, 10 mg	2.5–10 mg/day	Same as above

Loop

Name	Availability	Dosage Range	Side Effects
Bumetanide (p. 144) (Bumex)	**T:** 0.5 mg, 1 mg, 2 mg **I:** 0.25 mg/ml	5–10 mg/day	Orthostatic hypotension
Ethacrynic acid (p. 429) (Edecrin)	**T:** 25 mg, 50 mg **I:** 50 mg vial	50–200 mg/day	Same as above
Furosemide (p. 499) (Lasix)	**T:** 20 mg, 40 mg, 80 mg **OS:** 10 mg/ml, 40 mg/5 ml **I:** 10 mg/ml	**HTN:** 40–80 mg/day **Edema:** Up to 600 mg/day	Same as above
Torsemide (p. 1108) (Demadex)	**T:** 5 mg, 10 mg, 20 mg, 100 mg **I:** 10 mg/ml	**Edema:** 10–200 mg/day **HTN:** 5–10 mg/day	Constipation, dizziness, headaches, stomach upset

Potassium-Sparing

Name	Availability	Dosage Range	Side Effects
Amiloride (p. 44) (Midamor)	**T:** 5 mg	5–20 mg/day	Hyperkalemia
Spironolactone (p. 1028) (Aldactone)	**T:** 25 mg, 50 mg, 100 mg	25–100 mg/day	Hyperkalemia, nausea, vomiting, cramps, diarrhea
Triamterene (p. 1124) (Dyrenium)	**C:** 50 mg, 100 mg	Up to 300 mg/day	Same as amiloride

C: capsules; **I:** injection, **HTN:** hypertension; **OS:** oral solution; **S:** suspension; **T:** tablets.

Fertility Agents

Infertility is defined as a decreased ability to reproduce as opposed to sterility, the inability to reproduce. Infertility may be due to reproduction dysfunction of the male, female, or both.

Female infertility can be due to disruption of any phase of the reproductive process. The most critical phases include follicular maturation, ovulation, transport of the ovum through the fallopian tubes, fertilization of the ovum, nidation and growth/development of the conceptus. Causes of infertility include the following:

Anovulation, failure of follicular maturation: Absence of adequate hormonal stimulation; ovarian follicles do not ripen, and ovulation will not occur.

Unfavorable cervical mucus: Normally the cervical glands secrete large volumes of thin, watery mucus, but if the mucus is unfavorable (scant, thick, or sticky), sperm is unable to pass through to the uterus.

Hyperprolactinemia: Excessive prolactin secretion may cause amenorrhea, galactorrhea, and infertility.

Luteal phase defect: Progesterone secretion by the corpus luteum is insufficient to maintain endometrial integrity.

Endometriosis: Endometrial tissue is implanted in abnormal locations (e.g., uterine wall, ovary, extragenital sites).

Androgen excess: May decrease fertility (the most common condition is polycystic ovary).

Male infertility is due to decreased density or motility of sperm or semen of abnormal volume or quality. The most obvious manifestation of male infertility is impotence (inability to achieve erection). Whereas in female infertility an identifiable endocrine disorder can be found, most cases of male infertility are not associated with an identifiable endocrine disorder.

MEDICATIONS TO INDUCE OVULATION

Name	Category	Availability	Uses	Side Effects
Cetrorelix (p. 220) (Cetrotide)	GnRH antagonist	**I:** 0.25 mg, 3 mg	Inhibition of premature LH surges in women undergoing ovarian hyperstimulation	**OHSS:** abdominal pain, indigestion, bloating, decreased urine, nausea, vomiting, diarrhea, rapid weight gain, shortness of breath, swelling of lower legs. Headaches, nausea, pain/redness at injection site

(continued)

Fertility Agents *(continued)*

MEDICATIONS TO INDUCE OVULATION *(continued)*

Name	Category	Availability	Uses	Side Effects
Chorionic gonadotorpin (p. 237) (APL, Pregnyl, Profasi, Profasi HP)	Gonadotropin	**I:** 5,000 units, 10,000 units, 20,000 units	In conjunction with clomiphene, human menotropins or urofollitropin to stimulate ovulation	**OHSS:** abdominal pain, indigestion, bloating, decreased urine, nausea, vomiting, diarrhea, rapid weight gain, shortness of breath, swelling of lower legs. Ovarian enlargement, ovarian cyst formation
Clomiphene (Clomid, Milophene, Serophene)	Antiestrogen	**T:** 50 mg	Anovulation, oligo-ovulation with intact pituitary/ovarian response and endogenous estrogen	Ovarian cyst formation, ovarian enlargement, visual disturbances, premenstrual syndrome, hot flashes
Follitropin alpha (p. 490) (Gonal-F)	Gonadotropin	**I:** 37.5 IU FSH, 75 IU FSH, and 150 IU FSH	In conjunction with HCG to stimulate ovarian follicular development in pts with ovulatory dysfunction not due to primary ovarian failure (e.g., anovulation, oligo-ovulation)	**OHSS:** abdominal pain, indigestion, bloating, decreased urine, nausea, vomiting, diarrhea, rapid weight gain, shortness of breath, swelling of lower legs. Flulike symptoms, upper respiratory tract infections, bleeding between menstrual periods, nausea, ovarian enlargement, ovarian cysts, acne, breast pain/tenderness
Follitropin beta (Follistem)	Gonadotropin	**I:** 75 IU FSH	Same as above	**OHSS:** abdominal pain, indigestion, bloating, decreased urine, nausea, vomiting, diarrhea, rapid weight gain, shortness of breath, swelling of lower legs. Flulike symptoms, breast tenderness, dry skin, rash, dizziness, fever, headaches, nausea, unusual tiredness.
Ganirelex (p. 507) (Antagon)	GnRH antagonist	**I:** 250 mcg/0.5 ml	Inhibition of premature LH surges in women undergoing ovarian hyperstimulation	Same as cetrorelix

Goserelin (p. 535) (Zoladex)	GnRH agonist	**Implant:** 3.6 mg	Endometriosis, adjunct to menotropins/HCG for ovulation induction	Hot flashes, amenorrhea, blurred vision, edema, headaches, nausea, vomiting, breast tenderness, weight gain
Leuprolide (p. 651) (Lupron)	GnRH agonist	5 mg/ml for SC injection	Endometriosis, adjunct to menotropins/HCG for ovulation induction	Same as goserelin
Menotropins (p. 704) (Humegon, Pergonal)	Gonadotropin	**FSH:** 75 units, 150 units **LH activity:** 75 units, 150 units	In conjunction with HCG for ovulation stimulation in pts with ovulatory dysfunction due to primary ovarian failure	Same as chorionic gonadotropin
Nafarelin (p. 777) (Synarel)	GnRH agonist	**Nasal Spray:** 2 mg/ml	Same as leuprolide	Loss of bone mineral density, breast enlargement, bleeding between regular menstrual periods, acne, mood swings, seborrhea, hot flashes
Urofollitropin (Fertinex, Metrodin)	Gonadotropin	**FSH activity:** 75 units, 150 units	In conjunction with HCG for ovulation stimulation in pts with polycystic ovary syndrome who have elevated LH:FSH ratio and have failed clomiphene therapy	Same as chorionic gonadotropin

HCG: human chorionic gonadotropin; **I:** injection; **OHSS:** ovarian hyperstimulation syndrome; **T:** tablets.

H₂ Antagonists

USES

Short-term treatment of duodenal ulcer (DU), active benign gastric ulcer (GU); maintenance therapy of duodenal ulcer; pathologic hypersecretory conditions (e.g., Zollinger-Ellison syndrome); gastroesophageal reflux disease (GERD); and prevention of upper GI bleeding in critically ill pts.

H₂ Antagonists *(continued)*

ACTION

Inhibit gastric acid secretion by interfering with histamine at the histamine H₂ receptors in parietal cells. Also inhibit acid secretion caused by gastrin. Inhibition occurs with basal (fasting), nocturnal, food-stimulated, or fundic distention secretion. H₂ antagonists decrease both the volume and H₂ concentration of gastric juices.

H₂ ANTAGONISTS

Name	Availability	Dosage Range	Side Effects
Cimetidine (p. 241) (Tagamet)	**T:** 200 mg, 300 mg, 400 mg, 800 mg **L:** 300 mg/5 ml **I:** 150 mg/ml	**Treatment of DU:** 800 mg/at bedtime, 400 mg 2 times/day or 300 mg 4 times/day **Maintenance of DU:** 400 mg/at bedtime **Treatment of GU:** 800 mg/at bedtime or 300 mg 4 times/day **GERD:** 1,600 mg/day **Hypersecretory:** 1,200–2,400 mg/day	Headaches, fatigue, dizziness, confusion, diarrhea, gynecomastia
Famotidine (p. 442) (Pepcid)	**T:** 10 mg, 20 mg, 40 mg **T (chewable):** 10 mg **T (DT):** 20 mg, 40 mg **Gelcap:** 10 mg **OS:** 40 mg/5 ml **I:** 10 mg/ml	**Treatment of DU:** 40 mg/day **Maintenance of DU:** 20 mg/day **Treatment of GU:** 40 mg/day **GERD:** 40–80 mg/day **Hypersecretory:** 80–640 mg/day	Headaches, dizziness, diarrhea, constipation, abdominal pain, tinnitus
Nizatidine (p. 819) (Axid)	**T:** 75 mg **C:** 150 mg, 300 mg	**Treatment of DU:** 300 mg/day **Maintenance of DU:** 150 mg/day	Fatigue, urticaria, abdominal pain, constipation, nausea
Ranitidine (p. 965) (Zantac)	**T:** 75 mg, 150 mg, 300 mg **C:** 150 mg, 300 mg **Syrup:** 15 mg/ml **Granules:** 150 mg **I:** 0.5 mg/ml, 25 mg/ml	**Treatment of DU:** 300 mg/day **Maintenance of DU:** 150 mg/day **Treatment of GU:** 300 mg/day **GERD:** 300 mg/day **Hypersecretory:** 0.3–6 g/day	Blurred vision, constipation, nausea, abdominal pain

C: capsules; **DT:** disintegrating tablets; **I:** injection; **L:** liquid; **OS:** oral suspension; **T:** tablets.

Hematinic Preparations

USES

Prevention or treatment of iron deficiency resulting from improper diet, pregnancy, impairment of absorption, or prolonged blood loss.

ACTION

Iron supplements are provided to assure adequate supplies for the formation of hemoglobin, which is needed for erythropoiesis and O_2 transport.

HEMATINIC (IRON) PREPARATIONS

Name	Availability	Elemental Iron	Side Effects
Ferrous fumarate (p. 452) (FemIron, Ircon, Feostat, Vitron C)	**T:** 63 mg, 200 mg, 324 mg **S:** 100 mg/5 ml **D:** 45 mg/0.6 ml	33	Constipation, nausea, vomiting, diarrhea, abdominal pain/cramping
Ferrous gluconate (p. 452) (Fergon)	**T:** 240 mg, 325 mg	12	Same as above
Ferrous sulfate (p. 452) (Fer-Iron, Fer-In-Sol, Feosol)	**T:** 325 mg **Syrup:** 90 mg/5 ml **E:** 220 mg/5 ml **D:** 75 mg/0.6 ml	20	Same as above
Ferrous sulfate exsiccated (p. 452) (Slow FE, Feosol, Feratab)	**T:** 187 mg, 200 mg **T (SR):** 160 mg **C (ER):** 160 mg	30	Same as above

C: caplets; **D:** drops; **E:** elixir; **ER:** extended-release, **SR:** sustained-release; **S:** suspension; **T:** tablets.

Hormones

Functions of the body are regulated by two major control systems: the nervous system and endocrine (hormone) system. Together they maintain homeostasis and control different metabolic functions in the body.

Hormones are concerned with control of different metabolic functions in the body (e.g., rates of chemical reactions in cells, transporting substances through cell membranes, cellular metabolism [growth/secretions]). By definition, a hormone is a chemical substance secreted into body fluids by cells and has control over other cells in the body. Hormones can be local or general:

• *Local hormones* have specific local effects (e.g., acetylcholine, which is secreted at parasympathetic and skeletal nerve endings).

• *General hormones* are mostly secreted by specific endocrine glands (e.g., epinephrine/norepinephrine are secreted by the adrenal medulla in response to sympathetic stimulation), transported in the blood to all parts of the body, causing many different reactions.

Some general hormones affect all or almost all cells of the body (e.g. thyroid hormone from the thyroid gland increases the rate of most chemical reactions in almost all cells of the body); other general hormones affect only specific tissue (e.g. ovarian hormones are specific to female sex organs and secondary sexual characteristics of the female).

ACTION

Endocrine hormones almost never directly act intracellularly affecting chemical reactions. They first combine with hormone receptors either on the cell surface or inside the cell (cell cytoplasm or nucleus). The combination of hormone and receptors alters the function of the receptor, and the receptor is the direct cause of the hormone effects. Altered receptor function may include the following: *Altered cell permeability*, which causes a change in protein structure of the receptor, usually opening or closing a channel for one or more ions. The movement of these ions causes the effect of the hormone. *Activation of intracellular enzymes* immediately inside the cell membrane: e.g., hormone combines with receptor that then becomes the activated enzyme adenyl cyclase, which causes formation of cAMP.

Note: Camp has effects inside the cell. It is not the hormone but cAMP that causes these effects.

ACTION *(cont.)*

Regulation of hormone secretion is controlled by an internal control system, the negative feedback system:

- Endocrine gland oversecretes.
- Hormone exerts more and more of its effect.
- Target organ performs its function.
- Too much function in turn feeds back to endocrine gland to decrease secretory rate.

The endocrine system contains many glands and hormones. A summary of the important glands and their hormones secreted are as follows:

The pituitary gland (hypophysis) is a small gland found in the sella turcica at the base of the brain. The pituitary is divided into two portions physiologically: the anterior pituitary (adenohypophysis) and the posterior pituitary (neurohypophysis). Six important hormones are secreted from the anterior pituitary and two from the posterior pituitary.

Anterior pituitary hormones:

- Growth hormone.
- Adrenocorticotropin (corticotropin).

- Thyroid-stimulating hormone (thyrotropin).
- Follicle-stimulating hormone (FSH).
- Luteinizing hormone (LH).
- Prolactin.

Posterior pituitary hormones:

- Antidiuretic hormone (vasopressin).
- Oxytocin.

Almost all secretions of the pituitary hormones are controlled by hormonal or nervous signals from the hypothalamus. The hypothalamus is a center of information concerned with the well-being of the body, which in turn is used to control secretions of the important pituitary hormones just listed. Secretions from the posterior pituitary are controlled by nerve signals originating in the hypothalamus; anterior pituitary hormones are controlled by hormones secreted within the hypothalamus. These hormones are as follows:

- Thyrotropin-releasing hormone (TRH) releasing thyroid-stimulating hormone.
- Corticotropin-releasing hormone (CRH) releasing adrenocorticotropin.
- Growth hormone-releasing hormone

(GHRH) releasing growth hormone and growth hormone inhibitory hormone (GHIH) (also same as somatostatin).

- Gonadotropin-releasing hormone (GnRH) releasing the two gonadotropic hormones LH and FSH.
- Prolactin inhibitory factor (PIF) causing inhibition of prolactin and prolactin-releasing factor.

ANTERIOR PITUITARY HORMONES

All anterior pituitary hormones (except growth hormone) have as their principal effect stimulating target glands.

GROWTH HORMONE (GH)

Growth hormone affects almost all tissues of the body. GH (somatropin) causes growth in almost all tissues of the body (increases cell size, increases mitosis with increased number of cells, and differentiates certain types of cells). Metabolic effects include increased rate of protein synthesis, mobilization of fatty acids from adipose tissue, decreased rate of glucose utilization.

Hormones *[continued]*

ACTION *[cont.]*

THYROID-STIMULATING HORMONE (TSH)

Thyroid-stimulating hormone controls secretion of the thyroid hormones. The thyroid gland is located immediately below the larynx on either side of and anterior to the trachea and secretes two significant hormones, thyroxine (T4) and tri-iodothyroxine (T3), which have a profound effect on increasing the metabolic rate of the body. The thyroid gland also secretes calcitonin, an important hormone for calcium metabolism. Calcitonin promotes deposition of calcium in the bones, which decreases calcium concentration in the extracellular fluid.

ADRENOCORTICOTROPIN

Adrenocorticotropin causes the adrenal cortex to secrete adrenocortical hormones. The adrenal glands lie at the superior poles of the two kidneys. Each gland is composed of two distinct parts,

the adrenal medulla and cortex. The adrenal medulla, related to the sympathetic nervous system, secretes the hormones epinephrine and norepinephrine. When stimulated, they cause constriction of blood vessels, increased activity of the heart, inhibitory effects on the GI tract, and dilation of the pupils. The adrenal cortex secretes corticosteroids, of which there are two major types: mineralocorticoids and glucocorticoids. Aldosterone, the principal mineralocorticoid, primarily affects electrolytes of the extracellular fluids. Cortisol, the principal glucocorticoid, affects glucose, protein, and fat metabolism.

LUTEINIZING HORMONE (LH)

Luteinizing hormone plays an important role in ovulation and causes secretion of female sex hormones by the ovaries and testosterone by the testes.

FOLLICLE-STIMULATING HORMONE (FSH)

Follicle-stimulating hormone causes growth of follicles in the ovaries prior to ovulation and promotes formation of sperm in the testes.

Ovarian sex hormones are estrogens and progestins. Estradiol is the most important estrogen; progesterone, the most important progestin.

Estrogens mainly promote proliferation and growth of specific cells in the body and are responsible for development of most of the secondary sex characteristics. Primarily cause cellular proliferation and growth of tissues of sex organs/other tissue related to reproduction. Ovaries, fallopian tubes, uterus, vagina increase in size. Estrogen initiates growth of breast and milk-producing apparatus, external appearance.

Progesterone stimulates secretion of the

uterine endometrium during the latter half of the female sexual cycle, preparing the uterus for implantation of the fertilized ovum. Decreases the frequency of uterine contractions (helps prevent expulsion of the implanted ovum). Progesterone promotes development of breasts, causing alveolar cells to proliferate, enlarge, and become secretory in nature.

Testosterone is secreted by the testes and formed by the interstitial cells of Leydig. Testosterone production increases under the stimulus of the anterior pituitary gonadotropic hormones. It is responsible for distinguishing characteristics of the masculine body (stimulates the growth of male sex organs and promotes the development of male secondary sex characteristics: e.g., distribution of body hair, effect on voice, protein formation, and muscular development).

PROLACTIN

Prolactin promotes the development of breasts and secretion of milk.

POSTERIOR PITUITARY HORMONES

ANTIDIURETIC HORMONE (ADH) (VASOPRESSIN)

Antidiuretic hormone can cause antidiuresis (decreased excretion of water by the kidneys). In the presence of ADH the permeability of the renal-collecting ducts and tubules to water increases, which allows water to be absorbed, conserving water in the body. ADH in higher concentrations is a very potent vasoconstrictor, constricting arterioles everywhere in the body, increasing B/P.

OXYTOCIN

Oxytocin contracts the uterus during the birthing process, esp. toward the end of the pregnancy, helping to expel the baby. Oxytocin also contracts myoepithelial cells in the breasts, causing milk to be expressed from the alveoli into the ducts so the baby can obtain it by suckling.

PANCREAS

The pancreas is composed of two tissue types: *acini* (secrete digestive juices in the duodenum) and *islets of Langerhans* (secrete insulin/glucagon directly into the blood). The islets of Langerhans contain three cells: alpha, beta, and delta. Alpha cells secrete glucagon, beta cells secrete insulin, and delta cells secrete somatostatin.

Insulin promotes glucose entry into most cells, thus controlling the rate of metabolism of most carbohydrates. Insulin also affects fat metabolism.

Glucagon effects are opposite those of insulin, the most important of which is increasing blood glucose concentration by releasing it from the liver into the circulating body fluids.

Somatostatin (same chemical as secreted by the hypothalamus) has multiple inhibitory effects: depresses secretion of insulin and glucagon, decreases GI motility, decreases secretions/absorption of the GI tract.

Human Immunodeficiency Virus (HIV) Infection

USES	ACTION
Antiretroviral agents are used in the treatment of HIV infection.	*Antiretroviral agents* are classified as nucleoside analogues, non-nucleoside analogues, nucleotide analogues, and protease inhibitors. Nucleoside and non-nucleoside analogues act by inhibiting HIV reverse transcriptase, which is responsible for viral replication early in the virus life cycle. Protease inhibitors block protease, an enzyme required for viral replication late in the virus life cycle. Usually combinations of these agents may be most effective in suppressing viral replication.

ANTIRETROVIRAL AGENTS FOR TREATMENT OF HIV INFECTION

Name	Availability	Dosage Range	Side Effects
Nucleoside Analogues			
Abacavir (p. 1) (Ziagen)	**T:** 300 mg **OS:** 20 mg/ml	**A:** 300 mg 2 times/day	Nausea, vomiting, malaise, rash, fever, headaches, asthenia, fatigue
Didanosine (p. 342) (Videx)	**T:** 25 mg, 50 mg, 100 mg, 150 mg, 200 mg **C:** 125 mg, 200 mg, 250 mg, 400 mg **OS:** 100 mg, 167 mg, 250 mg	**T (>60 kg):** 200 mg 2 times/day **(<60 kg):** 125 mg 2 times/day **OS (>60 kg):** 250 mg 2 times/day **(<60 kg):** 167 mg 2 times/day	Peripheral neuropathy, pancreatitis, diarrhea, nausea, vomiting, headaches, insomnia, rash, hepatitis, seizures

Lamivudine (p. 640) (Epivir)	**T:** 100 mg, 150 mg **OS:** 5 mg/ml, 10 mg/ml	**A:** 150 mg 2 times/day **C:** 4 mg/kg 2 times/day	Diarrhea, malaise, fatigue, headaches, nausea, vomiting, abdominal pain, peripheral neuropathy, arthralgia, myalgia, skin rash
Stavudine (p. 1030) (Zerit)	**C:** 15 mg, 20 mg, 30 mg, 40 mg **OS:** 1 mg/ml	**A:** 40 mg 2 times/day (20 mg 2 times/day if peripheral neuropathy occurs)	Peripheral neuropathy, anemia, leukopenia, neutropenia
Zalcitabine (p. 1173) (Hivid)	**T:** 0.375 mg, 0.75 mg	**A (>60 kg):** 0.75 mg 3 times/day **(<60 kg):** 0.375 mg 3 times/day	Peripheral neuropathy, stomatitis, granulocytopenia, leukopenia
Zidovudine (p. 1177) (Retrovir)	**C:** 100 mg **T:** 300 mg **Syrup:** 50 mg/5ml, 10 mg/ml	**A:** 500–600 mg/day (100 mg 5 times/day or 300 mg 2 times/day)	Anemia, granulocytopenia, myopathy, nausea, malaise, fatigue, insomnia

Nucleotide Analogues

Tenofovir (p. 1061) (Viread)	**T:** 300 mg	**A:** 300 mg/day	Nausea, vomiting, diarrhea

Non-Nucleoside Analogues

Delavirdine (p. 316) (Rescriptor)	**T:** 100 mg, 200 mg	**A:** 200 mg 3 times/day for 14 days, then 400 mg 3 times/day	Rash, nausea, headaches, elevations in liver function tests
Efavirenz (p. 392) (Sustiva)	**C:** 50 mg, 100 mg, 200 mg	**A:** 600 mg/day **C:** 200–600 mg/day based on weight	Headaches, dizziness, insomnia, fatigue, rash, nightmares
Nevirapine (p. 802) (Viramune)	**T:** 200 mg	**A:** 200 mg/day for 14 days, then 200 mg 2 times/day	Rash, nausea, fatigue, fever, headaches, abnormal liver function tests

(continued)

Human Immunodeficiency Virus (HIV) Infection *(continued)*

ANTIRETROVIRAL AGENTS FOR TREATMENT OF HIV INFECTION *(continued)*

Name	Availability	Dosage Range	Side Effects
Protease Inhibitors			
Amprenavir (p. 67) (Agenerase)	**C:** 50 mg, 150 mg **OS:** 15 mg/ml	**A:** 1200 mg 2 times/day **C (4–16 yrs, <50 kg):** 20 mg/kg 2 times/day or 15 mg/kg 3 times/day	Rash, diarrhea, headaches, nausea, vomiting, numbness, abdominal pain, fatigue
Indinavir (p. 584) (Crixivan)	**C:** 200 mg, 400 mg	**A:** 800 mg q8h	Nephrolithiasis, hyperbilirubinemia, abdominal pain, asthenia, fatigue, flank pain, nausea, vomiting, diarrhea, headaches, insomnia, dizziness, altered taste
Lopinavir/ritonavir (p. 677) (Kaletra)	**C:** 133/33 mg **OS:** 80/20 mg	**A:** 400/100 mg/day **C (4–12 yrs):** 10–13 mg/kg 2 times/day	Diarrhea, nausea, vomiting, abdominal pain, headaches, rash
Nelfinavir (p. 796) (Viracept)	**T:** 250 mg **Oral Powder:** 50 mg/g	**A:** 750 mg q8h **C:** 20–25 mg/kg q8h	Diarrhea, fatigue, asthenia, headaches, hypertension, decreased ability to concentrate
Ritonavir (p. 985) (Norvir)	**C:** 100 mg **OS:** 80 mg/ml	**A:** Titrate up to 600 mg 2 times/day	Nausea, vomiting, diarrhea, altered taste sensation, fatigue, elevated liver function tests and triglyceride levels
Saquinavir (p. 999) (Invirase, Fortovase)	**C:** 200 mg	**A:** 600 mg 3 times/day	Diarrhea, elevations in liver function tests, hypertriglycerides, cholesterol, abnormal fat accumulation, hyperglycemia

A: adults; **C:** capsules; **C** (dosage): children; **OS:** oral solution; **T:** tablets.

Immunizations

RECOMMENDATIONS FOR IMMUNIZATION OF INFANTS/CHILDREN

	Birth	1 Mo	2 Mos	4 Mos	6 Mos	12 Mos	15 Mos	18 Mos	4–6 Yrs
Diphtheria[1]			X	X	X			X	X
Tetanus[1]			X	X	X			X	X
Pertussis[1]			X	X	X			X	X
Measles[2]							X		X
Mumps[2]							X		X
Rubella[2]							X		X
Haemophilus[3]			X	X	X		X		
Hepatitis A[4]									X
Hepatitis B[5,6]									
HBsAg-negative mothers	X	X			X				
HBsAg-positive mothers	X	X			X				
Poliovirus[7]			X	X	X	X			
Pneumococcal (PCV7)[8]			X	X	X		X		
Varicella[9]						X			

[1] Diphtheria-tetanus (DT) toxoids with acellular pertussis vaccine is the preferred vaccine for all doses, including completion of the vaccination series in those receiving one or more doses of diphtheria and tetanus toxoids with whole-cell pertussis vaccine.

[2] Trivalent measles, mumps, and rubella vaccine. The second dose is routinely recommended at 4–6 years, but should be completed no later than 11–12 years.

(continued)

Immunizations *(continued)*

[3]Haemophilus influenza type b (HIB) conjugate vaccine schedules depend on the vaccine formulation used. If PedvaxHIB is given at ages 2 and 4 mos, the 6 mo dose is not required.

[4]Hepatitis A vaccine is recommended for children ≥2 years in states and localities where hepatitis incidence exceeds 20 cases per 100,000 population.

[5]Hepatitis B vaccine is routine for infants, with at least 30 days elapsing between the first two doses and the third dose, given at least 2 mos after the second dose but not before age 6 mos. Those not receiving three doses as noted should initiate or complete the series at age 11 or 12 mos.

[6]In newborns of hepatitis B surface antigen-positive mothers, give 0.5 ml hepatitis B immune globulin (HBIG) within 12 hrs of birth, plus the first dose of vaccine at a separate site. Booster vaccine doses are given on days 30 and 180.

[7]The preferred vaccine is inactivated polio virus vaccine.

[8]Pneumococcal conjugate 7-valent vaccine is recommended for all children age <24 mos.

[9]Varicella vaccine is recommended at any visit on or before the first birthday for susceptible children (e.g., those lacking reliable history of chicken pox).

Laxatives

USES

Short-term treatment of constipation; colon evacuation before rectal/bowel examination; prevent straining (e.g., after anorectal surgery, myocardial infarction); reduce painful elimination (e.g., episiotomy, hemorrhoids, anorectal lesions); modify effluent from ileostomy, colostomy; prevent fecal impaction; remove ingested poisons.

ACTION

Laxatives ease or stimulate defecation. Mechanisms by which this is accomplished include (1) attracting, retaining fluid in colonic contents due to hydrophilic or osmotic properties; (2) acting directly or indirectly on mucosa to decrease absorption of water and NaCl; or (3) increasing intestinal motility, decreasing absorption of water and NaCl by virtue of decreased transit time.

Bulk-forming: Act primarily in small/large intestine. Retains water in stool, may bind water, ions in colonic lumen (soften feces, increase bulk); may increase colonic bacteria growth (increases fecal mass). Produce soft stool in 1–3 days.

Lubricant: Mineral oil is the only agent in this group. Promotes stool passage by coating the fecal surface with an oil layer that retains fecal fluid and prevents absorpiton of fecal water by the colon.

Hyperosmotic agents: Acts in colon. Similar to saline laxatives. Osmotic action may be enhanced in distal ileum/colon by bacterial metabolism to lactate, others organic acids. This decrease in pH increases motility, secretion. Produces soft stool in 1–3 days.

Saline: Acts in small/large intestine, colon (sodium phosphate). Poorly, slowly absorbed, causes hormone cholecystokinin release from duodenum (stimulates

fluid secretion, motility), possesses osmotic properties, produces watery stool in 2–6 hrs (low doses produce semifluid stool in 6–12 hrs)

Stimulant: Act in colon. Enhance accumulation of water/electrolytes in colonic lumen, enhance intestinal motility. May act directly on intestinal mucosa. Produce semifluid stool in 6–12 hrs.

Note: Bisacodyl suppository acts in 15–60 min.

Surfactants: Act in small/large intestine. Hydrate and soften stools by their surfactant action, facilitating penetration of fat and water into stool. Produce soft stool in 1–3 days.

LAXATIVES

Name	Onset of Action	Uses
Bulk		
Psyllium (p. 946) (Metamucil, Konsyl)	12–24 hrs up to 3 days	First line for postpartum women, elderly, pts with diverticulosis, irritable bowel syndrome, hemorrhoids Safe for chronic use

(continued)

LAXATIVES *(continued)*

Name	Onset of Action	Indications
Bulk *(continued)*		
Methylcellulose (p. 723) (Citrucel)	12–24 hrs up to 3 days	First line for postpartum women, elderly, pts with diverticulosis, irritable bowel syndrome, hemorrhoids Safe for chronic use
Polycarbophil (p. 904) (Fibercon, Mitrolan)	Same as above	Same as above
Surfactant		
Docusate sodium (p. 370) (Colace)	1–3 days	Aid in passage of hard, painful feces Prevents straining
Docusate calcium (p. 370) (Surfak)	Same as above	Same as above
Docusate potassium (p. 370) (Dialose)	Same as above	Same as above
Lubricant		
Mineral oil (Kondremul)	6–8 hrs	Prevents straining
Saline		
Magnesium citrate (p. 689) (Citro-Nesia)	30 min to 3 hrs	Bowel evacuation for colonic procedures/exams, fecal impaction, hepatic coma

Magnesium hydroxide	Same as above	Same as above
Sodium phosphate (Fleets Phospho-soda)	5–15 min	Same as above

Hyperosmotic

Glycerin	<30 min	Short-term relief of constipation
Lactulose (p. 638) (Chronulac)	1–3 days	Hepatic comas
Polyethylene glycol electrolyte solution (p. 905) (GoLYTELY)	30–60 min	Bowel evacuation for colonic procedures/exams

Stimulant

Bisacodyl (p. 126) (Dulcolax)	**PO:** 6–12 hrs **Rectal:** 15–60 min	Same as above
Casanthranol *(in Peri-Colace)*	6–12 hrs	Same as above
Cascara sagrada (p. 179)	6–12 hrs	Bowel evacuation for colonic procedures/exams
Castor oil	6–12 hrs	Same as above
Senna (p. 1006) (Senokot)	6–12 hrs	Same as above

Neuromuscular Blockers

USES

Adjuvant in surgical anesthesia to obtain relaxation of skeletal muscle (esp. abdominal wall) for surgery (allows lighter level of anesthesia, valuable in orthopedic procedures). Neuromuscular blocking agents of short duration often used to facilitate intubation with endotracheal tube; facilitate laryngoscopy, bronchoscopy, and esophagoscopy in combination with general anesthetics. Provide muscle relaxation in pts undergoing mechanical ventilation, muscle relaxation in diagnosis of myasthenia gravis. Prevent convulsive movements during electroconvulsive therapy.

ACTION

Paralysis results from the blocking of the normal neuromuscular transmission. Succinylcholine, a depolarizing agent, attaches to the acetylcholine (Ach) receptor on the motor end plate, causing depolarization. It prevents the binding of Ach to the receptor. Nondepolarizing agents also bind to the receptor at the motor end plate, but competitively block Ach from attaching to the receptor. These agents also block presynaptic channels that cause the release of Ach.

NEUROMUSCULAR BLOCKERS

Name	Class	Intubation Dose	ICU Dose	Side Effects
Atracurium (p. 90) (Tracrium)	Short	0.4–0.5 mg/kg	0.4–0.5 mg/kg bolus, then 4–12 mcg/kg/min	Flushed skin, hives
Cisatracurium (p. 246) (Nimbex)	Intermediate	0.2 mg/kg	0.15–0.2 mg/kg bolus, then 0.5–10 mcg/kg/min	Skin rash, flushing
Doxacurium (p. 379) (Nuromax)	Long	0.05 mg/kg	0.1 mg/kg bolus	Injection site reaction, urticaria
Mivacurium (p. 759) (Mivacron)	Short	0.15–0.2 mg/kg	0.15–0.25 mg/kg bolus, then 9–10 mcg/kg/min	Flushing, hypotension, dizziness, muscle spasm

Pancuronium (p. 858) (Pavulon)	Long	0.1 mg/kg	0.05–0.1 mg/kg bolus, then 0.02–0.1 mg/kg/hr	Increased B/P, increased salivation, itching of skin
Rocuronium (p. 991) (Zemuron)	Intermediate	0.45–1.2 mg/kg	0.6–1.2 mg/kg bolus, then 4–16 mcg/kg/min	Pain at injection site, hyper- or hypotension
Succinylcholine (p. 1038) (Anectine, Quelicin)	Ultrashort	1–2 mg/kg	—	Increased intraocular pressure, postop muscle pain, weakness, increased salivation, bradycardia, cardiac arrhythmias
Tubocurarine (p. 1136)	Intermediate	0.5–0.6 mg/kg		Decreased B/P
Vecuronium (p. 1149) (Norcuron)	Intermediate	0.08–0.1 mg/kg	0.1 mg/kg bolus, then 0.05–0.1 mg/kg/hr	Skeletal muscle weakness with prolonged use

Nitrates

USES

Sublingual: Acute relief of angina pectoris. *Oral, topical:* Long-term prophylactic treatment of angina pectoris. *Intravenous:* Adjunctive treatment in CHF associated with acute myocardial infarction. Produce controlled hypotension during surgical procedures; control B/P in perioperative hypertension, angina unresponsive to organic nitrates or beta blockers.

ACTION

Relax most smooth muscles, including arteries and veins. Effect is primarily on veins (decrease left/right ventricular end-diastolic pressure). In angina, nitrates decrease myocardial work and O_2 requirements (decrease preload by venodilation and afterload by arteriodilation). Nitrates also appear to redistribute blood flow to ischemic myocardial areas improving perfusion without increase in coronary blood flow.

Nitrates (continued)			

NITRATES

Name	Availability	Dosage Range	Side Effects
Isosorbide (p. 619) (Isordil, Sorbitrate)	**T:** 5 mg, 10 mg, 20 mg 30 mg, 40 mg, **T (ER):** 30 mg, 40 mg, 60 mg, 120 mg **SL:** 2.5 mg, 5 mg **T (chewable):** 5 mg, 10 mg **C (SR):** 40 mg	**SL:** 2.5-10 mg q2-3h **PO:** 10-40 mg q6h **PO (SR):** 40-80 mg q8-12h	Flushing, headaches, nausea, vomiting, orthostatic hypotension, restlessness, tachycardia
Nitroglycercin (p. 815) (Nitrostat, Nitrobid, Nitroglyn, Minitran, Nitro-Dur, Nitrodisc, Transderm-Nitro)	**SL:** 0.4 mg **T (SR):** 2.6 mg, 6.5 mg, 9 mg **C (SR):** 2.5 mg, 6.5 mg, 9 mg, 13 mg **Topical:** 2% ointment **Trans:** 0.1 mg/hr, 0.2 mg/hr, 0.3 mg/hr, 0.4 mg/hr, 0.6 mg/hr, 0.8 mg/hr **I:** 0.5 mg/ml, 5 mg/ml **Infusion:** 100 mcg/ml, 200 mcg/ml	**SL:** 0.4 mg up to 3 times q15min **SR:** 2.5-26 mg 3-4 times/day **Trans:** 0.1-0.8 mg/hr **T:** 1-2 inches up to 4-5 inches q4h	Same as above

C: capsules; **ER:** extended-release; **I:** injection; **SL:** sublingual; **SR:** sustained-release; **T:** tablets; **Trans:** transdermal.

Nonsteroidal Anti-Inflammatory Drugs (NSAIDs)

USES

Provide symptomatic relief from *pain/ inflammation* in the treatment of musculoskeletal disorders (e.g., rheumatoid arthritis, osteoarthritis, ankylosing spondylitis); *analgesic* for low to moderate pain; *reduce fever* (many agents not suited for routine/prolonged therapy due to toxicity). By virtue of its action on platelet function, aspirin is used in treatment or prophylaxis of diseases associated with hypercoagulability (reduces risk of stroke/heart attack).

ACTION

Exact mechanism for anti-inflammatory, analgesic, antipyretic effects unknown. Inhibition of enzyme cyclo-oxygenase, the enzyme responsible for prostaglandin synthesis, appears to be a major mechanism of action. May inhibit other mediators of inflammation (e.g., leukotrienes). Direct action on hypothalamus heat-regulating center may contribute to antipyretic effect.

NSAIDS

Name	Availability	Dosage Range	Side Effects
Aspirin (p. 83)	**T:** 81 mg, 160 mg, 325 mg **Supplement:** 300 mg, 600 mg	**P (A):** 325–650 mg q4h as needed **C:** up to 60–80 mg/kg/day **Arthritis:** 3.2–6 g/day **JRA:** 60–110 mg/kg/day **RF (A):** 5–8 g/day **C:** 75–100 mg/kg/day **TIA:** 1,300 mg/day **MI:** 81–325 mg/day	GI upset, dizziness, headaches

(continued)

NSAIDS *(continued)*

Name	Availability	Dosage Range	Side Effects
Celecoxib (p. 216) (Celebrex)	**C:** 100 mg, 200 mg	**OA:** 200 mg/day **RA:** 100–200 mg 2 times/day **FAP:** 400 mg 2 times/day	Diarrhea, back pain, dizziness, heartburn, headaches, nausea, stomach pain
Diclofenac (p. 338) (Voltaren)	**T:** 25 mg, 50 mg, 75 mg, 100 mg	**Arthritis:** 100–200 mg/day	Indigestion, constipation, diarrhea, nausea, headaches, fluid retention, abdominal cramps
Diflunisal (p. 346) (Dolobid)	**T:** 250 mg, 500 mg	**Arthritis:** 0.5–1 g/day **P:** 0.5 g q8–12h	Headaches, abdominal cramps, indigestion, diarrhea, nausea
Etodolac (p. 433) (Lodine)	**T:** 400 mg, 500 mg **T (ER):** 400 mg, 500 mg, 600 mg **C:** 200 mg, 300 mg	**Arthritis:** 600–800 mg/day **P:** 200–400 mg q6–8h	Indigestion, dizziness, headaches, bloated feeling, diarrhea, nausea, weakness, abdominal cramps
Fenoprofen (p. 448) (Nalfon)	**C:** 200 mg, 300 mg **T:** 600 mg	**Arthritis:** 300–600 mg 3–4 times/day **P:** 200 mg q4–6h as needed	Nausea, indigestion, nervousness, constipation, shortness of breath, heartburn
Flurbiprofen (p. 481) (Ansaid)	**T:** 50 mg, 100 mg	**Arthritis:** 200–300 mg/day	Indigestion, nausea, fluid retention, headaches, abdominal cramps, diarrhea
Ibuprofen (p. 567) (Motrin, Advil)	**T:** 100 mg, 200 mg, 400 mg, 600 mg, 800 mg **T (chewable):** 50 mg, 100 mg **C:** 200 mg **S:** 100 mg/5 ml, 100 mg/2.5 ml **Drops:** 40 mg/ml	**Arthritis:** 1.2–3.2 g/day **P:** 400 mg q4–6h as needed **Fever:** 200 mg q4–6h as needed **JA:** 30–40 mg/kg/day	Dizziness, abdominal cramps, stomach pain, heartburn, nausea
Indomethacin (p. 586) (Indocin)	**C:** 25 mg, 50 mg **C (SR):** 75 mg **S:** 25 mg/5 ml **Supplement:** 50 mg	**Arthritis:** 50–200 mg/day **Bursitis/tendonitis:** 75–150 mg/day **GA:** 150 mg/day	Fluid retention, dizziness, headaches, abdominal pain, indigestion, nausea
Ketoprofen (p. 631) (Orudis)	**T:** 12.5 mg **C:** 25 mg, 50 mg, 75 mg **C (ER):** 100 mg, 150 mg, 200 mg	**Arthritis:** 150–300 mg/day **P:** 25–50 mg q6–8h as needed	Headaches, nervousness, abdominal pain, bloated feeling, constipation, diarrhea, nausea

Drug	Dosage Forms	Dosage	Side Effects
Ketorolac (p. 633) (Toradol)	**T:** 10 mg **I:** 15 mg/ml, 30 mg/ml	**P (PO):** 10 mg q4–6h as needed **(IM/IV):** 60–120 mg/day	Fluid retention, abdominal pain, diarrhea, dizziness, headaches, nausea
Meloxicam (p. 701) (Mobic)	**C:** 7.5 mg	**Arthritis:** 7.5–15 mg/day	Heartburn, indigestion, nausea, diarrhea, headaches
Nabumetone (p. 774) (Relafen)	**T:** 500 mg, 750 mg	**Arthritis:** 1–2 g/day	Fluid retention, dizziness, headaches, abdominal pain, constipation, diarrhea, nausea
Naproxen (p. 788) (Anaprox, Naprosyn)	**T:** 200 mg, 250 mg, 375 mg, 500 mg **T (CR):** 375 mg **S:** 125 mg/5 ml	**Arthritis:** 250–550 mg/day **P:** 250 mg q6–8h **JA:** 10 mg/kg/day **GA:** 750 mg once, then 250 mg q8h	Tinnitus, fluid retention, shortness of breath, dizziness, drowsiness, headaches, abdominal pain, constipation, heartburn, nausea
Oxaprozin (p. 843) (Daypro)	**C:** 600 mg	**Arthritis:** 600–1,800 mg/day	Constipation, diarrhea, nausea, indigestion
Piroxicam (p. 900) (Feldene)	**C:** 10 mg, 20 mg	**Arthritis:** 20 mg/day	Abdominal pain, stomach pain, nausea
Rofecoxib (p. 991) (Vioxx)	**T:** 12.5 mg, 25 mg, 50 mg	**OA:** 12.5–25 mg/day **P:** 25–50 mg/day	Weakness, diarrhea, dizziness, nausea, fluid retention, stomach pain
Sulindac (p. 1042) (Clinoril)	**T:** 150 mg, 200 mg	**Arthritis:** 300 mg/day **GA:** 400 mg/day	Dizziness, abdominal pain, constipation, diarrhea, nausea
Tolmetin (p. 1100) (Tolectin)	**T:** 200 mg, 600 mg **C:** 400 mg	**Arthritis:** 600–1800 mg/day **JA:** 15–30 mg/kg/day	Fluid retention, dizziness, headaches, weakness, abdominal pain, diarrhea, indigestion, nausea, vomiting
Valdecoxib (Bextra)	**T:** 10 mg, 20 mg	**Arthritis:** 10 mg/day **Primary dysmenorrhea:** 20 mg 2 times/day	Dyspepsia, nausea, headaches

A: adults; **C:** capsules; **CR:** controlled-release; **C** (dosage): children; **ER:** extended-release; **FAP:** Familial adenomatous polyposis; **GA:** gouty arthritis; **I:** injection; **JA:** juvenile arthritis; **JRA:** juvenile rheumatoid arthritis; **MI:** myocardial infarction; **OA:** osteo arthritis; **P:** pain; **RA:** rheumatoid arthritis; **RF:** rheumatic fever; **S:** suspension; **TIA:** transient ischemic attack; **T:** tablets.

Nutrition: Enteral

INDICATIONS	ROUTES OF ENTERAL NUTRITION DELIVERY

Enteral nutrition (EN), also known as tube feedings, provides food/nutrients via the GI tract using special formulas, delivery techniques, and equipment. All routes of enteral nutrition consist of a tube through which liquid formula is infused.

Tube feedings are used in pts with major trauma, burns, undergoing radiation and/or chemotherapy, with liver failure, severe renal impairment, with physical or neurologic impairment, preop and postop to promote anabolism, prevent cachexia, malnutrition.

Nasogastric (NG):

INDICATIONS: Most common for short-term feeding in pts unable or unwilling to consume adequate nutrition by mouth. Requires at least a partially functioning GI tract. ***ADVANTAGES:*** Does not require surgical intervention and is fairly easily inserted. Allows full use of digestive tract. Decreases chance hyperosmolar solutions may cause distention, nausea, vomiting. ***DISADVANTAGES:*** Temporary. May be easily pulled out during routine nursing care. Has potential for pulmonary aspiration of gastric contents, risk of reflux esophagitis, regurgitation.

Nasoduodenal (ND), Nasojejunal (NJ):

INDICATIONS: Pts unable or unwilling to consume adequate nutrition by mouth. Requires at least a partially functioning GI tract. ***ADVANTAGES:*** Does

ROUTES OF ENTERAL NUTRITION DELIVERY *(cont.)*

not require surgical intervention and is fairly easily inserted. Preferred for pts at risk of aspiration. Valuable for pts with gastroparesis. **DISADVANTAGES:** Temporary. May be pulled out during routine nursing care. May be dislodged by coughing, vomiting. Small lumen size increases risk of clogging when medication is given through them, more susceptible to rupturing when using infusion device. Must be radiographed for placement, frequently extubated.

GASTROSTOMY:

INDICATIONS: Pts with esophageal obstruction or impaired swallowing, pts in whom NG, ND, or NJ not feasible, or when long-term feeding indicated. **ADVANTAGES:** Permanent feeding access. Tubing has larger bore, allowing noncontinuous (bolus) feeding (300–400 ml over 30–60 min q3–6h). May be inserted endoscopically using local anesthetic (procedure called percutaneous endoscopic gastrostomy [PEG]).

DISADVANTAGES: Requires surgery; may be inserted in conjunction with other surgery or endoscopically (see **ADVANTAGES**). Stoma care required. Tube may be inadvertently dislodged. Risk of aspiration, peritonitis, cellulitis, leakage of gastric contents.

JEJUNOSTOMY:

INDICATIONS: Pts with stomach or duodenal obstruction, impaired gastric motility, pts in whom NG, ND, or NJ not feasible, or when long-term feeding indicated. **ADVANTAGES:** Allows early postop feeding (small-bowel function is least affected by surgery). Risk of aspiration reduced. Rarely pulled out inadvertently. **DISADVANTAGES:** Requires surgery (laparotomy). Stoma care required. Risk of intraperitoneal leakage. Can be dislodged easily.

INITIATING ENTERAL NUTRITION

With continuous feeding, initiation of isotonic (about 300 mOsm/L) or moderately hypertonic feeding (up to 495 mOsm/L) can be given full strength, usually at a slow rate (30–50 ml/hr) and gradually increased (25 ml/hr q6–24h). Formulas with osmolality of >500 mOsm/L are generally started at half strength and gradually increased in rate, then concentration. Tolerance is increased if the rate and concentration are not increased simultaneously.

Nutrition: Enteral *(continued)*

SELECTION OF FORMULAS

Protein: Has many important physiologic roles and is the primary source of nitrogen in the body. Provides 4 kcal/g protein. Sources of protein in enteral feedings: sodium caseinate, calcium caseinate, soy protein, dipeptides.

Carbohydrate (CHO): Provides energy for the body and heat to maintain body temperature. Provides 3.4 kcal/g carbohydrate. Sources of carbohydrate (CHO) in enteral feedings: corn syrup, cornstarch, maltodextrin, lactose, sucrose, glucose.

Fat: Provides concentrated source of energy. Referred to as "kilocalorie dense" or "protein sparing." Provides 9 kcal/g fat. Sources of fat in enteral feedings: corn oil, safflower oil, medium chain triglycerides.

Electrolytes, vitamins, trace elements: Contained in formulas (not found in specialized products for renal and hepatic insufficiency).

All products containing protein, fat, carbohydrate, vitamin, electrolytes, trace elements are nutritionally complete and designed to be used by pts for long periods.

COMPLICATIONS

MECHANICAL: Usually associated with some aspect of the feeding tube.

Aspiration pneumonia: Caused by delayed gastric emptying, gastroparesis, gastroesophageal reflux, or decreased gag reflex. May be prevented or treated by reducing infusion rate, using lower fat formula, feeding beyond pylorus, checking residuals, using small-bore feeding tubes, elevating head of bed 30–45° during and for 30–60 min after intermittent feeding, and regularly checking tube placement.

Esophageal, mucosal, pharyngeal irritation, otitis: Caused by using large-bore NG tube. Prevented by use of small bore whenever possible.

Irritation, leakage at ostomy site: Caused by drainage of digestive juices from site. Prevented by close attention to skin/stoma care.

Tube, lumen obstruction: Caused by thickened formula residue, formation of formula-medication complexes. Pre-

COMPLICATIONS *[cont.]*

vented by frequently irrigating tube with clear water (also before and after giving formulas/medication), avoiding instilling medication if possible.

GASTROINTESTINAL: Usually associated with formula, rate of delivery, unsanitary handling of solutions or delivery system.

Diarrhea: Caused by low-residue formulas, rapid delivery, use of hyperosmolar formula, hypoalbuminemia, malabsorption, microbial contamination, or rapid GI transit time. Prevented by using fiber-supplemented formulas, decreasing rate of delivery, using dilute formula and gradually increasing strength.

Cramping, gas, abdominal distention: Caused by nutrient malabsorption, rapid delivery of refrigerated formula. Prevented by delivering formula by continuous methods, giving formulas at room temperature, decreasing rate of delivery.

Nausea, vomiting: Caused by rapid delivery of formula, gastric retention.

Prevented by reducing rate of delivery, using dilute formulas, selecting low-fat formulas.

Constipation: Caused by inadequate fluid intake, reduced bulk, inactivity. Prevented by supplementing fluid intake, using fiber-supplemented formula, encouraging ambulation.

METABOLIC: Fluid/electrolyte status should be monitored. Refer to monitoring section. Additionally, the very young and very old are at greater risk in developing complications such as dehydration or overhydration.

MONITORING

Daily: Estimate nutrient intake, fluid intake/output, weight of pt, clinical observations.

Weekly: Electrolytes (potassium, sodium, magnesium, calcium, phosphorus), blood glucose, BUN, creatinine, liver function tests (e.g., SGOT [AST], alkaline phosphatase), 24-hr urea and creatinine excretion, total iron-binding capacity (TIBC) or serum transferrin, triglycerides, cholesterol.

Monthly: Serum albumin.

Other: Urine glucose, acetone (when blood glucose >250), vital signs (temperature, respirations, pulse, B/P) q8h.

Nutrition: Parenteral

Parenteral nutrition (PN), also known as total parenteral nutrition (TPN) or hyperalimentation (HAL), provides required nutrients to pts by IV route of administration. The goal of PN is to maintain or restore nutritional status caused by disease, injury, or inability to consume nutrients by other means.

INDICATIONS

Conditions when pt is unable to use alimentary tract via oral, gastrostomy, or jejunostomy routes. Impaired absorption of protein caused by obstruction, inflammation, or antineoplastic therapy. Bowel rest necessary because of GI surgery or ileus, fistulas, or anastomotic leaks. Conditions with increased metabolic requirements (e.g., burns, infection, trauma). Preserve tissue reserves as in acute renal failure. Inadequate nutrition from tube feeding methods.

COMPONENTS OF PN

In order to meet IV nutritional requirements six essential categories in PN are needed for tissue synthesis and energy balance.

Protein: In the form of crystalline amino acids (CAA), primarily used for protein synthesis. Several products are designed to meet specific needs for pts with renal failure (e.g., NephrAmine), liver disease (e.g., HepatAmine), stress/trauma (e.g., Aminosyn HBC), use in neonates and pediatrics (e.g., Aminosyn PF, Troph-Amine). Calories: 4 kcal/g protein.

Energy: In the form of dextrose, available in concentrations of 5–70%. Dextrose <10% may be given peripherally; concentrations >10% must be given centrally. Calories: 3.4 kcal/g dextrose.

IV fat emulsion: Available in the form of 10 or 20% concentrations. Provides a concentrated source of energy/calories (9 kcal/g fat) and is a source of essential fatty acids. May be administered peripherally or centrally.

COMPONENTS OF PN _(cont.)_	ROUTE OF ADMINISTRATION
Electrolytes: Major electrolytes (calcium, magnesium, potassium, sodium; also acetate, chloride, phosphate). Doses of electrolytes are individualized, based on many factors (e.g., kidney and/or liver function, fluid status).	PN is administered via either peripheral or central vein.

Vitamins: Essential components in maintaining metabolism and cellular function; widely used in PN.

Trace elements: Necessary in long-term PN administration. Trace elements include zinc, copper, chromium, manganese, selenium, molybdenum, and iodine.

Miscellaneous: Additives include insulin, albumin, heparin, and histamine₂ blockers (e.g., cimetidine, rantidine, famotidine). Other medication may be included, but compatibility for admixture should be checked on an individual basis.

Peripheral: Usually involves 2–3 L/day of 5–10% dextrose with 3–5% amino acid solution along with IV fat emulsion. Electrolytes, vitamins, trace elements are added according to pt needs. Peripheral solutions provide about 2,000 kcal/day and 60–90 g protein/day. **ADVANTAGES:** Lower risks vs. central mode of administration. **DISADVANTAGES:** Peripheral veins may not be suitable (esp. in pts with illness of long duration); more susceptible to phlebitis (due to osmolalities >600 mOsm/L); veins may be viable only 1–2 wks; large volumes of fluid are needed to meet nutritional requirements, which may be contraindicated in many pts.

Central: Usually utilizes hypertonic dextrose (concentration range of 15–35%) and amino acid solution of 3–7% with IV fat emulsion. Electrolytes, vitamins, trace elements are added according to pt needs. Central solutions provide 2,000–4,000 kcal/day. Must be given through large central vein with high blood flow,

allowing rapid dilution, avoiding phlebitis/thrombosis (usually through percutaneous insertion of catheter into subclavian vein then advancement of catheter to superior vena cava). **ADVANTAGES:** Allows more alternatives/flexibility in establishing regimens; allows ability to provide full nutritional requirements without need of daily fat emulsion; useful in pts who are fluid restricted (increased concentration), those needing large nutritional requirements (e.g., trauma, malignancy), or those for whom PN indicated >7–10 days. **DISADVANTAGES:** Risk with insertion, use, maintenance of central line; increased risk of infection, catheter-induced trauma, and metabolic changes.

Nutrition: Parenteral *(continued)*

MONITORING

May vary slightly from institution to institution.

Baseline: CBC, platelet count, prothrombin time, weight, body length/head circumference (in infants), electrolytes, glucose, BUN, creatinine, uric acid, total protein, cholesterol, triglycerides, bilirubin, alkaline phosphatase, LDH, SGOT (AST), albumin, other tests as needed.

Daily: Weight, vital signs (TPR), nutritional intake (kcal, protein, fat), electrolytes (potassium, sodium chloride), glucose (serum, urine), acetone, BUN, osmolarity, other tests as needed.

2–3 times/wk: CBC, coagulation studies (PT, PTT), creatinine, calcium, magnesium, phosphorus, acid-base status, other tests as needed.

Weekly: Nitrogen balance, total protein, albumin, prealbumin, transferrin, liver function tests (SGOT [AST], SGPT [ALT]), alkaline phosphatase, LDH, bilirubin, Hgb, uric acid, cholesterol, triglycerides, other tests as needed.

COMPLICATIONS

Mechanical: Malfunction in system for IV delivery (e.g., pump failure, problems with lines, tubing, administration sets, catheter). Pneumothorax, catheter misdirection, arterial puncture, bleeding, hematoma formation may occur with catheter placement.

Infectious: Infections (pts often more susceptible to infections), catheter sepsis (e.g., fever, shaking chills, glucose intolerance) where no other site of infection is identified.

Metabolic: Includes hyperglycemia, elevated cholesterol and triglycerides, abnormal liver function tests.

Fluid, electrolyte, acid-base disturbances: May alter potassium, sodium, phosphate, magnesium levels.

Nutritional: Clinical effects seen may be due to lack of adequate vitamins, trace elements, essential fatty acids.

Opioid Analgesics

USES

Relief of moderate to severe pain associated with surgical procedures, myocardial infarction, burns, cancer, or other conditions. May be used as an adjunct to anesthesia, either as a preop medication or intraoperatively as a supplement to anesthesia. Also used for obstetrical analgesia. Codeine and hydrocodone have an antitussive effect. Opium tinctures, such as paregoric, are used for severe diarrhea. Methadone relieves severe pain, but is used primarily as part of heroin detoxification.

ACTION

Opioids refer to all drugs having actions similar to morphine and to receptors combining with these agents. Major effects are on the CNS (produce analgesia, drowsiness, mood changes, mental clouding, analgesia without loss of consciousness, nausea and vomiting) and gastrointestinal tract (decrease HCl secretion; diminish biliary, pancreatic, and intestinal secretions; diminish propulsive peristalsis). Also affects respiration (depressed) and cardiovascular system (peripheral vasodilation, decrease peripheral resistance, inhibit baroreceptor reflexes).

OPIOID ANALGESICS

Names	Availability	Analgesic Effect			Dosage Range
		Onset (min)	Peak (min)	Duration (hrs)	
Butorphanol (p. 151) (Stadol)	**I:** 1 mg/ml, 2 mg/ml	**IM:** 10–30 **IV:** 2–3	**IM:** 30–60 **IV:** 30	**IM:** 3–4 **IV:** 2–4	**IM:** 1–4 mg q3–4h **IV:** 0.5–2 mg q3–4h

(continued)

OPIOID ANALGESICS *(continued)*

Names	Availability	Analgesic Effect				Dosage Range
		Onset (min)	Peak (min)	Duration (hrs)		
Codeine (p. 271)	I: 30 mg, 60 mg T: 30 mg, 60 mg	**IM:** 10–30 **PO:** 30–45	**IM:** 30–60 **PO:** 60–120	**IM/PO:** 4–6		**IM/PO (A):** 15–60 mg q4–6h **(C):** 0.5 mg/kg q4–6h
Fentanyl (p. 450) (Sublimaze)	I: 50 mcg/ml	**IM:** 7–15 **IV:** 1–2	**IM:** 20–30 **IV:** 3–5	**IM:** 1–2 **IV:** 0.5–1		**IM:** 50–100 mcg q1–2h
Hydrocodone	Combination oral	10–30	30–60	4–6		5–10 mg q4–6h
Hydromorphone (p. 557) (Dilaudid)	T: 1 mg, 2 mg, 3 mg, 4 mg, 8 mg S: 3 mg I: 1 mg/ml, 2 mg/ml, 3 mg/ml, 4 mg/ml, 10 mg/ml	**PO:** 30 **IM:** 15 **IV:** 10–15	**PO:** 90–120 **IM:** 30–60 **IV:** 15–30	**PO:** 4–5 **IM:** 4–5 **IV:** 4		**PO:** 1–4 mg q3–6h **IM:** 1–4 mg q3–6h **IV:** 0.5–1 mg q3h **ER:** 3 mg q4–8h
Levorphanol (p. 658) (Levo-dromoran)	T: 2 mg I: 2 mg/ml	**PO:** 10–60 **IM:** —	**PO:** 90–120 **IM:** 60	4–5		**PO:** 2–4 mg q4h **IM:** 2–3 mg q4h
Meperidine (p. 704) (Demerol)	T: 50 mg, 100 mg I: 25 mg/ml, 50 mg/ml, 75 mg/ml, 100 mg/ml	**PO:** 15 **IM:** 10–15 **IV:** 1	**PO:** 60–90 **IM:** 30–60 **IV:** 5–7	2–4		**PO/IM (A):** 50–150 mg q3–4h **(C):** 1–1.8 mg/kg q3–4h
Methadone (p. 717) (Dolophine)	T: 5 mg, 10 mg OS: 5 mg/5 ml, 10 mg/5 ml I: 10 mg/ml	**PO:** 30–60 **IM:** 10–20 **IV:** —	**PO:** 90–120 **IM:** 60–120 **IV:** 15–30	**PO:** 4–6 **IM:** 4–5 **IV:** 3–4		**IM/PO:** 2.5–10 mg q3–4h
Morphine (p. 764) (Roxanol, MS Contin)	T (ER): 15 mg, 30 mg, 60 mg, 100 mg, 200 mg OS: 10 mg/5 ml, 20 mg/5 ml, 20 mg/ml I: 4 mg/ml, 10 mg/ml, 15 mg/ml	**PO:** 30–60 **IM:** 10–30 **IV:** —	**PO:** 90 **IM:** 30–60 **IV:** 20	**PO:** 4 **IM/IV:** 4–5		**PO:** 10–30 mg q4h **IM:** 5–20 mg q4h **IV:** 0.05–0.1 mg/kg q4h
Nalbuphine (p. 780) (Nubain)	I: 10 mg/ml, 20 mg/ml	**IM:** 2–15 **IV:** 2–3	**IM:** 60 **IV:** 30	**IM:** 3–6 **IV:** 3–4		**IM/IV:** 10–20 mg q3–6h

| Oxycodone (p. 849) (Roxicodone) | **T:** 15 mg, 30 mg **OS:** 5 mg/5 ml, 20 mg/ml **T (ER):** 10 mg, 20 mg, 40 mg, 80 mg, 160 mg | 30 | 60 | 3–4 | 4–6 | 5–15 mg or 5 ml q4–6h **(ER):** q12h (dose titrated) |
| Propoxyphene (p. 938) (Darvon) | **T:** 100 mg | 15–60 | 60–120 | | | **PO:** 100 mg q4–6h |

A: adults; **C:** children; **ER:** extended-release; **OS:** oral solution; **I:** injection; **S:** supplement; **T:** tablets.

Opioid Antagonists

USES

Primarily used to reverse respiratory depression induced by narcotic overdosage. Naloxone is the drug of choice for reversal of respiratory depression.

ACTION

Prevents/reverses effects of mu (μ) receptor opioid agonists (e.g., increases respiration, reverses sedative effect).

OPIOID ANTAGONISTS

Name	Availability	Dosage Range	Side Effects
Nalmefene (p. 782) (Revex)	**I:** 100 mcg/ml, 1 mg/ml	**IV/IM/SubQ:** Titrated individually	Nausea, vomiting, tachycardia, hypertension

(continued)

OPIOID ANTAGONISTS

Name	Availability	Dosage Range	Side Effects
Naloxone (p. 783) (Narcan)	**I:** 0.02 mg/ml, 0.4 mg/ml, 1 mg/ml	**IV/IM/SubQ (A):** 0.4–2 mg May repeat at 2–3 min intervals **(C):** 0.01 mg/kg May give subsequent doses of 0.1 mg/kg	Same as above
Naltrexone (p. 785) (Depade, ReVia)	**T:** 50 mg	**PO:** 50 mg/day or 100 mg every other day or 150 mg every third day	Abdominal pain, anxiety, diarrhea, tachycardia, increased sweating, loss of appetite, nausea

A: adults; **C** (dosage): children; **I:** injection; **T:** tablets.

Oral Contraceptives

ACTION

Combination oral contraceptives decrease fertility primarily by inhibition of ovulation. Additionally, they can promote thickening of the cervical mucus, thereby creating a physical barrier for the passage of sperm. Also, they can modify the endometrium, making it less favorable for nidation.

CLASSIFICATION

Oral contraceptives either contain both an estrogen and a progestin (combination oral contraceptives) or contain only a progestin (progestin-only oral contraceptives). The combination oral contraceptives have four subgroups:

Monophasic: Daily estrogen and progestin dosage remains constant.

Biphasic: Estrogen remains constant, but the progestin dosage increases during the second half of the cycle.

Triphasic: Progestin changes for each phase of the cycle.

Estrophasic: Progestin remains constant, and the estrogen dose gradually increases through the monthly cycle.

ORAL CONTRACEPTIVES

Monophasic

Brand Names	Estrogen (mcg)	Progestin (mg)
Genora 1/50	50 mestranol	1 norethindrone
Nelova 1/50M		
Norethin 1/50M		
Norinyl 1+ 50		
Ortho-Novum 1/50		
Ovcon-50	50 ethinyl estradiol	1 norethindrone
Demulen 1/50	50 ethinyl estradiol	1 ethynodiol diacetate
Ovral	50 ethinyl estradiol	0.5 norgestrel
Genora 1/35	35 ethinyl estradiol	1 norethindrone
Nelova 1/35E		
Norethin 1/35E		
Norinyl 1+35		
Ortho-Novum 1/35		
Brevicon	35 ethinyl estradiol	0.5 norethindrone
Genora 0.5/35		
Ortho Evra	0.02 ethinyl estradiol	0.15 norelgestromin
NuvaRing	2.7 ethinyl estradiol	11.7 etonogestrel

Monophasic

Brand Names	Estrogen (mcg)	Progestin (mg)
Modicon		
Nelova 0.5/35E		
Ovcon-35	35 ethinyl estradiol	0.4 norethindrone
Ortho-Cyclen	35 ethinyl estradiol	0.25 norgeestimate
Demulen 1/35	35 ethinyl estradiol	1 ethynodiol diacetate
Loestrin 21 1.5/30	30 ethinyl estradiol	1.5 norethindrone acetate
Loestrin Fe 1.5/30		
Lo/Ovral	30 ethinyl estradiol	0.3 norgestrel
Desogen	30 ethinyl estradiol	0.15 desogestrel
Ortho-Cept		
Levlen	30 ethinyl estradiol	0.15 levonorgestrel
Levora		
Nordette		
Loestrin 21 1/20	20 ethinyl estradiol	1 norethindrone acetate
Yasmin	30 ethinyl estradiol	3 drospirenone

ORAL CONTRACEPTIVES *(continued)*

Biphasic

	Phase 1	Phase 2
Jenest-28	0.5 mg norethindrone 35 mcg ethinyl estradiol	1 mg norethindrone 35 mcg ethinyl estradiol
Nelova 10/11	0.5 mg norethindrone 35 mcg ethinyl estradiol	1 mg norethindrone 35 mcg ethinyl estradiol
Ortho-Novum 10/11	0.5 mg norethindrone 35 mcg ethinyl estradiol	1 mg norethindrone 35 mcg ethinyl estradiol

Triphasic

	Phase 1	Phase 2	Phase 3
Estrastep	1 mg norethindrone 20 mcg ethinyl estradiol	1 mg norethindrone 30 mcg ethinyl estradiol	1 mg norethindrone 35 mcg ethinyl estradiol
Tri-Norinyl	0.5 mg norethindrone 35 mcg ethinyl estradiol	1 mg norethindrone 35 mcg ethinyl estradiol	0.5 mg norethindrone 35 mcg ethinyl estradiol
OrthoNovum 7/7/7	0.5 mg norethindrone 35 mcg ethinyl estradiol	0.75 mg norethindrone 35 mcg ethinyl estradiol	1 mg norethindrone 35 mcg ethinyl estradiol
Tri-Levlen Triphasil	0.05 mg levonorgestrel 30 mcg ethinyl estradiol	0.075 mg levonorgestrel 40 mcg ethinyl estradiol	0.125 mg levonorgestrel 30 mcg ethinyl estradiol
Ortho Tri-Cyclen	0.18 mg norgestimate 35 mcg ethinyl estradiol	0.215 mg norgestimate 35 mcg ethinyl estradiol	0.25 mg norgestimate 35 mcg ethinyl estradiol

Progestin Only

Micronor Nor Q D	0.35 mg norethindrone
Ovrette	0.075 mg norgestrel

Oxytocics

USES

To induce, augment labor when maternal or fetal medical need exists; control of postpartum hemorrhage; cause uterine contraction after cesarean section or during other uterine surgery; induce therapeutic abortion.

ACTION

Oxytocics (Pitocin) stimulate frequency/force of contraction of uterine smooth muscle. Responsiveness of uterus increases closer to term. Stimulates breast (contracting of myoepithelial cells surrounding mammary gland) to release milk.

See Oxytocin individual monograph

Proton Pump Inhibitors

USES

Treatment of various gastric disorders, including gastric and duodenal ulcers, GERD, pathologic hypersecretory conditions.

ACTION

Suppress gastric acid secretion by specific inhibition of the hydrogen-potassium adenosine triphophatase (H^+/K^+ ATPase) enzyme system, which transports the acid at the gastric parietal cells. These agents do not have anticholinergic or histamine receptor antagonistic properties.

Proton Pump Inhibitors *(continued)*

PROTON PUMP INHIBITORS

Name	Availability	Dosage Range	Side Effects
Esomeprazole (p. 419) (Nexium)	**C:** 20 mg, 40 mg	20–40 mg/day	Headaches, diarrhea, abdominal pain, nausea
Lansoprazole (p. 644) (Prevacid)	**C:** 15 mg, 30 mg	15–30 mg/day	Diarrhea, skin rash, itching, headaches
Omeprazole (p. 836) (Prilosec)	**C:** 10 mg, 20 mg, 40 mg	20–40 mg/day	Headaches, diarrhea, abdominal pain, nausea
Rabeprazle (p. 961) (Aciphex)	**T:** 20 mg	20 mg/day	Headaches
Pantoprazole (p. 858) (Protonix)	**T:** 20 mg, 40 mg **I:** 40 mg	40 mg/day	Diarrhea, headaches

C: capsules; **I:** injection; **T:** tablets.

Sedative-Hypnotics

USES

Treatment of insomnia, e.g., difficulty falling asleep initially, frequent awakening, awakening too early.

ACTION

Sedatives decrease activity, moderate excitement, and have calming effects. Hypnotics produce drowsiness, enhance onset/maintenance of sleep (resembling natural sleep). Benzodiazepines are the most widely used agents (largely replace barbiturates): greater safety, lower incidence of drug dependence.

ACTION *(cont.)*

Benzodiazepines potentiate gamma-aminobutyric acid, which inhibits impulse transmission in the CNS reticular formation in brain. Benzodiazepines decrease sleep latency, number of awakenings, and time spent in awake stage of sleep; increase total sleep time. Schedule IV drugs.

SEDATIVE-HYPNOTICS

Name	Availability	Dosage Range	Side Effects
Benzodiazepines			
Estazolam (p. 421) (ProSom)	**T:** 1 mg, 2 mg	**A:** 1–2 mg **E:** 0.5–1 mg	Daytime sedation, memory and psychomotor impairment, tolerance, withdrawal reactions, rebound insomina, dependence
Flurazepam (p. 480) (Dalmane)	**C:** 15 mg, 30 mg	**A/E:** 15–30 mg	Same as above
Quazepam (p. 952) (Doral)	**T:** 7.5 mg, 15 mg	**A:** 7.5–15 mg **E:** 7.5 mg	Same as above
Temazepam (p. 1054) (Restoril)	**C:** 7.5 mg, 15 mg, 30 mg	**A:** 15–30 mg **E:** 7.5–15 mg	Same as above
Triazolam (p. 1125) (Halcion)	**T:** 0.125 mg, 0.25 mg	**A:** 0.125–0.25 mg **E:** 0.125 mg	Same as above

(continued)

SEDATIVE-HYPNOTICS (continued)

Non-Benzodiazepines

Name	Availability		Dosage Range	Side Effects
Zaleplon (p. 1174) (Sonata)	**C:** 5 mg, 10 mg	**A:** 5–10 mg **E:** 5 mg		Headaches, dizziness, myalgia, somnolence, asthenia, abdominal pain
Zolpidem (p. 1184) (Ambien)	**T:** 5 mg, 10 mg	**A:** 10 mg **E:** 5 mg		Dizziness, daytime drowsiness, headaches, confusion, depression, hangover, asthenia

A: adults; **C:** capsules; **E:** elderly; **T:** tablets.

Sympathomimetics

USES

Stimulation of alpha₁-receptors: Induce vasoconstriction primarily in skin and mucous membranes; nasal decongestion; combine with local anesthetics to delay anesthetic absorption; increases B/P in certain hypotensive states; produce mydriasis, facilitating eye exams, ocular surgery.

Stimulation of beta₁-receptors: Treatment of cardiac arrest, heart failure, shock, AV block.

Stimulation of beta₂-receptors: Treatment of asthma.

Stimulation of dopamine receptors: Treatment of shock.

ACTION

The sympathetic nervous system (SNS) is involved in maintaining homeostasis (involved in regulation of heart rate, force of cardiac contractions, B/P, bronchial airway tone, carbohydrate, fatty acid metabolism). The SNS is mediated by neurotransmitters (primarily norepinephrine, epinephrine, and dopamine), which act on adrenergic receptors. These receptors include beta₁, beta₂, alpha₁, alpha₂, and dopaminergic. Sympathomimetics differ widely in their actions based on their specificity to affect these receptors.

• *Alpha₁:* Mydriasis, constriction of arterioles, veins.

• *Alpha₂:* Inhibits transmitter release.

• *Beta₁:* Increases rate, force of contraction, conduction velocity of heart; releases renin from kidney.

• *Beta₂:* Dilates arterioles, bronchi, relaxes uterus.

• *Dopamine:* Dilates kidney vasculature.

SYMPATHOMIMETICS

Name	Availability	Receptor Specificity	Uses	Dosage Range
Dobutamine (p. 365) (Dobutrex)	I: 12.5 mg/ml, 500 mg/250 ml	Beta$_1$, beta$_2$ alpha$_1$	Inotropic support in cardiac decompensation	**IV infusion:** 2.5–10 mcg/kg/min
Dopamine (p. 376) (Intropin)	I: 40 mg, 80 mg, 160 ml vials, 800 mcg/ml, 1,600 mcg/ml	Beta$_1$, alpha$_1$, dopaminergic	Vasopressor, cardiac stimulant	**Dopaminergic:** 0.5–3 mcg/kg/min **Beta$_1$:** 2–10 mcg/kg/min **Alpha$_1$:** >10 mcg/kg/min
Epinephrine (p. 401) (Adrenalin)	I: 0.1 mg/ml, 1 mg/ml	Beta$_1$, beta$_2$ alpha$_1$	Cardiac arrest, anaphylactic shock	**Vasopressor:** 1–10 mcg/min **Cardiac arrest:** 1 mg q3–5min during resuscitation
Norepinephrine (p. 821) (Levophed)	I: 1 mg/ml	Beta$_1$, alpha$_1$	Vasopressor	**IV:** 0.5–1 mcg/min up to 2–12 mcg/min
Phenylephrine (p. 886) (Neo-Synephrine)	I: 10 mg/ml	Alpha$_1$	Vasopressor	**IV:** Initially, 10–180 mcg/min, then 40–60 mcg/min

I: injection.

Thyroid

USES

Treatment of primary or secondary hypothyroidism, myxedema, cretinism, or simple goiter.

Thyroid (continued)

ACTION

Thyroid hormone (T$_4$ [thyroxine] and T$_3$ [triiodothyroxine]) are essential for normal growth, development, and energy metabolism. *Promotes growth/development:* Controls DNA transcription and protein synthesis. Necessary in development of nervous system. *Stimulates energy use:* Increases basal metabolic rate (increases O$_2$ consumption, heat production). *Cardiovascular:* Stimulates heart by increased rate, force of contraction, cardiac output.

THYROID

Name	Availability	Dosage Average	Side Effects
Levothyroxine (p. 660) (Levoxyl, Synthroid)	**T:** 25 mcg, 50 mcg, 75 mcg, 88 mcg, 100 mcg, 112 mcg, 150 mcg, 175 mcg, 200 mcg, 300 mcg	75–100 mcg/day	Weight loss, palpitations, increased appetite, tremors, nervousness, tachycardia, increased B/P, headaches, insomnia, menstrual irregularities
Liothyronine (p. 666) (Cytomel)	**T:** 5 mcg, 25 mcg, 50 mcg	25–50 mcg/day	Same as above
Liotrix (Thyrolar)	**T:** 1/4 grain, 1/2 grain, 1 grain, 2 grains, 3 grains	1/2–1 grain/day	Same as above
Thyroid (p. 1080)	**T:** 15 mg, 30 mg, 60 mg, 90 mg, 120 mg, 180 mg, 240 mg, 300 mg	60–120 mg/day	Same as above

T: tablets.

Vitamins

INTRODUCTION

Vitamins are organic substances required for growth, reproduction, and maintainance of health and are obtained from food or supplementation in small quantities (vitamins cannot be synthesized by the body or the rate of synthesis is too slow/inadequate to meet metabolic needs). Vitamins are essential for energy transformation and regulation of metabolic processes. They are catalysts for all reactions using proteins, fats, carbohydrates for energy, growth, and cell maintenance.

WATER SOLUBLE

Water-soluble vitamins include vitamin C (ascorbic acid), B_1 (thiamine), B_2 (riboflavin), niacin, B_6 (pyridoxine), folic acid, B_{12} (cyanocobalamin). Water-soluble vitamins act as co-enzymes for almost every cellular reaction in the body. B-complex vitamins differ from one another in both structure and function, but are grouped together because they first were isolated from the same source (yeast and liver).

FAT SOLUBLE

Fat-soluble vitamins include vitamins A, D, E, and K. They are soluble in lipids and are usually absorbed into the lymphatic system of the small intestine and then into the general circulation. Absorption is facilitated by bile. These vitamins are stored in the body tissue when excessive quantities are consumed. May be toxic when taken in large doses (see sections on individual vitamins).

VITAMINS

Name	Uses	RDA	Side Effects
Vitamin A (p. 1162)	Required for normal growth, bone development, vision, reproduction, maintenance of epithelial tissue	**M:** 1,000 mcg **F:** 800 mcg	**High doses:** Liver toxicity, cheilitis, facial dermatitis, photosensitivity, mucosal dryness
Vitamin B₁ (Thiamine) (p. 1074)	Important in red blood cell formation, carbohydrate metabolism, neurologic function, myocardial contractility, growth, energy production	**M:** 1.5 mg **F:** 1.1 mg	**Large parenteral doses:** May cause pain on injection
Vitamin B₂ (Riboflavin)	Necessary for function of coenzymes in oxidation-reduction reactions, essential for normal cellular growth, assists in absorption of iron and pyridoxine	**M:** 1.7 mg **F:** 1.3 mg	Orange-yellow discoloration in urine

(continued)

VITAMINS *(continued)*

Name	Uses	RDA	Side Effects
Vitamin B₃ (Niacin) (p. 803)	Coenzyme for many oxidation-reduction reactions	**M:** 19 mg **F:** 15 mg	**High dose (>500 mg):** Nausea, vomiting, diarrhea, gastritis, liver toxicity, skin rash, facial flushing, headaches
Vitamin B₅ (Pantothenic acid)	Precursor to coenzyme A, important in synthesis of cholesterol, hormones, fatty acids	**M:** 4–7 mg **F:** 4–7 mg	Occasional GI problems (e.g., diarrhea)
Vitamin B₆ (Pyridoxine) (p. 951)	Enzyme cofactor for amino acid metabolism, essential for erythrocyte production, hemoglobin synthesis	**M:** 2 mg **F:** 1.6 mg	**High doses:** May cause sensory neuropathy
Vitamin B₁₂ (Cyanocobalamin) (p. 287)	Coenzyme in cells, including bone marrow, CNS, and GI tract, necessary for lipid metabolism, formation of myelin	**M:** 2 mcg **F:** 2 mcg	Skin rash, diarrhea, pain at injection site
Vitamin C (Ascorbic acid) (p. 80)	Cofactor in various reactions Necessary for collagen formation, acts as an antioxidant	**M:** 60 mg **F:** 60 mg (increased with smoking, pregnancy, lactation)	**High doses:** May cause calcium oxalate crystalluria, esophagitis, diarrhea
Vitamin D (Calciferol) (p. 1163)	Necessary for proper formation of bone, calcium, mineral homeostasis, regulation of parathyroid hormone, calcitonin, phosphate	**M:** 200–400 units **F:** 200–400 units	Hypercalcemia, kidney stones, renal failure, hypertension, psychosis, diarrhea, nausea, vomiting, anorexia, fatigue, headaches, mental changes
Vitamin E (Tocopherol) (p. 1165)	Antioxidant	**M:** 10 mg **F:** 8 mg	**High doses:** GI complaints, malaise, headache

M: males; **F:** females.

abacavir

ah-bah-**kay**-veer
(Ziagen)

FIXED-COMBINATION(S)

With lamivudine and zidovu-dine, antivirals **(Trizivir)**

▶CLASSIFICATION

PHARMACOTHERAPEUTIC:
Antiretroviral agent. ***CLINICAL:***
Antiviral (see pp. 57C, 94C)

ACTION/*THERAPEUTIC EFFECT*

Inhibits activity of HIV-1 reverse transcriptase by competing with natural substrate dGTP and by its incorporation into viral DNA, *inhibiting viral DNA growth.*

PHARMACOKINETICS

Rapidly, extensively absorbed following PO administration. Protein binding: 50%. Widely distributed including CSF and erythrocytes. Metabolized in liver to inactive metabolites. Primarily excreted in urine. Unknown if removed by hemodialysis. Half-life: 1.5 hrs.

USES

Treatment of HIV infection, in combination with other agents.

PRECAUTIONS

CONTRAINDICATIONS: Hypersensitivity to any component. ***CAUTIONS:*** Liver disease.

▷***LIFESPAN CONSIDERATIONS:***
Pregnancy/Lactation: Unknown if drug crosses placenta or is excreted in breast milk. Recommend not to breast-feed while taking abacavir (may increase potential for HIV transmission, adverse effects). **Pregnancy Category C. Children:** No safety issues noted in those 3–13 yrs of age. **Elderly:** Caution due to increased risk of liver, renal, cardiac function, concomitant diseases, other drug therapy.

INTERACTIONS

DRUG: Alcohol may increase concentration and half-life. ***HERBAL:*** **St. John's wort** may decrease concentration, effect. ***FOOD:*** None known. ***LAB VALUES:*** May increase SGPT (ALT), SGOT (AST), GGT, blood glucose, triglycerides.

AVAILABILITY (Rx)

TABLETS: 300 mg. ***ORAL SOLUTION:*** 20 mg/ml.

ADMINISTRATION/HANDLING

PO:

• May give without regard to food.
• Oral solution may be refrigerated. Do not freeze.

INDICATIONS/ROUTES/DOSAGE

HIV (in combination):

PO: **Adults:** 300 mg 2 times/day. **Children (3 mos–16 yrs):** 8 mg/kg 2 times/day. **Maximum:** 300 mg 2 times/day.

SIDE EFFECTS

Note: Side effects occurred in 3-drug combination (abacavir, lamivudine, zidovudine).

Adult: *FREQUENT:* Nausea (47%), nausea with vomiting (16%), diarrhea (12%), decreased appetite (11%). ***OCCASIONAL*** (7%): Insomnia. **Children: *FREQUENT:*** Nausea with vomiting (39%), fever (19%), headache, diarrhea (16%), rash (11%). ***OCCASIONAL:*** Decreased appetite (9%).

ADVERSE REACTIONS/TOXIC EFFECTS

Hypersensitivity reaction (may be life threatening). Symptoms include fever, rash, fatigue, intractable nausea and vomiting, severe diarrhea, abdominal pain, cough, pharyngitis, dyspnea. May include life-threatening hypotension. Lactic acidosis, severe hepatomegaly may occur.

NURSING IMPLICATIONS

BASELINE ASSESSMENT:

Question for possibility of pregnancy. Obtain baseline laboratory testing, esp. liver function tests, before beginning therapy and at periodic intervals during therapy. Offer emotional support.

INTERVENTION/EVALUATION:

Assess for nausea, vomiting. Determine pattern of bowel activity and stool consistency. Assess eating pattern; monitor for weight loss. Monitor lab values carefully, particularly liver function.

PATIENT/FAMILY TEACHING:

Do not take any medications, including OTC drugs without consulting physician. Small, frequent meals may offset anorexia, nausea. Abacavir is not a cure for HIV infection, nor does it reduce risk of transmission to others.

abciximab

ab-**six**-ih-mab
(c7E3 Fab, ReoPro✦)
►CLASSIFICATION

PHARMACOTHERAPEUTIC:
GP IIb/IIIa receptor inhibitor.
CLINICAL: Antiplatelet; antithrombotic (see p. 29C)

ACTION/*THERAPEUTIC EFFECT*

Produces rapid inhibition of platelet aggregation by preventing the binding of fibrinogen to GP IIb/IIIa receptor sites on platelets. *Prevents closure of treated coronary arteries. Prevents acute cardiac ischemic complications.*

PHARMACOKINETICS

Clears rapidly from plasma. Following IV bolus administration, half-life decreases <10 min, second phase of half-life within 30 min. Platelet function recovers after 48 hrs. At end of infusion, bleeding time returns to <12 min within 12 hrs in 75% of pts, within 24 hrs in 90% of pts.

USES

Adjunct to aspirin and heparin therapy to prevent cardiac ischemic complications in pts undergoing percutaneous coronary intervention (PCI) and those with unstable angina not responding to conventional medical therapy when PCI is planned within 24 hrs.

PRECAUTIONS

CONTRAINDICATIONS: Active internal bleeding, recent (within 6 wks) GI or GU bleeding, history of CVA <2 yrs or CVA with residual neurologic defect, oral anticoagulants <7 days unless prothrombin time <1.2 × control, thrombocytopenia (<100,000 cells/mcl), recent surgery or trauma (within 6 wks), intracranial neoplasm, arteriovenous malformation or aneurysm, severe uncontrolled hypertension, history of vasculitis, prior IV dextran use before or during PTCA. ***CAUTIONS:*** Pts who weigh <75 kg, those >65 yrs, those with history of GI disease, those receiving thrombolytics, heparin, aspirin, PTCA <12 hrs of onset of symptoms for acute MI, prolonged PTCA (>70 min), failed PTCA.
▷***LIFESPAN CONSIDERATIONS:***
Pregnancy/Lactation: Unknown

if drug causes fetal harm or can affect reproduction capacity. Unknown if distributed in breast milk. **Pregnancy Category C. Children:** Safety and efficacy not established. **Elderly:** Major bleeding risk increased.

INTERACTIONS

DRUG: **Anticoagulants, heparin** may increase risk of hemorrhage. **Platelet aggregation inhibitors (e.g., aspirin, dextran, thrombolytic agents)** may increase risk of bleeding. *HERBAL:* None known. *FOOD:* None known. *LAB VALUES:* Increases clotting time (ACT), prothrombin time (PT), activated partial thromboplastin time (APTT); decreases platelet count.

AVAILABILITY (Rx)

INJECTION: 2 mg/ml (5 ml vials).

ADMINISTRATION/HANDLING

IV 🖩

Storage:

• Store vials in refrigerator. Solution appears clear, colorless. Do not shake. Discard any unused portion left in vial or if preparation contains *any* opaque particles.

Reconstitution:

• Use 0.2–0.22 micron filter; filtering may be done during preparation or at administration. • Bolus dose may be given undiluted. • Withdraw desired dose and further dilute in 250 ml of 0.9% NaCl or D_5W (e.g., 10 mg in 250 ml equals concentration of 40 mcg/ml).

Rate of administration:

• See Indications/Dosage/Routes.

Administration precautions:

• Give in separate IV line; do not add any other medication to infusion. • For bolus injection and continuous infusion, use sterile, nonpyrogenic, low protein-binding 0.2 or 0.22 micron filter. • While vascular sheath is in position, maintain pt on complete bed rest with head of bed elevated at 30°. • Maintain affected limb in straight position. • Following sheath removal, apply femoral pressure for 30 min, either manually or mechanically, then apply pressure dressing.

IV INCOMPATIBILITY ⊘

Administer in separate line; no other medication should be added to infusion solution.

INDICATIONS/ROUTES/DOSAGE

Percutaneous coronary intervention (PCI):

IV BOLUS: **Adults:** 0.25 mg/kg given 10–60 min before angioplasty or atherectomy, then 12 hr IV infusion of 0.125 mcg/kg/min. **Maximum:** 10 mcg/min.

PCI (unstable angina):

IV BOLUS: **Adults:** 0.25 mg/kg, followed by 18–24 hr infusion of 10 mcg/min, concluding 1 hr after procedure.

SIDE EFFECTS

FREQUENT: Nausea (16%), hypotension (12%). *OCCASIONAL* (9%): Vomiting. *RARE* (3%): Bradycardia, abnormal thinking, dizziness, pain, peripheral edema, urinary tract infection.

ADVERSE REACTIONS/TOXIC EFFECTS

Major bleeding complications may occur; stop infusion immediately. Hypersensitivity reaction may occur. Atrial fibrillation/flutter, pulmonary edema, complete AV block occurs occasionally.

NURSING IMPLICATIONS

BASELINE ASSESSMENT:

Heparin should be discontinued 4 hrs prior to arterial sheath removal. Maintain pt on bed rest for 6–8 hrs following sheath removal or drug discontinuation, whichever is later. Check platelet count, PT, APTT before med infusion (assess for pre-existing blood abnormalities), 2–4 hrs after treatment, and at 24 hrs or before discharge, whichever is first. Check insertion site, distal pulse of affected limb while femoral artery sheath is in place, and then routinely for 6 hrs after femoral artery sheath removal. Minimize need for numerous injection sites, blood drawings, intubations, catheters.

INTERVENTION/EVALUATION:

Stop abciximab and/or heparin infusion if any serious bleeding occurs that is uncontrolled by pressure. Assess skin for bruises, petechiae, particularly femoral arterial access, also catheter insertion, arterial and venous puncture, cutdown, needle site, gastrointestinal sites. Handle pt carefully and as infrequently as possible to prevent bleeding. Do not obtain B/P in lower extremities (possible deep vein thrombi). Assess for decrease in B/P, increase in pulse rate, complaint of abdominal/back pain, severe headache, evidence of hemorrhage, ACT, PT, APTT, platelet count. Question for increase in discharge during menses. Assess urine output for hematuria. Monitor for any occurring hematoma. Use care in removing any dressing, tape.

acarbose

ah-**car**-bose
(Prandase✦, Precose)

►CLASSIFICATION

PHARMACOTHERAPEUTIC:
Alpha glucosidase inhibitor.
CLINICAL: Antidiabetic: Oral (see p. 39C)

ACTION/*THERAPEUTIC EFFECT*

Delays glucose absorption and digestion of carbohydrates, *resulting in smaller rise in blood glucose concentration after meals, lowering postprandial hyperglycemia.* Does not enhance insulin secretion.

USES

Used either alone or in combination with a sulfonylurea, insulin, or metformin to lower blood glucose in pts with type 2 diabetes mellitus when diet plus either acarbose or sulfonylurea do not give adequate control.

PRECAUTIONS

CONTRAINDICATIONS: Significant renal dysfunction (serum creatinine >2 mg/dl), hypersensitivity to drug, diabetic ketoacidosis or cirrhosis, inflammatory bowel disease, colonic ulceration, partial intestinal obstruction or predisposition to intestinal obstruction, chronic intestinal diseases associated with marked disorders of digestion or absorption, conditions that may deteriorate as result of increased gas formation in the intestine. ***CAUTIONS:*** Elderly, malnourished, or debilitated, those with renal or hepatic dysfunction, cardiac disease. Increased risk for hypoglycemia when given in combination with insulin.

INTERACTIONS

DRUG:* Digestive enzymes, intestinal absorbents (e.g., charcoal)** reduce acarbose effect. Do not use concurrently. **Sulfonylureas** may produce hypoglycemia. **Diuretics, corticosteroids, phenytoin, sympathomimetics, phenothiazines, nicotinic acid, thyroid hormones, estrogens, oral contraceptives, calcium channel blockers, isoniazid** may produce hyperglycemia. ***HERBAL: None known. ***FOOD:*** None known. ***LAB VALUES:*** May increase serum transaminase levels and slightly reduce hematocrit.

AVAILABILITY (Rx)

TABLETS: 25 mg, 50 mg, 100 mg.

ADMINISTRATION/HANDLING

PO:

• Give with the first bite of each main meal.

INDICATIONS/ROUTES/DOSAGE

Diabetes mellitus:

***PO:* Adults, elderly:** Initially, 25 mg 3 times/day at the start (with first bite) of each main meal. **Range:** 50–100 mg 3 times/day. **Maximum: <60 kg:** 50 mg 3 times/day; **>60 kg:** 100 mg 3 times/day.

SIDE EFFECTS

FREQUENT: Transient GI disturbances: Flatulence (77%), diarrhea (33%), abdominal pain (21%). Symptoms tend to diminish in frequency and intensity over time.

ADVERSE REACTIONS/TOXIC EFFECTS

None significant.

NURSING IMPLICATIONS

BASELINE ASSESSMENT:

Check blood glucose level. Discuss lifestyle to determine extent of learning, emotional needs.

INTERVENTION/EVALUATION:

Monitor blood glucose and food intake. Assess for hypoglycemia (cool wet skin, tremors, dizziness, anxiety, headache, tachycardia, numbness in mouth, hunger, diplopia) or hyperglycemia (polyuria, polyphagia, polydipsia, nausea, vomiting, dim vision, fatigue, deep rapid breathing). Be alert to conditions that alter glucose requirements: fever, increased activity or stress, surgical procedure.

PATIENT/FAMILY TEACHING:

Do not skip or delay meals. Check with physician when glucose demands are altered (e.g., fever, infection, trauma, stress, heavy physical activity). Avoid alcoholic beverages. Weight control, exercise, hygiene (including foot care), and nonsmoking are an essential part of therapy.

acebutolol

ah-see-**beaut**-oh-lol
(Monitan✤, Sectral)

▶ **CLASSIFICATION**

PHARMACOTHERAPEUTIC: Beta₁-adrenergic blocker. ***CLINICAL:*** Antihypertensive, antiarrhythmic (see pp. 13C, 60C)

ACTION/*THERAPEUTIC EFFECT*

Predominantly blocks beta₁-adrenergic receptors in cardiac tissue, *slowing sinus heart rate, decreasing cardiac output, decreasing B/P.* Large doses may block beta$_2$ receptors, *increasing airway resistance.* Exhibits antiarrhythmic activity, slows AV conduction, reduces rate of spontaneous firing of sinus pacemaker.

PHARMACOKINETICS

Onset	Peak	Duration
PO (hypotensive)		
1–1.5 hrs	2–8 hrs	24 hrs
PO (antiarrhythmic)		
1 hr	4–6 hrs	10 hrs

Well absorbed from GI tract. Protein binding: 26%. Undergoes extensive first-pass liver metabolism to active metabolite. Eliminated via bile, secreted into GI tract via intestine, excreted in urine. Removed by hemodialysis. Half-life: 3–4 hrs; metabolite: 8–13 hrs.

USES/*UNLABELED*

Management of mild to moderate hypertension. Used alone or in combination with diuretics, esp. thiazide type. Management of cardiac arrhythmias (primarily PVCs). *Treatment of chronic angina, pectoris, hypertrophic cardiomyopathy, myocardial infarction, pheochromocytoma, tremors, anxiety, thyrotoxicosis, syndrome of mitral valve prolapse.*

PRECAUTIONS

CONTRAINDICATIONS: Overt cardiac failure, cardiogenic shock, heart block greater than first degree, severe bradycardia. ***CAUTIONS:*** Impaired renal or hepatic function, peripheral vascular disease, hyperthyroidism, diabetes, inadequate cardiac function, bronchospastic disease.

▷***LIFESPAN CONSIDERATIONS:*** **Pregnancy/Lactation:** Readily crosses placenta; distributed in breast milk. May produce bradycardia, apnea, hypoglycemia, hypothermia during delivery, small birth weight infants. **Pregnancy Category B. Children:** No age-related precautions noted. Dosage not established. **Elderly:** Age-related peripheral vascular disease requires caution.

INTERACTIONS

DRUG: **Diuretics,** other **hypotensives** may increase hypotensive effect; **sympathomimetics, xanthines** may mutually inhibit effects; may mask symptoms of hypoglycemia, prolong hypoglycemic effect of **insulin, oral hypoglycemics; NSAIDs** may decrease antihypertensive effect; **cimetidine** may increase concentration. ***HERBAL:*** None known. ***FOOD:*** None known. ***LAB VALUES:*** May increase ANA titer, SGOT (AST), SGPT (ALT), alkaline phosphatase, LDH, bilirubin, BUN, creatinine, K, uric acid, lipoproteins, triglycerides.

AVAILABILITY (Rx)

CAPSULES: 200 mg, 400 mg.

ADMINISTRATION/HANDLING
PO:

• May be given without regard to meals.

INDICATIONS/ROUTES/DOSAGE
Mild to moderate hypertension:

PO: Adults: Initially, 400 mg/day in 1–2 divided doses. **Maintenance:** 400–800 mg/day. **Range: Adults:** Up to 1,200 mg/day in 2 divided doses.

Ventricular arrhythmias:

PO: Adults: Initially, 200 mg q12h. Increase gradually up to 600–1,200 mg/day in 2 divided doses.

Usual elderly dosage:

PO: Initially, 200–400 mg/day. **Maximum:** 800 mg/day.

Dosage in renal impairment:

Creatinine Clearance	% of Normal Dosage
<50 ml/min	50
<25 ml/min	25

SIDE EFFECTS

Generally well tolerated, with mild and transient effects. ***FREQUENT:*** Hypotension manifested as dizziness, nausea, diaphoresis, headache, cold extremities, fatigue, constipation/diarrhea. ***OCCASIONAL:*** Insomnia, flatulence, urinary frequency, impotence or decreased libido. ***RARE:*** Rash, arthralgia, myalgia, confusion (esp. elderly), change in taste.

ADVERSE REACTIONS/TOXIC EFFECTS

Overdosage may produce profound bradycardia, hypotension. Abrupt withdrawal may result in sweating, palpitations, headache, tremulousness. May precipitate CHF, MI in pts with cardiac disease, thyroid storm in those with thyrotoxicosis, peripheral ischemia in those with existing peripheral vascular disease. Hypoglycemia may occur in previously controlled diabetics. Thrombocytopenia (unusual bruising, bleeding) occurs rarely.

NURSING IMPLICATIONS

BASELINE ASSESSMENT:

Assess B/P, apical pulse immediately before drug is administered. (If pulse is 60/min or below, or systolic B/P is below 90 mm Hg, withhold medication, contact physician.)

INTERVENTION/EVALUATION:

Monitor B/P for hypotension, respiration for shortness of breath. Assess pulse for strength/weakness, irregular rate, bradycardia. Monitor EKG for cardiac arrhythmias, particularly shortening of QT interval, prolongation of PR interval. Assess frequency and consistency of stools. Assess for evidence of CHF: dyspnea (particularly on exertion or lying down), night cough, peripheral edema, distended neck veins, decreased urine output, weight gain. Assess for nausea, diaphoresis, headache, fatigue.

PATIENT/FAMILY TEACHING:

Do not abruptly discontinue medication. Compliance with therapy regimen is essential to control hypertension, arrhythmias. Report shortness of breath, excessive fatigue, weight gain, prolonged dizziness or headache. Do not use nasal decongestants, OTC cold preparations (stimulants) without physician approval. Restrict salt, alcohol intake.

acetaminophen

ah-see-tah-**min**-oh-fen
(Abenol✤, Apo-Acetaminophen✤, Atasol✤, Feverall, Tempra, Tylenol)

FIXED-COMBINATION(S)

With butabarbital, a sedative-hypnotic; with caffeine, a stimulant **(Fioricet);** codeine, a narcotic analgesic **(Tylenol with codeine);** with hydrocodone, a narcotic analgesic **(Vicodin, Zydone);** with oxycodone, a narcotic analgesic **(Percocet, Tylox);** with propoxyphene, an analgesic **(Darvocet);** with tramadol, an analgesic **(Ultracet).**

▶CLASSIFICATION

PHARMACOTHERAPEUTIC:
Central analgesic. **CLINICAL:**
Non-narcotic analgesic, anti-pyretic

ACTION/*THERAPEUTIC EFFECT*

Exact mechanism unknown, but appears to inhibit prostaglandin synthesis in CNS and, to a lesser extent, by blocking pain impulse through peripheral action, *resulting in analgesia.* Acts centrally on hypothalamic heat-regulating center, producing peripheral vasodilation (skin erythema, sweating, heat loss), *resulting in antipyresis.*

PHARMACOKINETICS

Onset	Peak	Duration
PO		
15–30 min	1–1.5 hrs	4–6 hrs

Rapidly, completely absorbed from GI tract; rectal absorption variable. Widely distributed to most body tissues. Metabolized in liver; excreted in urine. Removed by hemodialysis. Half-life: 1–4 hrs (half-life increased in hepatic disease, elderly, neonates; decreased in children).

USES

Relief of mild to moderate pain, fever.

PRECAUTIONS

CONTRAINDICATIONS: Hypersensitivity to acetaminophen. **CAUTIONS:** Impaired hepatic function, anemia.

▷**LIFESPAN CONSIDERATIONS:**
Pregnancy/Lactation: Crosses placenta; distributed in breast milk. Routinely used in all stages of pregnancy, appears safe for short-term use. **Pregnancy Category B. Children/Elderly:** No age-related precautions noted.

INTERACTIONS

DRUG: Alcohol (chronic use), **liver enzymes inducers (e.g., cimetidine), hepatotoxic medications (e.g., phenytoin)** may increase risk of hepatotoxicity with prolonged high dose or single toxic dose. May increase risk of bleeding with **warfarin** with regular use. **HERBAL:** None known. **FOOD:** None known. **LAB VALUES:** May increase SGOT (AST), SGPT (ALT), bilirubin, prothrombin levels (may indicate hepatotoxicity). Therapeutic blood serum level: 10–30 mcg/ml; toxic blood serum level: >200 mcg/ml.

AVAILABILITY (OTC)

CAPSULES: 500 mg. **ELIXIR:** 120 mg/5 ml, 160 mg/5 ml, 325 mg/5 ml. **LIQUID:** 160 mg/5 ml. **SOLUTION:** 100 mg/ml, 120 mg/2.5 ml. **SUPPOSITORY:** 120 mg, 325 mg, 650 mg. **TABLETS (chewable):** 80 mg. **TABLETS:** 160 mg, 325 mg, 500 mg, 650 mg.

ADMINISTRATION/HANDLING
PO:
• Give without regard to meals. • Tablets may be crushed.

Rectal:
• Moisten suppository with cold water before inserting well up into rectum.

INDICATIONS/ROUTES/DOSAGE
Analgesia, antipyresis:
Note: Children may repeat doses 4–5 times/day; maximum of 5 doses/24 hrs.

PO: Adults, elderly: 325–650 mg q4–6h or 1 gram 3–4 times/day. **Maximum:** 4 g/day. **Children (11 yrs):** 480 mg/dose; **(9–10 yrs):** 400 mg/dose; **(6–8 yrs):** 320 mg/dose; **(4–5 yrs):** 240 mg/dose; **(2–3 yrs):** 160 mg/dose; **(1–2 yrs):** 120 mg/dose; **(4–11 mos):** 80 mg/dose;

(0–3 mos): 40 mg/dose. **Neonates:** 10–15 mg/kg/dose q6–8 h.

RECTAL: **Adults:** 650 mg q4–6h. **Maximum:** 6 doses/24 hrs. **Children (6–12 yrs):** 325 mg q4–6h. **Maximum:** 2.6 g/24 hrs. **Children (3–6 yrs):** 120 mg q4–6h. **Maximum:** 720 mg/24 hrs. **Children (1–3 yrs):** 80 mg q4h. **Children (3–11 mos):** 80 mg q6h. **Children (<3 mos):** Consult physician.

SIDE EFFECTS

Well tolerated. *RARE:* Hypersensitivity reaction.

ADVERSE REACTIONS/TOXIC EFFECTS

Early signs of acetaminophen toxicity: anorexia, nausea, diaphoresis, generalized weakness within first 12–24 hrs. *Later signs of toxicity:* vomiting, right upper quadrant tenderness, elevated liver function tests within 48 to 72 hrs after ingestion. *Antidote:* Acetylcysteine.

NURSING IMPLICATIONS

BASELINE ASSESSMENT:

If given for analgesia, assess onset, type, location, and duration of pain. Effect of medication is reduced if full pain recurs before next dose. *Fixed-combination:* Obtain vital signs before giving medication. If respirations are 12/min or lower (20/min or lower in children), withhold medication, contact physician.

INTERVENTION/EVALUATION:

Assess for clinical improvement and relief of pain, fever. Therapeutic blood serum level: 10–30 mcg/ml; toxic serum level: >200 mcg/ml.

PATIENT/FAMILY TEACHING:

Consult physician for use in children <3 yrs, oral use >5 days (children), >10 days (adults), or fever >3 day duration. Severe/recurrent pain or high/continuous fever may indicate serious illness.

acetazolamide

ah-seat-ah-**zole**-ah-myd
(Apo-Acetazolamide✤, Dazamide, Diamox)

▶**CLASSIFICATION**

PHARMACOTHERAPEUTIC: Carbonic anhydrase inhibitor. *CLINICAL:* Antiglaucoma, anticonvulsant, diuretic, urinary alkalinizer (see p. 46C)

ACTION/*THERAPEUTIC EFFECT*

Reduces formation of hydrogen and bicarbonate ions from carbon dioxide and water by inhibiting, in proximal renal tubule, the enzyme carbonic anhydrase, thereby promoting renal excretion of sodium, potassium, bicarbonate, water. **Ocular:** Reduces rate of aqueous humor formation, *lowers intraocular pressure.* **Diamox only:** Increases CO_2 tension, retards neuronal conduction, *producing anticonvulsant activity.*

USES/*UNLABELED*

Treatment of open-angle, secondary or angle closure glaucoma, adjunct in managing absence seizures (e.g., petit mal), tonic-clonic, simple partial and myoclonic seizures. Prophylaxis/treatment of altitude sickness. *Lowers intraocular pressure in treatment of malignant glaucoma, treatment of toxicity of weakly acidic medications, prevents uric acid/renal calculi by alkalinizing the urine.*

PRECAUTIONS

CONTRAINDICATIONS: Hypersensitivity to sulfonamides, severe renal disease, adrenal insufficiency, hypochloremic acidosis. **CAUTIONS:** History of hypercalcemia, diabetes mellitus, gout, digitalized patients, obstructive pulmonary disease.

INTERACTIONS

DRUG: May increase **digoxin** toxicity (due to hypokalemia). May increase effects/toxicity of **amphetamines**; may decrease effects of **methenamine. HERBAL:** None known. **FOOD:** None known. **LAB VALUES:** May increase ammonia, bilirubin, glucose, chloride, uric acid, calcium; may decrease bicarbonate, potassium.

AVAILABILITY (Rx)

CAPSULES (sustained-release): 500 mg. **TABLETS:** 125 mg, 250 mg. **INJECTION:** 500 mg.

INDICATIONS/ROUTES/DOSAGE

Glaucoma:

PO: Adults, elderly: 250 mg 1–4 times/day. **EXTENDED-RELEASE:** 500 mg 2 times/day. **Children:** 10–15 mg/kg/day in divided doses q8h. **IV: Adults, elderly:** 500 mg; may repeat in 2–4 hrs, then continue with oral therapy. **Children:** 5–10 mg/kg q6h. **Maximum:** 1 g/day.

Epilepsy:

PO: Adults, elderly, children: 375–1,000 mg/day in up to 4 divided doses.

Altitude sickness:

PO: Adults, elderly: 250 mg 2–4 times/day. If possible, begin 24–48 hrs before ascent; continue for at least 48 hrs at high altitude as needed to control symptoms.

SIDE EFFECTS

FREQUENT: Unusually tired/weak, diarrhea, increased urination/frequency, decreased appetite/weight, altered taste (metallic), nausea, vomiting, numbness in extremities, lips, mouth. **OCCASIONAL:** Depression, drowsiness. **RARE:** Headache, photosensitivity, confusion, tinnitus, severe muscle weakness, loss of taste.

ADVERSE REACTIONS/TOXIC EFFECTS

Long-term therapy may result in acidotic state. Nephrotoxicity/hepatotoxicity occurs occasionally, manifested as dark urine/stools, pain in lower back, jaundice, dysuria, crystalluria, renal colic/calculi. Bone marrow depression may be manifested as aplastic anemia, thrombocytopenia, thrombocytopenic purpura, leukopenia, agranulocytosis, hemolytic anemia.

NURSING IMPLICATIONS

BASELINE ASSESSMENT:

Glaucoma: Assess affected pupil for dilation, response to light. *Epilepsy:* Obtain history of seizure disorder (length, intensity, duration of seizure, presence of aura, LOC.

INTERVENTION/EVALUATION:

Monitor for acidosis (headache, lethargy progressing to drowsiness, CNS depression, Kussmaul's respiration).

PATIENT/FAMILY TEACHING:

Report presence of tingling or tremor in hands or feet, unusual bleeding/bruising, unexplained fever, sore throat, flank pain.

acetohexamide

(Dymelor)

See Classification section under: Antidiabetic (p.39C)

acetylcysteine (*N*-acetylcysteine) *

ah-sea-tyl-**sis**-teen
(Mucomyst, Mucosil,
Parvolex♣)

▶CLASSIFICATION

PHARMACOTHERAPEUTIC:
Respiratory inhalant, intratracheal. **CLINICAL:** Mucolytic,
antidote

ACTION/*THERAPEUTIC EFFECT*

Splits linkage of mucoproteins, *reducing viscosity of pulmonary secretions, facilitates removal by coughing, postural drainage, mechanical means. Maintains/restores hepatic concentration of glutathione* (necessary for inactivation of hepatotoxic acetaminophen toxicity).

USES/*UNLABELED*

Adjunctive treatment for abnormally viscid mucous secretions present in acute and chronic bronchopulmonary disease and pulmonary complication of cystic fibrosis, tracheostomy care; treatment of acetaminophen overdose. *Prevention of renal damage from dyes given during certain diagnostic tests (e.g., CT scans).*

PRECAUTIONS

CONTRAINDICATIONS: None significant. **CAUTIONS:** Bronchial asthma, elderly, debilitated with severe respiratory insufficiency.

INTERACTIONS

DRUG: None known. **HERBAL:** None known. **FOOD:** None known. **LAB VALUES:** None known.

AVAILABILITY (Rx)

SOLUTION: 10%, 20%.

INDICATIONS/ROUTES/DOSAGE

Bronchopulmonary,
tracheostomy:

NEBULIZATION: Adults, elderly, children: (20% solution): 3–5 ml 3–4 times daily. **Range:** 1–10 ml q2–6h. **Adults, elderly, children: (10% solution):** 6–10 ml 3–4 times daily. **Range:** 2–20 ml q2–6h. **Infants:** 1–2 ml (20%) or 2–4 ml (10%) 3–4 times daily.

INTRATRACHEAL INSTILLATION: Adults, children: 1–2 ml of 10–20% solution instilled into tracheostomy q1–4h.

Acetaminophen overdose:

ORAL SOLUTION (5%): Adults, elderly, children: Loading dose of 140 mg/kg, followed in 4 hrs by maintenance dose of 70 mg/kg q4h for 17 additional doses (unless acetaminophen assay reveals nontoxic level).

Prevention of renal damage:

PO: Adults, elderly: 600 mg 2 times daily for 4 doses starting the day before the procedure.

SIDE EFFECTS

FREQUENT: Inhalation: Stickiness on face, transient unpleasant odor. **OCCASIONAL: Inhalation:** Increased bronchial secretions, irritated throat, nausea, vomiting, rhinorrhea. **RARE: Inhalation:** Skin rash. **Oral:** Facial edema, bronchospasm, wheezing.

ADVERSE REACTIONS/TOXIC EFFECTS

Large dosage may produce severe nausea, vomiting.

NURSING IMPLICATIONS

BASELINE ASSESSMENT:
Mucolytic: Assess pretreatment respirations for rate, depth, rhythm.

INTERVENTION/EVALUATION:

If bronchospasm occurs, treatment should be discontinued and physician notified; bronchodilator may be added to therapy. Monitor rate, depth, rhythm, type of respiration (abdominal, thoracic). Check sputum for color, consistency, amount.

PATIENT/FAMILY TEACHING:

A slight, disagreeable odor from solution may be noticed during initial administration but disappears quickly. Explain importance of adequate hydration. Teach proper coughing and deep breathing.

acitretin

ah-sa-**tree**-tin
(Soriatane)

▶CLASSIFICATION

PHARMACOTHERAPEUTIC:
Second-generation retinoid. ***CLINICAL:*** Antipsoriatic

ACTION/*THERAPEUTIC EFFECT*

Adjusts factors influencing epidermal proliferation, RNA/DNA synthesis, controls glycoprotein formation, governs immune response, *regulating keratinocyte growth and differentiation.*

USES/*UNLABELED*

Treatment of severe psoriasis, including erythodermic and generalized pustule types. Reduces severity of scaling, erythema, and epidermal induration. *Treatment of Darier's disease, palmoplantar pustulosis, lichen planus; children with lameliar ichthyosis, nonbullous and bullous ichthyosiform erythroderma, Sjögren-Larsson syndrome.*

PRECAUTIONS

CONTRAINDICATIONS: Pregnancy (Pregnancy Category X) or those who intend to become pregnant within 3 yrs following discontinuation of therapy (teratogenic, embryotoxic effects), sensitivity to parabens (used as preservative in gelatin capsule). ***CAUTIONS:*** Impaired hepatic/renal function, those with elevated cholesterol/triglycerides.

INTERACTIONS

DRUG: Concurrent use of **methotrexate** increases risk of hepatotoxicity. **Alcohol** prevents elimination of acitretin. Interferes with contraceptive effect of **"minipill" oral contraceptive. *HERBAL:*** None known. ***FOOD:*** None known. ***LAB VALUES:*** May increase triglycerides, SGOT (AST), SGPT (ALT). May decrease LDH (high-density lipoprotein).

AVAILABILITY (Rx)

CAPSULES: 10 mg, 25 mg.

INDICATIONS/ROUTES/DOSAGE
Psoriasis:

PO: Adults, elderly: 25–50 mg/day as a single dose with main meal. May increase to 75 mg/day if necessary and dose tolerated. **Maintenance:** 25–50 mg/day after the initial response is noted. Continue until lesions have resolved.

SIDE EFFECTS

FREQUENT (>75%): Lip inflammation, (50–75%): Alopecia, skin peeling, (25–50%): Shakiness, dry eyes, rash, hyperesthesia, paresthesia, sticky skin, dry mouth, epistaxis, dryness/thickening of conjunctiva. ***OCCASIONAL*** (1–10%): Eye irritation, brow and lash loss, sweating, chills, sensation of cold, flushing, edema, blurred vision, diarrhea, nausea, thirst.

ADVERSE REACTIONS/TOXIC EFFECTS

Benign intracranial hypertension (pseudotumor cerebri) occurs rarely.

NURSING IMPLICATIONS

BASELINE ASSESSMENT:

Inform women of childbearing potential of fetal risk if pregnancy occurs. A negative pregnancy test should be obtained and pt has begun her menstrual period before therapy begins.

INTERVENTION/EVALUATION:

Monitor liver function tests. Triglycerides should be monitored at 1–2 wk intervals until response to drug is established.

PATIENT/FAMILY TEACHING:

Pregnancy must be avoid during therapy and for 3 yrs after treatment has stopped. Avoid exposure to sun/sunlamps (effects of UV light is enhanced). May experience decreased tolerance to contact lenses. Transient worsening of psoriasis sometimes occurs during initial treatment.

---

acyclovir

aye-**sigh**-klo-veer
(Avirax✦, Zovirax)

►**CLASSIFICATION**

PHARMACOTHERAPEUTIC:
Synthetic nucleoside. ***CLINICAL:*** Antiviral (see p. 57C)

ACTION/*THERAPEUTIC EFFECT*

Converted to acyclovir triphosphate, becoming part of DNA chain, *interfering with DNA synthesis and viral replication.* Virustatic.

PHARMACOKINETICS

Poorly absorbed from GI tract; minimal absorption following topical application. Protein binding: 9–36%. Widely distributed. Partially metabolized in liver. Excreted primarily in urine. Removed by hemodialysis. Half-life: 2.5 hrs (increased in impaired renal function).

USES/*UNLABELED*

Treatment of herpes zoster (shingles), varicella zoster (chickenpox), herpes simplex encephalitis, neonatal simplex. Treatment of initial and recurrent episodes of genital herpes, mucocutaneous herpes simplex. *Herpes simplex ocular infections, infectious mononucleosis.* **Topical:** Initial episodes of genital herpes, immunocompromised pts with limited nonthreatening herpes simplex infections.

PRECAUTIONS

CONTRAINDICATIONS: Acyclovir reconstituted with bacteriostatic water containing benzyl alcohol should not be used in neonates. ***CAUTIONS:*** Renal or hepatic impairment, dehydration, fluid/electrolyte imbalance, concurrent use of nephrotoxic agents, neurologic abnormalities.

▷***LIFESPAN CONSIDERATIONS:***
Pregnancy/Lactation: Crosses placenta; distributed in breast milk. **Pregnancy Category C. Children:** Safety and efficacy in children <2 yrs not established (<1 yr for IV use). **Elderly:** Age-

related decrease in renal function may require decreased dosage.

INTERACTIONS

DRUG: Probenecid may increase half-life. Nephrotoxic medications (e.g., **aminoglycosides**) may increase nephrotoxicity. **HERBAL:** None known. **FOOD:** None known. **LAB VALUES:** May increase BUN, serum creatinine concentrations.

AVAILABILITY (Rx)

TABLETS: 400 mg, 800 mg. **CAPSULES:** 200 mg. **ORAL SUSPENSION:** 200 mg/5 ml. **POWDER FOR INJECTION:** 500 mg, 1,000 mg. **OINTMENT.**

ADMINISTRATION/HANDLING

PO:

• May give without regard to food. • Do not crush or break capsules. • Store capsules at room temperature.

Topical:

• Avoid eye contact. • Use finger cot or rubber glove to prevent autoinoculation.

IV 🕮

Storage:

• Store vials at room temperature. • Solutions of 50 mg/ml stable for 12 hrs at room temperature; may form precipitate when refrigerated. Potency not affected by precipitate and redissolution. • IV infusion (piggyback) stable for 24 hrs at room temperature. Yellow discoloration does not affect potency.

Reconstitution:

• Add 10 ml Sterile Water for Injection to each 500 mg vial (50 mg/ml). Do not use bacteriostatic water for injection containing benzyl alcohol or parabens (will cause precipitate). • Shake well until solution clear. • Further dilute with at least 100 ml D_5W or 0.9% NaCl. Final concentration should be 7 mg/ml or less.

Rate of administration:

• Infuse for at least 1 hr (renal tubular damage may occur with too rapid rate). • Maintain adequate hydration, esp. during urine concentration that occurs 2 hrs following IV administration.

IV INCOMPATIBILITIES ⊘

Amifostine (Ethylol), aztreonam (Azactam), cefipime (Maxipime), diltiazem (Cardizem), dobutamine (Dobutrex), dopamine (Intropin), fludarabine (Fludara), foscarnet (Foscavir), gemcitabine (Gemzar), idarubicin (Idamycin), meperidine (Demerol), meropenem (Merrem IV), morphine, ondansetron (Zofran), piperacillin-tazobactam (Zosyn), sagramostim (Leukine), vinorelbine (Navelbine).

IV COMPATIBILITIES

Heparin, hydromorphone (Dilaudid), lorazepam (Ativan), magnesium, morphine, multivitamins, potassium chloride, propofol (Diprivan).

INDICATIONS/ROUTES/DOSAGE

GENITAL HERPES:

Initial episode:

PO: Adults, elderly: 200 mg q4h (5 times/day) for 10 days. **IV: Adults, elderly:** 5 mg/kg q8h for 5 days. **Children:** 250 mg/m² q8h for 5 days.

Recurrent episode:

PO: Adults, elderly: 200 mg q4h (5 times/day) for 5 days.

SHINGLES (HERPES ZOSTER):

PO: Adults, elderly: 800 mg q4h (5 times/day) for 7–10 days.

CHICKENPOX (VARICELLA ZOSTER):

PO: Adults, children: 800 mg 4

times/day for 5 days. **Children (2–12 yrs, <40 kg):** 20 mg/kg/dose (**Maximum:** 800 mg) 4 times/day for 5 days.

MUCOCUTANEOUS HERPES SIMPLEX:

IV: **Adults, elderly:** 5 mg/kg q8h for 7 days. **Children:** 10 mg/kg q8h for 7 days.

HERPES SIMPLEX ENCEPHALITIS:

IV: **Adults, elderly:** 10 mg/kg q8h for 10 days. **Children (3 mos–12 yrs):** 20 mg/kg q8h for 10 days.

HERPES SIMPLEX NEONATAL:

IV: 10 mg/kg q8h for 10 days.

Usual topical dosage:

TOPICAL: **Adults, elderly:** 3–6 times/day for 7 days.

Dosage in renal impairment:

Dose/frequency is modified based on severity of infection, degree of renal impairment.

PO: Creatinine clearance of 10 ml/ 1.73 m^2 or less: 200 mg q12h.

IV

Creatinine Clearance (ml/min)	Dosage Percent	Dosage Interval
>50	100	8 hrs
25–50	100	12 hrs
10–25	100	24 hrs
<10	50	24 hrs

SIDE EFFECTS

FREQUENT: Parenteral (7–9%): Phlebitis/inflammation at IV site, nausea, vomiting. *Topical* (28%): Burning, stinging. *OCCASIONAL: Parenteral* (3%): Itching, rash, hives. *PO* (6–12%): Malaise, nausea, headache. *Topical* (4%): Itching. *RARE: Parenteral* (1–2%): Confusion, hallucinations, seizures, tremors. *Topical* (<1%): Skin rash. *PO* (1–3%): Vomiting, rash, diarrhea, headache.

ADVERSE REACTIONS/TOXIC EFFECTS

Rapid parenteral administration, excessively high doses, or fluid/electrolyte imbalance may produce renal failure (abdominal pain, decreased urination, decreased appetite, increased thirst, nausea, vomiting). Toxicity not reported with oral or topical use.

NURSING IMPLICATIONS

BASELINE ASSESSMENT:

Question history of allergies, particularly to acyclovir. Assess herpes simplex lesions before treatment to compare baseline with treatment effect.

INTERVENTION/EVALUATION:

Assess IV site for phlebitis (heat, pain, red streaking over vein). Evaluate cutaneous lesions. Assure adequate ventilation. Manage chickenpox and disseminated herpes zoster with strict isolation. Provide analgesics and comfort measures; esp. exhausting to elderly. Encourage fluids.

PATIENT/FAMILY TEACHING:

Drink adequate fluids. Do not touch lesions with fingers to avoid spreading infection to new site. *Genital herpes:* Continue therapy for full length of treatment. Space doses evenly. Use finger cot or rubber glove to apply topical ointment. Avoid sexual intercourse during duration of lesions to prevent infecting partner. Acyclovir does not cure herpes. Pap smear should be done at least annually due to increased risk of cancer of cervix in women with genital herpes.

adenosine

ah-**den**-oh-seen
(Adenocard)

►CLASSIFICATION

PHARMACOTHERAPEUTIC:
Cardiac agent, diagnostic aid.
CLINICAL: Antiarrhythmic

ACTION/*THERAPEUTIC EFFECT*

Slows impulse formation in SA node, slows conduction time through AV node, *depressing left ventricular function and restoring normal sinus rhythm.*

USES

Treatment of paroxysmal supraventricular tachycardia, including those associated with accessory bypass tracts (Wolff-Parkinson-White syndrome). Adjunct in diagnosis in myocardial perfusion imaging or stress echocardiography.

PRECAUTIONS

CONTRAINDICATIONS: Second- or third-degree AV block or sick sinus syndrome (with functioning pacemaker), atrial flutter or fibrillation, ventricular tachycardia. **CAUTIONS:** Heart block, arrhythmias at time of conversion, asthma, hepatic/renal failure.

INTERACTIONS

DRUG: Methylxanthines (e.g., caffeine, theophylline) may decrease effect. **Dipyridamole** may increase effect. **Carbamazepine** may increase degree of heart block caused by adenosine. **HERBAL:** None known. **FOOD:** None known. **LAB VALUES:** None known.

AVAILABILITY (Rx)
INJECTION: 3 mg/ml.

ADMINISTRATION/HANDLING
IV 💉
Storage:
• Store at room temperature. Solution appears clear. • Crystallization occurs if refrigerated; if crystallization occurs, dissolve crystals by warming to room temperature. Discard unused portion.

Rate of administration:
• Administer very rapidly (over 1–2 sec) undiluted directly into vein, or if using IV line, use closest port to insertion site. If IV line is infusing any fluid other than 0.9% NaCl, flush line first. • After rapid bolus injection, follow with rapid 0.9% NaCl flush.

IV INCOMPATIBILITIES ⊘
Any other drug or solution other than 0.9% NaCl or D_5W.

INDICATIONS/ROUTES/DOSAGE
Usual adult dosage:
RAPID IV BOLUS: Adults, elderly: Initially, 6 mg (over 1–2 sec). If first dose does not convert within 1–2 min, give 12 mg; may repeat 12 mg dose in 1–2 min if no response has occurred.

Diagnostic testing:
IV INFUSION: Adults: 140 mcg/kg/min for 6 min.

SIDE EFFECTS

FREQUENT (12–18%): Facial flushing, shortness of breath/dyspnea. **OCCASIONAL** (2–7%): Headache, nausea, lightheadedness, chest pressure. **RARE** (≤1%): Numbness/tingling in arms, dizziness, sweating, hypotension, palpitations, chest/jaw/neck pain.

ADVERSE REACTIONS/TOXIC EFFECTS

May produce short-lasting heart block.

NURSING IMPLICATIONS

BASELINE ASSESSMENT:

Identify arrhythmia per cardiac monitor and apical pulse.

INTERVENTION/EVALUATION:

Assess cardiac performance per continuous EKG. Monitor B/P, apical pulse (rate, rhythm, and strength), and respirations. Monitor I&O; assess for fluid retention. Check electrolytes.

albendazole

all-**ben**-dah-zole
(Albenza)

▶**CLASSIFICATION**
CLINICAL: Anthelmintic

ACTION/*THERAPEUTIC EFFECT*

Vermicidal. Degrades parasite cytoplasmic microtubules, irreversibly blocks cholinesterase secretion, glucose uptake in helminth and larvae (depletes glycogen, decreases ATP production, depletes energy). *Immobilizes and kills worms.*

USES

Treatment of parenchymal neurocysticercosis due to active lesions caused by larval forms of pork tapeworm, *Taenia solium.* Treatment of cystic hydatid disease of liver, lung, and peritoneum caused by larval form of dog tapeworm. *Treatment of Echinococcus granulosus.*

PRECAUTIONS

CONTRAINDICATIONS: None significant. ***CAUTIONS:*** Hepatic function impairment.

INTERACTIONS

DRUG: **Dexamethasone, praziquantel** increases albendazole concentration. ***HERBAL:*** None known. ***FOOD:*** None known. ***LAB VALUES:*** May decrease total WBC count.

AVAILABILITY (Rx)
TABLETS: 400 mg.

INDICATIONS/ROUTES/DOSAGE
Neurocysticercosis:

PO: Adults, elderly, >60 kg: 400 mg 2 times/day. **<60 kg:** 15 mg/kg/day. Continue for 8–30 days.

Cystic hydatid:

PO: Adults, elderly, >60 kg: 400 mg 2 times/day. **<60 kg:** 15 mg/kg/day. Continue for 28 days, rest 14 days, repeat cycle 3 times.

SIDE EFFECTS

FREQUENT (3–10%): *Neurocysticercosis:* Nausea, vomiting, headache. *Hydatid:* Abnormal liver function tests, abdominal pain, nausea, vomiting. ***OCCASIONAL*** (1–3%): *Neurocysticercosis:* Increased intracranial pressure, meningeal signs. *Hydatid:* Headache, dizziness, alopecia, fever.

ADVERSE REACTIONS/TOXIC EFFECTS

Pancytopenia occurs rarely. In presence of cysticerosis, drug may produce retinal damage in presence of retinal lesions.

NURSING IMPLICATIONS

BASELINE ASSESSMENT:

Treatment should not be initiated until after a negative pregnancy test is obtained.

albumin, human

al-**byew**-min
(Albuminar, Albutein, Buminate, Plasbumin)

►CLASSIFICATION
PHARMACOTHERAPEUTIC:
Plasma protein fraction. ***CLINICAL:*** Blood derivative

ACTION/*THERAPEUTIC EFFECT*

Regulates circulating blood volume, tissue fluid balance and maintains pressure, *restoring intravascular volume, plasma volume, and maintaining cardiac output.* Binds and functions as carrier of intermediate metabolites (hormones, enzymes, drugs) in transport and exchange of tissue products.

PHARMACOKINETICS

Distributed throughout extracellular water. Onset of action: 15 min provided patient is well hydrated. Half-life: 15–20 days.

USES

Treatment of hypovolemia with or without shock (restores intravascular volume, maintains cardiac output and colloid oncotic pressure), severe burns (maintains plasma volume, prevents intravascular hemoconcentration), neonatal hyperbilirubinemia, respiratory distress syndrome (ARDS) to correct fluid volume overload, cardiopulmonary bypass treatment adjunct to provide hemodilution, ascites to maintain cardiovascular function, acute nephrosis or nephrotic syndrome to control edema, hemodialysis (long term in those susceptible to shock or hypotension), pancreatic, intra-abdominal infection to treat shock associated with acute hemorrhage, acute liver failure, RBC resuspension.

PRECAUTIONS

CONTRAINDICATIONS: Severe anemia, cardiac failure, history of allergic reaction to albumin, hypervolemia, pulmonary edema, no albumin deficiency. ***CAUTIONS:*** Hypertension, normal serum albumin concentration, low cardiac reserve, pulmonary disease, hepatic or renal failure.

▷***LIFESPAN CONSIDERATIONS:***
Pregnancy/Lactation: Unknown if drug crosses placenta or is distributed in breast milk. **Pregnancy Category C. Children/Elderly:** No age-related precautions noted.

INTERACTIONS

DRUG: None significant. ***HERBAL:*** None known. ***FOOD:*** None known. ***LAB VALUES:*** May increase serum alkaline phosphatase concentrations.

AVAILABILITY (Rx)

INJECTION: 5%, 25%.

ADMINISTRATION/HANDLING
IV 🜉

Storage:

• Store at room temperature. Appears as clear, brownish, odorless, moderate viscous fluid. • Do not use if solution has been frozen, solution appears turbid, or contains sediment, or if not used within 4 hrs of opening vial.

Reconstitution:

• 5% solution may be made from

25% solution by adding 1 volume 25% to 4 volumes 0.9% NaCl or D_5W (NaCl preferred). Do note use sterile water for injection (life-threatening hemolysis, acute renal failure can result).

Rate of administration:

• Give by IV infusion. Rate is variable, depends on use, blood volume, concentration of solute. • 5%: usually given at 5–10 ml/min; 25%: usually at 2–3 ml/min. • 5% administered undiluted; 25% may be administered undiluted or diluted with 0.9% NaCl or D_5W. NaCl preferred. • May give without regard to pt blood group or Rh factor.

IV INCOMPATIBILITIES ⊘

Midazolam (Versed), vancomycin (Vancocin), verapamil (Isoptin).

IV COMPATIBILITIES

Diltiazem (Cardizem), lorazepam (Ativan).

INDICATIONS/ROUTES/DOSAGE

Note: Dosage based on pt's condition; duration of administration based on pt's response.

Hypovolemia:

IV: Adults, elderly: 25 g (5% or 25%) by infusion. May be repeated in 15–30 min. **Maximum:** 2 g/kg/24 hrs. **Children:** 2.5–12.5 g or 0.5–1 g/kg. May be repeated in 15–30 min. **Neonates:** 0.5 g/kg/dose.

Hypoproteinemia:

IV: Adults, elderly: 50–75 g as 25% injection at rate of 100 ml over 30–40 min. **Children:** 0.5–1 g/kg/dose; may repeat q1–2 days.

Burns:

IV: Adults, elderly, children: Initially, begin with administration of large volumes of crystalloid injection to maintain plasma volume. After 24 hrs, an initial dose of 25 g with dose adjusted to maintain plasma albumin concentration of 2–2.5 g/100 ml.

Cardiopulmonary bypass:

IV: Adults, elderly: 5% or 25%: With crystalloid to maintain plasma albumin concentration of 2.5 g/100 ml.

Acute nephrosis, nephrotic syndrome:

IV: Adults, elderly: 25 g of 25% injection, with diuretic once a day for 7–10 days.

Renal dialysis:

IV: Adults, elderly: 25%: 100 ml (25 g).

Hyperbilirubinemia, erythroblastosis fetalis:

IV: Infants: 1 g/kg 1–2 hrs before transfusion.

SIDE EFFECTS

OCCASIONAL: Hypotension. **RARE:** High dose, repeated therapy may result in altered vital signs; chills, fever, increased salivation, nausea, vomiting, urticaria, tachycardia.

ADVERSE REACTIONS/TOXIC EFFECTS

Fluid overload (headache, weakness, blurred vision, behavioral changes, incoordination, isolated muscle twitching) and CHF (rapid breathing, rales, wheezing, coughing, increased B/P, distended neck veins) may occur.

NURSING IMPLICATIONS

BASELINE ASSESSMENT:

Obtain B/P, pulse, respirations immediately before administration. There should be adequate hydration before albumin is administered.

INTERVENTION/EVALUATION:

Monitor B/P for hypo/hypertension. Assess frequently for evidence of fluid overload, pulmonary edema (see Adverse Reaction/Toxic Effects). Check skin for flushing, urticaria. Monitor I&O ratio (watch for decreased output). Assess for therapeutic response (increased B/P, decreased edema).

albuterol 🖊

ale-**beut**-er-all
(Proventil, Proventil HFA, Ventolin [inhalation]), Ventolin HFA
Do not confuse with atenolol.

albuterol sulfate

(AccuNeb, Airomir🍁, Novosalmol🍁, Proventil, Ventolin [syrup, tablets, nebulization], Volmax)

FIXED-COMBINATION(S)

With ipratropium, a bronchodilator **(Combivent, DuoNeb, Duovent).**

▶CLASSIFICATION

PHARMACOTHERAPEUTIC: Sympathomimetic (adrenergic agonist). **CLINICAL:** Bronchodilator (see p. 62C)

ACTION/THERAPEUTIC EFFECT

Stimulates beta₂-adrenergic receptors in the lungs resulting in relaxation of bronchial smooth muscle. *Relieves bronchospasm, reduces airway resistance.*

PHARMACOKINETICS

	Onset	Peak	Duration
Inhalation	5 min	0.5 hr	3–6 hrs
PO	30 min	2–3 hrs	4–6 hrs

Rapid, well absorbed from GI tract; gradual absorption from bronchi following inhalation. Metabolized in liver. Primarily excreted in urine. Half-life: 3.8 hrs; oral: 3.7–5 hrs inhalation. Unknown if removed by hemodialysis.

USES

Relief of bronchospasm due to reversible obstructive airway disease, exercise-induced bronchospasm.

PRECAUTIONS

CONTRAINDICATIONS: History of hypersensitivity to sympathomimetics. **CAUTIONS:** Hypertension, cardiovascular disease, hyperthyroidism, diabetes mellitus.

▷**LIFESPAN CONSIDERATIONS: Pregnancy/Lactation:** Appears to cross placenta; unknown if distributed in breast milk. May inhibit uterine contractility. **Pregnancy Category C. Children:** Safety and efficacy not established in children <2 yrs (syrup) or <6 yrs (tablets). **Elderly:** May be more sensitive to tremor or tachycardia due to age-related increased sympathetic sensitivity.

INTERACTIONS

DRUG: Beta-adrenergic blocking agents (beta-blockers) antagonize effects. May increase risk of arrhythmias **with digoxin. MAO inhibitors, tricyclic antidepressants** may potentiate cardiovascular effects. **HERBAL:** None known. **FOOD:** None known. **LAB VALUES:**

May decrease serum potassium levels, increase glucose levels.

AVAILABILITY (Rx)

TABLETS: 2 mg, 4 mg. ***TABLETS (extended-release):*** 4 mg, 8 mg. ***SYRUP:*** 2 mg/5 ml. ***AEROSOL:*** Metered dose inhaler. ***SOLUTION FOR INHALATION:*** 0.83 mg/ml, 5 mg/ml. ***CAPSULES FOR INHALATION:*** 200 mcg.

ADMINISTRATION/HANDLING

PO:

• Do not crush or break extended-release tablets. • May give without regard to food.

Inhalation:

• Shake container well, exhale completely through mouth; place mouthpiece into mouth and close lips, holding inhaler upright. • Inhale deeply through mouth while fully depressing the top of canister. Hold breath as long as possible before exhaling slowly. • Wait 2 min before inhaling second dose (allows for deeper bronchial penetration). • Rinse mouth with water immediately after inhalation (prevents mouth/throat dryness).

Nebulization:

• Dilute 0.5 ml of 0.5% solution to final volume of 3 ml with 0.9% NaCl to provide 2.5 mg. • Administer over 5–15 min. • Nebulizer should be used with compressed air or O_2 at rate of 6–10 liters/min.

INDICATIONS/ROUTES/DOSAGE

Bronchospasm:

***INHALATION (Aerosol):* Adults, elderly, children >12 yrs:** 2 inhalations q4–6h. One inhalation q4h may be sufficient in some pts. Wait 1–2 min before administering second inhalation.

***INHALATION (Capsules):* Adults, elderly, children >4 yrs:** 200–400 mcg q4–6h.

***INHALATION (Solution):* Adults, elderly:** 2.5 mg 3–4 times/day by nebulization.

***TABLETS:* Adults, children >12 yrs:** 2 or 4 mg 3–4 times/day. Gradually increased to maximum dose of 8 mg 4 times/day (32 mg/day). **Children 6–12 yrs:** Initially, 2 mg 3–4 times/day. Gradually increase to maximum dose of 24 mg/day in divided doses. **Elderly:** 2 mg 3–4 times/day. Gradually increased to maximum dose of 8 mg 3–4 times/day.

***SYRUP:* Adults, children >14 yrs:** 2–4 mg 3–4 times/day. Maximum: 32 mg/day. **Children 6–14 yrs:** 2 mg 3–4 times/day. Dosage may be gradually increased to 24 mg/day in divided doses. **Children 2–6 yrs:** Initially, 0.1 mg/kg 3 times/day (do not exceed 2 mg 3 times/day). Gradually increased to 0.2 mg/kg 3 times/day (do not exceed 4 mg 3 times/day).

***EXTENDED-RELEASE:* Adults, children >12 yrs:** 4 or 8 mg q12h. May be gradually increased to 16 mg daily.

Exercise-induced bronchospasm:

***INHALATION:* Adults, elderly, children >12 yrs:** 2 inhalations 30 min before exercise.

SIDE EFFECTS

FREQUENT: Headache (27%), nausea (15%), restlessness, nervousness, trembling (20%), dizziness (<7%), throat dryness/irritation, pharyngitis (<6%), B/P changes/hypertension (3–5%), heartburn, transient wheezing (<5%). ***OCCASIONAL*** (2–3%): Insomnia, weakness, unusual/bad taste or taste/smell change. ***Inhalation:*** Dry, irritated mouth or throat, coughing, bronchial irritation.

RARE: Drowsiness, diarrhea, dry mouth, flushing, sweating, anorexia.

ADVERSE REACTIONS/TOXIC EFFECTS

Excessive sympathomimetic stimulation may produce palpitations, extrasystoles, tachycardia, chest pain, slight increase in B/P followed by substantial decrease, chills, sweating, blanching of skin. Too frequent or excessive use may lead to loss of bronchodilating effectiveness and/or severe, paradoxical bronchoconstriction.

NURSING IMPLICATIONS

BASELINE ASSESSMENT:

Offer emotional support (high incidence of anxiety due to difficulty in breathing and sympathomimetic response to drug).

INTERVENTION/EVALUATION:

Monitor rate, depth, rhythm, type of respiration; quality and rate of pulse, EKG, serum potassium, ABG determinations. Assess lung sounds for wheezing (bronchoconstriction) and rales.

PATIENT/FAMILY TEACHING:

Instruct on proper use of inhaler. Increase fluid intake (decreases lung secretion viscosity). Do not take more than 2 inhalations at any one time (excessive use may produce paradoxical bronchoconstriction or a decreased bronchodilating effect). Rinsing mouth with water immediately after inhalation may prevent mouth/throat dryness. Avoid excessive use of caffeine derivatives (chocolate, coffee, tea, cola, cocoa).

alclometasone

(Aclovate)

See Classification section under: Corticosteroid: topical (p. 80C)

aldesleukin

all-des-**lyew**-kin
(Interleukin-2, IL-2, Proleukin)
See Interleukin-2, pp. 67C, 602

alemtuzumab

al-lem-**two**-zoo-mab
(Campath)

▶CLASSIFICATION

PHARMACOTHERAPEUTIC: Monoclonal antibody. ***CLINICAL:*** Antineoplastic (see p. 67C)

ACTION/*THERAPEUTIC EFFECT*

Binds to CD52, a cell surface glycoprotein, found on surface of all B and T lymphocytes, most monocytes, macrophages, NK cells, and granulocytes, *producing cytotoxicity, reducing tumor size.*

PHARMACOKINETICS

Half-life: Approximately 12 days. Peak and trough levels rise during first few wks of therapy, approach steady state by about wk 6.

USES

Treatment of B-cell chronic lymphocytic leukemia (B-CLL) in pts who have been treated with alkylating agents and who have failed fludarabine (Fludara) therapy.

PRECAUTIONS

CONTRAINDICATIONS: Active systemic infections, immunosuppression, known hypersensitivity or anaphylactic reaction. ***CAUTIONS:*** None significant.
▷***LIFESPAN CONSIDERATIONS:***
Pregnancy/Lactation: Has potential to cause fetal B and T lymphocyte depletion. Discontinue breast-feeding during treatment and for ≥3 mos following last dose. **Pregnancy Category C. Children:** Safety and efficacy not established. **Elderly:** No age-related precautions noted.

INTERACTIONS

DRUG: None known. ***HERBAL:*** None known. ***FOOD:*** None known. ***LAB VALUES:*** May decrease white blood cell count, hemoglobin, platelet count.

AVAILABILITY (Rx)

SOLUTION FOR INJECTION: 30 mg/3 ml.

ADMINISTRATION/HANDLING
IV 💉

Storage:
Note: Do not give by IV push or bolus.
• Prior to dilution, refrigerate ampules. Do not freeze. • Use within 8 hrs after dilution. Diluted solution may be stored at room temperature or refrigerated. • Discard if particulate matter is present or if solution is discolored.

Reconstitution:
• Withdraw needed amount from ampule into a syringe. • Using a low-protein binding, nonfiber-releasing 5 μm filter, inject into 100 ml 0.9% NaCl or D$_5$W. • Invert bag to mix; do not shake.

Rate of administration:
• Give the 100 ml solution as a 2-hr IV infusion.

IV INCOMPATIBILITY ⊘

Do not mix with any other medications.

INDICATIONS/ROUTES/DOSAGE

Note: Pretreatment with 650 mg acetaminophen and 50 mg diphenhydramine before each infusion may prevent infusion-related effects.

Chronic lymphocytic leukemia (B-CLL):

IV INFUSION: **Adults, elderly:** Initially, 3 mg/day given as a 2-hr infusion. When the 3 mg daily dose is tolerated (low grade or no infusion-related toxicities), increase daily dose to 10 mg. When the 30 mg/day dose is tolerated, maintenance dose of 30 mg/day may be initiated. **Maintenance dose:** 30 mg/day 3 times/wk on alternate days (Mon.-Wed.-Fri. or Tues.-Thurs.-Sat.) for ≤12 wks (increase to 30 mg/day is usually achieved in 3–7 days).

SIDE EFFECTS

FREQUENT: Rigors (86%), fever (85%), nausea (54%), vomiting (41%), rash (40%), fatigue, (34%), hypotension (32%), urticaria (30%), pruritus, skeletal pain, headache (24%), diarrhea (22%), anorexia (20%). ***OCCASIONAL*** (<10%): Myalgia, dizziness, abdominal pain, throat irritation, vomiting, neutropenia, rhinitis, bronchospasm, urticaria.

ADVERSE REACTIONS/TOXIC EFFECTS

Neutropenia occurs in 85%; anemia in 80%, thrombocytopenia in 72%, rash in 40%. Respiratory toxicity (16–26%) manifested as dyspnea, cough, bronchitis, pneumonitis, pneumonia.

NURSING IMPLICATIONS

BASELINE ASSESSMENT:

Pretreatment with acetaminophen and diphenhydramine before each infusion may prevent infusion-related effects. CBC, platelet count should be obtained frequently during and following therapy to assess for neutropenia, anemia, thrombocytopenia.

INTERVENTION/EVALUATION:

Monitor for an infusion-related symptoms complex consisting mainly of rigors, fever, chills, hypotension, generally occurring 30 min to 2 hrs from beginning of first infusion. Slowing drip rate or slowing infusion resolves symptoms. Monitor for hematologic toxicity (fever, sore throat, signs of local infection, easy bruising, or unusual bleeding from any site), symptoms of anemia (excessive tiredness, weakness).

PATIENT/FAMILY TEACHING:

Avoid crowds, those with known infection. Avoid contact with anyone who recently received live virus vaccine; do not receive vaccinations.

alendronate sodium

ah-**len**-drew-nate
(Fosamax)
Do not confuse with Flomax.

▶CLASSIFICATION

PHARMACOTHERAPEUTIC:
Biphosphonate. **CLINICAL:** Bone resorption inhibitor, calcium regulator

ACTION/*THERAPEUTIC EFFECT*

Inhibits normal and abnormal bone resorption, without retarding mineralization, *leading to significant increased bone mineral density, reversing the progression of osteoporosis.*

PHARMACOKINETICS

Poorly absorbed following PO administration. Protein binding: 78%. After PO administration, rapidly taken into bone, with uptake greatest at sites of active bone turnover. Excreted in urine. Terminal half-life: >10 yrs (reflects release from skeleton as bone is resorbed).

USES/*UNLABELED*

Treatment of osteoporosis, glucocorticoid-induced osteoporosis, Paget's disease; prevention of osteoporosis, vertebral compression fractures in postmenopausal women. *Treatment of breast cancer.*

PRECAUTIONS

CONTRAINDICATIONS: Renal impairment when serum creatinine >5 mg/dl, hypocalcemia. Concurrent use with hormone replacement therapy not recommended. **CAUTIONS:** Gastrointestinal diseases (duodenitis, dysphagia, esophagitis, gastritis, ulcers) (drug may exacerbate these conditions), vitamin D deficiency.

▷**LIFESPAN CONSIDERATIONS:**
Pregnancy/Lactation: Possible incomplete fetal ossification, decreased maternal weight gain, delay in delivery. Excretion in breast milk unknown. Do not give to nursing women. **Pregnancy Category C. Children:** Safety and efficacy not established. **Elderly:** No age-related precautions noted.

INTERACTIONS

DRUG: Concurrent dietary supplements, food, beverages may interfere with alendronate absorption. IV **ranitidine** may double drug bioavailability. **Aspirin** may increase GI disturbances. ***HERBAL:*** None known. ***FOOD:*** None known. ***LAB VALUES:*** Reduces serum calcium, phosphate concentrations. Significant decrease in serum alkaline phosphatase noted in those with Paget's disease.

AVAILABILITY (Rx)

TABLETS: 5 mg, 10 mg, 40 mg, 35 mg, 70 mg.

ADMINISTRATION/HANDLING

PO:

• Give first thing in morning, at least 30 min before first food, beverage, or medication of the day. • Give with 6–8 oz plain water only (mineral water, coffee, tea, juice will decrease absorption). • Instruct patient *not* to lie down for at least 30 min after administering medication and until eating first food of the day (plain water and not lying down allows medication to reach stomach quickly, minimizes esophageal irritation).

INDICATIONS/ROUTES/DOSAGE

Note: Take with full glass plain water only, 30 min before first food, beverage, or medication.

Treatment of osteoporosis, prevention of fractures:

PO: Adults, elderly: 10 mg once daily, in the morning or 70 mg once/wk.

Paget's disease:

PO: Adults, elderly: 40 mg once daily, in the morning.

Prevention of osteoporosis:

PO: Adults, elderly: 5 mg once daily, in the morning or 35 mg once/week.

SIDE EFFECTS

FREQUENT (7–8%): Back pain, abdominal pain. ***OCCASIONAL*** (2–3%): Nausea, abdominal distension, constipation/diarrhea, flatulence. ***RARE*** (<2%): Skin rash, esophageal irritation.

ADVERSE REACTIONS/TOXIC EFFECTS

Hypocalcemia, hypophosphatemia, significant GI disturbances result from overdosage.

NURSING IMPLICATIONS

BASELINE ASSESSMENT:

Hypocalcemia, vitamin D deficiency must be corrected before therapy

INTERVENTION/EVALUATION:

Check electrolytes (esp. calcium and alkaline phosphatase serum levels).

PATIENT/FAMILY TEACHING:

Instruct pt that expected benefits occur only when medication is taken with full glass (6–8 oz) of plain water, first thing in the morning and at least 30 min before first food, beverage, or medication of the day is taken. Any other beverage (mineral water, orange juice, coffee) significantly reduces absorption of medication. Do not lie down for at least 30 min after taking medication (potentiates delivery to stomach, reduces risk of esophageal irritation). Consider weight-bearing exercises, modify behavioral factors (e.g., cigarette smoking, alcohol consumption).

alfentanil

(Alfenta)

See Classification section under: Opioid analgesics

alitretinoin

al-**lee**-tret-ih-nown
(Panretin)

▶CLASSIFICATION

PHARMACOTHERAPEUTIC: Second-generation retinoid. **CLINICAL:** Antineoplastic (see p. 67C)

ACTION/*THERAPEUTIC EFFECT*

Binds to and activates all known retinoid receptors. Once activated, receptors act as transcription factors, regulating genes that control cellular differentiation and proliferation, *inhibiting growth of Kaposi's sarcoma cells.*

USES/*UNLABELED*

Topical treatment of cutaneous lesions in those with AIDS-related Kaposi's sarcoma. *Breast, cervical, ovarian, prostatic carcinomas, myelodysplastic syndrome, psoriasis.*

PRECAUTIONS

CONTRAINDICATIONS: When systemic therapy is required (>10 new Kaposi's sarcoma [KS] lesions in previous month), symptomatic pulmonary KS, symptomatic visceral involvement, symptomatic lymphedema. **CAUTIONS:** None known.

INTERACTIONS

DRUG: Increased risk of toxicity to products containing DEET (component of insect repellent). **HERBAL:** None known. **FOOD:** None known. **LAB VALUES:** None known.

AVAILABILITY (Rx)

GEL: 0.1%.

INDICATIONS/ROUTES/DOSAGE

Kaposi's sarcoma:

TOPICAL: Adults: Initially, apply 2 times/day to lesions. May increase to 3–4 times/day. Allow gel to dry 3–5 min before covering with clothing.

SIDE EFFECTS

FREQUENT (>5%): Rash (erythema, scaling, irritation, redness, dermatitis), itching, exfoliative dermatitis (flaking, peeling, desquamation, exfoliation), stinging, tingling, edema skin disorders (scabbing, crusting, drainage).

ADVERSE REACTIONS/TOXIC EFFECTS

Severe local skin reaction (intense erythema, edema, vesiculation) may limit treatment.

NURSING IMPLICATIONS

PATIENT/FAMILY TEACHING:

Do not apply dressings over medication gel. Do not apply gel to healthy skin surrounding lesions or apply gel on or near mucosal surfaces. If severe irritation occurs, frequency of application can be reduced or discontinued for a few days until symptoms subside.

allopurinol

al-low-**pure**-ih-nawl
(Aloprim, Apo-Allopurinol✤, Purinol✤, Zyloprim)

►CLASSIFICATION

PHARMACOTHERAPEUTIC:
Xanthine oxidase inhibitor. ***CLIN-ICAL:*** Antigout

ACTION/*THERAPEUTIC EFFECT*

Decreases uric acid production by inhibition of xanthine oxidase, an enzyme, *reducing uric acid concentrations in both serum and urine.*

PHARMACOKINETICS

Well absorbed from GI tract. Widely distributed. Metabolized in liver to active metabolite. Excreted primarily in urine. Removed by hemodialysis. Half-life: 1–3 hrs; metabolite: 12–30 hrs.

USES/*UNLABELED*

Treatment of chronic gouty arthritis, uric acid nephropathy. Prevents or treats hyperuricemia secondary to blood dyscrasias, cancer chemotherapy. Prevents recurrence of uric acid or calcium stone formation. **Aloprim:** Management of elevated uric acid in cancer pts unable to tolerate oral therapy. *Used in mouthwash following fluorouracil therapy to prevent stomatitis.*

PRECAUTIONS

CONTRAINDICATIONS: Asymptomatic hyperuricemia. ***CAUTIONS:*** Impaired renal, hepatic function, CHF, diabetes, mellitus, hypertension.
▷***LIFESPAN CONSIDERATIONS:***
Pregnancy/Lactation: Unknown if drug crosses placenta or is distributed in breast milk. **Pregnancy Category C. Children/Elderly:** No age-related precautions noted.

INTERACTIONS

DRUG: **Thiazide diuretics** may decrease effect. May increase effect of **oral anticoagulants.** May increase effect, toxicity of **azathioprine, mercaptopurine. Ampicillin, amoxicillin** may increase incidence of skin rash. ***HERBAL:*** None known. ***FOOD:*** None known. ***LAB VALUES:*** May increase alkaline phosphatase, SGOT (AST), SGPT (ALT), BUN, creatinine.

AVAILABILITY (Rx)

TABLETS: 100 mg, 300 mg. ***POWDER FOR INJECTION:*** 500 mg.

ADMINISTRATION/HANDLING

PO:
• May give with or immediately after meals or milk. • Instruct pt to drink at least 10–12 eight oz glasses of water/day. • Doses >300 mg/day to be administered in divided doses.

IV 🏶

Storage:
• Store unreconstituted vials at room temperature. • May store reconstituted solution at room temperature and give within 10 hrs. Do not use if precipitate forms or solution is discolored.

Reconstitution:
• Reconstitute 500 mg vial with 25 ml sterile water for injection giving a clear, almost colorless solution (concentration of 20 mg/ml). • Further dilute with 0.9% NaCl or D_5W (19 ml of added diluent yields 1 mg/ml, 9 ml yields 2 mg/ml, 2.3 ml yields maximum concentration of 6 mg/ml).

Rate of administration:
• Infuse over 30–60 min.

IV INCOMPATIBILITIES ⊘

Amikacin (Amikin), carmustine (BiCNU), cefotaxime (Claforan), chlorpromazine (Thorazine), cimetidine (Tagamet), clindamycin (Cleocin), cytarabine (Ara-C), dacarbazine (DTIC), diphenhydramine (Benadryl), doxorubicin (Adriamycin), doxycycline (Vibramycin), droperidol (Inapsine), fludarabine (Fludara), gentamicin (Garamycin), haloperidol (Haldol), hydroxyzine (Vistaril), idarubicin (Idamycin), imipenem-cilastatin (Primaxin), meperidine (Demerol), methylprednisolone (Solu Medrol), metoclopramide (Reglan), ondansetron (Zofran), prochlorperazine (Compazine), promethazine (Phenergan), streptozocin (Zanosar), tobramycin (Nebcin), vinorelbine (Navelbine).

IV COMPATIBILITIES

Bumetanide (Bumex), calcium gluconate, furosemide (Lasix), heparin, hydromorphone (Dilaudid), lorazepam (Ativan), morphine, potassium chloride.

INDICATIONS/ROUTES/DOSAGE

Antigout:

PO: **Adults, children >10 yrs:** Initially, 100 mg/day; may increase by 100 mg/day at weekly intervals. **Maximum:** 800 mg/day. **Maintenance:** 100–200 mg 2–3 times/day or 300 mg/day.

Neoplastic disease therapy:

PO: **Adults:** Initially, 600–800 mg/day starting 2–3 days prior to initiation of chemotherapy or radiation therapy. **Children 6–10 yrs:** 100 mg 3 times/day or 300 mg once daily. **Children <6 yrs:** 50 mg 3 times/day.

IV: **Adults:** 200–400 mg/m²/day beginning 24–48 hrs prior to initiation of chemotherapy. **Children:** 200 mg/m²/day. **Maximum:** 600 mg/day.

Uric acid calculi:

PO: **Adults:** 100–200 mg 1–4 times/day or 300 mg once daily.

Calcium oxalate calculi:

PO: **Adults:** 200–300 mg/day.

Usual elderly dosage:

PO: Initially, 100 mg/day, gradually increased to optimal uric acid level.

Dosage in renal impairment:

Creatinine Clearance (ml/min)	Dosage Adjustment
>50	No change
10–50	50%
<10	30%

SIDE EFFECTS

OCCASIONAL: PO: Drowsiness, unusual hair loss. ***IV:*** Rash, nausea, vomiting. ***RARE:*** Diarrhea, headache.

ADVERSE REACTIONS/TOXIC EFFECTS

Pruritic maculopapular rash should be considered a toxic reaction. May be accompanied by malaise, fever, chills, joint pain, nausea, vomiting. Severe hypersensitivity may follow appearance of rash. Bone marrow depression, hepatotoxicity, peripheral neuritis, or acute renal failure occurs rarely.

NURSING IMPLICATIONS

BASELINE ASSESSMENT:

Instruct pt to drink 10–12 glasses (8 oz) of fluid daily while on medication.

INTERVENTION/EVALUATION:

Discontinue medication immediately if rash or other evidence of allergic reaction appears. Encourage high fluid intake (3,000 ml/day). Monitor I&O (output should be at least 2,000 ml/day). Assess CBC, uric acid and liver function serum levels. Assess urine for cloudiness, unusual color, odor. Assess for therapeutic response (reduced joint tenderness, swelling, redness, limitation of motion).

PATIENT/FAMILY TEACHING:

May take 1 or more wks for full therapeutic effect. Encourage drinking 10–12 glasses (8 oz) of fluid daily while on medication. Avoid tasks that require alertness, motor skills until response to drug is established.

almotriptan malate

ale-moe-**trip-tan**
(Axert)

▶CLASSIFICATION

PHARMACOTHERAPEUTIC:
Serotonin receptor agonist. ***CLINICAL:*** Antimigraine (see p. 53C)

ACTION/*THERAPEUTIC EFFECT*

Binds selectively to vascular receptors, producing a vasoconstrictive effect on cranial blood vessels, *producing relief of migraine headache.*

PHARMACOKINETICS

Well absorbed following PO administration. Metabolized by the liver, excreted in urine.

USES

Acute treatment of migraine headache with or without aura.

PRECAUTIONS

CONTRAINDICATIONS: Coronary artery disease, uncontrolled hypertension, ischemic heart disease (angina pectoris, history of MI, silent ischemia), Prinzmetal's angina, concurrent use (or within 24 hrs) of ergotamine-containing preparations, concurrent (or

within 2 wks) of MAO therapy, hemiplegic or basilar migraine, within 24 hrs of another serotonin receptor agonist, Wolff-Parkinson-White syndrome, arrhythmias associated with cardiac conduction pathways disorders. ***CAUTIONS:*** Mild-to-moderate renal/hepatic impairment, pt profile suggesting cardiovascular risks, controlled hypertension, history of CVA.

▷*LIFESPAN CONSIDERATIONS:*
Pregnancy/Lactation: Unknown if distributed in breast milk. **Pregnancy Category C. Children:** Safety and efficacy not established in pts <12 yrs. **Elderly:** No age-related precautions noted.

INTERACTIONS

DRUG: **Ergotamine-containing drugs** may produce vasospastic reaction. **Monoamine oxidase inhibitors** may increase concentration. Combined use of **fluoxetine, fluvoxamine, paroxetine, sertraline** may produce weakness, hyperreflexia, incoordination. Avoid taking **ketokonazole, itraconaole, ritonavir, erythromycin** in last 7 days. ***HERBAL:*** None significant. ***FOOD:*** None significant. ***LAB VALUES:*** None significant

AVAILABILITY (Rx)
TABLETS: 6.5 mg, 12.5 mg.

ADMINISTRATION/HANDLING
PO:
• Swallow tablets whole. • Take with full glass of water.

INDICATIONS/ROUTES/DOSAGE
Migraine headache:
***PO:* Adults, elderly:** 6.25–12.5 mg. If headache returns, dose may be repeated after 2 hrs. **Maximum:** No more than 2 doses within 24 hrs.

SIDE EFFECTS

FREQUENT: Nausea, dry mouth, paresthesia, flushing. **OCCASIONAL:** Sensation of warm/hot, weakness, dizziness.

ADVERSE REACTIONS/TOXIC EFFECTS

Excessive dosage may produce tremor, redness of extremities, reduced respirations, cyanosis, seizures, chest pain. Serious arrhythmias occur rarely, but particularly in pts with hypertension, obesity, smokers, diabetics, and those with strong family history of coronary artery disease.

NURSING IMPLICATIONS

BASELINE ASSESSMENT:

Question pt regarding history of peripheral vascular disease. Question pt regarding onset, location, and duration of migraine and possible precipitating symptoms.

INTERVENTION/EVALUATION:

Evaluate for relief of migraine headache and resulting photophobia, phonophobia (sound sensitivity), nausea, and vomiting.

PATIENT/FAMILY TEACHING:

Take a single dose as soon as symptoms of an actual migraine attack appear. Medication is intended to relieve migraine, not to prevent or reduce number of attacks. Lie down in quiet, dark room for additional benefit after taking medication. Avoid tasks that require alertness, motor skills until response to drug is established. If heart throbbing, pain/tightness in chest or throat, or pain or weakness of extremities occurs, contact physician immediately.

alpha$_1$-proteinase inhibitor (human, alpha$_1$-PI)

(Prolastin)

▶CLASSIFICATION

PHARMACOTHERAPEUTIC: Proteinase inhibitor. **CLINICAL:** Alveolar protectant

ACTION/*THERAPEUTIC EFFECT*

Protects alveolar epithelial lining of lower respiratory tract by alleviating imbalance between elastase (enzyme capable of degrading elastin tissue in lower respiratory tract) and alpha$_1$-proteinase inhibitor (inhibits neutrophil elastase), *allowing for subsequent protection from degradation of elastin tissue.*

USES

Chronic replacement therapy in those with clinically demonstrable panacinar emphysema. Do not use in patients with PiMZ or PiMS phenotypes (small risk of panacinar emphysema).

PRECAUTIONS

CONTRAINDICATIONS: Pts with known antibody reaction against IgA (may experience severe reaction, including anaphylaxis). **CAUTIONS:** Those at risk for circulatory overload.

INTERACTIONS

DRUG: None significant. **HERBAL:** None known. **FOOD:** None known. **LAB VALUES:** None significant.

AVAILABILITY (Rx)

POWDER FOR INJECTION: 500 mg, 1,000 mg.

ADMINISTRATION/HANDLING

IV

Storage:

• Refrigerate vials. Do not exceed 77° F. • Do not freeze. Do not refrigerate once reconstituted. • After reconstitution, administer within 3 hrs.

Reconstitution:

• Reconstitute with Sterile Water for Injection (supplied by manufacturer).

Rate of administration:

• Rate of 0.08 ml/kg/min as IV infusion.

IV INCOMPATIBILITY ⊘

Do not mix with any other medication.

INDICATIONS/ROUTES/DOSAGE

Replacement therapy:

IV INFUSION: Adults, elderly: 60 mg/kg once weekly at rate of at least 0.08 ml/kg/min.

SIDE EFFECTS

RARE (<1%): Delayed fever, light-headedness, dizziness.

ADVERSE REACTIONS/TOXIC EFFECTS

Mild leukocytosis occurs rarely.

NURSING IMPLICATIONS

BASELINE ASSESSMENT:

All pts should be immunized against hepatitis B before initial dose is given.

INTERVENTION/EVALUATION:

Maintain blood levels of alpha$_1$-Pl at 80 mg/dl. Monitor respiratory status throughout therapy.

PATIENT/FAMILY TEACHING:

Explain purpose of medication, importance of hepatitis B vaccine, periodic pulmonary function tests. Avoid smoking.

alprazolam 🖉

ale-**praz**-oh-lam
(Apo-Alpraz ✤, Novo-Alprazol ✤, Xanax)
Do not confuse with Zantac.

▶CLASSIFICATION

PHARMACOTHERAPEUTIC:
Benzodiazepine **(Schedule IV)**.
CLINICAL: Antianxiety (see p. 10C)

ACTION/*THERAPEUTIC EFFECT*

Enhances action of inhibitory neurotransmitters in the brain, *producing anxiolytic effect due to CNS depressant action.*

PHARMACOKINETICS

Well absorbed from GI tract. Protein binding: 80%. Metabolized in liver. Primarily excreted in urine. Minimal removal by hemodialysis. Half-life: 11–16 hrs.

USES/*UNLABELED*

Management of anxiety disorders associated with depression, panic disorder. *Improves mood, relieves cramps, prevents insomnia with premenstrual syndrome, management of irritable bowel syndrome.*

PRECAUTIONS

CONTRAINDICATIONS: Acute narrow-angle glaucoma, acute alcohol intoxication with depressed vital signs, severe chronic obstructive pulmonary disease, myasthenia gravis, ketoconazole, itraconazole. **CAUTIONS:** Impaired renal/hepatic function.

Pregnancy/Lactation: Crosses placenta; distributed in breast milk. Chronic ingestion during pregnancy may produce withdrawal symptoms, CNS depression in neonates. **Pregnancy Category D. Children:** Safety and efficacy not established. **Elderly:** Use small initial doses with gradual increase to avoid ataxia (muscular incoordination) or excessive sedation.

INTERACTIONS

DRUG: Potentiated effects when used with other **CNS depressants (including alcohol). Ketoconazole, nefazodone, fluvoxamine** may inhibit liver metabolism, increase serum concentrations. **HERBAL: Kava kava, valerian** may increase CNS depressant effect. **FOOD: Grapefruit juice** may inhibit metabolism. **LAB VALUES:** None significant.

AVAILABILITY (Rx)

TABLETS: 0.25 mg, 0.5 mg, 1 mg, 2 mg. **ORAL SOLUTION:** 0.5 mg/5 ml, 1 mg/ml.

ADMINISTRATION/HANDLING

PO:

• May be given without regard to meals. • Tablets may be crushed.

INDICATIONS/ROUTES/DOSAGE

Anxiety disorders:

PO: Adults >18 yrs: Initially, 0.25–0.5 mg 3 times daily. Titrate to maximum of 4 mg daily in divided doses. **Elderly/debilitated/liver disease/low serum albumin:** Initially, 0.25 mg 2–3 times daily. Gradually increase to optimum therapeutic response.

Panic disorder:

PO: Adults: Initially, 0.5 mg 3 times/day. May increase at 3–4 day intervals at no more than 1 mg/day. **Range:** 1–10 mg/day.

Usual elderly dosage:

PO: Initially, 0.125–0.25 mg 2 times/day; may increase in 0.125 mg increments until desired effect attained.

Premenstrual syndrome:

PO: Adults: 0.25 mg 3 times/day.

SIDE EFFECTS

FREQUENT: Muscular incoordination (ataxia), lightheadedness, transient mild drowsiness, slurred speech (particularly in elderly, debilitated). **OCCASIONAL:** Confusion, depression, blurred vision, constipation/diarrhea, dry mouth, headache, nausea. **RARE:** Behavioral problems (e.g., anger), impaired memory, paradoxical reaction (insomnia, nervousness, irritability).

ADVERSE REACTIONS/TOXIC EFFECTS

Abrupt or too rapid withdrawal may result in pronounced restlessness, irritability, insomnia, hand tremors, abdominal/muscle cramps, sweating, vomiting, seizures. Overdosage results in somnolence, confusion, diminished reflexes, coma. Blood dyscrasias noted rarely.

NURSING IMPLICATIONS

BASELINE ASSESSMENT:

Offer emotional support to anxious pt. Assess motor responses (agitation, trembling, tension) and autonomic responses (cold, clammy hands, sweating).

INTERVENTION/EVALUATION:

For those on long-term therapy, liver/renal function tests, blood counts should be performed periodically. Assess for paradoxical reaction, particularly during early therapy. Evaluate for therapeutic response: calm facial expression, decreased restlessness and/or insomnia.

PATIENT/FAMILY TEACHING:

Drowsiness usually disappears during continued therapy. If dizziness occurs, change positions slowly from recumbent to sitting position before standing. Avoid tasks that require alertness, motor skills until response to drug is established. Smoking reduces drug effectiveness. Sour hard candy, gum, or sips of tepid water may relieve dry mouth. Do not abruptly withdraw medication after long-term therapy. Avoid alcohol. Do not take other medications without consulting physician.

alprostadil (prostaglandin E₁; PGE₁)

ale-**pros**-tah-dill
(Caverject, Edex, Muse, Prostin VR✤, Prostin VR Pediatric)

▶**CLASSIFICATION**

PHARMACOTHERAPEUTIC: Prostaglandin. **CLINICAL:** Patent ductus arteriosus agent, anti-impotence

ACTION/*THERAPEUTIC EFFECT*

Vasodilator having direct effect on vascular smooth muscle, ductus arteriosus. *Relaxes cavernous smooth muscle, dilates penile arteries, increases arterial blood flow to penis. Prevents closure of ductus arteriosus.*

USES/*UNLABELED*

Temporarily maintains patency of ductus arteriosus until surgery is performed in those with congenital heart defects and dependent on patent ductus for survival (e.g., pulmonary atresia or stenosis). Treatment of erectile dysfunction due to neurogenic, vasculogenic, psychogenic causes, adjunct in diagnosis of erectile dysfunction. *Treatment of atherosclerosis, gangrene, pain due to severe peripheral arterial occlusive disease.*

PRECAUTIONS

CONTRAINDICATIONS: Respiratory distress syndrome (hyaline membrane disease). Conditions predisposing to priaprism, anatomical deformation of penis, penile implants. **CAUTIONS:** Severe liver disease, coagulation defects, leukemia, multiple myeloma, polycythemia, sickle cell disease, thrombocythenia.

INTERACTIONS

DRUG: Anticoagulants, heparin, thrombolytics may increase risk of bleeding. **Sympathomimetics** may decrease effect. **Vasodilators** may increase risk of hypotension. **HERBAL:** None known. **FOOD:** None known. **LAB VALUES:** May increase bilirubin. May decrease calcium, glucose, potassium.

AVAILABILITY (Rx)

INJECTION: 500 mcg/ml. **POWDER FOR INJECTION:** 5 mcg, 10 mcg, 20 mcg, 40 mcg. **URETHRAL PELLET (Muse):** 125 mcg, 250 mcg, 500 mcg, 1,000 mcg.

ADMINISTRATION/HANDLING

Urethral pellet:

Storage:

• Refrigerate pellet unless used within 14 days.

IV 🔢

Storage:

• Store parenteral form in refrigerator. • Must dilute before use. • Prepare fresh q24h. • Discard unused portions.

Reconstitution:

• Dilute 500 mcg ampoule with D$_5$W or 0.9% NaCl to volume dependent on infusion pump capabilities.

Rate of administration:

• Infuse for shortest time, lowest dose possible. • If significant decrease in arterial pressure is noted via umbilical artery catheter, auscultation, or Doppler transducer, decrease infusion rate immediately. • Discontinue infusion immediately if apnea or bradycardia occurs (overdosage).

IV INCOMPATIBILITY ⃠

No information available via Y-site administration.

INDICATIONS/ROUTES/DOSAGE

Note: Give by continuous IV infusion or through umbilical artery catheter placed at ductal opening.

Maintain patency ductus arteriosus:

IV INFUSION: Neonates: Initially, 0.05–0.1 mcg/kg/min. After therapeutic response achieved, use lowest dose to maintain response. **Maximum:** 0.4 mcg/kg/min.

Impotence:

PELLET, INTRACAVERNOSAL: Individualized.

SIDE EFFECTS

FREQUENT: Intracavernosal (1–4%): Penile pain (37%), prolonged erection, hypertension, local pain, penile fibrosis, injection site hematoma/ecchymosis, headache, respiratory infection, flulike symptoms. **Intra-**urethral (3%): Penile pain (36%), urethral pain/burning, testicular pain, urethral bleeding, headache, dizziness, respiratory infection, flulike symptoms. **Systemic** (>1%): Fever, seizures, flushing, bradycardia, hypotension, tachycardia, apnea, diarrhea, sepsis. **OCCASIONAL: Intracavernosal** (<1%): Hypotension, pelvic pain, back pain, dizziness, cough, nasal congestion. **Intraurethral** (<3%): Fainting, sinusitis, back/pelvic pain. **Systemic** (<1%): Jitteriness, lethargy, stiffness, arrhythmias, respiratory depression, anemia, bleeding, thrombocytopenia, hematuria.

ADVERSE REACTIONS/TOXIC EFFECTS

Overdosage manifested as apnea, flushing of face/arms, bradycardia. Cardiac arrest, sepsis occur rarely.

NURSING IMPLICATIONS

INTERVENTION/EVALUATION:

Patent ductus arteriosus: Monitor arterial pressure by umbilical artery catheter, auscultation, or Doppler transducer. If significant decrease in arterial pressure occurs, decrease infusion rate immediately. Maintain continuous cardiac monitoring. Assess heart sounds, femoral pulse (circulation to lower extremities), and respiratory status frequently. Monitor symptoms of hypotension, B/P, arterial blood gases, temperature. If apnea or bradycardia occurs, discontinue infusion and notify physician.

PATIENT/FAMILY TEACHING:

Patent ductus arteriosus: Explain purpose of this palliative therapy to parents. **Impotence:** Erection is to occur within 2–5 min. Do not use if female is pregnant (unless using condom barrier). Inform physician if erection lasts >4 hrs or becomes painful.

alteplase, recombinant

all-teh-place
(Activase, Activase tPA❧, Cathflo Activase)

▶CLASSIFICATION

PHARMACOTHERAPEUTIC:
Tissue plasminogen activator (tPA). ***CLINICAL:*** Thrombolytic (see p. 30C).

ACTION/*THERAPEUTIC EFFECT*

An enzyme, binds to fibrin in a thrombus and converts entrapped plasminogen to plasmin, initiating fibrinolysis, *degrading fibrin clots, fibrinogen, other plasma proteins.* Appears to be more readily clot selective binding within a clot than circulating fibrinogen.

PHARMACOKINETICS

Rapidly metabolized in liver. Primarily excreted in urine. Half-life: 35 min.

USES/*UNLABELED*

Management of acute myocardial infarction (AMI) for lysis of thrombi obstructing coronary arteries and management of acute massive pulmonary embolus for lysis of acute pulmonary emboli. Treatment acute ischemic stroke (within 3 hrs of symptoms). Clears thrombin in central venous catheters. *Coronary thrombolysis, decrease ischemic events in unstable angina.*

PRECAUTIONS

CONTRAINDICATIONS: Active internal bleeding, recent (within 2 mos) cerebrovascular accident, intracranial or intraspinal surgery or trauma, intracranial neoplasm, arteriovenous malformation or aneurysm, bleeding diathesis, severe uncontrolled hypertension. ***CAUTIONS:*** Recent (10 days) major surgery or GI bleeding, OB delivery, organ biopsy, recent trauma (cardiopulmonary resuscitation, left heart thrombus, endocarditis, severe hepatic/renal disease, pregnancy, elderly, cerebrovascular disease, diabetic retinopathy, thrombophlebitis, occluded AV cannula at infected site).

▷*LIFESPAN CONSIDERATIONS:*
Pregnancy/Lactation: Use only when benefit outweighs potential risk to fetus. Unknown if drug crosses placenta or is distributed in breast milk. **Pregnancy Category C. Children:** Safety and efficacy not established. **Elderly:** Risk of thrombolytic therapy increased, careful patient selection, monitoring recommended.

INTERACTIONS

DRUG:* Anticoagulants, heparin, cefotetan, plicamycin, valproic acid** may increase risk of hemorrhage. **Platelet aggregation inhibitors (e.g., aspirin), NSAIDs, ticlodipine** may increase risk of bleeding. ***HERBAL: None known. ***FOOD:*** None known. ***LAB VALUES:*** Decreases plasminogen and fibrinogen level during infusion, decreasing clotting time (confirms presence of lysis). Decreases hemoglobin and hematocrit.

AVAILABILITY (Rx)

POWDER FOR INJECTION: 2 mg, 50 mg, 100 mg.

ADMINISTRATION/HANDLING

IV 💉

Storage:

• Store vials at room temperature. • After reconstitution, solutions appear

---

colorless to pale yellow. • Solution is stable for 8 hrs after reconstitution. Discard unused portions.

Reconstitution:

• Reconstitute immediately prior to use with Sterile Water for Injection. • Reconstitute 100 mg vial with 100 ml Sterile Water for Injection (50 mg vial with 50 ml sterile water) without preservative to provide a concentration of 1 mg/ml. May be further diluted with 50 ml D_5W or 0.9% NaCl to provide a concentration of 0.5 mg/ml. • Avoid excessive agitation; gently swirl or slowly invert vial to reconstitute.

Rate of administration:

• Give by IV infusion via infusion pump. See individual dosages. • If minor bleeding occurs at puncture sites, apply pressure for 30 sec; if unrelieved, apply pressure dressing. • If uncontrolled hemorrhage occurs, discontinue infusion immediately (slowing rate of infusion may produce worsening hemorrhage). • Avoid undue pressure when drug is injected into catheter (can rupture catheter or expel clot into circulation).

IV INCOMPATIBILITIES ⊘

Do not add any other medication to the container of alteplase solution or administer other medications through the same intravenous line.

IV COMPATIBILITIES

Lidocaine, metoprolol (Lopressor), propranolol (Inderal).

INDICATIONS/ROUTES/DOSAGE

Acute myocardial infarction:

IV INFUSION: Adults: 100 mg over 90 min **(>67 kg):** 15 mg bolus given over 1–2 min; then 50 mg over 30 min; then 35 mg over 60 min. **(<67 kg):** 15 mg bolus, then 0.75 mg/kg over next 30 min (**Maximum:** 50

mg), then 0.5 mg/kg over 60 min (**Maximum:** 35 mg). **THREE-HOUR INFUSION (>67 kg):** 60 mg over first hr (6–10 mg as bolus over 1–2 min), 20 mg over second hr and 20 mg over third hr. **(<67 kg):** 1.25 mg/kg given over 3 hrs as 60% of dose over first hr (6–10% as 1–2 min bolus), 20% over second hr and 20% over third hr.

Acute pulmonary emboli:

IV INFUSION: Adults: 100 mg over 2 hrs. Institute or reinstitute heparin near end or immediately after infusion (when PTT or thrombin time returns to twice normal or less).

Acute ischemic stroke:

IV INFUSION: Adults: 0.9 mg/kg over 60 min (10% total dose as initial IV bolus over 1 min).

Catheter clearance:

IV: Adults, elderly: 2 mg; may repeat in >120 min.

SIDE EFFECTS

FREQUENT: Superficial bleeding at puncture sites, decreased B/P. **OCCASIONAL:** Allergic reaction (rash, wheezing), bruising.

ADVERSE REACTIONS/TOXIC EFFECTS

Severe internal hemorrhage may occur. Lysis of coronary thrombi may produce atrial or ventricular dysrhythmias, stroke.

NURSING IMPLICATIONS

BASELINE ASSESSMENT:

Obtain baseline B/P, apical pulse. Record weight. Evaluate 12-lead EKG, CPK, CPK-MB, electrolytes. Assess hematocrit, platelet count, thrombin (TT), activated thromboplastin (APTT), prothrombin time (PT), fibrinogen level, before therapy is instituted. Type and hold blood.

INTERVENTION/EVALUATION:
Continuous cardiac monitoring for arrhythmias, B/P, pulse and respirations q15min until stable, then hourly. Check peripheral pulses, heart and lung sounds. Monitor chest pain relief and notify physician of continuation or recurrence (note location, type, and intensity). Assess for bleeding: overt blood, blood in any body substance. Monitor PTT per protocol. Maintain B/P; avoid any trauma that might increase risk of bleeding (injections, shaving, etc.). Assess neurologic status.

---

altretamine (hexamethylmelamine)

(Hexalen)

See Classification section under: Antineoplastics (p. 67C)

---

aluminum carbonate

(Basaljel)

aluminum hydroxide

(Alternagel, Alu-Cap, Alu-Tab, Amphojel, Basaljel✦, Dialume)

FIXED-COMBINATION(S)

With magnesium, an antacid **(Aludrox, Delcid, Gaviscon, Maalox);** with magnesium and simethicone, an antiflatulent **(DiGel, Gelusil, Maalox Plus, Mylanta, Silain-Gel);** with magnesium and calcium, an antacid **(Camalox)**

▶**CLASSIFICATION**
CLINICAL: Antacid (p. 8C)

ACTION/*THERAPEUTIC EFFECT*
Reduces gastric acid, *thereby neutralizing or increasing gastric pH.* Binds with phosphate in intestine, then excreted in feces *(reduces phosphates in urine, preventing formation of phosphate urinary stones; reduces serum phosphate levels).* May increase absorption of calcium (due to decreased serum phosphate levels). Astringent, adsorbent properties *(decreases fluidity of stools).*

USES
Symptomatic relief of upset stomach associated with hyperacidity (heartburn, acid indigestion, sour stomach). Hyperacidity associated with gastric, duodenal ulcers. Symptomatic treatment of gastroesophageal reflux disease. Prophylactic treatment of GI bleeding secondary to gastritis and stress ulceration. In conjunction with low phosphate diet, prevents formation of phosphate urinary stones, reduces elevated phosphate levels.

PRECAUTIONS
CONTRAINDICATIONS: Intestinal obstruction, very young. ***CAUTIONS:*** Impaired renal function, gastric outlet obstruction, elderly, dehydration, fluid restriction, Alzheimer's disease, symptoms of appendicitis, GI/rectal bleeding, constipation, fecal impaction, chronic diarrhea.

INTERACTIONS
DRUG: May decrease excretion of **quinidine, anticholinergics.** May decrease effects of **methenamine.** May increase **salicylate** excretion. May decrease absorption of **quinolones, iron preparations, isoniazid, ketoconazole, tetracyclines.** ***HERBAL:*** None known. ***FOOD:***

None known. ***LAB VALUES:*** May increase gastrin, systemic/urinary pH. May decrease serum phosphate.

AVAILABILITY (OTC)

Aluminum carbonate: TABLETS: 500 mg. ***CAPSULES:*** 500 mg. ***SUSPENSION:*** 400 mg/5 ml.

Aluminum hydroxide: TABLETS: 300 mg, 500 mg, 600 mg. ***CAPSULES:*** 400 mg, 500 mg. ***SUSPENSION:*** 320 mg/5 ml, 450 mg/5 ml, 675 mg/5 ml. ***LIQUID:*** 600 mg/5 ml.

ADMINISTRATION/HANDLING
PO:

• Usually administered 1–3 hrs after meals. • Individualize dose (based on neutralizing capacity of antacids). • Chewable tablets: Thoroughly chew tablets before swallowing (follow with glass of water or milk). • If administering suspension, shake well before use.

INDICATIONS/ROUTES/DOSAGE
Note: Usual dose is 30–60 ml.

ALUMINUM CARBONATE:
Antacid:
PO: Adults, elderly: 2 capsules or 10 ml q2h up to 12 times/day.

Hyperphosphatemia:
PO: Adults, elderly: 2 capsules or 12.5 ml 3–4 times/day with meals.

ALUMINUM HYDROXIDE:
Antacid:
PO: Adults, elderly: 500–1,800 mg (5–30 ml) 3–6 times/day between meals and bedtime.

Hyperphosphatemia:
PO: Adults: 1.9–4.8 g 3–4 times/day. **Children:** 50–150 mg/kg/24 hrs in divided doses q4–6h.

SIDE EFFECTS
FREQUENT: Chalky taste, mild constipation, stomach cramps. ***OCCASIONAL:*** Nausea, vomiting, speckling/whitish discoloration of stools.

ADVERSE REACTIONS/TOXIC EFFECTS

Prolonged constipation may result in intestinal obstruction. Excessive or chronic use may produce hypophosphatemia (anorexia, malaise, muscle weakness, bone pain) resulting in osteomalacia, osteoporosis. Prolonged use may produce urinary calculi.

NURSING IMPLICATIONS

BASELINE ASSESSMENT:
Do not give other oral medication within 1–2 hrs of antacid administration.

INTERVENTION/EVALUATION:
Assess pattern of daily bowel activity and stool consistency. Monitor serum phosphate, calcium, uric acid, aluminum levels. Assess for relief of gastric distress.

PATIENT/FAMILY TEACHING:
Chewable tablets: Chew tablets thoroughly before swallowing (may be followed by water or milk). Tablets may discolor stool. Maintain adequate fluid intake.

amantadine hydrochloride

ah-**man**-tih-deen
(Symmetrel)

▶CLASSIFICATION

PHARMACOTHERAPEUTIC: Dopaminergic agonist. *CLINICAL:* Antiviral, antiparkinson (see p. 57C)

ACTION/*THERAPEUTIC EFFECT*

Antiviral action against influenza A virus believed *to prevent uncoating of virus, penetration of host cells, release of nucleic acid into host cells.* Antiparkinsonism *due to increased release of dopamine.* Virustatic.

PHARMACOKINETICS

Rapidly, completely absorbed from GI tract. Protein binding: 67%. Widely distributed. Primarily excreted in urine. Minimally removed by hemodialysis. Half-life: 11–15 hrs (half-life increased in elderly, decreased in impaired renal function).

USES/*UNLABELED*

Prevention, treatment of respiratory tract infections due to influenza virus, Parkinson's disease, drug-induced extrapyramidal reactions. *Treatment of fatigue associated with multiple sclerosis, AHDH.*

PRECAUTIONS

CONTRAINDICATIONS: None significant. *CAUTIONS:* History of seizures, orthostatic hypotension, CHF, peripheral edema, liver disease, recurrent eczematoid dermatitis, cerebrovascular disease, renal dysfunction, those receiving CNS stimulants.

▷*LIFESPAN CONSIDERATIONS:* **Pregnancy/Lactation:** Unknown if drug crosses placenta; distributed in breast milk. **Pregnancy Category C. Children:** No age-related precautions noted in those >1 yr. **Elderly:** May exhibit increased sensivity to anticholinergic effects. Age-related decreased renal function may require dosage adjustment.

INTERACTIONS

DRUG: **Tricyclic antidepressants, antihistamines, phenothiazine, anticholinergics** may increase anticholinergic effects. **Hydrochlorothiazide, triamterene** may increase concentration, toxicity. *HERBAL:* None known. *FOOD:* None known. *LAB VALUES:* None significant.

AVAILABILITY (Rx)

CAPSULES: 100 mg. *SYRUP:* 50 mg/5 ml.

ADMINISTRATION/HANDLING
PO:
• May give without regard to food.
• Administer nighttime dose several hours before bedtime (prevents insomnia).

INDICATIONS/ROUTES/DOSAGE

Prophylaxis, symptomatic treatment respiratory illness due to influenza A virus:

Note: Give as single or in 2 divided doses.

PO: **Adults (10–64 yrs):** 200 mg daily. **Adults (>64 yrs):** 100 mg daily. **Children (9–12 yrs):** 100 mg 2 times/day. **Children (1–9 yrs):** 5 mg/kg/day (up to 150 mg/day).

Parkinson's disease, extrapyramidal symptoms:

PO: **Adults, elderly:** 100 mg 2 times/day. May increase up to 300 mg/day in divided doses.

Dosage in renal impairment:

Dose and/or frequency is modified based on creatinine clearance (Ccr).

Creatinine Clearance	Dosage
30–50 ml/min	200 mg first day; 100 mg/day thereafter
15–29 ml/min	200 mg first day; 100 mg on alternate days
<15 ml/min	200 mg every 7 days

SIDE EFFECTS

FREQUENT (5–10%): Nausea, dizziness, poor concentration, insomnia, nervousness. **OCCASIONAL (1–5%):** Orthostatic hypotension, anorexia, headache, livedo reticularis (reddish blue, netlike blotching of skin), blurred vision, urinary retention, dry mouth/nose. **RARE:** Vomiting, depression, irritation/swelling of eyes, rash.

ADVERSE REACTIONS/TOXIC EFFECTS

CHF, leukopenia, neutropenia occur rarely. Hyperexcitability, convulsions, ventricular arrhythmias may occur.

NURSING IMPLICATIONS

BASELINE ASSESSMENT:

When treating infections caused by influenza A virus, obtain specimens for viral diagnostic tests before giving first dose (therapy may begin before results are known).

INTERVENTION/EVALUATION:

Monitor I&O, renal function tests if ordered; check for peripheral edema. Evaluate food tolerance, vomiting. Assess skin for rash, blotching. Assess for dizziness. *Parkinsonism:* Assess for clinical re-

versal of symptoms (improvement of tremor of head/hands at rest, masklike facial expression, shuffling gait, muscular rigidity).

PATIENT/FAMILY TEACHING:

Continue therapy for full length of treatment. Doses should be evenly spaced. Do not take any medications without consulting physician. Avoid alcoholic beverages. Do not drive, use machinery, or engage in other activities that require mental acuity if experiencing dizziness, blurred vision. Get up slowly from a sitting or lying position. Inform physician of new symptoms, especially blotching, rash, dizziness, blurred vision, nausea/vomiting. Take nighttime dose several hours before bedtime to prevent insomnia.

amcinonide

(Cyclocort)

See Classification section under: Corticosteroid: topical (p. 80C)

amifostine

am-ih-**fos**-teen
(Ethyol)

►CLASSIFICATION

PHARMACOTHERAPEUTIC: Antineoplastic adjunct. **CLINICAL:** Protective agent

ACTION/THERAPEUTIC EFFECT

Converted by alkaline phosphatase in tissues, allowing its ability to protect normal tissue relative to tumor tissue, *reducing the toxic effect of chemotherapeutic agent cisplatin.*

USES/*UNLABELED*

Reduces cumulative renal toxicity associated with repeated administration of cisplatin in those with advanced ovarian cancer. Treatment of postop radiation-induced dry mouth in pts with head or neck cancer. *Protects lung fibroblasts from damaging effects of chemotherapeutic agent paclitaxel.*

PRECAUTIONS

CONTRAINDICATIONS: Sensitivity to aminothiol compounds or mannitol. ***CAUTION:*** Uncorrected dehydration or hypotensive pts, those receiving antihypertensive therapy that cannot be interrupted prior to 24 hrs before amifostine treatment, preexisting cardiovascular or cerebrovascular conditions, (i.e., ischemic heart disease, arrhythmias, CHF, history of stroke or TIA), pts receiving chemotherapy for malignancies that are potentially curable (e.g., certain malignancies of germ cell origin).

INTERACTIONS

DRUG: Pts receiving **antihypertensive medication** or drugs that may potentiate hypotension. ***HERBAL:*** None known. ***FOOD:*** None known. ***LAB VALUES:*** May reduce calcium serum levels, esp. those with nephrotic syndrome.

AVAILABILITY (Rx)

POWDER FOR INJECTION: 500 mg (10 ml single-use vial).

ADMINISTRATION/HANDLING

IV 🔲

Storage:
• Reconstituted solution stable for 5 hrs at room temperature, 24 hrs under refrigeration. • Do not use if discolored or contains particulate matter.

Reconstitution:
• Reconstitute with 9.7 ml 0.9% NaCl.
• Further dilute with 0.9% NaCl for a concentration of 5–40 mg/ml.

Rate of administration:
• Administer over 15 min (30 min prior to chemotherapy). • If hypotension requires interruption of therapy, place pt in Trendelenburg position; give an infusion of normal saline using a separate IV line. • An antiemetic, dexamethasone 20 mg IV and serotonin $5HT_3$ (receptor antagonist) should be given prior to and concurrently with amifostine.

IV INCOMPATIBILITY ⊘

Do not mix in solution other than 0.9% NaCl.

IV COMPATIBILITIES

Mannitol, potassium chloride.

INDICATIONS/ROUTES/DOSAGE

Cytoprotective (chemotherapy):

IV INFUSION: Adults: 910 mg/m^2 once daily as 15 min infusion, beginning 30 min prior to chemotherapy (15 min infusion is better tolerated than extended infusions). If full dose cannot be administered, dose for subsequent cycles should be 740 mg/m^2.

Treatment of dry mouth:

IV INFUSION: Adults: 200 mg/m^2 once daily as 3 min infusion, starting 15–30 min before radiation therapy.

SIDE EFFECTS

FREQUENT (62%): Transient reduction in B/P (with onset 14 min into infusion and lasts about 6 min). B/P generally returns to normal in 5–15 min; severe nausea, vomiting. ***OCCASIONAL*** (10–20%): Flushing/feeling of warmth or chills/feeling of coldness, dizziness, hiccups, sneezing, somnolence. **RARE** (<1%): Clinically relevant hypocalcemia, mild skin rash.

ADVERSE REACTIONS/TOXIC EFFECTS

A pronounced drop in B/P may require temporary cessation of amifostine.

NURSING IMPLICATIONS

BASELINE ASSESSMENT:

Be sure pt is adequately hydrated prior to infusion. Pt should maintain supine position during the infusion. Monitor B/P q5min during infusion. Interrupt infusion if systolic B/P decreases significantly from baseline (for baseline of <100, B/P drop by 20 mm Hg; for baseline of 100–119, a drop by 25 mm Hg; for baseline of 120–139, a drop by 30 mm Hg; for baseline of 140–179, a drop by 40 mm Hg; for baseline of >180, a drop by 50 mm Hg). If B/P returns to normal within 5 min and pt appears asymptomatic, begin infusion again so full dose can be administered.

INTERVENTION/EVALUATION:

Carefully monitor pt for fluid balance, adequate hydration. Monitor serum calcium levels in those at risk of hypocalcemia (nephrotic syndrome). Monitor B/P q5min during infusion.

amikacin sulfate

am-ih-**kay**-sin
(Amikin)
Do not confuse with Amicar.

►CLASSIFICATION

PHARMACOTHERAPEUTIC: Aminoglycoside. **CLINICAL:** Antibiotic (see p. 17C)

ACTION/*THERAPEUTIC EFFECT*

Irreversibly binds to protein on bacterial ribosome, *interfering in protein synthesis of susceptible microorganisms.*

PHARMACOKINETICS

Rapid, complete absorption after IM administration. Protein binding: 0–10%. Widely distributed (does not cross blood-brain barrier, low concentrations in CSF). Excreted unchanged in urine. Removed by hemodialysis. Half-life: 2–4 hrs (increased in reduced renal function, neonates; decreased in cystic fibrosis, burn or febrile pts).

USES

Treatment of skin/skin structure, bone, joint, respiratory tract, intra-abdominal and complicated urinary tract infections; postop, burns, septicemia, meningitis.

PRECAUTIONS

CONTRAINDICATIONS: Sulfite sensitivity (may result in anaphylaxis, esp. in asthmatics). **CAUTIONS:** Possible cross-sensitivity to other aminoglycosides. Elderly, neonates (potential for renal insufficiency or immaturity); neuromuscular disorders (potential for respiratory depression), prior hearing loss, vertigo, renal impairment.

▷*LIFESPAN CONSIDERATIONS:*
Pregnancy Lacatation: Readily crosses placenta; small amounts distributed in breast milk. May produce fetal nephrotoxicity. **Pregnancy Category C. Children:**

Neonates, premature infants may be more susceptible to toxicity due to immature renal function. **Elderly:** Higher risk of toxicity due to age-related renal impairment, increase risk of hearing loss.

INTERACTIONS

DRUG: Other **aminoglycosides, nephrotoxic- and ototoxic-producing medications** may increase toxicity. May increase effects of **neuromuscular blocking agents. HERBAL:** None known. **FOOD:** None known. **LAB VALUES:** May increase BUN, SGPT (ALT), SGOT (AST), bilirubin, creatinine, LDH concentrations; may decrease serum calcium, magnesium, potassium, sodium concentrations. Therapeutic blood serum level: Peak: 20–30 mcg/ml; toxic serum level: >30 mcg/ml; Trough: 1–9 mcg/ml; toxic serum level: >10 mcg/ml.

AVAILABILITY (Rx)

INJECTION: 50 mg/ml, 250 mg/ml.

ADMINISTRATION/HANDLING
IM:

• To minimize discomfort, give deep IM slowly. • Less painful if injected into gluteus maximus rather than lateral aspect of thigh.

IV 🎔
Storage:

• Store vials at room temperature. • Solutions appear clear but may become pale yellow (does not affect potency). • Intermittent IV infusion (piggyback) is stable for 24 hrs at room temperature. • Discard if precipitate forms or dark discoloration occurs.

Reconstitution:

• Dilute each 500 mg with 100 ml 0.9% NaCl or D$_5$W.

Rate of administration:

• Infuse over 30–60 min for adults, older children, and over 60–120 min for infants, young children.

IV INCOMPATIBILITIES ⊘

Allopurinal (Zyloprim), amphotericin (Fungizone), propofol (Diprivan).

IV COMPATIBILITIES

Cisatracurium (Nimbex), diltiazem (Cardizem), lorazepam (Ativan), midazolam (Versed), potassium chloride.

INDICATIONS/ROUTES/DOSAGE

Note: Space doses evenly around the clock. Dosage based on ideal body weight. Peak, trough serum level is determined periodically to maintain desired serum concentrations (minimizes risk of toxicity).

Uncomplicated urinary tract infections:

IM/IV: Adults, elderly: 250 mg q12h.

Moderate to severe infections:

IM/IV: Adults, elderly, children: 15 mg/kg/day in divided doses q8–12h. Do not exceed 15 mg/kg or 1.5 g/day. **Neonates: Loading dose:** 10 mg/kg, then 7.5 mg/kg q12h.

Dosage in renal impairment:

Dose and/or frequency is modified based on degree of renal impairment, serum concentration of drug. After loading dose of 5–7.5 mg/kg, maintenance dose/frequency based on serum creatinine or creatinine clearance.

SIDE EFFECTS

FREQUENT: Pain, induration at IM injection site; phlebitis, thrombophlebitis with IV administration. **OCCASIONAL:** Hypersensitivity reactions (rash, fever, urticaria, pruritus). **_RARE:_** Neuromuscular blockade (difficulty breathing, drowsiness, weakness).

ADVERSE REACTIONS/TOXIC EFFECTS

Frequently occurring nephrotoxicity (evidenced by increased BUN and serum creatinine, decreased creatinine clearance) may be reversible if drug stopped at first sign of symptoms; irreversible ototoxicity (tinnitus, dizziness, ringing/roaring in ears, reduced hearing) and neurotoxicity (headache, dizziness, lethargy, tremors, visual disturbances) occur occasionally. Risk is greater with higher dosages, prolonged therapy. Superinfections, particularly with fungi, may result from bacterial imbalance.

NURSING IMPLICATIONS

BASELINE ASSESSMENT:

Dehydration must be treated before aminoglycoside therapy. Establish pt's baseline hearing acuity before beginning therapy. Question for history of allergies, especially to aminoglycosides and sulfite. Obtain specimen for culture, sensitivity before giving the first dose (therapy may begin before results are known).

INTERVENTION/EVALUATION:

Monitor I&O (maintain hydration), urinalysis (casts, RBC, WBC, decrease in specific gravity). Monitor results of peak/trough blood tests. Be alert to ototoxic and neurotoxic symptoms (see Adverse Reactions/Toxic Effects). Check IM injection site for pain, induration. Evaluate IV site for phlebitis (heat, pain, red streaking over vein). Assess for skin rash. Assess

for superinfection, particularly genital/anal pruritus, changes of oral mucosa, diarrhea. When treating those with neuromuscular disorders, assess respiratory response carefully. Therapeutic blood serum level: Peak: 20–30 mcg/ml; toxic serum level: >30 mcg/ml; Trough: 1–9 mcg/ml; toxic serum level: >10 mcg/ml.

PATIENT/FAMILY TEACHING:

Continue antibiotic for full length of treatment. Space doses evenly. Discomfort may occur with IM injection. Notify physician in event of any hearing, visual, balance, urinary problems even after therapy is completed. Do not take other medication without consulting physician. Lab tests are essential part of therapy.

amiloride hydrochloride

ah-**mill**-or-ride
(Midamor)

FIXED-COMBINATION(S)

With hydrochlorothiazide, a thiazide diuretic **(Moduretic)**

▶**CLASSIFICATION**

PHARMACOTHERAPEUTIC: Guanidine derivative. **_CLINICAL:_** Potassium-sparing diuretic, antihypertensive, antihypokalemic (see p. 84C)

ACTION/_THERAPEUTIC EFFECT_

Directly interferes with sodium reabsorption in distal tubule, _increasing sodium and water excretion and decreasing potassium excretion._ Initial decrease in B/P occurs by decreasing plasma and extracellular fluid volume.

PHARMACOKINETICS

	Onset	Peak	Duration
PO	2 hrs	6–10 hrs	24 hrs

Incompletely absorbed from GI tract. Protein binding: minimal. Primarily excreted in urine; partially eliminated in feces. Half-life: 6–9 hrs.

USES/*UNLABELED*

Adjunctive therapy in treatment of diuretic-induced hypokalemia in those with CHF or hypertension. Used when maintenance of serum potassium levels is necessary (digitalized patients, cardiac arrhythmias). *Reduction of lithium-induced polyuria; slows pulmonary function reduction in cystic fibrosis; treatment of edema associated with CHF, hepatic cirrhosis, nephrotic syndrome; hypertension.*

PRECAUTIONS

CONTRAINDICATIONS: Serum potassium >5.5 mEq/L, pts on other potassium-sparing diuretics, anuria, acute or chronic renal insufficiency, diabetic nephropathy. ***CAUTIONS:*** Those with BUN >30 mg/dl or serum creatinine >1.5 mg/dl, elderly, debilitated, hepatic insufficiency, those with cardiopulmonary disease, diabetes mellitus.

▷***LIFESPAN CONSIDERATIONS:*** **Pregnancy/Lactation:** Unknown if drug crosses placenta or is distributed in breast milk. **Pregnancy Category B. Children:** No age-related precautions noted. **Elderly:** Increased risk of hyperkalemia, age-related decreased renal function may require caution.

INTERACTIONS

DRUG: May decrease effect of **anticoagulants, heparin. NSAIDs** may decrease antihypertensive effect. **ACE inhibitors (e.g., captopril), potassium-containing diuretics, potassium supplements** may increase potassium. May decrease **lithium** clearance, increase toxicity. ***HERBAL:*** None known. ***FOOD:*** None known. ***LAB VALUES:*** May increase BUN, calcium excretion, creatinine, glucose, magnesium, potassium, uric acid. May decrease sodium.

AVAILABILITY (Rx)

TABLETS: 5 mg.

ADMINISTRATION/HANDLING

PO:

• Give with food to avoid GI distress.

INDICATIONS/ROUTES/DOSAGE

PO: Adults, children >20 kg: Initially, 5 mg daily. May be increased to 10 mg daily, as single dose or in divided doses. If hypokalemia persists, dose may be increased to 15 mg, then to 20 mg, with electrolyte monitoring. **Children 6–20 kg:** 0.625 mg/kg/day. **Maximum:** 10 mg/day.

Usual elderly dosage:

PO: Initially, 5 mg/day or every other day.

SIDE EFFECTS

FREQUENT (3–8%): Headache, nausea, diarrhea, vomiting, decreased appetite. ***OCCASIONAL*** (<3%): Dizziness, constipation, abdominal pain, weakness, fatigue, cough, impotence. ***RARE*** (<1%): Tremors, vertigo, confusion, nervousness, insomnia, thirst, dry mouth, heartburn, shortness of breath, increased urination, hypotension, rash.

ADVERSE REACTIONS/TOXIC EFFECTS

Severe hyperkalemia may produce irritability, anxiety, heaviness of legs, paresthesia of hands/face/lips, hypotension, bradycardia, tented T waves, widening of QRS, ST depression.

NURSING IMPLICATIONS

BASELINE ASSESSMENT:

Assess baseline electrolytes, particularly for low potassium. Assess renal/hepatic functions. Assess edema (note location, extent), skin turgor, mucous membranes for hydration status. Assess muscle strength, mental status. Note skin temperature, moisture. Obtain baseline weight. Initiate strict I&O. Note pulse rate/regularity.

INTERVENTION/EVALUATION:

Monitor B/P, vital signs, electrolytes (particularly potassium), I&O, weight. Note extent of diuresis. Watch for changes from initial assessment; hyperkalemia may result in muscle strength changes, tremor, muscle cramps, change in mental status (orientation, alertness, confusion), cardiac arrhythmias. Monitor potassium level, particularly during initial therapy. Weigh daily. Assess lung sounds for rales, wheezing.

PATIENT/FAMILY TEACHING:

Expect increase in volume and frequency of urination. Therapeutic effect takes several days to begin and can last for several days when drug is discontinued. High-potassium diet/potassium supplements can be dangerous, especially if pt has renal/hepatic problems. Avoid foods high in potassium such as whole grains (cereals), legumes, meat, bananas, apricots, orange juice, potatoes (white, sweet), raisins.

Contact physician if confusion, irregular heartbeat, nervousness, numbness of hands/feet/lips, difficulty breathing, unusual tiredness, weakness in legs occur (hyperkalemia).

aminocaproic acid ✳

ah-meen-oh-kah-**pro**-ick
(Amicar)
Do not confuse with Amikin.

▶CLASSIFICATION

PHARMACOTHERAPEUTIC: Systemic hemostatic. **CLINICAL:** Antifibrinolytic, antihemorrhagic

ACTION/THERAPEUTIC EFFECT

Inhibits activation of plasminogen activator substances *preventing fibrin clots from forming.*

USES/UNLABELED

Treatment of excessive bleeding from hyperfibrinolysis or urinary fibrinolysis as noted in anemia, abruptio placentae, cirrhosis, carcinoma of prostate, lung, stomach, cervix. *Prevents reoccurrence of subarachnoid hemorrhage. Prevents hemorrhage in hemophiliacs following dental surgery.*

PRECAUTIONS

CONTRAINDICATIONS: Evidence of active intravascular clotting process, disseminated intravascular coagulation without concurrent heparin therapy, hematuria of upper urinary tract origin (unless benefits outweigh risk). *Parenteral:* Newborns. **EXTREME CAUTION:** Impaired cardiac, hepatic, or renal disease, those with hyperfibrinolysis.

INTERACTIONS

DRUG: None significant. **HERBAL:** None known. **FOOD:** None known. **LAB VALUES:** May elevate serum potassium level.

ADMINISTRATION/HANDLING

IV 🏺

Reconstitution:

• Dilute each 1 g in up to 50 ml 0.9% NaCl, D_5W, Ringer's or Sterile Water for Injection (do not use Sterile Water for Injection in those with subarachnoid hemorrhage).

Rate of administration:

• Give only by IV infusion. • Infuse ≤5 g over first hr in 250 ml of solution; give each succeeding 1 g over 1 hr in 50–100 ml solution.

Administration precautions:

• Monitor for hypotension during infusion. Rapid infusion may produce bradycardia, arrhythmias.

IV INCOMPATIBILITY ⊘

Sodium lactate. Do not mix with other medications.

INDICATIONS/ROUTES/DOSAGE

Note: Reduce dosage in presence of cardiac, renal, or hepatic impairment.

Acute bleeding:

PO/IV INFUSION: Adults, elderly: Initially, 4–5 g over 1 hr, then 1–1.25 g/hr. Continue for 8 hrs or until bleeding is controlled. **Maximum:** Up to 30 g/24 hrs. **Children:** 3 g/m^2 over first hr, then 1 g/m^2/hr. **Maximum:** 18 g/m^2/24 hrs.

SIDE EFFECTS

OCCASIONAL: Nausea, diarrhea, cramps, decreased urination, decreased B/P, dizziness, headache, muscle fatigue/weakness (myopathy), bloodshot eyes.

ADVERSE REACTIONS/TOXIC EFFECTS

Too rapid IV administration produces tinnitus, skin rash, arrhythmias, unusual tiredness, weakness. Rarely, grand mal seizure occurs, generally preceded by weakness, dizziness, headache.

NURSING IMPLICATIONS

INTERVENTION/EVALUATION:

Question any change in skeletal strength as noted by pt (consider possibility of cardiac damage as a result). Skeletal myopathy characterized by increase in creatine kinase, SGOT (AST) serum levels. Monitor these lab results frequently. Monitor heart rhythm. Assess for decrease in B/P, increase in pulse rate, abdominal or back pain, severe headache (may be evidence of hemorrhage). Assess peripheral pulses, skin for bruises, petechiae. Question for increase in amount of discharge during menses. Check for excessive bleeding from minor cuts, scratches. Assess gums for erythema, gingival bleeding. Assess urine output for hematuria.

PATIENT/FAMILY TEACHING:

Report any sign of red/dark urine, black/red stool, coffee-ground vomitus, red-speckled mucus from cough.

aminophylline (theophylline ethylenediamine) ✳

am-in-**ah**-phil-lin
(Aminophylline, Phyllocontin)

theophylline

(SloBid, Theo-Dur, Theolair, Uniphyl)
Immediate-release: **Aerolate, Theolair.** Extended-release: **Theo-24, Uniphyl**

▶CLASSIFICATION

PHARMACOTHERAPEUTIC: Xanthine derivative. *CLINICAL:* Bronchodilator (see p. 60C)

ACTION/*THERAPEUTIC EFFECT*

Directly relaxes smooth muscle of bronchial airway, pulmonary blood vessels, *relieving bronchospasm, increasing vital capacity. Produces cardiac, skeletal muscle stimulation.*

USES/*UNLABELED*

Symptomatic relief, prevention of bronchial asthma, reversible bronchospasm due to chronic bronchitis, emphysema, or COPD. *Treatment of apnea in neonates.*

PRECAUTIONS

CONTRAINDICATIONS: History of hypersensitivity to xanthine, caffeine. *CAUTIONS:* Impaired cardiac, renal, or hepatic function, hypertension, hyperthyroidism, diabetes mellitus, peptic ulcer, glaucoma, severe hypoxemia, underlying seizure disorder.

INTERACTIONS

DRUG: **Glucocorticoids** may produce hypernatremia. **Phenytoin, primidone, rifampin** may increase metabolism. **Beta-blockers** may decrease effects. **Cimetidine, ciprofloxacin, erythromycin, norfloxacin** may increase concentration, toxicity. Smoking may decrease concentration. *HERBAL:* None known. *FOOD:* None known. *LAB VALUES:* None significant.

AVAILABILITY (Rx)

CAPSULES (immediate-release): 100 mg, 200 mg. *CAPSULES (extended-release):* 50 mg, 60 mg, 75 mg, 100 mg, 125 mg, 200 mg, 250 mg, 300 mg. *TABLETS (immediate-release):* 100 mg, 125 mg, 200 mg, 250 mg, 300 mg. *TABLETS (extended-release):* 100 mg, 200 mg, 250 mg, 300 mg, 400 mg, 450 mg, 500 mg. *ELIXIR:* 80 mg/15 ml. *SOLUTION:* 80 mg/15 ml, 150 mg/15 ml. *SYRUP:* 80 mg/15 ml, 150 mg/15 ml. *INJECTION:* 25 mg/ml.

ADMINISTRATION/HANDLING
PO:

• Give with food to avoid GI distress. • Do not crush or break extended-release forms.

IV 🍴
Storage:

• Store at room temperature. • Discard if solution contains a precipitate.

Dilution:

• Give loading dose diluted in 100–200 ml of D_5W or 0.9% NaCl. Prepare maintenance dose in larger volume parenteral infusion.

Rate of administration:

• Do not exceed flow rate of 1 ml/min (25 mg/min) for either piggyback or infusion. • Administer loading dose over 20–30 min. • Use infusion pump or microdrip to regulate IV administration.

IV INCOMPATIBILITIES ⊘

Amiodarone (Cordarone), ciprofloxacin (Cipro), dobutamine (Dobutrex), ondansetron (Zofran).

IV COMPATIBILITIES

Aztreonam (Azactam), ceftazidime

(Fortaz), fluconazole (Diflucan), heparin, morphine, potassium chloride.

INDICATIONS/ROUTES/DOSAGE

Note: Dosage calculated on basis of lean body weight. Dosage based on peak serum theophylline concentrations, clinical condition, presence of toxicity.

Chronic bronchospasm:

PO: Adults, elderly, children: Initially, 16 mg/kg or 400 mg/day (whichever is less) in 2–4 divided doses (6–12 hr intervals). May increase by 25% every 2–3 days up to maximum of 24 mg/kg/day **(1–9 yrs);** 20 mg/kg/day **(9–12 yrs);** 18 mg/kg/day **(12–16 yrs);** 13 mg/kg/day **(>16 yrs).** Doses above maximum based on serum theophylline concentrations, clinical condition, presence of toxicity.

Acute bronchospasm in pts not currently on theophylline:

IV LOADING DOSE: Adults, children (>1 yr): Initially, 6 mg/kg (aminophylline), then begin maintenance aminophylline dosage based on patient group:

Pt Group	Maintenance Aminophylline Dosage
Neonates	Not recommended
Children (1–12 mos)	Not recommended
Children (6 mos–9 yrs)	1–1.2 mg/kg/hr
Children (9–16 yrs), young adult smokers	0.8–1 mg/kg/hr
Older pts, pts with cor pulmonale	0.3–0.6 mg/kg/hr
CHF, liver disease	0.1–0.5 mg/kg/hr

PO/LOADING DOSE: Adults, children >1 yr: Initially, 5 mg/kg (theophylline), then begin maintenance theophylline dosage based on patient group.

Pt Group	Maintenance Theophylline Dosage
Children (1–9 yrs)	4 mg/kg q6h
Children (9–16 yrs), young adult smokers	3 mg/kg q6h
Healthy, nonsmoking adults	3 mg/kg q8h
Older pts, pts with cor pulmonale	2 mg/kg q8h
Pts with CHF, liver disease	1–2 mg/kg q12h

Acute bronchospasm in pts currently on theophylline:

PO/IV: Adults, children >1 yr: Obtain serum theophylline level. If not possible and pt in respiratory distress and not experiencing toxicity, may give 2.5 mg/kg dose. **Maintenance:** Dosage based on peak serum theophylline concentrations, clinical condition, presence of toxicity.

SIDE EFFECTS

FREQUENT: Momentary change in sense of smell during IV administration; shakiness, restlessness, tachycardia, trembling. ***OCCASIONAL:*** Heartburn, vomiting, headache, mild diuresis, insomnia, nausea.

ADVERSE REACTIONS/TOXIC EFFECTS

Too rapid rate of IV administration may produce marked fall in B/P with accompanying faintness and lightheadedness, palpitations, tachycardia, hyperventilation, nausea, vomiting, angina-like pain, seizures, ventricular fibrillation, cardiac standstill.

NURSING IMPLICATIONS

BASELINE ASSESSMENT:
Offer emotional support (high incidence of anxiety due to diffi-

culty in breathing and sympath-omimetic response to drug). Peak serum concentration should be taken 1 hr after IV, 1–2 hrs following immediate-release dose, 3–8 hrs following extended-release. Take trough level just before next dose.

INTERVENTION/EVALUATION:

Monitor rate, depth, rhythm, type of respiration; quality and rate of pulse. Assess lung sounds for rhonchi, wheezing, rales. Monitor arterial blood gases. Observe lips, fingernails for blue or dusky color in light-skinned pts; gray in dark-skinned pts. Observe for clavicular retractions, hand tremor. Evaluate for clinical improvement (quieter, slower respirations, relaxed facial expression, cessation of clavicular retractions). Monitor theophylline blood serum levels (therapeutic serum level range: 10–20 mcg/ml).

PATIENT/FAMILY TEACHING:

Increase fluid intake (decreases lung secretion viscosity). Avoid excessive use of caffeine derivatives (chocolate, coffee, tea, cola, cocoa). Smoking, charcoal-broiled food, high-protein, low-carbohydrate diet may decrease theophylline level.

amiodarone hydrochloride

ah-me-**oh**-dah-roan
(Cordarone, Pacerone)

▶CLASSIFICATION

PHARMACOTHERAPEUTIC:
Cardiac agent. **_CLINICAL:_** Antiarrhythmic (see p. 13C)

ACTION/_THERAPEUTIC EFFECT_

Prolongs myocardial cell action potential duration and refractory period by direct action on all cardiac tissue, _decreasing AV conduction, sinus node function._

PHARMACOKINETICS

Slowly, variably absorbed from GI tract. Protein binding: 96%. Extensively metabolized in liver to active metabolite. Excreted via bile; not removed by hemodialysis. Half-life: 26–107 days; metabolite: 61 days.

USES/_UNLABELED_

Treatment of documented, life-threatening, recurrent ventricular fibrillation, and recurrent, hemodynamically unstable ventricular tachycardia in those who have not responded adequately to other antiarrhythmic agents. _Treatment/prophylaxis of supraventricular arrhythmias refractory to conventional treatment, symptomatic atrial flutter._

PRECAUTIONS

CONTRAINDICATIONS: Severe sinus-node dysfunction, second- and third-degree AV block, bradycardia-induced syncope (except in presence of pacemaker), severe hepatic disease. **_CAUTIONS:_** Thyroid disease.

▷**_LIFESPAN CONSIDERATIONS:_**
Pregnancy/Lactation: Crosses placenta; distributed in breast milk. May adversely affect fetal development. **Pregnancy Category D. Children:** Safety and efficacy not established. **Elderly:** May be more sensitive to effects on thyroid function. May experience increased incidence ataxia, other neurotoxic effects.

INTERACTIONS

DRUG: May increase cardiac effects with **other antiarrhythmics.** May increase effect of **beta-blockers, oral anticoagulants.** May increase concentration, toxicity of **digoxin, phenytoin. HERBAL:** None known. **FOOD:** None known. **LAB VALUES:** May increase SGOT (AST), SGPT (ALT), alkaline phosphatase, ANA titer. May cause changes in EKG, thyroid function tests. Therapeutic blood serum level: 0.5–2.5 mcg/ml; toxic serum level: not established.

AVAILABILITY (Rx)

TABLETS: 200 mg. **INJECTION:** 50 mg/ml.

ADMINISTRATION/HANDLING

PO:

• Give with meals to reduce GI distress. • Tablets may be crushed.

IV 🜹

Storage:

• Store at room temperature. • Use in PVC containers within 2 hrs of dilution; within 24 hrs with glass or polyolefin containers.

Reconstitution:

• Use glass or polyolefin containers for dilution. • Dilute loading dose (150 mg) in 100 ml D_5W (1.5 mg/ml). • Dilute maintenance dose (900 mg) in 500 ml D_5W (1.8 mg/ml). Concentrations >3 mg/ml causes peripheral vein phlebitis.

Rate of administration:

• Does not need protection from light during administration. • Administer through central venous catheter (CVC) if possible, using in-line filter. • Bolus over 10 min (15 mg/min) not to exceed 30 mg/min; then 1 mg/min over 6 hrs; then 0.5 mg/min over 18 hrs. • Infusions >1 hr, concentration not to exceed 2 mg/ml (unless CVC used).

IV INCOMPATIBILITIES ⊘

Aminophylline (Theophylline), cefazolin (Ancef), heparin, sodium bicarbonate.

IV COMPATIBILITIES

Amikacin (Amikin), dobutamine (Dobutrex), dopamine (Intropin), labetolol (Normodyne), lidocaine, midazolam (Versed), nitroglycerin, nor-epinephrine (Levophed), phenylephrine (Neo-Synephrine), potassium chloride.

INDICATIONS/ROUTES/DOSAGE

Life-threatening ventricular arrhythmias:

PO: Adults, elderly: Initially, 800–1,600 mg/day in 1–2 divided doses for 1–3 wks. After arrhythmias controlled or side effects occur, reduce to 600–800 mg/day for about 4 wks. **Maintenance:** 200–600 mg/day. **Children:** Initially, 10–15 mg/kg/day for 4–14 days, then 5 mg/kg/day for several wks. **Maintenance:** 2.5 mg/kg minimal dose for 5 of 7 days/wk.

IV INFUSION: Adults: Initially, 1,050 mg over 24 hrs: 150 mg over 10 min, follow by 360 mg over 6 hrs, follow by 540 mg over 18 hrs. May continue at 0.5 mg/min up to 2–3 wks regardless of age, renal or left ventricular function.

SIDE EFFECTS

Corneal microdeposits are noted in almost all pts treated for >6 mos (can lead to blurry vision). **FREQUENT (>3%): Parenteral:** Hypotension, nausea, fever, bradycardia. **PO:** Constipation, headache, decreased appetite, nausea, vomiting, numbness of fingers/toes, photosensitivity, muscular incoordination.

OCCASIONAL (<3%): ***PO:*** Bitter/metallic taste, decreased sexual ability/interest, dizziness, facial flushing, blue-gray coloring of skin of face, arms, neck, blurred vision, slow heartbeat, asymptomatic corneal deposits. ***RARE*** (<1%): ***PO:*** Skin rash, vision loss, blindness.

ADVERSE REACTIONS/TOXIC EFFECTS

Serious, potentially fatal pulmonary toxicity (alveolitis, pulmonary fibrosis, pneumonitis, adult respiratory distress syndrome) may begin with progressive dyspnea and cough with rales, decreased breath sounds, pleurisy. CHF, hepatotoxicity may be noted. May worsen existing arrhythmias or produce new arrhythmias.

NURSING IMPLICATIONS

BASELINE ASSESSMENT:

Obtain baseline pulmonary function tests, chest x-ray, liver enzyme tests, SGOT (AST), SGPT (ALT), alkaline phosphatase. Assess B/P, apical pulse immediately before drug is administered (if pulse is 60/min or below, or systolic B/P is below 90 mm Hg, withhold medication, contact physician).

INTERVENTION/EVALUATION:

Monitor for symptoms of pulmonary toxicity (progressively worsening dyspnea, cough). Dosage should be discontinued or reduced if toxicity occurs. Assess pulse for strength/weakness, irregular rate, bradycardia. Monitor EKG for cardiac changes, particularly widening of QRS, prolongation of PR and QT intervals. Notify physician of any significant interval changes. Assess for nausea, fatigue, paresthesia, tremor. Monitor for

signs of hypothyroidism (periorbital edema, lethargy, pudgy hands/feet, cool/pale skin, vertigo, night cramps) and hyperthyroidism (hot/dry skin, bulging eyes [exophthalmos], frequent urination, eyelid edema, weight loss, breathlessness). Monitor SGOT (AST), SGPT (ALT), alkaline phosphatase for evidence of liver toxicity. Assess skin, cornea for bluish discoloration in those who have been on drug therapy longer than 2 mos. Monitor liver function tests, thyroid test results. If elevated liver enzymes, dose reduction or discontinuation is evident. Monitor for therapeutic serum level (1.5–2.5 mcg/ml). Therapeutic blood serum level: 0.5–2.5 mcg/ml; toxic serum level: not established.

PATIENT/FAMILY TEACHING:

Protect against photosensitivity reaction on skin exposed to sunlight. Bluish skin discoloration gradually disappears when drug is discontinued. Report shortness of breath, cough. Outpatients should monitor pulse before taking medication. Do not abruptly discontinue medication. Compliance with therapy regimen is essential to control arrhythmias. Restrict salt, alcohol intake. Recommend ophthalmic exams q6mos. Report any vision changes.

amitriptyline hydrochloride

a-me-**trip**-tih-leen
(Apo-Amitriptyline✶, Elavil, Endep)
Do not confuse with Melliril.

(see p. 34C)

FIXED-COMBINATION(S)

With chlordiazepoxide, an antianxiety **(Limbitrol)**; with perphenazine, an antipsychotic **(Etrafon, Triavil)**

►CLASSIFICATION

PHARMACOTHERAPEUTIC: Tricyclic. ***CLINICAL:*** Antidepressant, antineuralgic, antibulimic (see p. 34C)

ACTION/*THERAPEUTIC EFFECT*

Blocks reuptake of neurotransmitters (norepinephrine, serotonin) at presynaptic membranes, increasing synaptic concentration at postsynaptic receptor sites, *resulting in antidepressant effect.* Has strong anticholinergic activity.

PHARMACOKINETICS

Rapid, well absorbed from GI tract. Protein binding: 90%. Metabolized in liver, undergoes first-pass metabolism. Primarily excreted in urine. Minimal removal by hemodialysis. Half-life: 10–26 hrs.

USES/*UNLABELED*

Treatment of various forms of depression, exhibited as persistent, prominent dysphoria (occurring nearly every day for at least 2 wks) manifested by 4 of 8 symptoms: appetite change, sleep pattern change, increased fatigue, impaired concentration, feelings of guilt or worthlessness, loss of interest in usual activities, psychomotor agitation or retardation, suicidal tendencies. *Relieves neuropathic pain (e.g., diabetic neuropathy, postherpetic neuralgia, treatment of bulimia nervosa).*

PRECAUTIONS

CONTRAINDICATIONS: Acute recovery period following MI, within 14 days of MAO inhibitor ingestion. ***CAUTIONS:*** Prostatic hypertrophy, history of urinary retention or obstruction, glaucoma, diabetes mellitus, , history of seizures, hyperthyroidism, cardiac/hepatic/renal disease, schizophrenia, increased intraocular pressure, hiatal hernia.
▷***LIFESPAN CONSIDERATIONS:*** **Pregnancy/Lactation:** Crosses placenta; minimally distributed in breast milk. **Pregnancy Category D. Children:** More sensitive to increased dosage, toxicity. **Elderly:** Increased risk of toxicity. Increased sensitivity to anticholinergic effects. Cautions in those with cardiovascular disease.

INTERACTIONS

DRUG: **CNS depressants** (including **alcohol, barbiturates, phenothiazines, sedative-hypnotics, anticonvulsants)** may increase sedation, respiratory depression, hypotensive effects. **Antithyroid agents** may increase risk of agranulocytosis. **Phenothiazines** may increase sedative, anticholinergic effects. **Cimetidine, valproic acid** may increase concentration, toxicity. May decrease effects of **clonidine, guanadrel.** May increase cardiac effects with **sympathomimetics.** May increase risk of hypertensive crisis, hyperpyretic, convulsions with **MAO inhibitors. *HERBAL:*** None known. ***FOOD:*** None known. ***LAB VALUES:*** May alter EKG readings (flattens T wave), glucose. Therapeutic blood serum level: Peak: 120–250 ng/ml; toxic serum level: >500 ng/ml.

AVAILABILITY (Rx)

TABLETS: 10 mg, 25 mg, 50 mg, 75 mg, 100 mg, 150 mg. ***INJECTION:*** 10 mg/ml.

ADMINISTRATION/HANDLING
PO:
* Give with food or milk if GI distress occurs.

IM:
* Give by IM only if oral administration is not feasible. * Crystals may form in injection. Redissolve by immersing ampule in hot water for 1 min. * Give deep IM slowly.

INDICATIONS/ROUTES/DOSAGE
Depression:

PO: Adults: Initially, 25 mg 2–4 times/day; adjust as needed. **Maximum:** *Out-patient:* 150 mg. *In-patient:* 300 mg. **Elderly:** Initially, 25 mg at bedtime up to 10 mg 3 times/day and 20 mg at bedtime. **Maximum:** 100 mg/day. **Children 6–12 yrs:** 1–5 mg/kg/day in 2 divided doses.

IM: Adults: 20–30 mg 4 times/day.

SIDE EFFECTS
FREQUENT: Dizziness, drowsiness, dry mouth, orthostatic hypotension, headache, increased appetite/weight, nausea, unusual tiredness, unpleasant taste. ***OCCASIONAL:*** Blurred vision, confusion, constipation, hallucinations, delayed micturation, eye pain, arrhythmias, fine muscle tremors, Parkinsonian syndrome, nervousness, diarrhea, increased sweating, heartburn, insomnia. ***RARE:*** Hypersensitivity, alopecia, tinnitus, breast enlargement.

ADVERSE REACTIONS/TOXIC EFFECTS
High dosage may produce confusion, seizures, severe drowsiness, fast/slow/irregular heartbeat, fever, hallucinations, agitation, shortness of breath, vomiting, unusual tiredness/weakness. Abrupt withdrawal from prolonged therapy may produce headache, malaise, nausea, vomiting, vivid dreams. Rarely, blood dyscrasias, cholestatic jaundice noted.

NURSING IMPLICATIONS

BASELINE ASSESSMENT:

Observe/record behavior. Assess psychological status, thought content, sleep patterns, appearance, interest in environment. For those on long-term therapy, liver/renal function tests, blood counts should be performed periodically.

INTERVENTION/EVALUATION:

Supervise suicidal risk pt closely during early therapy (as depression lessens, energy level improves, increasing suicide potential). Assess appearance, behavior, speech pattern, level of interest, mood. Monitor B/P, pulse for hypotension, arrhythmias. Therapeutic blood serum level: Peak: 120–250 ng/ml; toxic serum level: >500 ng/ml.

PATIENT/FAMILY TEACHING:

Change positions slowly to avoid hypotensive effect. Tolerance to postural hypotension, sedative and anticholinergic effects usually develops during early therapy. Maximum therapeutic effect may be noted in 2–4 wks. Sensitivity to sun may occur. Report visual disturbances. Do not abruptly discontinue medication. Avoid tasks that require alertness, motor skills until response to drug is established.

amlexanox

am-**lecks**-ah-knocks
(Apthasol)

▶CLASSIFICATION

PHARMACOTHERAPEUTIC:
Mouth agent. **CLINICAL:** Antiulcer

ACTION/*THERAPEUTIC EFFECT*

Has antiallergic and anti-inflammatory properties. Appears to inhibit
formation and/or release of inflammatory mediators (e.g., histamine)
from mast cells, neutrophils, mono-
nuclear cells, *alleviating signs/
symptoms of ahpthous ulcers.*

USES

Treatment of signs/symptoms aphthous ulcer in those with normal
immune system.

PRECAUTIONS

CONTRAINDICATIONS: None
known. **CAUTIONS:** None known.

INTERACTIONS

DRUG: None known. **HERBAL:**
None known. **FOOD:** None known.
LAB VALUES: None known.

INDICATIONS/ROUTES/DOSAGE

Aphthous ulcers:

TOPICAL: Adults, elderly: Administer ¼ inch directly to ulcers
4 times/day (after meals and at
bedtime) following oral hygiene.

SIDE EFFECTS

RARE (1–2%): Stinging, burning at
administration site, rash.

ADVERSE REACTIONS/TOXIC
EFFECTS

Ingestion of a full tube would result in nausea, vomiting, diarrhea.

NURSING IMPLICATIONS

PATIENT/FAMILY TEACHING:
If rash occurs, discontinue use.

amlodipine

am-**low**-dih-peen
(Norvasc)

FIXED-COMBINATION(S)

With benazepril, an angiotensin-
converting enzyme inhibitor
(Lotrel)

▶CLASSIFICATION

PHARMACOTHERAPEUTIC:
Calcium channel blocker. **CLIN-
ICAL:** Antihypertensive, antiang-
inal (see p. 65C).

ACTION/*THERAPEUTIC EFFECT*

Inhibits calcium movement across
cell membranes of cardiac and
vascular smooth muscle, *dilates
coronary arteries, peripheral ar-
teries/arterioles. Decreases total
peripheral vascular resistance by
vasodilation.*

PHARMACOKINETICS

	Onset	Peak	Duration
PO	—	—	24 hrs

Slowly absorbed from GI tract. Undergoes first-pass metabolism in
liver. Excreted primarily in urine.
Not removed by hemodialysis.
Half-life: 30–50 hrs (half-life increased in elderly, those with hepatic cirrhosis).

USES

Management of hypertension,
chronic stable angina, vasospastic
(Prinzmetal's or variant) angina.
May be used alone or with other
antihypertensives or antianginals.

PRECAUTIONS

CONTRAINDICATIONS: Severe
hypotension. **CAUTIONS:** Im-

paired hepatic function, aortic stenosis, CHF.

▷ *LIFESPAN CONSIDERATIONS:*

Pregnancy/Lactation: Unknown if drug crosses placenta or is distributed in breast milk. **Pregnancy Category C. Children:** Safety and efficacy not established. **Elderly:** Half-life may be increased, more sensitive to hypotensive effects.

INTERACTIONS

DRUG: None significant. *HERBAL:* None known. *FOOD:* Grapefruit/grapefruit juice may increase concentration, hypotensive effects. *LAB VALUES:* None significant.

AVAILABILITY (Rx)

TABLETS: 2.5 mg, 5 mg, 10 mg.

ADMINISTRATION/HANDLING

PO:

• May give without regard to food.
• Grapefruit juice may increase concentration.

INDICATIONS/ROUTES/DOSAGE

Note: Dosage should be titrated >7–14 days.

Hypertension:

PO: **Adults:** Initially, 5 mg/day as single dose. **Maximum:** 10 mg/day.

PO: **Small frame, fragile, elderly:** Initially, 2.5 mg/day as single dose.

Angina (chronic stable or vasospastic):

PO: **Adults:** 5–10 mg. **Elderly, hepatic insufficiency:** 5 mg.

SIDE EFFECTS

FREQUENT (>5%): Peripheral edema, headache, flushing. *OCCASIONAL* (<5%): Dizziness, palpitations, nausea, unusual tiredness/weakness (asthenia). *RARE* (<1%): Chest pain, slow heartbeat, orthostatic hypotension.

ADVERSE REACTIONS/TOXIC EFFECTS

Overdosage may produce excessive peripheral vasodilation, marked hypotension w/reflex tachycardia.

NURSING IMPLICATIONS

BASELINE ASSESSMENT:

Assess baseline renal/liver function tests, B/P, and apical pulse.

INTERVENTION/EVALUATION:

Assess B/P (if systolic B/P is below 90 mm Hg, withhold medication, contact physician). Assess for peripheral edema behind medial malleolus (sacral area in bedridden pts). Assess skin for flushing. Question for headache, asthenia.

PATIENT/FAMILY TEACHING:

Do not abruptly discontinue medication. Compliance with therapy regimen is essential to control hypertension. Avoid tasks that require alertness, motor skills until response to drug is established. Avoid concomitant ingestion of grapefruit juice.

amoxicillin

ah-**mocks**-ih-sill-in
(Amoxil, Apo-Amoxi✚, Novamoxin✚, Polymox, Trimox, Wymox)
Do not confuse with Tylox.

▶CLASSIFICATION

PHARMACOTHERAPEUTIC: Penicillin. *CLINICAL:* Antibiotic (see p. 26C)

ACTION/*THERAPEUTIC EFFECT*

Bactericidal in susceptible microorganisms by *inhibition of cell wall synthesis.*

PHARMACOKINETICS

Well absorbed from GI tract. Protein binding: 20%. Partially metabolized in liver. Primarily excreted in urine. Removed by hemodialysis. Half-life: 1–1.3 hrs (half-life increased in reduced renal function).

USES/*UNLABELED*

Treatment of skin/skin structure, respiratory, GI, and genitourinary infections, otitis media, gonorrhea. Treatment of *H. pylori* associated with peptic ulcer; *Lyme disease; typhoid fever.*

PRECAUTIONS

CONTRAINDICATIONS: Infectious mononucleosis, hypersensitivity to any penicillin. ***CAUTIONS:*** History of allergies (esp. cephalosporins), antibiotic-associated colitis.

▷***LIFESPAN CONSIDERATIONS:***
Pregnancy/Lactation: Crosses placenta, appears in cord blood, amniotic fluid. Distributed in breast milk in low concentrations. May lead to allergic sensitization, diarrhea, candidiasis, skin rash in infant. **Pregnancy Category B. Children:** Immature renal function in neonate/young infant may delay renal excretion. **Elderly:** Age-related renal impairment may require dosage adjustment.

INTERACTIONS

DRUG: **Allopurinol** may increase incidence of rash. **Probenecid** may increase concentration, toxicity risk. May decrease effects of **oral contraceptives.** ***HERBAL:*** None known. ***FOOD:*** None known. ***LAB VALUES:*** May increase SGOT (AST), SGPT (ALT), LDH, bilirubin, creatinine, BUN. May cause positive Coombs' test.

AVAILABILITY (Rx)

TABLETS (chewable): 125 mg, 200 mg, 250 mg, 400 mg. ***TABLETS:*** 500 mg, 875 mg. ***CAPSULES:*** 250 mg, 500 mg. ***POWDER FOR PO SUSPENSION:*** 50 mg/ml, 125 mg/5 ml, 200 mg/ml, 250 mg/5 ml, 400 mg/5 ml.

ADMINISTRATION/HANDLING

PO:

• Store capsules, tablets at room temperature. • After reconstitution, oral solution is stable for 14 days at either room temperature or refrigerated. • Give without regard to meals. • Instruct pt to chew or crush chewable tablets thoroughly before swallowing.

INDICATIONS/ROUTES/DOSAGE

Ear, nose, throat, GU, skin/skin structure infections:

PO: **Adults, children >20 kg:** 250–500 mg q8h (or 500–875 mg tablets 2 times/day). **Children <20 kg:** 20–40 mg/kg/day in divided doses q8–12h.

Lower respiratory tract infections:

PO: **Adults, children >20 kg:** 500 mg q8h (or 875 mg tablets 2 times/day). **Children <20 kg:** 40 mg/kg/day in divided doses q8–12h.

Acute, uncomplicated gonorrhea, epididymo-orchitis:

PO: **Adults:** 3 g one time with 1 g probenecid. Follow with tetracycline or erythromycin therapy.

Acute otitis media:

PO: **Children:** 80–90 mg/kg/day.

H. pylori:

PO: **Adults (in combination):** 1 g 2 times/day for 10 days. **Neonates,**

children ≤3 mos: 20–30 mg/kg/day in divided doses q12h.

Renal function impairment:

Creatinine clearance 10–30: Administer q12h. **Creatinine clearance <10:** Administer q24h.

SIDE EFFECTS

FREQUENT: GI disturbances (mild diarrhea, nausea or vomiting), headache, oral/vaginal candidiasis. *OCCASIONAL:* Generalized rash, urticaria.

ADVERSE REACTIONS/TOXIC EFFECTS

Superinfections, potentially fatal antibiotic-associated colitis (abdominal cramps, watery severe diarrhea, fever) may result from altered bacterial balance. Severe hypersensitivity reactions including anaphylaxis, acute interstitial nephritis occur rarely.

NURSING IMPLICATIONS

BASELINE ASSESSMENT:

Question for history of allergies, esp. penicillins, cephalosporins.

INTERVENTION/EVALUATION:

Hold medication and promptly report rash or diarrhea (with fever, abdominal pain, mucus and blood in stool may indicate antibiotic-associated colitis). Be alert for superinfection: increased fever, sore throat onset, vomiting, diarrhea, black/hairy tongue, ulceration or changes of oral mucosa, anal/genital pruritus.

PATIENT/FAMILY TEACHING:

Continue antibiotic for full length of treatment. Space doses evenly. Take with meals if GI upset occurs. Thoroughly chew the chewable tablets before swallowing. Notify physician in event of rash, diarrhea, or other new symptom.

amoxicillin/clavulanate potassium   🔖

a-**mocks**-ih-sill-in/klah-view-**lan**-ate (<u>Augmentin</u>, Augmentin ES 600, Clavulin ✤)

▶CLASSIFICATION

PHARMACOTHERAPEUTIC: Penicillin. *CLINICAL:* Antibiotic (see p. 26C)

ACTION/*THERAPEUTIC EFFECT*

Amoxocillin is bactericidal in susceptible microorganisms *by inhibition of cell wall synthesis.* Clavulanate inhibits bacterial beta-lactamase, *protecting amoxicillin from enzymatic degradation.*

PHARMACOKINETICS

Well absorbed from GI tract. Protein binding: 20%. Partially metabolized in liver. Primarily excreted in urine. Removed by hemodialysis. Half-life: 1–1.3 hrs (half-life increased in reduced renal function).

USES/*UNLABELED*

Treatment of skin/skin structure, lower respiratory tract and urinary infections, otitis media, sinusitis. *Treatment of bronchitis, chancroid.*

PRECAUTIONS

CONTRAINDICATIONS: Infectious mononucleosis, hypersensitivity to any penicillin. *CAUTIONS:* History of allergies, esp. cephalosporins, antibiotic-associated colitis.

▷ *LIFESPAN CONSIDERATIONS:*
Pregnancy/Lactation: Crosses placenta, appears in cord blood, amniotic fluid. Distributed in breast milk in low concentrations. May lead to allergic sensitization, diarrhea, candidiasis, skin rash in infant. **Pregnancy Category B. Children:** Immature renal function in neonate/young infant may delay renal excretion. **Elderly:** Age-related renal impairment may require dosage adjustment.

INTERACTIONS

DRUG:* Allopurinol** may increase incidence of rash. **Probenecid** may increase concentration, toxicity risk. May decrease effects of **oral contraceptives. *HERBAL: None known. ***FOOD:*** None known. ***LAB VALUES:*** May increase SGOT (AST), SGPT (ALT). May cause positive Coombs' test.

AVAILABILITY (Rx)

TABLETS (chewable): 125 mg, 200 mg, 250 mg, 400 mg. ***TABLETS:*** 250 mg, 500 mg, 875 mg. ***POWDER FOR PO SUSPENSION:*** 125 mg/5 ml, 200 mg/5 ml, 250 mg/5 ml, 400 mg/5 ml.

ADMINISTRATION/HANDLING

PO:

• Store tablets at room temperature. • After reconstitution, oral solution is stable for 14 days at either room temperature or refrigeration. • Give without regard to meals. • Instruct pt to chew or crush chewable tablets thoroughly before swallowing.

INDICATIONS/ROUTES/DOSAGE

Note: Dosage expressed in terms of amoxicillin. Alternative dosing in adults: 500–875 mg 2 times/day;

in children: 200–400 mg 2 times/day.

Mild to moderate infections:

***PO:* Adults, elderly, children >40 kg:** 250 mg q8h. **Children <40 kg:** 20 mg/kg/day in divided doses q8h.

Respiratory tract infections, severe infections:

***PO:* Adults, elderly, children >40 kg:** 500 mg q8h. **Children <40 kg:** 40 mg/kg/day in divided doses q8h.

Otitis media, sinusitis, lower respiratory tract infections:

***PO:* Children <40 kg:** 40 mg/kg/day in divided doses q8h.

Usual neonate dosage:

***PO:* Neonates, children ≤ 3 mos:** 30 mg/kg/day in divided doses q12h..

Dosage in renal impairment:

Creatinine clearance 10–30: 250–500 mg q12h. **Creatinine clearance <10:** 250–500 mg q24h.

SIDE EFFECTS

FREQUENT: GI disturbances (mild diarrhea, nausea or vomiting), headache, oral/vaginal candidiasis. ***OCCASIONAL:*** Generalized rash, urticaria.

ADVERSE REACTIONS/TOXIC EFFECTS

Superinfections, potentially fatal antibiotic-associated colitis (abdominal cramps, watery severe diarrhea, fever) may result from altered bacterial balance. Severe hypersensitivity reactions including anaphylaxis, acute interstitial nephritis occur rarely.

NURSING IMPLICATIONS

BASELINE ASSESSMENT:

Question for history of allergies, esp. penicillins, cephalosporins.

INTERVENTION/EVALUATION:

Hold medication and promptly report rash or diarrhea (with fever, abdominal pain, mucus and blood in stool may indicate antibiotic-associated colitis). Be alert for superinfection: increased fever, sore throat onset, vomiting, diarrhea, black/hairy tongue, ulceration or changes of oral mucosa, anal/genital pruritus.

PATIENT/FAMILY TEACHING:

Continue antibiotic for full length of treatment. Space doses evenly. Take with meals if GI upset occurs. Thoroughly chew the chewable tablets before swallowing. Notify physician in event of rash, diarrhea, or other new symptom.

amphotericin B

am-foe-**tear**-ih-sin
(Abelcet, AmBisome, Amphotec, Fungizone)

▶CLASSIFICATION

CLINICAL: Antifungal, antiprotozoal

ACTION/*THERAPEUTIC EFFECT*

Generally fungistatic but may be fungicidal with high dosage or very susceptible microorganisms. Binds to sterols in fungal cell membrane, *increasing membrane permeability, allowing loss of potassium, other cellular components.*

PHARMACOKINETICS

Protein binding: 90%. Widely distributed. Metabolic fate unknown. Cleared by nonrenal pathways. Minimal removal by hemodialysis. Half-life: 24 hrs (half-life increased in neonates, children). **Amphotec:** Half-life: 26–28 hrs. Not dialyzable. **Abelcet:** Half-life: 7.2 days. Not dialyzable. **AmBisome:** Half-life: 100–153 hrs.

USES

Fungizone: Treatment of Cryptococcosis, blastomycosis, systemic candidiasis, disseminated forms of moniliasis, coccidioidomycosis, and histoplasmosis, zygomycosis, sporotrichosis, aspergillosis. **Abelcet:** Treatment of invasive fungal infections refractory or intolerant to Fungizone. **Amphotec:** Treatment of invasive aspergillosis in pts with renal impairment or toxicity or prior treatment failure with Fungizone. **AmBisome:** Empiric treatment for fungal infection in febrile neutropenic pts. Aspergillus, Candida, or Cryptococcus infections refractory to Fungizone or pts with renal impairment or toxicity with Fungizone. Treatment of visceral leishmaniasis. **Topical:** Treatment of cutaneous/mucocutaneous infections caused by *Candida albicans* (paronychia, oral thrush, perleche, diaper rash, intertriginous candidiasis).

PRECAUTIONS

CONTRAINDICATIONS: Hypersensitivity to amphotericin B, sulfite. **CAUTIONS:** Renal impairment, in combination with antineoplastic therapy. Give only for progressive, potentially fatal fungal infection.
▷**LIFESPAN CONSIDERATIONS:**
Pregnancy/Lactation: Crosses placenta; unknown if distributed in breast milk. **Pregnancy Category B. Children:** Safety and efficacy not established but use the least amount for therapeutic regimen. **Elderly:** No age-related precautions noted.

INTERACTIONS

DRUG:* Steroids** may cause severe hypokalemia. **Bone marrow depressants** may increase anemia. May increase **digoxin** toxicity (due to hypokalemia). **Nephrotoxic medications** may increase nephrotoxicity. ***HERBAL: None known. ***FOOD:*** None known. ***LAB VALUES:*** May increase SGOT, SGPT, alkaline phosphatase, BUN, serum creatinine. May decrease calcium, magnesium, potassium.

AVAILABILITY (Rx)

INJECTION: 50 mg, 100 mg (Amphotec), 50 mg (Ambisone). ***SUSPENSION FOR INJECTION:*** 5 mg/ml (lipid complex: Abelcet). ***CREAM, LOTION, OINTMENT.***

ADMINISTRATION/HANDLING

IV 🏛

Storage:

• ***AmBisome:*** Refrigerate unreconstituted solution. Reconstituted solution of 4 mg/ml is stable for 24 hrs. Concentration of 1–2 mg/ml is stable for 6 hrs. • ***Fungizone:*** Refrigerate unreconstituted solution. Reconstituted solution is stable for 24 hrs at room temperature or 7 days if refrigerated. Diluted solution ≤0.1 mg/ml to be used promptly. Do not use if cloudy or contains a precipitate. • ***Amphotec:*** Store unreconstituted solution at room temperature. Reconstituted solution stable for 24 hrs. • ***Abelcet:*** Refrigerate unreconstituted solution. Reconstituted solution is stable for 48 hrs if refrigerated; 6 hrs at room temperature.

Reconstitution:

ABELCET:

• Shake 20 ml (100 mg) vial gently until contents are dissolved. Withdraw required dose using 5-micron filter needle (supplied by manufac-turer). • Inject dose into D_5W; 4 ml D_5W required for each 1 ml (5 mg) to final concentration of 1 mg/ml. Reduce dose by half for pediatric, fluid-restricted pts (2 mg/ml).

AMBISOME:

• Reconstitute each 50 mg vial with 12 ml Sterile Water for Injection to provide concentration of 4 mg/ml. • Shake vial vigorously for 30 secs. Withdraw required dose and empty syringe contents through a 5-micron filter into an infusion of D_5W to provide final concentration of 1–2 mg/ml.

AMPHOTEC:

• Add 10 ml Sterile Water for Injection to each 50 mg vial to provide concentration of 5 mg/ml. Shake gently. • Further dilute *only* with D_5W using specific amount recommended by manufacturer to provide concentration of 0.16 to 0.83 mg/ml.

FUNGIZONE:

• Rapidly inject 10 ml Sterile Water for Injection to each 50 mg vial to provide concentration of 5 mg/ml. Immediately shake vial until solution is clear. • Further dilute each 1 mg in at least 10 ml D_5W to provide a concentration of 0.1 mg/ml.

Rate of administration:

• Give by slow IV infusion. Infuse conventional amphoterecin or Fungisone over 2–6 hrs; Abelcet over 2 hrs (shake contents if infusion >2 hrs); Amphotec over 2–4 hrs; AmBisome over 1–2 hrs.

ADMINISTRATION PRECAUTIONS

• Monitor B/P, temperature, pulse, respirations; assess for adverse reactions q15min twice, then q30min for 4 hrs of initial infusion. • Potential for thrombophlebitis may be less with use of pediatric scalp vein needles or (with physician order) adding dilute heparin solution. • Observe strict aseptic technique, since no bacteriostatic agent or preservative is present in diluent.

IV INCOMPATIBILITIES ⊘

FUNGIZONE:

Allopurinol (Aloprim), amifostine (Ethyol), aztreonam (Azactam), cefepime (Maxipime), docetaxel (Taxotere), doxorubicin (Adriamycin), enalapril (Vasotec), etoposide (VP-16), filgrastim (Neupogen), fluconazole (Diflucan), fludarabine (Fludara), foscarnet (Foscavir), gemcitabine (Gemzar), meropenem (Merrem IV), ondansetron (Zofran), paclitaxel (Taxol), piperacillin/tazobactam (Zosyn), propofol (Diprivan), vinorelbine (Navelbine).

ABELCET/AMPHOTEC/AMBISOME:

Do not mix with any other drug, diluent, or solution.

IV COMPATIBILITIES

None known; do not mix with other medications or electrolytes.

INDICATIONS/ROUTES/DOSAGE

Usual parenteral dosage:

IV INFUSION: **Adults, elderly:** Dosage based on pt tolerance, severity of infection. Initially, 1 mg test dose is given over 20–30 min. If test dose is tolerated, 5 mg dose may be given the same day. Subsequently, increases of 5 mg/dose are made q12–24h until desired daily dose is reached. Alternatively, if test dose is tolerated, a dose of 0.25 mg/kg is given same day; increased to 0.5 mg/kg the second day. Dose increased until desired daily dose reached. **Total**

daily dose: 1 mg/kg/day up to 1.5 mg/kg every other day. Do not exceed maximum total daily dose of 1.5 mg/kg.

Usual AmbiSome dosage:

IV INFUSION: **Adults, children:** 3–5 mg/kg over 1 hr.

Usual Amphotec dosage:

IV INFUSION: **Adults, children:** 3–4 mg/kg over 2–4 hrs.

Usual Abelcet dosage:

IV INFUSION: **Adults, children:** 5 mg/kg at rate of 2.5 mg/kg/hr.

Cutaneous infections:

TOPICAL: **Adults, elderly, children:** Apply liberally and rub in 2–4 times/day.

SIDE EFFECTS

FREQUENT (>10%): *Fungizone:* Fever, chills, headache, anemia, hypokalemia, hypomagnesemia, anorexia, malaise, generalized pain, nephrotoxicity. *Abelcet:* Chills, fever, increased serum creatinine, multiple organ failure. *Amphotec:* Chills, fever, hypotension, tachycardia, increased creatinine, hypokalemia, bilirubinemia. *AmBisome:* Hypokalemia, hypomagnesemia, hyperglycemia, hypocalcemia, edema, abdominal pain, back pain, chills, chest pain, hypotension, diarrhea, nausea, vomiting, headache, fever, rigors, insomnia, dyspnea, epistaxis, increased liver/renal function tests. *Topical:* Local irritation, dry skin. *RARE: Topical:* Skin rash.

ADVERSE REACTIONS/TOXIC EFFECTS

Each alternative formulation is less nephrotoxic than conventional amphotericin (Fungizone). Cardiovascular toxicity (hypotension, ventricular fibrillation), anaphylactic reaction occur rarely. Vision and hearing alterations, seizures, hepatic failure, coagulation defects, multiple organ failure, sepsis may be noted.

NURSING IMPLICATIONS

BASELINE ASSESSMENT:

Question for history of allergies, esp. to amphotericin B, sulfite. Avoid, if possible, other nephrotoxic medications. Check for/obtain orders to reduce adverse reactions during IV therapy (antipyretics, antihistamines, antiemetics, or small doses of corticosteroids given before or during amphotericin administration may control reactions).

INTERVENTION/EVALUATION:

Monitor B/P, temperature, pulse, respirations; assess for adverse reactions q15min twice, then q30min for 4 hrs of initial infusion (fever, shaking, chills, anorexia, nausea, vomiting, abdominal pain). If symptoms occur, slow infusion and administer medication for symptomatic relief. For severe reaction or without symptomatic relief orders, stop infusion and notify physician. Evaluate IV site for phlebitis (heat, pain, red streaking over vein). Monitor I&O, renal function tests for nephrotoxicity. Check potassium and magnesium levels, hematologic and hepatic function test results. *Topical:* Assess for itching, irritation, burning.

PATIENT/FAMILY TEACHING:

Prolonged therapy (weeks or months) is usually necessary. Fever reaction may decrease with continued therapy. Muscle weakness may be noted during therapy (due to hypokalemia). *Topi-*

cal: Application may cause staining of skin or nails; soap and water or dry cleaning will remove fabric stains. Do not use other preparations or occlusive coverings without consulting physician. Keep areas clean, dry; wear light clothing. Separate personal items with direct contact to area.

ampicillin sodium

amp-ih-**sill**-in
(Apo-Ampi✿, Novo-Ampicillin✿, Nu-Ampi✿, Omnipen, Polycillin, Principen)

▶**CLASSIFICATION**

PHARMACOTHERAPEUTIC:
Penicillin. ***CLINICAL:*** Antibiotic (see p. 27C)

ACTION/*THERAPEUTIC EFFECT*

Inhibits cell wall synthesis in susceptible microorganisms *producing bactericidal effect.*

PHARMACOKINETICS

Moderately absorbed from GI tract. Protein binding: 28%. Widely distributed. Partially metabolized in liver. Primarily excreted in urine. Removed by hemodialysis. Half-life: 1–1.5 hrs (half-life increased in impaired renal function).

USES

Treatment of respiratory, GI and GU tract, skin/skin structure, bone and joint infections, otitis media, gonorrhea, endocarditis, meningitis, septicemia, mild to moderate typhoid fever, perioperative prophylaxis.

PRECAUTIONS

CONTRAINDICATIONS: Infectious mononucleosis, hypersensitivity to any penicillin. ***CAUTIONS:*** History of allergies, particularly cephalosporins, antibiotic-associated colitis.

▷***LIFESPAN CONSIDERATIONS:***
Pregnancy/Lactation: Readily crosses placenta; appears in cord blood, amniotic fluid. Distributed in breast milk in low concentrations. May lead to allergic sensitization, diarrhea, candidiasis, skin rash in infant. **Pregnancy Category B. Children:** Immature renal function in neonates/young infants may delay renal excretion. **Elderly:** Age-related renal impairment may require dose adjustment.

INTERACTIONS

DRUG: **Allopurinol** may increase incidence of rash. **Probenecid** may increase concentration, toxicity risk. May decrease effects of **oral contraceptives. HERBAL:** None known. ***FOOD:*** None known. ***LAB VALUES:*** May increase SGOT (AST), SGPT (ALT). May cause positive Coombs' test.

AVAILABILITY (Rx)

CAPSULES: 250 mg, 500 mg. ***POWDER FOR ORAL SUSPENSION:*** 125 mg/5 ml, 250 mg/5 ml, 500 mg/5 ml. ***POWDER FOR INJECTION:*** 125 mg, 250 mg, 500 mg, 1 g, 2 g.

ADMINISTRATION/HANDLING

PO:

• Store capsules at room temperature. • Oral suspension, after reconstituted, is stable for 7 days at room temperature, 14 days if refrigerated. • Give orally 1 hr before or 2 hrs after meals for maximum absorption.

IM:

• Reconstitute each vial with Sterile Water for Injection or Bacteriostatic Water for Injection (consult individual vial for specific volume of diluent). • Stable for 1 hr. • Give deeply in large muscle mass.

IV 🖾

Storage:

• The IV solution, diluted with 0.9% NaCl, is stable for 2–8 hrs at room temperature or 3 days if refrigerated. • If diluted with D_5W, is stable for 2 hrs at room temperature or 3 hrs if refrigerated. • Discard if precipitate forms.

Reconstitution:

• For IV injection, dilute each vial with 5 ml Sterile Water for Injection (10 ml for 1 and 2 g vials). • For intermittent IV infusion (piggyback), further dilute with 50–100 ml 0.9% NaCl or D_5W.

Rate of administration:

• For IV injection, give over 3–5 min (10–15 min for 1–2 g dose). • For intermittent IV infusion (piggyback), infuse over 20–30 min. • Due to potential for hypersensitivity/anaphylaxis, start initial dose at few drops per minute, increase slowly to ordered rate; stay with pt first 10–15 min, then check q10min. • Change to oral route as soon as possible.

IV INCOMPATIBILITIES ⊘

Calcium gluconate, diltiazem (Cardizem), epinephrine, fluconazole (Diflucan), ondansetron (Zofran), sargramostim (Leukine), verapamil (Calan), vinorelbine (Navelbine).

IV COMPATIBILITIES

Heparin, insulin, magnesium, potassium chloride.

INDICATIONS/ROUTES/DOSAGE

Respiratory tract, skin/ skin structure infections:

PO: Adults, elderly, children >20

kg: 250–500 mg q6h. **Children <20 kg:** 50 mg/kg/day in divided doses q6h.

IM/IV: **Adults, elderly, children >40 kg:** 250–500 mg q6h. **Children <40 kg:** 25–50 mg/kg/day in divided doses q6–8h.

Bacterial meningitis, septicemia:

IM/IV: **Adults, elderly:** 2 g q4h or 3 g q6h. **Children:** 100–200 mg/kg/day in divided doses q4h.

Gonococcal infections:

PO: **Adults:** 3.5 g one time with 1 g probenecid plus tetracycline, erythromycin, or ampicillin.

Perioperative prophylaxis:

IM/IV: **Adults, elderly:** 2 g 30 min prior to procedure. May repeat in 8 hrs. **Children:** 50 mg/kg using same dosage regimen.

Usual dosage (neonates):

Note: Higher doses may be needed for neonatal meningitis.

IM/IV: **Neonates 7–28 days:** 75 mg/kg/day in divided doses q8h up to 200 mg/kg/day in divided doses q6h. **Neonates 0–7 days:** 50 mg/kg/day in divided doses q12h up to 150 mg/kg/day in divided doses q8h.

SIDE EFFECTS

FREQUENT: Pain at IM injection site, GI disturbances (mild diarrhea, nausea or vomiting), oral/vaginal candidiasis. *OCCASIONAL:* Generalized rash, urticaria, phlebitis, thrombophlebitis with IV administration, headache. *RARE:* Dizziness, seizures esp. with IV therapy.

ADVERSE REACTIONS/TOXIC EFFECTS

Superinfections, potentially fatal antibiotic-associated colitis (abdominal cramps, watery severe diarrhea, fever) may result from altered bacterial balance. Severe hypersensitivity reactions including anaphylaxis, acute interstitial nephritis occur rarely.

NURSING IMPLICATIONS

BASELINE ASSESSMENT:

Question for history of allergies, esp. penicillins, cephalosporins.

INTERVENTION/EVALUATION:

Hold medication and promptly report rash (although common with ampicillin, may indicate hypersensitivity) or diarrhea (with fever, abdominal pain, mucus and blood in stool may indicate antibiotic-associated colitis). Evaluate IV site for phlebitis (heat, pain, red streaking over vein). Check IM injection site for pain, induration. Monitor I&O, urinalysis, renal function tests. Assess for signs of superinfection: increased fever, sore throat onset, vomiting, diarrhea, anal/genital pruritus, changes in oral mucosa, black/hairy tongue.

PATIENT/FAMILY TEACHING:

Space doses evenly. Take antibiotic for full length of treatment. More effective if taken 1 hr before or 2 hrs after food/beverages. Discomfort may occur with IM injection. Notify physician of rash, diarrhea, or other new symptom.

ampicillin/sulbactam sodium

amp-ih-**sill**-in/sull-**bak**-tam (Unasyn)

►CLASSIFICATION

PHARMACOTHERAPEUTIC:
Penicillin. *CLINICAL:* Antibiotic
(see p. 27C)

ACTION/*THERAPEUTIC EFFECT*

Ampicillin is bactericidal in susceptible microorganisms *by inhibition
of cell wall synthesis.* Sulbactam: inhibits bacterial beta-lactamase,
*protecting ampicillin from enzymatic
degradation.*

PHARMACOKINETICS

Moderately absorbed from GI tract.
Protein binding: 28–38%. Widely
distributed. Partially metabolized in
liver. Primarily excreted in urine.
Removed by hemodialysis. Half-life:
1 hr (half-life increased in impaired
renal function).

USES

Treatment of intra-abdominal,
skin/skin structure, gynecologic
infections.

PRECAUTIONS

CONTRAINDICATIONS: Infectious mononucleosis, hypersensitivity to any penicillin. *CAUTIONS:*
History of allergies, particularly to
cephalosporins, antibiotic-associated colitis.

▷*LIFESPAN CONSIDERATIONS:*
Pregnancy/Lactation: Readily
crosses placenta; appears in cord
blood, amniotic fluid. Distributed in
breast milk in low concentrations.
May lead to allergic sensitization,
diarrhea, candidiasis, skin rash in
infant. **Pregnancy Category B.
Children:** Safety and efficacy not
established in children <1 yr. **Elderly:** Age-related renal impairment may require dose adjustment.

INTERACTIONS

DRUG: **Allopurinol** may increase

incidence of rash. **Probenecid**
may increase concentration, toxicity risk. May decrease effects of
oral contraceptives. *HERBAL:*
None known. *FOOD:* None known.
LAB VALUES: May increase SGOT
(AST), SGPT (ALT), alkaline phosphatase, LDH, creatinine. May
cause positive Coombs' test.

AVAILABILITY (Rx

POWDER FOR INJECTION: 1.5 g,
3 g.

ADMINISTRATION/HANDLING

IM:

• Reconstitute each 1.5 g vial with
3.2 ml Sterile Water for Injection to
provide concentration of 250 mg
ampicillin/125 mg sulbactam/ml. •
Give deeply into large muscle
mass within 1 hr after preparation.

IV 🔟

Storage:

• When reconstituted with 0.9%
NaCl, IV solution is stable for 8 hrs
at room temperature, 48 hrs if refrigerated. Stability may be different with other diluents. • Discard if
precipitate forms.

Reconstitution:

• For IV injection, dilute with
10–20 ml sterile water for injection. • For intermittent IV infusion
(piggyback), further dilute with
50–100 ml D_5W or 0.9% NaCl..

Rate of administration:

• For IV injection, give slowly over
minimum of 10–15 min. • For intermittent IV infusion (piggyback),
infuse over 15–30 min. • Due to
potential for hypersensitivity/ana-
phylaxis, start initial dose at few
drops per min, increase slowly to
ordered rate; stay with pt first
10–15 min, then check q10min. •
Change to oral antibiotic as soon
as possible.

IV INCOMPATIBILITIES $\oslash$

Diltiazem (Cardizem), idarubicin (Idamycin), ondansetron (Zofran), sargramastim (Leukine).

IV COMPATIBILITIES

Heparin, insulin.

INDICATIONS/ROUTES/DOSAGE

Skin/skin structure, intra-abdominal, gynecologic infections:

IM/IV: Adults, elderly: 1.5 g (1 g ampicillin/500 mg sulbactam) to 3 g (2 g ampicillin/1 g sulbactam) q6h.

Skin/skin structure infections:

IV: Children 1–12 yrs: 300 mg/kg/day in divided doses q6h.

Dosage in renal impairment:

Modification of dose and/or frequency based on creatinine clearance and/or severity of infection.

Creatinine Clearance	Dosage
>30 ml/min	.5–3 g q6–8h
15–29 ml/min	1.5–3 g q12h
5–14 ml/min	1.5–3 g q24h
<5 ml/min	Not recommended

SIDE EFFECTS

FREQUENT: Diarrhea and rash (most common), urticaria, pain at IM injection site; thrombophlebitis with IV administration; oral/vaginal candidiasis. ***OCCASIONAL:*** Nausea, vomiting, headache, malaise, urinary retention.

ADVERSE REACTIONS/TOXIC EFFECTS

Severe hypersensitivity reactions, including anaphylaxis, acute interstitial nephritis, blood dyscrasias may be noted. Superinfections, potentially fatal antibiotic-associated colitis (abdominal cramps, watery severe diarrhea, fever) may result from altered bacterial balance. Overdose may produce seizures.

NURSING IMPLICATIONS

BASELINE ASSESSMENT:

Question for history of allergies, esp. penicillins, cephalosporins.

INTERVENTION/EVALUATION:

Hold medication and promptly report rash (although common with ampicillin, may indicate hypersensitivity) or diarrhea (with fever, mucus and blood in stool, abdominal pain may indicate antibiotic-associated diarrhea). Evaluate IV site for phlebitis (heat, pain, red streaking over vein). Check IM injection site for pain, induration. Monitor I&O, urinalysis, renal function tests. Assess for initial signs of superinfection: increased fever, sore throat onset, vomiting, diarrhea, anal/genital pruritus, ulceration or changes of oral mucosa.

PATIENT/FAMILY TEACHING:

Space doses evenly. Take antibiotic for full length of treatment. Discomfort may occur with IM injection. Notify physician of rash, diarrhea, or other new symptom.

amprenavir

am-**prenn**-ah-veer
(Agenerase)

▶**CLASSIFICATION**

PHARMACOTHERAPEUTIC: Antiviral. ***CLINICAL:*** Protease inhibitor (see pp. 57C, 96C)

ACTION/*THERAPEUTIC EFFECT*

Inhibits HIV-1 protease by binding to active site of HIV-1 protease, preventing processing of viral precursors and forming immature noninfectious viral particles. This produces *impairment of HIV viral replication and proliferation.*

PHARMACOKINETICS

Rapidly absorbed following PO administration. Protein binding: 90%. Metabolized in the liver. Primarily excreted in feces. Half-life: 7.1–10.6 hrs.

USES

Treatment of HIV-1 infection in combination with other antiretroviral agents.

PRECAUTIONS

CONTRAINDICATIONS: None significant. ***CAUTIONS:*** Liver function impairment, diabetes mellitus, hemophilia, hypersensitivity to sulfas, vitamin K deficiency due to anticoagulant/malabsorption.
▷***LIFESPAN CONSIDERATIONS:***
Pregnancy/Lactation: Unknown if drug crosses placenta or distributed in breast milk. **Pregnancy Category C. Children:** Safety and efficacy not established in those <4 yrs. **Elderly:** Age-related liver impairment may require decreased dosage.

INTERACTIONS

DRUG: May interfere with metabolism of **amiodarone, lidocaine, oral contraceptives, midazolam, triazolam, tricyclic antidepressants, qinidine, bepridil, ergotamine. Antacids, didanosine** may decrease absorption. **Carbamazepine, phenobarbital, phenytoin, rifampin** may decrease concentration.

Amprenavir may increase concentration of **clozapine, HMG-CoA reductase inhibitors (-statins), warfarin.** ***HERBAL:*** St. John's wort may decrease concentration. ***FOOD:*** High-fat meal may decrease absorption. ***LAB VALUES:*** May increase glucose, cholesterol, triglycerides.

AVAILABILITY (Rx)

CAPSULES: 50 mg, 150 mg. ***ORAL SOLUTION:*** 15 mg/ml.

ADMINISTRATION/HANDLING

PO:
* May give without regard to food.

INDICATIONS/ROUTES/DOSAGE

HIV-1 infection:

PO: **Adults, children 13–16 yrs:** *Capsules:* 1,200 mg 2 times/day. **Children 4–12 yrs, 13–16 yrs <50 kg:** 20 mg/kg 2 times/day or 15 mg/kg 3 times/day. **Maximum:** 2,400 mg/day. *Oral solution:* **Children 4–12, 13–16 yrs <50 kg:** 22.5 mg/kg/day (1.5 ml/kg) 2 times/day or 17 mg/kg/day (1.1 ml/kg) 3 times/day. **Maximum:** 2,800 mg/day.

SIDE EFFECTS

FREQUENT: Diarrhea/loose stools (56%), nausea (38%), oral paresthesia (30%), rash (25%), vomiting (20%). ***OCCASIONAL:*** Rash (18%), peripheral paresthesia (12%), depression (4%).

ADVERSE REACTIONS/TOXIC EFFECTS

Severe hypersensitivity reactions, Stevens-Johnson syndrome (blisters, peeling of skin, loosening skin/mucous membranes, fever).

BASELINE ASSESSMENT:

Obtain baseline laboratory testing before beginning therapy and at periodic intervals during therapy. Offer emotional support.

INTERVENTION/EVALUATION:

Assess for nausea, vomiting. Determine pattern of bowel activity and stool consistency. Assess eating pattern; monitor for weight loss. Assess tingling/numbness of peripheral extremities. Assess skin for rash.

PATIENT/FAMILY TEACHING:

Avoid high-fat meals (decreases drug absorption). Small, frequent meals may offset anorexia, nausea. Amprenavir is not a cure for HIV infection, nor does it reduce risk of transmission to others.

anagrelide

an-ah-**gree**-lide
(Agrylin)

▶CLASSIFICATION

PHARMACOTHERAPEUTIC:
Hematological agent. ***CLINICAL:*** Antiplatelet (see p. 29C)

ACTION/*THERAPEUTIC EFFECT***

Reduces platelet production and preventing platelet shape changes caused by platelet aggregating agents, *thereby inhibiting platelet aggregation.*

PHARMACOKINETICS

Following PO administration, peak plasma concentration occurs within 1 hr. Extensively metabo-lized. Primarily excreted in urine. Half-life: approximately 3 days.

USES

Treatment of essential thrombocythemia, reducing elevated platelet count and risk of thrombosis. Treatment of thrombocythemia due to myeloproliferative disorders.

PRECAUTIONS

CONTRAINDICATIONS: None significant. ***CAUTIONS:*** Cardiac disease, renal, liver impairment.
▷***LIFESPAN CONSIDERATIONS:***
Pregnancy/Lactation: Unknown if crosses placenta or distributed in breast milk. May cause fetal harm. **Pregnancy Category C. Children:** Safety and efficacy in those <16 yrs not established. **Elderly:** Age-related decreased renal/liver function, cardiac disease requires caution.

INTERACTIONS

DRUG: None significant. ***HERBAL:*** None known. ***FOOD:*** None known. ***LAB VALUES:*** May increase liver enzymes (rare).

AVAILABILITY (Rx
CAPSULES: 0.5 mg, 1 mg.

ADMINISTRATION/HANDLING
PO:
• May give without regard to food.

INDICATIONS/ROUTES/DOSAGE
Thrombocythemia:

***PO:* Adults, elderly:** Initially, 0.5 mg 4 times/day or 1 mg 2 times/day. Adjust dose to lowest effective dose, increasing by ≤0.5 mg/day in any 1 week. **Maximum:** 10 mg/day or 2.5 mg/dose.

SIDE EFFECTS

FREQUENT (≥5%): Headache, palpitations, diarrhea, abdominal pain, nausea, flatulence, bloating, asthenia (loss of strength and energy), pain, dizziness. **_OCCASIONAL_** (<5%): Tachycardia, chest pain, vomiting, paresthesia, peripheral edema, anorexia, dyspepsia, rash. **_RARE:_** Confusion, insomnia.

ADVERSE REACTIONS/TOXIC EFFECTS

Angina, heart failure, arrhythmias occur rarely.

NURSING IMPLICATIONS

BASELINE ASSESSMENT:

Assess platelet count, hemoglobin, hematocrit, WBC, prior to treatment and q2days during first week of treatment and weekly thereafter until therapeutic range is achieved. Ask if pt is breast-feeding, pregnant, or planning to become pregnant (may cause fetal harm).

INTERVENTION/EVALUATION:

Monitor liver function test results, BUN, creatinine, and those with suspected heart disease. Assess skin for bruises, petechiae, also catheter insertion site, needle site, GI sites.

PATIENT/FAMILY TEACHING:

Platelet count responds within 7–14 days. Not recommended in women who are pregnant. Use contraceptives while taking anagrelide.

anakinra

(Kineret)
See New Drug Supplement.

anastrozole

ah-**nas**-trow-zole
(Arimidex)
Do not confuse with Imitrex.

▶CLASSIFICATION

PHARMACOTHERAPEUTIC: Aromatase inhibitor. **_CLINICAL:_** Antineoplastic, hormone (see p. 67C).

ACTION/_THERAPEUTIC EFFECT_

Decreases circulating estrogen by inhibiting aromatase, an enzyme that catalyzes the final step in estrogen production. Since growth of many breast cancers are stimulated by estrogens, *drug significantly lowers serum estradiol (estrogen) concentration.*

PHARMACOKINETICS

Well absorbed into systemic circulation. Protein binding: 40%. Food does not affect extent of absorption. Extensively metabolized. Eliminated by hepatic metabolism and, to a lesser extent, renal excretion. Mean half-life: 50 hrs in postmenopausal women. Plasma concentrations reach steady state levels at about 7 days.

USES

Treatment of advanced breast cancer in postmenopausal women who have developed progressive disease while receiving tamoxifen therapy. First-line therapy in advanced/metastatic breast cancer.

PRECAUTIONS

CONTRAINDICATIONS: None significant. **_CAUTIONS:_** None significant.

▷**LIFESPAN CONSIDERATIONS:**
Pregnancy/Lactation: Crosses placenta; may cause fetal harm. Unknown if excreted in breast milk. **Pregnancy Category D. Children:** Safety and efficacy not established. **Elderly:** No age-related precautions noted.

INTERACTIONS

DRUG: None significant. **HERBAL:** None known. **FOOD:** None known. **LAB VALUES:** May elevate serum GGT level in those with liver metastases. May increase SGOT (AST), SGPT (ALT), alkaline phosphate, total cholesterol, LDL cholesterol.

AVAILABILITY (Rx)
TABLETS: 1 mg.

ADMINISTRATION/HANDLING
PO:
• May give without regard to food.

INDICATIONS/ROUTES/DOSAGE
Breast cancer:
PO: Adults, elderly: 1 mg once daily.

SIDE EFFECTS

FREQUENT (8–16%): Asthenia (loss of strength/energy), nausea, headache, hot flashes, back pain, vomiting, cough, diarrhea. **OCCASIONAL** (4–6%): Constipation, abdominal pain, anorexia, bone pain, pharyngitis, dizziness, rash, dry mouth peripheral edema, pelvic pain, depression, chest pain, paresthesia. **RARE** (1–2%): Weight gain, sweating.

ADVERSE REACTIONS/TOXIC EFFECTS

Thrombophlebitis, anemia, leukopenia occur rarely. Vaginal hemorrhage occurs rarely (2%).

NURSING IMPLICATIONS

INTERVENTION/EVALUATION:

Monitor for and assist with amubulation if asthenia/dizziness occurs. Assess for headache. Offer antiemetic for nausea/vomiting. Monitor for onset of diarrhea; offer antidiarrheal medication.

PATIENT/FAMILY TEACHING:

Notify physician if nausea, asthenia, hot flashes become unmanageable.

anistreplase

(Eminase)

See Classification section under: Thrombolytics (p. 30C)

antihemophilic factor (factor VIII, AHF)

(Alphanate, Hyate C, Bioclate, Helixate, Humate-P, Koate-DVI✦, Koate-HP, Kogenate, Monoclate-P)

▶CLASSIFICATION

PHARMACOTHERAPEUTIC: Antihemophilic agent. **CLINICAL:** Hemostatic

ACTION/THERAPEUTIC EFFECT

Assists in conversion of prothrombin to thrombin (essential for blood coagulation), *increasing clotting time.* Replaces missing clotting factor, *correcting or preventing bleeding episodes.*

USES/*UNLABELED*

Treatment, prevention of bleeding in patients with hemophilia A factor XIII deficiency, von Willebrand disease, hypofibrinogenemia. *Treatment of disseminated intravascular coagulation (DIC).*

PRECAUTIONS

CONTRAINDICATIONS: None known. ***CAUTIONS:*** Hepatic disease, those with blood type A, B, AB.

INTERACTIONS

DRUG: None known. ***HERBAL:*** None known. ***FOOD:*** None known. ***LAB VALUES:*** None known.

AVAILABILITY (Rx)

INJECTION: Actual number of AHF units listed on each vial.

ADMINISTRATION/HANDLING
IV 📺

Storage:

• Refer to individual vials for specific storage requirements.

Reconstitution:

• Warm concentrate and diluent to room temperature. • To dissolve, gently agitate or rotate. Do not shake vigorously. Complete dissolution may take 5–10 min. • Filter before administration. Use only plastic syringes for IV injection (solution may stick to glass surface).

Rate of administration:

• Administer IV at rate of approx. 2 ml/min. Can give up to 10 ml/min.

Administration precautions:

• Check pulse rate before and during administration. If pulse rate increases, reduce or stop administration. • After administration, apply prolonged pressure on venipuncture site. • Monitor IV site for oozing q5–15min for 1–2 hrs after administration.

IV INCOMPATIBILITY ⊘

Do not mix antihemophilic factor with other IV solutions or medications.

INDICATIONS/ROUTES/DOSAGE

Note: Dosage is highly individualized, based on pt weight, severity of bleeding, coagulation studies.

Prophylaxis of spontaneous hemorrhage:

IV: Adults, elderly, children: 10 AHF/IU/kg as a single infusion.

Moderate hemorrhage, minor surgery:

IV: Adults, elderly, children: Initially, 15–25 AHF/IU/kg. **Maintenance:** 10–15 IU/kg q8–12h.

Severe hemorrhage (near vital organ):

IV: Adults, elderly, children: Initially, 40–50 AHF/IU/kg. **Maintenance:** 20–25 IU/kg q8–12h.

Major surgery:

IV: Adults, elderly, children: 40–50 AHF/IU/kg 1 hr prior to surgery, 20–25 IU/kg 5 hrs later, then 10–15 IU/kg/day for 10–14 days.

Von Willebrand disease:

IV: Adults: 40–80 IU/kg q8–12h.

SIDE EFFECTS

OCCASIONAL: Allergic reaction (fever, chills, urticaria [hives], wheezing, slight hypotension, nausea, feeling of chest tightness), stinging at injection site, dizziness, dry mouth, headache, unpleasant taste.

ADVERSE REACTIONS/TOXIC EFFECTS

There is a risk of transmitting viral hepatitis and a slight risk of transmitting AIDS. Possibility of intravascular hemolysis is present if large or frequent doses used in those with blood group A, B, or AB.

NURSING IMPLICATIONS

BASELINE ASSESSMENT:

When monitoring B/P, avoid over-inflation of cuff. Remove adhesive tape from any pressure dressing very carefully and slowly.

INTERVENTION/EVALUATION:

After IV administration, apply prolonged pressure on venipuncture site. Monitor IV site for oozing q5–15min for 1–2 hrs after administration. Assess for allergic reaction. Report any evidence of hematuria or change in vital signs immediately. Assess for decrease in B/P, increase in pulse rate, complaint of abdominal or back pain, severe headache (may be evidence of hemorrhage). Question for increase in amount of discharge during menses. Assess skin for bruises, petechiae. Check for excessive bleeding from minor cuts, scratches. Assess gums for erythema, gingival bleeding. Assess urine for hematuria. Evaluate for therapeutic relief of pain, reduction of swelling, and restricted joint movement.

PATIENT/FAMILY TEACHING:

Use electric razor, soft toothbrush to prevent bleeding. Report any sign of red or dark urine, black or red stool, coffee-ground vomitus, red-speckled mucus from cough.

antithymocyte globulin

an-tie-**thigh**-mow-site
(Atgam)

▶CLASSIFICATION
PHARMACOTHERAPEUTIC:
Biologic response modifier.
CLINICAL: Immunosuppressant

ACTION/THERAPEUTIC EFFECT

Lymphocyte selective immunosuppressant; reduces number of circulating thymus-dependent lymphocytes (T-lymphocytes), altering function of T-lymphocytes, which are responsible for cell-mediated and humoral immunity. Stimulates release of hematopoietic growth factors. *Allows increase of graft survival rate.*

USES/UNLABELED

Management of allograft rejection in renal transplant patients, increasing frequency of resolution of acute rejection period. Treatment of moderate to severe aplastic anemia in patients not suited for bone marrow transplants. *Immunosuppressant in liver, bone marrow, heart transplants, treatment of multiple sclerosis, myasthenia gravis, pure red cell aplasia, scleroderma.*

PRECAUTIONS

CONTRAINDICATIONS: Systemic hypersensitivity reaction to previous injection of antithymocyte globulin. **CAUTIONS:** Concurrent immunosuppressive therapy.

INTERACTIONS

DRUG: None known. **HERBAL:** None known. **FOOD:** None known. **LAB VALUES:** May alter renal function tests.

ADMINISTRATION/HANDLING

IV 💉

Storage:

• Keep refrigerated before and after dilution. • Discard diluted solution after 24 hrs.

Reconstitution:

• Total daily dose must be further diluted with 0.9% NaCl (do not use D_5W). • Gently rotate diluted solution. Do not shake. • Final concentration must not exceed 4 mg/ml.

Rate of administration:

• Use 0.2 to 1 micron filter. • Give total daily dose over minimum of 4 hrs.

IV INCOMPATIBILITY ⊘

No information available via Y-site administration.

INDICATIONS/ROUTES/DOSAGE

Renal allograft recipients:

IV INFUSION: Adults: 10–30 mg/kg/day. **Children:** 5–25 mg/kg/day. *Delay of onset of rejection:* 15 mg/kg/day for 14 days, then 15 mg/kg/day every other day for 14 days. Give first dose within 24 hrs before or after transplant. *Treatment of rejection:* 10–15 mg/kg/day for 14 days. May continue with alternate-day therapy up to 21 doses.

Aplastic anemia:

IV INFUSION: Adults: 10–20 mg/kg/day for 8–14 days. May continue alternate-day therapy up to 21 doses.

SIDE EFFECTS

FREQUENT: Fever (51%), thrombocytopenia (30%), rash (2%), chills (16%), leukopenia (14%), systemic infection (13%). **OCCASIONAL** (5–10%): Serum sickness–like symptoms, dyspnea, apnea, arthralgia, chest/back/flank pain, nausea, vomiting, diarrhea, phlebitis.

ADVERSE REACTIONS/TOXIC EFFECTS

Thrombocytopenia occurs but is generally transient. Severe hypersensitivity reaction, including anaphylaxis, occurs rarely.

NURSING IMPLICATIONS

BASELINE ASSESSMENT:

Use of high-flow vein (CVL, PICC, Groshong catheter) may prevent chemical phlebitis that may occur if peripheral vein is used.

INTERVENTION/EVALUATION:

Monitor frequently for chills, fever, erythema, itching. Obtain order for prophylactic antihistamines or corticosteroids.

apraclonidine

(Iopidine)

See Classification section under: Antiglaucoma agents (p. 45C)

aprotinin

ah-**pro**-tih-nin
(Trasylol)

►CLASSIFICATION

PHARMACOTHERAPEUTIC: Natural proteinase inhibitor. **CLINICAL:** Antifibrinolytic; antihemorrhagic

ACTION/*THERAPEUTIC EFFECT*

Pts undergoing cardiac surgery with use of a heart-lung machine normally develop adverse changes in blood components. These changes produce hemostatic defect, generally resulting in diffuse bleeding. Aprotinin inhibits coagulation, *directly preventing fibrinolysis, preserving platelet function, thereby decreasing bleeding.*

USES/*UNLABELED*

For prophylactic, perioperative use to reduce blood loss and need for transfusions in pts undergoing cardiopulmonary bypass in repeat coronary artery bypass graft (CABG) surgery and in primary CABG surgery in pts with high risk of bleeding or where access to blood is unavailable or unacceptable. *For reduction in bleeding and transfusion requirements in liver transplant, total hip replacement, colorectal surgery, peripheral vascular surgery, heart and heart-lung transplants.*

PRECAUTIONS

CONTRAINDICATIONS: Allergy to aprotinin. ***EXTREME CAUTION:*** History of allergies, previous aprotinin therapy, those undergoing deep hypothermic circulatory arrest, >65 yrs, surgery of aortic arch.

INTERACTIONS

DRUG: May block hypotensive effect of **ACE inhibitors (e.g., captopril),** inhibits effects of **fibrinolytic agents (alteplase, anistreplase, streptokinase, urokinase),** increases effect of **heparin** (prolonging activated clotting time). ***HERBAL:*** None known. ***FOOD:*** None known. ***LAB VALUES:*** Prolongs whole blood clotting time of heparinized blood, significantly prolongs activated clotting time (ACT), partial thromboplastin time (PTT), increases serum creatine kinase (CK) levels, serum creatinine, serum transaminase.

AVAILABILITY (Rx)

INJECTION: 10,000 KIU/ml.

INDICATIONS/ROUTES/DOSAGE

Note: Give loading dose over 20–30 min after anesthesia induction but before sternotomy (rapid administration can produce fall in B/P). When loading dose is complete, follow by continuous IV infusion until surgery is completed and pt leaves operating room.

Regimen A (high dose):

IV: Adults, elderly: Initially, 2 million KIU loading dose, 2 million KIU into pump prime volume, then continuous IV infusion of 500,000 KIU/hr of operation.

Regimen B (low dose):

IV: Adults, elderly: Initially, 1 million KIU loading dose, 1 million KIU into pump prime volume, then continuous IV infusion of 250,000 KIU/hr of operation.

SIDE EFFECTS

Side effects reported are frequently seen in open-heart surgery and not necessarily attributed to aprotinin.

ADVERSE REACTIONS/TOXIC EFFECTS

Even after uneventful test dose, loading dose may produce anaphylaxis. Stop infusion immediately and initiate emergency treatment for anaphylaxis. Treatment: parenteral epinephrine, O_2, antihistamines, corticosteroids, airway management (including intubation).

NURSING IMPLICATIONS

BASELINE ASSESSMENT:

Question pt regarding previous use of aprotinin (increased risk of anaphylactic reaction to drug).

INTERVENTION/EVALUATION:

Assess for decrease in B/P, increase in pulse rate, abdominal or back pain, severe headache (may be evidence of hemorrhage). Assess peripheral pulses; skin for bruises, petechiae. Question for increase in amount of discharge during menses. Check for excessive bleeding from minor cuts, scratches. Assess gums for erythema, gingival bleeding. Assess urine output for hematuria.

---

argatroban

our-ga-**trow**-ban
(Acova)

►CLASSIFICATION

PHARMACOTHERAPEUTIC:
Thrombin inhibitor. **CLINICAL:**
Anticoagulant

ACTION/*THERAPEUTIC EFFECT*

A direct thrombin inhibitor that reversibly binds to thrombin active site. Exerts its effect by inhibiting thrombin catalyzed or induced reactions, *producing anticoagulation.*

PHARMACOKINETICS

Following IV administration, distributed primarily in extracellular fluid. Metabolized in the liver. Primarily excreted in the feces, presumably through biliary secretion. Half-life: 39–51 min.

USES

Prophylaxis or treatment of thrombosis in heparin-induced thrombocytopenia (HIT).

PRECAUTIONS

CONTRAINDICATIONS: Overt major bleeding. **CAUTIONS:** Severe hypertension, immediately following lumbar puncture, spinal anesthesia, major surgery, patients with congenital or acquired bleeding disorders, ulcerations, liver function impairment.

▷**LIFESPAN CONSIDERATIONS:**
Pregnancy/Lactation: Unknown if excreted in breast milk. **Pregnancy Category B. Children:** Safety and efficacy not established in those <18 yrs of age. **Elderly:** No age-related precautions noted.

INTERACTIONS

DRUG: Antiplatelet agents, thrombolytics, other anticoagulants may increase risk of bleeding. **HERBAL:** None known. **FOOD:** None known. **LAB VALUES:** Increased APTT, prothrombin time, INR.

AVAILABILITY (Rx)

INJECTION: 100 mg/ml.

ADMINISTRATION/HANDLING

IV 🜄

Storage:

• Discard if solution appears cloudy or an insoluble precipitate is noted. • Following reconstitution, stable for 24 hrs at room temperature, 48 hrs if refrigerated. • Avoid direct sunlight.

Reconstitution:

• Must be diluted 100 fold prior to infusion in 0.9% NaCl, D₅W, or lactated Ringer's to provide a final concentration of 1 mg/ml. • The

---

solution must be mixed by repeated inversion of the diluent bag for 1 min. • After reconstitution, solution may show a brief haziness due to formation of microprecipitates that rapidly dissolve upon mixing.

Rate of administration:

• Rate of administration is based on body weight at 2 mcg/kg/min (for example, 50 kg patient infuse at 6 ml/hr).

IV INCOMPATIBILITY ⊘

Do not mix with any other medications or solutions.

INDICATIONS/ROUTES/DOSAGE

HIT:

IV INFUSION: **Adults, elderly:** Initially, 2 mcg/kg/min administered as a continuous infusion. **Liver impairment:** Initially, 0.5 mcg/kg/min. After initial infusion, dose may be adjusted until steady state APTT is 1.5–3 times initial baseline value not to exceed 100 sec.

SIDE EFFECTS

FREQUENT (3–8%): Dyspnea, hypotension, fever, diarrhea, nausea, pain, vomiting, infection, cough.

ADVERSE REACTIONS/TOXIC EFFECTS

Ventricular tachycardia, atrial fibrillation occur occasionally. Major bleeding, sepsis occur rarely.

NURSING IMPLICATIONS

BASELINE ASSESSMENT:

Assess CBC, including platelet count. Check PT, PTT. Determine initial B/P. Minimize need for numerous injection sites, blood drawings, catheters.

INTERVENTION/EVALUATION:

Assess for any sign of bleeding: bleeding at surgical site, hematuria, blood in stool, bleeding from gums, petechiae, bruising, bleeding from injection sites. Handle pt carefully and as infrequently as possible to prevent bleeding. Do not obtain B/P in lower extremities (possible deep vein thrombi). Assess for decrease in B/P, increase in pulse rate, complaint of abdominal/back pain, severe headache (evidence of hemorrhage), ACT, PT, APTT, platelet count. Question for increase in discharge during menses. Assess urine output for hematuria. Monitor for any occurring hematoma. Use care in removing any dressing, tape.

PATIENT/FAMILY TEACHING:

Use electric razor, soft toothbrush to prevent bleeding. Report any sign of red or dark urine, black or red stool, coffee-ground vomitus, red-speckled mucus from cough.

arsenic trioxide

are-sih-nic try-**ox**-ide
(Trisenox)

▶CLASSIFICATION

CLINICAL: Antineoplastic (see p. 68C)

ACTION/*THERAPEUTIC EFFECT*

Produces morphological changes and DNA fragmentation in promyelocytic leukemia cells, *thereby producing cell death.*

USES

Induction of remission and consolidations in pts with acute promyelocytic leukemia (APL) who are refractory to or have relapsed from retinoid and anthracycline chemotherapy.

PRECAUTIONS

CONTRAINDICATIONS: None known. ***CAUTIONS:*** Renal impairment, cardiac abnormalities.

INTERACTIONS

DRUG: May prolong QT interval in those taking **antiarrhythmics, thiordazine. Diuretics, amphotericin B** may produce electrolyte abnormalities. ***HERBAL:*** None known. ***FOOD:*** None known. ***LAB VALUES:*** May decrease white blood cell count, Hgb, platelet count, magnesium, calcium. May increase SGOT, SGPT. Higher risk of hypokalemia than hyperkalemia, hyperglycemia than hypoglycemia.

AVAILABILITY (Rx)

INJECTION: 1 mg/ml.

ADMINISTRATION/HANDLING

IV 🟥

Note: A central venous line is not required for drug administration.

Storage:

• Store at room temperature. • Diluted solution is stable for 24 hrs at room temperature, 48 hrs if refrigerated.

Reconstitution:

• After withdrawing drug from ampule, dilute with 100–250 ml D_5W or 0.9% NaCl.

Rate of administration:

• Transfuse over 1–2 hrs. Duration of infusion may be extended up to 4 hrs.

IV INCOMPATIBILITY ⊘

Do not mix with any other medications.

INDICATIONS/ROUTES/DOSAGE

Acute promyelocytic leukemia (APL), induction treatment:

IV: Adults, elderly: 0.15 mg/kg/day until bone marrow suppression occurs. Total induction dose should not exceed 60 doses.

Acute promyelocytic leukemia (APL), consolidation treatment:

IV: Adults, elderly: Consolidation treatment should begin 3–6 wks after completion of induction therapy. Give dose of 0.15 mg/kg/day for 25 doses up to 5 wks.

SIDE EFFECTS

COMMON (50–75%): Nausea, cough, fatigue, fever, headache, vomiting, abdominal pain, tachycardia, diarrhea, dyspnea. ***FREQUENT*** (30–43%): Dermatitis, insomnia, edema, rigors, prolonged QT interval, sore throat, pruritus, arthralgia, paresthesia, anxiety. ***OCCASIONAL*** (20–28%): Constipation, myalgia, hypotension, epistaxis, anorexia, dizziness, sinusitis. ***OCCASIONAL*** (8–15%): Ecchymosis, nonspecific pain, weight gain, herpes simplex, wheezing, flushing, increased sweating, tremor, hypertension, palpitations, dyspepsia, eye irritation, blurred vison, weakness., decreased breath sounds, rales. ***RARE:*** Confusion, petechiae, dry mouth oral candidiasis, incontinence, rhonchi.

ADVERSE REACTIONS/TOXIC EFFECTS

Seizures, GI hemorrhage, renal impairment or failure, pleural or pericardial effusion, hemoptysis, sepsis occur rarely. Prolonged QT interval, complete AV block, unexplained fever, dyspnea, weight gain, effusion are evidence of arsenic toxicity. Treatment should be halted and steroid treatment instituted.

NURSING IMPLICATIONS

BASELINE ASSESSMENT:

Assess platelet count, Hgb, Hct, WBC prior to and frequently during treatment. Ask if pt is breast-feeding, pregnant, or planning to become pregnant (may cause fetal harm).

INTERVENTION/EVALUATION:

Monitor liver function test results, CBC, serum values. Monitor for arsenic toxicity syndrome (fever, dyspnea, weight gain, confusion, muscle weakness, seizures).

PATIENT/FAMILY TEACHING:

Avoid crowds, those with known infection. Avoid contact with anyone who recently received live virus vaccine; do not receive vaccinations.

artificial tears

(Isopto Tears, Liquifilm Forte, Hypotears, Neo-Tears, Just Tears, Tears Naturale, Lacril, Murocel, Lyteers, Isopto Plain, Ultra Tears, Moisture Drops)

▶**CLASSIFICATION**

PHARMACOTHERAPEUTIC: Ophthalmic lubricant

ACTION/*THERAPEUTIC EFFECT*

Stabilizes/thickens precorneal tear film, lengthening tear film breakup time. *Protects and lubricates the eyes.*

USES/*UNLABELED*

Relief of dryness and irritation due to deficient tear production; ocular lubricant for artificial eyes; some products may be used with hard contact lenses. *Treatment of recurrent corneal erosions, decreased corneal sensitivity.*

PRECAUTIONS

CONTRAINDICATIONS: Hypersensitivity to any component of preparation. ***CAUTIONS:*** None known.

INTERACTIONS

DRUG: None known. ***HERBAL:*** None known. ***FOOD:*** None known. ***LAB VALUES:*** None known.

INDICATIONS/ROUTES/DOSAGE

Ophthalmic lubricant:

Adults, elderly: 1–2 drops 3–4 times/day as needed.

SIDE EFFECTS

OCCASIONAL: Eye irritation, blurred vision, stickiness of eyelashes.

ADVERSE REACTIONS/TOXIC EFFECTS

None known.

NURSING IMPLICATIONS

BASELINE ASSESSMENT:

Determine extent of dryness, irritation.

INTERVENTION/EVALUATION:

Monitor for increased irritation or discomfort. Assess therapeutic response.

PATIENT/FAMILY TEACHING:

Wash hands thoroughly before use. Do not touch the tip of the dropper or container to any surface.

ascorbic acid (vitamin C)

(Apo-C✦, Cecon, Redoxon✦)

▶CLASSIFICATION

CLINICAL: Vitamin (see p. 128C)

ACTION/*THERAPEUTIC EFFECT*

Nutritional supplement necessary for collagen formation, tissue repair, oxidation-reduction reactions. *Involved in metabolism, carbohydrate utilization, synthesis of lipids, proteins, carnitine. Preserves blood vessel integrity.*

PHARMACOKINETICS

Readily absorbed from GI tract. Protein binding: 25%. Metabolized in liver. Excreted in urine. Removed by hemodialysis.

USES/*UNLABELED*

Prophylaxis, treatment of vitamin C deficiency. Increased requirement may be needed in GI disease, malignancy, peptic ulcer, tuberculosis, smokers, oral contraceptive users, hyperthyroidism, prolonged stress, burns, infection, chronic fever, parenteral hyperalimentation, hemodialysis. *Prevention of common cold, urinary acidifier, control of idiopathic methemoglobinemia.*

PRECAUTIONS

CONTRAINDICATIONS: None significant. *CAUTIONS:* Those on sodium restriction, daily salicylate treatment, warfarin therapy, diabetes mellitus, history of renal stones.

▷*LIFESPAN CONSIDERATIONS:*
Pregnancy/Lactation: Crosses placenta, excreted in breast milk. Large doses during pregnancy may produce scurvy in neonates. **Pregnancy Category C. Children/Elderly:** No age-related precautions noted.

INTERACTIONS

DRUG: May increase iron toxicity with **deferoxamine.** *HERBAL:* None known. *FOOD:* None known. *LAB VALUES:* May decrease bilirubin, urinary pH. May increase uric acid, urine oxalate.

AVAILABILITY (OTC)

TABLETS: 100 mg, 250 mg, 500 mg, 1,000 mg. *TABLETS (chewable):* 100 mg, 250 mg, 500 mg. *TABLETS (time-release):* 500 mg, 1,000 mg, 1,500 mg. *CAPSULES (time-release):* 500 mg. *SOLUTION:* 100 mg/ml. *SYRUP:* 250 mg/ml. *INJECTION:* 250 mg/ml, 500 mg/ml.

ADMINISTRATION/HANDLING
PO:
• May give without regard to food.
IV 💉
Storage:
• Store at room temperature. • Protect from freezing/light.

Rate of administration:
• May give undiluted or dilute in D_5W, 0.9% NaCl, lactated Ringer's. • For IV push, give 100 mg over 1 min. • For IV solution, infuse over 4–12 hrs.

IV INCOMPATIBILITY ⊘

No information available via Y-site administration.

INDICATIONS/ROUTES/DOSAGE
Dietary supplement:

PO: Adults, elderly: 45–60 mg/day. **Children >4 yrs:** 30–40 mg/day.

Deficiency:

***PO/IM/IV:* Adults, elderly:** 75–150 mg/day.

Scurvy:

***PO:* Adults, elderly:** 300 mg–1 g/day.

Burns:

***PO:* Adults, elderly:** Up to 2 g/day.

Enhance wound healing:

***PO:* Adults, elderly:** 300–500 mg/day for 7–10 days.

SIDE EFFECTS

RARE: Abdominal cramps, nausea, vomiting, diarrhea, increased urination with doses exceeding 1 g. ***Parenteral:*** Flushing, headache, dizziness, sleepiness or insomnia, soreness at injection site.

ADVERSE REACTIONS/TOXIC EFFECTS

May produce urine acidification leading to crystalluria. Large doses given IV may lead to deep vein thrombosis. Prolonged use of large doses may result in scurvy when dosage is reduced to normal.

NURSING IMPLICATIONS

INTERVENTION/EVALUATION:

Assess for clinical improvement (improved sense of well-being and sleep patterns). Observe for reversal of deficiency symptoms (gingivitis, bleeding gums, poor wound healing, digestive difficulties, joint pain).

PATIENT/FAMILY TEACHING:

Abrupt vitamin C withdrawal may produce rebound deficiency. Reduce dosage gradually. Foods rich in vitamin C include rose hips, guava, black currant jelly, brussel sprouts, green peppers, spinach, watercress, strawberries, citrus fruits.

asparaginase

ah-spa-**raj**-in-ace
(Elspar, Kidrolase✤)

▶CLASSIFICATION

PHARMACOTHERAPEUTIC: Enzyme. ***CLINICAL:*** Antineoplastic (see p. 68C)

ACTION/*THERAPEUTIC EFFECT*

Breaks down extracellular supplies of amino acid, asparagine (necessary for survival of these cells), *interfering with DNA, RNA, protein synthesis in leukemic cells.* Cell cycle-specific for G_1 phase of cell division.

PHARMACOKINETICS

Metabolized via slow sequestration by reticuloendothelial system. Half-life: 39–49 hrs IM; 8–30 hrs IV.

USES/*UNLABELED*

Treatment of acute lymphocytic leukemia (in combination with other agents). *Treatment of acute myelocytic leukemia, acute myelomonocytic leukemia, chronic lymphocytic leukemia, Hodgkin's disease, lymphosarcoma, reticulum cell sarcoma, melanosarcoma.*

PRECAUTIONS

CONTRAINDICATIONS: Previous anaphylactic reaction, pancreatitis, history of pancreatitis. ***CAUTIONS:*** Existing or recent chickenpox, herpes zoster, diabetes mellitus, gout, infection, liver function impairment, recent cytotoxic/radiation therapy.

✤ - Canadian trade name   ✳ - see also www.wbsaunders.com/SIMON/SaundersNDH

▷**LIFESPAN CONSIDERATIONS:**
Pregnancy/Lactation: If possible, avoid use during pregnancy, esp. first trimester. Breast feeding not recommended. **Pregnancy Category C. Children/Elderly:** No age-related precautions noted.

INTERACTIONS

DRUG: Steroids, vincristine may increase hyperglycemia, risk of neuropathy, disturbances of erythropoiesis. May decrease effect of **antigout medications.** May block effects of **methotrexate. Live virus vaccines** may potentiate virus replication, increase vaccine side effects, decrease pt's antibody response to vaccine. **HERBAL:** None known. **FOOD:** None known. **LAB VALUES:** May increase blood ammonia, BUN, uric acid, glucose, partial thromboplastin time (PTT), platelet count, prothrombin time (PT), thrombin time (TT), SGOT (AST), SGPT (ALT), alkaline phosphatase, bilirubin. May decrease blood clotting factors (plasma fibrinogen, antithrombin, plasminogen), albumin, calcium, cholesterol.

AVAILABILITY (Rx)

POWDER FOR INJECTION: 10,000 IU.

ADMINISTRATION/HANDLING

Note: May be carcinogenic, mutagenic, or teratogenic. Handle with extreme care during preparation/administration. Handle voided urine as infectious waste. Powder, solution may irritate skin on contact. Wash area for 15 min if contact occurs.

IM:

• Add 2 ml 0.9% NaCl injection to 10,000 IU vial to provide a concentration of 5,000 IU/ml. • Administer no more than 2 ml at any one site.

IV 🎇

Storage:

• Refrigerate powder for injection. • Reconstituted solutions stable for 8 hrs if refrigerated. • Gelatinous fiberlike particles may develop (remove via 5-micron filter during administration).

Reconstitution:

Note: Administer intradermal test dose (2 IU) prior to initiating therapy or when more than 1 wk has elapsed between doses. Observe pt for 1 hr for appearance of wheal or erythema.

Test Solution: Reconstitute 10,000 IU vial with 5 ml Sterile Water for Injection or 0.9% NaCl. Shake to dissolve. Withdraw 0.1 ml, inject into vial containing 9.9 ml same diluent for concentration of 20 IU/ml.

• Reconstitute 10,000 IU vial with 5 ml Sterile Water for Injection or 0.9% NaCl to provide a concentration of 2,000 IU/ml. • Shake gently to assure complete dissolution (vigorous shaking produces foam, some loss of potency).

Rate of administration:

• For IV injection, administer into tubing of freely running IV solution of D$_5$W or 0.9% NaCl over at least 30 min. • For IV infusion, further dilute with up to 1,000 ml D$_5$W or 0.9% NaCl.

IV INCOMPATIBILITY ⊘

None known. Consult pharmacy.

INDICATIONS/ROUTES/DOSAGE

Note: Dosage individualized based on clinical response, tolerance to adverse effects. When used in combination therapy, consult specific protocols for optimum dosage, sequence of drug administration.

Acute lymphocytic leukemia:

IV: **Adults, elderly, children:** Single agent: 200 IU/kg/day for 28 days.

IV: **Children:** Combination (with prednisone, vincristine): 1,000 IU/kg/day for 10 days beginning day 22 of treatment period.

IM: **Children:** Combination (with prednisone, vincristine): 6,000 IU/m^2 on days 4, 7, 10, 13, 16, 19, 22, 25, 28.

SIDE EFFECTS

FREQUENT: Allergic reaction (rash, urticaria, arthralgia, facial edema, hypotension, respiratory distress), pancreatitis (severe stomach pain with nausea/vomiting). **OCCASIONAL:** CNS effects (confusion, drowsiness, depression, nervousness, tiredness), stomatitis (sores in mouth/lips), hypoalbuminemia/uric acid nephropathy (swelling of feet or lower legs), hyperglycemia. **RARE:** Hyperthermia (fever or chills), thrombosis, seizures.

ADVERSE REACTIONS/TOXIC EFFECTS

Hepatotoxicity usually occurs within 2 wks of initial treatment. Increased risk of allergic reaction, including anaphylaxis, after repeated therapy, severe bone marrow depression.

NURSING IMPLICATIONS

BASELINE ASSESSMENT:

Before giving medication, agents for adequate airway and allergic reaction (antihistamine, epinephrine, O$_2$, IV corticosteroid) should be readily available. Hepatic, renal, pancreatic, CBC, blood chemistry, CNS functions should be performed before therapy begins and when a week or more has elapsed between doses.

INTERVENTION/EVALUATION:

Determine serum amylase concentration frequently during therapy. Discontinue medication at first sign of renal failure, pancreatitis (abdominal pain, nausea, vomiting). Monitor for hematologic toxicity (fever, sore throat, signs of local infection, easy bruising, unusual bleeding), symptoms of anemia (excessive tiredness, weakness).

PATIENT/FAMILY TEACHING:

Increase fluid intake (protects against renal impairment). Nausea may decrease during therapy. Do not have immunizations without physician's approval (drug lowers body's resistance). Avoid contact with those who have recently taken live virus vaccine.

aspirin (acetylsalicylic acid, ASA)

ass-purr-in
(Ascriptin, Bayer, Bufferin, Ecotrin, Entrophen✤, Halfprin, Novasen✤)

FIXED-COMBINATION(S)

With butabarbital, a barbiturate, and codeine, a narcotic **(Fiorinal);** with dipyridamole, an antiplatelet agent **(Aggrenox);** with oxycodone, a narcotic **(Percodan);** with pentazocine, an analgesic **(Talwin Cmpd);** with caffeine, a stimulant **(Anacin, Midol).**

►CLASSIFICATION

PHARMACOTHERAPEUTIC: Nonsteroidal salicylate ***CLINICAL:*** Anti-inflammatory, antipyretic, anticoagulant (see pp. 29C, 105C)

ACTION/*THERAPEUTIC EFFECT*

Produces analgesic, anti-inflammatory effect by inhibiting prostaglandin synthesis, *reducing inflammatory response and intensity of pain stimulus reaching sensory nerve endings.* Antipyresis produced by drug's effect on hypothalamus, producing vasodilation, *thereby decreasing elevated body temperature.* Inhibits platelet aggregation.

PHARMACOKINETICS

Rapidly, completely absorbed from GI tract; enteric-coated absorption delayed; rectal absorption delayed, incomplete. Protein binding: High. Widely distributed. Rapidly hydrolyzed to salicylate. Half-life: 15–20 min (aspirin); salicylate: 2–3 hrs at low dose; >20 hrs at high dose.

USES/*UNLABELED*

Treatment of mild to moderate pain, fever, inflammatory conditions. Treatment of transient ischemic attack, ischemic stroke, angina, acute myocardial infarction (MI), recurrent MI, specific revascularization procedures, rheumatologic diseases. *Prophylaxis against thromboembolism, treatment of Kawasaki disease.*

PRECAUTIONS

CONTRAINDICATIONS: Chickenpox or flu in children/teenagers, GI bleeding or ulceration, bleeding disorders, history of hypersensitivity to aspirin or NSAIDs, allergy to tartrazine dye, impaired hepatic function. ***CAUTIONS:*** Vitamin K deficiency, chronic renal insufficiency, those with "aspirin triad" (rhinitis, nasal polyps, asthma).

▷***LIFESPAN CONSIDERATIONS:*** **Pregnancy/Lactation:** Readily crosses placenta; distributed in breast milk. May prolong gestation and labor, decrease fetal birth weight, increase incidence of stillbirths, neonatal mortality, hemorrhage. Avoid use during last trimester (may adversely affect fetal cardiovascular system: premature closure of ductus arteriosus). **Pregnancy Category C (Category D** if full dose used in third trimester). **Children:** Caution in children with acute febrile illness (Reye's syndrome). **Elderly:** May be more susceptible to toxicity, lower doses recommended.

INTERACTIONS

DRUG: **Alcohol, NSAIDs** may increase risk of GI effects (e.g., ulceration). **Urinary alkalinizers, antacids** increase excretion. **Anticoagulants, heparin, thrombolytics** increase risk of bleeding. Large dose may increase effect **of insulin, oral hypoglycemics. Valproic acid, platelet aggregation inhibitors** may increase risk of bleeding. May increase toxicity of **methotrexate, zidovudine. Ototoxic medications, vancomycin** may increase ototoxicity. May decrease effect of **probenecid, sulfinpyrazone. HERBAL:** None known. **FOOD:** None known. **LAB VALUES:** May alter SGOT (AST), SGPT (ALT), alkaline phosphatase, uric acid; prolong prothrombin time, bleeding time. May decrease cholesterol, potassium, T_3, T_4.

AVAILABILITY (OTC)

TABLETS: 325 mg, 500 mg. ***TABLETS (chewable):*** 81 mg. ***TABLETS (enteric-coated):*** 81 mg, 165 mg, 325 mg, 500 mg, 650 mg, 975 mg. ***TABLETS (controlled-release):*** 650 mg, 800 mg. ***SUPPOSITORY:*** 120 mg, 200 mg, 300 mg, 600 mg.

ADMINISTRATION/HANDLING

PO:

• Do not crush or break enteric-coated or sustained-release form.
• May give with water, milk, or meals if GI distress occurs.

Rectal:

• Refrigerate suppositories. • If suppository is too soft, chill for 30 min in refrigerator or run cold water over foil wrapper. • Moisten suppository with cold water before inserting well up into rectum.

INDICATIONS/ROUTES/DOSAGE

Pain, fever:

***PO/RECTAL:* Adults, elderly:** 325–650 mg q4h as needed, up to 4 g/day.

Rheumatoid arthritis, osteoarthritis, other inflammatory conditions:

***PO:* Adults, elderly:** 3.2–6 g/day in divided doses.

Juvenile arthritis:

***PO:* Children:** 60–110 mg/kg/day in divided doses (q6–8h). May increase dose at 5–7 day intervals.

Acute rheumatic fever:

***PO:* Adults, elderly:** 5–8 g/day. **Children:** 100 mg/kg/day, then decrease to 75 mg/kg/day for 4–6 wks.

Thrombosis (decrease TIAs):

***PO:* Adults, elderly:** 1.3 g/day in 2–4 divided doses.

Thrombosis (decrease MI):

***PO:* Adults, elderly:** 300–325 mg/day.

Usual pediatric dosage:

***PO/RECTAL:* Children:** 10–15 mg/kg/dose q4h up to 60–80 mg/kg/day.

SIDE EFFECTS

OCCASIONAL: GI distress (cramping, heartburn, abdominal distention, mild nausea), allergic reaction (pruritus, urticaria, bronchospasm).

ADVERSE REACTIONS/TOXIC EFFECTS

High doses may produce GI bleeding and/or gastric mucosal lesions. Low-grade toxicity characterized by ringing in ears, generalized pruritus (may be severe), headache, dizziness, flushing, tachycardia, hyperventilation, sweating, thirst. Febrile, dehydrated children can reach toxic levels quickly. Marked intoxication manifested by hyperthermia, restlessness, abnormal breathing pattern, convulsions, respiratory failure, coma.

NURSING IMPLICATIONS

BASELINE ASSESSMENT:

Do not give to children/teenagers who have flu or chickenpox (increases risk of Reye's syndrome). Do not use if vinegarlike odor is noted (indicates chemical breakdown). Assess type, location, duration of pain, inflammation. Inspect appearance of affected joints for immobility, deformities, skin condition. Therapeutic serum level for antiarthritic effect: 20–30 mg/dl (toxicity occurs if levels are over 30 mg/dl).

INTERVENTION/EVALUATION:

Monitor urinary pH (sudden acidification, pH from 6.5 to 5.5), may result in toxicity. Assess skin for evidence of bruising. If given as antipyretic, assess temperature directly before and 1 hr after giving medication. Evaluate for therapeutic response: relief of pain, stiffness, swelling, increase in joint mobility, reduced joint tenderness, improved grip strength.

PATIENT/FAMILY TEACHING:

Do not crush or chew sustained-release or enteric-coated form. Report ringing in ears or persistent GI pain. Therapeutic anti-inflammatory effect noted in 1–3 wks.

atenolol   *💊*

ay-**ten**-oh-lol
(Apo-Atenol✢, Tenormin)
Do not confuse with albuterol.

FIXED-COMBINATION(S)

With chlorthalidone, a diuretic **(Tenoretic)**

▶CLASSIFICATION

PHARMACOTHERAPEUTIC:
Beta₁-adrenergic blocker. **CLINICAL:** Antihypertensive, antianginal, antiarrhythmic (see p. 60C)

ACTION/*THERAPEUTIC EFFECT*

Blocks beta₁-adrenergic receptors in cardiac tissue, *slowing sinus heart rate, decreasing cardiac output, decreasing B/P.* Large doses may block beta₂-adrenergic receptors, increasing airway resistance. *Decreases myocardial O₂ demand.*

PHARMACOKINETICS

Onset	Peak	Duration
PO (antiarrhythmic)		
1 hr	2–4 hrs	24 hrs
PO (antihypertensive)		
—	—	24 hrs

Incompletely absorbed from GI tract. Protein binding: 6–16%. Minimal liver metabolism. Primarily excreted unchanged in urine. Removed by hemodialysis. Half-life: 6–7 hrs (half-life increased in impaired renal function).

USES/*UNLABELED*

Management of mild to moderate hypertension. Used alone or in combination with diuretics, esp. thiazide type. Management of chronic stable angina pectoris. Reduces cardiovascular mortality in those with definite or suspected acute MI. *Hypertrophic cardiomyopathy, pheochromocytoma, prophylaxis of migraine, tremors, thyrotoxicosis, syndrome of mitral valve prolapse. Improves survival in diabetics with heart disease.*

PRECAUTIONS

CONTRAINDICATIONS: Overt cardiac failure, cardiogenic shock, heart block greater than first degree, severe bradycardia. **CAUTIONS:** Impaired renal or hepatic function, peripheral vascular disease, hyperthyroidism, diabetes, inadequate cardiac function, bronchospastic disease.

▷*LIFESPAN CONSIDERATIONS:*
Pregnancy/Lactation: Readily crosses placenta; distributed in breast milk. Avoid use during first trimester. May produce bradycardia, apnea, hypoglycemia, hypothermia during delivery, small birth weight infants. **Pregnancy Category D. Children:** No age-

💊 - see color pill atlas   <u>underscored</u> - top 100 prescribed drug

related precautions noted. **Elderly:** Age-related peripheral vascular disease, renal function requires caution.

INTERACTIONS

DRUG: Diuretics, other hypotensives may increase hypotensive effect; **sympathomimetics, xanthines** may mutually inhibit effects; may mask symptoms of hypoglycemia, prolong hypoglycemic effect of **insulin, oral hypoglycemics; NSAIDs** may decrease antihypertensive effect; **Cimetidine** may increase concentration. **HERBAL:** None known. **FOOD:** None known. **LAB VALUES:** May increase ANA titer, BUN, creatinine, potassium, uric acid, lipoproteins, triglycerides.

AVAILABILITY (Rx)

TABLETS: 25 mg, 50 mg, 100 mg. **INJECTION:** 5 mg/10 ml.

ADMINISTRATION/HANDLING
PO:

• May give without regard to meals. • Tablets may be crushed.

IV 🕮
Storage:

• Store at room temperature. • After reconstitution, parenteral form is stable for 48 hrs at room temperature.

Reconstitution:

• May give undiluted or dilute in 10–50 ml 0.9% NaCl or D_5W.

Rate of administration:

• Give IV push over 5 min. • Give IV infusion over 15 min.

IV INCOMPATIBILITIES ⊘

Amphotericin complex (AmbiSome, Abelcet, Amphotec).

INDICATIONS/ROUTES/DOSAGE
Hypertension:

PO: Adults: Initially, 25–50 mg once/day. May increase up to 100 mg once/day.

Angina pectoris:

PO: Adults: Initially, 50 mg once daily. May increase up to 200 mg once daily.

Usual elderly dosage:

PO: Initially, 25 mg/day for angina/hypertension.

Acute myocardial infarction:

IV: Give 5 mg over 5 min, may repeat in 10 min. In those who tolerate full 10 mg IV dose, begin 50 mg tablets 10 min after last IV dose followed by another 50 mg oral dose 12 hrs later. Thereafter, give 100 mg once/day or 50 mg twice/day for 6–9 days. (Alternatively, for those who do not tolerate full IV dose, give 50 mg orally 2 times/day or 100 mg once/day for at least 7 days.)

Dosage in renal impairment:

Creatinine Clearance	Dosage
15–35 ml/min	50 mg daily
<15 ml/min	50 mg every other day

SIDE EFFECTS

Generally well tolerated, with mild and transient side effects. **FREQUENT:** Hypotension manifested as dizziness, nausea, diaphoresis, headache, cold extremities, fatigue, constipation/diarrhea. **OCCASIONAL:** Insomnia, flatulence, urinary frequency, impotence or decreased libido. **RARE:** rash, arthralgia, myalgia, confusion (esp. in elderly), change in taste.

ADVERSE REACTIONS/TOXIC EFFECTS

Overdosage may produce profound bradycardia, hypotension. Abrupt withdrawal may result in sweating, palpitations, headache, tremulousness. May precipitate CHF, MI in those with cardiac disease, thyroid storm in those with thyrotoxicosis, peripheral ischemia in those with existing peripheral vascular disease. Hypoglycemia may occur in previously controlled diabetics. Thrombocytopenia (unusual bruising, bleeding) occurs rarely.

NURSING IMPLICATIONS

BASELINE ASSESSMENT:

Assess B/P, apical pulse immediately before drug is administered (if pulse is 60/min or below, or systolic B/P is below 90 mm Hg, withhold medication, contact physician). *Antianginal:* Record onset, type (sharp, dull, squeezing), radiation, location, intensity and duration of anginal pain, and precipitating factors (exertion, emotional stress). Assess baseline renal/liver function tests.

INTERVENTION/EVALUATION:

Monitor B/P for hypotension, pulse for bradycardia, respiration for shortness of breath. Assess pattern of daily bowel activity and stool consistency. Assess for evidence of CHF: dyspnea (particularly on exertion or lying down), night cough, peripheral edema, distended neck veins). Monitor I&O (increase in weight, decrease in urine output may indicate CHF). Assess extremities for coldness. Assist with ambulation if dizziness occurs.

PATIENT/FAMILY TEACHING:

Do not abruptly discontinue medication. Compliance with therapy essential to control hypertension, angina. To reduce hypotensive effect, rise slowly from lying to sitting position and permit legs to dangle from bed momentarily before standing. Avoid tasks that require alertness, motor skills until drug reaction is established. Report dizziness, depression, confusion, rash, unusual bruising or bleeding. Outpatients should monitor B/P, pulse before taking medication (teach correct technique). Restrict salt, alcohol intake. Therapeutic antihypertensive effect noted in 1–2 wks.

atorvastatin

ah-tore-**vah**-stah-tin
(Lipitor)

►CLASSIFICATION

PHARMACOTHERAPEUTIC: HMG-CoA reductase inhibitor. **CLINICAL:** Antihyperlipidemic (see p. 50C)

ACTION/THERAPEUTIC EFFECT

Inhibits HMG-CoA reductase, the enzyme that catalyzes the early step in cholesterol synthesis. *Decreases LDL cholesterol, VLDL cholesterol, and plasma triglycerides, increases HDL cholesterol.*

PHARMACOKINETICS

Poorly absorbed from GI tract. Protein binding: >98%. Metabolized in liver. Minimally eliminated in urine. Plasma levels markedly increased with chronic alcoholic liver disease, unaffected by renal disease. Half-life: 14 hrs.

USES

Adjunct to diet therapy to decrease elevated total and LDL cholesterol concentrations in those with primary hypercholesterolemia (types IIa and IIb) and in those with combined hypercholesterolemia and hypertriglyceridemia.

PRECAUTIONS

CONTRAINDICATIONS: Active liver disease, unexplained elevated liver function tests, pregnancy, lactation. ***CAUTIONS:*** Anticoagulant therapy, history of liver disease, substantial alcohol consumption, major surgery, severe acute infection, trauma, hypotension, severe metabolic, endocrine, or electrolyte disorders, uncontrolled seizures.

▷***LIFESPAN CONSIDERATIONS:*** **Pregnancy/Lactation:** Distributed in breast milk. Contraindicated during pregnancy. May produce skeletal malformation. **Pregnancy Category X. Children:** Safety and efficacy not established. **Elderly:** No age-related precautions noted.

INTERACTIONS

DRUG: **Antacids, colestipol, propranolol** decreases atorvastin activity. **Warfarin, digoxin, oral contraceptives, itraconazole** levels may increase concentration, producing severe muscle pain, inflammation, weakness. Increased risk of rhabdomyolysis, acute renal failure with **cyclosporine, erythromycin, gemfibrizol, nicotinic acid. *HERBAL:*** None known. ***FOOD:*** May be given without regard to meals. ***LAB VALUES:*** May increase creatinine kinase, serum transaminase concentrations.

AVAILABILITY (Rx)

TABLETS: 10 mg, 20 mg, 40 mg, 80 mg.

ADMINISTRATION/HANDLING

PO:

• May be given without regard to food. • Do not break film-coated tablets.

INDICATIONS/ROUTES/DOSAGE

Hyperlipidemia:

PO: Adults, elderly: Initially, 10 mg/day given as a single daily dose. **Dose range:** Increase at 2–4 wk intervals up to maximum of 80 mg/day.

SIDE EFFECTS

Generally well tolerated. Side effects usually mild and transient. ***FREQUENT*** (16%): Headache. ***OCCASIONAL*** (2–5%): Myalgia, rash/pruritus, allergy. ***RARE:*** Flatulence, dyspepsia.

ADVERSE REACTIONS/TOXIC EFFECTS

Potential for cataracts, photosensitivity.

NURSING IMPLICATIONS

BASELINE ASSESSMENT:

Question for possibility of pregnancy before initiating therapy (Pregnancy Category X). Assess baseline lab results: cholesterol, triglycerides, liver function tests.

INTERVENTION/EVALUATION:

Monitor for headache. Assess for rash, pruritus, malaise. Monitor cholesterol and triglyceride lab results for therapeutic response.

PATIENT/FAMILY TEACHING:

Follow special diet (important part of treatment). Periodic lab tests are essential part of therapy. Do not take other medications without physician's knowledge.

atovaquone ✳

ah-**tow**-vah-quon
(Mepron)

▶CLASSIFICATION

PHARMACOTHERAPEUTIC:
Systemic anti-infective. ***CLINI-CAL:*** Antiprotozoal

ACTION/*THERAPEUTIC EFFECT*

Inhibits mitochondrial electron-transport system at the cytochrome bc_1 complex (Complex III), *interrupting nucleic acid and ATP synthesis.*

USES

Treatment or prevention of mild to moderate *Pneumocystis carinii pneumonia* (PCP) in those intolerant to trimethoprim-sulfamethoxazole (TMP-SMZ).

PRECAUTIONS

CONTRAINDICATIONS: Development or history of potentially life-threatening allergic reaction to drug. ***CAUTIONS:*** Elderly, pts with severe PCP, chronic diarrhea, malabsorption syndromes.

INTERACTIONS

DRUG: **Rifampin** may decrease concentration, **atovaquone** may increase rifampin concentration. ***HERBAL:*** None known. ***FOOD:*** None known. ***LAB VALUES:*** May elevate SGOT (AST), SGPT (ALT), alkaline phosphatase, amylase. May decrease sodium.

INDICATIONS/ROUTES/DOSAGE

Pneumocystis carinii pneumonia (PCP):

PO: **Adults:** 750 mg with food 2 times/day for 21 days.

Prevention of PCP:
PO: **Adults:** 1,500 mg once daily with food.

Usual pediatric dosage:
PO: 40 mg/kg/day.

SIDE EFFECTS

FREQUENT (>10%): Rash, nausea, diarrhea, headache, vomiting, fever, insomnia, cough. ***OCCASIONAL*** (<10%): Abdominal discomfort, thrush, asthenia (loss of strength, energy), anemia, neutropenia.

ADVERSE REACTIONS/TOXIC EFFECTS

None significant.

NURSING IMPLICATIONS

INTERVENTION/EVALUATION:

Assess for GI discomfort, nausea, vomiting. Check consistency and frequency of stools. Assess skin for rash. Monitor I&O, renal function tests, hemoglobin. Monitor elderly closely because of decreased hepatic, renal, and cardiac function.

PATIENT/FAMILY TEACHING:

Continue therapy for full length of treatment. Do not take any other medication unless approved by physician. Notify physician in event of rash, diarrhea, or other new symptom.

atracurium

(Tracrium)

See Classification section under: Neuromuscular blockers (p. 102C)

atropine sulfate

ah-trow-peen
(Atropine Sulfate, Atropisol✤)

FIXED-COMBINATION(S)

With diphenoxylate, a constipating meperidine derivative **(Lomotil);** with hyoscyamine, scopolamine, an anticholinergic, and phenobarbital, a sedative-hypnotic **(Donnatal).**

▶CLASSIFICATION

PHARMACOTHERAPEUTIC: Belladonna alkaloid. **CLINICAL:** Anticholinergic, antispasmotic, antiarrhythmic, antidote (see p. 27C)

ACTION/*THERAPEUTIC EFFECT*

Inhibits action of acetylcholine on structures innervated by postganglionic sites (smooth/cardiac muscle, SA/AV nodes, exocrine glands). Larger doses may *decrease motility, secretory activity of GI system, tone of ureter, urinary bladder.*

USES

Prevents/reduces salivation and respiratory tract secretions in anesthesia. Treatment of cardiac arrhythmias, sinus bradycardia.

PRECAUTIONS

CONTRAINDICATIONS: Narrow-angle glaucoma, severe ulcerative colitis, toxic megacolon, obstructive disease of GI tract, paralytic ileus, intestinal atony, bladder neck obstruction due to prostatic hypertrophy, myasthenia gravis in those not treated with neostigmine, tachycardia secondary to cardiac insufficiency or thyrotoxicosis, cardiospasm, unstable cardiovascular status in acute hemorrhage. **EX-TREME CAUTION:** Autonomic neuropathy, known or suspected GI infections, diarrhea, mild to moderate ulcerative colitis. **CAUTIONS:** Hyperthyroidism, hepatic or renal disease, hypertension, tachyarrhythmias, CHF, coronary artery disease, gastric ulcer, esophageal reflux or hiatal hernia associated with reflux esophagitis, infants, elderly, systemic administration in those with COPD.

INTERACTIONS

DRUG: **Antacids, antidiarrheals** may decrease absorption. **Anticholinergics** may increase effects. May decrease absorption of **ketoconazole.** May increase severity of GI lesions with **KCl (wax matrix).** **HERBAL:** None known. **FOOD:** None known. **LAB VALUES:** None significant.

AVAILABILITY [Rx

INJECTION: 0.05 mg/ml, 0.3 mg/ml, 0.4 mg/ml, 0.5 mg/ml, 0.8 mg/ml, 1 mg/ml.

ADMINISTRATION/HANDLING

IM:
• May be given SubQ or IM.

IV 🔟
• Must be given rapidly (prevents paradoxical slowing of heart rate).

IV INCOMPATIBILITY ⊘
Pentothol (Thiopental).

IV COMPATIBILITIES
Heparin, potassium chloride, propofol (Diprivan).

INDICATIONS/ROUTES/DOSAGE

Anti-arrhythmic:

IV: Adults, elderly: 0.4–1 mg q1–2h as needed. **Maximum:** 2 mg. **Children:** 0.01–0.03 mg/kg. **Minimum:** 0.1 mg. **Maximum:** 0.5 mg (1 mg in adolescents).

Preoperative:

SubQ/IM/IV: **Adults, elderly, children >20 kg:** 0.4 mg (range: 0.2–0.6 mg) 30–60 min prior to time of induction of anesthesia or other preanesthetic medications. **Children (3 kg):** 0.1 mg; **(7–9 kg):** 0.2 mg; **(12–16 kg):** 0.3 mg.

Antisecretory:

IM: **Adults:** 0.2–0.6 mg 30–60 min before surgery. **Children:** 0.01–0.02 mg/kg/dose 30–60 min before surgery. **Maximum:** 0.4 mg.

SIDE EFFECTS

Note: Discontinue medication immediately if dizziness, increased pulse, or blurring of vision occurs. *FREQUENT:* Dry mouth/nose/throat (may be severe), decreased sweating, constipation, irritation at SubQ/IM injection site. *OCCASIONAL:* Swallowing difficulty, blurred vision, bloated feeling, impotence, urinary hesitancy. *RARE:* Allergic reaction (rash, urticaria), mental confusion/excitement (particularly children), fatigue.

ADVERSE REACTIONS/TOXIC EFFECTS

Overdosage may produce tachycardia, palpitations, hot/dry/flushed skin, absence of bowel sounds, increased respiratory rate, nausea, vomiting, confusion, drowsiness, slurred speech, CNS stimulation, psychosis (agitation, restlessness, rambling speech, visual hallucinations, paranoid behavior, delusions), followed by depression.

NURSING IMPLICATIONS

BASELINE ASSESSMENT:

Before giving medication, instruct pt to void (reduces risk of urinary retention).

INTERVENTION/EVALUATION:

Monitor changes in B/P, pulse, temperature. Assess skin turgor, mucous membranes to evaluate hydration status (encourage adequate fluid intake unless NPO for surgery), bowel sounds for peristalsis. Be alert for fever (increased risk of hyperthermia). Monitor I&O, palpate bladder for urinary retention. Assess stool frequency and consistency.

PATIENT/FAMILY TEACHING:

Take oral form 30 min before meals (food decreases absorption of medication). Avoid becoming overheated during exercise in hot weather (may result in heat stroke). Avoid hot baths, saunas. Avoid tasks that require alertness, motor skills until response to drug is established. Sugarless gum, sips of tepid water relieve dry mouth. Do not take antacids or medicine for diarrhea within 1 hr of taking this medication (decreased effectiveness). For preop use, explain that warm, dry, flushing feeling may occur. Remind pt to remain in bed and not eat or drink anything.

auranofin

aur-an-**oh**-fin
(Ridaura)
Do not confuse with Cardura.

aurothioglucose

ah-row-thigh-oh-**glue**-cose
(Solganal)

▶CLASSIFICATION

PHARMACOTHERAPEUTIC: Gold compound. *CLINICAL:* Antirheumatic

ACTION

Alters cellular mechanisms, enzyme systems, immune responses, collagen biosynthesis, *suppressing synovitis of the active stage of rheumatoid arthritis.*

PHARMACOKINETICS

Auranofin (29% Gold): Moderately absorbed from GI tract. Protein binding: 60%. Rapidly metabolized. Primarily excreted in urine. Half-life: 21–31 days. ***Aurothioglucose (≈ 50% Gold):*** Slow, erratic absorption after IM administration. Protein binding: High. Primarily excreted in urine. Half-life: 3–27 days (half-life increased with increased number of doses).

USES/*UNLABELED*

Management of rheumatoid arthritis in those with insufficient therapeutic response to NSAIDs. *Treatment of pemphigus, psoriatic arthritis.*

PRECAUTIONS

CONTRAINDICATIONS: History of gold-induced pathologies (necrotizing enterocolitis, exfoliative dermatitis, pulmonary fibrosis, blood dyscrasias), bone marrow aplasia, severe blood dyscrasias, serious adverse effects with previous gold therapy. ***CAUTIONS:*** Renal/hepatic disease, marked hypertension, compromised cerebral or cardiovascular circulation. Blood dyscrasias, severe debilitation, history of sensitivity to gold compounds, Sjörgren's syndrome in rheumatoid arthritis, systemic lupus erythematosus, eczema.

▷*LIFESPAN CONSIDERATIONS:* **Pregnancy/Lactation:** Crosses placenta; distributed in breast milk. Use only when benefits outweigh hazard to fetus. **Pregnancy Category C. Children:** No age-related precautions noted. **Elderly:** Age-related decreased renal function may require caution.

INTERACTIONS

DRUG:* Bone marrow depressants, hepatotoxic, nephrotoxic medications** may increase toxicity. **Penicillamine** may increase risk of hematologic or renal adverse effects. ***HERBAL: None known. ***FOOD:*** None known. ***LAB VALUES:*** May decrease hemoglobin, hematocrit, platelets, WBC. May alter liver function tests. May increase urine protein.

AVAILABILITY (Rx)

CAPSULES: 3 mg. ***INJECTION:*** 50 mg/ml suspension.

ADMINISTRATION/HANDLING
PO:

• Give without regard to food.

IM:

• Give in upper outer quadrant of gluteus.

INDICATIONS/ROUTES/DOSAGE
Rheumatoid arthritis:

Note: Give as weekly injections.

IM: Adults, elderly: Initially, 10 mg, then 25 mg for 2 doses, then 50 mg weekly thereafter until total dose of 0.8–1 g given. If pt is improved and there are no signs of toxicity, may give 50 mg at 3–4 wk intervals for many months. **Children (6–12 yrs):** Initially, 2.5 mg, then 6.25 mg for 2 doses, then 12.5 mg weekly thereafter until total dose of 200–250 mg given; thereafter, 6.25–12.5 mg q3–4 wks.

PO: Adults, elderly: 6 mg/day in 1 or 2 divided doses. If there is no response in 6 mos, may increase to 9 mg/day (in 3 divided doses).

If response is still inadequate, discontinue.

SIDE EFFECTS

FREQUENT: Auranofin: Diarrhea (50%), pruritic rash (26%), abdominal pain (14%), stomatitis (13%), nausea (10%). **Aurothioglucose:** Rash (39%), stomatitis (19%), diarrhea (13%). **OCCASIONAL:** Nausea, vomiting, anorexia, abdominal cramps.

ADVERSE REACTIONS/TOXIC EFFECTS

Signs of gold toxicity: decreased hemoglobin, leukopenia (WBC below 4,000/mm³), reduced granulocyte counts (below 150,000/mm³), proteinuria, hematuria, stomatitis (ulcers, sores, white spots in mouth, throat), blood dyscrasias (anemia, leukopenia, thrombocytopenia, eosinophilia), glomerulonephritis, nephrotic syndrome, cholestatic jaundice.

NURSING IMPLICATIONS

BASELINE ASSESSMENT:

Rule out pregnancy before beginning treatment. CBC, urinalysis, platelet count, renal and liver function tests should be performed before therapy begins.

INTERVENTION/EVALUATION:

Monitor daily bowel activity and stool consistency. Assess urine tests for proteinuria, hematuria. Monitor CBC, blood chemistries, renal and hepatic function studies. Question for pruritus (may be first sign of impending rash). Assess skin daily for rash, purpura or ecchymoses. Assess oral mucous membranes, borders of tongue, palate, pharynx for ulceration, complaint of metallic taste sensation (sign of stomati-

tis). Evaluate for therapeutic response: relief of pain, stiffness, swelling, increase in joint mobility, reduced joint tenderness, improved grip strength.

PATIENT/FAMILY TEACHING:

Therapeutic response may be expected in 3–6 mos. Avoid exposure to sunlight (gray to blue pigment may appear). Contact physician if pruritus, rash, sore mouth, indigestion, or metallic taste occurs. Maintain diligent oral hygiene.

azathioprine

asia-**thigh**-oh-preen
(Imuran)
Do not confuse with Imferon.

▶CLASSIFICATION

PHARMACOTHERAPEUTIC:
Immunologic agent. **CLINICAL:**
Immunosuppressant

ACTION

Antagonizes metabolism, inhibits RNA, DNA and protein synthesis, *suppressing cell-mediated hypersensitivities, alters antibody production, immune response in transplant recipients. Reduces arthritis severity.*

USES/UNLABELED

Adjunct in prevention of rejection in kidney transplantation; treatment of rheumatoid arthritis in those unresponsive to conventional therapy. *Treatment of inflammatory bowel disease, chronic active hepatitis, biliary cirrhosis, systemic lupus erythematosus, glomerulonephritis, nephrotic syndrome, inflammatory myopathy, myasthenia gravis, polymyositis, pemphigus, pemphigoid.*

PRECAUTIONS

CONTRAINDICATIONS: Pregnant rheumatoid arthritis pts. ***CAUTIONS:*** Immunosuppressed pts, those previously treated for rheumatoid arthritis with alkylating agents (cyclophosphamide, chlorambucil, melphalan), chickenpox (current or recent), herpes zoster, gout, decreased liver/renal function, infection.

INTERACTIONS

DRUG: **Allopurinol** may increase activity, toxicity. **Bone marrow depressants** may increase bone marrow depression. Other **immunosuppressants** may increase risk of infection or development of neoplasms. **Live virus vaccines** may potentiate virus replication, increase vaccine side effects, decrease pt's antibody response to vaccine. ***HERBAL:*** None known. ***FOOD:*** None known. ***LAB VALUES:*** May decrease hemoglobin, albumin, uric acid. May increase SGPT (ALT), SGOT (AST), alkaline phosphatase, amylase, bilirubin.

AVAILABILITY (Rx

TABLETS: 50 mg. ***INJECTION:*** 100 mg vial.

ADMINISTRATION/HANDLING
PO:

• Give during or after meal to reduce potential for GI disturbances. • Store oral form at room temperature.

IV ▥
Storage:

• Store parenteral form at room temperature. • After reconstitution, IV solution stable for 24 hrs.

Reconstitution:

• Reconstitute 100 mg vial with 10 ml Sterile Water for Injection to provide concentration of 10 mg/ml. • Swirl vial gently to mix and dissolve solution. • May further dilute in 50 ml D_5W or 0.9% NaCl.

Rate of administration:

• Infuse over 30–60 min. **Range:** 5 min–8 hours.

IV INCOMPATIBILITIES ⊘

Methyl and propyl parabens, phenol.

INDICATIONS/ROUTES/DOSAGE

Note: May give in divided doses if GI disturbance occurs.

Kidney transplantation:

IV: Adults, elderly, children: Initially, 3–5 mg/kg/day as single dose on day of transplant. ***PO:*** 3–5 mg/kg/day before or at the time of surgery. **Maintenance:** 1–3 mg/kg/day.

Rheumatoid arthritis:

PO: Adults: Initially, 1 mg/kg/day as single or in 2 divided doses. May increase by 0.5 mg/kg/day after 6–8 wks at 4 wk intervals up to maximum dose of 2.5 mg/kg/day. **Maintenance:** Lowest effective dose. May decrease dose by 0.5 mg/kg or 25 mg/day q4wks (other therapy maintained). **Elderly:** Initially, 1 mg/kg/day (50–100 mg); may increase by 25 mg/day until response or toxicity.

SIDE EFFECTS

FREQUENT: Nausea, vomiting, anorexia, particularly during early treatment and with large doses. ***OCCASIONAL:*** Rash. ***RARE:*** Severe nausea, vomiting with diarrhea, stomach pain, hypersensitivity reaction.

ADVERSE REACTIONS/TOXIC EFFECTS

Increased risk of neoplasia (new, abnormal growth tumors). Significant leukopenia, thrombocytopenia may occur, particularly in those undergoing kidney rejection. Hepatotoxicity occurs rarely.

NURSING IMPLICATIONS

BASELINE ASSESSMENT:

Arthritis: Assess onset, type, location and duration of pain, fever, or inflammation. Inspect appearance of affected joints for immobility, deformities, and skin condition.

INTERVENTION/EVALUATION:

CBC, platelet count, liver function studies should be performed weekly during first month of therapy, twice monthly during second and third months of treatment, then monthly thereafter. If rapid fall in WBC occurs, dosage should be reduced or discontinued. Assess particularly for delayed bone marrow suppression. Routinely watch for any change from normal. ***Arthritis:*** Evaluate for therapeutic response: relief of pain, stiffness, swelling, increase in joint mobility, reduced joint tenderness, improved grip strength.

PATIENT/FAMILY TEACHING:

Contact physician if unusual bleeding or bruising, sore throat, mouth sores, abdominal pain, or fever occurs. Therapeutic response in rheumatoid arthritis may take up to 12 wks. Women of childbearing age must avoid pregnancy.

azelaic acid   ✳

aye-zeh-**lay**-ick acid
(Azelex, Finevin)

▶CLASSIFICATION

PHARMACOTHERAPEUTIC:
Hypopigmentation agent. ***CLINICAL:*** Antiacne

ACTION/*THERAPEUTIC EFFECT*

Possesses antimicrobial action by inhibiting cellular protein synthesis in aerobic and anaerobic microorganisms, *improving acne vulgaris, normalizing keratin process.* Interrupts hyperactivity of normal melanocytes and their resulting growth in melasma, *reducing macular hyperpigmentation of facial or nuchal (back of neck) hair.*

USES/*UNLABELED*

Treatment of mild to moderate acne vulgaris. **Finevin:** Treatment of mild to moderate inflammatory acne vulgaris. *Treatment of melasma (hyperfunctioning melanocytes).*

PRECAUTIONS

CONTRAINDICATIONS: None significant. ***CAUTIONS:*** None significant.

INTERACTIONS

DRUG: None significant. ***HERBAL:*** None known. ***FOOD:*** None known. ***LAB VALUES:*** None significant.

AVAILABILITY (Rx)

CREAM: 20%.

INDICATIONS/ROUTES/DOSAGE

Antiacne, hypopigmentation:

TOPICAL: Adults, adolescents: Apply topically to affected area 2 times/day (morning and evening).

𝒪 - see color pill atlas

SIDE EFFECTS

OCCASIONAL (1–5%): Pruritus, stinging, burning, tingling. ***RARE*** (<1%): Erythema, dryness, rash, peeling, irritation, contact dermatitis.

ADVERSE REACTIONS/TOXIC EFFECTS

None significant.

NURSING IMPLICATIONS

INTERVENTION/EVALUATION:

Assess skin for erythema, dryness. Question pt regarding possible inflammatory reaction (burning, stinging, tingling of skin).

PATIENT/FAMILY TEACHING:

Inform pt mild burning, stinging, tingling of skin, and itching may occur at beginning of each treatment, may last 5–20 min but lessens with continued use. Contact physician if acne worsens, does not improve in first 4 wks, or if medication produces excessive redness, dryness, or peeling of skin. Avoid occlusive dressings. Keep away from mouth, eyes, other mucous membranes. Report abnormal changes in skin color or if skin irritation persists. Therapeutic improvement noted in about 4 wks.

azelastine

aye-zeh-**las**-teen
(Astelin, Optivar)

▶CLASSIFICATION

PHARMACOTHERAPEUTIC: Antihistamine. ***CLINICAL:*** Antiallergy

ACTION/*THERAPEUTIC EFFECT*

Prevents activation of basophils, mast cells, eosinophils, macrophages, and monocytes. Blocks synthesis, release, or target receptors of several mediators of immediate inflammatory response (e.g., histamine), *relieving allergic rhinitis.*

PHARMACOKINETICS

Onset	Peak	Duration
Nasal spray		
—	2–3 hrs	12 hrs
Ophthalmic		
—	3 min	8 hrs

Well absorbed through nasal mucosa. Primarily excreted in feces. Half-life: 22 hrs.

USES

Treatment of symptoms of seasonal allergic rhinitis (e.g., rhinorrhea, sneezing, nasal pruritus). Treatment of symptoms of vasomotor rhinitis (e.g., nasal congestion). Treatment of itching of eye associated with allergin conjunctivitis.

PRECAUTIONS

CONTRAINDICATIONS: History of hypersensitivity to antihistamines, newborn or premature infants, nursing mothers, third trimester of pregnancy. ***CAUTIONS:*** Renal function impairment.

▷***LIFESPAN CONSIDERATIONS:*** **Pregnancy/Lactation:** Unknown if drug crosses placenta or is distributed in breast milk. Do not use during third trimester. **Pregnancy Category C. Children:** Safety and efficacy not established in those <12 yrs of age. **Elderly:** No age-related precautions noted.

INTERACTIONS

DRUG: Alcohol, CNS depressants may increase CNS depression. **Cimetidine** may increase plasma concentration. **HERBAL:** None known. **FOOD:** None known. **LAB VALUES:** May suppress wheal and flare reaction to antigen skin testing unless drug is discontinued 4 days before testing. May increase SGPT (AST).

AVAILABILITY (Rx)

NASAL SPRAY: 137 mcg. **OPHTHALMIC SOLUTION:** 0.05%.

ADMINISTRATION/HANDLING

Nasal:

• Clear nasal passages as much as possible before use. • Tilt head slightly forward. • Insert spray tip into nostril, pointing toward nasal passage, away from nasal septum. • Spray into nostril while holding the other nostril closed and concurrently inhale though nose to permit medication as high into nasal passages as possible.

Ophthalmic:

• Tilt pt's head back; place solution in conjunctival sac. • Have pt close eyes; press gently on lacrimal sac for 1 min.

INDICATIONS/ROUTES/DOSAGE

Allergic rhinitis:

NASAL: Adults, elderly, children ≥5 yrs: 1–2 sprays into each nostril 2 times/day.

Vasomotor rhinitis:

NASAL: Adults, elderly, children ≥12 yrs: 2 sprays twice daily.

Allergic conjunctivitis:

OPHTHALMIC: Adults, elderly: 1 drop twice daily.

SIDE EFFECTS

FREQUENT (15–20%): Headache, bitter taste. **RARE:** Nasal burning, paroxysmal sneezing. **Ophthalmic:** Transient eye burning/stinging, bitter taste, headache.

ADVERSE REACTIONS/TOXIC EFFECTS

Epistaxis (nosebleed) occurs rarely.

NURSING IMPLICATIONS

BASELINE ASSESSMENT:

Question for hypersensitivity to antihistamines.

INTERVENTION/EVALUATION:

Assess therapeutic response to medication.

azithromycin

aye-**zith**-row-my-sin
(<u>Zithromax</u>)

▶CLASSIFICATION

PHARMACOTHERAPEUTIC: Macrolide. **CLINICAL:** Antibiotic (see p. 23C)

ACTION/*THERAPEUTIC EFFECT*

Binds to ribosomal receptor sites of susceptible organisms, *inhibiting protein synthesis.*

PHARMACOKINETICS

Rapidly absorbed from GI tract. Protein binding: Moderate. Widely distributed. Eliminated primarily unchanged via biliary excretion. Half-life: 68 hrs.

USES/*UNLABELED*

Treatment of mild to moderate infections of upper respiratory tract (pharyngitis, tonsillitis), lower respiratory tract (acute bacterial exacerbations, COPD, pneumonia), uncomplicated skin/skin structure infections, and sexually transmitted diseases (nongonococcal urethritis, cervicitis due to *Chlamydia trachomatis*), gonorrhea, chancroid. Prevents disseminated mycobacterium avium complex (MAC). Treatment of mycoplasma pneumonia. **Injection:** Community-acquired pneumonia, PID, acne. *Uncomplicated gonococcal infections of cervix, urethra, rectum; gonococcal pharyngitis, chlamydial infections.*

PRECAUTIONS

CONTRAINDICATIONS: Hypersensitivity to azithromycin, erythromycins, any macrolide antibiotic. **CAUTIONS:** Hepatic/renal dysfunction.

▷**LIFESPAN CONSIDERATIONS:** **Pregnancy/Lactation:** Unknown if distributed in breast milk. **Pregnancy Category B. Children:** Safety and efficacy not established in those <16 yrs for IV use and <6 mos for oral use. **Elderly:** No age related precautions in those with normal renal function.

INTERACTIONS

DRUG: May increase serum concentrations of **carbamazepine, cyclosporine, theophylline, warfarin. Aluminum/magnesium-containing antacids** may decrease concentration (give 1 hr before or 2 hrs after antacid). **HERBAL:** None known. **FOOD:** None known. **LAB VALUES:** May increase serum CPK, SGOT (AST), SGPT (ALT).

AVAILABILITY (Rx)

TABLETS: 250 mg, 600 mg. **INJEC-** **TION:** 500 mg. **ORAL SUSPEN-SION:** 100 mg/5 ml, 200 mg/5 ml.

ADMINISTRATION/HANDLING
PO:
• May give without regard to food.
• May store suspension at room temperature. Stable for 10 days after reconstitution. • Do not administer oral suspension with food. Give at least 1 hr before or 2 hrs after meals.

IV ▥
Storage:
• Store vials at room temperature.
• Following reconstitution, is stable for 24 hrs at room temperature or 7 days if refrigerated.

Reconstitution:
• Reconstitute each 500 mg vial with 4.8 ml Sterile Water for Injection to provide concentration of 100 mg/ml. • Shake well to ensure dissolution. • Further dilute with 250 or 500 ml 0.9% NaCl or D_5W or any combination thereof, including 20 mEq KCl or lactated Ringer's to provide final concentration of 2 mg with 250 ml diluent or 1 mg/ml with 500 ml diluent.

Rate of administration:
• Infuse over 60 min.

IV INCOMPATIBILITY ⊘
Information not available.

IV COMPATIBILITIES
None known; do not mix with other medication.

INDICATIONS/ROUTES/DOSAGE
Lower/upper respiratory tract, skin/skin structure infections:

PO: Adults, elderly: Initially, 500 mg on first day, then 250 mg on days 2–5 (total dose 1.5 g).

Prevention of MAC:

PO: Adults: 1,200 mg once/week.

Nongonococcal urethritis, cervicitis due to C. trachomatis:

PO: Adults: 1 g as a single dose.

Usual parenteral dosage:

IV: Adults: 500 mg/day followed by oral therapy.

Usual pediatric dosage:

PO: 10 mg/kg (**Maximum:** 500 mg) on day 1; then 5 mg/kg on days 2–5 (**Maximum:** 250 mg).

SIDE EFFECTS

OCCASIONAL: Nausea, vomiting, diarrhea, abdominal pain. **RARE:** Headache, dizziness, allergic reaction.

ADVERSE REACTIONS/TOXIC EFFECTS

Superinfections, esp. antibiotic-associated colitis (abdominal cramps, watery severe diarrhea, fever) may result from altered bacterial balance. Acute interstitial nephritis occurs rarely.

NURSING IMPLICATIONS

BASELINE ASSESSMENT:

Question pt for history of allergies to azithromycin, erythromycins, hepatitis.

INTERVENTION/EVALUATION:

Check for GI discomfort, nausea, vomiting. Determine pattern of bowel activity and stool consistency. Monitor hepatic function tests, assess for hepatotoxicity: malaise, fever, abdominal pain, GI disturbances. Evaluate for superinfection: genital/anal pruritus, sore mouth or tongue, moderate to severe diarrhea.

PATIENT/FAMILY TEACHING:

Continue therapy for full length of treatment. Doses should be evenly spaced. Take oral medication with 8 oz water at least 1 hr before or 2 hrs after food/beverage.

aztreonam

az-**tree**-oh-nam
(Azactam)

▶CLASSIFICATION

PHARMACOTHERAPEUTIC: Monobactam. **CLINICAL:** Antibiotic

ACTION/THERAPEUTIC EFFECT

Bactericidal effects due to inhibition of cell wall synthesis, *producing cell lysis, death.*

PHARMACOKINETICS

Completely absorbed following IM administration. Protein binding: 56–60%. Partially metabolized by hydrolysis. Primarily excreted unchanged in urine. Removed by hemodialysis. Half-life: 1.4–2.2 hrs (half-life increased in reduced renal, liver function).

USES/UNLABELED

Lower respiratory tract, skin/skin structure, intra-abdominal, gynecologic, complicated/uncomplicated urinary tract infections; septicemia. *Treatment of bone/joint infections.*

PRECAUTIONS

CONTRAINDICATIONS: None known. **CAUTIONS:** History of allergy, especially antibiotics, hepatic or renal impairment.

▷**LIFESPAN CONSIDERATIONS:**
Pregnancy/Lactation: Crosses

placenta, distributed in amniotic fluid; low concentration in breast milk. **Pregnancy Category B. Children:** Safety and efficacy not established in children <9 mos of age. **Elderly:** Age-related renal impairment may require dosage adjustment.

INTERACTIONS

DRUG: None known. **HERBAL:** None known. **FOOD:** None known. **LAB VALUES:** Positive Coombs' test. May increase SGOT (AST), SGPT (ALT), LDH, alkaline phosphatase, creatinine.

AVAILABILITY (Rx)

INJECTION: 500 mg, 1 g, 2 g.

ADMINISTRATION/HANDLING
IM:

• Shake immediately, vigorously after adding diluent. • Inject deeply into large muscle mass. • Following reconstitution for IM injection, solution is stable for 48 hrs at room temperature, or 7 days if refrigerated.

IV 🔲

Storage:

• Store vials at room temperature. • Solution appears colorless to light yellow. • Following reconstitution, solution is stable for 48 hrs at room temperature, or 7 days if refrigerated. • Discard if precipitate forms. Discard unused portions.

Reconstitution:

• For IV push, dilute each g with 6–10 ml Sterile Water for Injection. • For intermittent IV infusion, further dilute with 50–100 ml D_5W or 0.9% NaCl.

Rate of administration:

• For IV push, give over 3–5 min. • For IV infusion, administer over 20–60 min.

IV INCOMPATIBILITIES ⊘

Acyclovir (Zovirax), amphotericin (Fungizone), daunorubicin (Cerubidine), ganciclovir (Cytovene), lorazepam (Ativan), metronidazole (Flagyl), vancomycin (Vancocin).

IV COMPATIBILITIES

Aminophyllin, bumetanide (Bumex), diltiazem (Cardizem), dobutamine (Dobutrex), dopamine (Intropin), heparin, insulin, potassium chloride, propofol (Diprivan).

INDICATIONS/ROUTES/DOSAGE
Urinary tract infections:
IM/IV: Adults, elderly: 500 mg to 1 g q8–12h.

Moderate to severe systemic infections:
IM/IV: Adults, elderly: 1–2 g q8–12h.

Severe or life-threatening infections:
IV: Adults, elderly: 2 g q6–8h.

Usual pediatric dosage:
IV: 30 mg/kg q6–8h. **Maximum:** 120 mg/kg/day.

Dosage in renal impairment:
Dose and/or frequency is modified based on creatinine clearance, severity of infection:

Creatinine Clearance	Dosage
10–30 ml/min	1–2 g initially; then ½ the usual dose at usual intervals
<10 ml/min	1–2 g initially; then ¼ the usual dose at usual intervals

SIDE EFFECTS

OCCASIONAL (<3%): Discomfort/swelling at IM injection site, nausea, vomiting, diarrhea, rash. **RARE** (<1%): Phlebitis/thrombophlebitis at IV injection site, abdominal cramps, headache, hypotension.

ADVERSE REACTIONS/TOXIC EFFECTS

Superinfection, antibiotic-associated colitis (abdominal cramps, watery severe diarrhea, fever) may result from altered bacterial balance. Severe hypersensitivity reactions including anaphylaxis occur rarely.

NURSING IMPLICATIONS

BASELINE ASSESSMENT:

Question pt for history of allergies, esp. to aztreonam, other antibiotics.

INTERVENTION/EVALUATION:

Evaluate for phlebitis (heat, pain, red streaking over vein), pain at IM injection site. Assess for GI discomfort, nausea, vomiting. Monitor stool frequency and consistency. Assess skin for rash. Be alert for superinfection: increased temperature, sore throat, vomiting, diarrhea, black/hairy tongue, ulceration or changes of oral mucosa, anal/genital pruritus.

PATIENT/FAMILY TEACHING:

Report nausea, vomiting, diarrhea, rash.

bacampicillin

(Spectrobid)

See Classification section under: Antibiotic: penicillins

bacitracin

bah-cih-**tray**-sin
(Baciguent, Bacitracin, Baci-IM)

FIXED-COMBINATION(S)

With polymixin B, an antibiotic **(Polysporin);** with polymixin B and neomycin, antibiotics **(Mycitracin, Neosporin)**

▶**CLASSIFICATION**

PHARMACOTHERAPEUTIC: Anti-infective. ***CLINICAL:*** Antibiotic

ACTION/*THERAPEUTIC EFFECT*

Interferes with plasma membrane permeability in susceptible microorganisms, *inhibiting cell wall synthesis.* Bacteriostatic.

PHARMACOKINETICS

No information available for irrigation.

USES

Ophthalmic: Superficial ocular infections (conjunctivitis, keratitis, corneal ulcers, blepharitis). ***Topical:*** Minor skin abrasions, superficial infections. ***Irrigation:*** Treatment, prophylaxis of surgical procedures.

PRECAUTIONS

CONTRAINDICATIONS: None significant. ***CAUTIONS:*** None significant.

▷***LIFESPAN CONSIDERATIONS:*** **Pregnancy/Lactation:** Avoid parenteral use during pregnancy. **Pregnancy Category C. Children/Elderly:** No age-related precautions noted.

INTERACTIONS

DRUG: None significant. ***HERBAL:*** None known. ***FOOD:*** None known. ***LAB VALUES:*** None significant.

AVAILABILITY (Rx)

POWDER FOR IRRIGATION: 50,000 U. ***OPHTHALMIC OINTMENT. (OTC) TOPICAL OINTMENT.***

ADMINISTRATION/HANDLING

Ophthalmic:

• Place finger on lower eyelid and pull out until a pocket is formed between eye and lower lid. Place $1/4$–$1/2$ inch ointment in pocket. • Close eye gently for 1–2 min, rolling eyeball (increases contact area of drug to eye). Remove excess ointment around eye with tissue.

INDICATIONS/ROUTES/DOSAGE

Usual ophthalmic dosage:

Adults: $1/2$-inch ribbon in conjunctival sac q3–4h.

Usual topical dosage:

Adults, children: Apply 1–5 times/day to affected area.

Irrigation:

Adults, elderly: 50,000–150,000 units, as needed.

SIDE EFFECTS

Note: It is important to know side effects of components when bacitracin is used in fixed-combination. ***RARE: Topical:*** Hypersensitivity reaction (itching, burning, inflammation), allergic contact dermatitis. ***Ophthalmic:*** Burning, itching, redness, swelling, pain.

ADVERSE REACTIONS/TOXIC EFFECTS

Severe hypersensitivity reaction (hypotension, apnea) occurs rarely.

NURSING IMPLICATIONS

INTERVENTION/EVALUATION:

Topical: Evaluate for hypersensitivity: itching, burning, inflammation. With preparations containing corticosteroids, consider masking effect on clinical signs. ***Ophthalmic:*** Assess eye for therapeutic response or increased redness, swelling, burning, itching (hypersensitivity reaction).

PATIENT/FAMILY TEACHING:

Continue therapy for full length of treatment. Doses should be evenly spaced. Report burning, itching, rash, or increased irritation.

baclofen

back-low-fin (Apo-Baclofen❧, Lioresal, Liotec❧)

▶CLASSIFICATION

PHARMACOTHERAPEUTIC: Skeletal muscle relaxant. ***CLINICAL:*** Antispastic, analgesic in trigeminal neuralgia (see p. 117C)

ACTION/*THERAPEUTIC EFFECT*

Acts at spinal cord level *(decreases frequency/amplitude of muscle spasms in pts with spinal cord lesions)*.

PHARMACOKINETICS

Well absorbed from GI tract. Protein binding: 30%. Partially metabolized in liver. Primarily excreted in urine. Half-life: 2.5–4 hrs. Intrathecal: 1.5 hrs..

USES/*UNLABELED*

Relief of signs and symptoms of spasticity due to spinal cord injuries or diseases and multiple sclerosis, esp. flexor spasms, concomitant pain, clonus, and muscular rigidity. *Treatment of trigeminal neuralgia.*

❧ - Canadian trade name ✳ - see also www.wbsaunders.com/SIMON/SaundersNDH

PRECAUTIONS

CONTRAINDICATIONS: Skeletal muscle spasm due to rheumatic disorders, stroke, cerebral palsy, Parkinson's disease. ***CAUTIONS:*** Impaired renal function, CVA, diabetes mellitus, epilepsy, preexisting psychiatric disorders.

▷***LIFESPAN CONSIDERATIONS:*** **Pregnancy/Lactation:** Unknown if drug crosses placenta or is distributed in breast milk. **Pregnancy Category C. Children:** Safety and efficacy not established in those <12 yrs of age. **Elderly:** Increased risk of CNS toxicity (hallucinations, sedation, confusion, mental depression); age-related renal impairment may require decreased dosage.

INTERACTIONS

DRUG: Potentiated effects when used with other **CNS depressants** (including **alcohol**). ***HERBAL:*** None known. ***FOOD:*** None known. ***LAB VALUES:*** May increase SGOT (AST), SGPT (ALT), alkaline phosphatase, blood sugar.

AVAILABILITY (Rx)

TABLETS: 10 mg, 20 mg. ***AMPS:*** 500 mcg/ml, 2,000 mcg/ml.

ADMINISTRATION/HANDLING
PO:

• Give without regard to meals. • Tablets may be crushed.

INDICATIONS/ROUTES/DOSAGE
Musculoskeletal spasm:

***PO:* Adults:** Initially, 5 mg 3 times/day. May increase by 15 mg/day at 3 day intervals. **Range:** 40–80 mg/day. Total dose not to exceed 80 mg/day.

Usual elderly dosage:

PO: Initially, 5 mg 2–3 times/day. May gradually increase dose.

Usual intrathecal dosage:

Adults, elderly, children >12 yrs: 300–800 mcg/day. **Children ≤12 yrs:** 100–300 mcg/day.

SIDE EFFECTS

FREQUENT (>10%): Transient drowsiness, weakness, dizziness, lightheadedness, nausea, vomiting. ***OCCASIONAL*** (2–10%): Headache, paresthesia of hands/feet, constipation, anorexia, hypotension, confusion, nasal congestion. ***RARE*** (<1%): Paradoxical CNS excitement/restlessness, slurred speech, tremor, dry mouth, diarrhea, nocturia, impotence.

ADVERSE REACTIONS/TOXIC EFFECTS

Abrupt withdrawal may produce hallucinations, seizures. Overdosage results in blurred vision, convulsions, myosis, mydriasis, severe muscle weakness, strabismus, respiratory depression, vomiting.

NURSING IMPLICATIONS

BASELINE ASSESSMENT:

Record onset, type, location, and duration of muscular spasm. Check for immobility, stiffness, swelling.

INTERVENTION/EVALUATION:

Assess for paradoxical reaction. Assist with ambulation at all times. For those on long-term therapy, liver/renal function tests, blood counts should be performed periodically. Evaluate for therapeutic response: decreased intensity of skeletal muscle pain. Be alert to signs of infection.

✐ - see color pill atlas

PATIENT/FAMILY TEACHING:

Drowsiness usually diminishes with continued therapy. Avoid tasks that require alertness, motor skills until response to drug is established. Do not abruptly withdraw medication after long-term therapy. Avoid alcohol and CNS depressants.

balsalazide disodium

ball-**sall**-ah-zide
(Colazal)

►CLASSIFICATION

PHARMACOTHERAPEUTIC:
GI anti-inflammatory agent

ACTION/*THERAPEUTIC EFFECT*

Changes intestinal microflora, altering prostaglandin production, inhibiting function of natural killer cells, mast cells, neutrophils, macrophages, *diminishing inflammatory effect in colon.*

USES

Treatment of ulcerative colitis.

PRECAUTIONS

CONTRAINDICATIONS: Hypersensitivity to salicylates. ***CAUTIONS:*** Renal/liver impairment.

INTERACTIONS

DRUG: None significant. ***HERBAL:*** None known. ***FOOD:*** None known. ***LAB VALUES:*** May increase SGOT (AST); SGPT (ALT), alkaline phosphatase, bilirubin, LDH.

AVAILABILITY (Rx)

CAPSULES: 750 mg.

INDICATIONS/ROUTES/DOSAGE

Ulcerative colitis:

PO: Adults, elderly: Three 750 mg capsules 3 times/day for duration of 8 wks.

SIDE EFFECTS

FREQUENT (6–8%): Headache, abdominal pain, nausea, diarrhea. ***OCCASIONAL*** (2–4%): Vomiting, arthralgia, rhinitis, insomnia, fatigue, flatulence, coughing, dyspepsia.

ADVERSE REACTIONS/TOXIC EFFECTS

Hepatotoxicity occurs rarely.

NURSING IMPLICATIONS

INTERVENTION/EVALUATION:

Assess bowel sounds for peristalsis. Monitor daily bowel activity and stool consistency (watery, loose, soft, semisolid, solid). Assess for abdominal discomfort. Monitor blood serum chemistries for liver test abnormalities.

basiliximab

bay-zul-**ix**-ah-mab
(Simulect)

►CLASSIFICATION

PHARMACOTHERAPEUTIC:
Monoclonal antibody. ***CLINICAL:*** Immunosuppressive

ACTION/*THERAPEUTIC EFFECT*

Binds and blocks interleukin-2 receptor chains found on surface of activated T-lymphocytes, *inhibiting lymphocytic activity, thereby preventing cellular immune response involved in allograft rejection.*

PHARMACOKINETICS

Half-life: adults: 4–10 days, children: 5–17 days.

USES

Adjunct with cyclosporine, corticosteroids in the prophylaxis of acute organ rejection in pts receiving renal transplant.

PRECAUTIONS

CONTRAINDICATIONS: None significant. ***CAUTIONS:*** Infection, history of malignancy.
▷***LIFESPAN CONSIDERATIONS:***
Pregnancy/Lactation: Unknown if crosses placenta, distributed in breast milk. **Pregnancy Category B. Children/Elderly:** No age-related precautions noted.

INTERACTONS

DRUG: None significant. ***HERBAL:*** None known. ***FOOD:*** None known. ***LAB VALUES:*** Alters calcium, glucose, potassium, hemoglobin, hematocrit. Increases cholesterol, BUN, serum creatinine, uric acid. Decreases magnesium, phosphate, platelet count.

AVAILABILITY (Rx)

POWDER FOR INJECTION: 20 mg.

ADMINISTRATION/HANDLING

IV 🏮

Storage:

• Refrigerate. • Use within 4 hrs (24 hrs if refrigerated) • Discard if precipitate forms.

Reconstitution:

• Reconstitute with 5 ml Sterile Water for Injection. • Shake gently to dissolve. • Further dilute with 50 ml 0.9% NaCl or D_5W. Gently invert to avoid foaming.

Rate of administration:

• Infuse over 20–30 min.

IV INCOMPATIBILITY ⊘

Specific information not available. Other medications should not be added simultaneously through same IV line.

INDICATIONS/ROUTES/DOSAGE
Prophylaxis of organ rejection:

IV: **Adults, elderly:** Two doses of 20 mg each in reconstituted volume of 50 ml given as IV infusion over 20–30 min. Give first dose of 20 mg within 2 hrs before transplant surgery and the second dose of 20 mg 4 days after transplant. **Children:** 12 mg/m^2 as above.

SIDE EFFECTS

FREQUENT (>10%): GI disturbances (constipation, diarrhea, dyspepsia), CNS (headache, tremor, dizziness, insomnia), respiratory infection, dysuria, acne, leg/back pain, peripheral edema, hypertension. ***OCCASIONAL*** (3–10%): Angina, neuropathy, abdominal distention, tachycardia, rash, hypotension, urinary disturbances (hematuria, frequent micturation, genital edema), joint pain, increased hair growth, muscle pain.

ADVERSE REACTIONS/TOXIC EFFECTS

None significant.

NURSING IMPLICATIONS

BASELINE ASSESSMENT:

Obtain baseline BUN, creatinine, potassium, uric acid, glucose, calcium, phosphatase blood serum levels and vital signs, particularly B/P, pulse rate. Breast feeding not recommended.

INTERVENTION/EVALUATION:

Diligently monitor all blood serum levels. Assess B/P for hypertension/hypotension; pulse for evidence of tachycardia. Question for GI disturbances, CNS effects, urinary changes. Monitor for presence of wound infection, CBC, signs of infection (fever, sore throat, unusual bleeding/bruising).

PATIENT/FAMILY TEACHING:

Report difficulty in breathing or swallowing, rapid heartbeat, rash, or itching, swelling of lower extremities and weakness. Avoid pregnancy.

BCG, intravesical

(Immu Cyst ✦, Pacis, TheraCys, Tice BCG)

▶CLASSIFICATION

PHARMACOTHERAPEUTIC: Antineoplastic

ACTION/*THERAPEUTIC EFFECT*

Promotes local inflammation reaction with histiocytic and leukocytic infiltration in urinary bladder. *Inflammatory effects associated with apparent elimination/reduction of superficial cancerous lesions of urinary bladder.*

USES

Treatment of carcinoma in situ with or without associated papillary tumors; therapy for pts with carcinoma in situ of bladder following failure to respond to other treatment regimens. *TheraCys:* Treatment of primary and relapsed carcinoma in situ of urinary bladder (eliminates residual tumor cells, reduces frequency of tumor recurrence). *Tice BCG:* Pri-

mary or secondary treatment in absence of invasive cancer in pts with contraindication to radical surgery.

PRECAUTIONS

CONTRAINDICATIONS: Those on immunosuppressive or corticosteroid therapy, those who have compromised immune system, positive HIV virus, undetermined fever or fever due to infection, urinary tract infection, positive Mantoux test, as immunizing agent for tuberculosis prevention, within 1–2 wks following transurethral resection. *CAUTIONS:* None significant.

INTERACTIONS

DRUG: **Bone marrow depressants, immunosuppressants** may decrease immune response, increase risk of osteomyelitis of disseminated BCG infection. **Live virus vaccines** may potentiate virus replication, increase vaccine side effects, decrease pt's antibody response to vaccine. *HERBAL:* None known. *FOOD:* None known. *LAB VALUES:* None significant.

INDICATIONS/ROUTES/DOSAGE

Intravesical treatment and prophylaxis for carcinoma in situ of urinary bladder:

THERACYS:

INTRAVESICAL: **Adults, elderly:** Vials (in 50 ml saline) once weekly for 6 wks, then one treatment at 3, 6, 12, 18, 24 mos after initial treatment. Begin 7–14 days after biopsy or transurethral resection.

PACIS:

INTRAVESICAL: **Adults, elderly:** 1 amp in 50 ml saline/wk for 6 wks. May repeat once.

TICE BCG:

INTRAVESICAL: Adults, elderly: One amp in 50 ml preservative-free saline/wk for 6 wks. May repeat once. Thereafter, continue monthly for 6–12 mos.

SIDE EFFECTS

FREQUENT: Dysuria, urinary frequency, hematuria, hypersensitivity reaction manifested as malaise, fever, chills. **OCCASIONAL:** Cystitis, urinary urgency, nausea, vomiting, anorexia, diarrhea, myalgia/arthralgia. **RARE:** Urinary incontinence, cramping.

ADVERSE REACTIONS/TOXIC EFFECTS

Systemic BCG infection manifested as fever >103° or persistent fever >101° for more than 2 days or severe malaise has produced deaths. Infectious disease specialist should be notified and fast-acting antituberculosis therapy begun immediately.

NURSING IMPLICATIONS

BASELINE ASSESSMENT:
Pt symptoms usually begin 2–4 hrs after instillation and last 24–72 hrs.

INTERVENTION/EVALUATION:
Have pt sit to void after instillation. For 6 hrs postinstillation, urine should be disinfected with equal volume 5% hypochlorite solution (undiluted household bleach) before flushing. Diligently monitor renal status (assess for hematuria, urinary frequency, dysuria, urinalysis for bacterial urinary tract infection). Monitor closely for BCG systemic infection (see Adverse Reactions/Toxic Effects).

PATIENT/FAMILY TEACHING:
Contact physician/nurse if symptoms persist or increase or if any of the following occur: blood in urine, fever, chills, a frequent urge to urinate, joint pain, nausea and vomiting, or painful urination. Do not have immunizations without physician's approval (drug lowers body's resistance). Avoid contact with those who have recently taken live virus vaccine.

becaplermin

beh-**cap**-lear-min
(Regranex)

▶CLASSIFICATION

PHARMACOTHERAPEUTIC: Biological response modifier. **CLINICAL:** Growth factor

ACTION/*THERAPEUTIC EFFECT*

Platelet-derived growth factor that *stimulates body to grow new tissue* to heal open wounds.

USES

Treatment of lower extremity diabetic neuropathic ulcers extending into SubQ tissue or beyond.

PRECAUTIONS

CONTRAINDICATIONS: Skin neoplasms at site of application. **CAUTIONS:** Wounds showing exposed joints, tendons, ligaments or bones.

▷**LIFESPAN CONSIDERATIONS:** **Pregnancy/Lactation:** Unknown if distributed in breast milk. **Pregnancy Category C. Children:** Safety and efficacy not established in those <16 yrs of age. **Elderly:** No age-related precautions noted.

INTERACTIONS
DRUG: None significant. **HERBAL:** None known. **FOOD:** None known. **LAB VALUES:** None significant.

AVAILABILITY (Rx)
GEL: 100 mcg.

ADMINISTRATION/HANDLING
• Refrigerate gel. • Measure gel on a clean, nonabsorbable surface. • Transfer to ulcer and spread as a thin, continuous layer onto the ulcer. • With a gauze pad moistened with 0.9% NaCl, cover ulcer for 12 hrs; remove and wash any residual gel from ulcer and replace with new gauze pad moistened with 0.9% NaCl until time of next application.

INDICATIONS/ROUTES/DOSAGE
Ulcers:

TOPICAL: Adults, elderly: Apply once daily (spread evenly; cover with saline-moistened gauze dressing). After 12 hrs, rinse ulcer, recover with saline gauze.

SIDE EFFECTS
OCCASIONAL (2%): Local rash near ulcer.

ADVERSE REACTIONS/TOXIC EFFECTS
None significant.

NURSING IMPLICATIONS

INTERVENTION/EVALUATION:
Do not allow tip of tube to come in contact with the ulcer.

PATIENT/FAMILY TEACHING:
Dose requires recalculation weekly or biweeky, depending on rate of change in the width and length of ulcer.

beclomethasone dipropionate

B

beck-low-**meth**-ah-sewn (Beclodisk✤, Becloforte inhaler✤, Beclovent, Beconase, Beconase AQ, Qvar, Vancenase, Vancenase AQ [84 mcg], Vanceril, Vanceril Double Strength)
Do not confuse with baclofen.

▶CLASSIFICATION

PHARMACOTHERAPEUTIC: Adrenocorticosteroid. **CLINICAL:** Anti-inflammatory, immunosuppressant (see pp. 67C, 69C)

ACTION/THERAPEUTIC EFFECT
Inhalation: Decreases number, activity of inflammatory cells into bronchial wall, *inhibits bronchoconstriction, produces smooth muscle relaxation, decreases mucus secretion.* **Intranasal:** Inhibits early-phase allergic reaction, migration of inflammatory cells into nasal tissue, *decreasing response to seasonal and perennial rhinitis.*

PHARMACOKINETICS
Rapidly absorbed from pulmonary, nasal, and GI tissue. Protein binding: 87%. Metabolized in liver, undergoes extensive first-pass effect. Primarily eliminated in feces. Half-life: 15 hrs.

USES/UNLABELED
Inhalation: Control of bronchial asthma in those requiring chronic steroid therapy. **Intranasal:** Relief of seasonal/perennial rhinitis; prevention of nasal polyps from recurring after surgical removal; treatment of nonallergic rhinitis. *Nasal: Prophylaxis of seasonal rhinitis.*

✤ - Canadian trade name   ✳ - see also www.wbsaunders.com/SIMON/SaundersNDH

PRECAUTIONS

CONTRAINDICATIONS: Hypersensitivity to any corticosteroid, primary treatment of status asthmaticus, systemic fungal infections, persistently positive sputum cultures for *Candida albicans*, untreated localized infection involving nasal mucosa. ***CAUTIONS:*** Adrenal insufficiency, cirrhosis, glaucoma, hypothyroidism, untreated infection, osteoporosis, tuberculosis, sensitivity to beclomethasone.

▷***LIFESPAN CONSIDERATIONS:*** **Pregnancy/Lactation:** Unknown if drug crosses placenta or is distributed in breast milk. **Pregnancy Category C. Children:** Prolonged treatment/high doses may decrease short-term growth rate, cortisol secretion. **Elderly:** No age-related precautions noted.

INTERACTIONS

DRUG: None significant. ***HERBAL:*** None known. ***FOOD:*** None known. ***LAB VALUES:*** None significant.

AVAILABILITY (Rx)

AEROSOL FOR INHALATION. INTRANASAL: 42 mcg, 84 mcg per spray.

ADMINISTRATION/HANDLING

Inhalation:

• Shake container well, exhale completely, place mouthpiece between lips, inhale and hold breath as long as possible before exhaling. • Allow at least 1 min between inhalations. • Rinse mouth after each use to decrease dry mouth and hoarseness.

Intranasal:

• Clear nasal passages as much as possible. • Insert spray tip into nostril, pointing toward nasal passages, away from nasal septum. • Spray into nostril while holding other nostril closed and concurrently inspire through nose to permit medication as high into nasal passages as possible.

INDICATIONS/ROUTES/DOSAGE

Usual inhalation dosage:

INHALATION: **Adults, elderly children >12 yrs:** *(42 mcg):* 2 inhalations 3–4 times/day. **Maximum:** 20 inhalations/day. *(84 mcg):* 2 inhalations 2 times/day. **Maximum:** 10 inhalations/day. **Children 6–12 yrs:** *(42 mcg):* 1–2 inhalations 3–4 times/day. **Maximum:** 10 inhalations/day. *(84 mcg):* 2 inhalations 2 times/day. **Maximum:** 5 inhalations/day.

Usual intranasal dosage:

INTRANASAL: **Adults, children >12 yrs:** 1–2 sprays in each nostril 1–2 times/day. **Maximum:** 12 sprays/day. **Children 6–12 yrs:** 1–2 sprays in each nostril once daily.

SIDE EFFECTS

FREQUENT: Inhalation (4–14%): Throat irritation, dry mouth, hoarseness, cough. ***Intranasal:*** Burning, dryness inside nose. ***OCCASIONAL: Inhalation*** (2–3%): Localized fungal infection (thrush). ***Intranasal:*** Nasal-crusting nosebleed, sore throat, ulceration of nasal mucosa. ***RARE: Inhalation:*** Transient bronchospasm, esophageal candidiasis. ***Intranasal:*** Nasal/pharyngeal candidiasis, eye pain.

ADVERSE REACTIONS/TOXIC EFFECTS

Acute hypersensitivity reaction (urticaria, angioedema, severe bronchospasm) occurs rarely. Transfer from systemic to local steroid therapy may unmask previously suppressed bronchial asthma condition.

NURSING IMPLICATIONS

BASELINE ASSESSMENT:
Question for hypersensitivity to any corticosteroids.

INTERVENTION/EVALUATION:
In those receiving bronchodilators by inhalation concomitantly with inhalation of steroid therapy, advise pt to use bronchodilator several minutes before corticosteroid aerosol (enhances penetration of steroid into bronchial tree).

PATIENT/FAMILY TEACHING:
Do not change dose schedule or stop taking drug; must taper off gradually under medical supervision. **Inhalation:** Maintain careful mouth hygiene. Rinse mouth with water immediately after inhalation (prevents mouth/throat dryness, fungal infection of mouth). Contact physician/nurse if sore throat or mouth occurs. **Intranasal:** Contact physician if no improvement in symptoms, sneezing or nasal irritation occur. Clear nasal passages prior to use. Improvement noted in several days.

benazepril

ben-**ayz**-ah-prill
(Lotensin)

FIXED-COMBINATION(S)
With hydrochlorothiazide, a diuretic **(Lotensin-HCT)**; with amlodipine, a calcium channel blocker **(Lotrel)**

Do not confuse with Loniten, lovastatin.

▶ **CLASSIFICATION**
PHARMACOTHERAPEUTIC: Angiotensin-converting enzyme (ACE) inhibitor. *CLINICAL:* Antihypertensive (see p. 7C)

B

ACTION/*THERAPEUTIC EFFECT*
Decreases rate of conversion of angiotensin I to angiotensin II, a potent vasoconstrictor. Reduces peripheral arterial resistance, *lowers B/P.*

PHARMACOKINETICS

	Onset	Peak	Duration
PO	1 hr	2–4 hrs	24 hrs

Partially absorbed from GI tract. Protein binding: 97%. Metabolized in liver to active metabolite. Primarily excreted in urine. Minimal removal by hemodialysis. Half-life: 35 min; metabolite: 10–11 hrs.

USES/*UNLABELED*
Treatment of hypertension. Used alone or in combination with other antihypertensives. *Treatment of CHF.*

PRECAUTIONS
CONTRAINDICATIONS: History of angioedema with previous treatment with ACE inhibitors. *CAUTIONS:* Renal impairment, those with sodium depletion or on diuretic therapy, dialysis, hypovolemia, coronary or cerebrovascular insufficiency, liver impairment, diabetes mellitus.

▷*LIFESPAN CONSIDERATIONS:* **Pregnancy/Lactation:** Crosses placenta; unknown if distributed in breast milk. May cause fetal-neonatal mortality/morbidity. **First Trimester: Pregnancy Category C; Second and Third Trimester:**

Pregnancy Category D. Children: Safety and efficacy not established. **Elderly:** May be more sensitive to hypotensive effects.

INTERACTIONS

DRUG: Alcohol, diuretics, hypotensive agents may increase effects. **NSAIDs** may decrease effect. **Potassium-sparing diuretics, potassium supplements** may cause hyperkalemia. May increase **lithium** concentration, toxicity. **HERBAL:** None known. **FOOD:** None known. **LAB VALUES:** May increase potassium, SGOT (AST), SGPT (ALT), alkaline phosphatase, bilirubin, BUN, creatinine. May decrease sodium. May cause positive ANA titer.

AVAILABILITY (Rx)

TABLETS: 5 mg, 10 mg, 20 mg, 40 mg.

ADMINISTRATION

• May give without regard to food.

INDICATIONS/ROUTES/DOSAGE

Hypertension (used alone):

PO: Adults: Initially, 10 mg/day. **Maintenance:** 20–40 mg/day as single dose. **Maximum:** 80 mg/day.

Usual elderly dosage:

PO: Initially, 10 mg/day. **Range:** 20–40 mg/day.

Hypertension (combination therapy):

Note: Discontinue diuretic 2–3 days prior to initiating benazepril therapy.

PO: Adults: Initially, 5 mg/day titrated to pt's needs.

Dosage in renal impairment (Ccr <30 ml/min):

Initially, 5 mg/day titrated up to maximum of 40 mg/day.

SIDE EFFECTS

FREQUENT (3–6%): Cough, headache, dizziness. **OCCASIONAL** (2%): Fatigue, somnolence/drowsiness, nausea. **RARE** (<1%): Skin rash, fever, joint pain, diarrhea, loss of taste.

ADVERSE REACTIONS/TOXIC EFFECTS

Excessive hypotension ("first-dose syncope") may occur in those with CHF, severe salt/volume depletion. Angioedema (swelling of face/lips), hyperkalemia occur rarely. Agranulocytosis, neutropenia may be noted in those with impaired renal function or collagen vascular disease (systemic lupus erythematosus, scleroderma). Nephrotic syndrome may be noted in those with history of renal disease.

NURSING IMPLICATIONS

BASELINE ASSESSMENT:

Obtain B/P immediately before each dose, in addition to regular monitoring (be alert to fluctuations). If excessive reduction in B/P occurs, place pt in supine position with legs elevated. In those with renal impairment, autoimmune disease, or taking drugs that affect leukocytes or immune response, CBC should be performed before therapy begins and q2wks for 3 mos, then periodically thereafter.

INTERVENTION/EVALUATION:

Assist with ambulation if dizziness occurs. Monitor B/P, renal function, urinary protein, leukocyte count.

PATIENT/FAMILY TEACHING:

To reduce hypotensive effect,

rise slowly from lying to sitting position and permit legs to dangle from bed momentarily before standing. Full therapeutic effect may take 2–4 wks. Skipping doses or voluntarily discontinuing drug may produce severe, rebound hypertension.

benzocaine

(Americaine, Anbesol, Cetacaine, Chloroseptic Lozenges, Dermoplast, Hurricane, Orajel)
See Classification section under: Anesthetics: local

benzonatate

ben-**zow**-nah-tate
(Tessalon Perles)

▶CLASSIFICATION
PHARMACOTHERAPEUTIC: Non-narcotic antitussive. **CLINI-CAL:** Anticough

ACTION/*THERAPEUTIC EFFECT*
Anesthetizes stretch receptors in respiratory passages, lungs, and pleura, *thereby reducing cough production.*

USES
Relief of nonproductive cough including acute cough of minor throat/bronchial irritation.

PRECAUTIONS
CONTRAINDICATIONS: None significant. **CAUTIONS:** Productive cough.

INTERACTIONS
DRUG: CNS depressants may increase effect. **HERBAL:** None known. **FOOD:** None known. **LAB VALUES:** None significant.

AVAILABILITY (Rx)
CAPSULES: 100 mg.

ADMINISTRATION/HANDLING
PO:
• Give without regard to meals. • Swallow whole, do not chew/dissolve in mouth (may produce temporary local anesthesia/choking).

INDICATIONS/ROUTES/DOSAGE
Antitussive:
PO: Adults, elderly, children >10 yrs: 100 mg 3 times/day, up to 600 mg/day.

SIDE EFFECTS
OCCASIONAL: Mild drowsiness, mild dizziness, constipation, GI upset, skin eruptions, nasal congestion.

ADVERSE REACTIONS/TOXIC EFFECTS
Paradoxical reaction (restlessness, insomnia, euphoria, nervousness, tremors) has been noted.

NURSING IMPLICATIONS

BASELINE ASSESSMENT:
Assess type, severity, frequency of cough, and production.

INTERVENTION/EVALUATION:
Initiate deep breathing and coughing exercises, particularly in those with impaired pulmonary function. Monitor for paradoxical reaction. Increase fluid intake and environmental humidity to lower viscosity of

lung secretions. Assess for clinical improvement and record onset of relief of cough.

PATIENT/FAMILY TEACHING:
Avoid tasks that require alertness, motor skills until response to drug is established. Dry mouth, drowsiness, dizziness may be an expected response of drug.

benztropine mesylate ✳

benz-**trow**-peen
(Apo-Benztropine ✦, Cogentin)

►CLASSIFICATION

PHARMACOTHERAPEUTIC:
Anticholinergic. **CLINICAL:** Antiparkinson

ACTION/THERAPEUTIC EFFECT
Selectively blocks central cholinergic receptors, assists in balancing cholinergic/dopaminergic activity. *Reduces incidence, severity of akinesia, rigidity, and tremor.*

USES
Treatment of Parkinson's disease, drug-induced extrapyramidal reactions, except tardive dyskinesia.

PRECAUTIONS
CONTRAINDICATIONS: Angle closure glaucoma, GI obstruction, paralytic ileus, intestinal atony, severe ulcerative colitis, prostatic hypertrophy, myasthenia gravis, megacolon, children <3 yrs. **CAUTIONS:** Treated open-angle glaucoma, heart disease, hypertension, pts with tachycardia, arrhythmias, prostatic hypertrophy, liver/renal impairment, obstructive diseases of the GI or GU tract, urinary retention.

INTERACTIONS
DRUG: Alcohol, CNS depressants may increase sedation. **Amantadine, anticholinergics, MAO inhibitors** may increase effects. **Antacids, antidiarrheals** may decrease absorption, effects. **HERBAL:** None known. **FOOD:** None known. **LAB VALUES:** None significant.

AVAILABILITY (Rx)
TABLETS: 0.5 mg, 1 mg, 2 mg. **INJECTION:** 1 mg/ml.

INDICATIONS/ROUTES/DOSAGE
Idiopathic Parkinsonism:
PO/IM: Adults: Initially, 0.5–1 mg/day at bedtime up to 6 mg/day.

Postencephalitic Parkinsonism:
PO/IM: Adults: 2 mg/day as single or divided dose.

Drug-induced extrapyramidal symptoms:
PO/IM: Adults: 1–4 mg 1–2 times/day.

Acute dystonic reactions:
IM/IV: Adults: 1–2 mg, then 1–2 mg PO 2 times/day to prevent recurrence.

Usual elderly dosage:
PO: Initially, 0.5 mg 1–2 times/day, may increase by 0.5 mg q5–6days. **Maximum:** 6 mg/day.

SIDE EFFECTS
Note: Elderly (>60 yrs) tend to develop mental confusion, disorientation, agitation, psychotic-like symptoms.

FREQUENT: Drowsiness, dry mouth, blurred vision, constipation, decreased sweating/urination, GI upset, photosensitivity. ***OCCASIONAL:*** Headache, memory loss, muscle cramping, nervousness, peripheral paresthesia, orthostatic hypotension, abdominal cramping. ***RARE:*** Rash, confusion, eye pain.

ADVERSE REACTIONS/TOXIC EFFECTS

Overdosage may vary from severe anticholinergic effects (unsteadiness, severe drowsiness, severe dryness of mouth/nose/throat, tachycardia, shortness of breath, skin flushing). Also produces severe paradoxical reaction (hallucinations, tremor, seizures, toxic psychosis).

NURSING IMPLICATIONS

BASELINE ASSESSMENT:

Assess mental status for confusion, disorientation, agitation, psychotic-like symptoms (medication frequently produces such side effects in those >60 yrs).

INTERVENTION/EVALUATION:

Be alert to neurologic effects: headache, lethargy, mental confusion, agitation. Assess for clinical reversal of symptoms (improvement of tremor of head/hands at rest, masklike facial expression, shuffling gait, muscular rigidity).

PATIENT/FAMILY TEACHING:

Avoid tasks that require alertness, motor skills until response to drug is established. Dry mouth, drowsiness, dizziness may be an expected response of drug. Avoid alcoholic beverages during therapy. Drowsiness tends to diminish or disappear with continued therapy.

bepridil hydrochloride B

beh-prih-dill
(Bepadin, Vascor)
Do not confuse with Prepidil.

▶CLASSIFICATION

PHARMACOTHERAPEUTIC:
Calcium channel blocker. ***CLINICAL:*** Antianginal (see p. 61C)

ACTION/*THERAPEUTIC EFFECT*

Inhibits calcium ion entry across cell membranes of cardiac and vascular smooth muscle *(dilates coronary arteries, peripheral arteries/arterioles);* decreases heart rate, myocardial contractility, slows SA and AV conduction.

PHARMACOKINETICS

Rapidly, completely absorbed from GI tract. Protein binding: >99%. Undergoes first-pass metabolism in liver to active metabolite. Primarily excreted in urine. Not removed by hemodialysis. Half-life: <24 hrs.

USES

Treatment of chronic stable angina (effort-associated angina) in those who have failed to respond or are intolerant to other antianginal drugs. May be used alone or concurrently with beta-blockers, nitrates.

PRECAUTIONS

CONTRAINDICATIONS: Sick sinus syndrome/second- or third-degree AV block (except in presence of pacemaker), severe hypotension (<90 mm Hg, systolic), history of serious ventricular arrhythmias, uncompensated cardiac insufficiency, congenital QT interval prolongation, use with other drugs prolonging QT interval. **CAUTIONS:** Impaired renal/hepatic function, CHF.

▷**LIFESPAN CONSIDERATIONS:**
Pregnancy/Lactation: Unknown if drug crosses placenta. Distributed in breast milk. **Pregnancy Category C. Children:** No age-related precautions noted. **Elderly:** Age-related renal impairment may require caution.

INTERACTIONS

DRUG: Beta-blockers may have additive effect. May increase **digoxin** concentration. **Procainamide, quinidine** may increase risk of QT interval prolongation. **Hypokalemia-producing agents** may increase risk of arrhythmias. **HERBAL:** None known. **FOOD: Grapefruit juice** may increase serum levels, effect. **LAB VALUES:** QT interval may be increased.

AVAILABILITY (Rx)

TABLETS: 200 mg, 300 mg, 400 mg.

ADMINISTRATION/HANDLING
PO:

• Do not crush or break film-coated tablets. • May give without regard to food. May give with meals and at bedtime (decreases risk of nausea).

INDICATIONS/ROUTES/DOSAGE
Chronic stable angina:

PO: Adults, elderly: Initially, 200 mg/day; after 10 days, dosage may be adjusted. **Maintenance:** 200–400 mg/day.

SIDE EFFECTS

FREQUENT (9–27%): Dizziness, lightheadedness, nervousness, headache, asthenia (loss of strength), hand tremor, nausea, diarrhea. **OCCASIONAL** (3–8%): Drowsiness, insomnia, tinnitus, abdominal discomfort, palpitations, dry mouth, shortness of breath, wheezing, anorexia, constipation. **RARE** (<2%): Peripheral edema, anxiety, flatulence, nasal congestion, paresthesia.

ADVERSE REACTIONS/TOXIC EFFECTS

Can induce serious arrhythmias. CHF, second- and third-degree AV block occur rarely. Overdosage produces nausea, drowsiness, confusion, slurred speech, profound bradycardia.

NURSING IMPLICATIONS

BASELINE ASSESSMENT:

Record onset, type (sharp, dull, squeezing), radiation, location, intensity, and duration of anginal pain, and precipitating factors (exertion, emotional stress). Assess pulse rate, EKG for arrhythmias before drug is administered.

INTERVENTION/EVALUATION:

Assist with ambulation if lightheadedness, dizziness, drowsiness occur. Question for asthenia, headache, ringing/roaring in ears. Assess EKG for arrhythmias, lung sounds for rales, wheezing.

PATIENT/FAMILY TEACHING:

Do not abruptly discontinue medication. Compliance with therapy regimen is essential to control anginal pain. To avoid hypotensive effect, rise slowly from lying to sitting position, wait momentarily before standing. Avoid tasks that require alertness, motor skills until response to drug is established. Contact physician/nurse if irregular heartbeat, shortness of breath, pronounced dizziness, nausea, dyspepsia, ringing/roaring in ears, or constipation occurs. Avoid grapefruit/grapefruit juice.

beractant

burr-**act**-tant
(Survanta)
Do not confuse with Sufenta.

▶CLASSIFICATION

PHARMACOTHERAPEUTIC:
Natural bovine lung extract.
CLINICAL: Pulmonary surfactant

ACTION/*THERAPEUTIC EFFECT*

Lowers surface tension on alveolar surfaces during respiration, stabilizes alveoli vs. collapse that may occur at resting transpulmonary pressures. *Replenishes surfactant, restores surface activity to lungs.*

PHARMACOKINETICS

Not absorbed systemically.

USES

Prevention/treatment (rescue) of respiratory distress syndrome (RDS—hyaline membrane disease) in premature infants. Oxygenation improves within minutes of administration.

PRECAUTIONS

CONTRAINDICATIONS: None significant. ***CAUTIONS:*** Those at risk for circulatory overload.
▷*LIFESPAN CONSIDERATIONS:*
Neonate: No age-related precautions noted for neonate.

INTERACTIONS

DRUG: None significant. ***HERBAL:*** None known. ***FOOD:*** None known. ***LAB VALUES:*** None significant.

AVAILABILITY (Rx)

SUSPENSION: 25 mg/ml vial.

ADMINISTRATION/HANDLING
Intratracheal:
Storage:
• Refrigerate vials. • Warm by standing vial at room temperature for 20 min or warm in hand 8 min. • If settling occurs, gently swirl vial (do not shake) to redisperse. • After warming, may return to refrigerator within 8 hrs one time only. • Each vial should be injected with a needle only one time; discard unused portions. • Color appears off-white to light brown.

Administration:
• Instill through catheter inserted into infant's endotracheal tube. Do not instill into main stem bronchus. • Monitor for bradycardia, decreased O_2 saturation during administration. Stop dosing procedure if these effects occur; begin appropriate measures before reinstituting therapy.

INDICATIONS/ROUTES/DOSAGE
Usual dosage:
INTRATRACHEAL: **Infants:** 100 mg of phospholipids/kg birth weight (4 ml/kg). Give within 15 min of birth if infant <1,250 g with evidence of surfactant deficiency; give within 8 hrs when RDS confirmed by x-ray and requiring mechanical ventilation. May repeat no sooner than 6 hrs after preceding dose.

SIDE EFFECTS
FREQUENT: Transient bradycardia, O_2 desaturation; increased CO_2 tension. ***OCCASIONAL:*** Endotracheal tube reflux. ***RARE:*** Apnea, endotracheal tube block-

age, hypo/hypertension, pallor, vasoconstriction.

ADVERSE REACTIONS/TOXIC EFFECTS

Nosocomial sepsis may occur associated with increased mortality).

NURSING IMPLICATIONS

BASELINE ASSESSMENT:

Drug must be administered in highly supervised setting. Clinicians in care of neonate must be experienced with intubation, ventilator management. Offer emotional support to parents.

INTERVENTION/EVALUATION:

Monitor infant with arterial or transcutaneous measurement of systemic O_2 and CO_2. Assess lung sounds for rales and moist breath sounds.

betamethasone

bay-tah-**meth**-a-sone
(Alphatrex, Beben♣, Betaderm♣, Betatrex, , Beta-Val, Betnesol♣ Celestone, Cel-U-Jec, Diprolene, Diprosone, Luxig Foam, Selestoject, Uticort, Valisone)

FIXED-COMBINATION(S)

Betamethasone sodium phosphate with betamethasone acetate **(Celestone Soluspan)**. Betamethasone dipropionate with clotrimazole, an antifungal **(Lotrisone)**

▶CLASSIFICATION

PHARMACOTHERAPEUTIC: Adrenocorticosteroid. ***CLINI-CAL:*** Anti-inflammatory, immunosuppressant (see pp. 67C, 69C)

ACTION/*THERAPEUTIC EFFECT*

Systemic: Inhibits accumulation of inflammatory cells at inflammation sites, inhibits synthesis of mediators of inflammation, *decreases tissue response to inflammatory process.* **Topical:** Forms complexes that enter cell nucleus stimulating formation of enzymes, *reducing inflammatory effect.*

PHARMACOKINETICS

Rapidly, completely absorbed after PO, IM administration. Metabolized in liver, kidneys, tissue. Primarily excreted in urine. Half-life: 3–5 hrs.

USES

Substitution therapy in *deficiency states:* acute/chronic adrenal insufficiency, congenital adrenal hyperplasia, adrenal insufficiency secondary to pituitary insufficiency. *Nonendocrine disorders:* arthritis, rheumatic carditis, allergic, collagen, intestinal tract, liver, ocular, renal, and skin diseases, bronchial asthma, cerebral edema, malignancies. **Topical:** Relief of inflammatory and pruritic dermatoses. **Foam:** Relief of inflammation, itching associated with dermatosis.

PRECAUTIONS

CONTRAINDICATIONS: Hypersensitivity to any corticosteroid or sulfite, systemic fungal infection, peptic ulcers (except life-threatening situations). Avoid live virus vaccine such as smallpox. **Topical:** Marked circulation impairment. ***CAUTIONS:*** Hypothyroidism, cirrhosis, ocular herpes simplex, history of tuberculosis (may reactivate disease), nonspecific ulcerative colitis, CHF, hypertension, psychosis, renal insufficiency. Prolonged therapy should be discontinued slowly. **Topical:** Do not apply to extensive areas.

> **LIFESPAN CONSIDERATIONS:**
Pregnancy/Lactation: Drug crosses placenta, distributed in breast milk. May cause cleft palate (chronic use first trimester). Nursing contraindicated. **Pregnancy Category C. Children:** Prolonged treatment/high dose may decrease short-term growth rate, cortisol secretion. **Elderly:** More likely to develop hypertension, osteoporosis.

INTERACTIONS

DRUG: Amphotericin may increase hypokalemia. May decrease effect of **oral hypoglycemics, insulin, diuretics, potassium supplements.** May increase **digoxin** toxicity (due to hypokalemia). **Hepatic enzyme inducers** may decrease effect. **Live virus vaccines** may potentiate virus replication, increase vaccine side effects, decrease pt's antibody response to vaccine. **HERBAL:** None known. **FOOD:** None known. **LAB VALUES:** May decrease calcium, potassium, thyroxine. May increase cholesterol, lipids, glucose, sodium, amylase.

AVAILABILITY (Rx)

TABLETS: 0.6 mg. **SYRUP:** 0.6 mg/5 ml. **INJECTION, CREAM:** 0.025%, 0.05%, 0.01%, 0.1%. **LOTION:** 0.025%, 0.05%, 0.1%. **GEL:** 0.025%. **OINTMENT:** 0.05%, 0.1%. **AEROSOL:** 0.1%.

ADMINISTRATION/HANDLING
PO:

• Give with milk or food (decreases GI upset). • Give single doses prior to 9 AM; multiple doses should be given at evenly spaced intervals.

Topical:

• Gently cleanse area prior to application. • Use occlusive dressings only as ordered. • Apply sparingly and rub into area thoroughly. • When using aerosol, spray area 3 sec from 15 cm distance; avoid inhalation.

IM:

• Celestone Soluspan should not be mixed with diluent or anesthetics containing preservatives.

INDICATIONS/ROUTES/DOSAGE
Usual dosage:

PO: Adults, elderly: 0.6–7.2 mg/day. **Children:** 0.063–0.25 mg/kg/day in 3–4 divided doses.

IM/IV: Up to 9 mg/day.

Usual topical dosage:

Adults, elderly: 2–4 times/day. **FOAM:** Apply twice daily.

SIDE EFFECTS

FREQUENT: Systemic: Increased appetite, abdominal distention, nervousness, insomnia, false sense of well-being. **Foam:** Burning, stinging, pruritus. **OCCASIONAL: Systemic:** Dizziness, facial flushing, diaphoresis, decreased/blurred vision, mood swings. **Topical:** Allergic contact dermatitis, purpura (blood-containing blisters, thinning of skin with easy bruising), telangiectasis (raised dark red spots on skin). **RARE: Systemic:** General allergic reaction (rash, hives), pain/redness/swelling at injection site, hallucinations, mental depression.

ADVERSE REACTIONS/TOXIC EFFECTS

High-dose or long-term therapy: acne, Cushing syndrome (moon face), muscle wasting (esp. arms, legs), osteoporosis, bone fractures, cataracts, glaucoma, psychosis, diabetes mellitus, pancreatitis, peptic ulcer, amenorrhea, poor healing, hypercalcemia, hypokalemia. Abrupt withdrawal following long-term therapy: anorexia, nausea, fever, headache, joint pain, rebound inflammation, fatigue, weakness, lethargy, dizziness, orthostatic hypotension.

NURSING IMPLICATIONS

BASELINE ASSESSMENT:

Question for hypersensitivity to any of the corticosteroids, sulfite. Obtain baselines for height, weight, B/P, glucose, electrolytes. Check results of initial tests (e.g., TB skin test, x-rays, EKG).

INTERVENTION/EVALUATION:

Monitor I&O, daily weight; assess for edema. Check lab results for blood coagulability and clinical evidence of thromboembolism. Be alert to infection: sore throat, fever, or vague symptoms. Monitor electrolytes. Assess for hypocalcemia (muscle twitching, cramps, positive Trousseau's or Chvostek's signs) or hypokalemia (weakness and muscle cramps, numbness/tingling esp. lower extremities, nausea and vomiting, irritability, EKG changes). Assess emotional status, ability to sleep.

PATIENT/FAMILY TEACHING:

Take with food or milk. Do not change dose/schedule or stop taking drug; must taper off gradually under medical supervision. Notify physician of fever, sore throat, muscle aches, sudden weight gain/swelling. Maintain careful personal hygiene, avoid exposure to disease or trauma. Severe stress (serious infection, surgery, or trauma) may require increased dosage. Inform dentist or other physicians of betamethasone therapy now or within past 12 mos. **Topical:** Apply after shower or bath for best absorption. Do not cover unless physician orders; do not use tight diapers, plastic pants or coverings. Do not expose treated area to sunlight.

betaxolol   ✴

beh-**tax**-oh-lol
(Kerlone, Betoptic)

▶CLASSIFICATION

PHARMACOTHERAPEUTIC:
Beta-adrenergic blocker. ***CLINICAL:*** Antihypertensive; antiglaucoma (see p. 58C)

ACTION/*THERAPEUTIC EFFECT*

Systemic: Predominantly blocks beta$_1$-adrenergic receptors in cardiac tissue by binding to receptor sites, *slowing sinus heart rate, decreasing cardiac output, decreasing B/P.* Large doses may block beta$_2$ receptors, *increasing airway resistance.* **Ophthalmic:** Reduces aqueous humor production, *decreasing intraocular pressure.*

USES/*UNLABELED*

Management of mild to moderate hypertension. Used alone or in combination with diuretics, esp. thiazide type. Reduces intraocular pressure (IOP) in management of chronic open-angle glaucoma, ocular hypertension. *With miotics, decreases IOP in acute/chronic angle closure glaucoma, treatment of secondary glaucoma, malignant glaucoma, angle closure glaucoma during/after iridectomy.*

PRECAUTIONS

CONTRAINDICATIONS: Sinus bradycardia, overt cardiac failure, cardiogenic shock, heart block greater than first degree. **CAUTIONS:** Impaired renal or hepatic function, peripheral vascular disease, hyperthyroidism, diabetes, inadequate cardiac function.

INTERACTIONS

DRUG: Diuretics, other hypotensives may increase hypotensive effect; **sympathomimetics, xanthines** may mutually inhibit effect; may mask symptoms of hypoglycemia, prolong hypoglycemic effect of **insulin, oral hypoglycemics; NSAIDs** may decrease antihypertensive effect; **cimetidine** may increase concentration. **HERBAL:** None known. **FOOD:** None known. **LAB VALUES:** May increase ANA titer, BUN, creatinine, potassium, uric acid, lipoproteins, triglycerides.

AVAILABILITY (Rx)

TABLETS: 10 mg, 20 mg. **OPHTHALMIC SOLUTION:** 0.5%. **OPHTHALMIC SUSPENSION:** 0.25%.

INDICATIONS/ROUTES/DOSAGE

Hypertension:

PO: Adults: Initially, 10 mg/day alone or added to diuretic therapy. Dose may be doubled if no response in 7–14 days. If used alone, addition of another antihypertensive to be considered.

Usual elderly dosage:

PO: Initially, 5 mg/day.

Dosage in renal impairment (dialysis):

Initially 5 mg/day, increase by 5 mg/day q2wks. **Maximum:** 20 mg/day.

Glaucoma:

EYEDROPS: Adults, elderly: 1 drop 2 times/day.

SIDE EFFECTS

Generally well tolerated, with mild and transient side effects. **FREQUENT: Systemic:** Hypotension manifested as dizziness, nausea, diaphoresis, headache, fatigue, constipation/diarrhea; shortness of breath. **Ophthalmic:** Eye irritation, visual disturbances. **OCCASIONAL: Systemic:** Insomnia, flatulence, urinary frequency, impotence or decreased libido. **Ophthalmic:** Increased light sensitivity, watering of eye. **RARE: Systemic:** Rash, arrhythmias, arthralgia, myalgia, confusion, change in taste, increased urination. **Ophthalmic:** Dry eye, conjunctivitis, eye pain.

ADVERSE REACTIONS/TOXIC EFFECTS

Oral form may produce profound bradycardia, hypotension, bronchospasm. Abrupt withdrawal may result in sweating, palpitations, headache, tremulousness. May precipitate CHF, MI in those with cardiac disease, thyroid storm in those with thyrotoxicosis, peripheral ischemia in those with existing peripheral vascular disease. Hypoglycemia may occur in previously controlled diabetics. Ophthalmic overdosage may produce bradycardia, hypotension, bronchospasm, acute cardiac failure.

NURSING IMPLICATIONS

BASELINE ASSESSMENT:

PO: Assess baseline renal/liver function tests. Assess B/P, apical pulse immediately before drug is administered (if pulse is 60/min or below, or systolic B/P is below 90 mm Hg, withhold medication, contact physician).

INTERVENTION/EVALUATION:

Monitor B/P for hypotension. Assess pulse for strength/weakness, irregular rate, bradycardia. Monitor daily bowel activity and stool activity. Assist with ambulation if dizziness occurs. Assess for evidence of CHF: dyspnea (particularly on exertion or lying down), night cough, peripheral edema, distended neck veins, increase in weight, decrease in urine output. Assess for nausea, diaphoresis, headache, fatigue.

PATIENT/FAMILY TEACHING:

Do not abruptly discontinue medication. Compliance with therapy regimen is essential to control glaucoma, hypertension. To avoid hypotensive effect, rise slowly from lying to sitting position, wait momentarily before standing. Avoid tasks that require alertness, motor skills until response to drug is established. Report shortness of breath, excessive fatigue, prolonged dizziness, or headache. Do not use nasal decongestants, OTC cold preparations (stimulants) without physician approval. Restrict salt, alcohol intake.

bethanechol chloride

be-**than**-eh-coal
(Duvoid, Myotonachol✤, Urecholine)

▶**CLASSIFICATION**

PHARMACOTHERAPEUTIC:
Cholinergic

ACTION/*THERAPEUTIC EFFECT*

Acts directly at cholinergic receptors of smooth muscle of urinary bladder and GI tract. Increases tone of detrusor muscle, *may initiate micturition, bladder emptying. Stimulates gastric, intestinal motility.*

USES/*UNLABELED*

Treatment of acute postop and postpartum nonobstructive urinary retention, neurogenic atony of bladder with retention. *Treatment of postop gastric atony, congenital megacolon, gastroesophageal reflux.*

PRECAUTIONS

CONTRAINDICATIONS: Hyperthyroidism, peptic ulcer, latent or active bronchial asthma, mechanical GI and urinary obstruction or recent GI resection, acute inflammatory GI tract conditions, anastomosis, bladder wall instability, pronounced bradycardia, hypotension, hypertension, cardiac disease, coronary artery disease, vasomotor instability, epilepsy, Parkinsonism. ***CAUTIONS:*** None significant.

INTERACTIONS

DRUG:* Cholinesterase inhibitors** may increase effects/toxicity. **Procainamide, quinidine** may decrease effect. ***HERBAL: None known. ***FOOD:*** None known. ***LAB VALUES:*** May increase amylase, lipase, SGOT (AST).

AVAILABILITY (Rx)

TABLETS: 5 mg, 10 mg, 25 mg, 50 mg. ***INJECTION:*** 5 mg/ml.

INDICATIONS/ROUTES/DOSAGE

Postop/postpartum urinary retention, atony of bladder:

PO: Adults, elderly: 10–50 mg

3–4 times/day. Minimum effective dose determined by initially giving 5–10 mg, and repeating same amount at 1 hr intervals until desired response achieved, or maximum of 50 mg reached. **Children:** 0.6 mg/kg/day in 3–4 divided doses.

***SubQ:* Adults, elderly:** Initially, 2.5–5 mg. Minimum effective dose determined by giving 2.5 mg (0.5 ml), repeating same amount at 15–30 min intervals up to a maximum of 4 doses. Minimum dose repeated 3–4 times/day. **Children:** 0.2 mg/kg/day in 3–4 divided doses.

SIDE EFFECTS

Note: Effects more noticeable with SubQ administration.

OCCASIONAL: Belching, change in vision, blurred vision, diarrhea, frequent urinary urgency. ***RARE: (SubQ):*** Shortness of breath, tight chest, bronchospasm.

ADVERSE REACTIONS/TOXIC EFFECTS

Overdosage produces CNS stimulation (insomnia, nervousness, orthostatic hypotension), cholinergic stimulation (headache, increased salivation/sweating, nausea, vomiting, flushed skin, stomach pain, seizures).

NURSING IMPLICATIONS

BASELINE ASSESSMENT:
Violent cholinergic reaction if given IM or IV (circulatory collapse, severe hypotension, bloody diarrhea, shock, cardiac arrest). ***Antidote:*** 0.6–1.2 mg atropine sulfate.

INTERVENTION/EVALUATION:
Assess for cholinergic reaction:

GI discomfort/cramping, feeling of facial warmth, excessive salivation and sweating, lacrimation, pallor, urinary urgency, blurred vision. Question for complaints of difficulty chewing, swallowing, progressive muscle weakness (see Adverse Reactions/Toxic Effects).

PATIENT/FAMILY TEACHING:
Report nausea, vomiting, diarrhea, sweating, increased salivary secretions, irregular heartbeat, muscle weakness, severe abdominal pain, or difficulty in breathing.

bexarotene

becks-**aye**-row-teen
(Targretin)

▶CLASSIFICATION

PHARMACOTHERAPEUTIC: Retinoid. ***CLINICAL:*** Antineoplastic (see p. 49C)

ACTION/*THERAPEUTIC EFFECT*
Binds to and activates retinoid X receptor subtypes that regulate the genes that control cellular differentiation and proliferation, *inhibiting growth of tumor cell lines of hematopoietic and squamous cell and inducing tumor regression.*

PHARMACOKINETICS
Metabolized in liver. Moderately absorbed from GI tract. Protein binding: >99%. Primarily eliminated through hepatobiliary system. Half-life: 7 hrs.

USES/*UNLABELED*

Treatment of cutaneous T-cell lymphoma (CTCL) in those refractory to at least one prior systemic therapy. *Treatment of diabetes mellitus, head, neck, lung, renal cell carcinomas, Kaposi's sarcoma.*

PRECAUTONS

CONTRAINDICATIONS: None significant. **CAUTIONS:** Liver impairment, diabetes mellitus, lipid abnormalities.

▷**LIFESPAN CONSIDERATIONS:**
Pregnancy/Lactation: May cause fetal harm. Unknown if distributed in breast milk. **Pregnancy Category X. Children:** Safety and efficacy not established. **Elderly:** No age-related precautions noted.

INTERACTIONS

DRUG: Phenytoin, rifampin may decrease concentrations. **Erythromycin, ketoconazole, itraconazole** may increase concentrations, bexarotene may enhance effect of **antidiabetic agents. HERBAL:** None known. **FOOD: Grapefruit juice** may increase concentration/toxicity. **LAB VALUES:** CA-125 in ovarian cancer may be increased. May produce abnormal liver function tests, increase cholesterol, triglycerides, total and LDL cholesterol, decrease HDL cholesterol.

AVAILABILITY (Rx)

CAPSULES. SOFT GELATIN: 75 mg.

ADMINISTRATION/HANDLING
PO:

• Give with food.

INDICATIONS/ROUTES/DOSAGE
CTCL:

PO: Adults: 300 mg/m^2/day. If no response and initial dose well tolerated, may be increased to 400 mg/m^2/day.

SIDE EFFECTS

FREQUENT: Hyperlipemia (79%), headache (30%), hypothyroidism (29%), asthenia (loss of strength and energy) (20%). **OCCASIONAL:** Rash (17%), nausea (15%), peripheral edema (13%), dry skin, abdominal pain (11%), chills, exfoliative dermatitis (10%), diarrhea (7%).

ADVERSE REACTIONS/TOXIC EFFECTS

Pancreatitis, liver failure, pneumonia occur rarely.

NURSING IMPLICATIONS

BASELINE ASSESSMENT:

Assess baseline lipid profile, WBC, liver function, thyroid function. Question possibility of pregnancy (Pregnancy Category X). Inform women of childbearing potential of risk to fetus if pregnancy occurs. Instruct in need for use of two reliable forms of contraceptives concurrently during therapy and for 1 mo after discontinuation of therapy, even in infertile, premenopausal woman.

INTERVENTION/EVALUATION:

Monitor cholesterol, triglycerides, liver and thyroid function tests, CBC.

PATIENT/FAMILY TEACHING:

Do not use medicated, drying, or abrasive soaps; wash with bland soap. Inform physician if you are pregnant or are planning to become pregnant (Pregnancy Category X).

bicalutamide

by-kale-**yew**-tah-myd
(Casodex)

▶CLASSIFICATION

PHARMACOTHERAPEUTIC:
Antiandrogen hormone. ***CLINI-CAL:*** Antineoplastic (see p.49C)

ACTION/*THERAPEUTIC EFFECT*

Competitively inhibits androgen action by binding to androgen receptors in target tissue, d*ecreasing growth of prostatic carcinoma.*

PHARMACOKINETICS

Well absorbed from GI tract. Protein binding: 96%. Metabolized in liver to inactive metabolite. Excreted in urine and feces. Not removed by hemodialysis. Half-life: 5.8 days.

USES

Treatment of advanced metastatic prostatic carcinoma (in combination with LHRH agonistic analogues—i.e., leuprolide). Treatment with both drugs must be started at same time.

PRECAUTIONS

CONTRAINDICATIONS: None significant. ***CAUTIONS:*** Moderate to severe liver impairment..
▷***LIFESPAN CONSIDERATIONS:***
Pregnancy/Lactation: May inhibit spermatogenesis, not used in women. **Pregnancy Category X. Children:** Safety and efficacy not established. **Elderly:** No age-related precautions noted.

INTERACTIONS

DRUG: May displace **warfarin** from protein-binding sites, in-crease warfarin effect. ***HERBAL:*** None known. ***FOOD:*** None known. ***LAB VALUES:*** May increase SGOT (AST), SGPT (ALT), alkaline phosphatase, serum creatinine, bilirubin, BUN. May increase WBC, hemoglobin.

AVAILABILITY (Rx)

TABLETS: 50 mg.

ADMINISTRATION/HANDLING

PO:

• May be given without regard to food. • Take at same time each day.

INDICATIONS/ROUTES/DOSAGE

Prostatic carcinoma:

PO: Adults, elderly: 50 mg once daily (morning or evening). Use concurrently with a leuteinizing hormone-releasing hormone analog or after surgical castration.

SIDE EFFECTS

FREQUENT: Hot flashes (49%), breast pain (38%), muscle pain (27%), constipation (17%), diarrhea (10%), asthenia (15%), nausea (11%). ***OCCASIONAL*** (8–9%): Nocturia, abdominal pain, peripheral edema. ***RARE*** (3–7%): Vomiting, weight loss, dizziness, insomnia, rash, impotence, gynecomastia.

ADVERSE REACTIONS/TOXIC EFFECTS

Sepsis, CHF, hypertension, iron deficiency anema may be noted.

NURSING IMPLICATIONS

INTERVENTION/EVALUATION:

Check for diarrhea, nausea, and vomiting.

PATIENT/FAMILY TEACHING:

Do not stop taking medication

(both drugs must be continued). Take medications at same time each day. Explain possible expectancy of frequent side effects. Contact physician if vomiting continues at home.

bimatoprost

(Lumigan)

See Classification section under: Antiglaucoma agents

bisacodyl

bise-ah-**co**-dahl
(Apo-Bisacodyl♣, Dacody, Dulcolax)

▶CLASSIFICATION

PHARMACOTHERAPEUTIC: GI stimulant. **CLINICAL:** Laxative (see p. 94C)

ACTION/*THERAPEUTIC EFFECT*

Increases peristalsis by direct effect on colonic smooth musculature (stimulates intramural nerve plexi). *Promotes fluid and ion accumulation in colon to increase laxative effect.*

PHARMACOKINETICS

	Onset	Peak	Duration
PO	6–12 hrs	—	—
Rectal	15–60 min	—	—

Minimal absorption following PO, rectal administration. Absorbed drug excreted in urine; remainder eliminated in feces.

USES

Facilitates defecation in those with diminished colonic motor response; for evacuation of colon for rectal, bowel examination, elective colon surgery.

PRECAUTIONS

CONTRAINDICATIONS: Abdominal pain, nausea, vomiting, appendicitis, intestinal obstruction, undiagnosed rectal bleeding. ***CAUTIONS:*** None significant.

▷*LIFESPAN CONSIDERATIONS:*
Pregnancy/Lactation: Unknown if drug crosses placenta or is distributed in breast milk. **Pregnancy Category C. Children:** Avoid in children <6 yrs (usually unable to describe symptoms or more severe side effects). **Elderly:** Repeated use may cause weakness, orthostatic hypotension due to electrolyte loss.

INTERACTIONS

DRUG:* Antacids, cimetidine, ranitidine, famotidine; milk** may cause rapid dissolution of bisacodyl (produces abdominal cramping, vomiting). May decrease transit time of concurrently administered oral medication, decreasing absorption. ***HERBAL: None known. ***FOOD:*** None known. **LAB VALUES:** None significant.

AVAILABILITY (OTC)

TABLETS (enteric-coated): 5 mg. ***SUPPOSITORY:*** 10 mg.

ADMINISTRATION/HANDLING

PO:

• Give on empty stomach (faster action). • Offer 6–8 glasses of water/day (aids stool softening). • Administer tablets whole; do not chew or crush. • Avoid giving within 1 hr of antacids, milk, other oral medication.

Rectal:
• If suppository is too soft, chill for 30 min in refrigerator or run cold water over foil wrapper. • Moisten suppository with cold water before inserting well up into rectum.

INDICATIONS/ROUTES/DOSAGE
Laxative:
PO: Adults: 5–15 mg as needed. **Children 3–12 yrs:** 5–10 mg (0.3 mg/kg) at bedtime or after breakfast.

RECTAL: Adults, children ≥12 yrs: 10 mg to induce bowel movement. **Children 2–11 yrs:** 5–10 mg as a single dose. **Children <2 yrs:** 5 mg.

Usual elderly dosage:
PO: Initially, 5 mg/day.
RECTAL: 5–10 mg/day.

SIDE EFFECTS
FREQUENT: Some degree of abdominal discomfort, nausea, mild cramps, griping, faintness. **OCCASIONAL:** Rectal administration may produce burning of rectal mucosa, mild proctitis.

ADVERSE REACTIONS/TOXIC EFFECTS
Long-term use may result in laxative dependence, chronic constipation, loss of normal bowel function. Chronic use or overdosage may result in electrolyte disturbances (hypokalemia, hypocalcemia, metabolic acidosis, or alkalosis), persistent diarrhea, malabsorption, weight loss. Electrolyte disturbance may produce vomiting, muscle weakness.

NURSING IMPLICATIONS

INTERVENTION/EVALUATION:
Encourage adequate fluid intake. Assess bowel sounds for peristalsis. Monitor daily bowel activity and stool consistency (watery, loose, soft, semisolid, solid) and record time of evacuation. Assess for abdominal disturbances. Monitor serum electrolytes in those exposed to prolonged, frequent, or excessive use of medication.

PATIENT/FAMILY TEACHING:
Institute measures to promote defecation: increase fluid intake, exercise, high-fiber diet. Do not take antacids, milk, or other medication within 1 hr of taking medication (decreased effectiveness). Report unrelieved constipation, rectal bleeding, muscle pain or cramps, dizziness, weakness.

bismuth subsalicylate

bis-muth sub-sal-**ih**-sah-late (Bismed♣, Pepto-Bismol)

FIXED-COMBINATION(S)

With ranitidine, an H-2 antagonist **(Tritec);** kit with metronidazole and tetracycline, anti-infectives **(Helidac)**

▶**CLASSIFICATION**

PHARMACOTHERAPEUTIC:
Antisecretory, antimicrobial. **CLINICAL:** Antidiarrheal, antinauseant, antiulcer (see p. 38C).

ACTION/THERAPEUTIC EFFECT
Inhibits synthesis of prostaglandins responsible for intestinal inflamma-

---

tion and hypermotility. Binds toxins produced by *Escherichia coli*. Absorbs fluid and electrolytes across intestinal wall, *preventing diarrhea.*

USES/UNLABELED

Control of diarrhea. Treatment of indigestion, nausea; relieves gas pain/abdominal cramps, *Helicobacter pylori*–associated duodenal ulcer, gastritis. *Prevents traveler's diarrhea.*

PRECAUTIONS

CONTRAINDICATIONS: Bleeding ulcers, hemorrhagic states, gout, hemophilia, renal function impairment. ***CAUTIONS:*** Elderly, diabetic pts.

INTERACTIONS

DRUG: **Anticoagulants, heparin, thrombolytics** may increase risk of bleeding. Large dose may increase **oral hypoglycemic, insulin** effects. Other **salicylates** may increase toxicity. May decrease absorption of **tetracyclines.** ***HERBAL:*** None known. ***FOOD:*** None known. ***LAB VALUES:*** May alter SGPT (ALT), SGOT (AST), alkaline phosphatase, uric acid. May decrease potassium. May prolong prothrombin time.

AVAILABILITY (OTC)

TABLETS: 262 mg. ***SUSPENSION:*** 262 mg/5 ml, 525 mg/5 ml.

INDICATIONS/ROUTES/DOSAGE

Diarrhea, gastric distress:

PO: Adults, elderly: 2 tablets (30 ml) q30–60min up to 8 doses/24 hrs. **Children 9–12 yrs:** 1 tablet or 15 ml q30–60min up to 8 doses/24 hrs. **Children 6–9 yrs:** $2/3$ tablet or 10 ml q30–60min up to 8 doses/24 hrs. **Children 3–6 yrs:** $1/3$ tablet or 5 ml q30–60min up to 8 doses/24 hrs.

***H. pylori*–associated duodenal ulcer, gastritis:**

PO: Adults, elderly: 525 mg 4 times/day (with 500 mg amoxicillin and 500 mg metronidazole 3 times/day after meals) for 7–14 days.

SIDE EFFECTS

FREQUENT: Grayish black stools. ***RARE:*** Constipation.

ADVERSE REACTIONS/TOXIC EFFECTS

Debilitated pts and infants may develop impaction.

NURSING IMPLICATIONS

INTERVENTION/EVALUATION:

Encourage adequate fluid intake. Assess bowel sounds for peristaltic activity. Monitor stool frequency and consistency (watery, loose, soft, semisolid, solid).

PATIENT/FAMILY TEACHING:

Stool may appear gray/black. Chew tablets thoroughly before swallowing.

bisoprolol fumarate

bye-**sew**-prow-lol
(Zebeta)

FIXED-COMBINATION(S)

With hydrochlorothiazide, a diuretic **(Ziac)**

Do not confuse with Diabeta.

▶CLASSIFICATION

PHARMACOTHERAPEUTIC: Beta-adrenergic blocker. ***CLINICAL:*** Antihypertensive (see p. 58C)

ACTION/*THERAPEUTIC EFFECT*

Predominantly blocks beta$_1$-adrenergic receptors in cardiac tissue by binding to receptor sites, *slowing sinus heart rate, decreasing cardiac output, decreasing B/P.* Large doses may block beta$_2$ receptors, *increasing airway resistance.*

PHARMACOKINETICS

Well absorbed from GI tract. Protein binding: 26–33%. Metabolized in liver. Primarily excreted in urine. Not removed by hemodialysis. Half-life: 9–12 hrs (half-life increased in impaired renal function).

USES

Management of hypertension, alone or in combination with diuretics, other medications.

PRECAUTIONS

CONTRAINDICATIONS: Overt cardiac failure, cardiogenic shock, heart block greater than first degree. ***CAUTIONS:*** Impaired renal or hepatic function, peripheral vascular disease, hyperthyroidism, diabetes, inadequate cardiac function, bronchospastic disease.

▷***LIFESPAN CONSIDERATIONS:*** **Pregnancy/Lactation:** Readily crosses placenta; distributed in breast milk. Avoid use during first trimester. May produce bradycardia, apnea, hypoglycemia, hypothermia during delivery, small birth weight infants. **Pregnancy Category C. Children:** Safety and efficacy not established. **Elderly:** Age-related peripheral vascular disease may increase risk of decreased peripheral circulation.

INTERACTIONS

DRUG: **Diuretics, other hypotensives** may increase hypotensive effect; **sympathomimetics, xan-** **thines** may mutually inhibit effects; may mask symptoms of hypoglycemia, prolong hypoglycemic effect of **insulin, oral hypoglycemics; NSAIDs** may decrease antihypertensive effect; **cimetidine** may increase concentration. ***HERBAL:*** None known. ***FOOD:*** None known. ***LAB VALUES:*** May increase ANA titer, BUN, creatinine, potassium, uric acid, lipoproteins, triglycerides.

AVAILABILITY (Rx)

TABLETS: 5 mg, 10 mg.

ADMINISTRATION/HANDLING

PO:

• May give without regard to food.
• Scored tablet may be crushed.

INDICATIONS/ROUTES/DOSAGE

Hypertension:

PO: **Adults, elderly:** Initially, 2.5–5 mg/day as single dose either alone or in combination with a diuretic. May increase gradually up to 20 mg/day.

PO: **Renal impairment (<40 ml/min), hepatic impairment (cirrhosis, hepatitis):** Initially, 2.5 mg.

SIDE EFFECTS

Generally well tolerated, with mild and transient side effects. ***FREQUENT:*** Hypotension manifested as dizziness, nausea, diaphoresis, headache, cold extremities, fatigue, constipation/diarrhea. ***OCCASIONAL:*** Insomnia, flatulence, urinary frequency, impotence or decreased libido. ***RARE:*** Rash, arthralgia, myalgia, confusion (esp. elderly), change in taste.

ADVERSE REACTIONS/TOXIC EFFECTS

Overdosage may produce profound bradycardia, hypotension.

Abrupt withdrawal may result in sweating, palpitations, headache, tremulousness. May precipitate CHF, MI in those with cardiac disease, thyroid storm in those with thyrotoxicosis, peripheral ischemia in those with existing peripheral vascular disease. Hypoglycemia may occur in previously controlled diabetics. Thrombocytopenia (unusual bruising, bleeding) occurs rarely.

NURSING IMPLICATIONS

BASELINE ASSESSMENT:

Assess baseline renal/liver function tests. Assess B/P, apical pulse immediately before drug is administered (if pulse is 60/min or below, or systolic B/P is below 90 mm Hg, withhold medications, contact physician).

INTERVENTION/EVALUATION:

Assess pulse for strength/weakness, irregular rate, bradycardia. Assist with ambulation if dizziness occurs. Assess for peripheral edema of hands, feet (usually, first area of lower extremity swelling is behind medial malleolus in ambulatory, sacral area in bedridden). Monitor stool frequency and consistency.

PATIENT/FAMILY TEACHING:

Do not abruptly discontinue medication. Compliance with therapy regimen is essential to control hypertension. If dizziness occurs, sit or lie down immediately. Avoid tasks that require alertness, motor skills until response to drug is established. Teach pts how to take pulse properly before each dose and to report excessively slow pulse rate (<60 beats/min), peripheral numbness, dizziness. Do not use nasal decongestants, OTC cold preparations (stimulants) without physician approval. Restrict salt, alcohol intake.

bitolterol mesylate

by-**toll**-ter-all
(Tornalate)

▶CLASSIFICATION

PHARMACOTHERAPEUTIC:
Sympathomimetic (adrenergic agonist). ***CLINICAL:*** Bronchodilator (see pp. 60C, 119C)

ACTION/*THERAPEUTIC EFFECT*

Stimulates beta$_2$-adrenergic receptors in lungs, *relaxing bronchial smooth muscle. Relieves bronchospasm, reduces airway resistance.*

USES

Prophylaxis, symptomatic treatment of bronchial asthma, acute bronchitis, reversible obstructive airway disease.

PRECAUTIONS

CONTRAINDICATIONS: History of hypersensitivity to sympathomimetics. ***CAUTIONS:*** Hypertension, cardiovascular disorders, hyperthyroidism, seizure disorders, diabetes mellitus.

INTERACTIONS

DRUG: May decrease effects of **beta-blockers.** May increase risk of arrhythmias with **digoxin.** ***HERBAL:*** None known. ***FOOD:*** None known. ***LAB VALUES:*** May decrease potassium.

AVAILABILITY (Rx)

AEROSOL: 0.8%. ***SOLUTION FOR INHALATION:*** 0.2%.

INDICATIONS/ROUTES/DOSAGE

Symptomatic relief:

INHALATION: **Adults, elderly, children >12 yrs:** 2 inhalations, separated by 1–3 min interval. Third inhalation may be needed.

Prophylaxis:

INHALATION: **Adults, elderly, children >12 yrs:** 2 inhalations q8h. Do not exceed 3 inhalations q6h, or 2 inhalations q4h.

Nebulization:

CONTINUOUS FLOW: **Adults, children ≥12 yrs:** 1.5–3.5 mg diluted and delivered over 10–15 min, 3–4 times/day, at least 4 hrs apart.

INTERMITTENT FLOW: 0.5–1.5 mg as above.

SIDE EFFECTS

FREQUENT (9–14%): Tremor. *OCCASIONAL* (3–5%): Cough, dry or irritated mouth/throat, headache, nausea, vomiting. *RARE* (<1%): Dizziness, vertigo, palpitations, insomnia.

ADVERSE REACTIONS/TOXIC EFFECTS

Although tolerance to the bronchodilating effect has not been observed, prolonged or too frequent use may lead to tolerance. Severe paradoxical bronchoconstriction may occur with excessive use.

NURSING IMPLICATIONS

BASELINE ASSESSMENT:

Offer emotional support (high incidence of anxiety due to difficulty in breathing and sympathomimetic response to drug).

INTERVENTION/EVALUATION:

Monitor rate, depth, rhythm, type of respiration; quality and rate of pulse. Assess lung sounds for wheezing. Observe lips, fingernails for blue or dusky color in light-skinned patients; gray in dark-skinned patients. Observe for clavicular retractions, hand tremor. Evaluate for clinical improvement (quieter, slower respirations, relaxed facial expression, cessation of clavicular retractions).

PATIENT/FAMILY TEACHING:

Increase fluid intake (decreases lung secretion viscosity). Rinsing mouth with water immediately after inhalation may prevent mouth/throat dryness.

bivalirudin

bye-**vail**-ih-rhu-din
(Angiomax)

▶CLASSIFICATION

PHARMACOTHERAPEUTIC: Thrombin inhibitor. *CLINICAL:* Anticoagulant (see p. 000)

ACTION/THERAPEUTIC EFFECT

Inhibits thrombogenic action of thrombin by *prolonging activated partial thromboplastin time (APTT) and prothrombin (PY) time.*

PHARMACOKINETICS

Primarily eliminated by kidneys. Half-life: 25 min (half-life increased with moderate to severe renal function). 25% is removed by hemodialysis.

USES

Anticoagulant in pts with unstable angina undergoing percutaneous transluminal coronary angioplasty (PTCA).

PRECAUTIONS

CONTRAINDICATIONS: Active major bleeding. ***CAUTIONS:*** Conditions associated with increased risk of bleeding (e.g., bacterial endocarditis, recent major bleeding, CVA, stroke, intracerebral surgery, hemorrhagic diathesis, severe hypertension, severe renal/liver function impairment, recent major surgery).
▷***LIFESPAN CONSIDERATIONS:***
Pregnancy/Lactation: Unknown if distributed in breast milk or crosses placenta. **Pregnancy Category B. Children:** Safety and efficacy not established. **Elderly:** Age-related renal function impairment may require dosage adjustment.

INTERACTIONS

DRUG: Warfarin, platelet aggregation inhibitors other than aspirin, thrombolytics may increase risk of bleeding complications. ***HERBAL:*** Ginkgo biloba may increase risk of bleeding. ***FOOD:*** None significant. ***LAB VALUES:*** Prolongs APTT, PT time.

AVAILABILITY (Rx)

INJECTION, LYOPHILIZED: 250 mg.

ADMINISTRATION/HANDLING

IV 🏛

Storage:
* Store unreconstituted vials at room temperature. * Reconstituted solution may be refrigerated for ≤24 hrs. * Diluted drug with a concentration of 0.5–5 mg/ml is stable at room temperature for ≤24 hrs.

Reconstitution:
* To each 250 mg vial add 5 ml

Sterile Water for Injection. * Gently swirl until all material is dissolved. * Further dilute each vial in 50 ml D_5W or 0.9% NaCl to yield final concentration of 5 mg/ml (1 vial in 50 ml, 2 vials in 100 ml, 5 vials in 250 ml). * If low-rate infusion is used after the initial infusion, reconstitute the 250 mg vial with added 5 ml Sterile Water for Injection. * Gently swirl until all material is dissolved. * Further dilute each vial in 500 ml D_5W or 0.9% NaCl to yield final concentration of 0.5 mg/ml. * Produces a clear, colorless solution (do not use if cloudy or contains a precipitate).

Rate of administration:
* Adjust IV infusion based on APTT or pt's body weight.

IV INCOMPATIBILITY ⊘

Do not mix with any other medication.

INDICATIONS/ROUTES/DOSAGE

Note: Intended for use with aspirin (300–325 mg daily).

Anticoagulant:

Note: Treatment should be initiated just prior to angioplasty.

***IV:* Adults, elderly:** 1 mg/kg given as IV bolus followed by a 4-hr IV infusion at rate of 2.5 mg/kg/hr. After initial 4-hr infusion is completed, give additional IV infusion at rate of 0.2 mg/kg/hr for ≤20 hrs, if necessary.

SIDE EFFECTS

FREQUENT (42%): Back pain. ***OC-CASIONAL*** (12–15%): Nausea, headache, hypotension, generalized pain. ***RARE*** (4–8%): Injection site pain, insomnia, hypertension, anxiety, vomiting, pelvic/abdominal pain, bradycardia, nervousness, dyspepsia, fever, urinary retention.

B

ADVERSE REACTIONS/TOXIC EFFECTS
A hemorrhagic event occurs rarely and is characterized by fall in B/P or hematocrit.

NURSING IMPLICATIONS

BASELINE ASSESSMENT:
Assess CBC, bleeding time. Determine initial B/P. Assess renal function.

INTERVENTION/EVALUATION:
Monitor APTT hematocrit, urine/stool culture for occult blood, renal function studies. Assess for decrease in B/P, increase in pulse rate. Question for increase in amount of discharge during menses. Assess urine output for hematuria.

---

black cohosh

Also known as baneberry, bugbane, bugwort, fairy candles
(Black Cohosh Softgel, Remifemin)

▶CLASSIFICATION
HERBAL

ACTION/EFFECT
Mechanism of action unknown. A phytoestrogen that may have estrogen-like effects, *reducing symptoms of menopause (e.g., hot flashes).*

USES
Treatment of symptoms of menopause, inducing labor in pregnant women. May reduce lipids and/or blood pressure (esp. when combined with prescription medications). Mild sedative action.

PRECAUTIONS
CONTRAINDICATIONS: Pregnancy (has menstrual and uterine stimulant effects that may increase risk of miscarriage). Not to be taken longer than 6 mos. **CAUTIONS:** Patients with breast, uterine, ovarian cancer; endometriosis, uterine fibroids.

▷**LIFESPAN CONSIDERATIONS:**
Pregnancy/Lactation: Contraindicated. **Children:** Safety and efficacy not established. **Elderly:** No age-related precautions noted.

INTERACTIONS
DRUG: May have additive antiproliferative effect with **tamoxifen.** May increase action of **antihypertensives. HERBAL:** None significant. **FOOD:** None significant. **LAB VALUES:** May decrease serum LH concentration.

AVAILABILITY
SOFTGEL CAPSULES: 40 mg. **TABLETS:** 20 mg.

INDICATIONS/ROUTES/DOSAGE
Menopause, inducing labor, lipids and/or blood pressure, sedative:
PO: Adults, elderly: 20–80 mg 2 times/day.

SIDE EFFECTS
Nausea, headache, dizziness, increase in weight, visual changes, migraines.

ADVERSE REACTIONS/TOXIC EFFECTS
Overdose may cause nausea/vomiting, decreased heart rate, perspiration.

NURSING IMPLICATIONS

BASELINE ASSESSMENT:
Assess if pt is pregnant/breastfeeding (contraindicated).

INTERVENTION/EVALUATION:

Monitor blood pressure, lipid levels.

PATIENT/FAMILY TEACHING:

Inform physician if pregnancy occurs or planning to become pregnant, breast-feeding. Do not take longer than 6 mos.

bleomycin sulfate

blee-oh-**my**-sin
(Blenoxane)

▶CLASSIFICATION

PHARMACOTHERAPEUTIC:
Glycopeptide antibiotic. **CLINI-CAL:** Antineoplastic, sclerosing agent (see p. 49C).

ACTION/*THERAPEUTIC EFFECT*

Mechanism of action unknown but appears *to inhibit DNA synthesis and, to a lesser extent, RNA and protein synthesis.* Most effective in G_2 phase of cell division.

USES/*UNLABELED*

Treatment of lymphomas: Hodgkin's disease, reticulum cell sarcoma, lymphosarcoma and squamous cell carcinomas: head and neck, including mouth, tongue, tonsil, nasopharynx, oropharynx, sinus, palate, lip, buccal mucosa, gingiva, epiglottis, larynx. Treatment of testicular carcinoma, choriocarcinoma. Treatment of malignant pleural effusions, prevention of recurrent pleural effusions. *Treatment of renal carcinoma, soft tissue sarcoma, osteosarcoma, ovarian tumors, mycosis fungoides.*

PRECAUTIONS

CONTRAINDICATIONS: Previous allergic reaction. ***EXTREME CAUTION:*** Severe renal/pulmonary impairment.

INTERACTIONS

DRUG: Other antineoplastics may increase toxicity. **Cisplatin**-induced renal impairment may decrease clearance, increase toxicity. ***HERBAL:*** None known. ***FOOD:*** None known. ***LAB VALUES:*** None significant.

AVAILABILITY (Rx)

POWDER FOR INJECTION: 15 units, 30 units.

ADMINISTRATION/HANDLING

Note: May be carcinogenic, mutagenic, or teratogenic. Handle with extreme care during preparation/administration.

Storage:

• Refrigerate powder. • After reconstitution with 0.9% NaCl, solution is stable for 24 hrs at room temperature.

SubQ/IM:

Reconstitution:

• Reconstitute 15 unit vial with 1–5 ml (30 unit vial with 2–10 ml) Sterile Water for Injection, 0.9% NaCl injection, or Bacteriostatic Water for Injection to provide concentration of 3–15 units/ml. Do not use D_5W.

IV 🏥

Reconstitution:

• Reconstitute 15 unit vial with at least 5 ml (30 unit vial with at least 10 ml) 0.9% NaCl to provide a concentration not greater than 3 units/ml.

Rate of administration:

• Administer over at least 10 min for IV injection.

IV INCOMPATIBILITY ⃠

None known via Y-site administration.

IV COMPATIBILITIES

Cytarabine (ARA-C, Cytosar), cyclophosphamide (Cytoxan), doxorubicin (Adriamycin, Rubex), Etoposide (Vepesid), methotrexate, vincristine (Oncovin).

INDICATIONS/ROUTES/DOSAGE

Note: Dosage individualized based on clinical response, tolerance to adverse effects. When used in combination therapy, consult specific protocols for optimum dosage, sequence of drug administration. Cumulative doses >400 units increase risk of pulmonary toxicity. Test doses of 2 units or less for first 2 doses recommended, due to increased possibility of anaphylactoid reaction in lymphoma pts.

Squamous cell carcinoma, non-Hodgkin's lymphoma, testicular carcinoma:

IV/IM/SUBQ:* Adults, elderly, children >12 yrs:** 0.25–0.5 units/kg 1–2 times/wk, or ***IV INFUSION: 0.25 units/kg/day over 24 hrs for 4–5 days.

Hodgkin's lymphoma:

***IV/IM/SUBQ:* Adults, elderly, children >12 yrs:** Initially, 0.25–0.5 units/kg 1–2 times/wk. **Maintenance:** 1 unit/day or 5 units/wk.

Squamous cell carcinoma of head, neck, or uterine cervix:

***REGIONAL ARTERIAL INFUSION:* Adults, children >12 yrs:** 30–60 units/day over 1–24 hrs.

SIDE EFFECTS

FREQUENT: Anorexia, weight loss, erythematous skin swelling, urticaria, rash, striae (streaking),

vesiculation (small blisters), hyperpigmentation (particularly at areas of pressure, skin folds, nail cuticles, IM injection sites, scars), mucosal lesions of lips, tongue (stomatitis). Usually evident 1–3 wks after initial therapy. May also be accompanied by decreased skin sensitivity followed by hypersensitivity of skin, nausea, vomiting, alopecia, fever/chills with parenteral form (particularly noted few hours after large single dose, lasts 4–12 hrs).

ADVERSE REACTIONS/TOXIC EFFECTS

Interstitial pneumonitis occurs in 10% of pts, occasionally progressing to pulmonary fibrosis. Appears to be dose/age related (over 70 years, those receiving total dose more than 400 units). Renal, hepatic toxicity occur infrequently.

NURSING IMPLICATIONS

BASELINE ASSESSMENT:

Obtain chest x-rays q1–2wks.

INTERVENTION/EVALUATION:

Monitor lung sounds for pulmonary toxicity (dyspnea, fine lung rales). Monitor hematologic, pulmonary function studies, hepatic, renal function tests. Assess skin daily for cutaneous toxicity. Monitor for stomatitis (burning/erythema of oral mucosa at inner margin of lips), hematologic toxicity (fever, sore throat, signs of local infection, easy bruising, unusual bleeding), symptoms of anemia (excessive tiredness, weakness).

PATIENT/FAMILY TEACHING:

Fever/chills reaction occurs less

frequently with continued therapy. Improvement of Hodgkin's disease, testicular tumors noted within 2 wks, squamous cell carcinoma within 3 wks. Do not have immunizations without doctor's approval (drug lowers body's resistance). Avoid contact with those who have recently taken live virus vaccine.

bosentan

(Tracleer)
See New Drug Supplement.

botulinum toxin Type A

botch-you-lin-em toxin
(Botox)

►CLASSIFICATION

PHARMACOTHERAPEUTIC: Neurotoxin. *CLINICAL:* Neuromuscular conduction blocker

ACTION/*THERAPEUTIC EFFECT*

Blocks neuromuscular conduction by binding to receptor sites on motor nerve endings, entering the nerve terminals, inhibiting release of acetylcholine, producing denervation of the muscle, *resulting in reduction of muscle activity.*

USES/*UNLABELED*

Treatment of cervical dystonia (CD) in adults to decrease severity of abnormal head position and neck pain associated with CD. *Treatment of hemifacial spasms, oromandibular dystonia, spasmoditic torticollis, laryngeal dystonia, writer's cramp, focal task-spe-*

cific dystonia, head and neck tremor unresponsive to drug therapy, dynamic muscle contracture in pediatric cerebral palsy pts.

PRECAUTIONS

CONTRAINDICATIONS: Presence of infection at proposed injection site(s). *CAUTIONS:* Pts with neuromuscular junctional disorders (amyotrophic lateral sclerosis, motor neuropathy, myasthenia gravis, Lambert-Eaton syndrome) may experience significant systemic effects (severe dysphagia, respiratory compromise).

INTERACTIONS

DRUG: **Aminoglycoside antbiotics,** other drugs that interfere with neuromuscular transmission **(curare-like compounds)** may potentiate effect of botulinum toxin. *HERBAL:* None significant. *FOOD:* None significant. *LAB VALUES:* None significant.

AVAILABILITY (Rx)

INJECTION: 100 units.

ADMINISTRATION/HANDLING

IM:

Storage:

• Store in freezer. • Administer within 4 hrs after removal from freezer and reconstituted. • May store reconstituted solution in refrigerator for up to 4 hrs. • Appears as a clear, colorless solution (discard if particulate matter is present).

Reconstitution:

• 0.9% NaCl is recommended diluent. • For resulting dose of U/0.1 ml, draw up 1 ml diluent to provide 10 U, 2 ml to provide 5 U, 4 ml to provide 2.5 U, or 8 ml to provide 1.25 U. • Slowly and gently inject diluent into the vial, avoid bubbles and rotate vial gently to mix.

Rate of administration:

• Administer within 4 hrs after reconstitution. • To be injected into affected muscle using 25-, 27-, or 30-gauge needle for superficial muscles and a 22-gauge needle for deeper musculature.

INDICATIONS/ROUTES/DOSAGE

Note: To be administered into affected muscle by physician.

Cervical dystonia, pts with known history of tolerating toxin:

IM: **Adults, elderly:** Mean dose is 236 U with range of 198–300 U divided among the affected muscles, based on pt's head and neck position, localization of pain, muscle hypertrophy, pt response, adverse event history.

Cervical dystonia, pts without prior use:

IM: **Adults, elderly:** Administer at lower dose than with pts with known history of tolerance.

SIDE EFFECTS

Note: Side effects usually occur within first wk following injection. **FREQUENT** (11–15%): Localized pain, tenderness, bruising at injection site, localized weakness of injection muscle, upper respiratory tract infection, neck pain, headache. **OCCASIONAL** (2–10%): Increased cough, flu syndrome, back pain, rhinitis, dizziness, hypertonia, soreness at injection site, asthenia, dry mouth, nausea, drowsiness. **RARE:** Stiffness, numbness, double vision, ptosis (drooping of upper eyelid).

ADVERSE REACTIONS/TOXIC EFFECTS

Dysphagia, mild to moderate in severity, occurs in approximately 20% of pts. Cardiac arrhythmias, severe dysphagia manifested as aspiration, dyspnea, pneumonia occur rarely. Overdose produces systemic weakness, muscle paralysis.

NURSING IMPLICATIONS

BASELINE ASSESSMENT:

Assess onset, type, location, and duration of dystonia.

INTERVENTION/EVALUATION:

Clinical improvement begins within first 2 wks after injection. Maximum benefit appears at approximately 6 wks postinjection.

PATIENT/FAMILY TEACHING:

Resume activity slowly and carefully. Seek medical attention immediately if swallowing, speech, or respiratory difficulties appear.

botulinum toxin Type B

botch-you-lin-em toxin
(Myobloc)

▶CLASSIFICATION

PHARMACOTHERAPEUTIC: Neurotoxin. **CLINICAL:** Neuromuscular conduction blocker

ACTION/*THERAPEUTIC EFFECT*

Inhibits acetycholine release at the neuromuscular junction by binding, internalization and translocation of the toxin where it acts as a endoprotease, an enzyme, splitting polypeptides *essential for neurotransmitter release.*

USES

Treatment of cervical dystonia (CD) to reduce severity of abnor-

---

mal head position and neck pain associated with CD.

PRECAUTIONS

CONTRAINDICATIONS: None nignificant. **CAUTIONS:** Pts with neuromuscular junctional disorders (amyotrophic lateral sclerosis, motor neuropathy, myasthenia gravis, Lambert-Eaton syndrome) may experience significant systemic effects (severe dysphagia, respiratory compromise).

INTERACTIONS

DRUG: Aminoglycoside antbiotics, other drugs that interfere with neuromuscular transmission **(curare-like compounds)** may potentiate effect of botulinum toxin. **HERBAL:** None significant. **FOOD:** None significant. **LAB VALUES:** None significant.

AVAILABILITY (Rx)

INJECTION: 5,000 units.

ADMINISTRATION/HANDLING
IM:

Storage:

• May be refrigerated for up to 21 mos. Do not freeze. • Administer within 4 hrs after removal from freezer and reconstituted. • May store reconstituted solution in refrigerator for up to 4 hrs. • Appears as a clear, colorless solution (discard if particulate matter is present).

Reconstitution:

• 0.9% NaCl is recommended diluent. • Slowly and gently inject diluent into the vial; avoid bubbles and rotate vial gently to mix.

Rate of administration:

• Administer within 4 hrs after reconstitution. • To be injected into affected muscle using 25-, 27-, or 30-gauge needle for superficial muscles and a 22-gauge needle for deeper musculature.

INDICATIONS/ROUTES/DOSAGE

Note: To be administered into affected muscle by physician.

Cervical dystonia in pts with history of tolerating toxin:
IM: Adults, elderly: 2,500–5,000 U divided among the affected muscles.

Cervical dystonia, pts without prior use:
IM: Adults, elderly: Administer at lower dose than with pts with known history of tolerance.

SIDE EFFECTS

Note: Side effects usually occur within first week following injection. **FREQUENT** (12–19%): Infection, neck pain, headache, injection site pain, dry mouth. **OCCASIONAL** (4–10%): Flu syndrome, generalized pain, increased cough, back pain, myasthenia. **RARE:** Dizziness, nausea, rhinitis, headache, vomiting, edema, allergic reaction.

ADVERSE REACTIONS/TOXIC EFFECTS

Dysphagia, mild to moderate in severity, occurs in approximately 10% of pts. Cardiac arrhythmias, severe dysphagia manifested as aspiration, dyspnea, pneumonia occur rarely. Overdose produces systemic weakness, muscle paralysis.

NURSING IMPLICATIONS

BASELINE ASSESSMENT:
Assess onset, type, location, and duration of dystonia.

INTERVENTION/EVALUATION:
Duration of effect lasts between 12 and 16 wks at doses of 5,000 U or 10,000 U.

bretylium tosylate

bre-**till**-ee-um
(Bretylate❧, Bretylol)

▶CLASSIFICATION
CLINICAL: Antiarrhythmic (see p. 12C)

ACTION/THERAPEUTIC EFFECT
Directly affects myocardial cell membrane. Initially, releases norepinephrine, then inhibits its release, *contributing to suppression of ventricular tachycardia.*

USES
Prophylaxis and treatment of ventricular fibrillation in those with life-threatening ventricular tachyarrhythmias who have not responded to conventional antiarrhythmic therapy.

PRECAUTIONS
CONTRAINDICATIONS: None significant. **EXTREME CAUTION:** Digitalis-induced arrhythmias, fixed cardiac output (severe pulmonary hypertension, aortic stenosis). **CAUTIONS:** Impaired renal function, sinus bradycardia. Risk of orthostatic hypotension in the elderly.

INTERACTIONS
DRUG: May increase **digoxin** toxicity (due to initial norepinephrine release). **Procainamide, quinidine** may decrease inotropic effect, increase hypotension. **HERBAL:** None known. **FOOD:** None known. **LAB VALUES:** None significant.

AVAILABILITY (Rx)
INJECTION: 50 mg/ml. **PREMIX SOLUTIONS:** 500 mg/250 ml, 1,000 mg/250 ml.

ADMINISTRATION/HANDLING
IM:
• Do not dilute. • Do not give more than 5 ml into one site (over 3 ml may cause pain at injection site). • Rotate injection sites (same-site injection may cause muscular atrophy and necrosis).

IV 🔟
Storage:
• Store solution at room temperature.

Reconstitution:
• Dilute vials with at least 50 ml D_5W or 0.9% NaCl.

Rate of administration:
• For injection, give undiluted over 1 min. • For intermittent IV infusion (piggyback), infuse over at least 8 min (too rapid IV produces nausea, vomiting). • For IV infusion, give 1–2 mg per minute of diluted solution.

IV INCOMPATIBILITIES ⊘
Amphotericin B complex (Abelcet, Ambisome, Amphotec), propofol (Diprivan).

IV COMPATIBILITIES
Amiodarone (Cordarone), diltiazem (Cardizem), dobutamine (Dobutrex), propofol (Diprivan).

INDICATIONS/ROUTES/DOSAGE
Ventricular arrhythmias, immediate, life threatening:
IV: Adults, elderly: 5 mg/kg undiluted over 1 min. May increase to 10

mg/kg, repeat as needed. **Maintenance:** 5–10 mg/kg diluted over >8 min, q6h or IV infusion at 1–2 mg/min. **Children:** 5 mg/kg, then 10 mg/kg at 15–30 min interval. **Maximum:** 30 mg/kg total dose. **Maintenance:** 5–10 mg/kg q6h.

Ventricular arrhythmias, other:

IM: **Adults, elderly:** 5–10 mg/kg undiluted, may repeat at 1–2 hr intervals. **Maintenance:** 5–10 mg/kg q6–8h.

IV: **Adults, elderly:** 5–10 mg/kg diluted over >8 min, may repeat at 1–2 hr intervals. **Maintenance:** 5–10 mg/kg q6h or IV infusion at 1–2 mg/min. **Children:** 5–10 mg/kg/dose diluted q6h.

SIDE EFFECTS

FREQUENT: Transitory hypertension followed by postural and supine hypotension in 50% of pts observed as dizziness, lightheadedness, faintness, vertigo. *OCCASIONAL* (1–3%): Diarrhea, loose stools, nausea, vomiting. *RARE* (<1%): Angina, bradycardia.

ADVERSE REACTIONS/TOXIC EFFECTS

Respiratory depression from possible neuromuscular blockade.

NURSING IMPLICATIONS

BASELINE ASSESSMENT:

Have pt in area with equipment and personnel for constant cardiac and B/P monitoring.

INTERVENTION/EVALUATION:

Assess for conversion of ventricular arrhythmias and absence of new arrhythmias. Constantly monitor B/P, pulse. Notify physician of systolic B/P <75 mm Hg (dopamine or norepinephrine may be needed, or blood, plasma, or volume correction). Keep pt supine (risk of hypotension) during life-threatening therapy and during infusion until tolerance develops. Provide emotional support to pt and family.

PATIENT/FAMILY TEACHING:

Tolerance to hypotensive effect usually occurs within several days after initial therapy. One hr after dose administration, may rise slowly from lying to sitting position and permit legs to dangle from bed for at least 5 min before standing.

brimonidine

(Alphagan)

See Classification section under: Antiglaucoma agents

brinzolamide

(Azopt)

See Classification section under: Antiglaucoma agents

bromocriptine mesylate

brom-oh-**crip**-teen
(Apo-Bromocriptine✤, Parlodel)

▶CLASSIFICATION

PHARMACOTHERAPEUTIC: Dopamine agonist. *CLINICAL:* Infertility therapy adjunct, antihyperprolactinemic, lactation inhibitor, antidyskinetic, growth hormone suppressant (see p. 74C)

ACTION/*THERAPEUTIC EFFECT*

Activated at postsynaptic dopamine receptors. Directly inhibits prolactin secretion, *reduces elevated growth hormone concentration, suppresses galactorrhea and reinitiates the ovulatory menstrual cycle.*

PHARMACOKINETICS

Onset	Peak	Duration
PO (growth hormone reduction)		
1–2 hrs	—	4–5 hrs
PO (prolactin reduction)		
2 hrs	8 hrs	24 hrs

Minimal absorption from GI tract. Protein binding: 90–96%. Metabolized in liver. Excreted in feces via biliary secretion. Half-life: 15 hrs.

USES/*UNLABELED*

Treatment of hyperprolactinemia conditions (amenorrhea with or without galactorrhea, prolactin-secreting adenomas, infertility). Treatment of Parkinson's disease, acromegaly. *Treatment of neuroleptic malignant syndrome, cocaine addiction, hyperprolacemia associated with pituitary adenomas.*

PRECAUTIONS

CONTRAINDICATIONS: Pregnancy, peripheral vascular disease, severe ischemic heart disease, uncontrolled hypertension, hypersensitivity to ergot alkaloids. ***CAUTIONS:*** Impaired hepatic/cardiac function, hypertension, psychiatric disorders.

▷*LIFESPAN CONSIDERATIONS:*
Pregnancy/Lactation: Not recommended during pregnancy or while breast feeding. **Children:** Safety and efficacy not established. **Pregnancy Category B. Elderly:** CNS effects may occur more frequently.

INTERACTIONS

DRUG: Disulfiram reaction (chest pain, confusion, flushed face, nausea, vomiting) may occur with **alcohol. Estrogens, progestins** may decrease effects. **Phenothiazines, haloperidol, MAO inhibitors** may decrease prolactin effect. **Hypotensive agents** may increase hypotension. **Levodopa** may increase effects. **Erythromycin, ritonavir** may increase concentration, toxicity. **Risperidone** may increase serum prolactin concentrations, interfere with bromocriptine effects. ***HERBAL:*** None known. ***FOOD:*** None known. ***LAB VALUES:*** May increase plasma concentration of growth hormone.

AVAILABILITY (Rx)

TABLETS: 2.5 mg. ***CAPSULES:*** 5 mg.

ADMINISTRATION/HANDLING

PO:
• Pt should be lying down before administering first dose. • Give after food intake (decreases incidence of nausea).

INDICATIONS/ROUTES/DOSAGE

Hyperprolactinemia:

PO: Adults, elderly: Initially, 1.25–2.5 mg/day. May increase by 2.5 mg/day at 3–7 day intervals. **Range:** 2.5–15 mg/day.

Parkinson's disease:

PO: Adults, elderly: Initially, 1.25 mg 2 times/day. Increase by 2.5 mg/day q14–28days. **Range:** 10–40 mg/day.

Acromegaly:

PO: Adults, elderly: Initially, 1.25–2.5 mg/day at bedtime for 3 days. May increase by 1.25–2.5 mg/day q3–7days. **Range:** 20–30 mg/day. **Maximum:** 100 mg/day.

SIDE EFFECTS

Note: Incidence of side effects is high, esp. at beginning of therapy or with high dosage. *FREQUENT:* Nausea (49%), headache (19%), dizziness (17%). *OCCASIONAL* (3–7%): Fatigue, lightheadedness, vomiting, abdominal cramps, diarrhea, constipation, nasal congestion, drowsiness, dry mouth. *RARE:* Muscle cramping, urinary hesitancy.

ADVERSE REACTIONS/TOXIC EFFECTS

Visual or auditory hallucinations noted in Parkinsonism syndrome. Long-term, high-dose therapy may produce continuing runny nose, fainting, GI hemorrhage, peptic ulcer, severe abdominal/stomach pain.

NURSING IMPLICATIONS

BASELINE ASSESSMENT:

Evaluation of pituitary (rule out tumor) should be done prior to treatment for hyperprolactinemia with amenorrhea/galactorrhea and infertility. Obtain pregnancy test.

INTERVENTION/EVALUATION:

Assist with ambulation if dizziness is noted after administration. Assess for therapeutic response (decrease in engorgement, decrease in Parkinsonism symptoms). Monitor for constipation.

PATIENT/FAMILY TEACHING:

To reduce lightheadedness, rise slowly from lying to sitting position and permit legs to dangle momentarily before standing. Avoid sudden posture changes. Avoid tasks that require alertness, motor skills until response to drug is established. Must use contraceptive measures (other than oral) during treatment. Report any watery nasal discharge to physician.

brompheniramine

(Bromphen, Dimetane)

See Classification section under: Antihistamines

budesonide

byew-**des**-oh-nyd
(Entocort✦, Pulmicort, Rhinocort, Rhinocort Aqua)

▶CLASSIFICATION

PHARMACOTHERAPEUTIC: Glucocorticosteroid. *CLINICAL:* Anti-inflammatory, antiallergy (see p. 67C)

ACTION/*THERAPEUTIC EFFECT*

Decreases/prevents tissue response to inflammatory process, *inhibits accumulation of inflammatory cells.*

PHARMACOKINETICS

Minimally absorbed from nasal tissue, moderately absorbed from inhalation. Protein binding: 88%. Primarily metabolized in liver. Half-life: 2–3 hrs.

USES/*UNLABELED*

Management of symptoms of seasonal or perennial allergic rhinitis in adults and children and nonallergic perennial rhinitis in adults. Maintenance treatment of asthma. *Capsule:* Treatment of Crohn's disease. *Treatment of vasomotor rhinitis.*

PRECAUTIONS

CONTRAINDICATIONS: Hypersensitivity to any corticosteroid or components, primary treatment of status asthmaticus, systemic fungal infections, persistently positive sputum cultures for *Candida albicans,* untreated localized infection involving nasal mucosa. ***CAUTIONS:*** Adrenal insufficiency, cirrhosis, glaucoma, hypothyroidism, untreated infection, osteoporosis, tuberculosis.

▷***LIFESPAN CONSIDERATIONS:***
Pregnancy/Lactation: Unknown if drug crosses placenta or is distributed in breast milk. **Pregnancy Category C. Children:** Prolonged treatment/high doses may decrease short-term growth rate, cortisol secretion. **Elderly:** No age-related precautions noted.

INTERACTIONS

DRUG: None significant. ***HERBAL:*** None known. ***FOOD:*** None known. ***LAB VALUES:*** None significant.

AVAILABILITY (Rx)

AEROSOL FOR INTRANASAL: 32 mcg/activation. ***DRY POWDER FOR ORAL INHALATION:*** 200 mcg. ***SUSPENSION FOR NEBULIZATION:*** 0.25 mg/2 ml, 0.5 mg/2 ml. ***CAPSULES:*** 3 mg.

ADMINISTRATION/HANDLING

Inhalation:

• Shake container well, exhale completely, place mouthpiece between lips, inhale and hold breath as long as possible before exhaling. • Allow at least 1 min between inhalations. • Rinse mouth after each use to decrease dry mouth and hoarseness.

Intranasal:

• Clear nasal passages before use. • Tilt head slightly forwared. • Insert spray tip into nostril, pointing toward nasal passages, away from nasal septum. • Spray into 1 nostril while holding other nostril closed and concurrently inspire through nostril to allow medication as high into nasal passages as possible.

INDICATIONS/ROUTES/DOSAGE

INTRANASAL: **Adults, elderly, children ≥6 yrs:** *(Rhinocort):* 2 sprays to each nostril 2 times/day or 4 sprays to each nostril in morning. *(Rhinocort Aqua):* 1 spray to each nostril once daily. **Maximum:** *(Adults, children >12 yrs)):* 8 sprays/day. *(Children <12 yrs):* 4 sprays/day.

NEBULIZATION: **Children 1–8 yrs:** 0.25–1 mg/day titrated to lowest effective dose..

INHALATION: **Adults, elderly, children ≥6 yrs:** Initially, 200–400 mcg 2 times/day. **Maximum:** 400 mcg 2 times/day.

Crohn's disease:

PO: **Adults, elderly:** 9 mg once daily for up to 8 wks.

SIDE EFFECTS

FREQUENT (>3%): ***Nasal:*** Mild nasopharyngeal irritation, burning, stinging, dryness, headache, cough. ***Inhalation:*** Flulike syndrome, headache, pharyngitis. ***OCCASIONAL*** (1–3%): ***Nasal:*** Dry mouth, dyspepsia, rebound congestion, rhinorrhea, loss of sense of taste. ***Inhalation:*** Back pain, vomiting, altered taste/voice, abdominal pain, nausea, dyspepsia.

ADVERSE REACTIONS/TOXIC EFFECTS

Acute hypersensitivity reaction (urticaria, angioedema, severe bronchospasm) occurs rarely.

NURSING IMPLICATIONS

BASELINE ASSESSMENT:

Question for hypersensitivity to any corticosteroids, components.

PATIENT/FAMILY TEACHING:

Improvement noted in 24 hrs; but full effect may take 3–7 days. Contact physician if no improvement in symptoms, sneezing or nasal irritation occurs.

bumetanide

byew-**met**-ah-nide
(Bumex, Burinex✦)

▶CLASSIFICATION

PHARMACOTHERAPEUTIC:
Loop. *CLINICAL:* Diuretic (see p. 71C)

ACTION/*THERAPEUTIC EFFECT*

Enhances excretion of sodium, chloride, and, to lesser degree, potassium, by direct action at ascending limb of loop of Henle and in the proximal tubule, *producing diuresis.*

PHARMACOKINETICS

Onset	Peak	Duration
PO		
30–60 min	60–120 min	4–6 hrs
IM		
40 min	60–120 min	4–6 hrs
IV		
Rapid	15–30 min	2–3 hrs

Completely absorbed from GI tract (absorption decreased in CHF, nephrotic syndrome). Protein binding: 94–96%. Partially metabolized in liver. Primarily excreted in urine. Not removed by hemodialysis. Half-life: 1–1.5 hrs.

USES/*UNLABELED*

Treatment of edema associated with CHF, chronic renal failure including nephrotic syndrome, hepatic cirrhosis with ascites; treatment of acute pulmonary edema. *Treatment of hypertension, hypercalcemia.*

PRECAUTIONS

CONTRAINDICATIONS: Anuria, hepatic coma, severe electrolyte depletion. *CAUTIONS:* Hypersensitivity to sulfonamides, impaired renal or hepatic function, diabetes mellitus, elderly/debilitated.

▷*LIFESPAN CONSIDERATIONS:*
Pregnancy/Lactation: Unknown if drug is distributed in breast milk. **Pregnancy Category C. Children:** Safety and efficacy not established. **Elderly:** May be more sensitive to hypotension/electrolyte effects. Increased risk for circulatory collapse or thrombolic episode. Age-related renal impairment may require reduced or extended dosage interval.

INTERACTIONS

DRUG: **Amphotericin, ototoxic, nephrotoxic agents** may increase toxicity. May decrease effect of **anticoagulants, heparin. Hypokalemia-causing agents** may increase risk hypokalemia. May increase risk of **lithium** toxicity. *HERBAL:* None known. *FOOD:* None known. *LAB VALUES:* May increase glucose, BUN, uric acid, urinary phosphate. May decrease calcium, chloride, magnesium, potassium, sodium.

AVAILABILITY [Rx]

TABLETS: 0.5 mg, 1 mg, 2 mg. *INJECTION:* 0.25 mg/ml.

ADMINISTRATION/HANDLING

PO:

* Give with food to avoid GI upset,

preferably with breakfast (may prevent nocturia).

IV 🖳

Storage:

• Store at room temperature. • Stable for 24 hrs if diluted.

Rate of administration:

• May give undiluted but is compatible with D₅W, 0.9% NaCl, or lactated Ringer's. • Administer IV push >1–2 min. • May give through Y tube or 3-way stop-cock. • May give as continuous infusion.

IV INCOMPATIBILITIES ⊘

Dobutamine (Dobutrex), midazolam (Versed), milrinone (Primacor).

IV COMPATIBILITIES

Cisatracurium (Nimbex), diltiazem (Cardizem), lorazepam (Ativan), milrinore (Primacor), propofol (Diprivan).

INDICATIONS/ROUTES/DOSAGE

Edema:

PO: **Adults >18 yrs:** 0.5–2 mg given as single dose in AM. May repeat at 4–5 hr intervals. **Elderly:** 0.5 mg/day, increase as needed.

IM/IV: **Adults, elderly:** 0.5–1 mg given as single dose. May be repeated at 2–3 hr intervals.

Usual pediatric dose:

IV/IM/PO: 0.015–0.1 mg/kg/dose q6–24h.

SIDE EFFECTS

EXPECTED: Increase in urine frequency/volume. ***FREQUENT:*** Orthostatic hypotension, dizziness. ***OCCASIONAL:*** Blurred vision, diarrhea, headache, anorexia, premature ejaculation, impotence, GI upset. ***RARE:*** Rash, urticaria, pruritus, weakness, muscle cramps, nipple tenderness.

ADVERSE REACTIONS/TOXIC EFFECTS

Vigorous diuresis may lead to profound water/electrolyte depletion, resulting in hypokalemia, hyponatremia, dehydration, coma, circulatory collapse. Acute hypotensive episodes may occur. Ototoxicity manifested as deafness, vertigo, tinnitus (ringing/roaring in ears) may occur, esp. in pts with severe renal impairment or who are on other ototoxic drugs. Blood dyscrasias have been reported.

NURSING IMPLICATIONS

BASELINE ASSESSMENT:

Check vital signs, esp. B/P for hypotension prior to administration. Assess baseline electrolytes; particularly check for low potassium. Assess edema, skin turgor, mucous membranes for hydration status. Initiate I&O.

INTERVENTION/EVALUATION:

Continue to monitor B/P, vital signs, electrolytes, I&O, weight. Note extent of diuresis. Watch for changes from initial assessment (hypokalemia may result in muscle strength changes, tremor, muscle cramps, change in mental status, cardiac arrhythmias; hyponatremia may result in confusion, thirst, cold/clammy skin).

PATIENT/FAMILY TEACHING:

Expect increased frequency and volume of urination, hearing abnormalities (such as sense of fullness in ears, ringing/roaring in ears). Eat foods high in potassium such as whole grains (cereals), legumes, meat, bananas, apricots, orange juice, potatoes (white, sweet), raisins. Get up slowly from sitting/lying position.

bupivacaine

(Marcaine, Sensorcaine)
See Classification section under: Anesthetics: local

buprenorphine

(Buprenex)
See Classification section under: Opioid analgesics

bupropion

byew-**pro**-peon
(<u>Wellbutrin</u>, Wellbutrin SR ✚, Zyban)

▶**CLASSIFICATION**

PHARMACOTHERAPEUTIC: Aminoketone. ***CLINICAL:*** Antidepressant, smoking cessation aid (see p. 33C)

ACTION/*THERAPEUTIC EFFECT*

Blocks reuptake of neurotransmitters (serotonin, norepinephrine) at CNS presynaptic membranes, increasing availability at postsynaptic receptor sites. Resulting enhancement of synaptic activity *produces antidepressant effect.* Reduces firing rate of noradrenergic neurons, elim-

inating nicotine withdrawal symptoms.

PHARMACOKINETICS

Rapidly absorbed from GI tract. Crosses blood-brain barrier. Protein binding: 84%. Extensive first-pass metabolism in liver to active metabolite. Primarily excreted in urine. Half-life: 14 hrs.

USES/*UNLABELED*

Treatment of depression, particularly endogenous depression, exhibited as persistent and prominent dysphoria (occurring nearly every day for at least 2 wks) manifested by 4 of 8 symptoms: change in appetite, change in sleep pattern, increased fatigue, impaired concentration, feelings of guilt/worthlessness, loss of interest in usual activities, psychomotor agitation/retardation, or suicidal tendencies. Also use as assist in smoking cessation. *Attention deficit hyperactivity disorder in adults, children.*

PRECAUTIONS

CONTRAINDICATIONS: Pts with seizure disorder, current or prior diagnosis of bulimia or anorexia nervosa, concurrent use of MAO inhibitor. ***CAUTIONS:*** History of seizure, cranial trauma; those currently taking antipsychotics, antidepressants, impaired renal, hepatic function.

▷***LIFESPAN CONSIDERATIONS:*** **Pregnancy/Lactation:** Unknown if drug crosses placenta or is distributed in breast milk. **Pregnancy Category B. Children:** Safety and efficacy not established in those <18 yrs of age. **Elderly:** More sensitive to anticholinergic, sedative, cardiovascular effects. Age-related impaired renal function may require dosage adjustment.

INTERACTIONS

***DRUG:* Alcohol, tricyclic antidepressants, lithium, ritonavir, trazodone** may increase risk of seizures. May increase risk of acute toxicity with **MAO inhibitors.** *HERBAL:* None known. *FOOD:* None known. *LAB VALUES:* May decrease WBCs.

AVAILABILITY (Rx)

TABLETS: 75 mg, 100 mg. ***TABLETS (sustained-release):*** 50 mg, 100 mg, 150 mg.

ADMINISTRATION/HANDLING

PO:

• May take with or without food (take with food to reduce GI irritation). • Give at least 4 hr interval for immediate onset and 8 hr interval for sustained-release tablet to avoid seizures. • Avoid bedtime dosage (decreases risk of insomnia). • Do not crush sustained-release preparations.

INDICATIONS/ROUTES/DOSAGE

Depression:

Note: Gradually increase dose to minimize agitation, motor restlessness, insomnia.

***PO:* Adults:** *Immediate-release:* Initially 100 mg 2 times/day, may increase to 100 mg 3 times/day no sooner than 3 days after beginning therapy. **Maximum:** 450 mg/day. **Maintenance:** Lowest effective dose. *Sustained-release:* Initially, 150 mg/day as single dose in the morning. May increase to 300 mg/day at 150 mg 2 times/day as early as day 4 of dosing. **Maximum:** 400 mg/day. **Maintenance:** Lowest effective dose.

Smoking cessation:

***PO:* Adults:** Initially, 150 mg daily for 3 days; then 150 mg 2 times/day.

SIDE EFFECTS

Note: Fewer side effects noted with sustained-release form.

FREQUENT (18–32%): Constipation, weight gain or loss, nausea, vomiting, anorexia, dry mouth, headache, increased sweating, tremor, sedation, insomnia, dizziness, agitation. ***OCCASIONAL*** (5–10%): Diarrhea, akinesia, blurred vision, tachycardia, confusion, hostility, fatigue.

ADVERSE REACTIONS/TOXIC EFFECTS

Increased risk of seizures with increase in dosage greater than 150 mg/dose, in pts with history of bulimia or seizure disorders, of discontinuing agents that may lower seizure threshold.

NURSING IMPLICATIONS

BASELINE ASSESSMENT:

For those on long-term therapy, liver/renal function tests should be performed periodically.

INTERVENTION/EVALUATION:

Supervise suicidal risk pt closely during early therapy (as depression lessens, energy level improves, increasing suicide potential). Assess appearance, behavior, speech pattern, level of interest, mood.

PATIENT/FAMILY TEACHING:

Full therapeutic effect may be noted in 4 wks. Avoid tasks that require alertness, motor skills until response to drug is established.

buspirone hydrochloride

byew-spear-own
(BuSpar, Buspirex✦, Bustab✦)

▶CLASSIFICATION

PHARMACOTHERAPEUTIC:
Nonbarbiturate. ***CLINICAL:*** Antianxiety

ACTION/*THERAPEUTIC EFFECT*

Binds to serotonin, dopamine at presynaptic neurotransmitter receptors in the CNS, *producing antianxiety effect.*

PHARMACOKINETICS

Rapidly completely absorbed from GI tract. Protein binding: 95%. Undergoes extensive first-pass metabolism. Metabolized in liver to active metabolite. Primarily excreted in urine. Not removed by hemodialysis. Half-life: 2–3 hrs.

USES/*UNLABELED*

Short-term management (up to 4 wks) of anxiety disorders. *Management of symptoms of PMS (e.g., aches, pain, fatigue, irritability).*

PRECAUTIONS

CONTRAINDICATIONS: Severe renal/hepatic impairment, MAO inhibitor therapy. ***CAUTIONS:*** Renal/hepatic impairment.

▷***LIFESPAN CONSIDERATIONS:***
Pregnancy/Lactation: Unknown if drug crosses placenta or is distributed in breast milk. **Pregnancy Category B. Children:** Safety and efficacy not established. **Elderly:** No age-related precautions noted.

INTERACTIONS

DRUG:* Alcohol, CNS depressants** may increase sedation. **Erythromycin, itraconazole** may increase concentration, risk of toxicity. **MAO inhibitors** may increase B/P. ***HERBAL:* Kava** may increase sedation. ***FOOD:* Grapefruit/grapefruit juice** may increase concentration, toxicity. ***LAB VALUES: None significant.

AVAILABILITY (Rx)

TABLETS: 5 mg, 10 mg, 15 mg.

ADMINISTRATION/HANDLING

PO:

• Give without regard to meals. • Tablets may be crushed.

INDICATIONS/ROUTES/DOSAGE

***PO:* Adults:** 5 mg 2–3 times daily or 7.5 mg 2 times/day. May increase in 5 mg increments/day at intervals of 2–4 days. **Maintenance:** 15–30 mg/day in 2–3 divided doses. Do not exceed 60 mg/day.

Usual elderly dosage:

PO: Initially, 5 mg 2 times/day. May increase by 5 mg q2–3days. **Maximum:** 60 mg/day.

SIDE EFFECTS

FREQUENT (6–12%): Dizziness, drowsiness, nausea, headache. ***OCCASIONAL*** (2–5%): Nervousness, fatigue, insomnia, dry mouth, lightheadedness, mood swings, blurred vision, poor concentration, diarrhea, numbness in hands/feet. ***RARE:*** Muscle pain/stiffness, nightmares, chest pain, involuntary movements.

ADVERSE REACTIONS/TOXIC EFFECTS

No evidence of tolerance or psychologic and/or physical depen-

---

✐ - see color pill atlas

dence, no withdrawal syndrome. Overdosage may produce severe nausea, vomiting, dizziness, drowsiness, abdominal distention, excessive pupil contraction.

NURSING IMPLICATIONS

BASELINE ASSESSMENT:

Offer emotional support to anxious pt. Assess motor responses (agitation, trembling, tension) and autonomic responses (cold, clammy hands; sweating).

INTERVENTION/EVALUATION:

For those on long-term therapy, liver/renal function tests, blood counts should be performed periodically. Assist with ambulation if drowsiness, lightheadedness occur. Evaluate for therapeutic response: calm, facial expression, decreased restlessness and/or insomnia.

PATIENT/FAMILY TEACHING:

Improvement may be noted in 7–10 days, but optimum therapeutic effect generally takes 3–4 wks. Drowsiness usually disappears during continued therapy. If dizziness occurs, change position slowly from recumbent to sitting position before standing. Avoid tasks that require alertness, motor skills until response to drug is established.

busulfan

bew-**sull**-fan
(Busulfex, Myleran)
Do not confuse with Leukeran, Alkeran.

▶ **CLASSIFICATION**

PHARMACOTHERAPEUTIC: Alkylating agent. ***CLINICAL:*** Antineoplastic (see p. 49C)

ACTION/*THERAPEUTIC EFFECT*

Cell cycle-phase nonspecific. Interferes with DNA replication, RNA synthesis, *disrupting nucleic acid function. Myelosuppressant.*

PHARMACOKINETICS

Completely absorbed from GI tract. Protein binding: 33%. Metabolized in liver. Primarily excreted in urine. Minimal removal by hemodialysis. Half-life: 2.5 hrs.

USES/*UNLABELED*

Treatment of chronic myelogenous leukemia (CML). ***Injection:*** Combined with cyclophosphamide as conditioning regimen before allogeneic hematopoietic cell transplantation in pts with CML. *Treatment of acute myelocytic leukemia (AML).*

PRECAUTIONS

CONTRAINDICATIONS: Disease resistance to previous therapy with drug. ***EXTREME CAUTION:*** Compromised bone marrow reserve. ***CAUTIONS:*** Chickenpox, herpes zoster, infection, history of gout.

▷ ***LIFESPAN CONSIDERATIONS:*** **Pregnancy/Lactation:** If possible, avoid use during pregnancy, esp. first trimester. May cause fetal harm. Unknown if distributed in breast milk. Breast feeding not recommended. **Pregnancy Category D. Children/Elderly:** No age related precautions noted.

INTERACTIONS

DRUG: May decrease effect of

antigout medications. Bone marrow depressant may increase risk of bone marrow depression. **Live virus vaccines** may potentiate virus replication, increase vaccine side effects, decrease antibody response to vaccine. **HERBAL:** None known. **FOOD:** None known. **LAB VALUES:** May decrease magnesium, potassium, phosphates, sodium. May increase glucose, calcium, bilirubin, SGPT, creatinine, alkaline phosphatase, BUN.

AVAILABILITY (Rx)

TABLETS: 2 mg. **INJECTION:** 60 mg ampoule.

ADMINISTRATION/HANDLING

Note: May be carcinogenic, mutagenic, or teratogenic. Handle with extreme care during administration. Use of gloves recommended. If contact occurs with skin/mucosa, wash thoroughly with water.

PO:

• Give at same time each day. • Give on empty stomach if nausea/vomiting occur.

IV 🅦

Storage:

• Refrigerate ampoules. • Following dilution, stable for 8 hrs at room temperature, 12 hrs if refrigerated when diluted with 0.9% NaCl.

Reconstitution:

• Dilute with 0.9% NaCl or D_5W only. The diluent quantity must be 10 times the volume of busulfan (e.g., 9.3 ml busulfan must be diluted with 93 ml diluent). • Use filter to withdraw busulfan from ampoule. • Add busulfan to calculated diluent. • Use infusion pump to administer busulfan.

Rate of administration:

• Infuse over 2 hrs. • Prior to and after infusion, flush catheter line with 5 ml 0.9% NaCl or D_5W.

IV INCOMPATIBILITY ⊘

Do not mix with any other medications.

INDICATIONS/ROUTES/DOSAGE

Note: Dosage individualized based on clinical response, tolerance to adverse effects. When used in combination therapy, consult specific protocols for optimum dosage, sequence of drug administration.

Remission induction:

PO: Adults: 4–8 mg/day. Withdraw drug when WBC falls below 15,000/mm³. **Children:** 0.06–0.12 mg/kg once daily.

Maintenance therapy:

PO: Adults: Induction dose (4–8 mg/day) when total leukocyte count reaches 50,000/mm³. If remission occurs <3 mos, 1–3 mg/day may produce satisfactory response.

Usual elderly dosage:

PO: Initially, lowest dose for adults.

Usual parenteral dosage:

Note: Premedicate with phenytoin to decrease risk of seizures.

IV INFUSION: Adults: 0.8 mg/kg q6hrs (as 2 hr infusion) for total of 16 doses. **Children:** 60–120 mcg/kg/day or 1.8–4.6 mg/m²/day.

SIDE EFFECTS

VERY FREQUENT (72–98%): Nausea, stomatitis, vomiting, anorexia, insomnia, diarrhea, fever, abdominal pain, anxiety. **FREQUENT** (44–69%): Headache, rash, asthenia (loss of strength, energy), infection, chills, tachycardia, dyspepsia.

OCCASIONAL (16–38%): Constipation, dizziness, edema, pruritus, cough, dry mouth, depression, abdominal enlargement, pharyngitis, hiccups, back pain, alopecia, myalgia. ***RARE*** (5–13%): Injection site pain, arthralgia, confusion, hypotension, lethargy.

ADVERSE REACTIONS/TOXIC EFFECTS

Major adverse reaction is bone marrow depression resulting in hematologic toxicity (severe leukopenia, anemia, severe thrombocytopenia). Very high doses may produce blurred vision, muscle twitching, tonic-clonic seizures. Long-term therapy (>4 yrs) may produce pulmonary syndrome ("busulfan lung") characterized by persistent cough, congestion, rales, dyspnea. Hyperuricemia may produce uric acid nephropathy, renal stones, acute renal failure.

NURSING IMPLICATIONS

BASELINE ASSESSMENT:

Hemoglobin, hemocrit, WBC, differential, platelet count, hepatic and renal functions studies should be performed weekly (dosage based on hematologic values). Institute pt/family teaching regarding expected effects of treatment.

INTERVENTION/EVALUATION:

Monitor lab values diligently for evidence of bone marrow depression. Assess mouth for onset of stomatitis (redness/ulceration of oral mucous membranes, gum inflammation, difficulty swallowing). Initiate antiemetics to prevent nausea/vomiting. Monitor daily bowel activity and stool consistency.

PATIENT/FAMILY TEACHING:

Maintain adequate daily fluid intake (may protect against renal impairment). Report consistent cough, congestion, difficulty breathing. Promptly report fever, sore throat, signs of local infection, easy bruising or unusual bleeding from any site. Do not have immunizations without physician's approval (drug lowers body's resistance). Avoid contact with those who have recently taken live virus vaccine. Take at same time each day. Contraception is recommended during therapy.

butenafine

(Mentax)
See Classification section under: Antifungals: topical

butorphanol tartrate

byew-**tore**-phen-awl
(Stadol, Stadol NS)
Do not confuse with Haldol.

▶CLASSIFICATION

PHARMACOTHERAPEUTIC: Opioid **(Schedule IV). *CLINICAL:*** Analgesic, anesthesia adjunct (see p. 108C)

ACTION/*THERAPEUTIC EFFECT*

Binds at opiate receptor sites in CNS. Reduces intensity of pain stimuli incoming from sensory nerve endings, *altering pain perception and emotional response to pain.*

PHARMACOKINETICS

Onset	Peak	Duration
IM		
10–30 min	30–60 min	3–4 hrs
IV		
<1 min	30 min	2–4 hrs
Nasal		
15 min	1–2 hrs	4–5 hrs

Rapidly absorbed from IM injection. Protein binding: High. Extensively metabolized in liver. Primarily excreted in urine. Half-life: 2.5–4 hrs.

USES

Management of pain (including postop pain). *Nasal:* Migraine headache pain. *Parenteral:* Preop, preanesthetic medication, supplement balanced anesthesia, relief of pain during labor.

PRECAUTIONS

CONTRAINDICATIONS: CNS disease that affects respirations, pulmonary disease, preexisting respiratory depression, physical dependence on other opioid analgesics. *CAUTIONS:* Impaired hepatic/renal function, elderly, debilitated, head injury, hypertension, prior to biliary tract surgery (produces spasm of sphincter of Oddi), MI with nausea, vomiting.

▷*LIFESPAN CONSIDERATIONS:* **Pregnancy/Lactation:** Readily crosses placenta; distributed in breast milk (breast feeding not recommended). **Pregnancy Category B** (Category D if used for prolonged time, high dose at term). **Children:** Safety and efficacy not known in those <18 yrs of age. **Elderly:** May be more sensitive to effects; adjust dose and interval.

INTERACTIONS

DRUG: **Alcohol, CNS depressants** may increase CNS or respiratory depression, hypotension. **MAO inhibitors** may produce severe, fatal reaction (reduce dose to one-fourth usual dose). Effects may be decreased with **buprenorphine.** *HERBAL:* None known. *FOOD:* None known. *LAB VALUES:* None significant.

AVAILABILITY (Rx)

INJECTION: 1 mg/ml, 2 mg/ml. *NASAL SPRAY:* 10 mg/ml.

ADMINISTRATION/HANDLING

Intranasal:

• Instruct pt to blow nose to clear nasal passages as much as possible. • Tilt head slightly forward and insert spray tip into nostril, pointing toward nasal passages, away from nasal septum. • Spray into nostril while holding other nostril closed and concurrently inspire through nose to permit medication as high into nasal passages as possible.

IV ▩

Storage:

• Store at room temperature.

Rate of administration:

• May give undiluted. • Administer over 3–5 min.

IV INCOMPATIBILITIES ⊘

Amphotericin B complex (Abelcet, Ambisome, Amphotec).

IV COMPATIBILITIES

Esmolol (Brevibloc), propofol (Diprivan).

INDICATIONS/ROUTES/DOSAGE

Note: May be given by IM or IV push.

Analgesia:

IM: **Adults:** 1–4 mg q3–4h as needed.

IV: **Adults:** 0.5–2 mg q3–4h as needed.

Usual elderly dosage:

_IM/IV:_ 1 mg q4–6h as needed.

NASAL: Adults: 1 mg (1 spray in one nostril). May repeat in 60–90 min. May repeat 2 dose sequence q3–4h as needed. Alternatively, 2 mg (1 spray each nostril if pt remains recumbent), may repeat in 3–4h.

SIDE EFFECTS

FREQUENT: Parenteral: Drowsiness (43%), dizziness (19%). **_Nasal:_** Nasal congestion (13%), insomnia (11%). **_OCCASIONAL: Parenteral_** (3–9%): Confusion, sweating/clammy skin, lethargy, headache, nausea, vomiting, dry mouth. **_Nasal_** (3–9%): Vasodilation, constipation, unpleasant taste, dyspnea, epistaxis, nasal irritation, upper respiratory infection, tinnitus. **_RARE: Parenteral:_** Hypotension, pruritus, blurred vision, sensation of heat, CNS stimulation, insomnia. **_Nasal:_** Hypertension, tremor, ear pain, paresthesia, depression, sinusitis.

ADVERSE REACTIONS/TOXIC EFFECTS

Abrupt withdrawal after prolonged use may produce symptoms of narcotic withdrawal (abdominal cramping, rhinorrhea, lacrimation, anxiety, increased temperature, piloerection [goose bumps]). Overdosage results in severe respiratory depression, skeletal muscle flaccidity, cyanosis, extreme somnolence progressing to convulsions, stupor, coma. Tolerance to analgesic effect, physical dependence may occur with chronic use.

NURSING IMPLICATIONS

BASELINE ASSESSMENT:

Obtain vital signs before giving medication. If respirations are 12/min or lower (20/min or lower in children), withhold medica-

tion, contact physician. Assess onset, type, location, duration of pain. Effect of medication is reduced if full pain recurs before next dose. Protect from falls. During labor, assess fetal heart tones, uterine contractions.

INTERVENTION/EVALUATION:

Monitor for change in respirations, B/P, change in rate/quality of pulse. Initiate deep breathing and coughing exercises, particularly in those with impaired pulmonary function. Change pt's position q2–4h. Assess for clinical improvement and record onset of relief of pain.

PATIENT/FAMILY TEACHING:

Change positions slowly to avoid dizziness. Avoid tasks that require alertness, motor skills until response to drug is established. Instruct pt on proper use of nasal spray. Avoid use of alcohol or CNS depressants.

cabergoline

cab-**err**-go-leen
(Dostinex)

▶CLASSIFICATION
CLINICAL: Antihyperprolactemic

ACTION/THERAPEUTIC EFFECT

Agonist at dopamine D_2 receptors suppressing prolactin secretion. _Shrinks prolactinomas, restores gonadal function._

USES

Treatment of hyperprolactemic disorders, either idiopathic or due to pituitary adenomas.

PRECAUTIONS

CONTRAINDICATIONS: Uncontrolled hypertension, hypersensitivity to ergot alkaloids. ***CAUTIONS:*** Hepatic function impairment.

INTERACTIONS

DRUG: May increase hypotensive effect if given with other **antihypertensives. HERBAL:** None known. ***FOOD:*** None known. ***LAB VALUES:*** None significant.

INDICATIONS/ROUTES/DOSAGE

Hyperprolactemia:

***PO:* Adults, elderly:** 0.5 mg 2 times/week.

SIDE EFFECTS

FREQUENT (29%): Nausea. ***OCCASIONAL*** (5–20%): Headache, vertigo, dizziness, dyspepsia, postural hypotension, constipation. ***RARE*** (2–4%): Vomiting, dry mouth, diarrhea, flatulence.

ADVERSE REACTIONS/TOXIC EFFECTS

Overdosage may produce nasal congestion, syncope, or hallucinations.

NURSING IMPLICATIONS

BASELINE ASSESSMENT:

Obtain baseline liver function tests.

INTERVENTION/EVALUATION:

Monitor prolactin levels monthly until prolactin levels equalize.

PATIENT/FAMILY TEACHING:

To reduce hypotensive effect, rise slowly from lying to sitting position and permit legs to dangle momentarily before rising.

caffeine citrate

(Cafcit)

ACTION/*THERAPEUTIC EFFECT*

Stimulates medullary respiratory center. Appears to increase sensitivity of respiratory center to stimulatory effects of CO_2 *increasing alveolar ventilation, reducing severity and frequency of apneic episodes.*

USES

Short-term treatment of apnea in premature infants from 28 to <33 wks gestational age.

AVAILABILITY (Rx)

INJECTION: 20 mg/ml. ***ORAL SOLUTION:*** 20 mg/ml.

INDICATIONS/ROUTES/DOSAGE

Apnea:

IV: Loading dose of 1 ml/kg administered over 30 min.

PO/IV: Maintenance dose of 0.25 ml/kg/day over 10 min beginning 24 hrs after the loading dose.

SIDE EFFECTS

FREQUENT (5–10%): Feeding intolerance, rash.

ADVERSE REACTIONS/TOXIC EFFECTS

Sepsis, necrotizing enterocolitis may be noted.

NURSING IMPLICATIONS

INTERVENTION/EVALUATION:

Monitor respirations diligently. Assess skin for rash.

calcipotriene

kal-sih-**poe**-tree-in
(Dovonex)

▶CLASSIFICATION

CLINICAL: Antipsoriatic

ACTION/ *THERAPEUTIC EFFECT*

A synthetic vitamin D_3 analogue. Regulates skin cell (keratinocyte) production and development, *preventing abnormal growth and production of psoriasis (abnormal keratinocyte growth).*

USES

Treatment of mild to moderate plaque psoriasis. **Solution:** Treatment of chronic, moderately severe scalp psoriasis.

PRECAUTIONS

CONTRAINDICATIONS: Hypercalcemia or evidence of vitamin D toxicity, use on face. **CAUTIONS:** History of nephrolithiasis.

INTERACTIONS

DRUG: None significant. **HERBAL:** None known. **FOOD:** None known. **LAB VALUES:** Excessive use may increase serum calcium level.

AVAILABILITY (Rx)

CREAM: 0.005%. **OINTMENT:** 0.005%.

INDICATIONS/ROUTES/DOSAGE

Psoriasis:

TOPICAL: Adults, elderly, children >12 yrs: Apply thin layer to affected skin twice daily (morning and evening); rub in gently and completely. **SOLUTION:** Apply to lesions after combing hair.

SIDE EFFECTS

FREQUENT (10–15%): Burning, itching, skin irritation. **OCCASIONAL** (2–10%): Erythema, dry skin, peeling, rash, worsening of psoriasis, dermatititis. **RARE** (≤1%): Skin atrophy, hyperpigmentation, folliculitis.

ADVERSE REACTIONS/TOXIC EFFECTS

Potential for hypercalcemia (abdominal pain, depression, easy fatigability, high B/P, anorexia, nausea, thirst) may occur.

NURSING IMPLICATIONS

BASELINE ASSESSMENT:

Establish baseline electrolytes, particularly serum and urine calcium.

INTERVENTION/EVALUATION:

Assess skin for irritation, erythema, worsening of psoriasis (children, those >65 are at greater risk of reactions). If irritation of lesions or surrounding uninvolved skin develops or if serum calcium level increases outside normal range, medication should be discontinued.

PATIENT/FAMILY TEACHING:

Avoid contact with face or eyes. Wash hands after application. Report any sign of local reaction. Improvement noted usually beginning after 2 wks of therapy, marked improvement after 8 wks of therapy.

calcitonin-salmon

kal-sih-**toe**-nin
(Calcimar, Caltine♣, Miacalcin, Salmonine, Osteocalcin)

▶CLASSIFICATION

PHARMACOTHERAPEUTIC: Synthetic hormone. **CLINICAL:** Calcium regulator, bone resorption inhibitor, osteoporosis therapy

ACTION/*THERAPEUTIC EFFECT*

Reduces bone turnover by blocking bone resorption in Paget's disease; directly inhibits bone resorption, decreasing the number/function of osteoclasts in osteoporosis. *Reduces bone turnover, lowers serum calcium concentration.*

PHARMACOKINETICS

Injection: Rapidly metabolized (primarily in kidney). Primarily excreted in urine. Half-life: 70–90 min. *Nasal:* Rapid absorption. Half-life: 43 min.

USES/*UNLABELED*

Management of moderate to severe Paget's disease of bone, early treatment of hypercalcemic emergencies. Management of postmenopausal osteoporosis to prevent progressive loss of bone mass (with calcium, vitamin D). *Treatment of secondary osteoporosis due to hormone disturbance, drug therapy.*

PRECAUTIONS

CONTRAINDICATIONS: Data does not support use in children, protein allergy. *CAUTIONS:* History of allergy, renal dysfunction.
▷*LIFESPAN CONSIDERATIONS:*
Pregnancy/Lactation: Drug does not cross placenta; unknown if distributed in breast milk. Safe usage during lactation not established (inhibits lactation in animals). **Pregnancy Category C. Children:** Safety and efficacy not established. **Elderly:** No age-related precautions noted.

INTERACTIONS

DRUG: None significant. *HERBAL:* None known. *FOOD:* None known. *LAB VALUES:* None significant.

AVAILABILITY (Rx)

INJECTION: 200 IU/ml. *NASAL SPRAY:* 200 IU/activation.

ADMINISTRATION/HANDLING

Intranasal:

• Refrigerate. Nasal preparation can be stored at room temperature once pump is activated. • Clear nasal passages as much as possible. • Tilt head slightly forward and insert spray tip into nostril, pointing toward nasal passages, away from nasal septum. • Spray into nostril while holding other nostril closed and concurrently inspire through nose to permit medication as high into nasal passage as possible.

IM/SubQ

• May be administered SubQ or IM. No more than 2 ml dose should be given IM. • Skin test should be performed before therapy in pts suspected of sensitivity to calcitonin. • Bedtime administration may reduce nausea, flushing.

INDICATIONS/ROUTES/DOSAGE

Skin testing:

Prepare a 10 unit/ml dilution; withdraw 0.05 ml from 200 IU/ml vial solution in tuberculin syringe; fill up to 1 ml with 0.9% NaCl. Take 0.1 ml and inject intracutaneously on inner aspect of forearm. Observe after 15 min (positive response: appearance of more than mild erythema or wheal).

Paget's disease:

SubQ/IM: Adults, elderly: Initially, 100 IU/day (improvement in biochemical abnormalities, bone pain seen in first few months; in neurologic lesion, often longer than 1 yr). **Maintenance:** 50 IU/day or every other day. *INTRANASAL:* 200–400 units/day.

Postmenopausal osteoporosis:

SubQ/IM: **Adults, elderly:** 100 IU/day (with adequate calcium and vitamin D intake). *INTRANASAL:* 200 IU as single daily spray, alternating nostrils daily.

Hypercalcemia:

SubQ/IM: **Adults, elderly:** Initially, 4 IU/kg q12h; may increase to 8 IU/kg q12h if no response in 2 days; may further increase to 8 IU/kg q6h if no response in 2 days.

SIDE EFFECTS

FREQUENT: SubQ/IM (10%): Nausea (may occur 30 min after injection, usually diminishes with continued therapy), inflammation at injection site. *Nasal* (10–12%): Rhinitis, nasal irritation, redness, sores. *OCCASIONAL: SubQ/IM* (2–5%): Flushing of face or hands. *Nasal* (3–5%): Back pain, arthralgia, epistaxis (nosebleed), headache. *RARE: SubQ/IM:* Epigastric discomfort, dry mouth, diarrhea, floatulence. *Nasal:* Itching of earlobes, edema of feet, rash, increased sweating.

ADVERSE REACTIONS/TOXIC EFFECTS

Potential hypersensitivity reaction with protein allergy.

NURSING IMPLICATIONS

BASELINE ASSESSMENT:

Establish baseline electrolytes.

INTERVENTION/EVALUATION:

Assure rotation of injection sites; check for inflammation. Assess vertebral bone mass (document stabilization/improvement). Assess for allergic response: rash, urticaria, swelling, shortness of breath, tachycardia, hypotension.

PATIENT/FAMILY TEACHING:

Instruct pt/family on aseptic technique, proper injection of medication, including rotation of sites. Nausea is transient and usually decreases with continued therapy. Notify physician immediately if rash, itching, shortness of breath, significant nasal irritation occur.

calcium acetate

(Phos-Ex, PhosLo)

calcium carbonate

(Apo-Cal✤, Calsan✤, Caltrate✤, Dicarbasil, OsCal, Titralac, Tums)

calcium chloride

(Calcijex✤)

calcium citrate

(Citracal)

calcium glubionate

(NeoCalglucon)

calcium gluconate

Do not confuse with Asacol.

▶CLASSIFICATION

PHARMACOTHERAPEUTIC: Electrolyte replenisher. *CLINICAL:* Antacid, antihypocalcemic, antihyperkalemic, antihypermagnesemic, antihyperphosphatemic (see p. 9C)

ACTION/*THERAPEUTIC EFFECT*

Calcium is essential for function, integrity of nervous, muscular, skeletal systems. Important role in normal cardiac, renal function, respiration, blood coagulation, and cell membrane and capillary permeability. Assists in regulating release/storage of neurotransmitter/hormones. Neutralizes or reduces gastric acid (increase pH). *Calcium acetate:* Combines with dietary phosphate, forming insoluble calcium phosphate. *Replaces calcium in deficiency states, controls hyperphosphatemia in end-stage renal disease.*

PHARMACOKINETICS

Moderately absorbed from small intestine (dependent on presence of vitamin D metabolites, pH). Primarily eliminated in feces.

USES/UNLABELED

Parenteral: Acute hypocalcemia (e.g., neonatal hypocalcemic tetany, alkalosis), electrolyte depletion, cardiac arrest (strengthens myocardial contractions), hyperkalemia (reverses EKG, cardiac depression), hypermagnesemia (aids in reversing CNS depression). *PO:* Chronic hypocalcemia, calcium deficiency, antacid. *Calcium acetate:* Controls hyperphosphatemia in end-stage renal disease. *Calcium carbonate:* Treatment of hyperphosphatemia.

PRECAUTIONS

CONTRAINDICATIONS: Ventricular fibrillation, hypercalcemia, hypercalciuria, calcium renal calculi, sarcoidosis, digoxin toxicity. *Calcium acetate:* Hypoparathyroidism, decreased renal function. *CAUTIONS:* Dehydration, history of renal calculi, chronic renal impairment, decreased cardiac function, ventricular fibrillation during cardiac resuscitation.

▷ *LIFESPAN CONSIDERATIONS:*
Pregnancy/Lactation: Distributed in breast milk. Unknown whether calcium chloride or gluconate is distributed in breast milk. **Pregnancy Category C. Children:** Extreme irritation, possible tissue necrosis/sloughing; restrict use due to small vasculature. **Elderly:** Oral absorption may be decreased.

INTERACTIONS

DRUG: May antagonize **etidronate, gallium** effects. May decrease absorption of **ketoconazole, phenytoin, tetracyclines.** May decrease effects of **methenamine, parenteral magnesium.** May increase risk of arrhythmias with **digoxin.** *HERBAL:* None known. *FOOD:* None known. *LAB VALUES:* May increase calcium gastrin, pH. May decrease phosphate, potassium.

AVAILABILITY (OTC)

Calcium acetate: TABLETS: 250 mg, 667 mg, 1,000 mg. *CAPSULES:* 333.5 mg, 500 mg.

Calcium carbonate: TABLETS: 500 mg, 650 mg, 1,250 mg, 1,500 mg. *CHEWABLE TABLETS:* 350 mg, 500 mg, 750 mg, 1,250 mg. *CAPSULES:* 1,250 mg.

Calcium chloride (Rx): INJECTION: 10%.

Calcium citrate: TABLETS: 950 mg.

Calcium glubionate: SYRUP.

Calcium gluconate: TABLETS: 500 mg, 650 mg, 975 mg, 1,000 mg. *INJECTION: (Rx):* 10%.

ADMINISTRATION/HANDLING

PO:

• Take tablets with full glass of water 0.5–1 hr after meals. Give syrup before meals (increases absorption), diluted in juice or water.

• Chew chewable tablets well before swallowing.

IV 🍴

Storage:

Store at room temperature.

Dilution:

CALCIUM CHLORIDE:

• May give undiluted or may dilute with equal amount 0.9% NaCl or Sterile Water for Injection.

CALCIUM GLUCONATE:

• May give undiluted or may dilute in up to 1,000 ml NaCl.

Rate of administration:

CALCIUM CHLORIDE:

• Give by slow IV push: 0.5–1 ml/min (rapid administration may produce bradycardia, metallic or chalky taste, drop in B/P, sensation of heat, peripheral vasodilation).

CALCIUM GLUCONATE:

• Give by IV push: 0.5–1 ml/min (rapid administration may produce vasodilation, drop in B/P, arrhythmias, syncope, cardiac arrest). • Maximum rate for intermittent IV infusion is 200 mg/min (e.g., 10 ml/min when 1 g diluted with 50 ml diluent).

IV INCOMPATIBILITIES ⊘

Calcium chloride: Amphotericin B complex (Ambisome, Abelcet), propofol (Diprivan), sodium bicarbonate. ***Calcium gluconate:*** Amphotericin C complex (Ambisome, Abelcet), fluconazole (Diflucan).

IV COMPATIBILITIES

Cefazolin (Ancef), cefepime (Maxipime), ciprofloxacin (Cipro), cisatracuronium (Nimbex), dobutamine (Dobutrex), enalapril (Vasotec), famotidine (Pepcid), heparin, midazolam (Versed), multivitamins, potassium chloride, propofol (Diprivan).

INDICATIONS/ROUTES/DOSAGE

CALCIUM ACETATE

Hypophosphatemia:

PO: Adults, elderly: 2 tablets 3 times/day with meals.

CALCIUM CARBONATE

Antihypocalcemic, nutritional supplement:

PO: Adults, elderly: 0.5–1.25 g (500 mg calcium) 1–3 times/day.

Antacid:

PO: Adults, elderly: 0.5–1.25 g as needed.

CALCIUM GLUBIONATE

Antihypocalcemic:

PO: Adults, elderly: 15 ml 3–4 times/day. **Children 1–4 yrs:** 10 ml 3 times/day. **Children <1 yr:** 5 ml 5 times/day.

CALCIUM CHLORIDE

Hypocalcemia, electrolyte replenisher, cardiotonic:

IV: Adults, elderly: 500 mg–1 g at a rate not to exceed 0.5–1 ml/min. **Children:** 25 mg/kg given slowly (hypocalcemia, electrolyte replenisher).

CALCIUM GLUCONATE

Hypocalcemia, electrolyte replenisher:

IV: Adults, elderly: 1 g at a rate not to exceed 5 ml/min. May repeat. **Children:** 200–500 mg. May repeat.

Antihyperkalemia:

IV: Adults, elderly: 1–2 g.

SIDE EFFECTS

FREQUENT: Parenteral: Hypotension, flushing, feeling of warmth, nausea, vomiting; pain, rash, redness, burning at injection site; sweating, decreased B/P. **PO:** Chalky taste. **OCCASIONAL: PO:** Mild constipation, fecal impaction, swelling of hands/feet, metabolic alkalosis (muscle pain, restlessness, slow breathing, poor taste). **Calcium carbonate:** Milk-alkali syndrome (headache, decreased appetite, nausea, vomiting, unusual tiredness). **RARE: PO:** Difficult or painful urination.

ADVERSE REACTIONS/TOXIC EFFECTS

Hypercalcemia: *Early signs:* Constipation, headache, dry mouth, increased thirst, irritability, decreased appetite, metallic taste, fatigue, weakness, depression. *Later signs:* Confusion, drowsiness, increased B/P, increased light sensitivity, irregular heartbeat, nausea, vomiting, increased urination.

NURSING IMPLICATIONS

BASELINE ASSESSMENT:
Assess B/P, EKG readings, renal function, magnesium, phosphate, potassium concentrations.

INTERVENTION/EVALUATION:
Monitor B/P, EKG, renal function, magnesium, phosphate, potassium, serum and urine calcium concentrations. Monitor for signs of hypercalcemia.

PATIENT/FAMILY TEACHING:
Stress importance of diet. Take tablets with full glass of water, $\frac{1}{2}$–1 hr after meals. Give liquid before meals. Do not take within 1–2 hrs of other oral medications, fiber-containing foods. Avoid excessive alcohol, tobacco, caffeine.

---

calfactant

cal-**fact**-tant
(Infasurf)

▶CLASSIFICATION

PHARMACOTHERAPEUTIC:
Natural lung extract. **CLINICAL:**
Pulmonary surfactant

ACTION/*THERAPEUTIC EFFECT*

Modifies alveolar surface tension, stabilizing the alveoli, *restoring surface activity to infant lungs, improving lung compliance and respiratory gas exchange.*

PHARMACOKINETICS

No studies performed.

USES

Prevention of respiratory distress syndrome (RDS) in premature infants <29 wks of gestational age and for treatment of premature infants <72 hrs of age who develop RDS and require endotracheal intubation.

PRECAUTIONS

CONTRAINDICATIONS: None known. **CAUTIONS:** Hypersensitivity to calfactant.

▷**LIFESPAN CONSIDERATIONS:**
Used only in neonates. No age-related precautions noted.

INTERACTIONS

DRUG: None significant. **HERBAL:** None known. **FOOD:** None known. **LAB VALUES:** None significant.

AVAILABILITY (Rx)

INTRATRACHEAL SUSPENSION: 35 mg/ml vials.

𝒪 - see color pill atlas   <u>underscored</u> - top 100 prescribed drug

ADMINISTRATION/HANDLING
Intratracheal:
• Refrigerate. • Unopened, unused vials may be returned to refrigerator only once after having been warmed to room temperature. • Do not shake. • Enter only once, discard unused suspension.

INDICATIONS/ROUTES/DOSAGE
Respiratory distress syndrome (RDS):
INTRATRACHEAL: Infants: Instill 3 ml/kg of birth weight as soon as possible after birth, administered as 2 doses of 1.5 ml/kg. Repeat doses of 3 ml/kg of birth weight, up to a total of 3 doses, 12 hrs apart.

SIDE EFFECTS
FREQUENT: Cyanosis (65%), airway obstruction (39%), bradycardia (34%), reflux of surfactant into endotracheal tube (21%), requirement of manual ventilation (16%). ***OCCASIONAL*** (3%): Reintubation.

ADVERSE REACTIONS/TOXIC EFFECTS
Complications may occur as apnea, patent ductus arteriosus, intracranial hemorrhage, sepsis, pulmonary air leaks, pulmonary hemorrhage, necrotizing enterocolitis.

NURSING IMPLICATIONS

BASELINE ASSESSMENT:
Drug must be administered in highly supervised setting. Clinicians in care of neonate must be experienced with intubation, ventilator management. Offer emotional support to parents.

INTERVENTION/EVALUATION:
Monitor infant with arterial or transcutaneous measurement of systemic O_2 and CO_2. Assess lung sounds for rales and moist breath sounds.

C

candesartan cilexetil

can-deh-**sar**-tan sill-**ex**-eh-til
(Atacand)
FIXED-COMBINATION(S)
With hydrochlorothiazide, a diuretic **(Atacand HCT)**

▶CLASSIFICATION
PHARMACOTHERAPEUTIC:
Angiotensin II receptor antagonist.
CLINICAL: Antihypertensive
(see p. 7C)

ACTION/*THERAPEUTIC EFFECT*
Potent vasodilator. An angiotensin II receptor (type AT_1) antagonist; blocks vasoconstrictor and aldesterone-secreting effects of angiotensin II, inhibiting the binding of angiotensin II to the AT_1 receptors, *producing vasodilation, decreased peripheral resistance, decrease in B/P.*

PHARMACOKINETICS

Onset	Peak	Duration
PO		
30–60 min	3–4 hrs	24 hrs

Rapidly, completely absorbed. Protein binding: >99%. Undergoes minor hepatic metabolism to inactive metabolite. Excreted unchanged in urine and feces via biliary system. Not removed by hemodialysis. Half-life: 9 hrs.

USES/*UNLABELED*
Treatment of hypertension alone or in combination with other antihypertensives. *Treatment of heart failure.*

PRECAUTIONS

CONTRAINDICATIONS: None significant. ***CAUTIONS:*** Renal/hepatic function impairment, renal arterial stenosis.

▷***LIFESPAN CONSIDERATIONS:*** **Pregnancy/Lactation:** Unknown if distributed in breast milk. May cause fetal/neonatal morbidity/mortality. **Pregnancy Category C** (first trimester), **Category D** (second and third trimesters). **Children:** Safety and efficacy not established. **Elderly:** No age-related precautions noted.

INTERACTIONS

DRUG: None significant. ***HERBAL:*** None known. ***FOOD:*** None known. ***LAB VALUES:*** May increase BUN, serum creatinine, SGOT (AST), SGPT (ALT), alkaline phosphatase, bilirubin. May decrease Hemoglobin, hemocrit.

AVAILABILITY (Rx)

TABLETS: 4 mg, 8 mg, 16 mg, 32 mg.

ADMINISTRATION/HANDLING
PO:

• Give without regard to food.

INDICATIONS/ROUTES/DOSAGE

Note: If antihypertensive effect using once-daily dosing is inadequate, twice-daily regimen at same total daily dose or an increase in dose may provide therapeutic response. May be given concurrently with other antihypertensives. If B/P is not controlled by candesartan alone, a diuretic may be added.

Hypertension

PO: Adults, elderly, mildly impaired renal or hepatic function: Initially, 16 mg once daily in those who are not volume depleted. Can be given once or twice daily with total daily doses 8–32 mg. Give lower dose in those treated with diuretics, severe impaired renal function.

SIDE EFFECTS

OCCASIONAL (3–6%): Upper respiratory tract infection, dizziness, back and leg pain. ***RARE*** (1–2%): Pharyngitis, rhinitis, headache, fatigue, diarrhea, nausea, dry cough, peripheral edema.

ADVERSE REACTIONS/TOXIC EFFECTS

Overdosage may manifest as hypotension and tachycardia; bradycardia occurs less often. Institute supportive measures.

NURSING IMPLICATIONS

BASELINE ASSESSMENT:

Obtain B/P and apical pulse immediately before each dose, in addition to regular monitoring (be alert to fluctuations). If excessive reduction in B/P occurs, place pt in supine position, feet slightly elevated. Question possibility of pregnancy (see Pregnancy category). Assess medication history (esp. diuretic). Question for history of hepatic/renal impairment, renal artery stenosis. Obtain BUN, serum creatinine, SGOT (AST), SGPT (ALT), alkaline phosphatase, bilirubin, hemoglobin, hemocrit, and vital signs, particularly B/P, pulse rate.

INTERVENTION/EVALUATION:

Maintain hydration (offer fluids frequently). Assess for evidence of upper respiratory infection. Assist with ambulation if dizziness occurs. Monitor all blood serum levels. Assess B/P for hypertension/hypotension.

PATIENT/FAMILY TEACHING:

Inform female pt regarding consequences of second- and third-trimester exposure to candesartan. Report pregnancy to physician as soon as possible. Avoid tasks that require alertness, motor skills (possible dizziness effect). Report any sign of infection (sore throat, fever). Do not stop taking medication. Need for lifelong control. Caution against exercising during hot weather (risk of dehydration, hypotension).

capecitabine

cap-eh-**site**-ah-bean
(Xeloda)
Do not confuse with Xenical.

▶CLASSIFICATION

PHARMACOTHERAPEUTIC:
Antimetabolite. **CLINICAL:** Antineoplastic (see p. 68C).

ACTION/THERAPEUTIC EFFECT

Enzymatically converted to 5-fluorouracil. Inhibits enzymes necessary for synthesis of essential cellular components, *interfering with DNA synthesis, RNA processing, and protein synthesis.*

PHARMACOKINETICS

Readily absorbed from GI tract. Protein binding: <60%. Metabolized in the liver. Primarily excreted in urine. Half-life: 45 min.

USES

Treatment of metastatic breast cancer resistant to other therapy, colon cancer.

PRECAUTIONS

CONTRAINDICATIONS: None

significant. **CAUTIONS:** Liver impairment, history of coronary artery disease, sensitivity to capecitabine or 5-fluorouracil.

▷**LIFESPAN CONSIDERATIONS:**
Pregnancy/Lactation: May be harmful to fetus. Unknown if distributed in breast milk. **Pregnancy Category D. Children:** Safety and efficacy in those <18 yrs not established. **Elderly:** May be more sensitive to GI side effects.

INTERACTIONS

DRUG: May alter effects of **warfarin. HERBAL:** None known. **FOOD:** None known. **LAB VALUES:** May increase alkaline phosphatase, ALT, AST, billirubin. May decrease WBC, hemoglobin, hemocrit.

AVAILABILITY (Rx)

TABLETS: 150 mg, 500 mg.

ADMINISTRATION/HANDLING

• Give within 30 min of a meal.

INDICATIONS/ROUTES/DOSAGE

Metastatic breast cancer, colon cancer:

PO: Adults, elderly: Initially, 2,500 mg/m^2/day in two equally divided doses approximately 12 hrs apart for 2 wks. Follow with a 1 wk rest period given as 3 wk cycles.

SIDE EFFECTS

FREQUENT (>5%): Diarrhea (sometimes severe), nausea, vomiting, stomatitis (painful erythema, ulcers of mouth or tongue), hand and foot syndrome (painful palmar-plantar erythema amd swelling with paresthesia, tingling, blistering), fatigue, anorexia, dermatitis. **OCCASIONAL** (<5%): Constipation, dyspepsia, nail disorder, headache, dizziness, insomnia, edema, myalgia.

ADVERSE REACTIONS/TOXIC EFFECTS

Bone marrow depression (neutropenia, thrombocytopenia, anemia) cardiovascular toxicity noted as angina, cardiomyopathy, DVT lymphedema. Respiratory toxicity noted as dyspnea, epistaxis, pneumonia.

NURSING IMPLICATIONS

BASELINE ASSESSMENT:

Assess sensitivity to capcitabine or 5-fluorouracil. Obtain baseline hemoglobin, hemocrit, blood chemistries.

INTERVENTION/EVALUATION:

Monitor for severe diarrhea; if dehydration occurs, fluid and electrolyte replacement therapy should be ordered. Assess hands and feet for erythema (chemotherapy induced). Monitor CBC for evidence of bone marrow depression. Monitor for blood dyscrasias (fever, sore throat, signs of local infection, easy bruising, or unusual bleeding from any site), symptoms of anemia (excessive tiredness, weakness).

PATIENT/FAMILY TEACHING:

Inform pt of potential for, and notify physician if nausea, vomiting, possibly severe diarrhea and hand-and-foot syndrome, stomatitis occur. Do not have immunizations without physician's approval (drug lowers body's resistance). Avoid contact with those who have recently received live virus vaccine. Promptly report fever >100.5, sore throat, signs of local infection, easy bruising or unusual bleeding from any site.

capsaicin

cap-**say**-sin
(Zostrix)

▶CLASSIFICATION

PHARMACOTHERAPEUTIC:
Counterirritant.   ***CLINICAL:***
Topical analgesic

ACTION/*THERAPEUTIC EFFECT*

Depletes and prevents reaccumulation of the chemomediator of pain impulses (substance P) from peripheral sensory neurons to CNS, *relieving pain.*

USES/*UNLABELED*

Treatment of neuralgia (e.g., pain with shingles, painful diabetic neuropathy), osteoarthritis, rheumatoid arthritis. *Treatment of neurogenic pain.*

PRECAUTIONS

CONTRAINDICATIONS: None significant. ***CAUTIONS:*** For external use only.
▷***LIFESPAN CONSIDERATIONS:***
Pregnancy/Lactation: Unknown if distributed in breast milk. **Pregnancy Category C. Children:** Not recommended in those <2 yrs of age. **Elderly:** No age-related precautions noted.

INTERACTIONS

DRUG: None significant. ***HERBAL:*** None known. ***FOOD:*** None known. ***LAB VALUES:*** None significant.

AVAILABILITY (OTC)

CREAM: 0.025%, 0.075%.

INDICATIONS/ROUTES/DOSAGE
Usual topical dosage:
TOPICAL: Adults, elderly, chil-

C

dren >2 yrs: Apply directly to affected area 3–4 times/day. Continue for 14–28 days for optimal clinical response.

SIDE EFFECTS
FREQUENT (>30%): Burning, stinging, erythema at site of application.

ADVERSE REACTIONS/TOXIC EFFECTS
None significant.

NURSING IMPLICATIONS

PATIENT/FAMILY TEACHING:
Avoid contact with eyes, broken/irritated skin. Transient burning may occur on application; usually disappears after 72 hrs. Wash hands immediately after application. If there is no improvement or condition deteriorates after 28 days, discontinue use and consult physician.

captopril

cap-toe-prill
(Capoten, Novo-Captoril♣)
Do not confuse with Capitrol.

FIXED-COMBINATION(S)
With hydrochlorothiazide, a diuretic **(Capozide)**

▶CLASSIFICATION
PHARMACOTHERAPEUTIC:
Angiotensin-converting enzyme (ACE) inhibitor. **CLINICAL:** Antihypertensive, vasodilator (see p. 6C)

ACTION/*THERAPEUTIC EFFECT*
Suppresses renin-angiotensin-aldosterone system (prevents conversion of angiotensin I to angiotensin II, a potent vasoconstrictor; may also inhibit angiotensin II at local vascular and renal sites). Decreases plasma angiotensin II, increases plasma renin activity, decreases aldosterone secretion. *Reduces peripheral arterial resistance, pulmonary capillary wedge pressure, improves cardiac output, exercise tolerance.*

PHARMACOKINETICS

Onset	Peak	Duration
PO		
0.25 hrs	0.5–1.5 hrs	dose related

Rapidly, well absorbed from GI tract (decreased in presence of food). Protein binding: 25–30%. Metabolized in liver. Primarily excreted in urine. Removed by hemodialysis. Half-life: <3 hrs (increased with impaired renal function).

USES/*UNLABELED*
Treatment of hypertension alone or in combination with other antihypertensives. Adjunctive therapy for CHF (in combination with cardiac glycosides, diuretics). Reduces development of severe heart failure following MI in pts with impaired left ventricular (LV) function. Treats nephropathy/prevents kidney failure in type I diabetes. *Treatment of hypertension/ renal crises in scleroderma.*

PRECAUTIONS
CONTRAINDICATIONS: History of angioedema with previous treatment with ACE inhibitors. **CAUTIONS:** Renal impairment, those with sodium depletion or on diuretic therapy, dialysis, hypovolemia, coronary/cerebrovascular insufficiency.

▷*LIFESPAN CONSIDERATIONS:*
Pregnancy/Lactation: Crosses placenta; distributed in breast

milk. May cause fetal/neonatal mortality/morbidity. **Pregnancy Category D. Children:** Safety and efficacy not established. **Elderly:** May be more sensitive to hypotensive effects; caution recommended.

INTERACTIONS

DRUG: **Alcohol, diuretics, hypotensive agents** may increase effect. **NSAIDs** may decrease effect. **Potassium-sparing diuretics, potassium supplements** may cause hyperkalemia. May increase **lithium** concentration, toxicity. **HERBAL:** None known. **FOOD:** None known. **LAB VALUES:** May increase potassium, SGOT (AST), SGPT (ALT), alkaline phosphatase, bilirubin, BUN, creatinine. May decrease sodium. May cause positive ANA titer.

AVAILABILITY (Rx)

TABLETS: 12.5 mg, 25 mg, 50 mg, 100 mg.

ADMINISTRATION/HANDLING
PO:

• Best taken 1 hr before meals for maximum absorption (food significantly decreases drug absorption). • Tablets may be crushed.

INDICATIONS/ROUTES/DOSAGE
Hypertension:

PO: Adults, elderly: Initially, 12.5–25 mg 2–3 times/day. After 1–2 wks, may increase to 50 mg 2–3 times/day. Diuretic may be added if no response in additional 1–2 wks. If taken in combination with diuretic, may increase to 100–150 mg 2–3 times/day after 1–2 wks. **Maintenance:** 25–150 mg 2–3 times/day. **Maximum:** 450 mg/day.

CHF:

PO: Adults, elderly: Initially, 6.25–25 mg 3 times/day. Increase to 50 mg 3 times/day. After at least 2 wks, may increase to 50–100 mg 3 times/day. **Maximum:** 450 mg/day.

Post MI, impaired liver function:

PO: Adults, elderly: 6.25 mg once, then 12.5 mg 3 times/day. Increase to 25 mg 3 times/day over several days up to 50 mg 3 times/day over several weeks.

Nephropathy/prevention of kidney failure:

PO: Adults, elderly: 25 mg 3 times/day.

Usual pediatric dose:

PO: Newborns: 10 mcg/kg 2–3 times/day. **Children:** 150–300 mcg/kg 3 times/day.

SIDE EFFECTS

FREQUENT (4–7%): Rash. **OCCASIONAL** (2–4%): Pruritus, dysgeusia (change in sense of taste). **RARE** (0.5–<2%): Headache, cough, insomnia, dizziness, fatigue, paresthesia, malaise, nausea, diarrhea/constipation, dry mouth, tachycardia.

ADVERSE REACTIONS/TOXIC EFFECTS

Excessive hypotension ("first-dose syncope") may occur in those with CHF, severely salt/volume depleted. Angioedema (swelling of face/lips), hyperkalemia occur rarely. Agranulocytosis, neutropenia may be noted in those with impaired renal function or collagen vascular disease (systemic lupus erythematosus, scleroderma). Nephrotic syndrome may be noted in those with history of renal disease.

C

NURSING IMPLICATIONS

BASELINE ASSESSMENT:

Obtain B/P immediately before each dose, in addition to regular monitoring (be alert to fluctuations). If excessive reduction in B/P occurs, place pt in supine position with legs elevated. In pts with prior renal disease or receiving dosages higher than 150 mg/day, urine test for protein by dipstick method should be made with first urine of day before therapy begins and periodically thereafter. In those with renal impairment, autoimmune disease, or taking drugs that affect leukocytes or immune response, CBC should be performed before therapy begins and q2wks for 3 mos, then periodically thereafter.

INTERVENTION/EVALUATION:

Assess skin for rash, pruritus. Assist with ambulation if dizziness occurs. Monitor urinalysis for proteinuria. Assess for anorexia secondary to decreased taste perception. Monitor serum potassium levels in those on concurrent diuretic therapy.

PATIENT/FAMILY TEACHING:

Several weeks may be needed for full therapeutic effect of B/P reduction. Skipping doses or voluntarily discontinuing drug may produce severe, rebound hypertension. Avoid alcohol.

carbachol

(Isopto-Carbachol)

See Classification section under: Antiglaucoma (p. 44C)

carbamazepine

car-bah-**may**-zeh-peen
(Apo-Carbamazepine♣,
Carbatrol, Epitol, Tegretol)
Do not confuse with Toradol.

▶CLASSIFICATION

PHARMACOTHERAPEUTIC: Iminostilbene derivative. ***CLINICAL:*** Anticonvulsant, antineuralgic, antimanic, antipsychotic (see p. 32C)

ACTION/*THERAPEUTIC EFFECT*

Decreases sodium, calcium ion influx into neuronal membranes, reducing post-tetanic potentiation at synapse; *prevents repetitive discharge.*

PHARMACOKINETICS

Slowly, completely absorbed from GI tract. Protein binding: 75%. Metabolized in liver to active metabolite. Primarily excreted in urine. Not removed by hemodialysis. Half-life: 25–65 hrs (half-life decreased with chronic use).

USES/*UNLABELED*

Management of generalized tonic-clonic seizures (grand mal), complex partial seizures (temporal lobe, psychomotor), mixed seizures; treatment of trigeminal neuralgia (tic douloureux). *Treatment of neurogenic pain, bipolar disorder, diabetes insipidus, alcohol withdrawal, psychotic disorders.*

PRECAUTIONS

CONTRAINDICATIONS: History of bone marrow depression, history of hypersensitivity to tricyclic antidepressants, concomitant use of MAO inhibitors. ***CAUTIONS:***

♣ - Canadian trade name   ✳ - see also www.wbsaunders.com/SIMON/SaundersNDH

Impaired cardiac, hepatic, renal function.

▷**LIFESPAN CONSIDERATIONS:**
Pregnancy/Lactation: Crosses placenta; distributed in breast milk. Accumulates in fetal tissue. **Pregnancy Category C. Children:** Behavioral changes more likely to occur. **Elderly:** More susceptible to confusion, agitation, AV block, bradycardia, syndrome of inappropriate antidiuretic hormone.

INTERACTIONS

DRUG: May decrease effect of **steroids, anticoagulants.** May increase metabolism of **anticonvulsants, barbiturates, benzodiazepines, valproic acid. Tricyclic antidepressants, haloperidol, antipsychotics** may increase CNS depressant effects. **Cimetidine** may increase concentration, toxicity. May decrease effects of **estrogens, quinidine, clarithromycin, diltiazem, erythromycin, propoxyphene. Verapamil** may increase toxicity. May increase metabolism of **isoniazid** (hepatotoxicity). **Isoniazid** may increase concentration, toxicity. **MAO inhibitors** may cause hypertensive crises, convulsions. **HERBAL:** None known. **FOOD: Grapefruit** can increase absorption, concentration. **LAB VALUES:** May increase BUN, glucose, protein, SGOT (AST), SGPT (ALT), alkaline phosphatase, bilirubin, cholesterol, HDL, triglycerides. May decrease calcium, T_3, T_4, T_4 index. Therapeutic blood serum level: 4–12 mcg/ml; toxic serum level: >12 mcg/ml.

AVAILABILITY (Rx)

TABLETS (chewable): 100 mg.
TABLETS: 200 mg. **TABLETS (extended-release):** 100 mg, 200 mg, 300 mg, 400 mg. **ORAL SUSPENSION:** 100 mg/5 ml.

ADMINISTRATION/HANDLING
PO:

• Store oral suspension, tablets at room temperature. • Give with meals to reduce risk of GI distress. • Shake oral suspension well. Do not administer simultaneously with other liquid medicine. • Do not crush extended-release tablets.

INDICATIONS/ROUTES/DOSAGE

Note: When replacement by another anticonvulsant is necessary, decrease carbamazepine gradually as therapy begins with low replacement dose. When transferring from tablets to suspension, divide total tablet daily dose into smaller, more frequent doses of suspension. Administer extended-release tablets in 2 divided doses.

Seizure control:

PO: Adults, elderly, children >12 yrs: Initially, 200 mg 2 times/day. Increase dosage up to 200 mg/day at weekly intervals until response is attained. **Maintenance:** 800–1,200 mg/day. Do not exceed 1,000 mg/day in children 12–15 yrs, 1,200 mg/day in pts >15 yrs. **Children 6–12 yrs:** Initially, 100 mg 2 times/day. Increase by 100 mg/day until response is attained. **Maintenance:** 400–800 mg/day. Give dosage 200 mg or greater/day in 3–4 equally divided doses. **SYRUP: Children 6–12 yrs:** Initially, 50 mg 4 times/day. Increase dosage slowly (reduces sedation risk). **Children <6 yrs:** 10–20 mg/kg/day in 2–4 divided doses. **Maximum:** 35 mg/kg/day.

Trigeminal neuralgia:

PO: Adults, elderly: 100 mg 2 times/day on day 1. Increase by 100 mg q12h until pain is relieved. **Maintenance:** 200–1,200 mg/day. Do not exceed 1,200 mg/day.

SIDE EFFECTS

FREQUENT: Drowsiness, dizziness, nausea, vomiting. ***OCCASIONAL:*** Visual abnormalities (spots before eyes, difficulty focusing, blurred vision), dry mouth/pharynx, tongue irritation, headache, water retention, increased sweating, constipation/diarrhea.

ADVERSE REACTIONS/TOXIC EFFECTS

Toxic reactions appear as blood dyscrasias (aplastic anemia, agranulocytosis, thrombocytopenia, leukopenia, leukocytosis, eosinophilia), cardiovascular disturbances (CHF, hypo/hypertension, thrombophlebitis, arrhythmias), dermatologic effects (rash, urticaria, pruritus, photosensitivity). Abrupt withdrawal may precipitate status epilepticus.

NURSING IMPLICATIONS

BASELINE ASSESSMENT:

Seizures: Review history of seizure disorder (intensity, frequency, duration, LOC). Provide safety precautions, quiet, dark environment. CBC, serum iron determination, urinalysis, BUN should be performed before therapy begins and periodically during therapy.

INTERVENTION/EVALUATION:

Seizures: Observe frequently for recurrence of seizure activity. Assess for clinical improvement (decrease in intensity/frequency of seizures). Assess for clinical evidence of early toxic signs (fever, sore throat, mouth ulcerations, easy bruising, unusual bleeding, joint pain). ***Neuralgia:*** Avoid triggering tic douloureux (draft, talking, washing face, jarring bed, hot/warm/cold food or liquids). Therapeutic blood serum level: 4–12 mcg/ml; toxic serum level: >12 mcg/ml.

PATIENT/FAMILY TEACHING:

Do not abruptly withdraw medication following long-term use (may precipitate seizures). Strict maintenance of drug therapy is essential for seizure control. Drowsiness usually disappears during continued therapy. Avoid tasks that require alertness, motor skills until response to drug is established. Report visual abnormalities. Blood tests should be repeated frequently during first 3 mos of therapy and at monthly intervals thereafter for 2–3 yrs. Do not take liquid simultaneously with other liquid medicine. Do not take with grapefruit juice.

carbenicillin

(Geocillin)

See Classification section under: Antibiotic: penicillins (p. 27C)

carbidopa/levodopa

car-bih-dope-ah/**lev**-oh-dope-ah
(Sinemet)

▶CLASSIFICATION

PHARMACOTHERAPEUTIC: Dopamine precursor. ***CLINICAL:*** Antiparkinson

ACTION/*THERAPEUTIC EFFECT*

Converted to dopamine in basal ganglia. Increases dopamine concentration in brain, inhibiting hyperactive cholinergic activity, *reducing tremor.* Carbidopa prevents peripheral breakdown of levodopa, allowing more levodopa to be available for transport into brain.

PHARMACOKINETICS

Carbidopa: Rapidly, completely absorbed from GI tract. Widely distributed. Excreted primarily in urine. Half-life: 1–2 hrs. ***Levodopa:*** Converted to dopamine. Excreted primarily in urine. Half-life: 1–3 hrs.

USES

Treatment of idiopathic Parkinson's disease (paralysis agitans), postencephalitic parkinsonism, symptomatic parkinsonism following injury to nervous system by CO_2 poisoning, manganese intoxication.

PRECAUTIONS

CONTRAINDICATIONS: Narrow-angle glaucoma, those on MAO inhibitor therapy. ***CAUTIONS:*** History of MI, bronchial asthma (tartrazine sensitivity), emphysema; severe cardiac, pulmonary, renal, hepatic, endocrine disease; active peptic ulcer; treated open-angle glaucoma.

▷*LIFESPAN CONSIDERATIONS:*
Pregnancy/Lactation: Unknown if drug crosses placenta or is distributed in breast milk. May inhibit lactation. Do not nurse. **Pregnancy Category C. Children:** Safety and efficacy not established in those <18 yrs of age. **Elderly:** More sensitive to effects of levodopa. Anxiety, confusion, nervousness more common when receiving anticholinergics.

INTERACTIONS

DRUG: **Anticonvulsants, benzodiazepines, haloperidol, phenothiazines** may decrease effect. **MAO inhibitors** may increase risk of hypertensive crises. **Selegiline** may increase dyskinesias, nausea, orthostatic hypotension, confusion, hallucinations. ***HERBAL:*** None known. ***FOOD:*** None known. ***LAB VALUES:*** May increase alkaline phosphatase, SGOT (AST), SGPT (ALT), LDH, bilirubin, BUN.

AVAILABILITY (Rx)

TABLETS (expressed as carbidopa/levodopa): 10 mg/100 mg, 25 mg/100 mg, 25 mg/250 mg. ***TABLETS (extended-release):*** 50 mg/200 mg.

ADMINISTRATION/HANDLING

PO:

• Scored tablets may be crushed.
• May be given without regard to meals. • Do not crush sustained-release tablet; may cut in half.

INDICATIONS/ROUTES/DOSAGE

PARKINSONISM:

Not receiving levodopa:

PO: **Adults:** 25/100 mg tablet 3 times/day or 10/100 mg tablet 3–4 times/day. May increase by 1 tablet q1–2days up to 8 tablets/day.

Usual elderly dosage:

PO: Initially, 25/100 mg tablet 2 times/day, gradually increased as necessary.

Sustained-release:

Adults: 1 tablet 2 times/day no closer than 6 hrs between doses. **Range:** 2–8 tablets at 4–8 hr intervals. May increase dose at intervals not less than 3 days.

Receiving only levodopa:

Note: Discontinue levodopa at least 8 hrs prior to carbidopa/levodopa. Initiate with dose providing at least 25% of previous levodopa dosage.
PO: Adults (<1,500 mg levodopa/day): 1 tablet (25/100 mg) 3–4 times/day. **PO: Adults (>1,500 mg levodopa/day):** 1 tablet (25/250 mg) 3–4 times/day.

Sustained-release:

Adults: 1 tablet 2 times/day.

Receiving carbidopa/levodopa:

Adults: Provide about 10% more levodopa; may increase up to 30% more at 4–8 hr dosing intervals.

SIDE EFFECTS

FREQUENT (10–90%): Uncontrolled body movements (including face, tongue, arms, upper body), nausea and vomiting (80%), anorexia (50%). **OCCASIONAL:** Depression, anxiety, confusion, nervousness, difficulty urinating, irregular heartbeats, dizziness, lightheadedness, decreased appetite, blurred vision, constipation, dry mouth, flushed skin, headache, insomnia, diarrhea, unusual tiredness, darkening of urine. **RARE:** Hypertension, ulcer, hemolytic anemia (tiredness/weakness).

ADVERSE REACTIONS/TOXIC EFFECTS

High incidence of involuntary choreiform, dystonic, dyskinetic movements may be noted in pts on long-term therapy. Mental changes (paranoid ideation, psychotic episodes, depression) may be noted. Numerous mild to severe CNS, psychiatric disturbances may include reduced attention span, anxiety, nightmares, daytime somnolence, euphoria, fatigue, paranoia, hallucinations.

NURSING IMPLICATIONS

BASELINE ASSESSMENT:

Instruct pt to void before giving medication (reduces risk of urinary retention).

INTERVENTION/EVALUATION:

Be alert to neurologic effects: headache, lethargy, mental confusion, agitation. Monitor for evidence of dyskinesia (difficulty with movement). Assess for clinical reversal of symptoms (improvement of tremor of head/hands at rest, masklike facial expression, shuffling gait, muscular rigidity).

PATIENT/FAMILY TEACHING:

Avoid tasks that require alertness, motor skills until response to drug is established. Avoid alcoholic beverages during therapy. Sugarless gum, sips of tepid water may relieve dry mouth. Take with food to minimize GI upset. Effects may be delayed from several weeks to months. May cause darkening in urine/sweat (not harmful). Report any uncontrolled movement of face, eyelids, mouth, tongue, arms, hands, legs, mental changes, palpitations, irregular heartbeats, severe or continuing nausea/vomiting, difficulty in urinating.

carboplatin

car-bow-**play**-tin
(Paraplatin)

►CLASSIFICATION

PHARMACOTHERAPEUTIC:
Platinum coordination complex.
CLINICAL: Antineoplastic (see
p. 68C)

ACTION/*THERAPEUTIC EFFECT*

Inhibits DNA synthesis by cross-
linking with DNA strands, *prevent-*
ing cellular division, interfering
with DNA function. Cell cycle-
phase nonspecific.

PHARMACOKINETICS

Protein binding: Low. Hydrolyzed in
solution to active form. Primarily excreted in urine. Half-life: 2.6–5.9 hrs.

USES/*UNLABELED*

Treatment of recurrent ovarian
carcinoma in those previously
treated with chemotherapy, including cisplatin. Initial treatment of
advanced ovarian carcinoma.
Treatment of small cell, non small
cell carcinoma of lung, head/neck
carcinoma, testicular carcinoma.

PRECAUTIONS

CONTRAINDICATIONS: History of
severe allergic reaction to cisplatin,
platinum compounds, mannitol; severe myelosuppression, severe
bleeding. ***CAUTIONS:*** Infection,
chickenpox, herpes zoster, renal
function impairment.
▷*LIFESPAN CONSIDERATIONS:*
Pregnancy/Lactation: If possible, avoid use during pregnancy,
esp. first trimester. May cause fetal
harm. Unknown if distributed in
breast milk. Breast feeding not
recommended. **Pregnancy Cate-**
gory D. Children: Safety and efficacy not established. **Elderly:** Peripheral neurotoxicity increased,
myelotoxicity may be more severe. Age-related decreased renal

function may require decreased
dosage, more careful monitoring
of blood counts.

INTERACTIONS

DRUG: **Bone marrow depres-**
sants may increase bone marrow
depression. **Nephrotoxic-, oto-**
toxic-producing agents may
increase toxicity. **Live virus vac-**
cines may potentiate virus replication, increase vaccine side effects, decrease antibody response
to vaccine. ***HERBAL:*** None known.
FOOD: None known. ***LAB VALUES:***
May decrease electrolytes
(sodium, magnesium, calcium, potassium). High doses (above 4
times recommended dose) may
elevate alkaline phosphatase,
SGOT (AST), total bilirubin, BUN,
serum creatinine concentrations.

AVAILABILITY (Rx)

POWDER FOR INJECTION: 50
mg, 150 mg, 450 mg.

ADMINISTRATION/HANDLING

Note: May be carcinogenic, mutagenic, or teratogenic. Handle with
extreme care during preparation/
administration.

IV 🍴

Storage:
• Store vials at room temperature.
• After reconstitution, solution is
stable for 8 hrs. Discard unused
portion after 8 hrs.

Reconstitution:
• Reconstitute immediately before
use. • Do not use aluminum needles or administration sets that
come in contact with drug (may
produce black precipitate, loss of
potency). • Reconstitute each 50
mg with 5 ml Sterile Water for Injection, D_5W, or 0.9% NaCl to provide concentration of 10 mg/ml. •
May be further diluted with D_5W

C

or 0.9% NaCl to provide concentration as low as 0.5 mg/ml.

Rate of administration:

• Infuse over 15–60 min. • Rarely, anaphylactic reaction occurs minutes after administration. Use of epinephrine, corticosteroids alleviates symptoms.

IV INCOMPATIBILITIES ⊘

Amphotericin B complex (Ambisome, Amphotec, Abelcet).

IV COMPATIBILITIES

Etoposide (Vepesed), granisetron (Kytril), ondansetron (Zofran), paclitaxel (Taxol).

INDICATIONS/ROUTES/DOSAGE

Note: Dosage individualized based on clinical response, tolerance to adverse effects. Platelets must be >100,000 mm^3, neutrophils >2,000 mm^3 before giving any dosage.

Ovarian carcinoma (single agent):

IV: Adults: 360 mg/m^2 on day 1, q4wks. Do not repeat dose until neutrophil, platelet counts are within acceptable levels. Adjust dose in those previously treated based on lowest post-treatment platelet or neutrophil value.

Note: Make only one escalation, not >125% of starting dose.

Ovarian carcinoma (combination therapy):

IV: Adults: 300 mg/m^2 (with cyclophosphamide) on day 1, q4wks. Do not repeat dose until neutrophil, platelet counts are within acceptable levels.

Dosage in renal impairment:

Initial dose based on creatinine clearance; subsequent doses based on pt's tolerance, degree of myelosuppression.

Creatinine Clearance	Dosage Day 1
>60 ml/min	360 mg/m^2
41–59 ml/min	250 mg/m^2
16–40 ml/min	200 mg/m^2

Usual pediatric dosage:

IV: (Solid tumor): 300–600 mg/m^2 q4wks. (Brain tumor): 175 mg/m^2 q4wks.

SIDE EFFECTS

FREQUENT: Nausea (75–80%), vomiting (65%). **OCCASIONAL:** Generalized pain (17%), diarrhea/constipation (6%), peripheral neuropathy (4%). **RARE** (2–3%): Alopecia, asthenia (loss of energy, strength), hypersensitivity reaction (rash, urticaria, pruritus, erythema).

ADVERSE REACTIONS/TOXIC EFFECTS

Bone marrow suppression may be severe, resulting in anemia, infection, bleeding (GI bleeding, sepsis, pneumonia). Prolonged treatment may result in peripheral neurotoxicity.

NURSING IMPLICATIONS

BASELINE ASSESSMENT:

Offer emotional support. Treatment should not be repeated until WBC recovers from previous therapy. Transfusions may be needed in those receiving prolonged therapy (myelosuppression increased in those with previous therapy, impaired kidney function).

INTERVENTION/EVALUATION:

Monitor hematologic status, pulmonary function studies, hepatic and renal function tests. Monitor for fever, sore throat, signs of local infection, easy bruising or unusual bleeding from any site, symptoms of anemia (excessive tiredness, weakness).

PATIENT/FAMILY TEACHING:

Nausea, vomiting generally abates <24 hrs. Do not have immunizations without physician's approval (drug lowers body's resistance). Avoid contact with those who have recently received live virus vaccine.

carboprost ✳

kar-boe-prost
(Hemabate)

▶**CLASSIFICATION**

PHARMACOTHERAPEUTIC:
Prostaglandin. ***CLINICAL:*** Abortifacient, oxytocic

ACTION/*THERAPEUTIC EFFECT*

Direct action on myometrium. Stimulates contraction in gravid uterus, *produces cervical dilation and softening.*

USES/*UNLABELED*

To induce abortion between the 13th and 20th wk of pregnancy (as calculated from the first day of the last menstrual period), to treat postpartum hemorrhage related to uterine atony not responsive to conventional therapy. *Treatment of incomplete abortion, benign hydatiform mole, induction of labor, ripen cervix prior to abortion.*

PRECAUTIONS

CONTRAINDICATIONS: Hypersensitivity to carboprost or other prostaglandins; acute pelvic inflammatory disease; active cardiac, pulmonary, renal, or hepatic

disease. ***CAUTIONS:*** History of asthma, hypo/hypertension, anemia, jaundice, diabetes, epilepsy, compromised (scarred) uterus, cardiovascular, adrenal, or hepatic disease.

INTERACTIONS

DRUG: Oxytocin, oxytocics may cause uterine hypertonus, leading to uterine rupture or cervical lacerations. ***HERBAL:*** None known. ***FOOD:*** None known. ***LAB VALUES:*** None significant.

AVAILABILITY (Rx)

INJECTION: 250 mcg/ml.

INDICATIONS/ROUTES/DOSAGE
Abortion:

IM: Adults: Initially, 100–250 mcg, may repeat at 1.5–3.5 hr intervals. May increase up to 500 mcg if uterine contractility inadequate. **Maximum:** 12 mg total dose or continuous administration >2 days.

Postpartum hemorrhage:

IM: Adults: Initially, 250 mcg, may repeat at 15–90 min intervals. **Maximum:** 2 mg total dose.

SIDE EFFECTS

FREQUENT (33%): Nausea. ***OCCASIONAL*** (7%): Facial flushing. ***RARE:*** Vomiting, diarrhea.

ADVERSE REACTIONS/TOXIC EFFECTS

Excessive dosage may cause uterine hypertonicity with spasm and tetanic contraction, leading to cervical laceration/perforation, uterine rupture/hemorrhage.

NURSING IMPLICATIONS

BASELINE ASSESSMENT:

Assess any uterine activity/vaginal bleeding.

INTERVENTION/EVALUATION:

Check strength, duration, frequency of contractions and monitor vital signs q15min until stable, then hourly until abortion complete. Check resting uterine tone.

PATIENT/FAMILY TEACHING:

Report fever, chills, foul-smelling/increased vaginal discharge, uterine cramps/pain promptly.

carisoprodol

(Soma, Rela)

See Classification section under: Skeletal muscle relaxants

carmustine

car-**muss**-teen
(BiCNU, Gliadel)

▶CLASSIFICATION

PHARMACOTHERAPEUTIC: Alkylating agent, nitrosurea. *CLINICAL:* Antineoplastic (see p. 68C)

ACTION/*THERAPEUTIC EFFECT*

Inhibits DNA, RNA synthesis by cross-linking with DNA, RNA strands, preventing cellular division, *interfering with DNA/RNA function.* Cell cycle-phase nonspecific.

USES/*UNLABELED*

Treatment of primary and metastatic brain tumors, multiple myeloma, disseminated Hodgkin's disease, non-Hodgkin's lymphoma. *Gliadel Wafer:* Adjunct to surgery to prolong survival in recurrent glioblastoma multiforme. *Treatment of hepatic, GI carcinoma, malignant melanoma, mycosis fungoides.*

PRECAUTIONS

CONTRAINDICATIONS: None significant. *CAUTIONS:* Pts with decreased platelet, leukocyte, erythrocyte counts.

INTERACTIONS

DRUG: **Bone marrow depressants, cimetidine** may enhance myelosuppressive effect. **Hepatotoxic, nephrotoxic drugs** may enhance respective toxicities. **Live virus vaccines** may potentiate virus replication, increase vaccine side effects, decrease antibody response to vaccine. *HERBAL:* None known. *FOOD:* None known. *LAB VALUES:* May increase BUN, SGOT (AST), SGPT (ALT), alkaline phosphatase, bilirubin.

AVAILABILITY (Rx)

POWDER FOR INJECTION: 100 mg. *WAFER:* 7.7 mg.

ADMINISTRATION/HANDLING

Note: May be carcinogenic, mutagenic, or teratogenic. Wear protective gloves during preparation of drug; may cause transient burning, brown staining of skin.

IV 🗓

Storage:

• Refrigerate unopened vials of dry powder. • Reconstituted vials are stable for 8 hrs at room temperature or 24 hrs if refrigerated. • Solutions further diluted to 0.2 mg/ml with D_5W or 0.9% NaCl are stable for 48 hrs if refrigerated or an additional 8 hrs at room temperature. • Solutions appear clear, colorless to yellow. • Discard if precipitate forms, color change occurs, or oily film develops on bottom of vial.

Reconstitution:

• Reconstitute 100 mg vial with 3 ml sterile dehydrated (absolute) alcohol, followed by 27 ml Sterile Water for Injection to provide concentration of 3.3 mg/ml. • Further dilute with 50–250 ml D_5W or 0.9% NaCl.

Rate of administration:

• Infuse over 1–2 hrs (shorter duration may produce intense burning pain at injection site, intense flushing of skin, conjunctiva). • Flush IV line with 5–10 ml 0.9% NaCl or D_5W before and after administration to prevent irritation at injection site.

IV INCOMPATIBILITY ⊘

Allopurinol (Aloprim)

INDICATIONS/ROUTES/DOSAGE

Note: Dosage individualized based on clinical response, tolerance to adverse effects. When used in combination therapy, consult specific protocols for optimum dosage, sequence of drug administration.

Single agent in previously untreated pt:

IV INFUSION: **Adults, elderly:** 150–200 mg/m^2 as single dose or 75–100 mg/m^2 on 2 successive days. **Children:** 200–250 mg/m^2 q4–6wks as a single dose.

SIDE EFFECTS

FREQUENT: Nausea and vomiting within minutes to 2 hrs after administration (may last up to 6 hrs). *OCCASIONAL:* Diarrhea, esophagitis, anorexia, dysphagia. *RARE:* Thrombophlebitis.

ADVERSE REACTIONS/TOXIC EFFECTS

Hematologic toxicity, due to bone marrow depression, occurs frequently. Thrombocytopenia occurs at about 4 wks, lasts 1–2 wks; leukopenia evident at about 5–6 wks, lasts 1–2 wks. Anemia occurs less frequently, is less severe. Mild, reversible hepatotoxicity also occurs frequently. Prolonged therapy with high dosage may produce impaired renal function, pulmonary toxicity (pulmonary infiltrate and/or fibrosis).

NURSING IMPLICATIONS

BASELINE ASSESSMENT:

Perform liver function studies periodically during therapy. Perform blood counts weekly during and for at least 6 wks after therapy ends.

INTERVENTION/EVALUATION:

Monitor CBC, BUN, serum transaminase, alkaline phosphatase, bilirubin; pulmonary, renal function tests. Monitor for hematologic toxicity (fever, sore throat, signs of local infection, easy bruising, unusual bleeding from any site) or symptoms of anemia (excessive tiredness, weakness). Monitor lung sounds for pulmonary toxicity (dyspnea, fine lung rales).

PATIENT/FAMILY TEACHING:

Maintain adequate daily fluid intake (may protect against renal impairment). Do not have immunizations without doctor's approval (drug lowers body's resistance). Avoid contact with those who have recently received live virus vaccine. Contact physician if nausea/vomiting continues at home.

carteolol

(Cartrol, Ocupress)

See Classification section under: Beta adrenergic blockers (p. 61C)

carvedilol

car-**veh**-dih-lol
(Coreg)

▶CLASSIFICATION

PHARMACOTHERAPEUTIC:
Beta-adrenergic blocker. ***CLINICAL:*** Antihypertensive (see p. 61C)

ACTION/*THERAPEUTIC EFFECT*

Possesses nonselective beta-blocking and alpha-adrenergic blocking activity. *Reduces cardiac output, exercise-induced tachycardia, and reflex orthostatic tachycardia; causes vasodilation; reduces peripheral vascular resistance.*

PHARMACOKINETICS

	Onset	Peak	Duration
PO	30 min	1–2 hrs	24 hrs

Rapidly and extensively absorbed from GI tract. Protein binding: 98%. Metabolized in liver. Excreted primarily via bile into feces. Minimally removed by hemodialysis. Half-life: 7–10 hrs. Food delays rate of absorption.

USES/*UNLABELED*

Management of essential hypertension. Used alone or in combination with diuretics, esp. thiazide type. Treatment of CHF. *Treatment of angina pectoris, idiopathic cardiomyopathy.*

PRECAUTIONS

CONTRAINDICATIONS: Class IV decompensated cardiac failure, bronchial asthma or related bronchospastic conditions, second- or third-degree AV block, cardiogenic shock, severe bradycardia. ***CAUTIONS:*** CHF controlled with digitalis, diuretics, or angiotensin-converting enzyme inhibitor, peripheral vascular disease, anesthesia, diabetes mellitus, hypoglycemia, thyrotoxicosis, impaired hepatic function.

▷*LIFESPAN CONSIDERATIONS:*
Pregnancy/Lactation: Unknown if drug crosses placenta or is distributed in breast milk. May produce bradycardia, apnea, hypoglycemia, hypothermia during delivery, small birth weight infants. **Pregnancy Category C. Children:** Safety and efficacy not established. **Elderly:** Incidence of dizziness may be increased.

INTERACTIONS

DRUG:* Diuretics, other hypotensives** may increase hypotensive effect; may mask symptoms of hypoglycemia, prolong hypoglycemic effect of **insulin, oral hypoglycemics. Catapres** may potentiate B/P effects, **calcium blockers** increase risk of conduction disturbances, increases **digoxin** concentrations. **Cimetidine** may increase concentration, rifampin decreases concentration. ***HERBAL: None known. *FOOD:* None known. *LAB VALUES:* None significant.

AVAILABILITY (Rx)

TABLETS: 3.125 mg, 6.25 mg, 12.5 mg, 25 mg.

ADMINISTRATION/HANDLING
PO:

• Give with food (slows rate of absorption, reduces risk of orthostatic effects). • Take standing systolic B/P 1 hr after dosing as guide for tolerance.

INDICATIONS/ROUTES/DOSAGE
Hypertension:

PO: Adults, elderly: Initially, 6.25 mg twice daily. May double at 7–14 day intervals to highest tolerated dose. **Maximum:** 50 mg/day.

CHF:

PO: Adults, elderly: Initially, 3.125 mg twice daily. May double at 2 wk intervals to highest tolerated dose. **Maximum: <85 kg:** 25 mg twice daily; **>85 kg:** 50 mg twice daily.

SIDE EFFECTS

Generally well tolerated, with mild and transient side effects. *FREQUENT* (4–6%): Fatigue, dizziness. *OCCASIONAL* (2%): Diarrhea, bradycardia, rhinitis, back pain. *RARE* (<2%): Postural hypotension, somnolence, urinary tract infection, viral infection.

ADVERSE REACTIONS/TOXIC EFFECTS

Overdosage may produce profound bradycardia, hypotension, bronchospasm, cardiac insufficiency, cardiogenic shock, cardiac arrest. Abrupt withdrawal may result in sweating, palpitations, headache, tremulousness. May precipitate CHF, MI in those with cardiac disease, thyroid storm in those with thyrotoxicosis, peripheral ischemia in those with existing peripheral vascular disease. Hypoglycemia may occur in previously controlled diabetics.

NURSING IMPLICATIONS

BASELINE ASSESSMENT:

Assess B/P, apical pulse immediately before drug is administered (if pulse is 60/min or below, or systolic B/P is below 90 mm Hg, withhold medication, contact physician).

INTERVENTION/EVALUATION:

Monitor B/P for hypotension, respiration for breathlessness. Assess pulse for strength/weakness, irregular rate, bradycardia. Monitor EKG for cardiac arrhythmias. Assist with ambulation if dizziness occurs. Assess for evidence of CHF: dyspnea (particularly on exertion or lying down), night cough, peripheral edema, distended neck veins. Monitor I&O (increase in weight, decrease in urine output may indicate CHF).

PATIENT/FAMILY TEACHING:

Full antihypertensive effect noted 1–2 wks. Contact lens wearers may experience decreased lacrimation. Take with food. Do not abruptly discontinue medication. Compliance with therapy regimen is essential to control hypertension. Avoid tasks that require alertness, motor skills until response to drug is established. Report excessive fatigue, prolonged dizziness. Do not use nasal decongestants, OTC cold preparations (stimulants) without physician approval. Monitor B/P, pulse before taking medication. Restrict salt, alcohol intake.

cascara sagrada

cass-**care**-ah sah-**graud**-ah (Cascara Sagrada)

FIXED-COMBINATION(S)

With milk of magnesia, a saline laxative **(Same)**

▶CLASSIFICATION

PHARMACOTHERAPEUTIC: Stimulant. **CLINICAL:** Laxative (see p. 101C)

ACTION/THERAPEUTIC EFFECT

Increases peristalsis by direct effect on colonic smooth musculature (stimulates intramural nerve plexi). *Promotes fluid and ion accumulation in colon to increase laxative effect.*

USES

Facilitates defecation in those with diminished colonic motor response, for evacuation of colon for rectal, bowel examination, elective colon surgery.

PRECAUTIONS

CONTRAINDICATIONS: Abdominal pain, nausea, vomiting, appendicitis, intestinal obstruction. **CAUTIONS:** None significant.

INTERACTIONS

DRUG: May decrease transit time of concurrently administered oral medication, decreasing absorption. **HERBAL:** None known. **FOOD:** None known. **LAB VALUES:** May increase blood glucose. May decrease potassium, calcium.

AVAILABILITY (Rx)

TABLETS: 325 mg. **LIQUID:** (18% alcohol).

INDICATIONS/ROUTES/DOSAGE

Laxative:

PO: Adults, elderly: 1 tablet (or 5 ml) at bedtime. **Children 2–11 yrs:** 2.5 ml (1–3 ml) as a single dose. **Infants:** 1.25 ml (0.5–2 ml) as a single dose.

SIDE EFFECTS

FREQUENT: Pink-red, red-violet, red-brown, or yellow-brown discoloration of urine. **OCCASIONAL:** Some degree of abdominal discomfort, nausea, mild cramps, griping; faintness.

ADVERSE REACTIONS/TOXIC EFFECTS

Long-term use may result in laxative dependence, chronic constipation, loss of normal bowel function. Chronic use or overdosage may result in electrolyte disturbances (hypokalemia, hypocalcemia, metabolic acidosis or alkalosis), persistent diarrhea, malabsorption, weight loss. Electrolyte disturbance may produce vomiting, muscle weakness.

NURSING IMPLICATIONS

INTERVENTION/EVALUATION:

Encourage adequate fluid intake. Assess bowel sounds for peristalsis. Monitor daily bowel activity and stool consistency (watery, loose, soft, semisolid, solid) and record time of evacuation. Assess for abdominal disturbances. Monitor serum electrolytes in those exposed to prolonged, frequent, or excessive use of medication.

PATIENT/FAMILY TEACHING:
Urine may turn pink-red, red-violet, red-brown, or yellow-brown (only temporary and not harmful). Institute measures to promote defecation: increase fluid intake, exercise, high-fiber diet. Laxative effect generally occurs in 6–12 hrs, but may take 24 hrs. Do not use in presence of nausea, vomiting, abdominal pain longer than 1 wk. Do not take other oral medication within 1 hr of taking this medicine (decreased effectiveness due to increased peristalsis).

caspofungin acetate

cas-poe-**fun**-gin
(Cancidas)

▶CLASSIFICATION
CLINICAL: Antifungal

ACTION/THERAPEUTIC EFFECT
Inhibits synthesis of glucan (vital component of fungal cell formation), damaging fungal cell membrane. *Fungistatic.*

PHARMACOKINETICS
Distributed in tissue. Extensively bound to albumin. Slowly metabolized in liver to active metabolite. Primarily excreted in urine and to a lesser extent in feces. Not removed by hemodialysis. Half-life: 40–50 hrs

USES
Treatment of invasive aspergillosis in those who are refractory to or intolerant of other fungal therapies.

PRECAUTIONS
CONTRAINDICATIONS: None

significant. **CAUTIONS:** Hepatic function impairment.

▷**LIFESPAN CONSIDERATIONS:**
Pregnancy/Lactation: May be embryotoxic. Crosses placental barrier. Distributed in breast milk. **Pregnancy Category C**. **Children:** Safety and efficacy not established. **Elderly:** Age-related moderate renal impairment may require dosage adjustment.

INTERACTIONS
DRUG: May decrease effect of **tacrolimus. Cyclosporine, efavirenz, nelfinavir, nevirapine, phenytoin, rifampin, dexamethasone, or carbamazepine.** May increase concentration of caspofungin. **HERBAL:** None significant. **FOOD:** None significant. **LAB VALUES:** May increase SGOT (AST), SGPT (ALT), alkaline phosphatase, LDH, bilirubin, creatinine, serum uric acid, urine pH, urine protein, urine RBC's, urine WBC's, prothrombin time. May decrease serum albumin, serum bicarbonate, serum protein, potassium, Hgb, Hct, WBCs, platelet count.

AVAILABILITY (Rx)
POWDER FOR INJECTION: 50 mg, 70 mg vials.

ADMINISTRATION/HANDLING
IV 🏥
Storage:
• Store in refrigerator but warm to room temperature before preparing with diluent. • Reconstituted solution, prior to preparation of pt infusion solution, may be stored at room temperature for 1 hr prior to infusion. • Final infusion solution can be stored at room temperature for 24 hrs. • Discard if solution contains particulate or is discolored.

Reconstitution:

• For 50–70 mg loading dose, add 10.5 ml 0.9% NaCl to the vial. • Transfer 10 ml of reconstituted solution to 250 ml 0.9% NaCl. • For 35 mg dose in pts with moderate hepatic insufficiency, add 10.5 ml 0.9% NaCl to the vial. • Transfer 10 ml of reconstituted solution to 100 or 250 ml 0.9% NaCl for 50–70 mg daily dose. For moderate hepatic insufficiency transfer 7 ml to 100 or 250 ml 0.9% NaCl.

Rate of administration:

• Infuse over 60 min.

IV INCOMPATIBILITY ⊘

Do not mix with any other medication or use dextrose as a diluent.

INDICATIONS/ROUTES/DOSAGE

Aspergillosis:

IV: Adults, elderly: Give single 70 mg loading dose on day 1, followed by 50 mg daily thereafter.

SIDE EFFECTS

FREQUENT (26%): Fever. ***OCCASIONAL*** (4–11%): Headache, nausea, phlebitis. ***RARE*** (≤3%): Paresthesia, vomiting, diarrhea, abdominal pain, myalgia, chills, tremor, insomnia.

ADVERSE REACTIONS/TOXIC EFFECTS

Hypersensitivity reaction characterized by rash, facial swelling, pruritus, sensation of warmth.

NURSING IMPLICATIONS

BASELINE ASSESSMENT:

Determine baseline temperature, liver function tests. Assess allergies.

INTERVENTION/EVALUATION:

Assess for signs and symptoms of liver dysfunction and monitor hepatic enzyme test results in pts with preexisting liver dysfunction.

cefaclor

sef-ah-klor
(Apo-Cefaclor✤, Ceclor, Ceclor CD)

▶**CLASSIFICATION**

PHARMACOTHERAPEUTIC: Second-generation cephalosporin. ***CLINICAL:*** Antibiotic (see p. 19C)

ACTION/*THERAPEUTIC EFFECT*

Binds to bacterial membranes, *inhibiting synthesis of bacterial cell wall. Bactericidal.*

PHARMACOKINETICS

Well absorbed from GI tract. Protein binding: 25%. Widely distributed. Primarily excreted unchanged in urine. Moderately removed by hemodialysis. Half-life: 0.6–0.9 hrs (half-life increased with impaired renal function).

USES

Treatment of respiratory, skin/skin structure infections, otitis media, UTI. *Extended-Release:* Bacterial infections of acute, chronic bronchitis, skin/skin structure, pharyngitis, tonsillitis.

PRECAUTIONS

CONTRAINDICATIONS: History of hypersensitivity to cephalosporins, anaphylactic reaction to penicillins. ***CAUTIONS:*** Renal impairment, history of allergies or GI disease (esp. ulcerative colitis, antibiotic-associated colitis), concurrent use of nephrotoxic medications.

▷ *LIFESPAN CONSIDERATIONS:*
Pregnancy/Lactation: Readily crosses placenta. Distributed in breast milk. **Pregnancy Category B. Children:** No age related precautions noted in those >1 mo of age. **Elderly:** Age-related decreased renal function may require dosage adjustment.

INTERACTIONS

DRUG: **Probenecid** may increase serum concentrations of cefaclor. *HERBAL:* None known. *FOOD:* None known. *LAB VALUES:* Positive direct/indirect Coombs' test. May increase BUN, serum creatinine, SGPT (ALT), SGOT (AST), alkaline phosphatase, bilirubin, LDH concentrations.

AVAILABILITY (Rx)

CAPSULES: 250 mg, 500 mg. *TABLETS (extended-release):* 375 mg, 500 mg. *ORAL SUSPENSION:* 125 mg/5 ml, 187 mg/5 ml, 250 mg/5 ml, 375 mg/5 ml.

ADMINISTRATION/HANDLING

PO:
• After reconstitution, oral solution is stable for 14 days if refrigerated. • Shake oral suspension well before using. • Give without regard to meals; if GI upset occurs, give with food or milk. • Do not cut, crush, or chew extended-release tablets.

INDICATIONS/ROUTES/DOSAGE

Mild to moderate infections:
PO: **Adults, elderly:** 250 mg q8h. **Children >1 mo:** 20 mg/kg/day in divided doses q8h.

Severe infections:
PO: **Adults, elderly:** 500 mg q8h. **Maximum:** 4 g/day. **Children >1 mo:** 40 mg/kg/day in divided doses q8h. **Maximum:** 1 g/day.

Usual dosage for extended-release tablets:
PO: **Adults, children >16 yrs:** 375–500 mg q12hrs.

Otitis media:
PO: **Children >1 mo:** 40 mg/kg/day in divided doses q8h. **Maximum:** 1 g/day.

Dosage in renal impairment:
Reduced dosage may be necessary in those with creatinine clearance <40 ml/min.

SIDE EFFECTS

FREQUENT: Oral candidiasis (sore mouth/tongue), mild diarrhea, mild abdominal cramping, vaginal candidiasis (itching, discharge). *OCCASIONAL:* Nausea, serum sickness reaction [joint pain, fever] (usually occurs following second course of therapy, resolves after drug discontinuation). *RARE:* Allergic reaction (rash, pruritus, urticaria).

ADVERSE REACTIONS/TOXIC EFFECTS

Antibiotic-associated colitis (severe abdominal pain and tenderness, fever, watery and severe diarrhea), other superinfections may result from altered bacterial balance. Nephrotoxicity may occur, esp. with preexisting renal disease. Severe hypersensitivity reaction (severe pruritus, angioedema, bronchospasm, anaphylaxis), particularly in those with history of allergies, esp. penicillin.

C

NURSING IMPLICATIONS

BASELINE ASSESSMENT:

Question for history of allergies, particularly cephalosporins, penicillins.

INTERVENTION/EVALUATION:

Check mouth for white patches on mucous membranes, tongue. Monitor bowel activity and stool consistency carefully; mild GI effects may be tolerable, but increasing severity may indicate onset of antibiotic-associated colitis. Monitor I&O, renal function reports for nephrotoxicity. Be alert for superinfection: severe genital/anal pruritus, abdominal pain, severe mouth soreness, moderate to severe diarrhea.

PATIENT/FAMILY TEACHING:

Continue therapy for full length of treatment. Doses should be evenly spaced. May cause GI upset (may take with food or milk).

cefadroxil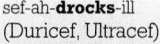

sef-ah-**drocks**-ill
(Duricef, Ultracef)

▶CLASSIFICATION

PHARMACOTHERAPEUTIC:
First-generation cephalosporin.
CLINICAL: Antibiotic (see p. 19C)

ACTION/*THERAPEUTIC EFFECT*

Binds to bacterial membranes, *inhibiting synthesis of bacterial cell wall*. Bactericidal.

PHARMACOKINETICS

Well absorbed from GI tract. Protein binding: 15–20%. Widely distributed. Primarily excreted unchanged in urine. Removed by hemodialysis. Half-life: 1.2–1.5 hrs (half-life increased with impaired renal function).

USES

Treatment of respiratory and GU tract, skin and soft tissue infections; follow-up to parenteral therapy.

PRECAUTIONS

CONTRAINDICATIONS: History of hypersensitivity to cephalosporins, anaphylactic reaction to penicillins. ***CAUTIONS:*** Renal impairment, history of allergies or GI disease (esp. ulcerative colitis, antibiotic-associated colitis), concurrent use of nephrotoxic medications.
▷*LIFESPAN CONSIDERATIONS:*
Pregnancy/Lactation: Readily crosses placenta. Distributed in breast milk. **Pregnancy Category B. Children:** No age-related precautions noted. **Elderly:** Age-related decreased renal function may require dosage adjustment.

INTERACTIONS

DRUG:* Probenecid** increases serum concentrations of cefadroxil. ***HERBAL: None known. ***FOOD:*** None known. ***LAB VALUES:*** Positive direct/indirect Coombs' test. May increase BUN, serum creatinine, SGPT (ALT), SGOT (AST), alkaline phosphatase, bilirubin, LDH concentrations.

AVAILABILITY (Rx)

CAPSULES: 500 mg. ***TABLETS:*** 1,000 mg. ***ORAL SUSPENSION:*** 125 mg/5 ml, 250 mg/5 ml, 500 mg/5 ml.

ADMINISTRATION/HANDLING

PO:

• After reconstitution, oral solution is stable for 14 days if refrigerated. • Shake oral suspension well before using. • Give without regard to meals; if GI upset occurs, give with food or milk.

INDICATIONS/ROUTES/DOSAGE

Note: Space doses evenly around the clock.

Urinary tract infections:

PO: **Adults, elderly:** 1–2 g/day in 1–2 divided doses.

Skin/skin structure infections, group A beta-hemolytic streptococcal pharyngitis, tonsillitis:

PO: **Adults, elderly:** 500 mg–1 g/day as single or 2 divided doses.

Usual dosage for children:

PO: **Children:** 30 mg/kg/day as single or 2 divided doses.

Dosage in renal impairment:

Dose and/or frequency is based on degree of renal impairment and/or severity of infection. After initial 1 g dose:

Creatinine Clearance	Dosage Interval
25–50 ml/min	500 mg q12h
10–25 ml/min	500 mg q24h
0–10 ml/min	500 mg q36h

SIDE EFFECTS

FREQUENT: Oral candidiasis (sore mouth/tongue), mild diarrhea, mild abdominal cramping, vaginal candidiasis (itching, discharge). **OCCASIONAL:** Nausea, unusual bruising/bleeding, serum sickness reaction [joint pain, fever] (usually occurs following second course of therapy, resolves after drug discontinuation). **RARE:** Allergic reaction (rash, pruritus, urticaria), thrombophlebitis (pain, redness, swelling at injection site).

ADVERSE REACTIONS/TOXIC EFFECTS

Antibiotic-associated colitis (severe abdominal pain and tenderness, fever, watery and severe diarrhea), other superinfections may result from altered bacterial balance. Nephrotoxicity may occur, esp. with preexisting renal disease. Severe hypersensitivity reaction (severe pruritus, angioedema, bronchospasm, anaphylaxis), particularly those with history of allergies, esp. penicillin.

NURSING IMPLICATIONS

BASELINE ASSESSMENT:

Question history of allergies, particularly cephalosporins, penicillins.

INTERVENTION/EVALUATION:

Check mouth for white patches on mucous membranes, tongue. Monitor bowel activity and stool consistency carefully; mild GI effects may be tolerable, but increasing severity may indicate onset of antibiotic-associated colitis. Monitor I&O, renal function reports for nephrotoxicity. Be alert for superinfection: genital/anal pruritus, moniliasis, abdominal pain, sore mouth or tongue, moderate to severe diarrhea.

PATIENT/FAMILY TEACHING:

Continue therapy for full length of treatment. Doses should be evenly spaced. May cause GI upset (may take with food or milk).

---

cefazolin sodium

cef-ah-**zoe**-lin
(Ancef, Kefzol)

▶CLASSIFICATION

PHARMACOTHERAPEUTIC:
First-generation cephalosporin.
CLINICAL: Antibiotic (see p.
19C)

ACTION/*THERAPEUTIC EFFECT*

Binds to bacterial membranes, *inhibiting synthesis of bacterial cell wall. Bactericidal.*

PHARMACOKINETICS

Widely distributed. Protein binding: 85%. Primarily excreted unchanged in urine. Moderately removed by hemodialysis. Half-life: 1.4–1.8 hrs (half-life increased with impaired renal function).

USES

Treatment of respiratory tract, skin, soft tissue, bone and joint, GU tract, serious intra-abdominal, biliary infections; septicemia. Preferred first-generation cephalosporin for perioperative prophylaxis.

PRECAUTIONS

CONTRAINDICATIONS: History of hypersensitivity to cephalosporins, anaphylactic reaction to penicillins. ***CAUTIONS:*** Renal impairment, history of allergies or GI disease (esp. ulcerative colitis, antibiotic-associated colitis), concurrent use of nephrotoxic medications.
▷*LIFESPAN CONSIDERATIONS:*
Pregnancy/Lactation: Readily crosses placenta; distributed in breast milk. **Pregnancy Category B. Children:** No age-related pre-

cautions noted. **Elderly:** Age-related renal impairment may require reduced dosage.

INTERACTIONS

DRUG:* Probenecid** increases serum concentrations of cefazolin. ***HERBAL: None known. ***FOOD:*** None known. ***LAB VALUES:*** Positive direct/indirect Coombs' test. May increase BUN, serum creatinine, SGPT (ALT), SGOT (AST), alkaline phosphatase, bilirubin, LDH concentrations.

AVAILABILITY (Rx)

INJECTION: 250 mg, 500 mg, 1 g. ***READY-TO-HANG INFUSION:*** 500 mg/50 ml, 1 g/50 ml.

ADMINISTRATION/HANDLING

Note: Give by IM injection, IV push, intermittent IV infusion (piggyback).

IM:

• To minimize discomfort, inject deep IM slowly. • Less painful if injected into gluteus maximus rather than lateral aspect of thigh.

IV 🔟

Storage:
• Solution appears light yellow to yellow. • IV infusion (piggyback) stable for 24 hrs at room temperature, 96 hrs if refrigerated. • Discard if precipitate forms.

Reconstitution:
• Reconstitute each 1 g with at least 10 ml Sterile Water for Injection. • May further dilute in 50–100 ml D_5W or 0.9% NaCl (decreases incidence of thrombophlebitis).

Rate of administration:
• For IV push, administer over 3–5

---

min. • For intermittent IV infusion (piggyback), infuse over 20–30 min.

IV INCOMPATIBILITIES ⊘

Amiodarone (Cordarone), amphotericin B complex (Ambisome, Abelcet), hetastarch (Hespan), pentamidine (Pentam IV), vancomycin (Vancocin), vinorelbine (Navelbine).

IV COMPATIBILITIES

Amiodarone (Cordarone), calcium gluconate, diltiazem (Cardizem), famotidine (Pepcid), heparin, lidocaine, magnesium, midazolam (Versed), multivitamins, propofol (Diprivan), vercuonium (Norcuron).

INDICATIONS/ROUTES/DOSAGE

Note: Space doses evenly around the clock.

Uncomplicated UTI:
IM/IV: **Adults, elderly:** 1 g q12h.

Mild to moderate infections:
IM/IV: **Adults, elderly:** 250–500 mg q8–12h.

Severe infections:
IM/IV: **Adults, elderly:** 0.5–1 g q6–8h.

Life-threatening infections:
IM/IV: **Adults, elderly:** 1–1.5 g q6h. **Maximum:** 12 g/day.

Perioperative prophylaxis:
IM/IV: **Adults, elderly:** 1 g 30–60 min before surgery, 0.5–1 g during surgery, and q6–8h for up to 24 hrs postop.

Usual pediatric dosage:
IM/IV: **Neonates ≤7 days:** 40 mg/kg/day in divided doses q12h. **>7 days:** 40–60 mg/kg/day in divided doses q8–12h. **Children:** 50–100 mg/kg/day in divided doses q8h.

Dosage in renal impairment:

Creatinine Clearance	Dosing Interval
10–30 ml/min	q12h
<10 ml/min	q24h

SIDE EFFECTS

FREQUENT: Discomfort with IM administration, oral candidiasis (sore mouth/tongue), mild diarrhea, mild abdominal cramping, vaginal candidiasis (itching, discharge). ***OCCASIONAL:*** Nausea, serum sickness reaction [joint pain, fever] (usually occurs following second course of therapy, resolves after drug discontinuation). ***RARE:*** Allergic reaction (rash, pruritus, urticaria), thrombophlebitis (pain, redness, swelling at injection site).

ADVERSE REACTIONS/TOXIC EFFECTS

Antibiotic-associated colitis (severe abdominal pain and tenderness, fever, watery and severe diarrhea), other superinfections may result from altered bacterial balance. Nephrotoxicity may occur, esp. with preexisting renal disease. Severe hypersensitivity reaction (severe pruritus, angioedema, bronchospasm, anaphylaxis), particularly those with history of allergies, esp. penicillin.

NURSING IMPLICATIONS

BASELINE ASSESSMENT:
Question for history of allergies, particularly cephalosporins, penicillins.

INTERVENTION/EVALUATION:
Evaluate IV site for phlebitis (heat, pain, red streaking over vein). Check mouth for white patches on mucous membranes,

C

tongue. Monitor bowel activity and stool consistency carefully; mild GI effects may be tolerable, but increasing severity may indicate onset of antibiotic-associated colitis. Monitor I&O, renal function reports for nephrotoxicity. Be alert for superinfection: severe genital/anal pruritus, abdominal pain, severe mouth soreness, moderate to severe diarrhea.

PATIENT/FAMILY TEACHING:

Discomfort may occur with IM injection. Doses should be evenly spaced. Continue antibiotic therapy for full length of treatment.

cefdinir

cef-din-ur
(Omnicef)

▶CLASSIFICATION

PHARMACOTHERAPEUTIC: Third-generation cephalosporin. ***CLINICAL:*** Antibiotic (see p. 20C)

ACTION/*THERAPEUTIC EFFECT*

Binds to bacterial membranes, *inhibiting synthesis of bacterial cell wall. Bactericidal.*

PHARMACOKINETICS

Moderately absorbed from GI tract. Protein binding: 60–70%. Widely distributed. Not appreciably metabolized. Primarily excreted unchanged in urine. Minimally removed by hemodialysis. Half-life: 1–2 hrs (half-life increased in those with impaired renal function).

USES/*UNLABELED*

Treatment of community-acquired pneumonia, acute exacerbation of chronic bronchitis, acute maxillary sinusitis, pharyngitis, tonsillitis, uncomplicated skin and skin structure infections, otitis media.

PRECAUTIONS

CONTRAINDICATIONS: Hypersensitivity to cephalosporins. ***CAUTIONS:*** Hypersensitivity to penicillins or other drugs; allergies; history of GI disease (e.g., colitis); renal impairment, impaired hepatic function.
▷*LIFESPAN CONSIDERATIONS:*
Pregnancy/Lactation: Crosses placenta; not detected in breast milk. **Pregnancy Category B. Children:** Newborn, infants may have lower renal clearance. **Elderly:** Age-related decrease in renal function in elderly may require decreased dose or increased dosage interval.

INTERACTIONS

DRUG: **Probenecid** increases serum concentration of cefdinir. **Antacids** decreases cefdinir plasma concentration. ***HERBAL:*** None known. ***FOOD:*** None known. ***LAB VALUES:*** May produce a false-positive reaction for ketones in urine. May increase SGOT (AST), SGOT (ALT), alkaline phosphatase, bilirubin, LDH concentrations.

AVAILABILITY (Rx)

CAPSULES: 300 mg. ***ORAL SUSPENSION:*** 125 mg/5 ml.

ADMINISTRATION/HANDLING
PO:

• Give without regard to meals. • To reconstitute oral suspension, for the 60 ml bottle, add 39 ml water; for the 120 ml bottle, add

65 ml water. • Shake oral suspension well before administering. • Store mixed suspension at room temperature. Discard unused portion after 10 days.

INDICATIONS/ROUTES/DOSAGE

Community-acquired pneumonia:

PO: **Adults, elderly, children ≥13 yrs:** 300 mg q12h for 10 days.

Acute exacerbation of chronic bronchitis:

PO: **Adults, elderly:** 300 mg q12h for 5 days.

Acute maxillary sinusitis:

PO: **Adults, elderly, children ≥13 yrs:** 300 mg q12h or 600 mg q24h for 10 days. **Children 6 mos–12 yrs:** 7 mg/kg q12h or 14 mg/kg q24h for 10 days.

Pharyngitis/tonsillitis:

PO: **Adults, elderly, children ≥13 yrs:** 300 mg q12h for 5–10 days or 600 mg q24h for 10 days. **Children 6 mos–12 yrs:** 7 mg/kg q12h for 5–10 days or 14 mg/kg q24h for 10 days.

Uncomplicated skin and skin structure infections:

PO: **Adults, elderly, children ≥13 yrs:** 300 mg q12h for 10 days. **Children 6 mos–12 yrs:** 7 mg/kg q12h for 10 days.

Acute bacterial otitis media:

PO: **Children 6 mos–12 yrs:** 7 mg/kg q12h or 14 mg/kg q24h for 10 days.

Oral suspension:

Pediatric <20 lbs: 2.5 ml (½ tsp) q12h or 5 ml (1 tsp) q24h. **Pediatric 20–40 lbs:** 5 ml (1 tsp) q12h or 10 ml (2 tsp) q24h. **Pediatric 41–60 lbs:** 7.5 ml (1½ tsp) q12h or 15 ml (3 tsp) q24h. **Pediatric 61–80 lbs:** 10 ml (2 tsp) q12h or 20 ml (4 tsp)

q24h. **Pediatric 81–95 lbs:** 12 ml (2½ tsp) q12h or 24 ml (5 tsp) q24h.

Dosage in renal impairment:

Creatinine clearance <30 ml/ min: 300 mg/day as single daily dose. *Hemodialysis pts:* 300 mg or 7 mg/kg dose every other day.

SIDE EFFECTS

FREQUENT: Oral candidiasis (sore mouth/tongue), mild diarrhea, mild abdominal cramping, vaginal candidiasis (itching, discharge). ***OCCASIONAL:*** Nausea, serum sickness reaction [joint pain, fever] (usually occurs following second course of therapy, resolves after drug discontinuation). ***RARE:*** Allergic reaction (rash, pruritus, urticaria).

ADVERSE REACTIONS/TOXIC EFFECTS

Antibiotic-associated colitis (severe abdominal pain and tenderness, fever, watery and severe diarrhea) may result from altered bacterial balance. Nephrotoxicity may occur, esp. with preexisting renal disease. Severe hypersensitivity reaction (severe pruritus, angioedema, bronchospasm, anaphylaxis), particularly those with history of allergies, esp. penicillin.

NURSING IMPLICATIONS

BASELINE ASSESSMENT:

Question for hypersensitivity to cefdinir or other cephalosporins, penicillins.

INTERVENTION/EVALUATION:

Monitor bowel activity and stool consistency carefully; mild GI effects may be tolerable, but increasing severity may indicate onset of antibiotic-associated colitis. Be alert for superinfection (e.g., genital-anal pruritus, ulceration or changes in oral mucosa, moderate to severe diarrhea, new or increased fever). Monitor hematology reports.

PATIENT/FAMILY TEACHING:

Take antacids 2 hrs before or after taking medication. Continue medication for full length of treatment; do not skip doses. Doses should be evenly spaced.

cefditoren

sef-dih-**tore**-inn
(Spectracef)

►**CLASSIFICATION**

PHARMACOTHERAPEUTIC: Third-generation cephalosporin. ***CLINICAL:*** Antibiotic (see p. 20C)

ACTION/*THERAPEUTIC EFFECT*

Bactericidal. Binds to bacterial membrane, *inhibiting bacterial cell wall synthesis.*

USES

Treatment of acute bacterial exacerbations of chronic bronchitis, pharyngitis/tonsillitis, and uncomplicated skin and skin structure infections.

PRECAUTIONS

CONTRAINDICATIONS: Known allergy to cephalosporins, carnitive deficiency (causes renal excretion of carnitine), inborn errors of metabolism, milk protein hypersensitivity. ***CAUTIONS:*** Diarrhea.

INTERACTIONS

DRUG: **Antacids** containing mag-

nesium and/or aluminum, **H₂ antagonists** may decrease absorption. **Probenecid** may increase absorption. ***HERBAL:*** None significant. ***FOOD:*** None significant. ***LAB VALUES:*** None significant.

AVAILABILITY (Rx)

TABLETS: 200 mg.

INDICATIONS/ROUTES/DOSAGE

Acute exacerbations of chronic bronchitis:

PO: Adults, elderly, children >12 yrs: 400 mg 2 times/day for 10 days.

Pharyngitis/tonsillitis, skin infections:

PO: Adults, elderly, children >12 yrs: 200 mg 2 times/day for 10 days.

Dosage in renal impairment:

Creatinine Clearance	Dosage
50–80 ml/min	No adjustment
30–49 ml/min	200 mg twice daily
<30 ml/min	200 mg once daily

SIDE EFFECTS

FREQUENT (>5%): Diarrhea, nausea, headache, abdominal pain, vaginal moniliasis, dyspepsia, vomiting.

ADVERSE REACTIONS/TOXIC EFFECTS

Antibiotic-associated colitis (severe abdominal pain and tenderness, fever, watery and severe diarrhea). Severe hypersensitivity reactions, esp. in pts with history of allergies, including penicillin.

NURSING IMPLICATIONS

BASELINE ASSESSMENT:

Question for history of allergies, particularly cephalosporins, penicillins. Assess if pt has a carnitine deficiency, inborn error of metabolism.

INTERVENTION/EVALUATION:

Check mouth for white patches on mucous membranes, tongue. Carefully monitor bowel activity and stool consistency; mild GI effects may be tolerable, but increasing severity may indicate onset of antibiotic-associated colitis. Monitor I&O, renal function reports. Be alert for superinfection: severe genital/anal pruritus, abdominal pain, severe mouth soreness, moderate to severe diarrhea. Monitor carnitine deficiency (muscle damage, hypoglycemia, fatigue, confusion).

PATIENT/FAMILY TEACHING:

Continue medication for full length of treatment; do not skip doses. May cause GI upset (may take with food).

cefepime

sef-eh-**peem**
(Maxipime)

▶CLASSIFICATION

PHARMACOTHERAPEUTIC: Fourth-generation cephalosporin. **CLINICAL:** Antibiotic (see p. 21C)

ACTION/*THERAPEUTIC EFFECT*

Binds to bacterial membranes, *inhibiting synthesis of bacterial cell wall. Bactericidal.*

PHARMACOKINETICS

Well absorbed after IM administration. Protein binding: 20%. Widely distributed. Primarily excreted unchanged in urine. Removed by hemodialysis. Half-life: 2–2.3 hrs (half-life increased with impaired renal function, elderly).

USES

Treatment of pneumonia, bronchitis, urinary tract, skin and skin structure, intra-abdominal infections, bacteremia, septicemia, fever and neutropenia in cancer pts, complicated intra-abdominal infections (with metronidazole).

PRECAUTIONS

CONTRAINDICATIONS: History of hypersensitivity to cephalosporins, anaphylactic reaction to penicillins. **CAUTIONS:** Renal impairment, history of allergies.

▷*LIFESPAN CONSIDERATIONS:* **Pregnancy/Lactation:** Unknown whether distributed in breast milk. **Pregnancy Category B. Children:** No age-related precautions noted in those >2 mos. **Elderly:** Age-related decreased renal function may require reduced dose or increased dosing interval.

INTERACTIONS

DRUG: Probenecid may increase concentration of cefepime. **HERBAL:** None known. **FOOD:** None known. **LAB VALUES:** Positive direct/indirect Coombs' test may occur. May increase SGOT (AST), SGPT (ALT), alkaline phosphatase, LDH, bilirubin.

AVAILABILITY (Rx)

POWDER FOR INJECTION: 500 mg, 1 g, 2 g.

ADMINISTRATION/HANDLING

Note: May give by IM injection, IV push, intermittent IV infusion (piggyback).

IM:

• Add 1.3 ml Sterile Water for Injection, 0.9% NaCl, or D_5W (2.4 ml for 1 g and 2 g vials) to 500 mg vial. •

Inject into a large muscle mass (e.g., upper gluteus maximus).

IV 🟦

Storage:
• Solution is stable for 24 hrs at room temperature or 7 days if refrigerated.

Reconstitution:
• Add 5 ml (10 ml for 1 g and 2 g vials) to 500 mg vial. • Further dilute with 50–100 ml 0.9% NaCl, or D_5W.

Rate of administration:
• For IV push, administer over 3–5 min. • For intermittent IV infusion (piggyback), infuse over 30 min.

IV INCOMPATIBILITIES ⊘

Acyclovir (Zovirax), amphotericin (Fungizone), cimetidine (Tagamet), ciprofloxacin (Cipro), cisplatin (Platinol), dacarbazine (DTIC), daunorubicin (Cerubidine), diazepam (Valium), diphenhydramine (Benadryl), dobutamine (Dobutrex), dopamine (Intropin), doxorubicin (Adriamycin), etoposide (Vepesid), droperidol (Inapsine), famotidine (Pepcid), ganciclovir (Cytovene), haloperidol (Haldol), mannitol, magnesium, meperidine (Demerol), metoclopramide (Reglan), morphine, ofloxacin (Floxin), ondansetron (Zofran), vancomycin (Vancocin).

IV COMPATIBILITIES

Bumetanide (Bumex), calcium gluconate, furosemide (Lasix), lorazepam (Ativan).

INDICATIONS/ROUTES/DOSAGE

Note: Space doses evenly around the clock.

Usual adult dosage:
IM/IV: 1–2 g q12h.

Urinary tract infections:
IM/IV: **Adults, elderly:** 500 mg q12h.

Empiric therapy for febrile neutropenia:
IV: **Adults:** 2 g q8h.

Usual pediatric dosage:
IM/IV: **Children (2 mos–16 yrs):** 50 mg/kg q8–12hrs. Do not exceed maximum adult dose.

Dosage in renal impairment:
Dose and/or frequency is based on degree of renal impairment (creatinine clearance) and/or severity of infection.

Creatinine Clearance	Dose
30–60 ml/min	0.5–2 g q24h
11–29 ml/min	0.5–1 g q24h
≤10 ml/min	0.25–0.5 g q24h

SIDE EFFECTS

FREQUENT: Discomfort with IM administration, oral candidiasis (sore mouth/tongue), mild diarrhea, mild abdominal cramping, vaginal candidiasis (itching, discharge). *OCCASIONAL:* Nausea, serum sickness reaction [joint pain, fever] (usually occurs following second course of therapy, resolves after drug discontinuation). *RARE:* Allergic reaction (rash, pruritus, urticaria), thrombophlebitis (pain, redness, swelling at injection site).

ADVERSE REACTIONS/TOXIC EFFECTS

Antibiotic-associated colitis (severe abdominal pain and tenderness, fever, watery and severe diarrhea), other superinfections may result from altered bacterial balance. Nephrotoxicity may occur, esp. with preexisting renal disease. Severe hypersensitivity reaction (severe pruritus, angioedema, bronchospasm, anaphylaxis), particularly those with history of allergies, esp. penicillin.

NURSING IMPLICATIONS

BASELINE ASSESSMENT:

Question history of allergies, particularly cephalosporins, penicillins.

INTERVENTION/EVALUATION:

Monitor IV site for phlebitis (heat, pain, red streaking over vein). Assess mouth for white patches on mucous membranes, tongue. Monitor bowel activity and stool consistency carefully; mild GI effects may be tolerable, but increasing severity may indicate onset of antibiotic-associated colitis. Monitor I&O, renal function reports for nephrotoxicity. Be alert for superinfection: severe genital/anal pruritus, abdominal pain, severe mouth soreness, moderate to severe diarrhea.

PATIENT/FAMILY TEACHING:

Discomfort may occur with IM injection. Continue therapy for full length of treatment. Doses should be evenly spaced.

---

cefixime

sef-ih-zeem
(Suprax)

▶CLASSIFICATION

PHARMACOTHERAPEUTIC:
Third-generation cephalosporin.
CLINICAL: Antibiotic (see p. 20C)

ACTION/*THERAPEUTIC EFFECT*

Binds to bacterial membranes, in-*hibiting synthesis of bacterial cell wall. Bactericidal.*

PHARMACOKINETICS

Moderately absorbed from GI tract. Protein binding: 65–70%. Widely distributed. Primarily excreted unchanged in urine. Minimally removed by hemodialysis. Half-life: 3–4 hrs (half-life increased with impaired renal function).

USES

Otitis media, acute bronchitis and acute exacerbations of chronic bronchitis, pharyngitis, tonsillitis, uncomplicated UTI, uncomplicated gonorrhea.

PRECAUTIONS

CONTRAINDICATIONS: Hypersensitivity to cephalosporins. ***CAUTIONS:*** Hypersensitivity to penicillins or other drugs; allergies; history of GI disease (e.g., colitis); renal impairment.

▷*LIFESPAN CONSIDERATIONS:*
Pregnancy/Lactation: Not recommended during labor and delivery. Excretion in breast milk not known. **Pregnancy Category B. Children:** Safety and efficacy not established in those <6 mos. **Elderly:** Age-related decreased renal function may require dosage adjustment.

INTERACTIONS

DRUG: Probenecid increases serum concentrations of cefixime. ***HERBAL:*** None known. ***FOOD:*** None known. ***LAB VALUES:*** Positive direct/indirect Coombs' test. May increase BUN, serum creatinine, SGPT (ALT), SGOT (AST), alkaline phosphatase, bilirubin, LDH concentrations.

AVAILABILITY (Rx)

TABLETS: 200 mg, 400 mg. ***ORAL SUSPENSION:*** 100 mg/5 ml.

C

ADMINISTRATION/HANDLING
PO:

• Give without regard to meals. • After reconstitution, oral suspension is stable for 14 days at room temperature. Do not refrigerate. • Shake oral suspension well before administering.

INDICATIONS/ROUTES/DOSAGE

Note: Use oral suspension to treat otitis media (achieves higher peak blood level).

Usual PO dosage:

PO: **Adults, elderly, children >50 kg:** 400 mg/day as single or 2 divided doses. **Children 6 mos–12 yrs <50 kg:** 8 mg/kg/day as single or 2 divided doses. **Maximum:** 400 mg.

Uncomplicated gonorrhea:

PO: **Adults:** 400 mg as single dose.

Dosage in renal impairment:

Creatinine Clearance (ml/min)	% of Standard Dose
21–60	75
<20	50

SIDE EFFECTS

FREQUENT: Oral candidiasis (sore mouth/tongue), mild diarrhea, mild abdominal cramping, vaginal candidiasis (itching, discharge). **OCCASIONAL:** Nausea, serum sickness reaction [joint pain, fever] (usually occurs following second course of therapy, resolves after drug discontinuation). **RARE:** Allergic reaction (rash, pruritus, urticaria).

ADVERSE REACTIONS/TOXIC EFFECTS

Antibiotic-associated colitis (severe abdominal pain and tenderness, fever, watery and severe diarrhea), other superinfections may result from altered bacterial balance. Nephrotoxicity may occur, esp. with preexisting renal disease. Severe hypersensitivity reaction (severe pruritus, angioedema, bronchospasm, anaphylaxis), particularly those with history of allergies, esp. penicillin.

NURSING IMPLICATIONS

BASELINE ASSESSMENT:
Question for hypersensitivity to cefixime or other cephalosporins, penicillins, other drugs.

INTERVENTION/EVALUATION:
Check mouth for white patches on mucous membranes, tongue. Monitor bowel activity and stool consistency carefully; mild GI effects may be tolerable, but increasing severity may indicate onset of antibiotic-associated colitis. Monitor I&O, renal function reports for nephrotoxicity. Be alert for superinfection:-severe genital/anal pruritus, abdominal pain, severe mouth soreness, moderate to severe diarrhea.

PATIENT/FAMILY TEACHING:
Continue medication for full length of treatment; do not skip doses. Doses should be evenly spaced. May cause GI upset (may take with food or milk).

cefmetazole sodium ✳

(Zefazone)

See Classification section under: Antibiotic: cephalosporins (p. 19C)

cefoperazone sodium

sef-o-**pear**-a-zone
(Cefobid)

▶CLASSIFICATION

PHARMACOTHERAPEUTIC:
Third-generation cephalosporin.
CLINICAL: Antibiotic

ACTION/*THERAPEUTIC EFFECT*

Binds to bacterial membranes, *inhibiting synthesis of bacterial cell wall. Bactericidal.*

USES

Treatment of intra-abdominal, biliary, pelvic inflammatory infections; respiratory, GU tract, skin and bone infections; septicemia.

PRECAUTIONS

CONTRAINDICATIONS: History of hypersensitivity to cephalosporins, anaphylactic reaction to penicillins. **CAUTIONS:** History of allergies, GI disease (esp. ulcerative colitis, antibiotic-associated colitis), hepatic or renal impairment.

INTERACTIONS

DRUG: Disulfiram reaction (facial flushing, nausea, sweating, headache, tachycardia) may occur when alcohol is ingested. May increase bleeding risk with anticoagulants, heparin, thrombolytics. **HERBAL:** None known. **FOOD:** None known. **LAB VALUES:** Positive direct/indirect Coombs' test may occur (interferes with hematologic tests, cross-matching procedures). Prothrombin times may be increased. May increase BUN, serum creatinine, SGOT (AST), SGPT

(ALT), alkaline phosphatase concentrations.

AVAILABILITY (Rx)
POWDER FOR INJECTION: 1 g, 2 g.

INDICATIONS/ROUTES/DOSAGE
Note: Space doses evenly around the clock.

Mild to moderate infections:
IM/IV: Adults, elderly: 2–4 g/day in divided doses q12h.

Severe or life-threatening infections:
IM/IV: Adults, elderly: Total daily dose and/or frequency may be increased to 6–12 g/day divided into 2, 3, or 4 equal doses of 1.5–4 g per dose.

Dosage in renal and/or hepatic impairment:
Do not exceed 4 g/day in those with liver disease and/or biliary obstruction. Modification of dose usually not necessary in those with renal impairment. Dose should not exceed 1–2 g/day in those with both hepatic and substantial renal impairment.

SIDE EFFECTS
FREQUENT: Discomfort with IM administration, oral candidiasis (sore mouth/tongue), mild diarrhea, mild abdominal cramping, vaginal candidiasis (itching, discharge). **OCCASIONAL:** Nausea, unusual bruising/bleeding, serum sickness reaction [joint pain, fever] (usually occurs following second course of therapy, resolves after drug discontinuation). **RARE:** Allergic reaction (rash, pruritus, urticaria), thrombophlebitis (pain, redness, swelling at injection site).

ADVERSE REACTIONS/TOXIC EFFECTS

Antibiotic-associated colitis (severe abdominal pain and tenderness, fever, watery and severe diarrhea), other superinfections may result from altered bacterial balance. Nephrotoxicity may occur, esp. with preexisting renal disease. Severe hypersensitivity reaction (severe pruritus, angioedema, bronchospasm, anaphylaxis), particularly those with history of allergies, esp. penicillin.

NURSING IMPLICATIONS

BASELINE ASSESSMENT:

Question for history of allergies, particularly cephalosporins, penicillins.

INTERVENTION/EVALUATION:

Evaluate IV site for phlebitis (heat, pain, red streaking over vein). Assess mouth for white patches on mucous membranes, tongue. Monitor bowel activity and stool consistency carefully; mild GI effects may be tolerable, but increasing severity may indicate onset of antibiotic-associated colitis. Monitor I&O, renal function reports for nephrotoxicity. Be alert for superinfection: severe genital/anal pruritus, abdominal pain, severe mouth soreness, moderate to severe diarrhea.

PATIENT/FAMILY TEACHING:

Discomfort may occur with IM injection. Doses should be evenly spaced. Continue antibiotic therapy for full length of treatment. Avoid alcohol and alcohol-containing preparations (salad dressings, sauces, cough syrups) during and for 72 hrs after last dose of cefoperazone.

---

cefotaxime sodium

seh-fo-**tax**-eem
(Claforan)
Do not confuse with cefuroxime.

▶CLASSIFICATION

PHARMACOTHERAPEUTIC:
Third-generation cephalosporin.
CLINICAL: Antibiotic (see p. 20C)

ACTION/*THERAPEUTIC EFFECT*

Binds to bacterial membranes, *inhibiting synthesis of bacterial cell wall. Bactericidal.*

PHARMACOKINETICS

Widely distributed (including CSF). Protein binding: 30–50%. Partially metabolized in liver to active metabolite. Primarily excreted in urine. Moderately removed by hemodialysis. Half-life: 1 hr (half-life increased with impaired renal function).

USES/*UNLABELED*

Treatment of respiratory, GU tract, skin and bone infections; septicemia, gonorrhea; gynecologic, intra-abdominal, biliary infections; meningitis; perioperative prophylaxis. *Treatment of Lyme disease.*

PRECAUTIONS

CONTRAINDICATIONS: History of hypersensitivity to cephalosporins, anaphylactic reaction to penicillins. **CAUTIONS:** Concurrent use of nephrotoxic medications, history of allergies or GI disease (esp. ulcerative colitis,

---

antibiotic-associated colitis), renal impairment with creatinine clearance <20 ml/min.

▷**LIFESPAN CONSIDERATIONS:**
Pregnancy/Lactation: Readily crosses placenta; distributed in breast milk. **Pregnancy Category B. Children:** No age-related precautions noted. **Elderly:** Age-related renal impairment may require dose adjustment.

INTERACTIONS

DRUG: Probenecid increases serum concentration of cefotaxime. **HERBAL:** None known. **FOOD:** None known. **LAB VALUES:** Positive direct/indirect Coombs' test may occur. May increase liver function tests.

AVAILABILITY (Rx)

POWDER FOR INJECTION: 500 mg, 1 g, 2 g.

ADMINISTRATION/HANDLING

Note: Give by IM injection, direct IV injection, intermittent IV infusion (piggyback).

IM:

• Reconstitute with Sterile Water for Injection or Bacteriostatic Water for Injection. • Add 2, 3, or 5 ml to 500 mg, 1 g, or 2 g vial, respectively, providing a concentration of 230 mg, 300 mg or 330 mg/ml, respectively. • To minimize discomfort, inject deep IM slowly. Less painful if injected into gluteus maximus rather than lateral aspect of thigh. For 2 g IM dose, give at 2 separate sites.

IV 🏺

Storage:

• Solution appears light yellow to amber. IV infusion (piggyback) may darken in color (does not indicate loss of potency). • IV infusion (piggyback) is stable for 24 hrs at room temperature, 5 days if refrigerated. • Discard if precipitate forms.

Reconstitution:

• Reconstitute with 10 ml Sterile Water for Injection to provide a concentration of 50 mg, 95 mg, or 180 mg/ml for 500 mg, 1 g, or 2 g vials, respectively. • May further dilute with 50–100 ml 0.9% NaCl or D_5W.

Rate of administration:

• For IV push, administer over 3–5 min. • For intermittent IV infusion (piggyback), infuse over 20–30 min.

IV INCOMPATIBILITIES ⊘

Allopurinol (Aloprim), filgrastim (Neupogen), fluconazole (Diflucan), hetastarch (Hespan), pentamidine (Pentam IV), vancomycin (Vancocin).

IV COMPATIBILITIES

Diltiazem (Cardizem), lorazepam (Ativan), magnesium, midazolam (Versed), propofol (Diprivan).

INDICATIONS/ROUTES/DOSAGE

Note: Space doses evenly around the clock.

Uncomplicated infections:
IM/IV: Adults, elderly: 1 g q12h.

Mild to moderate infections:
IM/IV: Adults, elderly: 1–2 g q8h.

Severe infections:
IM/IV: Adults, elderly: 2 g q6–8h.

Life-threatening infections:
IM/IV: Adults, elderly: 2 g q4h.

Uncomplicated gonorrhea:
IM: Adults: 1 g one time.

Perioperative prophylaxis:
IM/IV: Adults, elderly: 1 g 30–90 min before surgery.

Cesarean section:
IV: Adults: 1 g as soon as umbili-

cal cord is clamped, then 1 g 6 and 12 hrs after first dose.

Usual dosage for children:

IM/IV: **1 mo–12 yrs (<50 kg):** 100–200 mg/kg/day in divided doses q6–8h; **(≥50 kg):** 1–2 g q6–8h; *life-threatening infection:* 2 g q4h. **Maximum:** 12 g/day.

Dosage in renal impairment:

Creatinine clearance <20 ml/min: Give ½ dose at usual dosage intervals.

SIDE EFFECTS

FREQUENT: Discomfort with IM administration, oral candidiasis (sore mouth/tongue), mild diarrhea, mild abdominal cramping, vaginal candidiasis (itching, discharge). **OCCASIONAL:** Nausea, serum sickness reaction [joint pain, fever] (usually occurs following second course of therapy, resolves after drug discontinuation). **RARE:** Allergic reaction (rash, pruritus, urticaria), thrombophlebitis (pain, redness, swelling at injection site).

ADVERSE REACTIONS/TOXIC EFFECTS

Antibiotic-associated colitis (severe abdominal pain and tenderness, fever, watery and severe diarrhea), other superinfections may result from altered bacterial balance. Nephrotoxicity may occur, esp. with preexisting renal disease. Severe hypersensitivity reaction (severe pruritus, angioedema, bronchospasm, anaphylaxis), particularly those with history of allergies, esp. penicillin.

NURSING IMPLICATIONS

BASELINE ASSESSMENT:

Question for history of allergies, particularly cephalosporins, penicillins.

INTERVENTION/EVALUATION:

Evaluate IV site for phlebitis (heat, pain, red streaking over vein). Check IM injection sites for induration, tenderness. Check mouth for white patches on mucous membranes, tongue. Monitor bowel activity and stool consistency carefully; mild GI effects may be tolerable, but increasing severity may indicate onset of antibiotic-associated colitis. Monitor I&O, renal function reports for nephrotoxicity. Be alert for superinfection: severe genital/anal pruritus, abdominal pain, severe mouth soreness, moderate to severe diarrhea.

PATIENT/FAMILY TEACHING:

Discomfort may occur with IM injection. Doses should be evenly spaced. Continue antibiotic therapy for full length of treatment.

cefotetan disodium

seh-fo-**teh**-tan
(Cefotan)

▶**CLASSIFICATION**

PHARMACOTHERAPEUTIC: Second-generation cephalosporin. **CLINICAL:** Antibiotic (see p. 19C)

ACTION/*THERAPEUTIC EFFECT*

Binds to bacterial membranes, *inhibiting synthesis of bacterial cell wall.* Bactericidal.

PHARMACOKINETICS

Widely distributed. Protein binding: 78–91%. Primarily excreted unchanged in urine. Minimally removed by hemodialysis. Half-life:

3–4.6 hrs (half-life increased with impaired renal function).

USES

Treatment of respiratory, GU tract, skin, bone, gynecologic, intra-abdominal infections; perioperative prophylaxis.

PRECAUTIONS

CONTRAINDICATIONS: History of hypersensitivity to cephalosporins, anaphylactic reaction to penicillins. ***CAUTIONS:*** Renal impairment, history of allergies or GI disease (esp. ulcerative colitis, antibiotic-associated colitis), concurrent use of nephrotoxic medications.

▷***LIFESPAN CONSIDERATIONS:*** **Pregnancy/Lactation:** Readily crosses placenta. Distributed in breast milk. **Pregnancy Category B. Children:** Safety and efficacy not established. **Elderly:** Age-related renal impairment may require dosage adjustment.

INTERACTIONS

DRUG: Disulfiram reaction (facial flushing, nausea, sweating, headache, tachycardia) may occur when **alcohol** is ingested. May increase bleeding risk with **anticoagulants, heparin, thrombolytics.** ***HERBAL:*** None known. ***FOOD:*** None known. ***LAB VALUES:*** Positive direct/indirect Coombs' test may occur (interferes with hematologic tests, cross-matching procedures). Prothrombin times may be increased. May increase BUN, serum creatinine, SGOT (AST), SGPT (ALT), alkaline phosphatase concentrations.

AVAILABILITY [Rx]

POWDER FOR INJECTION: 1 g, 2 g.

ADMINISTRATION/HANDLING

Note: Give by IM injection, IV push, intermittent IV infusion (piggyback).

IM:

• Add 2, 3 ml Sterile Water for Injection or other appropriate diluent to 1 g, 2 g providing a concentration of 400 mg/ml or 500 mg/ml, respectively. • Less painful if injected deep IM slowly into gluteus maximus rather than lateral aspect of thigh.

IV 🍴

Storage:

• Solution appears colorless to light yellow. • Color change to deep yellow does not indicate loss of potency. • IV infusion (piggyback) is stable for 24 hrs at room temperature, 96 hrs if refrigerated. • Discard if precipitate forms.

Reconstitution:

• Reconstitute each 1 g with 10 ml Sterile Water for Injection to provide a concentration of 95 mg/ml. • May further dilute with 50–100 ml 0.9% NaCl or D_5W.

Rate of administration:

• For IV push, administer over 3–5 min. • For intermittent IV infusion (piggyback), infuse over 20–30 min.

IV INCOMPATIBILITY ⊘

Vancomycin (Vancocin).

IV COMPATIBILITIES

Diltiazem (Cardizem), heparin.

INDICATIONS/ROUTES/DOSAGE

Note: Space doses evenly around the clock.

Urinary tract infections:
***IM/IV:* Adults, elderly:** 1–2 g in divided doses q12–24h.

Mild to moderate infections:
***IM/IV:* Adults, elderly:** 1–2 g q12h.

Severe infections:
***IM/IV:* Adults, elderly:** 2 g q12h.

Life-threatening infections:

IM/IV: **Adults, elderly:** 3 g q12h.

Perioperative prophylaxis:

IV: **Adults, elderly:** 1–2 g 30–60 min before surgery.

Cesarean section:

IV: **Adults:** 1–2 g as soon as umbilical cord is clamped.

Usual pediatric dosage:

IM/IV: 40–80 mg/kg/day in divided doses q12h. **Maximum:** 6 g/day.

Dosage in renal impairment:

Dose and/or frequency modified on basis of creatinine clearance and/or severity of infection.

Creatinine Clearance	Dosage Interval
10–30 ml/min	Usual dose q24h
<10 ml/min	Usual dose q48h

SIDE EFFECTS

FREQUENT: Discomfort with IM administration, oral candidiasis (sore mouth/tongue), mild diarrhea, mild abdominal cramping, vaginal candidiasis (itching, discharge). **OCCASIONAL:** Nausea, unusual bruising/bleeding, serum sickness reaction [joint pain, fever] (usually occurs following second course of therapy, resolves after drug discontinuation). **RARE:** Allergic reaction (rash, pruritus, urticaria), thrombophlebitis (pain, redness, swelling at injection site).

ADVERSE REACTIONS/TOXIC EFFECTS

Antibiotic-associated colitis (severe abdominal pain and tenderness, fever, watery and severe diarrhea), other superinfections may result from altered bacterial balance. Nephrotoxicity may occur, esp. with preexisting renal disease. Severe hypersensitivity reaction (severe pruritus, angioedema, bronchospasm, anaphylaxis), particularly those with history of allergies, esp. penicillin.

NURSING IMPLICATIONS

BASELINE ASSESSMENT:

Question for history of allergies, particularly cephalosporins, penicillins.

INTERVENTION/EVALUATION:

Evaluate IV site for phlebitis (heat, pain, red streaking over vein). Check IM injection sites for induration, tenderness. Check mouth for white patches on mucous membranes, tongue. Monitor bowel activity and stool consistency carefully; mild GI effects may be tolerable, but increasing severity may indicate onset of antibiotic-associated colitis. Monitor I&O, renal function reports for nephrotoxicity. Be alert for superinfection: severe genital/anal pruritus, abdominal pain, severe mouth soreness, moderate to severe diarrhea.

PATIENT/FAMILY TEACHING:

Discomfort may occur with IM injection. Doses should be evenly spaced. Continue antibiotic therapy for full length of treatment. Avoid alcohol and alcohol-containing preparations (salad dressings, sauces, cough syrups) during and for 72 hrs after last dose of cefotetan.

cefoxitin sodium

seh-**fox**-ih-tin
(Mefoxin)

▶CLASSIFICATION

PHARMACOTHERAPEUTIC:
Second-generation cephalosporin. **CLINICAL:** Antibiotic
(see p. 19C)

ACTION/*THERAPEUTIC EFFECT*

Binds to bacterial membranes, *inhibiting synthesis of bacterial cell
wall*. Bactericidal.

PHARMACOKINETICS

Widely distributed. Protein binding:
70–80%. Primarily excreted unchanged in urine. Moderately removed by hemodialysis. Half-life:
0.7–1.1 hrs (half-life increased with
impaired renal function).

USES

Treatment of respiratory, GU tract,
skin, bone, intra-abdominal, gynecologic infections; gonorrhea, septicemia, perioperative prophylaxis.

PRECAUTIONS

CONTRAINDICATIONS: History of
hypersensitivity to cephalosporins,
anaphylactic reaction to penicillins.
CAUTIONS: Renal impairment, history of allergies or GI disease (esp.
ulcerative colitis, antibiotic-associated colitis), concurrent use of
nephrotoxic medications.
▷**LIFESPAN CONSIDERATIONS:**
Pregnancy/Lactation: Readily
crosses placenta. Distributed in
breast milk. **Pregnancy Category
B. Children:** In those >3 mos, high
doses associated with eosinophilia,
increased SGOT (AST). **Elderly:**
Age-related renal impairment may
require dosage adjustment.

INTERACTIONS

DRUG: Probenecid increases
serum concentrations of cefoxitin.
HERBAL: None known. **FOOD:**
None known. **LAB VALUES:** Positive direct/indirect Coombs' test
may occur (interferes with hematologic tests, cross-matching procedures). May increase BUN,
serum creatinine, SGOT (AST),
SGPT (ALT), alkaline phosphatase
concentrations.

AVAILABILITY (Rx)

POWDER FOR INJECTION: 1 g, 2 g.

ADMINISTRATION/HANDLING

Note: Give IM, IV push, or intermittent IV infusion (piggyback).

IM:

* Reconstitute each 1 g with 2 ml
Sterile Water for Injection or lidocaine to provide concentration of 400
mg/ml. * To minimize discomfort, inject deep IM slowly. Less painful if injected into gluteus maximus rather
than lateral aspect of thigh.

IV 💊

Storage:

* Solution appears colorless to
light amber but may darken (does
not indicate loss of potency). * IV
infusion (piggyback) is stable for
24 hrs at room temperature, 48 hrs
if refrigerated. * Discard if precipitate forms.

Reconstitution:

* Reconstitute each 1 g with 10 ml
Sterile Water for Injection to pro-
vide concentration of 95 mg/ml. *
May further dilute with 50–100 ml
0.9% Sterile Water for Injection,
NaCl, or D_5W.

Rate of administration:

* For IV push, administer over 3–5
min. * For intermittent IV infusion
(piggyback), infuse over 15–30 min.

IV INCOMPATIBILITIES ⊘

Filgrastim (Neupogen), pentamidine (Pentam IV), vancomycin
(Vancocin).

IV COMPATIBILITIES

Diltiazem (Cardizem), magnesium.

INDICATIONS/ROUTES/DOSAGE

Note: Space doses evenly around the clock.

Mild to moderate infections:

IM/IV: Adults, elderly: 1–2 g q6–8h.

Severe infections:

IM/IV: Adults, elderly: 1 g q4h or 2 g q6–8h up to 2 g q4h.

Uncomplicated gonorrhea:

IM: Adults: 2 g one time with 1 g probenecid.

Perioperative prophylaxis:

IM/IV: Adults, elderly: 2 g 30–60 min before surgery and q6h up to 24 hrs postop. **Children >3 mos:** 30–40 mg/kg 30–60 min before surgery and q6h postop for no more than 24 hrs.

Cesarean section:

IV: Adults: 2 g as soon as umbilical cord is clamped, then 2 g 4 and 8 hrs after first dose, then q6h for no more than 24 hrs.

Usual dosage for children:

IM/IV: Children >3 mos: 80–160 mg/kg/day in 4–6 divided doses. **Maximum:** 12 g/day. **Neonates:** 90–100 mg/kg/day in divided doses q6–8h.

Dosage in renal impairment:

After loading dose of 1–2 g, dosage and/or frequency is modified on basis of creatinine clearance and/or severity of infection.

Creatinine Clearance	Dosage
30–50 ml/min	1–2 g q8–12h
10–29 ml/min	1–2 g q12–24h
5–9 ml/min	500 mg–1 g q12–24h
<5 ml/min	500 mg–1 g q24–48h

SIDE EFFECTS

FREQUENT: Discomfort with IM administration, oral candidiasis (sore mouth/tongue), mild diarrhea, mild abdominal cramping, vaginal candidiasis (itching, discharge). **OCCASIONAL:** Nausea, serum sickness reaction [joint pain, fever] (usually occurs following second course of therapy, resolves after drug discontinuation). **RARE:** Allergic reaction (rash, pruritus, urticaria), thrombophlebitis (pain, redness, swelling at injection site).

ADVERSE REACTIONS/TOXIC EFFECTS

Antibiotic-associated colitis (severe abdominal pain and tenderness, fever, watery and severe diarrhea), other superinfections may result from altered bacterial balance. Nephrotoxicity may occur, esp. with preexisting renal disease. Severe hypersensitivity reaction (severe pruritus, angioedema, bronchospasm, anaphylaxis), particularly those with history of allergies, esp. penicillin.

NURSING IMPLICATIONS

BASELINE ASSESSMENT:

Question for history of allergies, particularly cephalosporins, penicillins.

INTERVENTION/EVALUATION:

Evaluate IV site for phlebitis (heat, pain, red streaking over vein). Check IM injection sites for induration, tenderness. Check mouth for white patches on mucous membranes, tongue. Monitor bowel activity and stool consistency carefully; mild GI effects may be tolerable, but increasing severity may indicate onset of antibiotic-associated colitis. Monitor I&O, renal function reports for nephrotoxicity. Be alert for superinfection: severe genital/anal pruritus, abdominal pain, severe mouth soreness, moderate to severe diarrhea.

PATIENT/FAMILY TEACHING:

Discomfort may occur with IM injection. Doses should be evenly spaced. Continue antibiotic therapy for full length of treatment.

cefpodoxime proxetil

sef-poe-**docks**-em
(Vantin)

▶CLASSIFICATION

PHARMACOTHERAPEUTIC: Second-generation cephalosporin. ***CLINICAL:*** Antibiotic (see p. 20C)

ACTION/*THERAPEUTIC EFFECT*

Binds to bacterial membranes, *inhibiting synthesis of bacterial cell wall. Bactericidal.*

PHARMACOKINETICS

Well absorbed from GI tract (food increases absorption). Protein binding: 21–40%. Widely distributed. Primarily excreted unchanged in urine. Partially removed by hemodialysis. Half-life: 2.3 hrs (half-life increased with impaired renal function, elderly).

USES

Treatment of lower respiratory tract infections (pneumonia, chronic bronchitis), upper respiratory tract (otitis media, pharyngitis/tonsillitis), acute maxillary sinusitis, sexually transmitted diseases (urethral and cervical gonorrhea, anorectal infection), skin and skin structure, urinary tract infections.

PRECAUTIONS

CONTRAINDICATIONS: History of hypersensitivity to cephalosporins, anaphylactic reaction to penicillins. ***CAUTIONS:*** Renal impairment, history of allergies or GI disease (esp. ulcerative colitis, antibiotic-associated colitis), concurrent use of nephrotoxic medications.

▷***LIFESPAN CONSIDERATIONS:*** **Pregnancy/Lactation:** Readily crosses placenta. Distributed in breast milk. **Pregnancy Category B. Children:** Safety and efficacy not established in those <5 mos. **Elderly:** Age-related renal impairment may require dosage adjustment.

INTERACTIONS

DRUG: **Antacids, H$_2$ antagonists** may decrease absorption. **Probenecid** may increase concentration. ***HERBAL:*** None known. ***FOOD:*** None known. ***LAB VALUES:*** Positive direct/indirect Coombs' test may occur. May increase SGOT (AST), SGPT (ALT), alkaline phosphatase, LDH, bilirubin, BUN, serum creatinine.

AVAILABILITY (Rx)

TABLETS: 100 mg, 200 mg. ***ORAL SUSPENSION:*** 50 mg/5 ml, 100 mg/5 ml.

ADMINISTRATION/HANDLING

PO:

• Administer with food to enhance absorption. • After reconstitution, oral suspension is stable for 14 days if refrigerated.

INDICATIONS/ROUTES/DOSAGE

Pneumonia, chronic bronchitis:

PO: Adults, elderly, children >13 yrs: 200 mg q12h for 10–14 days.

Gonorrhea, rectal gonococcal infection (women only):

PO: Adults, children >13 yrs: 200 mg as single dose.

Skin/skin structure infections:

PO: **Adults, elderly, children >13 yrs:** 400 mg q12h for 7–14 days.

Pharyngitis/tonsillitis:

PO: **Adults, elderly, children >13 yrs:** 100 mg q12h for 5–10 days. **Children 6 mos–12 yrs:** 5 mg/kg q12h for 5–10 days. **Maximum:** 100 mg/dose.

Acute maxillary sinusitis:

PO: **Adults, children >13 yrs:** 200 mg twice daily for 10 days. **Children 2 mos–12 yrs:** 5 mg/kg q12h for 10 days. **Maximum:** 400 mg/day.

Urinary tract infection:

PO: **Adults, elderly, children >13 yrs:** 100 mg q12h for 7 days.

Acute otitis media:

PO: **Children 2 mos–12 yrs:** 5 mg/kg q12h for 5 days. **Maximum:** 400 mg/dose.

Dosage in renal impairment:

Dose and/or frequency is based on degree of renal impairment (creatinine clearance). Creatinine clearance <30 ml/min: dose q24h; on hemodialysis: 3 times/wk after dialysis.

SIDE EFFECTS

FREQUENT: Oral candidiasis (sore mouth/tongue), mild diarrhea, mild abdominal cramping, vaginal candidiasis (itching, discharge). ***OCCASIONAL:*** Nausea, serum sickness reaction [joint pain, fever] (usually occurs following second course of therapy, resolves after drug discontinuation). ***RARE:*** Allergic reaction (rash, pruritus, urticaria).

ADVERSE REACTIONS/TOXIC EFFECTS

Antibiotic-associated colitis (severe abdominal pain and tenderness, fever, watery and severe diarrhea), other superinfections may result from altered bacterial balance.

Nephrotoxicity may occur, esp. with preexisting renal disease. Severe hypersensitivity reaction (severe pruritus, angioedema, bronchospasm, anaphylaxis), particularly those with history of allergies, esp. penicillin.

NURSING IMPLICATIONS

BASELINE ASSESSMENT:

Shake oral suspension well before using. Question history of allergies, particularly cephalosporins, penicillins.

INTERVENTION/EVALUATION:

Check mouth for white patches on mucous membranes, tongue. Monitor bowel activity and stool consistency carefully; mild GI effects may be tolerable, but increasing severity may indicate onset of antibiotic-associated colitis. Monitor I&O, renal function reports for nephrotoxicity. Be alert for superinfection: severe genital/anal pruritus, abdominal pain, severe mouth soreness, moderate to severe diarrhea.

PATIENT/FAMILY TEACHING:

Doses should be evenly spaced. Continue antibiotic therapy for full length of treatment. Take with food.

cefprozil

sef-**proz**-ill
(Cefzil)
Do not confuse with Ceftin.

▶CLASSIFICATION

PHARMACOTHERAPEUTIC: Second-generation cephalosporin. ***CLINICAL:*** Antibiotic (see p. 20C)

ACTION/*THERAPEUTIC EFFECT*

Binds to bacterial membranes, *inhibiting synthesis of bacterial cell wall. Bactericidal.*

PHARMACOKINETICS

Well absorbed from GI tract. Protein binding: 36–45%. Widely distributed. Primarily excreted unchanged in urine. Moderately removed by hemodialysis. Half-life: 1.3 hrs (half-life increased with impaired renal function).

USES

Treatment of pharyngitis/tonsillitis, otitis media, secondary bacterial infection of acute bronchitis and acute bacterial exacerbation of chronic bronchitis, uncomplicated skin/skin structure infections, acute sinusitis.

PRECAUTIONS

CONTRAINDICATIONS: History of hypersensitivity to cephalosporins, anaphylactic reaction to penicillins. ***CAUTIONS:*** Renal impairment, history of allergies or GI disease (esp. ulcerative colitis, antibiotic-associated colitis), concurrent use of nephrotoxic medications.

▷*LIFESPAN CONSIDERATIONS:* **Pregnancy/Lactation:** Readily crosses placenta. Distributed in breast milk. **Pregnancy Category B. Children:** Safety and efficacy not established in those <6 mos. **Elderly:** Age-related renal impairment may require dosage adjustment.

INTERACTIONS

DRUG: Probenecid increases serum concentrations of cefprozil. ***HERBAL:*** None known. ***FOOD:*** None known. ***LAB VALUES:*** Positive direct/indirect Coombs' test may occur (interferes with hematologic tests, cross-matching procedures). May increase liver function tests.

AVAILABILITY (Rx)

TABLETS: 250 mg, 500 mg. ***ORAL SUSPENSION:*** 125 mg/5 ml, 250 mg/5 ml.

ADMINISTRATION/HANDLING
PO:

• After reconstitution, oral suspension is stable for 14 days if refrigerated. • Shake oral suspension well before using. • Give without regard to meals; if GI upset occurs, give with food or milk.

INDICATIONS/ROUTES/DOSAGE

Note: Space doses evenly around the clock.

Pharyngitis, tonsillitis:

PO: **Adults, elderly:** 500 mg q24h for 10 days. **Children: (2–12 yrs):** 7.5 mg/kg q12h for 10 days.

Secondary bacterial infection of acute bronchitis; acute bacterial exacerbation of chronic bronchitis:

PO: **Adults, elderly:** 500 mg q12h for 10 days.

Skin/skin structure infections:

PO: **Adults, elderly:** 250–500 mg q12h for 10 days. **Children:** 20 mg/kg q24h.

Acute sinusitis:

PO: **Adults, elderly:** 250–500 mg q12h. **Children (6 mos–12 yrs):** 7.5–15 mg/kg q12h.

Otitis media:

PO: **Children (6 mos–12 yrs):** 15 mg/kg q12h for 10 days. **Maximum:** 1 g/day.

Dosage in renal impairment:

Dose and/or frequency is based on degree of renal impairment (creatinine clearance). Creatinine clearance <30 ml/min: 50% dosage at usual interval.

SIDE EFFECTS

FREQUENT: Oral candidiasis (sore mouth/tongue), mild diarrhea, mild abdominal cramping, vaginal candidiasis (itching, discharge). ***OCCASIONAL:*** Nausea, serum sickness reaction [joint pain, fever] (usually occurs following second course of therapy, resolves after drug discontinuation). ***RARE:*** Allergic reaction (rash, pruritus, urticaria).

ADVERSE REACTIONS/TOXIC EFFECTS

Antibiotic-associated colitis (severe abdominal pain and tenderness, fever, watery and severe diarrhea), other superinfections may result from altered bacterial balance. Nephrotoxicity may occur, esp. with preexisting renal disease. Severe hypersensitivity reaction (severe pruritus, angioedema, bronchospasm, anaphylaxis), particularly those with history of allergies, esp. penicillin.

NURSING IMPLICATIONS

BASELINE ASSESSMENT:
Question history of allergies, particularly cephalosporins, penicillins.

INTERVENTION/EVALUATION:
Check mouth for white patches on mucous membranes, tongue. Monitor bowel activity and stool consistency carefully; mild GI effects may be tolerable, but increasing severity may indicate onset of antibiotic-associated colitis. Monitor I&O, renal function reports for nephrotoxicity. Be alert for superinfection: severe genital/anal pruritus, abdominal pain, severe mouth soreness, moderate to severe diarrhea.

PATIENT/FAMILY TEACHING:
Doses should be evenly spaced. Continue antibiotic therapy for full length of treatment. May cause GI upset (may take with food or milk).

ceftazidime

sef-**taz**-ih-deem
(Ceptaz, Fortaz, Tazicef, Tazidime)

▶CLASSIFICATION
PHARMACOTHERAPEUTIC:
Third-generation cephalosporin. ***CLINICAL:*** Antibiotic (see p. 21C)

ACTION/THERAPEUTIC EFFECT

Binds to bacterial membranes, *inhibiting synthesis of bacterial cell wall. Bactericidal.*

PHARMACOKINETICS

Widely distributed (including CSF). Protein binding: 5–17%. Primarily excreted unchanged in urine. Removed by hemodialysis. Half-life: 2 hrs (half-life increased with impaired renal function).

USES

Treatment of intra-abdominal, biliary tract infections, respiratory, GU tract, skin, bone infections; meningitis, septicemia.

PRECAUTIONS

CONTRAINDICATIONS: History of hypersensitivity to cephalosporins, anaphylactic reactions to penicillins. ***CAUTIONS:*** Renal impairment, history of GI disease (esp. ulcerative colitis, antibiotic-associ-

---

♣ - Canadian trade name   ✳ - see also www.wbsaunders.com/SIMON/SaundersNDH

ated colitis) or allergies, concurrent use of nephrotoxic medications.

▷ *LIFESPAN CONSIDERATIONS:*
Pregnancy/Lactation: Readily crosses placenta. Distributed in breast milk. **Pregnancy Category B. Children:** No age-related precautions noted. **Elderly:** Age-related renal impairment may require dosage adjustment.

INTERACTIONS

DRUG: None significant. **HERBAL:** None known. **FOOD:** None known. **LAB VALUES:** Positive direct/indirect Coombs' test may occur (interferes with hematologic tests, cross-matching procedures). May increase BUN, serum creatinine, SGOT (AST), SGPT (ALT), alkaline phosphatase, LDH concentrations.

AVAILABILITY (Rx)

POWDER FOR INJECTION: 500 mg, 1 g, 2 g.

ADMINISTRATION/HANDLING

Note: Give by IM injection, direct IV injection, intermittent IV infusion (piggyback).

IM:

• For reconstitution, add 1.5 ml Sterile Water for Injection or lidocaine 1% to 500 mg or 3 ml to 1 g vial to provide a concentration of 280 mg/ml. • To minimize discomfort, inject deep IM slowly. Less painful if injected into gluteus maximus rather than lateral aspect of thigh.

IV 💊

Storage:

• Solution appears light yellow to amber, tends to darken (color change does not indicate loss of potency). • IV infusion (piggyback) stable for 18 hrs at room temperature, 7 days if refrigerated. • Discard if precipitate forms.

Reconstitution:

• Add 10 ml Sterile Water for Injection to each 1 g to provide concentration of 90 mg/ml. • May further dilute with 50–100 ml 0.9% NaCl, D_5W, or other compatible diluent.

Rate of administration:

• For IV push, administer over 3–5 min. • For intermittent IV infusion (piggyback), infuse over 15–30 min.

IV INCOMPATIBILITIES ⊘

Amphotericin B complex (Ambisome, Amphotec, Abelcet), doxorubicin liposome (Doxil), fluconazole (Diflucan), idarubicin (Idamycin), midazolam (Versed), pentamidine (Pentam IV), vancomycin (Vancocin).

IV COMPATIBILITIES

Cisatracurium (Nimbex), diltiazem (Cardizem), heparin, midazolam (Versed), propofol (Diprivan).

INDICATIONS/ROUTES/DOSAGE

Note: Space doses evenly around the clock.

Urinary tract infections:

IM/IV: **Adults:** 250–500 mg q8–12h.

Mild to moderate infections:

IM/IV: **Adults:** 1 g q8–12h.

Uncomplicated pneumonia, skin or skin structure infection:

IM/IV: **Adults:** 0.5–1 g q8h.

Bone and joint infection:

IM/IV: **Adults:** 2 g q12h.

Meningitis, serious gynecologic, intra-abdominal infections:

IM/IV: **Adults:** 2 g q8h.

Pseudomonal pulmonary infections in pts with cystic fibrosis:

IV: **Adults:** 30–50 mg/kg q8h. **Maximum:** 6 g/day.

Usual elderly dosage:

IM/IV: Normal renal function q12h.

Usual dosage for children:

IM/IV: **Children (1 mo–12 yrs):** 100–150 mg/kg/day in divided doses q8h. **Maximum:** 6 g/day. **Neonates (0–4 wks):** 100–150 mg/kg/day in divided doses q8–12h.

Dosage in renal impairment:

After initial 1 g dose, dose and/or frequency is modified on basis of creatinine clearance and/or severity of infection.

Creatinine Clearance (ml/min)	Dosage Interval
30–50	q12h
10–30	q24h
<10	q24–48h

SIDE EFFECTS

FREQUENT: Discomfort with IM administration, oral candidiasis (sore mouth/tongue), mild diarrhea, mild abdominal cramping, vaginal candidiasis (itching, discharge). ***OCCASIONAL:*** Nausea, serum sickness reaction [joint pain, fever] (usually occurs following second course of therapy, resolves after drug discontinuation). ***RARE:*** Allergic reaction (rash, pruritus, urticaria), thrombophlebitis (pain, redness, swelling at injection site).

ADVERSE REACTIONS/TOXIC EFFECTS

Antibiotic-associated colitis (severe abdominal pain and tenderness, fever, watery and severe diarrhea), other superinfections may result from altered bacterial balance. Nephrotoxicity may occur, esp. with preexisting renal disease. Severe hypersensitivity reaction (severe pruritus, angioedema, bronchospasm, anaphylaxis), particularly those with history of allergies, esp. penicillin.

NURSING IMPLICATIONS

BASELINE ASSESSMENT:

Question for history of allergies, particularly cephalosporins, penicillins.

INTERVENTION/EVALUATION:

Evaluate IV site for phlebitis (heat, pain, red streaking over vein). Check IM injection sites for induration, tenderness. Check mouth for white patches on mucous membranes, tongue. Monitor bowel activity and stool consistency carefully; mild GI effects may be tolerable, but increasing severity may indicate onset of antibiotic-associated colitis. Monitor I&O, renal function reports for nephrotoxicity. Be alert for superinfection: severe genital/anal pruritus, abdominal pain, severe mouth soreness, moderate to severe diarrhea.

PATIENT/FAMILY TEACHING:

Discomfort may occur with IM injection. Doses should be evenly spaced. Continue antibiotic therapy for full length of treatment.

ceftibuten

sef-tih-**byew**-ten
(Cedax)

►CLASSIFICATION

PHARMACOTHERAPEUTIC: Third-generation cephalosporin. ***CLINICAL:*** Antibiotic (see p. 21C)

ACTION/*THERAPEUTIC EFFECT*

Bactericidal. Binds to bacterial cell membranes, *inhibiting bacterial cell wall synthesis.*

USES

Binds to bacterial membranes, *inhibiting synthesis of bacterial cell wall. Bactericidal.*

PRECAUTIONS

CONTRAINDICATIONS: Hypersensitivity to cephalosporins. ***CAUTIONS:*** Hypersensitivity to penicillins or other drugs; allergies; history of GI disease (e.g., colitis); renal impairment.

INTERACTIONS

DRUG: **Probenecid** increases cephalosporin serum levels. Increased risk of nephrotoxicity with concurrent use of **aminoglycosides.** ***HERBAL:*** None known. ***FOOD:*** None known. ***LAB VALUES:*** Positive direct/indirect Coombs' test. May increase BUN, serum creatinine, SGPT (ALT), SGOT (AST), alkaline phosphatase, bilirubin, LDH concentrations.

AVAILABILITY (Rx)

CAPSULES: 400 mg. ***ORAL SUSPENSION:*** 90 mg/5 ml, 180 mg/5 ml.

INDICATIONS/ROUTES/DOSAGE

Note: Use oral suspension to treat otitis media (achieves higher peak blood level).

Usual PO dosage:

***PO:* Adults, elderly, children ≥12 yrs:** 400 mg/day as single daily dose for 10 days. **Children <12 yrs:** 9 mg/kg/day as single dose for 10 days. **Maximum:** 400 mg/day.

Dosage in renal impairment:

Based on creatinine clearance.

Creatinine Clearance	Dosage
>50 ml/min	400 mg or 9 mg/kg q24h
30–49 ml/min	200 mg or 4.5 mg/kg q24h
<30 ml/min	100 mg or 2.25 mg/kg q24h

SIDE EFFECTS

FREQUENT: Oral candidiasis (sore mouth/tongue), mild diarrhea, mild abdominal cramping, vaginal candidiasis (itching, discharge). ***OCCASIONAL:*** Nausea, serum sickness reaction [joint pain, fever] (usually occurs following second course of therapy, resolves after drug discontinuation). ***RARE:*** Allergic reaction (rash, pruritus, urticaria).

ADVERSE REACTIONS/TOXIC EFFECTS

Antibiotic-associated colitis (severe abdominal pain and tenderness, fever, watery and severe diarrhea), other superinfections may result from altered bacterial balance. Nephrotoxicity may occur, esp. with preexisting renal disease. Severe hypersensitivity reaction (severe pruritus, angioedema, bronchospasm, anaphylaxis), particularly in those with history of allergies, esp. penicillin.

BASELINE ASSESSMENT:

Question for history of allergies, particularly cephalosporins, penicillins.

INTERVENTION/EVALUATION:

Check mouth for white patches on mucous membranes, tongue. Monitor bowel activity and stool consistency carefully; mild GI effects may be tolerable, but increasing severity may indicate onset of antibiotic-associated colitis. Monitor I&O, renal function reports for nephrotoxicity. Be alert for superinfection: severe genital/anal pruritus, abdominal pain, severe mouth soreness, moderate to severe diarrhea.

PATIENT/FAMILY TEACHING:

Continue medication for full length of treatment; do not skip doses. Doses should be evenly spaced. May cause GI upset (may take with food or milk).

ceftizoxime sodium

cef-tih-**zox**-eem
(Cefizox)

▶CLASSIFICATION

PHARMACOTHERAPEUTIC:
Third-generation cephalosporin.
CLINICAL: Antibiotic (see p. 21C)

ACTION/THERAPEUTIC EFFECT

Binds to bacterial membranes, *inhibiting synthesis of bacterial cell wall. Bactericidal.*

PHARMACOKINETICS

Widely distributed (including CSF). Protein binding: 30%. Primarily excreted unchanged in urine. Moderately removed by hemodialysis. Half-life: 1.7 hrs (half-life increased with impaired renal function).

USES

Treatment of intra-abdominal, biliary tract, respiratory, GU tract, skin, bone infections; gonorrhea, meningitis, septicemia, pelvic inflammatory disease (PID).

PRECAUTIONS

CONTRAINDICATIONS: History of hypersensitivity to cephalosporins, anaphylactic reaction to penicillins. ***CAUTIONS:*** History of allergies, GI disease (esp. ulcerative colitis, antibiotic-associated colitis), hepatic and renal impairment.
▷***LIFESPAN CONSIDERATIONS:***
Pregnancy/Lactation: Readily crosses placenta; distributed in breast milk. **Pregnancy Category B. Children:** Associated with transient elevations of eosinophils, SGOT (AST), SGPT (ALT), or creatine kinase. **Elderly:** Age-related renal impairment may require dosage adjustment.

INTERACTIONS

DRUG: Probenecid increases serum concentration of ceftizoxime. ***HERBAL:*** None known. ***FOOD:*** None known. ***LAB VALUES:*** Positive direct/indirect Coombs' test may occur. May increase BUN, serum creatinine, SGOT (AST), SGPT (ALT), alkaline phosphatase concentrations.

AVAILABILITY (Rx)

POWDER FOR INJECTION: 1 g, 2 g.

ADMINISTRATION/HANDLING

Note: Give by IM injection, IV push, intermittent IV infusion (piggyback).

IM:

• Add 1.5 ml Sterile Water for Injection to each 0.5 g to provide concentration of 270 mg/ml. • Inject deep IM slowly to minimize discomfort. • When giving 2 g dose, divide dose and give in different large muscle masses.

IV 📷

Storage:

• Solutions appears clear to pale yellow. Color change from yellow to amber does not indicate loss of potency. • IV infusion (piggyback) is stable for 24 hrs at room temperature, 96 hrs if refrigerated. • Discard if precipitate forms.

Reconstitution:

• Add 5 ml Sterile Water for Injection to each 0.5 g to provide concentration of 95 mg/ml. • May further dilute with 50–100 ml 0.9% NaCl, D$_5$W, or other compatible fluid.

Rate of administration:

• For IV push, administer over 3–5 min. • For intermittent IV infusion (piggyback), infuse over 15–30 min.

IV INCOMPATIBILITY ⃠

Filgrastim (Neupogen).

IV COMPATIBILITY

Propofol (Diprivan).

INDICATIONS/ROUTES/DOSAGE

Uncomplicated UTI:

IM/IV: **Adults, elderly:** 500 mg q12h.

Mild to moderate to severe infection:

IM/IV: **Adults, elderly:** 1–2 g q8–12h.

PID:

IV: **Adults:** 2 g q4–8h.

Life-threatening infections:

IV: **Adults, elderly:** 3–4 g q8h, up to 2 g q4h.

Uncomplicated gonorrhea:

IM: **Adults:** 1 g one time.

Usual dosage for children:

IM/IV: **Children >6 mos:** 50 mg/kg q6–8h. **Maximum:** 12 g/day.

Dosage in renal impairment:

After loading dose of 0.5–1 g, dose and/or frequency is modified on basis of creatinine clearance and/or severity of infection.

Creatinine Clearance	Dosage Interval
50–80 ml/min	q8–12h
10–50 ml/min	q36–48h
<10 ml/min	q48–72h

SIDE EFFECTS

FREQUENT: Discomfort with IM administration, oral candidiasis (sore mouth/tongue), mild diarrhea, mild abdominal cramping, vaginal candidiasis (itching, discharge). **OCCASIONAL:** Nausea, serum sickness reaction [joint pain, fever] (usually occurs following second course of therapy, resolves after drug discontinuation). **RARE:** Allergic reaction (rash, pruritus, urticaria), thrombophlebitis (pain, redness, swelling at injection site).

ADVERSE REACTIONS/TOXIC EFFECTS

Antibiotic-associated colitis (severe abdominal pain and tenderness, fever, watery and severe diarrhea), other superinfections may result from altered bacterial balance. Nephrotoxicity may occur, esp. with preexisting renal disease. Severe hypersensitivity reaction (severe pruritus, angioedema, bronchospasm, anaphylaxis) particularly those with history of allergies, esp. penicillin.

NURSING IMPLICATIONS

BASELINE ASSESSMENT:

Question for history of allergies, particularly cephalosporins, penicillins.

C

INTERVENTION/EVALUATION:

Check mouth for white patches on mucous membranes, tongue. Monitor bowel activity and stool consistency carefully; mild GI effects may be tolerable, but increasing severity may indicate onset of antibiotic-associated colitis. Monitor I&O, renal function reports for nephrotoxicity. Be alert for superinfection: severe genital/anal pruritus, abdominal pain, severe mouth soreness, moderate to severe diarrhea.

PATIENT/FAMILY TEACHING:

Continue therapy for full length of treatment. Doses should be evenly spaced. Discomfort may occur with IM injection.

ceftriaxone sodium

cef-try-**ox**-zone
(Rocephin)

▶CLASSIFICATION

PHARMACOTHERAPEUTIC:
Third-generation cephalosporin.
CLINICAL: Antibiotic (see p. 21C)

ACTION/*THERAPEUTIC EFFECT*

Binds to bacterial membranes, *inhibiting synthesis of bacterial cell wall. Bactericidal.*

PHARMACOKINETICS

Widely distributed (including CSF). Protein binding: 83–96%. Primarily excreted unchanged in urine. Not removed by hemodialysis. Half-life: 4.3–4.6 hrs IV; 5.8–8.7 hrs IM (half-life increased with impaired renal function).

USES

Treatment of respiratory, GU tract, skin, bone, intra-abdominal, biliary tract infections; septicemia, meningitis, gonorrhea, Lyme disease, acute bacterial otitis media.

PRECAUTIONS

CONTRAINDICATIONS: History of hypersensitivity to cephalosporins, anaphylactic reactions to penicillins. *CAUTIONS:* Renal or hepatic impairment, history of GI disease (esp. ulcerative colitis, antibiotic-associated colitis), concurrent administration of nephrotoxic medications.

▷*LIFESPAN CONSIDERATIONS:*
Pregnancy/Lactation: Readily crosses placenta; distributed in breast milk. **Pregnancy Category B. Children:** May displace bilirubin from serum albumin. Caution in hyperbilirubinemic neonates. **Elderly:** Age-related renal impairment may require dosage adjustment.

INTERACTIONS

DRUG: None significant. *HERBAL:* None known. *FOOD:* None known. *LAB VALUES:* Positive direct/indirect Coombs' test may occur (interferes with hematologic tests, cross-matching procedures). May increase BUN, serum creatinine, SGOT (AST), SGPT (ALT), alkaline phosphatase, bilirubin concentrations.

AVAILABILITY (Rx)

POWDER FOR INJECTION: 1 g, 2 g.

ADMINISTRATION/HANDLING

Note: Give by IM injection, intermittent IV infusion (piggyback).

IM:

• Add 0.9 ml Sterile Water for Injection, 0.9% NaCl, D_5W, Bacteriostatic Water and 0.9% Benzyl Alcohol or lidocaine to each 250 mg to provide concentration of 250 mg/ml. • To minimize discomfort, inject deep IM slowly. Less painful if injected into gluteus maximus rather than lateral aspect of thigh.

IV 💊

Storage:

• Solution appears light yellow to amber. • IV infusion (piggyback) is stable for 3 days at room temperature, 10 days if refrigerated. • Discard if precipitate forms.

Reconstitution:

• Add 2.4 ml Sterile Water for Injection to each 250 mg to provide concentration of 100 mg/ml. • May further dilute with 50–100 ml 0.9% NaCl, D_5W, $D_{10}W$, or D_5W and 0.45% NaCl.

Rate of administration:

• For intermittent IV infusion (piggyback), infuse over 15–30 min for adults, 10–30 min in children, neonates. • Alternating IV sites, use large veins to reduce potential for phlebitis.

IV INCOMPATIBILITIES ⊘

Aminophylline, amphotericin B complex (Ambisome, Amphotec, Abelcet), filgrastim (Neupogen), fluconazole (Diflucan), labetalol (Normodyne), pentamidine (Pentam IV), vancomycin (Vancocin).

IV COMPATIBILITIES

Diltiazem (Cardizem), heparin, propofol (Diprivan).

INDICATIONS/ROUTES/DOSAGE

Mild to moderate infections:

IM/IV: **Adults, elderly:** 1–2 g given as single dose or 2 divided doses.

Serious infections:

IM/IV: **Adults, elderly:** Up to 4 g/day in 2 divided doses. **Children:** 50–75 mg/kg/day in divided doses q12h. **Maximum:** 2 g/day.

Skin/skin structure infections:

IM/IV: **Children:** 50–75 mg/kg/day as single or 2 divided doses. **Maximum:** 2 g/day.

Meningitis:

IV: **Children:** Initially, 75 mg/kg, then 100 mg/kg/day as single or in divided doses q12h. **Maximum:** 4 g/day.

Lyme disease:

IV: **Adults, elderly:** 2–4 g daily for 10–14 days.

Acute bacterial otits media:

IM: **Children:** 50 mg/kg daily for 3 days as single dose. **Maximum:** 1 g/day.

Perioperative prophylaxis:

IM/IV: **Adults, elderly:** 1 g 0.5–2 hrs before surgery.

Uncomplicated gonorrhea:

IM: **Adults:** 250 mg one time plus doxycycline.

Dosage in renal impairment:

Dosage modification usually unnecessary, but should be monitored in those with both renal and hepatic impairment or severe renal impairment.

SIDE EFFECTS

FREQUENT: Discomfort with IM administration, oral candidiasis (sore mouth/tongue), mild diarrhea, mild abdominal cramping, vaginal candidiasis (itching, discharge). ***OCCASIONAL:*** Nausea, serum sickness reaction [joint pain, fever] (usually occurs following second course of therapy, resolves after drug discontinuation). **RARE:** Allergic reaction (rash, pruritus, urticaria), thrombophlebitis (pain, redness, swelling at injection site).

ADVERSE REACTIONS/TOXIC EFFECTS

Antibiotic-associated colitis (severe abdominal pain and tenderness, fever, watery and severe diarrhea), other superinfections may result from altered bacterial balance. Nephrotoxicity may occur, esp. with preexisting renal disease. Severe hypersensitivity reaction (severe pruritus, angioedema, bronchospasm, anaphylaxis), particularly those with history of allergies, esp. penicillin.

NURSING IMPLICATIONS

BASELINE ASSESSMENT:

Question for history of allergies, particularly cephalosporins, penicillins.

INTERVENTION/EVALUATION:

Check mouth for white patches on mucous membranes, tongue. Monitor bowel activity and stool consistency carefully; mild GI effects may be tolerable, but increasing severity may indicate onset of antibiotic-associated colitis. Monitor I&O, renal function reports for nephrotoxicity. Be alert for superinfection: severe genital/anal pruritus, abdominal pain, severe mouth soreness, moderate to severe diarrhea.

PATIENT/FAMILY TEACHING:

Discomfort may occur with IM injection. Doses should be evenly spaced. Continue antibiotic therapy for full length of treatment.

cefuroxime axetil

sef-yur-**ox**-ime
(Ceftin)
Do not confuse with
cefotaxime, Cefzil.

cefuroxime sodium

(Kefurox, Zinacef)

▶CLASSIFICATION

PHARMACOTHERAPEUTIC:
Second-generation cephalosporin. ***CLINICAL:*** Antibiotic (see p. 20C)

ACTION/*THERAPEUTIC EFFECT*

Binds to bacterial membranes, *inhibiting synthesis of bacterial cell wall. Bactericidal.*

PHARMACOKINETICS

Rapidly absorbed from GI tract. Protein binding: 33–50%. Widely distributed (including CSF). Primarily excreted unchanged in urine. Moderately removed by hemodialysis. Half-life: 1.3 hrs (half-life increased with impaired renal function).

USES

Treatment of otitis media, respiratory, GU tract, gynecologic, skin, bone infections; septicemia, bacterial meningitis, gonorrhea and other gonococcal infections; ampicillin-resistant influenza, perioperative prophylaxis, impetigo, acute bacterial maxillary sinusitis, early Lyme disease.

PRECAUTIONS

CONTRAINDICATIONS: History of hypersensitivity to cephalosporins, anaphylactic reaction to penicillins.

CAUTIONS: Renal impairment, history of allergies or GI disease (esp. ulcerative colitis, antibiotic-associated colitis), concurrent use of nephrotoxic medications.

▷**LIFESPAN CONSIDERATIONS:**
Pregnancy/Lactation: Readily crosses placenta. Distributed in breast milk. **Pregnancy Category B. Children:** No age-related precautions noted. **Elderly:** Age-related renal impairment may require dosage adjustment.

INTERACTIONS

DRUG: Probenecid increases serum concentration of cefuroxime. **HERBAL:** None known. **FOOD:** None known. **LAB VALUES:** Positive direct/indirect Coombs' test may occur (interferes with hematologic tests, cross-matching procedures). May increase SGOT (AST), SGPT (ALT), alkaline phosphatase, bilirubin, LDH concentrations.

AVAILABILITY (Rx)

TABLETS: 125 mg, 250 mg, 500 mg. **ORAL SUSPENSION:** 125 mg/ 5 ml. **POWDER FOR INJECTION:** 750 mg, 1.5 g.

ADMINISTRATION/HANDLING

Note: Give PO, IM, IV push, intermittent IV infusion (piggyback).

PO:
• Give without regard to meals. If GI upset occurs, give with food or milk. • Tablets may be crushed, mixed with food. • Suspension must be given with food.

IM:
• To minimize discomfort, inject deep IM slowly. Less painful if injected into gluteus maximus rather than lateral aspect of thigh.

IV 💉

Storage:
• Solution appears light yellow to amber; may darken, but color change does not indicate loss of potency • IV infusion (piggyback) is stable for 24 hrs at room temperature, 7 days if refrigerated. • Discard if precipitate forms.

Reconstitution:
• Reconstitute 750 mg in 8 ml (1.5 g in 14 ml) Sterile Water for Injection to provide a concentration of 100 mg/ml. • For intermittent IV infusion (piggyback), further dilute with 50–100 ml 0.9% NaCl or D_5W.

Rate of administration:
• For IV push, administer over 3–5 min. • For intermittent IV infusion (piggyback), infuse over 15–60 min.

IV INCOMPATIBILITIES ⊘

Filgrastim (Neupogen), fluconazole (Diflucan), midazolam (Versed), vancomycin (Vancocin).

IV COMPATIBILITIES

Diltiazem (Cardizem), propofol (Diprivan).

INDICATIONS/ROUTES/DOSAGE

Pharyngitis/tonsillitis:
PO: Adults, elderly: 250 mg 2 times/ day. **Children:** 125 mg 2 times/day or 20 mg/kg/day in 2 divided doses.

Acute otitis media:
PO: Children: 250 mg 2 times/day or 30 mg/kg/day in 2 divided doses.

Acute/chronic bronchitis:
PO: Adults: 250–500 mg 2 times/ day.

Acute bacterial maxillary sinusitis:
PO: Adults, children >13 yrs: 250 mg 2 times/day for 10 days.

Children 3 mos–12 yrs: 30 mg/kg in 2 divided doses.

Impetigo:
PO: **Children:** 30 mg/kg/day in 2 divided doses.

Skin/skin structure infections:
PO: **Adults:** 250–500 mg 2 times/day.

IM/IV: **Adults:** 750 mg–1.5 g q8h.

Early Lyme disease:
PO: **Adults:** 500 mg 2 times/day.

Urinary tract infections:
PO: **Adults:** 125–250 mg 2 times/day.

IM/IV: **Adults:** 750 mg–1.5 g q8h.

Pneumonia:
IM/IV: **Adults:** 750 mg–1.5 g q8h.

Uncomplicated gonorrhea:
PO: **Adults:** 1 g as single dose.
IM: **Adults:** 1.5 g as single dose.

Disseminated gonococcal infection:
IM/IV: **Adults:** 750 mg to 1.5 g q8h.

Bone/joint infections:
IM/IV: **Adults, elderly:** 1.5 g q8h.

Life-threatening infections:
IV: **Adults, elderly:** 1.5 g q8h.
Children: 150 mg/kg/day in 3 divided doses.

Bacterial meningitis:
IV: **Adults:** Up to 3 g q8h. **Children:** Initially, 200–240 mg/kg/day in 3–4 divided doses; then, 100 mg/kg/day with clinical improvement.

Perioperative prophylaxis:
IV: **Adults, elderly:** 1.5 g 30–60 min before surgery and 750 mg q8h postop.

IM/IV: **Neonates:** 20–100 mg/kg/day in divided doses q12h.

Dosage in renal impairment:
Adult dosage is modified on basis of creatinine clearance and/or severity of infection.

Creatinine Clearance	Dosage Interval
10–20 ml/min	q12h
<10 ml/min	q24h

SIDE EFFECTS

FREQUENT: Discomfort with IM administration, oral candidiasis (sore mouth/tongue), mild diarrhea, mild abdominal cramping, vaginal candidiasis (itching, discharge). ***OCCASIONAL:*** Nausea, serum sickness reaction [joint pain, fever] (usually occurs following second course of therapy, resolves after drug discontinuation). ***RARE:*** Allergic reaction (rash, pruritus, urticaria), thrombophlebitis (pain, redness, swelling at injection site).

ADVERSE REACTIONS/TOXIC EFFECTS

Antibiotic-associated colitis (severe abdominal pain and tenderness, fever, watery and severe diarrhea), other superinfections may result from altered bacterial balance. Nephrotoxicity may occur, esp. with preexisting renal disease. Severe hypersensitivity reaction (severe pruritus, angioedema, bronchospasm, anaphylaxis), particularly those with history of allergies, esp. penicillin.

NURSING IMPLICATIONS

BASELINE ASSESSMENT:
Question for history of allergies, particularly cephalosporins, penicillins.

INTERVENTION/EVALUATION:
Check mouth for white patches on mucous membranes, tongue. Monitor bowel activity and stool consistency carefully; mild GI effects may be tolerable, but increasing severity may indicate onset of antibiotic-associated colitis. Monitor I&O, renal function reports for nephrotoxicity. Be alert for superinfection: severe genital/anal pruritus, abdominal pain, severe mouth soreness, moderate to severe diarrhea.

PATIENT/FAMILY TEACHING:
Discomfort may occur with IM injection. Doses should be evenly spaced. Continue antibiotic therapy for full length of treatment. May cause GI upset (may take with food or milk).

celecoxib

sell-eh-**cox**-ib
(Celebrex)
Do not confuse with Cerebyx.

▶**CLASSIFICATION**

PHARMACOTHERAPEUTIC:
Nonsteroidal anti-inflammatory.
CLINICAL: Anti-inflammatory (see p. 106C)

ACTION/THERAPEUTIC EFFECT
Inhibits cyclo-oxygenase-2, the enzyme responsible for producing prostaglandins that cause pain and inflammation, producing anti-inflammatory effects.

PHARMACOKINETICS
Widely distributed. Protein binding: 97%. Metabolized in the liver. Primarily eliminated in feces. Half-life: 11.2 hrs.

USES
Relief of signs and symptoms of osteoarthritis, rheumatoid arthritis in adults. Treatment of acute pain, menstrual pain. Used to reduce number of adenomatous colorectal polyps in familial adenomatous polyposis (FAP).

PRECAUTIONS
CONTRAINDICATIONS: Hypersensitivity to sulfonamides, NSAIDs, aspirin. **CAUTIONS:** Past history of peptic ulcer, >60 yrs, those receiving anticoagulant therapy, steroids, alcohol consumption, smoking.
▷**LIFESPAN CONSIDERATIONS:**
Pregnancy/Lactation: Unknown if drug crosses placenta or is distributed in breast milk. Avoid use during third trimester (may adversely affect fetal cardiovascular system: premature closure of ductus arteriosus). **Pregnancy Category C. Children:** Safety and efficacy not established in those <18 yrs of age. **Elderly:** No age-related precautions noted.

INTERACTIONS
DRUG: May increase risk of bleeding with **warfarin.** Significant interactions may occur with **lithium, fluconazole. HERBAL:** None known. **FOOD:** None known. **LAB VALUES:** May increase liver function test results.

AVAILABILITY (Rx)
CAPSULES: 100 mg, 200 mg.

ADMINISTRATION/HANDLING
PO:
• May give without regard to food.
• Do not crush or break capsules.

INDICATIONS/ROUTES/DOSAGE
Osteoarthritis:
PO: Adults, elderly: 200 mg/day as single dose or 100 mg twice daily.

Rheumatoid arthritis:

PO: Adults, elderly: 100–200 mg twice daily.

Familial edenomatous polyposis (FAP):

PO: Adults, elderly: 400 mg twice daily (give with food).

SIDE EFFECTS

FREQUENT (>5%): Diarrhea, dyspepsia, headache, upper respiratory tract infection. ***OCCASIONAL*** (1–5%): Abdominal pain, flatulence, nausea, back pain, peripheral edema, dizziness, rash.

ADVERSE REACTIONS/TOXIC EFFECTS

None significant.

NURSING IMPLICATIONS

BASELINE ASSESSMENT:

Assess onset, type, location, duration of pain/inflammation. Inspect appearance of affected joints for immobility, deformity, skin condition.

INTERVENTION/EVALUATION:

Evaluate for therapeutic response: pain relief, decreased stiffness, swelling, increased joint mobility, decreased tenderness, improved grip strength.

PATIENT/FAMILY TEACHING:

If GI upset occurs, take with food. Avoid aspirin, alcohol (increases risk of GI bleeding).

cephalexin

cef-ah-**lex**-in
(Apo-Cephalex✿, Novolexin✿, Keflet, Keflex)

cephalexin hydrochloride

(Keftab)

▶CLASSIFICATION

PHARMACOTHERAPEUTIC: First-generation cephalosporin. ***CLINICAL:*** Antibiotic (see p. 19C)

ACTION/*THERAPEUTIC EFFECT*

Binds to bacterial membranes, *inhibiting synthesis of bacterial cell wall. Bactericidal.*

PHARMACOKINETICS

Rapidly absorbed from GI tract. Widely distributed. Protein binding: 10–15%. Primarily excreted unchanged in urine. Moderately removed by hemodialysis. Half-life: 0.9–1.2 hrs (half-life increased with impaired renal function).

USES

Treatment of respiratory tract, GU tract, skin, soft tissue, bone infections; otitis media, rheumatic fever prophylaxis; follow-up to parenteral therapy.

PRECAUTIONS

CONTRAINDICATIONS: History of hypersensitivity to cephalosporins, anaphylactic reaction to penicillins. ***CAUTIONS:*** Renal impairment, history of allergies or GI disease (esp. ulcerative colitis, antibiotic-associated colitis), concurrent use of nephrotoxic medications.

▷*LIFESPAN CONSIDERATIONS:* **Pregnancy/Lactation:** Readily crosses placenta; distributed in breast milk. **Pregnancy Category B. Children:** No age-related precautions noted. **Elderly:** Age-related renal impairment may require dosage adjustment.

INTERACTIONS

DRUG: **Probenecid** increases serum concentration of cephalexin. *HERBAL:* None known. *FOOD:* None known. *LAB VALUES:* Positive direct/indirect Coombs' test may occur (interferes with hematologic test, cross-matching procedures). May increase SGOT (AST), SGPT (ALT), alkaline phosphatase concentrations.

AVAILABILITY (Rx)

CAPSULES: 250 mg, 500 mg. *TABLETS:* 250 mg, 500 mg, 1 g. *ORAL SUSPENSION:* 125 mg/5 ml, 250 mg/5 ml.

ADMINISTRATION/HANDLING

PO:

• After reconstitution, oral suspension is stable for 14 days if refrigerated. • Shake oral suspension well before using. • Give without regard to meals. If GI upset occurs, give with food or milk.

INDICATIONS/ROUTES/DOSAGE

Note: Space doses evenly around the clock.

Usual dosage for adults:

PO: **Adults, elderly:** 250–500 mg q6h up to 4 g/day.

Streptococcal pharyngitis, skin/skin structure infections, uncomplicated cystitis:

PO: **Adults, elderly:** 500 mg q12h.

Usual dosage for children:

PO: **Children:** 25–100 mg/kg/day in 2–4 divided doses.

Otitis media:

PO: **Children:** 75–100 mg/kg/day in 4 divided doses.

Dosage in renal impairment:

After usual initial dose, dose and/or frequency is modified on basis of creatinine clearance and/or severity of infection.

Creatinine Clearance	Dosage Interval
10–40 ml/min	q8–12h
<10 ml/min	q12–24h

SIDE EFFECTS

FREQUENT: Oral candidiasis (sore mouth/tongue), mild diarrhea, mild abdominal cramping, vaginal candidiasis (itching, discharge). *OCCASIONAL:* Nausea, serum sickness reaction [joint pain, fever] (usually occurs following second course of therapy, resolves after drug discontinuation). *RARE:* Allergic reaction (rash, pruritus, urticaria).

ADVERSE REACTIONS/TOXIC EFFECTS

Antibiotic-associated colitis (severe abdominal pain and tenderness, fever, watery and severe diarrhea), other superinfections may result from altered bacterial balance. Nephrotoxicity may occur, esp. with preexisting renal disease. Severe hypersensitivity reaction (severe pruritus, angioedema, bronchospasm, anaphylaxis), particularly in those with history of allergies, esp. penicillin.

NURSING IMPLICATIONS

BASELINE ASSESSMENT:

Question history of allergies, particularly cephalosporins, penicillins.

INTERVENTION/EVALUATION:

Check mouth for white patches on mucous membranes, tongue. Monitor bowel activity and stool consistency carefully; mild GI effects may be tolerable, but increasing severity may indicate onset of antibiotic-associated colitis. Monitor I&O, renal function reports for nephrotoxicity. Be alert for superinfection: severe genital/anal pruritus, abdominal pain, severe mouth soreness, moderate to severe diarrhea.

PATIENT/FAMILY TEACHING:

Continue therapy for full length of treatment. Doses should be evenly spaced. May cause GI upset (may take with food or milk).

cephalothin

(Keflin)

See Classification section under: Antibiotic: cephalosporins

cetirizine

sih-**tier**-eh-zeen
(Reactine ♣, Zyrtec)
Do not confuse with Zyprexa.

FIXED-COMBINATION(S)

With pseudoephedrine, a decongestant **(Zyrtec-D)**

▶**CLASSIFICATION**

PHARMACOTHERAPEUTIC:
Second-generation piperazine.
CLINICAL: Antihistamine (see p. 48C)

ACTION/*THERAPEUTIC EFFECT*

Competes with histamine at histaminic receptor sites on effector cells, *preventing allergic response* *(urticaria, pruritus). Also produces mild bronchodilation, blocks histamine-induced bronchoconstriction in asthmatic patients.* Minimal anticholinergic effects.

PHARMACOKINETICS

	Onset	Peak	Duration
PO	<1 hr	4–8 hr	<24 hrs

Rapidly, almost completely absorbed from GI tract. Protein binding: 93%. Food has no effect on absorption. Undergoes low first-pass metabolism; not extensively metabolized. Primarily excreted in urine (>80% as unchanged drug). Half-life: 6.5–10 hrs.

USES/*UNLABELED*

Relief of symptoms (sneezing, rhinorrhea, postnasal discharge, nasal pruritus, ocular pruritus, tearing) of seasonal and perennial allergic rhinitis (hay fever). Treatment of chronic urticaria (hives). *Treatment of bronchial asthma.*

PRECAUTIONS

CONTRAINDICATIONS: None significant. ***CAUTIONS:*** Impaired hepatic impairment, symptomatic prostatic hypertrophy, urinary retention, angle-closure glaucoma.

▷***LIFESPAN CONSIDERATIONS:***
Pregnancy/Lactation: Not recommended during early months of pregnancy. Unknown if excreted in breast milk (breast feeding not recommended). **Pregnancy Category B. Children:** Less likely to cause anticholinergic effects. **Elderly:** More sensitive to anticholinergic effects (e.g., dry mouth, urinary retention). Dizziness, sedation, confusion more likely to occur.

INTERACTIONS

DRUG: **Alcohol, CNS depres-**

sants may increase CNS depression. **HERBAL:** None known. **FOOD:** None known. **LAB VALUES:** May suppress wheal and flare reactions to antigen skin testing, unless antihistamines are discontinued 4 days before testing.

AVAILABILITY (Rx)

TABLETS: 5 mg, 10 mg. **SYRUP:** 5 mg/5 ml.

ADMINISTRATION/HANDLING
PO:

• Give without regard to meals.

INDICATIONS/ROUTES/DOSAGE

Allergic rhinitis, hives:

PO: Adults, elderly, 5–10 mg/day. May increase up to 20 mg/day.
Children 2–5 yrs: Initially, 2.5 mg once daily. **Maximum:** 5 mg once daily or 2.5 mg q12h. **Children 6–11 yrs:** 5–10 mg once daily.

Renal impairment (creatinine clearance 11–31 ml/min), hemodialysis (creatinine clearance <7 ml/min), hepatic impairment:

PO: Adults, elderly: 5 mg once daily.

SIDE EFFECTS

Minimal anticholinergic effects. **OCCASIONAL** (2–10%): Pharyngitis, dry mouth, nose, throat, nausea, vomiting, abdominal pain, headache, dizziness, fatigue, thickening mucus, drowsiness, increased sensitivity of skin to sun.

ADVERSE REACTIONS/TOXIC EFFECTS

Children may experience dominant paradoxical reaction (restlessness, insomnia, euphoria, nervousness, tremors). Dizziness, sedation, confusion more likely to occur in elderly pts.

NURSING IMPLICATIONS

BASELINE ASSESSMENT:

Assess lung sound, rhinitis, urticaria, or other symptoms, liver function tests.

INTERVENTION/EVALUATION:

For upper respiratory allergies, increase fluids to maintain thin secretions and offset thirst, loss of fluids from increased sweating. Monitor symptoms for therapeutic response.

PATIENT/FAMILY TEACHING:

Generally does not cause drowsiness; however, if blurred vision or eye pain occurs, do not drive or perform activities requiring visual acuity. Avoid alcohol during antihistamine therapy. Avoid prolonged exposure to sunlight.

cetrorelix

(Cetrotide)

See Classification section under: Fertility agents (p. 85C)

cevimeline

sev-ee-**me**-line
(Evoxac)

▶CLASSIFICATION

PHARMACOTHERAPEUTIC: Cholinergic agonist. **CLINICAL:** Mouth, throat agent

ACTION/THERAPEUTIC EFFECT

Binds to muscarinic receptors *increasing secretion of exocrine* glands (e.g., salivary glands), relieving dry mouth symptoms.

USES

Treatment of dry mouth symptoms in those with Sjögren's syndrome.

PRECAUTIONS

CONTRAINDICATIONS: Uncontrolled asthma, acute iritis, narrow angle glaucoma. ***CAUTIONS:*** Cholelithiasis, history of nephrolithiasis, cardiovascular disease, chronic bronchitis, COPD.

INTERACTIONS

DRUG: May interfere with effects of **antimuscarinic.** May increase effects of **parasympathomimetics.** May increase risk of conduction disturbances in those taking **beta-blockers.** ***HERBAL:*** None known. ***FOOD:*** Food decreases absorption rate. ***LAB VALUES:*** None significant.

AVAILABILITY (Rx)
CAPSULES: 30 mg.

INDICATIONS/ROUTES/DOSAGE
Dry mouth:
PO: Adults: 30 mg three times/day.

SIDE EFFECTS

FREQUENT (11–19%): Excessive sweating, headache, nausea, sinusitis rhinitis, upper respiratory tract infections, diarrhea. ***OCCASIONAL*** (3–10%): Dyspepsia, abdominal pain, coughing, urinary tract infection, vomiting, back pain, rash, dizziness, fatigue. ***RARE*** (1–2%): Skeletal pain, insomnia, hot flashes, excessive salivation, rigors, anxiety.

ADVERSE REACTIONS/TOXIC EFFECTS

May produce decreased visual acuity, esp. at night, and impairment of depth perceptions.

NURSING IMPLICATIONS

PATIENT/FAMILY TEACHING:
Advise caution while driving at night or performing hazardous duties in reduced lighting. Drink extra fluid to prevent possibility of dehydration.

---

chamomile

Also known as German chamomile, pinheads
(Blossom 120/jar, 45/jar, 30/jar)

▶**CLASSIFICATION**
HERBAL

ACTION/EFFECT

Anti-allergic, anti-inflammatory action due to inhibiting release of histamine. Possesses anti-allergic, antiflatulant, antispasmodic, mild sedative, anti-inflammatory action.

USES

Treatment of symptoms of flatulence, travel sickness, diarrhea, insomnia, gastrointestinal spasms. Topically used for hemorrhoids.

PRECAUTIONS

CONTRAINDICATIONS: Pregnancy, a teratogen, affects menstrual cycle, has uterine stimulant effects. ***CAUTIONS:*** Pts with asthma (may exacerbate condition) and those allergic to ragweed, aster, daisies, or chrysanthemums.

▷***LIFESPAN CONSIDERATIONS:***
Pregnancy/Lactation: Contraindicated. **Children:** Safety and

---

efficacy not established. **Elderly:** No age-related precautions noted.

INTERACTIONS

DRUG: May increase anticoagulation, risk of bleeding with **aspirin, clopidogrel, dalteparin, enoxaparin, heparin, warfarin.** May have additive effects with **benzodiazepines. HERBAL:** Sedative effects may increase with **ginseng, kava, St. John's wort, valerian.** May increase risk of bleeding with **feverfew, garlic, ginger, ginkgo, licorice. FOOD:** None significant. **LAB VALUES:** None significant.

AVAILABILITY

WHOLE FLOWERS: 120/jar; 45/jar; 30/jar (chamomile whole flowers) 120 g, 45 g, 30 g.

INDICATIONS/ROUTES/DOSAGE

Flatulence, travel sickness, diarrhea, insomnia, GI spasms:
PO: Adults, elderly: 2–8 g of dried flower heads 3 times/day or 1 cup of tea 3–4 times/day.

SIDE EFFECTS

Allergic reaction (e.g., contact dermatitis, severe hypersensitivity reaction, anaphylactic reaction), eye irritation.

ADVERSE REACTIONS/TOXIC EFFECTS

Anaphylactic reaction (bronchospasm, severe pruritus, angioedema).

NURSING IMPLICATIONS

BASELINE ASSESSMENT

Assess if pt is pregnant/breast-feeding/asthmatic. Assess if pt is taking other medications, esp. those that increase risk of bleeding or have sedative properties. Allergies to ragweed, aster, daisies, or chrysanthemums.

INTERVENTION/EVALUATION

Monitor for side effects (e.g., diarrhea, insomnia) to determine effectiveness. Monitor for signs of allergic reaction.

PATIENT/FAMILY TEACHING

Inform physician if pregnancy occurs or if planning to become pregnant, breast-feed. May cause sedation; do not drive or operate machinery until effect of herbal is known. Avoid use with other sedatives, alcohol.

---

charcoal, activated

(Actidose, Aqueous Charcodote✿, Charcocaps)

▶CLASSIFICATION
CLINICAL: Antidote

ACTION

Adsorbs (detoxifies) ingested toxic substances, irritants, intestinal gas.

USES

Emergency antidote in treatment of poisoning.

PRECAUTIONS

CONTRAINDICATIONS: None significant. **CAUTIONS:** None significant.

INTERACTIONS

DRUG: May decrease absorption, effects of orally administered medications. **HERBAL:** None known.

C

FOOD: None known. ***LAB VALUES:*** None significant.

AVAILABILITY (Rx)

TABLETS: 260 mg, 325 mg, 650 mg. ***CAPSULES:*** 250 mg, 260 mg. ***SUSPENSION:*** 12.5 g, 15 g, 25 g, 30 g, 50g.

INDICATIONS/ROUTES/DOSAGE

Antidote:

***PO:* Adults, elderly:** Can give 30–100 g as slurry (30 g in at least 8 oz H_2O) or 12.5–50 g in aqueous or sorbitol suspension. Usually given as single dose.

SIDE EFFECTS

OCCASIONAL: Diarrhea, GI discomfort, intestinal gas.

ADVERSE REACTIONS/TOXIC EFFECTS

None significant.

NURSING IMPLICATIONS

INTERVENTION/EVALUATION: Monitor vital signs, level of consciousness, and other clinical signs related to specific drug ingested.

---

chloral hydrate

klor-al **high**-drate
(Aquachloral Supprettes, Noctec, PMS-Chloral Hydrate ♣)

▶**CLASSIFICATION**

PHARMACOTHERAPEUTIC: Nonbarbiturate chloral derivative. ***CLINICAL:*** Sedative, hypnotic

ACTION/THERAPEUTIC EFFECT

Produces CNS depression. *Induces quiet, deep sleep, with only slight decrease in respiration, B/P.*

USES

Treatment of insomnia, adjunct to anesthesia preoperatively to produce sedation/relieve anxiety.

PRECAUTIONS

CONTRAINDICATIONS: Marked hepatic, renal impairment, severe cardiac disease, presence of gastritis. ***PO:*** Esophagitis, gastritis, gastric/duodenal ulcer. ***CAUTIONS:*** History of drug abuse, mental depression.

INTERACTIONS

DRUG: Alcohol, CNS depressants may increase effects. May increase effect of warfarin. IV furosemide given within 24 hrs following chloral hydrate may alter B/P, cause diaphoresis. ***HERBAL:*** None known. ***FOOD:*** None known. ***LAB VALUES:*** None significant.

AVAILABILITY (Rx)

CAPSULES: 250 mg, 500 mg. ***SYRUP:*** 250 mg/5 ml, 500 mg/5 ml. ***SUPPOSITORY:*** 324 mg, 500 mg, 648 mg.

INDICATIONS/ROUTES/DOSAGE

Premedication for dental/medical procedures:

***PO/RECTAL:* Adults:** 0.5–1 g. **Children:** 75 mg/kg up to 1 g total.

Premedication for EEG:

***PO/RECTAL:* Adults:** 0.5–1.5 g. **Children:** 25–50 mg/kg/dose.

SIDE EFFECTS

OCCASIONAL: Gastric irritation (nausea, vomiting, flatulence, diarrhea), rash, sleepwalking. ***RARE:*** Headache, paradoxical CNS hy-

---

peractivity/nervousness in children, excitement/restlessness in elderly (particularly noted when given in presence of pain).

ADVERSE REACTIONS/TOXIC EFFECTS

Overdosage may produce somnolence, confusion, slurred speech, severe incoordination, respiratory depression, coma. Tolerance and psychological dependence may occur by second week of therapy. Abrupt withdrawal of drug after long-term use may produce weakness, facial flushing, sweating, vomiting, tremor.

NURSING IMPLICATIONS

BASELINE ASSESSMENT:

Assess B/P, pulse, respirations immediately before administration. Raise bed rails. Provide environment conducive to sleep (back rub, quiet environment, low lighting).

INTERVENTION/EVALUATION:

Assess sleep pattern of pt. Assess elderly/children for paradoxical reaction. Evaluate for therapeutic response to insomnia: a decrease in number of nocturnal awakenings, increase in length of sleep.

PATIENT/FAMILY TEACHING:

Do not abruptly withdraw medication after long-term use. Tolerance, dependence may occur with prolonged use.

chlorambucil

klor-**am**-bew-sill
(Leukeran)
Do not confuse with Myleran, Alkeran.

▶CLASSIFICATION

PHARMACOTHERAPEUTIC:
Alkylating agent, nitrogen mustard. ***CLINICAL:*** Antineoplastic (see p. 68C)

ACTION/*THERAPEUTIC EFFECT*

Inhibits DNA, RNA synthesis by cross-linking with DNA and RNA strands, *interfering with nucleic acid function.* Cell cycle-phase nonspecific.

PHARMACOKINETICS

Rapidly, completely absorbed from GI tract. Protein binding: 99%. Rapidly metabolized in liver to active metabolite. Not removed by hemodialysis. Half-life: 1.5 hrs; metabolite: 2.5 hrs.

USES/*UNLABELED*

Palliative treatment of chronic lymphocytic leukemia, advanced malignant (non-Hodgkin's) lymphomas, lymphosarcoma, giant follicular lymphomas, advanced Hodgkin's disease. *Treatment of ovarian, testicular carcinoma, hairy cell leukemia, polycythemia vera, nephrotic syndrome.*

PRECAUTIONS

CONTRAINDICATIONS: Previous allergic reaction, disease resistance to previous therapy with drug. ***EXTREME CAUTION:*** Within 4 wks after full-course radiation therapy or myelosuppressive drug regimen.

▷***LIFESPAN CONSIDERATIONS:***
Pregnancy/Lactation: If possible, avoid use during pregnancy, esp. first trimester. Breast feeding not recommended. **Pregnancy Category D. Children:** No age-related precautions. When taken for nephritic syndrome, may in-

crease seizures. **Elderly:** No age-related precaution noted.

INTERACTIONS

DRUG: May decrease effect of **antigout medications. Bone marrow depressants** may increase bone marrow depression. Other **immunosuppressants (e.g., steroids)** may increase risk of infection or development of neoplasms. **Live virus vaccines** may potentiate virus replication, increase vaccine side effects, decrease antibody response to vaccine. ***HERBAL:*** None known. ***FOOD:*** None known. ***LAB VALUES:*** May increase SGOT (AST), alkaline phosphatase, uric acid.

AVAILABILITY (Rx)

TABLETS: 2 mg.

ADMINISTRATION/HANDLING

PO:
• Give without regard to food.

INDICATIONS/ROUTES/DOSAGE

Note: May be carcinogenic, mutagenic, or teratogenic. Handle with extreme care during administration. Dosage individualized on basis of clinical response, tolerance to adverse effects. When used in combination therapy, consult specific protocols for optimum dosage, sequence of drug administration.

Usual dosage (initial or short-course therapy):

PO: Adults, elderly, children: 0.1–0.2 mg/kg/day as single or divided dose for 3–6 wks. **Average dose:** 4–10 mg/day. **Single daily dose q2wks:** 0.4 mg/kg initially. Increase by 0.1 mg/kg q2wks until response and/or myelosuppression.

Usual dosage (maintenance):

PO: Adults, elderly, children: 0.03–0.1 mg/kg/day. **Average dose:** 2–4 mg/day.

SIDE EFFECTS

GI effects (nausea, vomiting, anorexia, diarrhea, abdominal distress) are generally mild, last less that 24 hrs, and occur only if single dose exceeds 20 mg. ***OCCASIONAL:*** Rash or dermatitis, pruritus, cold sores. ***RARE:*** Alopecia, urticaria (hives), erythema, hyperuricemia.

ADVERSE REACTIONS/TOXIC EFFECTS

Bone marrow depression manifested as hematologic toxicity (neutropenia, leukopenia, progressive lymphopenia, anemia, thrombocytopenia). After discontinuation of therapy, thrombocytopenia, leukopenia usually occur at 1–3 wks and lasts 1–4 wks. Neutrophil count decreases up to 10 days after last dose. Toxicity appears to be less severe with intermittent rather than continuous drug administration. Overdosage may produce seizures in children. Excessive uric acid level, hepatotoxicity occurs rarely.

NURSING IMPLICATIONS

BASELINE ASSESSMENT:

CBC should be performed each week during therapy, WBC count performed 3–4 days after each weekly CBC during first 3–6 wks of therapy (4–6 wks if pt on intermittent dosing schedule).

INTERVENTION/EVALUATION:

Monitor for hematologic toxicity (fever, sore throat, signs of local infection, easy bruising, or unusual bleeding from any site), symptoms of anemia (excessive tiredness, weakness). Assess skin for rash, pruritus, urticaria.

PATIENT/FAMILY TEACHING:

Increase fluid intake (may protect against hyperuricemia). Do not have immunizations without doctor's approval (drug lowers body's resistance). Avoid contact with those who have recently received live virus vaccine. Promptly report fever, sore throat, signs of local infection, easy bruising, or unusual bleeding from any site.

chloramphenicol

klor-am-**fen**-ih-call
(Chloromycetin, Chloroptic)

FIXED-COMBINATION(S)

With polymyxin B, an antibiotic, and hydrocortisone, acetate **(Ophthocort)**

▶CLASSIFICATION

PHARMACOTHERAPEUTIC: Dichloroacetic acid derivative. **CLINICAL:** Antibiotic

ACTION/THERAPEUTIC EFFECT

Bacteriostatic (may be bactericidal in high concentrations). Binds to ribosomal receptor sites, *inhibiting protein synthesis.*

USES

Intra-abdominal, soft tissue, or orificial infections, typhoid fever, osteomyelitis, septic arthritis, cellulitis, septicemia, meningitis; adjunctive therapy for cerebral abscesses or other CNS infections, rickettsial infections when tetracyclines are contraindicated.

Treatment of superficial ocular infections, superficial infections of external auditory canal.

PRECAUTIONS

CONTRAINDICATIONS: Prolonged treatment or frequent application should be avoided with topical application. **CAUTIONS:** Bone marrow depression, previous cytotoxic drug therapy, radiation therapy, hepatic or renal impairment, infants/children <2 yrs.

INTERACTIONS

DRUG: Anticonvulsants, bone marrow depressants may increase bone marrow depression. May increase effect of **oral hypoglycemics.** May antagonize effects of **clindamycin, erythromycin.** May increase concentration of **phenobarbital, phenytoin, warfarin. HERBAL:** None known. **FOOD:** None known. **LAB VALUES:** None significant. Therapeutic blood serum level: 10–20 mcg/ml; toxic serum level: >25 mcg/ml.

AVAILABILITY (Rx)

CAPSULES: 250 mg. **ORAL SUSPENSION:** 150 mg/5 ml. **POWDER FOR INJECTION:** 100 mg/ml. **OPHTHALMIC SOLUTION:** 5 mg/ml. **OPHTHALMIC OINTMENT:** 10 mg/g. **OTIC SOLUTION:** 0.5%.

INDICATIONS/ROUTES/DOSAGE

Mild to moderate infections:

PO/IV: Adults, elderly, children: 50 mg/kg/day in divided doses q6h.

Severe infections, infections due to moderately resistant organisms:

PO/IV: Adults, elderly, children: 50–100 mg/kg/day in divided doses q6h.

Dosage in renal or hepatic impairment:

Dosage is reduced on basis of degree of renal impairment, plasma concentration of drug. Initially, 1 g, then 500 mg q6h.

Usual dosage for neonates:

PO/IV: Newborn infants: 25 mg/kg/day in 4 doses q6h. **Infants >2 wks:** 50 mg/kg/day in 4 doses q6h. **Neonates <2 kg:** 25 mg/kg once daily. **Neonates <7days, >2 kg:** 25 mg/kg once daily. **Neonates >7 days, >2 kg:** 50 mg/kg/day in divided doses q12h.

Usual ophthalmic dosage:

OINTMENT: Adults, elderly, children: Apply thin strip to conjunctiva q3–4h.

DROPS: Adults, elderly, children: 1–2 drops 4–6 times/day.

Usual otic dosage:

OTIC: Adults, elderly, children: 2–3 drops into ear 3 times/day.

SIDE EFFECTS

OCCASIONAL: Systemic: Nausea, vomiting, diarrhea. **Ophthalmic:** Blurred vision, burning, stinging, hypersensitivity reaction. **Otic:** Hypersensitivity reaction. **RARE:** "Gray baby" syndrome [neonates]: (abdominal distention, blue gray skin color, cardiovascular collapse, unresponsiveness), rash, shortness of breath, confusion, headache, optic neuritis (eye pain, blurred vision), peripheral neuritis (numbness/weakness in hands/feet).

ADVERSE REACTIONS/TOXIC EFFECTS

Superinfection due to bacterial or fungal overgrowth. Narrow margin between effective therapy and toxic levels producing blood dyscrasias: Bone marrow depression with resulting aplastic anemia, hypoplastic anemia, pancytopenia (may occur weeks or months later).

NURSING IMPLICATIONS

BASELINE ASSESSMENT:
Avoid, if possible, other drugs that cause bone marrow depression. Establish baseline blood studies before therapy.

INTERVENTION/EVALUATION:
Assess for appetite, vomiting. Evaluate mental status. Check for visual disturbances. Assess skin for rash. Determine pattern of bowel activity and stool consistency. Watch for superinfection: diarrhea, anal/genital pruritus, change in oral mucosa, increased fever. Therapeutic blood serum level: 10–20 mcg/ml; toxic serum level: >25 mcg/ml.

PATIENT/FAMILY TEACHING:
Continue therapy for full length of treatment; ophthalmic treatment should continue at least 48 hrs after eye returns to normal appearance. Doses should be evenly spaced. Take oral doses on empty stomach, 1 hr before or 2 hrs after meals (may take with food if GI upset occurs, but not with iron or vitamins).

chlordiazepoxide ✳

klor-dye-az-eh-**pox**-eyd
(Libritabs)

chlordiazepoxide hydrochloride

(Apo-Chlordiazepoxide✦, Librium, Lipoxide, Novopoxide✦)

FIXED-COMBINATION(S)
With clidinium bromide, an anticholinergic **(Librax)**; with estrogen

(Menrium); with amitriptyline hydrochloride, an antidepressant **(Limbitrol)**.

▶CLASSIFICATION

PHARMACOTHERAPEUTIC: Benzodiazepine. *CLINICAL:* Antianxiety (see p. 10C)

ACTION/*THERAPEUTIC EFFECT*

Enhances action of gamma aminobutyric acid (GABA) neurotransmission at CNS, *producing anxiolytic effect.*

USES/*UNLABELED*

Management of anxiety disorders, acute alcohol withdrawal symptoms; short-term relief of symptoms of anxiety, preop anxiety, tension. *Treatment of panic disorder, tension headache, tremors.*

PRECAUTIONS

CONTRAINDICATIONS: Acute narrow-angle glaucoma, acute alcohol intoxication. *CAUTIONS:* Impaired kidney/liver function.

INTERACTIONS

DRUG: **Alcohol, CNS depressants** may increase CNS depressant effect. *HERBAL:* **Kava kava, valerian** may increase CNS depression. *FOOD:* None known. *LAB VALUES:* None significant. Therapeutic blood serum level: 1–3 mcg/ml; toxic serum level: >5 mcg/ml.

AVAILABILITY (Rx)

CAPSULES: 5 mg, 10 mg, 25 mg. *TABLETS:* 5 mg, 10 mg, 25 mg. *INJECTION:* 100 mg ampule.

INDICATIONS/ROUTES/DOSAGE

Note: Use smallest effective dose in elderly or debilitated, those with liver disease, low serum albumin.

PARENTERAL FORM: Do not exceed 300 mg/24 hrs.

Mild to moderate anxiety:

PO: **Adults:** 5–10 mg 3–4 times/day. **Elderly/debilitated:** 5 mg 2–4 times/day. Do not exceed 10 mg/day initially. **Children >6 yrs:** 5 mg 2–4 times/day. Do not exceed 10 mg/day initially.

Severe anxiety:

PO: **Adults:** 20–25 mg 3–4 times/day. *IM/IV:* **Adults:** Initially, 50–100 mg, then 25–50 mg 3–4 times/day. **Elderly:** 25–50 mg 3–4 times/day.

Preoperative:

IM/IV: **Adults:** 50–100 mg 1 hr before surgery. **Elderly/debilitated, children 12–18 yrs:** 25–50 mg 1 hr before surgery.

Alcohol withdrawal:

PO: **Adults:** 50–100 mg followed by repeated doses until agitation is controlled. Do not exceed 300 mg/day.

IM/IV: **Adults:** Initially, 50–100 mg. May repeat in 2–4 hrs, if necessary.

SIDE EFFECTS

FREQUENT: Pain with IM injection; drowsiness, ataxia, dizziness, confusion with oral dose, particularly in elderly, debilitated. *OCCASIONAL:* Rash, peripheral edema, GI disturbances. *RARE:* Paradoxical CNS hyperactivity/nervousness in children, excitement/restlessness in elderly (generally noted during first 2 wks of therapy, particularly noted in presence of uncontrolled pain).

ADVERSE REACTIONS/TOXIC EFFECTS

IV route may produce pain, swelling, thrombophlebitis, carpal tunnel syndrome. Abrupt or too rapid withdrawal may result in pronounced restlessness, irritability, insomnia, hand tremors, abdominal/muscle cramps, sweating, vomiting, seizures. Overdosage results in somnolence, confusion, diminished reflexes, coma.

NURSING IMPLICATIONS

BASELINE ASSESSMENT:

Assess B/P, pulse, respirations immediately before administration. Pt must remain recumbent for up to 3 hrs (individualized) after parenteral administration to reduce hypotensive effect.

INTERVENTION/EVALUATION:

Assess motor responses (agitation, trembling, tension) and autonomic responses (cold, clammy hands, sweating). Assess children, elderly for paradoxical reaction, particularly during early therapy. Assist with ambulation if drowsiness, ataxia occur. Therapeutic blood serum level: 1–3 mcg/ml; toxic serum level: >5 mcg/ml.

PATIENT/FAMILY TEACHING:

Discomfort may occur with M injection. Drowsiness usually disappears during continued therapy. If dizziness occurs, change positions slowly from recumbent to sitting before standing. Smoking reduces drug effectiveness. Do not abruptly withdraw medication after long-term therapy.

chloroprocaine

(Nesacaine)

See Classification section under: Anesthetics: local (p. 4C)

chloroquine hydrochloride

klor-oh-kwin
(Aralen hydrochloride)

chloroquine phosphate

(Aralen phosphate)

►CLASSIFICATION

PHARMACOTHERAPEUTIC: Amebecide. ***CLINICAL:*** Antimalarial

ACTION/*THERAPEUTIC EFFECT*

Concentrates in parasite acid vesicles, *increases pH (inhibits parasite growth).* May interfere with parasite protein synthesis.

USES/*UNLABELED*

Treatment of *Plasmodium falciparum* malaria (terminates acute attacks, cures nonresistant strains), suppression of acute attacks, prolongation of interval between treatment/relapse in *P. vivax, P. ovale, P. malariae* malaria. Adjunctive therapy for extraintestinal amebiasis (including liver abscess). In combination with primaquine, cure for *P. vivax* and *P. ovale* malaria. *Treatment of sarcoid-associated hypercalcemia, juvenile arthritis, rheumatoid arthritis, systemic lupus erythematosus, solar urticaria, chronic cutaneous vasculitis.*

PRECAUTIONS

CONTRAINDICATIONS: Hypersensitivity to 4-aminoquinolones, retinal or visual field changes, psoriasis, porphyria. ***CAUTIONS:*** Alcoholism, severe blood disorders, liver disease, neurologic disorders, G-6-PD deficiency. Children are esp. susceptible to chloroquine fatalities.

INTERACTIONS

DRUG: May increase concentration of penicillamine, increase risk of hematologic/renal or severe skin reaction. **HERBAL:** None known. **FOOD:** None known. **LAB VALUES:** Acute decrease in hemocrit, hemoglobin, RBC count may occur.

AVAILABILITY (Rx)

TABLETS: 500 mg. **INJECTION:** 50 mg/ml.

INDICATIONS/ROUTES/DOSAGE

Note: Chloroquine PO_4 500 mg = 300 mg base; chloroquine HCl 50 mg = 40 mg base.

CHLOROQUINE PHOSPHATE:

Treatment of malaria (acute attack): Dose (mg base):

Dose	Time	Adults	Children
Initial	Day 1	600 mg	10 mg/kg
Second	6 hrs later	300 mg	5 mg/kg
Third	Day 2	300 mg	5 mg/kg
Fourth	Day 3	300 mg	5 mg/kg

Suppression of malaria:

PO: Adults: 300 mg (base)/wk on same day each week beginning 2 wks before exposure; continue for 6–8 wks after leaving endemic area. **Children:** 5 mg base/kg/wk. If therapy is not begun prior to exposure, then: **PO: Adults:** 600 mg base initially given in 2 divided doses 6 hrs apart. **Children:** 10 mg base/kg.

Amebiasis:

PO: Adults: 1 g (600 mg base) daily for 2 days; then, 500 mg (300 mg base)/day for at least 2–3 wks.

CHLOROQUINE HCL:

Treatment of malaria:

IM: Adults: Initially, 160–200 mg base (4–5 ml), repeat in 6 hrs. **Maximum:** 800 mg base in first 24 hrs. Begin oral therapy as soon as possible and continue for 3 days until approximately 1.5 g base given. **Children:** Initially, 5 mg base/kg, repeat in 6 hrs. Do not exceed 10 mg base/kg/24 hrs.

Amebiasis:

IM: Adults: 160–200 mg base (4–5 ml) daily for 10–12 days. Change to oral therapy as soon as possible.

SIDE EFFECTS

FREQUENT: Discomfort with IM administration, mild transient headache, anorexia, nausea, vomiting. **OCCASIONAL:** Visual disturbances (blurring, difficulty focusing); nervousness, fatigue, pruritus esp. of palms, soles, scalp; bleaching of hair, irritability, personality changes, diarrhea, skin eruptions. **RARE:** Stomatitis (redness/burning of oral mucosa, gingivitis, glossitis), exfoliative dermatitis.

ADVERSE REACTIONS/TOXIC EFFECTS

Ocular toxicity (tinnitus), ototoxicity (reduced hearing). Prolonged therapy: peripheral neuritis and neuromyopathy, hypotension, EKG changes, agranulocytosis, aplastic anemia, thrombocytopenia, convulsions, psychosis. Overdosage: headache, vomiting, visual disturbance, drowsiness, convulsions, hypokalemia followed by cardiovascular collapse, death.

C

NURSING IMPLICATIONS

INTERVENTION/EVALUATION:

Check for and promptly report any visual disturbances. Evaluate for GI distress. Monitor hepatic function tests and check for fatigue, jaundice, or other signs of hepatic effects. Assess skin and buccal mucosa, inquire about pruritus. Check vital signs and be alert to signs/symptoms of overdosage (esp. with parental administration, children). Notify physician of tinnitus, reduced hearing. With prolonged therapy, test for muscle weakness.

PATIENT/FAMILY TEACHING:

IM administration may cause local pain. Continue drug for full length of treatment. Notify physician of *any* new symptom, visual difficulties or decreased hearing, tinnitus immediately. Periodic lab and visual tests are important part of therapy. Report blurred vision or any other change in vision.

chlorothiazide

(Diuril)

See Classification section under: Diuretics (p. 83C)

chlorpheniramine

(Teldrin, Chlor-Trimeton)

See Classification section under: Antihistamines (p. 47C)

chlorpromazine ✳

klor-**pro**-mah-zeen
(Thorazine)

chlorpromazine hydrochloride

(Chlorpromanyl✤, Largactil✤, Thorazine)

▶ CLASSIFICATION

PHARMACOTHERAPEUTIC:
Phenothiazine. **CLINICAL:** Antipsychotic, antiemetic, antianxiety, antineuralgia adjunct (see p. 55C)

ACTION/*THERAPEUTIC EFFECT*

Blocks dopamine neurotransmission at postsynaptic dopamine receptor sites. Possesses strong anticholinergic, sedative, antiemetic effects, moderate extrapyramidal effects, slight antihistamine action. *Reduces psychosis, relieves nausea and vomiting, controls intractable hiccups, porphyria.*

USES/*UNLABELED*

Management of psychotic disorders, manic phase of manic-depressive illness, severe nausea or vomiting, preop sedation, severe behavioral disturbances in children. Relief of intractable hiccups, acute intermittent porphyria. *Treatment of choreiform movement of Huntington's disease.*

PRECAUTIONS

CONTRAINDICATIONS: Severe CNS depression, comatose states, severe cardiovascular disease, bone marrow depression, subcortical brain damage. ***CAUTIONS:*** Im-

---

✤ - Canadian trade name   ✳ - see also www.wbsaunders.com/SIMON/SaundersNDH

paired respiratory/hepatic/renal/cardiac function, alcohol withdrawal, history of seizures, urinary retention, glaucoma, prostatic hypertrophy, hypocalcemia (increases susceptibility to dystonias).

INTERACTIONS

DRUG: **Alcohol, CNS depressants** may increase CNS, respiratory depression, hypotensive effects. **Tricyclic antidepressants, MAO inhibitors** may increase sedative, anticholinergic effects. **Antithyroid agents** may increase risk of agranulocytosis. Increased risk of extrapyramidal symptoms (EPS) with **EPS-producing medications. Hypotensives** may increase hypotension. May decrease **levodopa** effects. **Lithium** may decrease absorption, produce adverse neurologic effects. *HERBAL:* None known. *FOOD:* None known. *LAB VALUES:* May produce false-positive pregnancy test, phenylketonuria (PKU). EKG changes may occur, including Q and T wave disturbances. Therapeutic blood serum level: 50–300 mcg/ml; toxic serum level: >750 mcg/ml.

AVAILABILITY (Rx)

TABLETS: 10 mg, 25 mg, 50 mg, 100 mg, 200 mg. *INJECTION:* 25 mg/ml. *SUPPOSITORY:* 25 mg, 100 mg.

INDICATIONS/ROUTES/DOSAGE
Psychosis:

IM/IV: **Adults, elderly:** Initially, 25 mg; may repeat in 1–4 hrs. May gradually increase to 400 mg q4–6h. **Maximum:** 300–800 mg/day. **Children >6 mos:** 0.5–1 mg/kg q6–8h. **Maximum:** *(<5 yrs):* 40 mg/day. *(5–12 yrs):* 75 mg/day.

PO: **Adults, elderly:** 30–800 mg/day in 1–4 divided doses. **Children >6 mos:** 0.5–1 mg/kg q4–6h.

Nausea/vomiting:

IM/IV: **Adults, elderly:** 25–50 mg q4–6h. **Children:** 0.5–1 mg/kg q6–8h.

PO: **Adults, elderly:** 10–25 mg q4–6h. **Children:** 0.5–1 mg/kg q4–6h.

RECTAL: **Adults, elderly:** 50–100 mg q6–8h. **Children:** 1 mg/kg q6–8h.

Hiccups:

PO: **Adults:** 25–50 mg 3 times/day. May give IM/IV.

SIDE EFFECTS

FREQUENT: Drowsiness, blurred vision, hypotension, defective color vision, difficulty in night vision, dizziness, decreased sweating, constipation, dry mouth, nasal congestion. *OCCASIONAL:* Difficulty urinating, increased skin sensivity to sun, skin rash, decreased sexual ability, swelling or pain in breasts, weight gain, nausea, vomiting, stomach pain, tremors.

ADVERSE REACTIONS/TOXIC EFFECTS

Extrapyramidal symptoms appear dose related (particularly high dosage), and divided into 3 categories: akathisia (inability to sit still, tapping of feet, urge to move around); parkinsonian symptoms (masklike face, tremors, shuffling gait, hypersalivation); and acute dystonias: torticollis (neck muscle spasm), opisthotonos (rigidity of back muscles), and oculogyric crisis (rolling back of eyes). Dystonic reaction may also produce profuse sweating, pallor. Tardive dyskinesia (protrusion of tongue, puffing of cheeks, chewing/puckering of the mouth) occurs rarely (may be irreversible). Abrupt withdrawal after long-term therapy may precipitate nausea, vomiting, gastritis, dizziness, tremors. Blood dyscrasias, particularly agranulocytosis, mild leukopenia may occur. May lower seizure threshold.

NURSING IMPLICATIONS

BASELINE ASSESSMENT:

Avoid skin contact with solution (contact dermatitis). **Antiemetic:** Assess for dehydration (poor skin turgor, dry mucous membranes, longitudinal furrows in tongue). **Antipsychotic:** Assess behavior, appearance, emotional status, response to environment, speech pattern, thought content.

INTERVENTION/EVALUATION:

Monitor B/P for hypotension. Assess for extrapyramidal symptoms. Monitor WBC, differential count for blood dyscrasias. Monitor for fine tongue movement (may be early sign of tardive dyskinesia). Supervise suicidal risk pt closely during early therapy (as depression lessens, energy level improves, increasing suicide potential). Assess for therapeutic response (interest in surroundings, improvement in self-care, increased ability to concentrate, relaxed facial expression). Therapeutic blood serum level: 50–300 mcg/ml; toxic serum level: >750.

PATIENT/FAMILY TEACHING:

Full therapeutic response may take up to 6 wks. Urine may darken. Do not abruptly withdraw from long-term drug therapy. Report visual disturbances. Drowsiness generally subsides during continued therapy. Avoid tasks that require alertness, motor skills until response to drug is established. Avoid alcohol. Avoid exposure to sunlight.

chlorpropamide

(Diabinese)

See Classification section under: Antidiabetic agents (p. 39C)

C

chlorthalidone

klor-**thal**-ih-doan
(Apo-Chlorthalidone✦,
Hygroton, Thalitone)

FIXED-COMBINATION(S)

With clonidine, an antihypertensive **(Combipres);** with atenolol, an antihypertensive **(Tenoretic);** with reserpine, an antihypertensive **(Demi-Regroton, Regroton)**

▶CLASSIFICATION

PHARMACOTHERAPEUTIC: Thiazide. **CLINICAL:** Diuretic (see p. 83C)

ACTION/*THERAPEUTIC EFFECT*

Diuretic: Blocks reabsorption of sodium, potassium, chloride at distal convoluted tubule, *promoting renal excretion.* **Antihypertensive:** Reduces plasma, extracellular fluid volume, peripheral vascular resistance, *lowering B/P.*

PHARMACOKINETICS

Onset	Peak	Duration
PO (diuretic)		
2 hrs	2–6 hrs	Up to 36 hrs

Rapidly absorbed from GI tract. Excreted unchanged in urine. Half-life: 35–50 hrs. Onset antihypertensive effect: 3–4 days; optimal therapeutic effect: 3–4 wks.

✦ - Canadian trade name   ✳ - see also www.wbsaunders.com/SIMON/SaundersNDH

USES

Adjunctive therapy in edema associated with CHF, hepatic cirrhosis, corticoid or estrogen therapy, renal impairment. In treatment of hypertension, may be used alone or with other antihypertensive agents.

PRECAUTIONS

CONTRAINDICATIONS: History of hypersensitivity to sulfonamides or thiazide diuretics, renal decompensation, anuria. **CAUTIONS:** Severe renal disease, impaired hepatic function, diabetes mellitus, elderly/debilitated, gout, pts with hypercholesterolemia.
▷**LIFESPAN CONSIDERATIONS:**
Pregnancy/Lactation: Crosses placenta; small amount distributed in breast milk; nursing not advised. **Pregnancy Category B. Children:** No age-related precautions noted. **Elderly:** May be more sensitive to hypotensive and electrolyte effects.

INTERACTIONS

DRUG: Cholestyramine, colestipol may decrease absorption, effects. May increase **digoxin** toxicity (due to hypokalemia). May increase **lithium** toxicity. **HERBAL:** None known. **FOOD:** None known. **LAB VALUES:** May increase bilirubin, serum calcium, LDL, cholesterol, triglycerides, creatinine, glucose, uric acid. May decrease urinary calcium, magnesium, potassium, sodium.

AVAILABILITY (Rx)

TABLETS: 15 mg, 25 mg, 50 mg, 100 mg.

ADMINISTRATION/HANDLING
PO:
• Give with food or milk if GI upset occurs, preferably with breakfast (may prevent nocturia).
• Scored tablets may be crushed.

INDICATIONS/ROUTES/DOSAGE
Note: Fixed-combination medication should not be used for initial therapy but for maintenance therapy.

Edema:
PO: Adults: 50–100 mg 1 time/day in morning or 100 mg every other day. May require 150–200 mg every day or every other day. Reduce dose to lowest maintenance level when dry weight is achieved (nonedematous state).

Hypertension:
PO: Adults: Initially, 25 mg/day. May increase to 50 mg/day. **Maintenance:** 25–50 mg/day.

Usual elderly dosage:
PO: Initially, 12.5–25 mg/day or every other day.

SIDE EFFECTS
EXPECTED: Increase in urine frequency/volume. **FREQUENT:** Potassium depletion (rarely produces symptoms). **OCCASIONAL:** Anorexia, impotence, diarrhea, orthostatic hypotension, GI upset, photosensitivity. **RARE:** Rash.

ADVERSE REACTIONS/TOXIC EFFECTS
Vigorous diuresis may lead to profound water loss and electrolyte depletion, resulting in hypokalemia, hyponatremia, dehydration. Acute hypotensive episodes may occur. Hyperglycemia may be noted during prolonged therapy. Overdosage can lead to lethargy, coma without changes in electrolytes or hydration.

NURSING IMPLICATIONS

BASELINE ASSESSMENT:

Check vital signs, esp. B/P for hypotension before administration. Assess baseline electrolytes, particularly check for low potassium. Assess edema, skin turgor, mucous membranes for hydration status. Evaluate muscle strength, mental status.

INTERVENTION/EVALUATION:

Watch for electrolyte disturbances (hypokalemia may result in weakness, tremor, muscle cramps, nausea, vomiting, change in mental status, tachycardia; hyponatremia may result in confusion, thirst, cold/clammy skin). Periodically check blood sugar for hyperglycemia in prolonged therapy.

PATIENT/FAMILY TEACHING:

To reduce hypotensive effect, rise slowly from lying to sitting position and permit legs to dangle momentarily before standing. Eat foods high in potassium such as whole grains (cereals), legumes, meat, bananas, apricots, orange juice, potatoes (white, sweet), raisins. Avoid prolonged exposure to sunlight.

chlorzoxazone

(Paraflex, Parafon Forte DSC)

See Classification section under: Skeletal muscle relaxants

cholestyramine resin

C

coal-es-**tie**-rah-mean
(LoCHOLEST, Novo-Cholamine✿, Prevalite, Questran✿, Questran Lite)

▶CLASSIFICATION

PHARMACOTHERAPEUTIC:
Bile acid sequestrant. ***CLINICAL:*** Antihyperlipoproteinemic
(see p. 49C)

ACTION/*THERAPEUTIC EFFECT*

Binds with bile acids in intestine forming insoluble complex. Binding results in partial removal of bile acid from enterohepatic circulation, *removing low-density lipoproteins (LDL) and cholesterol from plasma.*

PHARMACOKINETICS

Not absorbed from GI tract. Decreases in LDL apparent in 5–7 days, serum cholesterol in 1 mo. Serum cholesterol returns to baseline levels about 1 mo after discontinuing drug.

USES/*UNLABELED*

Adjunct to dietary therapy to decrease elevated serum cholesterol levels in those with primary hypercholesterolemia. Relief of pruritus associated with partial biliary obstruction. *Treatment of diarrhea (due to bile acids); hyperoxaluria.*

PRECAUTIONS

CONTRAINDICATIONS: Hypersensitivity to cholestyramine or tartrazine (frequently seen in aspirin hypersensitivity), complete biliary obstruction. ***CAUTIONS:*** GI dysfunction (esp. constipation), hemorrhoids, bleeding disorders, osteoporosis.

▷**LIFESPAN CONSIDERATIONS:**
Pregnancy/Lactation: Not systemically absorbed. May interfere with maternal absorption of fat-soluble vitamins. **Pregnancy Category B. Children:** No age-related precautions noted. Limited experience in those <10 yrs of age. **Elderly:** Increased risk of GI side effects, adverse nutritional effects.

INTERACTIONS

DRUG: May increase effects of **anticoagulants** by decreasing vitamin K. May decrease **warfarin** absorption. May bind, decrease absorption of **digoxin, thiazides, penicillins, propranolol, tetracyclines, folic acid, thyroid hormones, other medications.** Binds, decreases effect of **oral vancomycin. HERBAL:** None known. **FOOD:** None known. **LAB VALUES:** May increase SGOT (AST), SGPT (ALT), alkaline phosphatase, magnesium. May decrease calcium, potassium, sodium. May prolong prothrombin time.

AVAILABILITY (Rx)
POWDER: 4 g.

ADMINISTRATION/HANDLING
PO:
• Give other drugs at least 1 hr before or 4–6 hrs after cholestyramine (capable of binding drugs in GI tract). • Do not give in dry form (highly irritating). Mix with 3–6 oz water, milk, fruit juice, soup. • Place powder on surface for 1–2 min (prevents lumping), then mix thoroughly. • Excessive foaming with carbonated beverages; use extra large glass and stir slowly. • Administer before meals.

INDICATIONS/ROUTES/DOSAGE
Primary hypercholesterolemia:
PO: Adults, elderly: 3–4 g 3–4 times/day. **Maximum:** 16–32 g/day in 2–4 divided doses. **Children >10 yrs:** 2 g/day up to 8 g/day. **Children ≤10 yrs:** Initially, 2 g/day. **Range:** 1–4 g/day.

SIDE EFFECTS
FREQUENT: Constipation (may lead to fecal impaction), nausea, vomiting, stomach pain, indigestion. **OCCASIONAL:** Diarrhea, belching, bloating, headache, dizziness. **RARE:** Gallstones, peptic ulcer, malabsorption syndrome.

ADVERSE REACTIONS/TOXIC EFFECT
GI tract obstruction, hyperchloremic acidosis, osteoporosis secondary to calcium excretion. High dosage may interfere with fat absorption, resulting in steatorrhea.

NURSING IMPLICATIONS

BASELINE ASSESSMENT:
Question for history of hypersensitivity to cholestyramine, tartrazine, aspirin. Obtain baseline serum cholesterol, triglycerides, electrolytes.

INTERVENTION/EVALUATION:
Determine pattern of bowel activity. Evaluate food tolerance, abdominal discomfort, and flatulence. Monitor blood chemistries. Encourage several glasses of water between meals.

PATIENT/FAMILY TEACHING:
Complete full course; do not omit or change doses. Take other drugs at least 1 hr before or 4–6 hrs after cholestyramine. Never take in dry form; mix with

3–6 oz water, milk, fruit juice, soup (place powder on surface for 1–2 min to prevent lumping, then mix well). Use extra large glass and stir slowly when mixing with carbonated beverages due to foaming. Take before meals and drink several glasses of water between meals. Eat high-fiber foods (whole grain cereals, fruits, vegetables) to reduce potential for constipation.

chorionic gonadotropin, hCG

kore-ee-**on**-ik goe-**nad**-oh-troe-pin (APL, Novarel, Pregnyl, Profasi HP)

▶CLASSIFICATION

PHARMACOTHERAPEUTIC: Sex hormone. **CLINICAL:** Androgen, progesterone stimulant (see p. 86C)

ACTION/*THERAPEUTIC EFFECT*

Stimulates production of gonadal steroid hormones by stimulating interstitial cells (Leydig cells) of the testes to produce androgen, and the corpus luteum of the ovary to produce progesterone. Androgen stimulation in the male *causes production of secondary sex characteristics and may stimulate descent of testes when no anatomic impediment exists.* In women of childbearing age with normally functioning ovaries, *causes maturation of corpus luteum and triggers ovulation.*

USES/*UNLABELED*

Treatment of prepubertal cryptorchidism without obstruction, se-

lected cases of hypogonadotropic hypogonadism. To induce ovulation and pregnancy in women with secondary anovulation (after pretreatment with menotropin). *Diagnosis of male hypogonadism, treatment of corpus luteum dysfunction.*

PRECAUTIONS

CONTRAINDICATIONS: Precocious puberty, carcinoma of the prostate or other androgen-dependent neoplasia. Not for adjunctive therapy in obesity. **CAUTIONS:** Prepubertal males, conditions aggravated by fluid retention (cardiac or renal disease, epilepsy, migraine, asthma).

INTERACTIONS

DRUG: None significant. **HERBAL:** None known. **FOOD:** None known. **LAB VALUES:** None significant.

AVAILABILITY (Rx)

POWDER FOR INJECTION: 5,000 unit, 10,000 unit, 20,000 unit vials.

INDICATIONS/ROUTES/DOSAGE

Prepubertal cryptorchidism, hypogonadotropic hypogonadism:

IM: Adults: Dosage is individualized based on indication, age and weight of pt, and physician preference.

Induction of ovulation and pregnancy:

IM: Adults: (After pretreatment with menotropins), 5,000–10,000 IU 1 day after last dose of menotropins.

SIDE EFFECTS

FREQUENT: Pain at injection site. **Induction of ovulation:** Ovarian cysts, uncomplicated ovarian enlargement. **OCCASIONAL:** Enlarged breasts, headache, irritability, fatigue, depression. **Induction**

of ovulation: Severe ovarian hyper-stimulation, peripheral edema. *Cryptorchidism:* Precocious puberty (acne, deepening voice, penile growth, pubic/axillary hair).

ADVERSE REACTIONS/TOXIC EFFECTS

When used with menotropins: increased risk of arterial thromboembolism, ovarian hyperstimulation with high incidence (20%) of multiple births (premature deliveries and neonatal prematurity), ruptured ovarian cysts.

NURSING IMPLICATIONS

BASELINE ASSESSMENT:

Obtain baseline weight, B/P.

INTERVENTION/EVALUATION:

Assess for edema: weigh every 2–3 days, report >5 lbs gain/wk; monitor B/P periodically during treatment; check for decreased urinary output, peripheral edema.

PATIENT/FAMILY TEACHING:

Promptly report abdominal pain, vaginal bleeding, signs of precocious puberty in males (deepening of voice; axillary, facial, and pubic hair; acne, penile growth) or signs of edema. In anovulation treatment, begin recording daily basal temperature; initiate intercourse daily beginning the day preceding hCG treatment. Possibility of multiple births.

ciclopirox

(Loprox, Penlac)

See Classification section under: Antifungals: Topical (p. 42C)

cidofovir

sid-dough-**foe**-vir
(Vistide)

▶CLASSIFICATION

PHARMACOTHERAPEUTIC: Anti-infective. *CLINICAL:* Antiviral (see p. 57C)

ACTION/*THERAPEUTIC EFFECT*

Suppresses cytomegalovirus (CMV) replication *by inhibition of viral DNA synthesis.* Incorporation of cidofovir in growing viral DNA chain *results in reduction in rate of viral DNA synthesis.*

PHARMACOKINETICS

Protein binding: <6%. Excreted primarily unchanged in urine. Effect of hemodialysis unknown. Elimination half-life: 1.4–3.8 hrs.

USES

Treatment of cytomegalovirus (CMV) retinitis in those with acquired immunodeficiency syndrome (AIDS).

PRECAUTIONS

CONTRAINDICATIONS: Hypersensitivity to cidofovir; history of clinically severe hypersensitivity to probenecid or other sulfa-containing medication; direct intraocular injection; renal function impairment (serum creatinine >1.5 mg/dl or creatinine clearance ≤55 ml/min or urine protein >100 mg/dl). *CAUTIONS:* Preexisting diabetes.

▷*LIFESPAN CONSIDERATIONS:*
Pregnancy/Lactation: Embryotoxic (reduced fetal body weight) in animals. Unknown if excreted in breast milk. Do not administer to nursing women. HIV-infected

women not to breast-feed. **Pregnancy Category C. Children:** Safety and efficacy not established. **Elderly:** Age-related renal impairment may require dosage adjustment.

INTERACTIONS

DRUG: Avoid concurrent administration of cidofovir and medication with nephrotoxic risk **(amphotericin B, aminoglycosides, foscarnet, IV pentamidine). HERBAL:** None known. **FOOD:** None known. **LAB VALUES:** May decrease neutrophil count, serum phosphate, uric acid, and bicarbonate; elevate serum creatinine.

AVAILABILITY (Rx)

INJECTION: 75 mg/ml (5 ml amp).

ADMINISTRATION/HANDLING

Note: Do not exceed the recommended dosage, frequency, or infusion rate.

IV 🔟

Storage:

• Store at controlled room temperature (68°–77°F). • Admixtures may be refrigerated for no more than 24 hrs. • Allow refrigerated admixtures to warm to room temperature before use.

Dilution:

• Dilute in 100 ml 0.9% NaCl.

Rate of administration:

• Infuse over 1 hr. • IV hydration with 0.9% NaCl and probenecid therapy *must* be used with each cidofovir infusion (minimizes risk of nephrotoxicity). • Ingestion of food before each dose of probenecid may reduce nausea and vomiting. An antiemetic may also reduce potential for nausea.

IV INCOMPATIBILITY ⊘

No information available via Y-site administration.

INDICATIONS/ROUTES/DOSAGE

Probenecid:

PO: Adults: Give 2 g 3 hrs prior to cidofovir dose, and 1 g given at 2 and again at 8 hrs after completion of the 1 hr cidofovir infusion (total of 4 g).

Hydration:

IV: Adults: 1 liter 0.9% NaCl given over 1–2 hrs immediately before cidofovir infusion. If tolerated, a second liter may be given at start or immediately after cidofovir infusion and infused over 1–3 hrs.

Usual dosage:

IV INFUSION: Adults: (Induction): 5 mg/kg at constant rate over 1 hr once weekly for 2 consecutive wks. **Maintenance:** 5 mg/kg at constant rate over 1 hr once every 2 wks.

Renal function impairment:

Dose based on creatinine clearance.

Creatinine Clearance	Induction Dose	Maintenance Dose
41–55 ml/min	2 mg/kg	2 mg/kg
30–40 ml/min	1.5 mg/kg	1.5 mg/kg
20–29 ml/min	1 mg/kg	1 mg/kg
≤19 ml/min	0.5 mg/kg	0.5 mg/kg

SIDE EFFECTS

FREQUENT: Nausea, vomiting (65%), fever (57%), asthenia (46%), rash (30%), diarrhea (27%), headache (27%), alopecia (25%), chills (24%), anorexia (22%), dyspnea (22%), abdominal pain (17%).

ADVERSE REACTIONS/TOXIC EFFECTS

Proteinuria (80%), nephrotoxicity (53%), neutropenia (31%), serum creatinine elevations (29%), infection (24%), anemia (20%), ocular hypotony (12%) (decrease in intraocular pressure), pneumonia (9%). Probenecid may produce hypersensitivity reaction (rash, fever, chills, anaphylaxis). Acute renal failure occurs rarely.

NURSING IMPLICATIONS

BASELINE ASSESSMENT:

For those taking zidovudine, temporarily discontinue zidovudine administration or decrease zidovudine dose by 50% on days of infusion (probenecid reduces metabolic clearance of zidovudine). Closely monitor renal function (urinalysis, serum creatinine) during therapy.

INTERVENTION/EVALUATION:

Monitor serum creatinine, urine protein, and WBC count prior to each dose. Monitor for proteinuria (may be early indicator of dose-dependent nephrotoxicity). Periodically monitor visual acuity and ocular symptoms.

PATIENT/FAMILY TEACHING:

Obtain regular follow-up ophthalmologic exams. Those of child-bearing age should use effective contraception during and for 1 mo following treatment. Men should practice barrier contraceptive methods during and for 3 mos following treatment. Must complete full course of probenecid with each cidofovir dose.

cilostazol

sill-oh-**stay**-zole
(Pletal)
Do not confuse with Plendil.

▶CLASSIFICATION

PHARMACOTHERAPEUTIC:
Phosphodiesterase III inhibitor.
CLINICAL: Antiplatelet

ACTION/*THERAPEUTIC EFFECT*

Inhibits platelet aggregation, dilation of vascular beds with greatest dilation in femoral beds, *improving walking distance in those with intermittent claudication.*

PHARMACOKINETICS

Moderately absorbed from GI tract. Protein binding: 95–98%. Extensively metabolized in the liver. Excreted primarily in the urine and, to a lesser extent, in the feces. Not removed by hemodialysis. Half-life: 11–13 hrs. Therapeutic effect noted in 2–4 wks but may take as long as 12 wks before beneficial effect is experienced.

USES

Reduction of symptoms of intermittent claudication indicated by increased walking distance without leg pain.

PRECAUTIONS

CONTRAINDICATIONS: CHF of any severity. ***CAUTIONS:*** None significant.
▷***LIFESPAN CONSIDERATIONS:***
Pregnancy/Lactation: Unknown if drug crosses placenta or is distributed in breast milk. **Pregnancy Category C. Children:** Safety and efficacy not established. **Elderly:** No age-related precautions noted.

INTERACTIONS

DRUG: None significant. ***HERBAL:*** None known. ***FOOD: Grapefruit juice*** may increase concentration, toxicity. ***LAB VALUES:*** May decrease hemoglobin, hemocrit. May increase creatinine, BUN.

AVAILABILITY (Rx)
TABLETS: 100 mg.

ADMINISTRATION/HANDLING
PO:
• Give at least 30 min before or 2 hrs after meals. • Do not take with grapefruit juice.

INDICATIONS/ROUTES/DOSAGE
Intermittent claudication:
PO: Adults, elderly: 100 mg 2 times/day at least 30 min before or 2 hrs after meals.

SIDE EFFECTS
FREQUENT (10–34%): Headache, diarrhea, palpitations, dizziness, pharyngitis. **OCCASIONAL** (3–7%): Nausea, rhinitis, back pain, peripheral edema, dyspepsia, abdominal pain, tachycardia, cough, flatulence, myalgia. **RARE** (1–2%): Leg cramps, paresthesia, rash, vomiting.

ADVERSE REACTIONS/TOXIC EFFECTS
Overdosage noted by severe headache, diarrhea, hypotension, cardiac arrhythmias.

NURSING IMPLICATIONS

BASELINE ASSESSMENT:
Assess platelet count, hemoglobin, hemocrit prior to treatment and periodically during treatment.

PATIENT/FAMILY TEACHING:
Take on an empty stomach (at least 30 min before or 2 hrs after meals). Do not take with grapefruit juice.

cimetidine

sih-**met**-ih-deen
(Apo-Cimetidine✿,
Novocimetine✿, Peptol✿,
Tagamet, Tagamet HB)

C

▶CLASSIFICATION

PHARMACOTHERAPEUTIC:
H$_2$ receptor antagonist. **CLINICAL:** Antiulcer, gastric acid secretion inhibitor (see p. 88C)

ACTION/*THERAPEUTIC EFFECT*

Inhibits histamine action at H$_2$ receptor sites of parietal cells, *inhibiting gastric acid secretion (fasting, nocturnal, or when stimulated by food, caffeine, insulin).*

PHARMACOKINETICS

Well absorbed from GI tract. Protein binding: 15–20%. Widely distributed. Metabolized in liver. Primarily excreted in urine. Not removed by hemodialysis. Half-life: 2 hrs (half-life increased with impaired renal function).

USES/*UNLABELED*

Short-term treatment of active duodenal ulcer. Prevention of duodenal ulcer recurrence, upper GI bleeding in critically ill pts. Treatment of active benign gastric ulcer, pathologic GI hypersecretory conditions, gastroesophageal reflux disease (GERD). *Treatment of upper GI bleeding, prophylaxis of aspiration pneumonia, acute urticaria, chronic warts.*

PRECAUTIONS

CONTRAINDICATIONS: None significant. **CAUTIONS:** Impaired renal/hepatic function, elderly.

✿ - Canadian trade name   ✳ - see also www.wbsaunders.com/SIMON/SaundersNDH

▷**LIFESPAN CONSIDERATIONS:**
Pregnancy/Lactation: Crosses placenta; distributed in breast milk. In infants, may suppress gastric acidity, inhibit drug metabolism, produce CNS stimulation. **Pregnancy Category B. Children:** Long-term use may induce cerebral toxicity, affect hormonal system. **Elderly:** More likely to experience confusion, esp. in those with impaired renal function.

INTERACTIONS

DRUG: Antacids may decrease absorption (do not give within ½–1 hr). May decrease absorption of **ketoconazole** (give at least 2 hrs after). May decrease metabolism, increase concentration of **oral anticoagulants, tricyclic antidepressants, oral hypoglycemics, metoprolol, metronidazole, phenytoin, propranolol, theophylline, calcium channel blockers, cyclosporine, lidocaine. HERBAL:** None known. **FOOD:** None known. **LAB VALUES:** Interferes with skin tests using allergen extracts. May increase creatinine, prolactin, transaminase. May decrease parathyroid hormone concentration.

AVAILABILITY (Rx)

TABLETS: 100 mg **(OTC),** 200 mg, 300 mg, 400 mg, 800 mg. **ORAL LIQUID:** 300 mg/5 ml. **INJECTION:** 300 mg/2 ml. **SUSPENSION:** 200 mg/5 ml.

ADMINISTRATION/HANDLING
PO:

• Give without regard to meals. Best given with meals and at bedtime. • Do not administer within 1 hr of antacids.

IM:

• Administer undiluted. • Inject deep into large muscle mass.

IV 🖩

Storage:

• Store at room temperature. • Reconstituted IV is stable for 48 hrs at room temperature.

Dilution:

• Dilute each 300 mg (2 ml) with 18 ml 0.9% NaCl, 0.45% NaCl, 0.2% NaCl, D_5W, $D_{10}W$, Ringer's solution, or lactated Ringer's to a total volume of 20 ml.

Rate of administration

• For IV push, administer over not less than 2 min (prevents arrhythmias, hypotension). • For intermittent IV (piggyback) administration, infuse over 15–20 min. • For IV infusion, dilute with 100–1,000 ml 0.9% NaCl, D_5W, or other compatible solution (see Dilution) and infuse over 24 hrs.

IV INCOMPATIBILITIES ⊘

Allopurinol (Aloprim), amphotericin B complex (Ambisome, Amphotec, Abelcet), cefepime (Maxipime).

IV COMPATIBILITIES

Diltiazem (Cardizem), heparin, midazolam (Versed), milrinone (Primacor), propofol (Diprivan).

INDICATIONS/ROUTES/DOSAGE
Active ulcer:

IM/IV: Adults, elderly: 300 mg q6h or 150 mg as single dose followed by 37.5 mg/hr continuous infusion.

PO: 300 mg 4 times/day or 400 mg 2 times/day or 800 mg at bedtime.

C

Prophylaxis duodenal ulcer:

PO: Adults, elderly: 400–800 mg at bedtime.

Gastric hypersectretory conditions:

IM/IV/PO: Adults, elderly: 300–600 mg q6h. **Maximum:** 2,400 mg/day.

GERD:

PO: Adults, elderly: 800 mg 2 times/day or 400 mg 4 times/day for 12 wks.

OTC use:

PO: Adults, elderly: 100 mg up to 30 min before meals. **Maximum:** 2 doses/day.

Prevention of upper GI bleeding:

IV INFUSION: Adults, elderly: 50 mg/hr.

Usual dosage for children:

IM/IV/PO: Children: 20–40 mg/kg/day in divided doses q6h. **Infants:** 10–20 mg/kg/day in divided doses q6–12h. **Neonates:** 5–10 mg/kg/day in divided doses q8–12h.

Dosage in renal impairment:

Based on 300 mg dose in adults.

Creatinine Clearance	Dosage Interval
>40 ml/min	q6h
20–40 ml/min	q8h or decrease dose by 25%
<20 ml/min	q12h or decrease dose by 50%

Give after hemodialysis and q12h between dialysis period.

SIDE EFFECTS

OCCASIONAL (2–4%): Headache. **Elderly, severely ill, impaired renal function:** Confusion, agitation, psychosis, depression, anxiety, disorientation, hallucinations (effects reverse 3–4 days after discontinuance). ***RARE*** (<2%): Diarrhea, dizziness, drowsiness, headache, nausea, vomiting, gynecomastia, rash, impotence.

ADVERSE REACTIONS/TOXIC EFFECTS

Rapid IV may produce cardiac arrhythmias, hypotension.

NURSING IMPLICATIONS

BASELINE ASSESSMENT:

Do not administer antacids concurrently (separate by 1 hr).

INTERVENTION/EVALUATION:

Monitor B/P for hypotension during IV infusion. Assess for GI bleeding: Hematemesis, blood in stool. Check mental status in elderly, severely ill, those with impaired renal function.

PATIENT/FAMILY TEACHING:

IM may produce transient discomfort at injection site. Do not take antacids within 1 hr of cimetidine administration. Avoid tasks that require alertness, motor skills until drug response is established. Avoid smoking. Report any blood in vomitus or stool, or dark, tarry stool.

ciprofloxacin hydrochloride

sip-row-**flocks**-ah-sin (Ciloxan, <u>Cipro</u>)

FIXED-COMBINATION(S)

With hydrocortisone, a glucocorticoid **(Cipro HC Otic)**

▶CLASSIFICATION

PHARMACOTHERAPEUTIC: Fluoroquinolone. ***CLINICAL:*** Anti-infective (see p. 22C)

ACTION/*THERAPEUTIC EFFECT*

Inhibits DNA enzyme in susceptible microorganisms, *interfering with bacterial DNA replication.* Bactericidal.

PHARMACOKINETICS

Well absorbed from GI tract (delayed by food). Protein binding: 20–40%. Widely distributed (including CSF). Metabolized in liver to active metabolite. Primarily excreted in urine. Minimal removal by hemodialysis. Half-life: 4–6 hrs (half-life increased with impaired renal function, elderly).

USES/*UNLABELED*

Treatment of infections of urinary tract, chronic bacterial prostatitis skin/skin structure, GI tract, bone/joint, lower respiratory tract, infectious diarrhea, uncomplicated gonorrhea, empiric treatment of febrile neutropenia, acute sinusitis. **Ophthalmic:** Conjunctival keratitis, keratoconjunctivitis, corneal ulcers, blepharitis, dacryocystitis, blepharoconjunctivitis, acute meibomianitis. *Treatment of chancroid.*

PRECAUTIONS

CONTRAINDICATIONS: Hypersensitivity to ciprofloxacin, quinolones. **Ophthalmic:** Vaccinia, varicella, epithelial herpes simplex, keratitis, mycobacterial infection, fungal disease of ocular structure. Not for use after uncomplicated removal of foreign body. ***CAUTIONS:*** Renal impairment, CNS disorders, seizures, those taking theophylline or caffeine. Suspension not for use in an NG tube.

▷*LIFESPAN CONSIDERATIONS:* **Pregnancy/Lactation:** Unknown if distributed in breast milk. If possible, do not use during pregnancy/lactation (risk of arthropathy to fetus/infant). **Pregnancy Category C. Children:** Safety and efficacy not established in those <18 yrs of age. **Elderly:** Age-related renal impairment may require dosage adjustment.

INTERACTIONS

DRUG: **Antacids, iron preparations, sucralfate** may decrease absorption. Decreases clearance, may increase concentration, toxicity of **theophylline.** May increase effects of **oral anticoagulants.** ***HERBAL:*** None known. ***FOOD:*** None known. ***LAB VALUES:*** May increase SGOT (AST), SGPT (ALT), alkaline phosphatase, LDH, bilirubin, BUN, creatinine.

AVAILABILITY (Rx)

TABLETS: 100 mg, 250 mg, 500 mg, 750 mg. ***ORAL SUSPENSION. INJECTION:*** 200 mg, 400 mg. ***OPHTHALMIC SOLUTION:*** 0.03%.

ADMINISTRATION/HANDLING
PO:

• May be given without regard to meals (preferred dosing time: 2 hrs after meals). • Do not administer antacids (aluminum, magnesium) within 2 hrs of ciprofloxacin. • Encourage cranberry juice, citrus fruits (acidifies urine). • Suspension may be stored for 14 days at room temperature.

IV 🔳

Storage:

• Store at room temperature. • Solution appears clear, colorless to slightly yellow.

Reconstitution:

• Available prediluted in infusion container ready for use.

Rate of administration:

• Infuse over 60 min.

Ophthalmic:

• Tilt pt's head back; place solution in conjunctival sac. • Have pt close eyes; press gently on lacrimal sac for 1 min. • Do not use ophthalmic solutions for injection. • Unless infection is very superficial, systemic administration generally accompanies ophthalmic.

IV INCOMPATIBILITIES ⊘

Aminophylline, ampicillin/sulbactam (Unasyn), cefepime (Maxipime), dexamethasone (Decadron), furosemide (Lasix), heparin, hydrocortisone (Solu-Cortef), methylprednisolone (Solu-Medrol), phenytoin (Dilantin), sodium bicarbonate.

IV COMPATIBILITIES

Calcium gluconate, diltiazem (Cardizem), dobutamine (Dobutrex), dopamine (Intropin), lidocaine, lorazepam (Ativan), midazolam (Versed), potassium chloride.

INDICATIONS/ROUTES/DOSAGE

Mild to moderate urinary tract infections:

PO: **Adults, elderly:** 250 mg q12h.

IV: **Adults, elderly:** 200 mg q12h.

Complicated urinary tract, mild to moderate respiratory tract infections, skin/skin structure, bones and joint, infectious diarrhea:

PO: **Adults, elderly:** 500 mg q12h.
IV: **Adults, elderly:** 400 mg q12h.

Severe, complicated infections:
PO: **Adults, elderly:** 750 mg q12h.
IV: **Adults, elderly:** 400 mg q12h.

Prostatitis:

PO: **Adults, elderly:** 500 mg q12h for 28 days.

Uncomplicated bladder infection:
PO: **Adults:** 100 mg 2 times/day for 3 days.

Acute sinusitis:
PO: **Adults:** 500 mg q12h.

Uncomplicated gonorrhea:
PO: **Adults:** 250 mg as single dose.

Usual dosage for children:

PO: 20–30 mg/kg/day in 2 divided doses. **Maximum:** 1.5 g/day.

IV: 20–30 mg/kg/day in 2 divided doses q12h. **Maximum:** 800 mg/day.

Dosage in renal impairment:

The dose and/or frequency is modified in pts based on severity of infection and degree of renal impairment.

Creatinine Clearance	Dosage Interval
<30 ml/min	q18h–24h

Hemodialysis, peritoneal dialysis 250–500 mg q24h (after dialysis)

Usual ophthalmic dosage:

Corneal ulcer: Adults, elderly: 2 drops q15min for 6 hrs, then 2 drops q30min remainder first day; 2 drops q1h second day; then q4h days 3–14.

Conjunctivitis: Adults, elderly: 1–2 drops q2h for 2 days, then q4h next 5 days.

SIDE EFFECTS

FREQUENT (2–5%): Nausea, diarrhea, dyspepsia, vomiting, constipation, flatulence, confusion, crystalluria. **Ophthalmic:** Burning, crusting in corner of eye. **OCCASIONAL** (<2%): Abdominal pain/discomfort, headache, rash. **Oph-**

thalmic: Bad taste, sense of something in eye, redness of eyelids, eyelid itching. *RARE* (<1%): Dizziness, confusion, tremors, hallucinations, hypersensitivity reaction, insomnia, dry mouth, paresthesia.

ADVERSE REACTIONS/TOXIC EFFECTS

Superinfection (esp. enterococcal, fungal), nephropathy, cardiopulmonary arrest, cerebral thrombosis may occur. Arthropathy may occur if given to children <18 yrs. *Ophthalmic:* Sensitization may contraindicate later systemic use of ciprofloxacin.

NURSING IMPLICATIONS

BASELINE ASSESSMENT:
Question for history of hypersensitivity to ciprofloxacin, quinolones.

INTERVENTION/EVALUATION:
Evaluate food tolerance. Determine pattern of bowel activity. Check for dizziness, headache, visual difficulties, tremors. Assess for chest, joint pain. *Ophthalmic:* Check for therapeutic response.

PATIENT/FAMILY TEACHING:
Do not skip dose; take full course of therapy. Take with 8 oz water; drink several glasses of water between meals. Eat/drink high sources of ascorbic acid to prevent crystalluria (cranberry juice, citrus fruits). Do not take antacids (reduces/destroys effectiveness). Shake suspension well before using; do not chew microcapsules in suspension. Sugarless gum or hard candy may relieve bad taste. *Ophthalmic:* Explain possibility of crystal precipitate forming, and usual resolution.

cisatracurium

(Nimbex)
See Classification section under: Neuromuscular blockers (p. 102C)

cisplatin

sis-**plah**-tin
(Platinol✚, Platinol-AQ)

▶**CLASSIFICATION**
PHARMACOTHERAPEUTIC:
Platinum coordination complex.
CLINICAL: Antineoplastic (see p. 69C)

ACTION/*THERAPEUTIC EFFECT*
Inhibits DNA, and to lesser extent, RNA, protein synthesis by crosslinking with DNA strands, *preventing cellular division.* Cell cyclephase nonspecific.

PHARMACOKINETICS
Widely distributed. Protein binding: >90%. Undergoes rapid nonenzymatic conversion to inactive metabolite. Excreted in urine. Removed by hemodialysis. Half-life: 58–73 hrs (half-life increased with impaired renal function).

USES/*UNLABELED*
Treatment of metastatic testicular tumors, metastatic ovarian tumors, advanced bladder carcinoma. *Treatment of carcinoma of breast, cervical, endometrial, gastric, lung, prostate, head/neck, neuroblastoma, germ cell tumors, osteosarcoma.*

PRECAUTIONS
CONTRAINDICATIONS: Myelo-

suppression, hearing impairment. **CAUTIONS:** Previous therapy with other antineoplastic agents, radiation.

▷**LIFESPAN CONSIDERATIONS:** **Pregnancy/Lactation:** If possible, avoid use during pregnancy, esp. first trimester. Breast feeding not recommended. **Pregnancy Category D. Children:** Ototoxic effects may be more severe. **Elderly:** Age-related renal impairment may require dosage adjustment.

INTERACTIONS

DRUG: May decrease effect of **antigout medications. Bone marrow depressants** may increase bone marrow depression. **Nephrotoxic, ototoxic agents** may increase toxicity. **Live virus vaccines** may potentiate virus replication, increase virus side effects, decrease pt's antibody response to vaccine. **HERBAL:** None known. **FOOD:** None known. **LAB VALUES:** May cause positive Coombs' test. May increase BUN, creatinine, uric acid, SGOT (AST). May decrease creatinine clearance, calcium, magnesium, phosphate, potassium, sodium.

AVAILABILITY (Rx)

INJECTION: 10 mg, 50 mg, 100 mg vials.

ADMINISTRATION/HANDLING

Note: Wear protective gloves during handling of cisplatin. Do not use aluminum needles or administration sets that may come in contact with drug; may cause formation of black precipitate, loss of potency. May be carcinogenic, mutagenic, or teratogenic. Handle with extreme care during preparation/administration.

IV 🔲

Storage:

• Following reconstitution, solution should appear clear, colorless. • Protect from direct bright sunlight; do not refrigerate (may precipitate). • Discard if precipitate forms. • Stable for 20 hrs at room temperature.

Reconstitution:

• Reconstitute 10 mg vial with 10 ml Sterile Water for Injection (50 ml for 50 mg vial) to provide concentration of 1 mg/ml. • For IV infusion, dilute desired dose in up to 1,000 ml D_5W, 0.33% or 0.45% NaCl containing 18.75 g mannitol/L.

Rate of administration:

• Infuse over 2–24 hrs. • Avoid rapid infusion (increases risk of nephrotoxicity, ototoxicity). • Monitor for anaphylactic reaction during first few minutes of IV infusion.

IV INCOMPATIBILITIES ⊘

Amifostine (Ethyol), amphotericin B complex (Ambisome, Amphotec, Abelcet), cefepime (Maxipime), piperacillin/tazobactam (Zosyn), thiotepa.

IV COMPATIBILITIES

Etoposide (Vepesed), granisetron (Kytril), ondansetron (Zofran).

INDICATIONS/ROUTES/DOSAGE

Note: Verify any cisplatin dose exceeding 120 mg/m^2 per course. Dosage individualized based on clinical response, tolerance to adverse effects. When used in combination therapy, consult specific protocols for optimum dosage, sequence of drug administration. Repeat courses should not be given more frequently than q3–4wks. Do not repeat unless auditory acuity within normal limits,

---

serum creatinine below 1.5 mg/dl, BUN below 25 mg/dl, circulating blood elements (platelets, WBC) are within acceptable levels.

Metastatic testicular tumors:

IV: Adults: (Combined with bleomycin, vinblastine): 20 mg/m^2/day for 5 days q3wks for 3–4 courses of therapy.

Metastatic ovarian tumors:

IV: Adults: (Combined with doxorubicin): 50 mg/m^2 once q3–4wks. *Single:* 100 mg/m^2 once q4wks.

Advanced bladder cancer:

IV: Adults: Single: 50–70 mg/m^2 q3–4wks.

SIDE EFFECTS

FREQUENT: Nausea, vomiting (begins 1–4 hrs after administration, generally last up to 24 hrs). Myelosuppression occurs in 25–30% of pts. Recovery can generally be expected in 18–23 days. ***OCCASIONAL:*** Peripheral neuropathy (numbness, tingling of fingers, toes, face) may occur with prolonged therapy (4–7 mos), pain/redness at injection site, loss of taste/appetite. ***RARE:*** Hemolytic anemia, blurred vision, stomatitis.

ADVERSE REACTIONS/TOXIC EFFECTS

Anaphylactic reaction (facial edema, wheezing, tachycardia, hypotension) may occur in first few minutes of IV administration in those previously exposed to cisplatin. Nephrotoxicity in 28–36% of pts treated with single dose of cisplatin, usually during second week of therapy. Ototoxicity (tinnitus, hearing loss) in 31% of pts treated with single dose of cisplatin (more severe in children). May become more frequent, severe with repeated doses.

NURSING IMPLICATIONS

BASELINE ASSESSMENT:

Pts should be well hydrated prior to and 24 hrs after medication to ensure good urinary output, decrease risk of nephrotoxicity.

INTERVENTION/EVALUATION:

Measure all vomitus (general guideline requiring immediate notification of physician: 750 ml/8 hrs, urinary output less than 100 ml/hr). Monitor I&O q1–2h beginning with pretreatment hydration, continue for 48 hrs after cisplatin therapy. Assess vital signs q1–2h during infusion. Monitor urinalysis, renal function reports for nephrotoxicity.

PATIENT/FAMILY TEACHING:

Report signs of ototoxicity (ringing/roaring in ears, hearing loss). Do not have immunizations without physician's approval (lowers body's resistance). Avoid contact with those who have recently taken oral polio vaccine. Contact physician if nausea/vomiting continues at home. Teach signs of peripheral neuropathy.

citalopram hydrobromide

sigh-**tail**-oh-pram high-dro-**broh**-mide

(Celexa)

Do not confuse with Zyprexa, Celebrex.

▶CLASSIFICATION

PHARMACOTHERAPEUTIC: Serotonin reuptake inhibitor. ***CLINICAL:*** Antidepressant (see p. 35C)

ACTION/*THERAPEUTIC EFFECT*

Blocks uptake of the neurotransmitter serotonin at CNS neuronal presynaptic membranes, increasing availability at post-synaptic receptor sites. Resulting enhancement of postsynaptic activity *produces antidepressant effect.*

PHARMACOKINETICS

Well absorbed following PO administration. Protein binding: 80%. Primarily metabolized in the liver. Primarily excreted in the feces with a lesser amount eliminated in the urine. Half-life: 35 hrs.

USES/*UNLABELED*

Treatment of major depressive disorder exhibited as persistent, prominent dysphoria (occurring nearly every day for at least 2 wks) manifested by 4 of 8 symptoms: appetite change, sleep pattern change, increased fatigue, impaired concentration, feelings of guilt or worthlessness, loss of interest in usual activities, psychomotor agitation or retardation, suicidal tendencies.

PRECAUTIONS

CONTRAINDICATIONS: Sensitivity to citalopram, concurrent use of MAO inhibitors. ***CAUTIONS:*** Liver/renal impairment, history of seizures, mania or hypomania.

▷***LIFESPAN CONSIDERATIONS:*** **Pregnancy/Lactation:** Distributed in breast milk. **Pregnancy Category C. Children:** May cause increased anticholinergic effects or hyperexcitability. **Elderly:** More sensitive to anticholinergic effects (e.g., dry mouth), more likely to experience dizziness, sedation, confusion, hypotension, hyperexcitability.

INTERACTIONS

DRUG: **MAO inhibitors** may cause serotonergic syndrome (excitement, diaphoresis, rigidity, hyperthermia, autonomic hyperactivity, coma). **Antifungals, macrolide antibiotics, cimetidine** may increase plasma levels; carbamazepine may decrease plasma levels. Increases **metoprolol** plasma levels. ***HERBAL:*** None known. ***FOOD:*** None known. ***LAB VALUES:*** May reduce serum sodium.

AVAILABILITY (Rx)

TABLETS: 20 mg, 40 mg. ***ORAL SOLUTION:*** 10 mg/5 ml.

ADMINISTRATION/HANDLING

PO:
• Give without regard to food. • Scored tablets may be crushed.

INDICATIONS/ROUTES/DOSAGE

Antidepressant:

PO: Adults: Initially, 20 mg once daily in the morning or evening. Dosage may be increased in increments of 20 mg at intervals of no less than 1 wk. **Maximum:** 60 mg/day. **Elderly, impaired hepatic function:** 20 mg/day. May titrate to 40 mg/day only for nonresponding pts.

SIDE EFFECTS

FREQUENT (11–21%): Nausea, dry mouth, somnolence, insomnia, excessive sweating. ***OCCASIONAL*** (4–8%): Tremor, diarrhea/loose stools, abnormal ejaculation, dyspepsia, fatigue, anxiety, vomiting, anorexia. ***RARE*** (2–3%): Sinusitis, sexual dysfunction, menstrual disorder, abdominal pain, agitation, decreased libido.

ADVERSE REACTIONS/TOXIC EFFECTS

Overdosage manifested as dizziness, drowsiness, tachycardia, severe somnolence, confusion, seizures.

NURSING IMPLICATIONS

BASELINE ASSESSMENT:

For those on long-term therapy, liver/renal function tests, blood counts should be performed periodically. Observe/record behavior. Assess psychological status, thought content, sleep pattern, appearance, interest in environment.

INTERVENTION/EVALUATION:

Supervise suicidal risk pt closely during early therapy (as energy level improves, suicide potential increases). Assess appearance, behavior, speech pattern, level of interest, mood.

PATIENT/FAMILY TEACHING:

Do not stop taking medication or increase dosage. Avoid use of alcohol. Avoid tasks that require alertness, motor skills until response to drug is established.

citrates

potassium citrate
(Urocit K)

potassium citrate and citric acid
(Polycitra-K)

sodium citrate and citric acid
(Bicitra)

tricitrates
(Polycitra syrup)

►CLASSIFICATION
CLINICAL: Alkalinizer

ACTION/*THERAPEUTIC EFFECT*

Increases urinary pH, increasing solubility of cystine in urine and ionization of uric acid to urate ion. Increasing urinary pH and urinary citrate decreases calcium ion activity and decreases saturation of calcium oxalate. Increases plasma bicarbonate, buffers excess hydrogen ion concentration, *increasing blood pH and reversing acidosis.*

USES

Treats/prevents uric acid/cystine lithiasis, prevents urate crystallization (increased urinary pH). Treats/prevents calcium phosphate, calcium oxalate or uric acid kidney stones (increase urinary citrate). Treats chronic metabolic acidosis. Neutralizes/buffers excess quantities of gastric hydrochloric acid.

PRECAUTIONS

CONTRAINDICATIONS: Aluminum toxicity, severe myocardial damage, heart failure, severe renal impairment, active urinary tract infection, hyperkalemia, peptic ulcer. ***CAUTIONS:*** Severe renal tubular acidosis.

INTERACTIONS

DRUG: May increase quinidine excretion. Antacids may increase risk of systemic alkalosis. NSAIDs, angiotensin-converting enzyme inhibitors, potassium-sparing diuretics, potassium-containing medication may increase risk of hyperkalemia. May decrease effect of methenamine. ***HERBAL:*** None known.

FOOD: None known. **LAB VALUES:** None significant.

AVAILABILITY (Rx)

TABLETS: 5 mEq, 10 mEq. **SYRUP. ORAL SOLUTION.**

INDICATIONS/ROUTES/DOSAGE

POTASSIUM CITRATE:

Antiurolithic, urinary alkalizer:

PO: Adults, elderly: 10 mEq 3 times/day up to 15 mEq 4 times/day or 20 mEq 3 times/day.

POTASSIUM CITRATE AND CITRIC ACID:

Antiurolithic, urinary/systemic alkalizer:

PO: Adults, elderly: 20–30 mEq 4 times/day. **Children:** 10–30 mEq 4 times/day.

SODIUM CITRATE AND CITRIC ACID:

Antiurolithic, urinary/systemic alkalizer:

PO: Adults, elderly: 10–30 mEq 4 times/day. **Maximum:** 150 mEq/day. **Children:** 5–15 mEq 4 times/day.

TRICITRATES:

Antiurolithic, urinary alkalizer:

PO: Adults, elderly: 15–30 mEq 4 times/day. **Children:** 5–10 mEq 4 times/day.

SIDE EFFECTS

OCCASIONAL: Diarrhea, mild abdominal pain, nausea, vomiting.

ADVERSE REACTIONS/TOXIC EFFECTS

Metabolic alkalosis, bowel obstruction/perforation, hyperkalemia, hypernatremia occur rarely.

NURSING IMPLICATIONS

INTERVENTION/EVALUATION:

Assess urinary pH, EKG in pts with cardiac disease, serum acid-base balance, CBC, hemoglobin, hematocrit, serum creatinine.

PATIENT/FAMILY TEACHING:

Take after meals. Mix in water or juice and follow with additional liquid if desired.

cladribine

clad-rih-bean
(Leustatin)

▶CLASSIFICATION

PHARMACOTHERAPEUTIC: Antimetabolite. **CLINICAL:** Antineoplastic (see p. 69C)

ACTION/THERAPEUTIC EFFECT

Disrupts cellular metabolism by incorporating into DNA of dividing cells. Cytotoxic to both actively dividing and quiescent lymphocytes and monocytes, *preventing DNA synthesis.*

PHARMACOKINETICS

Primarily excreted in urine. Half-life: 5.4 hrs.

USES/UNLABELED

Treatment for active hairy cell leukemia defined by clinically significant anemia, neutropenia, thrombocytopenia. *Chronic lymphocytic leukemia, non-Hodgkin's lymphoma, acute myeloid leukemia, autoimmune hemolytic anemia.*

PRECAUTIONS

CONTRAINDICATIONS: None significant. **CAUTIONS:** Renal/hepatic impairment, bone marrow suppression.

▷**LIFESPAN CONSIDERATIONS:**
Pregnancy/Lactation: May produce fetal harm; may be embryotoxic and fetotoxic; potential for serious reactions in nursing infants. **Pregnancy Category D.** **Children:** Safety and efficacy not established. **Elderly:** No age-related precautions noted.

INTERACTIONS

DRUG: Bone marrow depressants may increase bone marrow depression. High doses with **cyclophosphamide** and total body irradiation may cause severe, irreversible neurologic toxicity, acute renal dysfunction. **Nephrotoxic, neurotoxic medications** may increase toxicity. **Live virus vaccines** may potentiate virus replication, increase vaccine side effects, decrease pt's antibody response to vaccine. **HERBAL:** None known. **FOOD:** None known. **LAB VALUES:** None significant.

AVAILABILITY (Rx)

INJECTION: 1 mg/ml.

ADMINISTRATION/HANDLING

IV 🔲

Storage:

• Refrigerate unopened vials. • May refrigerate dilution solution for no more than 8 hrs before administration. • Solution is stable for at least 24 hrs at room temperature. • Discard unused portion.

Reconstitution:

• Must dilute before administration. • Wear gloves and protective clothing during handling; if contact with skin, rinse with copious amounts of water. • Add calculated dose (0.09 mg/kg) to 500 ml 0.9% NaCl. Avoid D_5W (increases degradation of medication).

Rate of administration:

• Monitor vital signs during infusion, esp. during first hour. Observe for hypotension or bradycardia (usually both do not occur during same course). • Immediately discontinue administration if severe hypersensitivity reaction occurs.

IV INCOMPATIBILITIES ⊘

Do not mix with other IV drugs, additives, or infuse concurrently via a common IV line.

INDICATIONS/ROUTES/DOSAGE

Hairy cell leukemia:

IV INFUSION: Adults, children: 0.09 mg/kg/day as continuous infusion for 7 days.

SIDE EFFECTS

FREQUENT: Fever (69%), fatigue (45%), nausea (28%), rash (27%), headache (22%), injection site reactions (19%), anorexia, anorexia (17%), vomiting (13%). **OCCASIONAL** (5–10%): Diarrhea, cough, purpura, chills, diaphoresis, constipation, dizziness, petechiae, myalgia, shortness of breath, malaise, pruritus, erythema, insomnia, edema, tachycardia, abdominal/trunk pain, epistaxis, arthralgia.

ADVERSE REACTIONS/TOXIC EFFECTS

Myelosuppression characterized as severe neutropenia (<500 cells/mm^3); severe anemia (hemoglobin <8.5 g/dl) and thrombocytopenia occur commonly. High-dose treatment may produce acute nephrotoxicity and/or neurotoxicity manifested as irreversible motor weakness of upper or lower extremities.

NURSING IMPLICATIONS

BASELINE ASSESSMENT:

Offer emotional support to pt

---

and family. Perform neurologic function tests before chemotherapy. Use strict asepsis and protect pt from infection.

INTERVENTION/EVALUATION:

Monitor temperature and report fever promptly. Assess for signs of infection. Assess skin for evidence of rash, purpure, petechaie.

PATIENT/FAMILY TEACHING:

Narrow margin between therapeutic and toxic response. Avoid crowds, persons with known infections; report signs of infection at once (fever, flulike symptoms). Do not have immunizations without physician's approval (drug lowers body's resistance). Avoid contact with those who have recently received live virus vaccine. Women of childbearing potential should not become pregnant during treatment.

---

clarithromycin ✐

clair-**rith**-row-my-sin
(<u>Biaxin</u>, Biaxin XL)

▶CLASSIFICATION

PHARMACOTHERAPEUTIC:
Macrolide. ***CLINICAL:*** Antibiotic (see p. 23C).

ACTION/THERAPEUTIC EFFECT

Bacteriostatic. Binds to ribosomal receptor sites, *inhibiting protein synthesis.* May be bactericidal with high dosage or very susceptible microorganisms.

PHARMACOKINETICS

Well absorbed from GI tract. Protein binding: 65–75%. Widely distributed. Metabolized in liver to active metabolite. Primarily excreted in urine. Not removed by hemodialysis. Half-life: 3–7 hrs; metabolite: 5–7 hrs (half-life increased with impaired renal function).

USES

Treatment of bacterial exacerbation of bronchitis, otitis media, acute maxillary sinusitis, Mycobacterium avium complex (MAC), pharyngitis, tonsillitis, *H. pylori* duodenal ulcer, bacterial pneumonia, skin/soft tissue infections. Prevention of MAC disease. ***Biaxin XL:*** Treatment of community-acquired pneumonia.

PRECAUTIONS

CONTRAINDICATIONS: Hypersensitivity to clarithromycin, erythromycins, any macrolide antibiotic. ***CAUTIONS:*** Hepatic and renal dysfunction, elderly with severe renal impairment.

▷***LIFESPAN CONSIDERATIONS:***
Pregnancy/Lactation: Unknown if distributed in breast milk. **Pregnancy Category C. Children:** Safety and efficacy not established in those <6 mos. **Elderly:** Age-related renal impairment may require dosage adjustment.

INTERACTIONS

DRUG: May increase concentration, toxicity of **carbamazepine, digoxin, theophylline.** May decrease concentration of **zidovudine.** May increase **warfarin** effects. **Rifampin** may decrease clarithromycin concentrations. ***HERBAL:*** None known. ***FOOD:*** None known. ***LAB VALUES:*** May rarely increase SGOT (AST), SGPT (ALT), BUN.

AVAILABILITY (Rx)

TABLETS: 250 mg, 500 mg. -

TABLETS (extended-release). ORAL SUSPENSION: 125 mg/5 ml, 250 mg/5 ml.

ADMINISTRATION/HANDLING
PO:
• Give without regard to food. • Do not crush/break tablets.

INDICATIONS/ROUTES/DOSAGE
Bronchitis (due to *H. influenzae*):
PO: **Adults, elderly:** 500 mg q12h for 7–14 days.

Bronchitis, pneumonia, skin/soft tissue infections:
PO: **Adults, elderly:** 250 mg for 7–14 days. *Extended-Release: (Community-acquired pneumonia):* 500 mg once daily for 7 days.

MAC prevention:
PO: **Adults, elderly:** 500 mg 2 times/day.

MAC treatment:
PO: **Adults, elderly:** 500 mg 2 times/day (in combination with other antimycobacterial agents).

Pharyngitis, tonsillitis:
PO: **Adults, elderly:** 250 mg q12h for 10 days.

Sinusitis:
PO: **Adults, elderly:** 500 mg q12h for 14 days.

H. pylori:
PO: **Adults:** 500 mg 2–3 times/day.

Usual pediatric dosage:
PO: **Children: (6 mos–12 yrs):** 7.5 mg/kg q12h. **Maximum:** 1 g/day.

Dosage in renal impairment:
Creatinine clearance <30 ml/min: Decrease dose by 50% and administer once or twice daily.

SIDE EFFECTS
OCCASIONAL (3–6%): Diarrhea, nausea, altered taste, abdominal pain. *RARE* (1–2%): Headache, dyspepsia.

ADVERSE REACTIONS/TOXIC EFFECTS
Antibiotic-associated colitis (severe abdominal pain and tenderness, fever, watery and severe diarrhea), other superinfections may result from altered bacterial balance. Hepatotoxicity, thrombocytopenia occur rarely.

NURSING IMPLICATIONS
BASELINE ASSESSMENT:
Question pt for history of hepatitis or allergies to clarithromycin, erythromycins.

INTERVENTION/EVALUATION:
Monitor bowel activity and stool consistency carefully; mild GI effects may be tolerable, but increasing severity may indicate onset of antibiotic-associated colitis. Be alert for superinfection: genital/anal pruritus, abdominal pain, mouth soreness, moderate to severe diarrhea.

PATIENT/FAMILY TEACHING:
Continue therapy for full length of treatment. Doses should be evenly spaced. Take medication with 8 oz water without regard to food.

clemastine fumarate

kleh-**mass**-teen
(Tavist, Tavist-1)

FIXED-COMBINATION(S)

With phenylpropanolamine, a nasal decongestant **(Tavist-D)**

▶CLASSIFICATION

PHARMACOTHERAPEUTIC:
Ethanolamine. **CLINICAL:** Antihistamine (see p. 48C)

ACTION/THERAPEUTIC EFFECT

Competes with histamine at histaminic receptor sites, *relieving allergic conditions (urticaria, pruritus)*. Anticholinergic effects cause drying of nasal mucosa.

PHARMACOKINETICS

Onset	Peak	Duration
PO		
15–60 min	5–7 hrs	10–12 hrs

Well absorbed from GI tract. Metabolized in liver. Excreted primarily in urine.

USES

Relief of allergic conditions (nasal allergies, allergic dermatitis), cold symptoms, hypersensitivity reaction.

PRECAUTIONS

CONTRAINDICATIONS: Acute asthmatic attack, those receiving MAO inhibitors. **CAUTIONS:** Narrow-angle glaucoma, peptic ulcer, prostatic hypertrophy, pyloroduodenal or bladder neck obstruction, asthma, COPD, increased intraocular pressure, cardiovascular disease, hyperthyroidism, hypertension, seizure disorders.

▷**LIFESPAN CONSIDERATIONS:**
Pregnancy/Lactation: Crosses placenta; detected in breast milk (may produce irritability in nursing infants). Increased risk of seizures in neonates, premature infants if used during third trimester of pregnancy. May pro-hibit lactation. **Pregnancy Category B. Children:** Safety and efficacy not established in those <6 yrs. **Elderly:** Age-related renal impairment may require dosage adjustment.

INTERACTIONS

DRUG: Alcohol, CNS depressants may increase CNS depressant effects. MAO inhibitors may increase anticholinergic, CNS depressant effects. **HERBAL:** None known. **FOOD:** None known. **LAB VALUES:** May suppress wheal, flare reactions to antigen skin testing, unless antihistamines discontinued 4 days prior to testing.

AVAILABILITY (Rx)

TABLETS: 1.34 mg, 2.68 mg. **SYRUP:** 0.67 mg/5 ml.

ADMINISTRATION/HANDLING

PO:

• Give without regard to meals. • Scored tablets may be crushed. Do not crush extended-release or film-coated forms.

INDICATIONS/ROUTES/DOSAGE

Allergic rhinitis:

PO: Adults, children >12 yrs: 1.34 mg 2 times/day. May increase dose to maximum 8.04 mg/day, if needed. **Children 6–11 yrs:** 0.67 mg 2 times/day. May increase dose to maximum 4.02 mg/day, if needed.

Allergic urticaria, angioedema:

PO: Adults, children >12 yrs: 2.68 1–3 times/day. Do not exceed 8.04 mg/day. **Children 6–11 yrs:** 1.34 mg 2 times/day. Do not exceed 4.02 mg/day.

Usual elderly dosage:

PO: 1.34 mg 1–2 times/day.

SIDE EFFECTS

Note: Fixed-combination form (Tavist-D) may produce mild CNS stimulation.

FREQUENT: Drowsiness, dizziness, dry mouth/nose/throat, urinary retention, thickening of bronchial secretions. **Elderly:** Sedation, dizziness, hypotension. ***OCCASIONAL:*** Epigastric distress, flushing, blurred vision, tinnitus, paresthesia, sweating, chills.

ADVERSE REACTIONS/TOXIC EFFECTS

Children may experience dominant paradoxical reaction (restlessness, insomnia, euphoria, nervousness, tremors). Overdosage in children may result in hallucinations, convulsions, death. Hypersensitivity reaction (eczema, pruritus, rash, cardiac disturbances, angioedema, photosensitivity) may occur. Overdosage may vary from CNS depression (sedation, apnea, cardiovascular collapse, death) to severe paradoxical reaction (hallucinations, tremor, seizures).

NURSING IMPLICATIONS

BASELINE ASSESSMENT:

If pt is undergoing allergic reaction, obtain history of recently ingested foods, drugs, environmental exposure, recent emotional stress. Monitor rate, depth, rhythm, type of respiration; quality and rate of pulse. Assess lung sounds for rhonchi, wheezing, rales.

INTERVENTION/EVALUATION:

Monitor B/P, esp. in elderly (increased risk of hypotension). Monitor children closely for paradoxical reaction.

📍 - see color pill atlas

PATIENT/FAMILY TEACHING:

Tolerance to antihistaminic effect generally does not occur; tolerance to sedative effect may occur. Avoid tasks that require alertness, motor skills until response to drug is established. Dry mouth, drowsiness, dizziness may be an expected response of drug. Avoid alcoholic beverages during antihistamine therapy. Coffee or tea may help reduce drowsiness.

clindamycin hydrochloride

klin-da-**my**-sin
(Cleocin HCL, Dalacin🍁)

clindamycin palmitate hydrochloride

(Cleocin Pediatric)

clindamycin phosphate

(Cleocin phosphate, Cleocin T)

▶CLASSIFICATION

PHARMACOTHERAPEUTIC: Lincosamide. ***CLINICAL:*** Antibiotic

ACTION/THERAPEUTIC EFFECT

Bacteriostatic. Binds to ribosomal receptor sites, *inhibiting protein synthesis.* Topically, decreases fatty acid concentration on skin, *preventing acne vulgaris breakout.*

PHARMACOKINETICS

Rapidly absorbed from GI tract. Widely distributed. Protein binding: 92–94%. Metabolized in liver to some active metabolites. Primarily excreted in urine. Not removed by hemodialysis. Half-life: 2.4–3 hrs (half-life increased with impaired renal function, premature infants).

C

USES/*UNLABELED*

Treatment of respiratory tract, skin/soft tissue, chronic bone/joint infections, septicemia, intra-abdominal, female GU infections, bacterial vaginosis, endocarditis. *Topical:* Acne vulgaris. *Treatment of malaria, otitis media, PCP, toxoplasmosis.*

PRECAUTIONS

CONTRAINDICATIONS: Hypersensitivity to clindamycin or lincomycin, known allergy to tartrazine dye, history of ulcerative colitis, regional enteritis, or antibiotic-associated colitis. ***CAUTIONS:*** Severe renal or hepatic dysfunction, concomitant use of neuromuscular blocking agents, neonates. Topical preparations should not be applied to abraded areas or near eyes.
▷*LIFESPAN CONSIDERATIONS:*
Pregnancy/Lactation: Readily crosses placenta; distributed in breast milk. **Pregnancy Category B.** *Topical/vaginal:* Unknown if distributed in breast milk. **Children:** Caution in those < 1 mo of age. **Elderly:** No age-related precautions noted.

INTERACTIONS

DRUG:* Adsorbent antidiarrheals** may delay absorption. **Chloramphenicol, erythromycin** may antagonize effects. May increase effect of **neuromuscular blockers.** ***HERBAL: None known. ***FOOD:*** None known. ***LAB VALUES:*** May increase SGOT (AST), SGPT (ALT), alkaline phosphatase.

AVAILABILITY (Rx)

CAPSULES: 75 mg, 150 mg, 300 mg. ***ORAL SOLUTION:*** 75 mg/5 ml. ***INJECTION:*** 150 mg/ml. ***VAGINAL CREAM:*** 2%. ***VAGINAL SUPPOSITORY. LOTION. TOPICAL SOLUTION.***

ADMINISTRATION/HANDLING

Note: Space doses evenly around the clock. May be given by IM injection, intermittent IV infusion (piggyback).

PO:

* Store capsules at room temperature. * After reconstitution, oral solution is stable for 2 wks at room temperature. * Do not refrigerate oral solution (avoids thickening). * Give with 8 oz water. May give without regard to food.

IM:

* Do not exceed 600 mg/dose. * Administer deep IM.

IV

Storage:
* IV infusion (piggyback) is stable for 16 days at room temperature.

Reconstitution:
* Dilute 300–600 mg with 50 ml D₅W or 0.9% NaCl (900–1,200 mg with 100 ml). * Never exceed concentration of 18 mg/ml.

Rate of administration:
* 50 ml (300–600 mg) piggyback is infused >10–20 min; 100 ml (900 mg–1.2 g) piggyback is infused >30–40 min. Severe hypotension/cardiac arrest can occur with too rapid administration. * No more than 1.2 g should be given in 1 infusion.

IV INCOMPATIBILITIES ⊘

Allopurinol (Aloprim), filgrastim (Neupogen), fluconazole (Diflucan), idarubicin (Idamycin).

IV COMPATIBILITIES

Amiodarone (Cordarone), diltiazem (Cardizem), heparin, magnesium, multivitamins, propofol (Diprivan).

INDICATIONS/ROUTES/DOSAGE

Usual adult dosage:

IM/IV: 300–600 mg q6–8h or 900 mg q8h. **Maximum:** 2.7 g/day.

PO: 150–300 mg q6h.

Usual dosage for children:

IM/IV: **(>1 mo):** 3.75–10 mg/kg q6h or 5–13.3 mg/kg q8h. **(<1 mo):** 3.75–5 mg/kg q6h or 5–6.7 mg/kg q8h.

PO: **(>1 mo):** 2–5 mg/kg q6h or 2.7–6.7 mg/kg q8h.

Bacterial vaginosis:

INTRAVAGINAL: **Adults:** One applicatorful at bedtime for 3–7 days or 1 suppository at bedtime for 3 days.

Acne vulgaris:

TOPICAL: **Adults:** Apply thin film 2 times/day to affected area.

SIDE EFFECTS

FREQUENT: Abdominal pain, nausea, vomiting, diarrhea. *Vaginal:* Vaginitis, itching. *Topical:* Dry scaly skin. *OCCASIONAL:* Phlebitis, thrombophlebitis with IV administration; pain, induration at IM injection site; allergic reaction, urticaria, pruritus. *Vaginal:* Headache, dizziness, nausea, vomiting, abdominal pain. *Topical:* Contact dermatitis, abdominal pain, mild diarrhea, stinging/burning. *RARE: Vaginal:* Hypersensitivity reaction.

ADVERSE REACTIONS/TOXIC EFFECTS

Antibiotic-associated colitis (severe abdominal pain and tenderness, fever, watery and severe diarrhea), during and several weeks after therapy (including topical), may occur. Blood dyscrasias (leukopenia, thrombocytopenia), nephrotoxicity (proteinuria, azotemia, oliguria) occur rarely.

NURSING IMPLICATIONS

BASELINE ASSESSMENT:

Question pt for history of allergies, particularly to clindamycin, lincomycin, aspirin. Avoid, if possible, concurrent use of neuromuscular blocking agents.

INTERVENTION/EVALUATION:

Monitor bowel activity, stool consistency; report diarrhea promptly due to potential for serious colitis (even with topical or vaginal). Assess skin for rash (dryness, irritation) with topical application. With all routes of administration, assess for superinfection: severe diarrhea, anal/genital pruritus, increased fever, change of oral mucosa.

PATIENT/FAMILY TEACHING:

Continue therapy for full length of treatment. Doses should be evenly spaced. Take oral doses with 8 oz water. Caution should be used when applying topical clindamycin concurrently with peeling, abrasive acne agents, soaps, or alcohol-containing cosmetics to avoid cumulative effect. Do not apply topical preparations near eyes or abraded areas. *Vaginal:* In event of accidental contact with eyes, rinse with copious amounts of cool tap water. Do not engage in sexual intercourse during treatment.

◊ - see color pill atlas

clobetasol

(Temovate)

See Classification section under: Corticosteroids; topical (p. 81C)

clofibrate

(Atromid-S)

See Classification section under: Antihyperlipidemics (p. 50C)

clomipramine hydrochloride

klow-**mih**-prah-meen
(Anafranil)

▶CLASSIFICATION

PHARMACOTHERAPEUTIC: Tricyclic. **CLINICAL:** Antidepressant (see p. 34C)

ACTION/*THERAPEUTIC EFFECT*

Blocks reuptake of neurotransmitters (norepinephrine, serotonin) at CNS presynaptic membranes, increasing availability at postsynaptic receptor sites, *reducing obsessive-compulsive behavior.* Strong anticholinergic activity.

USES/*UNLABELED*

Treatment of obsessive-compulsive disorder manifested as repetitive tasks producing marked distress, time-consuming, or significantly interfering with social or occupational behavior. *Treatment of men-tal depression, panic disorder, neurogenic pain, cataplexy associated with narcolepsy, bulimia.*

PRECAUTIONS

CONTRAINDICATIONS: Acute recovery period following MI, within 14 days of MAO inhibitor ingestion. **CAUTIONS:** Prostatic hypertrophy, history of urinary retention or obstruction, glaucoma, diabetes mellitus, history of seizures, hyperthyroidism, cardiac/hepatic/renal disease, schizophrenia, increased intraocular pressure, hiatal hernia.

INTERACTIONS

DRUG: Alcohol, CNS depressants may increase CNS, respiratory depression, hypotensive effects. Antithyroid agents may increase risk of agranulocytosis. Phenothiazines may increase sedative, anticholinergic effects. Cimetidine may increase concentration, toxicity. May decrease effects of clonidine, guanadrel. May increase cardiac effects with sympathomimetics. May increase risk of hypertensive crisis, hyperpyretic, convulsions with MAO inhibitors. **HERBAL:** None known. **FOOD:** None known. **LAB VALUES:** May alter EKG readings, glucose.

AVAILABILITY (Rx)

CAPSULES: 25 mg, 50 mg, 75 mg.

INDICATIONS/ROUTES/DOSAGE

Obsessive-compulsive disorder:

PO: Adults: Initially, 25 mg/day. Gradually increase over 2 wks to 100 mg/day in divided doses. May further increase over several weeks to 250 mg/day in divided doses. After titration, may give as single bedtime dose (reduces daytime sedation). **Children >10**

---

yrs: Initially, 25 mg/day. Gradually increase over 2 wks to 3 mg/kg or 100 mg/day in divided doses (whichever is less). May then increase over several weeks up to 3 mg/kg or 200 mg (whichever is less). **Maintenance:** Lowest effective dose.

SIDE EFFECTS

FREQUENT: Drowsiness, fatigue, dry mouth, blurred vision, constipation, sexual dysfunction (42%), ejaculatory failure (20%), impotence; weight gain (18%), delayed micturition, postural hypotension, excessive sweating, disturbed concentration, increased appetite, urinary retention. ***OCCASIONAL:*** GI disturbances (nausea, GI distress, metallic taste), asthenia, aggressiveness, muscle weakness. ***RARE:*** Paradoxical reactions (agitation, restlessness, nightmares, insomnia, extrapyramidal symptoms, particularly fine hand tremor), laryngitis, seizures.

ADVERSE REACTIONS/TOXIC EFFECTS

High dosage may produce cardiovascular effects (severe postural hypotension, dizziness, tachycardia, palpitations, arrhythmias) and seizures. May also result in altered temperature regulation (hyperpyrexia or hypothermia). Abrupt withdrawal from prolonged therapy may produce headache, malaise, nausea, vomiting, vivid dreams. Anemia has been noted.

NURSING IMPLICATIONS

INTERVENTION/EVALUATION:

Supervise suicidal risk pt closely during early therapy (as depression lessens, energy level improves, increasing suicide potential). Assess appearance, be-

havior, speech pattern, level of interest, mood.

PATIENT/FAMILY TEACHING:

Tolerance to postural hypotension, sedative, and anticholinergic effects usually develops during early therapy. Maximum therapeutic effect may be noted in 2–4 wks. Do not abruptly discontinue medication. Avoid tasks that require alertness, motor skills until response to drug is established. Avoid alcohol.

clonazepam

klon-**nah**-zih-pam
(Klonopin, Rivotril✦)
Do not confuse with clonidine.

▶CLASSIFICATION

PHARMACOTHERAPEUTIC: Benzodiazepine. ***CLINICAL:*** Anticonvulsant (see pp. 10C, 32C)

ACTION/*THERAPEUTIC EFFECT*

Elevates seizure threshold in response to electrical/chemical stimulation by enhancing presynaptic inhibition in CNS, *suppressing seizure activity.*

PHARMACOKINETICS

Well absorbed from GI tract. Protein binding: 85%. Metabolized in liver. Excreted in urine. Not removed by hemodialysis. Half-life: 18–50 hrs.

USES/*UNLABELED*

Adjunct in treatment of Lennox-Gastaut syndrome (petit mal variant epilepsy), akinetic, and myoclonic seizures, absence seizures (petit mal). Treatment of panic disorder. *Adjunct treatment of seizures, treatment of simple/complex partial seizures, tonic-clonic seizures.*

PRECAUTIONS

CONTRAINDICATIONS: Significant liver disease, narrow-angle glaucoma. ***CAUTIONS:*** Impaired kidney/liver function, chronic respiratory disease.

▷***LIFESPAN CONSIDERATIONS:***
Pregnancy/Lactation: Crosses placenta, may be distributed in breast milk. Chronic ingestion during pregnancy may produce withdrawal symptoms, CNS depression in neonates. **Pregnancy Category C. Children:** Long-term use may adversely affect physical/mental development. **Elderly:** Usually more sensitive to CNS effects (e.g., ataxia, dizziness, oversedation). Use low dose, increase gradually.

INTERACTIONS

DRUG:* Alcohol, CNS depressants** may increase CNS depressant effect. ***HERBAL:* Kava kava** may increase CNS sedation. ***FOOD: None known. ***LAB VALUES:*** None significant.

AVAILABILITY (Rx)

TABLETS: 0.125 mg, 0.25 mg, 0.5 mg, 1 mg, 2 mg.

ADMINISTRATION/HANDLING

PO:

• Give without regard to meals. • Tablets may be crushed.

INDICATIONS/ROUTES/DOSAGE

Anticonvulsant:

Note: When replacement by another anticonvulsant is necessary, decrease clonazepam gradually as therapy begins with low replacement dose.

***PO:* Adults, elderly:** 1.5 mg daily. Dosage may be increased in 0.5–1 mg increments at 3 day intervals until seizures are controlled. Do not exceed maintenance dose of 20 mg daily. **Infants, children <10 yrs, or <66 lbs:** 0.01–0.03 mg/kg daily in 2–3 divided doses. Dosage may be increased in up to 0.5 mg increments at 3 day intervals until seizures are controlled. Do not exceed maintenance dose of 0.2 mg/kg daily.

Panic disorder:

***PO:* Adults:** Initially 0.25 mg 2 times/day. Increase up to target dose of 1 mg/day after 3 days.

SIDE EFFECTS

FREQUENT: Mild, transient drowsiness, ataxia, behavioral disturbances (esp. in children) manifested as aggression, irritability, agitation. ***OCCASIONAL:*** Rash, ankle/facial edema, nocturia, dysuria, change in appetite/weight, dry mouth, sore gums, nausea, blurred vision. ***RARE:*** Paradoxical reaction (hyperactivity/nervousness in children, excitement/restlessness in elderly—particularly noted in presence of uncontrolled pain).

ADVERSE REACTIONS/TOXIC EFFECTS

Abrupt withdrawal may result in pronounced restlessness, irritability, insomnia, hand tremors, abdominal/muscle cramps, sweating, vomiting, status epilepticus. Overdosage results in somnolence, confusion, diminished reflexes, coma.

NURSING IMPLICATIONS

BASELINE ASSESSMENT:

Review history of seizure disorder (frequency, duration, intensity, level of consciousness). Implement safety measures and observe frequently for recurrence of seizure activity.

INTERVENTION/EVALUATION:
Assess children, elderly for paradoxical reaction, particularly during early therapy. Assist with ambulation if drowsiness, ataxia occur. For those on long-term therapy, liver/renal function tests, blood counts should be performed periodically. Evaluate for therapeutic response: a decrease in intensity/frequency of seizures.

PATIENT/FAMILY TEACHING:
Drowsiness usually diminishes with continued therapy. Avoid tasks that require alertness, motor skills until response to drug is established. Smoking reduces drug effectiveness. Do not abruptly withdraw medication after long-term therapy. Strict maintenance of drug therapy is essential for seizure control. Avoid alcohol.

clonidine

klon-ih-deen
(Catapres TTS, Dixarit✦)

clonidine hydrochloride

(Catapres, Duraclon)

FIXED-COMBINATION(S)
With chlorthalidone, a diuretic
(Combipres)
Do not confuse with Klonopin.

▶CLASSIFICATION

PHARMACOTHERAPEUTIC:
Antiandrenergic, sympatholytic.
CLINICAL: Antihypertensive
(see p. 51C)

ACTION/*THERAPEUTIC EFFECT*
Stimulates alpha$_2$-adrenergic receptors in CNS (inhibits sympathetic cardioaccelerator and vasoconstrictor center); decreases sympathetic outflow from CNS. *Reduces peripheral resistance, decreases B/P, heart rate.*

PHARMACOKINETICS

Onset	Peak	Duration
PO		
0.5–1 hr	2–4 hrs	up to 8 hrs

Well absorbed from GI tract. Transdermal best absorbed from chest, upper arm; least absorbed from thigh. Protein binding: 20–40%. Metabolized in liver. Primarily excreted in urine. Minimal removal by hemodialysis. Half-life: 12–16 hrs (half-life increased with impaired renal function).

USES/*UNLABELED*

Treatment of hypertension alone or in combination with other antihypertensive agents. Treatment of severe pain in cancer pts. *Diagnosis of pheochromocytoma, prevents migraine headaches, treatment of dysmenorrhea/menopausal flushing, opioid withdrawal. Attentiaon deficit hyperactivity disorder (ADHD).*

PRECAUTIONS

CONTRAINDICATIONS: None significant. *CAUTIONS:* Severe coronary insufficiency, recent MI, cerebrovascular disease, chronic renal failure, Raynaud's disease, thromboangiitis obliterans.

▷*LIFESPAN CONSIDERATIONS:*
Pregnancy/Lactation: Crosses placenta; distributed in breast milk. **Pregnancy Category C. Children:** More sensitive to effects, use caution. **Elderly:** May be more sensitive to hypotensive effect. Age-related renal impairment may require dosage adjustment.

C

INTERACTIONS

DRUG: **Tricyclic antidepressants** may decrease effect. Discontinuing concurrent **beta-blockers** may increase risk of clonidine-withdrawal hypertensive crisis. ***HERBAL:*** None known. ***FOOD:*** None known. ***LAB VALUES:*** None significant.

AVAILABILITY (Rx)

TABLETS: 0.1 mg, 0.2 mg, 0.3 mg. ***TRANSDERMAL PATCH:*** 2.5 mg (release at 0.1 mg/24 hrs), 5 mg (release at 0.2 mg/24 hrs), 7.5 mg (release at 0.3 mg/24 hrs). ***INJECTION:*** 100 mcg/ml, 500 mcg/ml

ADMINISTRATION/HANDLING

PO:

• Give without regard to food. • Tablets may be crushed. • Give last oral dose just before retiring.

Transdermal:

• Apply transdermal system to dry, hairless area of intact skin on upper arm or chest. • Rotate sites (prevents skin irritation). • Do not trim patch to adjust dose.

INDICATIONS/ROUTES/DOSAGE

Hypertension:

PO: **Adults:** Initially, 0.1 mg 2 times/day. Increase by 0.1–0.2 mg q2–4days. **Maintenance:** 0.2–1.2 mg/day in 2–4 divided doses up to maximum of 2.4 mg/day. **Children:** 5–25 mcg/kg/day in divided doses q6h; increase at 5–7 day intervals. **Maximum:** 0.9 mg/day.

TRANSDERMAL: **Adults, elderly:** System delivering 0.1 mg/24 hrs up to 0.6 mg/24 hrs every 7 days.

Usual elderly dosage:

PO: Initially, 0.1 mg at bedtime. May increase gradually.

ADHD:

PO: **Children:** 5 mcg/kg/day..

Severe pain:

EPIDURAL: **Adults, elderly:** 30–40 mcg/hr. **Children:** Initally, 0.5 mcq/kg/hr, not to exceed adult dose.

SIDE EFFECTS

FREQUENT: Dry mouth (40%), drowsiness (33%), dizziness (16%), sedation, constipation (10%). ***OCCASIONAL*** (1–5%): Depression, swelling of feet, loss of appetite, decreased sexual ability, itching eyes, dizziness, nausea, vomiting, nervousness. ***Transdermal:*** Itching, red skin, darkening of skin. ***RARE*** (<1%): Nightmares, vivid dreams, cold feeling in fingers/toes.

ADVERSE REACTIONS/TOXIC EFFECTS

Overdosage produces profound hypotension, irritability, bradycardia, respiratory depression, hypothermia, miosis (pupillary constriction), arrhythmias, apnea. Abrupt withdrawal may result in rebound hypertension associated with nervousness, agitation, anxiety, insomnia, hand tingling, tremor, flushing, sweating.

NURSING IMPLICATIONS

BASELINE ASSESSMENT:

Obtain B/P immediately before each dose is administered, in addition to regular monitoring (be alert to B/P fluctuations).

INTERVENTION/EVALUATION:

Monitor pattern of daily bowel activity and stool consistency. If clonidine is to be withdrawn, discontinue concurrent beta-blocker therapy several days before discontinuing clonidine (prevents clonidine withdrawal hypertensive crisis). Slowly reduce clonidine dose over 2–4 days.

PATIENT/FAMILY TEACHING:

Sugarless gum, sips of tepid water may relieve dry mouth. To reduce hypotensive effect, rise slowly from lying to sitting position and permit legs to dangle momentarily before standing. Skipping doses or voluntarily discontinuing drug may produce severe, rebound hypertension. Side effects tend to diminish during therapy.

clopidrogel

klow-**pih**-duh-grel
(Plavix)

▶CLASSIFICATION

PHARMACOTHERAPEUTIC: Thienopyridine derivative. **CLINICAL:** Antiplatelet (see p. 29C)

ACTION/THERAPEUTIC EFFECT

Inhibits binding of the enzyme adenosine phosphate (ADP) to its platelet receptor and subsequent ADP-mediated activation of a glycoprotein complex, *inhibiting platelet aggregation.*

PHARMACOKINETICS

	Onset	Peak	Duration
PO	1 hr	2 hrs	—

Rapidly absorbed. Protein binding: 98%. Extensively metabolized by the liver. Eliminated equally in the urine and feces. Half-life: 8 hrs.

USES

Reduction of myocardial infarction (MI), stroke, vascular death in pts with atherosclerosis documented by recent stroke, MI, or established peripheral arterial disease.

PRECAUTIONS

CONTRAINDICATIONS: Active pathologic bleeding (peptic ulcer, intracranial hemorrhage). **CAUTIONS:** Neutropenic pts, hepatic function impairment, those at risk of increased bleeding from trauma, surgery, or other pathologic conditions.

▷**LIFESPAN CONSIDERATIONS:**
Pregnancy/Lactation: Unknown if drug crosses placenta or is distributed in breast milk. **Pregnancy Category B. Children:** Safety and efficacy not established. **Elderly:** No age-related precautions noted.

INTERACTIONS

DRUG: May interfere with metabolism of **phenytoin, tamoxifen, tolbutamide, warfarin, torsemide, fluvastatin, other NSAIDs. HERBAL:** None known. **FOOD:** None known. **LAB VALUES:** Prolongs bleeding time.

AVAILABILITY (Rx)
TABLETS: 75 mg.

ADMINISTRATION/HANDLING
PO:

• Give without regard to food. •
Do not crush coated tablets.

INDICATIONS/ROUTES/DOSAGE
Inhibition of platelet aggregation:
PO: Adults, elderly: 75 mg once daily.

SIDE EFFECTS

FREQUENT (15%): Skin disorders. **OCCASIONAL** (6–8%): Upper respiratory tract infection, chest pain, flulike symptoms, headache, dizziness, arthralgia. **RARE** (3–5%): Fatigue, edema, hypertension, abdominal pain, dyspepsia, diarrhea, nausea, epistaxis, dyspnea, rhinitis.

ADVERSE REACTIONS/TOXIC EFFECTS

None significant.

NURSING IMPLICATIONS

BASELINE ASSESSMENT:

Perform platelet counts prior to drug therapy, q2days during the first week of treatment and weekly thereafter until therapeutic maintenance dose is reached. Abrupt discontinuation of drug therapy produces an elevation of platelet count within 5 days.

INTERVENTION/EVALUATION:

Monitor platelet count for evidence of thrombocytopenia. Assess BUN, creatinine, bilirubin, SGOT, SGPT, WBC, hemoglobin, blood tests, signs/symptoms of hepatic insufficiency during therapy.

PATIENT/FAMILY TEACHING:

Inform pt it may take longer to stop bleeding during drug therapy. Report any unusual bleeding. All physicians and dentists must be informed clopidogrel is being taken, esp. before surgery is scheduled or before taking any new drug.

---

clorazepate dipotassium ✳

klor-**az**-eh-payt
(Novoclopate ✦, Tranxene)

✦ - Canadian trade name

▶**CLASSIFICATION**

PHARMACOTHERAPEUTIC: Benzodiazepine. **CLINICAL:** Antianxiety, anticonvulsant (see p. 10C)

ACTION/THERAPEUTIC EFFECT

Enhances gamma-aminobutyric acid (GABA) neurotransmission at CNS, *producing anxiolytic effect.* Elevates seizure threshold in response to electrical/chemical stimulation by enhancing presynaptic inhibition in CNS, *suppressing seizure activity.*

USES

Management of anxiety disorders, short-term relief of anxiety symptoms, partial seizures, acute alcohol withdrawal symptoms.

PRECAUTIONS

CONTRAINDICATIONS: Acute narrow-angle glaucoma. **CAUTIONS:** Impaired renal/hepatic function, acute alcohol intoxication.

INTERACTIONS

DRUG: Alcohol, CNS depressants may increase CNS depressant effect. **HERBAL: Kava kava, valerian** may increase CNS depression. **FOOD:** None known. **LAB VALUES:** None significant. Therapeutic blood serum level: Peak: 0.12–1.5 mcg/ml; toxic serum level: >5 mcg/ml.

AVAILABILITY (Rx)

CAPSULES: 3.75 mg, 7.5 mg, 15 mg. **TABLETS:** 3.75 mg, 7.5 mg, 15 mg. **TABLETS (single dose):** 11.5 mg, 22.5 mg.

INDICATIONS/ROUTES/DOSAGE

Note: When replacement by another anticonvulsant is necessary, decrease clorazepate gradually as therapy begins with low-replacement dose.

Anxiety:

PO: Adults: 30 mg daily in divided doses. **Elderly, debilitated:** 7.5–15 mg in divided doses or single bedtime dose. **Daily dose range:** 15–60 mg.

Partial seizures:

PO: Adults, children >12 yrs: Initially, up to 7.5 mg 3 times daily. Do not increase dosage more than 7.5 mg/wk or exceed 90 mg/day. **Children 9–12 yrs:** 3.75–7.5 mg/dose 2 times/day. **Maximum:** 60 mg/day in 2–3 divided doses.

Alcohol withdrawal:

PO: Adults: Day 1: 30 mg followed by 30–60 mg in divided doses. **Day 2:** 45–90 mg in divided doses. **Day 3:** 22.5–45 mg in divided doses. **Day 4:** 15–30 mg in divided doses, then gradually reduce to 7.5–15 mg daily.

SIDE EFFECTS

FREQUENT: Drowsiness. **OCCASIONAL:** Dizziness, GI disturbances, nervousness, blurred vision, dry mouth, headache, confusion, ataxia, rash, irritability, slurred speech. **RARE:** Paradoxical CNS hyperactivity/nervousness in children, excitement/restlessness in elderly/debilitated (generally noted during first 2 wks of therapy, particularly noted in presence of uncontrolled pain).

ADVERSE REACTIONS/TOXIC EFFECTS

Abrupt or too rapid withdrawal may result in pronounced restlessness, irritability, insomnia, hand tremors, abdominal/muscle cramps, sweating, vomiting, seizures. Overdosage results in somnolence, confusion, diminished reflexes, coma.

NURSING IMPLICATIONS

BASELINE ASSESSMENT:

Anxiety: Assess autonomic response (cold, clammy hands, sweating) and motor response (agitation, trembling, tension). Offer emotional support to anxious pt. **Seizures:** Review history of seizure disorder (intensity, frequency, duration, LOC). Observe frequently for recurrence of seizure activity. Initiate seizure precautions.

INTERVENTION/EVALUATION:

Assess for paradoxical reaction, particularly during early therapy. Assist with ambulation if drowsiness, dizziness occur. Evaluate for therapeutic response: **Anxiety:** A calm facial expression; decreased restlessness. **Seizures:** A decrease in intensity or frequency of seizures. Therapeutic blood serum level: Peak: 0.12–1.5 mcg/ml; toxic serum level: >5 mcg/ml.

PATIENT/FAMILY TEACHING:

Do not abruptly withdraw medication following long-term use (may precipitate seizures). Strict maintenance of drug therapy is essential for seizure control. Drowsiness usually disappears during continued therapy. If dizziness occurs, change positions slowly from recumbent to sitting position before standing. Smoking reduces drug effectiveness. Avoid alcohol.

clotrimazole

kloe-**try**-mah-zole
(Canesten✚, Clotrimaderm✚, Gyne-Lotrimin, Lotrimin, Mycelex, Mycelex-G)

FIXED-COMBINATION(S)

With betamethasone dipropionate, a corticosteroid **(Lotrisone)**
Do not confuse with Myoflex.

▶CLASSIFICATION

PHARMACOTHERAPEUTIC:
Anti-infective. **CLINICAL:** Antifungal (see p. 42C)

ACTION/THERAPEUTIC EFFECT

Binds with phospholipids in fungal cell membrane. The altered cell membrane permeability *inhibits yeast growth.*

PHARMACOKINETICS

Poorly, erratically absorbed from GI tract. Bound to oral mucosa. Absorbed portion metabolized in liver. Eliminated in feces. **Topical:** Minimal systemic absorption (highest concentration in stratum corneum). **Intravaginal:** Small amount systemically absorbed.

USES/UNLABELED

Oral lozenges: Treatment/prophylaxis oropharyngeal candidiasis due to *Candida* sp. **Topical:** Treatment of tinea pedis, tinea cruris, tinea corporis, tinea versicolor, cutaneous candidiasis (moniliasis) due to *Candida albicans.* **Intravaginal:** Treatment of vulvovaginal candidiasis (moniliasis) due to *Candida* sp. **Topical:** *Treatment of paronychia, tinea barbae, tinea capitas.*

PRECAUTIONS

CONTRAINDICATIONS: Hypersensitivity to clotrimazole or any ingredient in preparation, children <3 yrs. **CAUTIONS:** Hepatic disorder with oral therapy.

▷**LIFESPAN CONSIDERATIONS:**
Pregnancy/Lactation: Pregnancy
Category B. Distribution in breast milk unknown. **Children:** No age-related precautions in those >5 yrs. **Elderly:** No age-related precautions noted.

INTERACTIONS

DRUG: None significant. **HERBAL:** None known. **FOOD:** None known. **LAB VALUES:** May increase SGOT (AST).

AVAILABILITY (Rx)

TROCHES: 10 mg. **VAGINAL TABLETS:** 100 mg, 500 mg. **VAGINAL CREAM:** 1%. **TOPICAL CREAM:** 1%. **TOPICAL SOLUTION:** 1%. **LOTION:** 1%.

ADMINISTRATION/HANDLING

PO:

• Lozenges must be dissolved in mouth >15–30 min for oropharyngeal therapy. • Swallow saliva.

Topical:

• Rub well into affected, surrounding areas. • Do not apply occlusive covering or other preparations.

Vaginal:

• Use vaginal applicator; insert high in vagina.

INDICATIONS/ROUTES/DOSAGE

Oral-local/oropharyngeal:

PO: Adults, elderly, children ≥3 yrs: 10 mg 5 times/day for 14 days.

Prophylaxis vs. oropharyngeal candidiasis:

PO: Adults, elderly: 10 mg 3 times/day.

Usual topical dosage:

TOPICAL: Adults, elderly, children ≥3 yrs: 2 times/day. Therapeutic effect may take up to 8 wks.

Vulvovaginal candidiasis:

VAGINAL: (tablets) Adults, elderly, children ≥12 yrs: 1 tablet (100 mg) at bedtime for 7 days; 2 tablets (200 mg) at bedtime for 3 days; or 500 mg tablet one time.

VAGINAL: (cream) Adults, elderly, children ≥12 yrs: 1 applicatorful at bedtime for 3–7 days.

SIDE EFFECTS

FREQUENT: PO: Nausea, vomiting, diarrhea, abdominal pain. **OCCASIONAL: Topical:** Itching, burning, stinging, erythema, urticaria. **Vaginal:** Mild burning (tablets/cream); irritation, cystitis (cream). **RARE: Vaginal:** Itching, rash, lower abdominal cramping, headache.

ADVERSE REACTIONS/TOXIC EFFECTS

None significant.

NURSING IMPLICATIONS

BASELINE ASSESSMENT:

Assess pt's ability to understand and follow directions regarding use of oral lozenges.

INTERVENTION/EVALUATION:

With oral therapy, assess for nausea, vomiting. Check skin for erythema, urticaria, blistering; inquire about itching, burning, stinging. With vaginal therapy, evaluate for vulvovaginal irritation, abdominal cramping, urinary frequency, discomfort.

PATIENT/FAMILY TEACHING:

Continue for full length of therapy. Inform physician of increased irritation. Avoid contact with eyes. **Topical:** Keep areas clean, dry; wear light clothing to promote ventilation. Separate personal items, linens. **Vaginal:** Continue use during menses. Refrain from sexual intercourse or advise partner to use condom during therapy.

cloxacillin

(Tegopen)

See Classification section under: Antibiotic: penicillins (p. 26C)

clozapine

klow-zah-peen
(Clozaril)
Do not confuse with Clinoril.

▶CLASSIFICATION

PHARMACOTHERAPEUTIC: Dibenzodiazepine derivative. **CLINICAL:** Antipsychotic (see p. 55C)

ACTION/THERAPEUTIC EFFECT

Interferes with the binding of dopamine at dopamine receptor sites (binds primarily at nondopamine receptor sites), *diminishing schizophrenic behavior.* Unlike other antipsychotics, produces few extrapyramidal effects.

USES

Management of severely ill schizophrenic pts who fail to respond to other antipsychotic therapy.

PRECAUTIONS

CONTRAINDICATIONS: Myeloproliferative disorders, history of clozapine-induced agranulocytosis or severe granulocytopenia, concurrent administration with other drugs having potential to suppress bone marrow function, severe CNS depression, comatose state. **CAUTIONS:** History of seizures, cardiovascular disease, impaired respiratory, hepatic, renal function, alcohol withdrawal, urinary retention, glaucoma, prostatic hypertrophy.

INTERACTIONS

DRUG: Alcohol, CNS depressants may increase CNS depressant effects. **Bone marrow depressants** may increase myelosuppression. **Lithium** may increase risk of seizures, confusion, dyskinesias. **Phenobarbital** decreases concentration. **HERBAL:** None known. **FOOD:** None known. **LAB VALUES:** None significant.

AVAILABILITY (Rx)

TABLETS: 25 mg, 100 mg.

ADMINISTRATION/HANDLING

PO:

• Give without regard to meals.

INDICATIONS/ROUTES/DOSAGE

Schizophrenic disorders:

PO: Adults: Initially, 25 mg 1–2 times/day. May increase by 25–50 mg/day over 2 wks until dose of 300–450 mg/day achieved. May further increase dose by 50–100 mg/day no more frequently than 1–2 times/wk. **Range:** 200–600 mg/day. **Maximum:** 900 mg/day.

Usual elderly dosage:

PO: Initially, 25 mg/day. May increase by 25 mg/day. **Maximum:** 450 mg/day.

SIDE EFFECTS

FREQUENT: Drowsiness (39%), salivation (31%), tachycardia (25%), dizziness (19%), constipation (14%). **OCCASIONAL:** Hypotension (9%), headache (7%); tremor, syncope, sweating, dry mouth (6%); nausea, visual disturbances (5%); nightmares, restlessness, akinesia, agitation, hypertension, abdominal discomfort/heartburn, weight gain (4%). **RARE:** Rigidity, confusion, fatigue, insomnia, diarrhea, rash.

ADVERSE REACTIONS/TOXIC EFFECTS

Seizures occur occasionally (3%). Overdosage produces CNS depression (sedation, coma, delirium), respiratory depression, hypersalivation. Blood dyscrasias, particularly agranulocytosis, mild leukopenia may occur.

NURSING IMPLICATIONS

BASELINE ASSESSMENT:

Obtain baseline WBC before initiating treatment and monitor WBC count every week for first 6 mos of continuous therapy, then biweekly for those with acceptable WBC counts. Assess behavior, appearance, emotional status, response to environment, speech pattern, thought content.

INTERVENTION/EVALUATION:

Monitor B/P for hyper/hypotension. Assess pulse for tachycardia (common side effect). Monitor CBC for blood dyscrasias. Supervise suicidal risk pt closely during early therapy (as depression lessens, energy level improves, increasing suicide potential). Assess for therapeutic response (interest in surroundings, improvement in self-care, increased ability to concentrate, relaxed facial expression).

PATIENT/FAMILY TEACHING:

Do not abruptly withdraw from

long-term drug therapy. Drowsiness generally subsides during continued therapy. Avoid tasks that require alertness, motor skills until response to drug is established. Avoid alcohol.

cocaine ✳

koe-**kane**
(Cocaine ♣, Cocaine HCl)

►**CLASSIFICATION**

PHARMACOTHERAPEUTIC: Amide. **CLINICAL:** Topical anesthetic

ACTION/THERAPEUTIC EFFECT

Blocks conduction of nerve impulses by decreasing membrane permeability, increases norepinephrine at postsynaptic receptor sites, producing intense vasoconstriction.

USES

Topical anesthesia for mucous membranes of oral laryngeal, nasal areas.

PRECAUTIONS

CONTRAINDICATIONS: Hypersensitivity to cocaine or local anesthetics, systemic or ophthalmic use. **CAUTIONS:** History of drug sensitivities or drug abuse (can cause strong psychologic dependence and some tolerance); has been abused for cortical stimulant effect. Severe trauma or sepsis in area to be anesthetized. Limit to office and surgical procedures; prolonged use can cause ischemic damage to nasal mucosa. Safety in children not established.

INTERACTIONS

DRUG: Tricyclic antidepressants, digoxin, methyldopa may increase arrhythmias. May decrease effects of beta-blockers. Cholinesterase inhibitors may increase effects, risk of toxicity. CNS stimulation-producing agents may increase effects. Sympathomimetics increase CNS stimulation, risk of cardiovascular effects. **HERBAL:** None known. **FOOD:** None known. **LAB VALUES:** None significant.

AVAILABILITY (Rx)

TOPICAL SOLUTION: 4%, 10%.

INDICATIONS/ROUTES/DOSAGE

Usual topical dosage:

TOPICAL: Adults, elderly: 1–10% solution. **Maximum single dose:** 1 mg/kg.

SIDE EFFECTS

FREQUENT: Loss of sense of smell/taste.

ADVERSE REACTIONS/TOXIC EFFECTS

Repeated nasal application may produce stuffy nose, chronic rhinitis. Early signs of overdosage produces increased B/P, increased pulse, irregular heartbeat, chills/fever, agitation, nervousness, confusion, inability to remain still, nausea, vomiting, abdominal pain, increased sweating, rapid breathing, large pupils. Advanced signs of overdosage produces arrhythmias, CNS hemorrhage, CHF, convulsions, delirium, hyperreflexia, loss of bladder/bowel control, respiratory weakness. Late signs of overdosage produces loss of reflexes, muscle paralysis, dilated pupils, LOC, cyanosis, pulmonary edema, cardiac/respiratory failure.

NURSING IMPLICATIONS

INTERVENTION/EVALUATION:

Monitor for anesthetic response. Be alert to CNS stimulation: assess for euphoria, restlessness, increased B/P, pulse, respirations. Be prepared to provide ventilatory support and emergency medications in event of progression of CNS response.

PATIENT/FAMILY TEACHING:

NPO until sensation returns when used for throat anesthesia. One time or infrequent use for procedures will not cause dependence. Report feelings of euphoria, restlessness, or rapid heartbeat if these develop during procedure.

---

codeine phosphate

koe-deen
(Codeine)

codeine sulfate

(Contin✤)

FIXED-COMBINATION(S)

With aspirin, butalbital, a barbiturate, and caffeine **(Fiorinal);** with acetaminophen **(Phenaphen, Tylenol with codeine);** with aspirin **(Empirin with codeine)**
Do not confuse with Lodine.

▶CLASSIFICATION

PHARMACOTHERAPEUTIC: Opioid agonist. **CLINICAL:** Analgesic: **Schedule II;** fixed-combination form: **Schedule III** (see p. 116C)

ACTION/*THERAPEUTIC EFFECT*

Binds at opiate receptor sites in CNS. *Reduces intensity of pain stimuli incoming from sensory nerve endings, suppresses cough reflex, decreases intestinal motility.*

USES/*UNLABELED*

Relief of mild to moderate pain and/or nonproductive cough. *Treatment of diarrhea.*

PRECAUTIONS

CONTRAINDICATIONS: None significant. **EXTREME CAUTION:** CNS depression, anoxia, hypercapnia, respiratory depression, seizures, acute alcoholism, shock, untreated myxedema, respiratory dysfunction. **CAUTIONS:** Increased intracranial pressure, impaired hepatic function, acute abdominal conditions, hypothyroidism, prostatic hypertrophy, Addison's disease, urethral stricture, COPD.

INTERACTIONS

DRUG: Alcohol, CNS depressants may increase CNS or respiratory depression, hypotension. **MAO inhibitors** may produce severe, fatal reaction (reduce dose to $1/4$ usual dose). **HERBAL:** None known. **FOOD:** None known. **LAB VALUES:** May increase amylase, lipase.

AVAILABILITY (Rx)

TABLETS: 15 mg, 30 mg, 60 mg. **SOLUBLE TABLETS:** 15 mg, 30 mg, 60 mg. **INJECTION:** 30 mg, 60 mg.

INDICATIONS/ROUTES/DOSAGE

Note: Reduce initial dosage in those with hypothyroidism, concurrent CNS depressants, Addison's disease, renal insufficiency, elderly/debilitated.

✤ - Canadian trade name   ✳ - see also www.wbsaunders.com/SIMON/SaundersNDH

Analgesia:

PO/SubQ/IM: Adults, elderly: 30 mg q4–6h. **Range:** 15–60 mg daily. **Children:** 0.5–1 mg/kg q4–6h. **Maximum:** 60 mg/dose.

Antitussive:

PO: Adults, elderly, children >12 yrs: 10–20 mg q4–6h. **Children 6–11 yrs:** 5–10 mg q4–6h. **Children 2–5 yrs:** 2.5–5 mg q4–6h.

SIDE EFFECTS

Note: Ambulatory pts, those not in severe pain may experience dizziness, nausea, vomiting, hypotension more frequently than those in supine position or with severe pain.

FREQUENT: Constipation, drowsiness, nausea, vomiting. ***OCCASIONAL:*** Paradoxical excitement, confusion, pounding heartbeat, facial flushing, decreased urination, blurred vision, dizziness, dry mouth, headache, hypotension, decreased appetite, redness/burning/pain at injection site. ***RARE:*** Hallucinations, depression, stomach pain, insomnia.

ADVERSE REACTIONS/TOXIC EFFECTS

Too frequent use may result in paralytic ileus. Overdosage results in cold/clammy skin, confusion, convulsions, decreased B/P, restlessness, pinpoint pupils, bradycardia, respiratory depression, LOC, severe weakness. Tolerance to analgesic effect, physical dependence may occur with repeated use.

NURSING IMPLICATIONS

BASELINE ASSESSMENT:

Analgesic: Assess onset, type, location, and duration of pain. Effect of medication is reduced if full pain recurs before next dose. ***Anti-***

tussive: Assess type, severity, frequency of cough, and production.

INTERVENTION/EVALUATION:

Increase fluid intake and environmental humidity to improve viscosity of lung secretions. Initiate deep breathing and coughing exercises. Assess for clinical improvement; record onset of relief of pain or cough.

PATIENT/FAMILY TEACHING:

Change positions slowly to avoid orthostatic hypotension. Avoid tasks that require alertness, motor skills until response to drug is established. Tolerance/dependence may occur with prolonged use of high doses. Avoid alcohol.

colchicine

coal-cheh-seen
(Colchicine)

▶CLASSIFICATION

PHARMACOTHERAPEUTIC: Alkaloid. ***CLINICAL:*** Antigout

ACTION/THERAPEUTIC EFFECT

Decreases leukocyte motility, phagocytosis, lactic acid production, *resulting in decreased urate crystal deposits, inflammatory process.*

PHARMACOKINETICS

Rapidly absorbed from GI tract. Highest concentration in liver, spleen, kidney. Protein binding: 30–50%. Reenters intestinal tract (biliary secretion), reabsorbed from intestines. Partially metabolized in liver. Eliminated primarily in feces.

USES/*UNLABELED*
Treatment of attacks of acute gouty arthritis, prophylaxis of recurrent gouty arthritis. *Reduce frequency of familial Mediterranean fever, treatment of acute attacks of calcium pyrophosphate deposition, sarcoid arthritis, amyloidosis, biliary cirrhosis, recurrent pericarditis.*

PRECAUTIONS
CONTRAINDICATIONS: Severe GI, renal, hepatic, or cardiac disorders; blood dyscrasias. ***CAUTIONS:*** Impaired hepatic function, elderly, debilitated.

▷***LIFESPAN CONSIDERATIONS:*** **Pregnancy/Lactation:** Unknown if drug crosses placenta or is distributed in breast milk. **Pregnancy Category D. Children:** Safety and efficacy not established. **Elderly:** May be more susceptible to cumulative toxicity. Age-related renal impairment may increase risk of myopathy.

INTERACTIONS
DRUG: **NSAIDs** may increase risk of neutropenia, thrombocytopenia, bone marrow depression. **Bone marrow depressants** may increase risk of blood dyscrasias. ***HERBAL:*** None known. ***FOOD:*** None known. ***LAB VALUES:*** May decrease platelet count. May increase SGOT (AST), alkaline phosphatase.

AVAILABILITY (Rx)
TABLETS: 0.5 mg, 0.6 mg. ***INJECTION:*** 1 mg.

ADMINISTRATION/HANDLING
PO:
• Give without regard to meals.

IV 🏮
Note: SubQ or IM administration produces severe local reaction. Use via IV route only.

Storage:
• Store at room temperature.

Reconstitution:
• May dilute with 0.9% NaCl or Sterile Water for Injection. • Do not dilute with D_5W.

Rate of administration:
• Administer over 2–5 min.

IV INCOMPATIBILITY ⊘
No information available via Y-site administration.

INDICATIONS/ROUTES/DOSAGE
Acute gouty arthritis:
PO: Adults, elderly: 0.5–1.2 mg, then 0.5–0.6 mg q1–2h or 1–1.2 mg q2h until pain relieved or nausea, vomiting, or diarrhea occurs. Total dose: 4–8 mg.

IV: Adults, elderly: Initially, 2 mg, then 0.5 mg q6h until satisfactory response. **Maximum:** 4 mg/24 hrs or 4 mg/one course of treatment. **Note:** If pain recurs, may give 1–2 mg/day for several days but no sooner than 7 days after a full course of IV therapy (4 mg).

Chronic gouty arthritis:
PO: Adults, elderly: 0.5–0.6 mg once weekly up to once daily (dependent on number of attacks per year).

SIDE EFFECTS
Note: Those with impaired renal function may exhibit myopathy and neuropathy manifested as generalized weakness.

FREQUENT: PO: Nausea, vomiting, abdominal discomfort. ***OCCASIONAL: PO:*** Anorexia. ***RARE:***

Hypersensitivity reaction, including angioedema. ***Parenteral only:*** Nausea, vomiting, diarrhea, abdominal discomfort, pain/redness at injection site, neuritis in injected arm.

ADVERSE REACTIONS/TOXIC EFFECTS

Bone marrow depression (aplastic anemia, agranulocytosis, thrombocytopenia) may occur with long-term therapy. Overdose: *Initially:* Burning feeling in throat/skin, severe diarrhea, abdominal pain. *Second stage:* Fever, seizures, delirium, renal damage (hematuria, oliguria). *Third stage:* Hair loss, leukocytosis, stomatitis.

NURSING IMPLICATIONS

BASELINE ASSESSMENT:

Instruct pt to drink 8–10 glasses (8 oz) of fluid daily while on medication. Medication should be discontinued if any GI symptoms occur.

INTERVENTION/EVALUATION:

Discontinue medication immediately if GI symptoms occur. Encourage high fluid intake (3,000 ml/day). Monitor I&O (output should be at least 2,000 ml/day). Assess serum uric acid levels. Assess for therapeutic response (reduced joint tenderness, swelling, redness, limitation of motion).

PATIENT/FAMILY TEACHING:

Encourage low-purine food intake, to drink 8–10 glasses (8 oz) of fluid daily while on medication. Report skin rash, sore throat, fever, unusual bruising/bleeding, weakness, tiredness, numbness. Stop medication as soon as gout pain is relieved or at first sign of nausea, vomiting, or diarrhea.

colesevelam

ko-leh-**sev**-eh-lam
(Welchol)

▶CLASSIFICATION

PHARMACOTHERAPEUTIC: Bile acid sequestrant. ***CLINICAL:*** Antihyperlipidemic agent (see p. 49C)

ACTION/*THERAPEUTIC EFFECT*

A nonsystemic polymer that binds with bile acids in the intestine, preventing their reabsorption and removing them from the body thereby *decreasing LDL cholesterol.*

USES

Adjunctive therapy to diet and exercise used either alone or in combination with an HMG-CoA reductase inhibitor (e.g., simvastatin) to decrease elevated LDL cholesterol in patients with primary hypercholesterolemia (Fredrickson type IIa).

PRECAUTIONS

CONTRAINDICATIONS: Hypersensitivity to colesevelam, complete biliary obstruction. ***CAUTIONS:*** History of constipation.

▷*LIFESPAN CONSIDERATIONS:* **Pregnancy/Lactation:** Not absorbed systematically, may decrease proper vitamin absorption and may have effect on nursing infants. **Children:** Safety and efficacy not established. **Elderly:** No age-related precautions noted.

INTERACTIONS

DRUG: May decrease absorption of **vitamin A, D, E, K, NSAIDs, aspirin, clindamycin, digoxin, furosemide, glipizide, hydrocortisone, imipramine, phenytoin, propranolol, tetracyclines, thi-**

azide diuretics. *HERBAL:* None known. *FOOD:* None known. *LAB VALUES:* None significant.

AVAILABILITY (Rx)
TABLETS: 625 mg.

INDICATIONS/ROUTES/DOSAGE
Cholesterol lowering:

PO: Adults, elderly: 3 tablets with meals 2 times/day or 6 tablets once daily with meal. May increase daily dose to 7 tablets/day.

SIDE EFFECTS
FREQUENT (8–12%): Flatulence, constipation, infection, dyspepsia.

ADVERSE REACTIONS/TOXIC EFFECTS
GI tract obstruction may be noted.

NURSING IMPLICATIONS

BASELINE ASSESSMENT:
Assess baseline lab results: cholesterol, triglycerides, liver function tests.

INTERVENTION/EVALUATION:
Monitor cholesterol and triglyceride lab results for therapeutic response. Assess bowel activity.

PATIENT/FAMILY TEACHING:
Follow special diet (important part of treatment). Periodic tests are essential part of therapy. Do not take other medications without physician's knowledge.

colestipol

(Cholestid)
See Classification section under: Antihyperlipidemics

colfosceril palmitate

kol-**foss**-er-ill
(Exosurf)

▶CLASSIFICATION
CLINICAL: Lung surfactant

ACTION/*THERAPEUTIC EFFECT*
Lowers surface tension on alveolar surfaces during respiration, stabilizes alveoli vs. collapse that may occur at resting pulmonary pressures. *Replenishes surfactant, restores surface activity to lungs.*

USES
Prophylactic use in infants <1,350 g at risk of developing RDS, infants >1,350 g with evidence of pulmonary immaturity; treatment in infants with RDS.

PRECAUTIONS
CONTRAINDICATIONS: None significant. *CAUTIONS:* Those at risk for circulatory overload.

INTERACTIONS
DRUG: None significant. *HERBAL:* None known. *FOOD:* None known. *LAB VALUES:* None significant.

AVAILABILITY (Rx)
POWDER FOR INJECTION: 108 mg.

ADMINISTRATION/HANDLING
Intratracheal:
Storage:
• Store vials at room temperature. After reconstitution, stable for 12 hrs.

Reconstitution:
• Reconstitute immediately prior to use with 8 ml preservative-free Sterile Water for Injection. Refer to manufacturer's instructions. • Do not use if vacuum in vial is not present.

Administration:

• Instill through catheter inserted into infant's endotracheal tube. Do not instill into main stem of bronchus. • Stop administration if reflux into endotracheal tube occurs. If needed, increase peak inspiratory pressure on ventilator by 4–5 cm H_2O until tube clears. • Stop administration if transcutaneous O_2 saturation decreases. If needed, increase peak inspiratory pressure on ventilator by 4–5 cm H_2O for 1–2 min. May also need to increase FiO_2 for 1–2 min.

INDICATIONS/ROUTES/DOSAGE

Prophylaxis for RDS:

***INTRATRACHEAL*: Neonates:** 5 ml/kg given as two 2.5 ml/kg doses as soon as possible after birth. May repeat 12 and 24 hrs later in infants remaining on mechanical ventilator.

RDS rescue:

***INTRATRACHEAL*: Neonates:** 5 ml/kg given as two 2.5 ml/kg doses. Repeat in 12 hrs in all infants remaining on ventilator.

SIDE EFFECTS

OCCASIONAL: Gagging. ***RARE:*** Apnea, bradycardia, tachycardia.

ADVERSE REACTIONS/TOXIC EFFECTS

Failure to reduce peak ventilator inspiratory pressures after chest expansion, after dosing, may result in lung overdistention and fatal pulmonary air leak. Failure to reduce transcutaneous O_2 saturation if in excess of 95% by decreasing FiO_2 in small but repeated steps until saturation is 90% to 95% may result in hyperoxia. Failure to reduce ventilator if arterial or transcutaneous CO_2 measurements are <30 may result in hypocarbia, reducing brain-blood flow.

NURSING IMPLICATIONS

BASELINE ASSESSMENT:

Clinicians in care of neonate must be experienced with intubation, ventilator management. Give emotional support to parents. Suctioning infant before dosing may decrease chance of mucous plugs obstructing endotracheal tube.

INTERVENTION/EVALUATION:

Monitor infant with arterial or transcutaneous measurement of systemic O_2 and CO_2. Maintain vigilant clinical attention to neonate prior to, during, and after drug administration. Assess lung sounds for rales and moist breath sounds. If chest expansion improves dramatically after dosing, reduce peak ventilator inspiratory pressures immediately (failure to do so may result in lung overdistention and fatal pulmonary air leak). If transcutaneous O_2 saturation >95% and neonate appears pink, reduce FiO_2 in small but repeated steps until saturation is 90% to 95% (failure to do so may result in hyperoxia). If arterial or transcutaneous CO_2 measurements are <30, reduce ventilator immediately (failure to do so may result in hypocarbia, reducing brain-blood flow).

conjugated estrogens 🖉

ess-troe-jenz
(Cenestin, C.E.S.🍁, Congest🍁, Premarin)

C

FIXED-COMBINATION(S)

With meprobamate, a tranquilizer **(Milprem);** Premarin with methyltestosterone, an androgen, with medroxyprogesterone, a progestin **(Premphase, Prempro)**

▶CLASSIFICATION

PHARMACOTHERAPEUTIC: Estrogen *CLINICAL:* Hormone

ACTION/*THERAPEUTIC EFFECT*

Increases synthesis of DNA, RNA, and various proteins in responsive tissues. Reduces release of gonadotropin-releasing hormone, reducing follicle-stimulating hormone (FSH) and leuteinizing hormone (LH). *Promotes vasomotor stability, maintains genitourinary function, normal growth, development of female sex organs. Prevents accelerated bone loss by inhibiting bone resorption, restoring balance of bone resorption and formation. Inhibits LH, decreases serum concentration of testosterone.*

PHARMACOKINETICS

Well absorbed from GI tract. Widely distributed. Protein binding: 50–80%. Metabolized in liver. Primarily excreted in urine.

USES/*UNLABELED*

Management of moderate to severe vasomotor symptoms associated with menopause. Treatment of atrophic vaginitis, kraurosis vulvae, female hypogonadism and castration, primary ovarian failure. Retardation of osteoporosis in postmenopausal women. Palliative treatment of inoperable, progressive cancer of the prostate in men and of the breast in postmenopausal women. *Prevents estrogen deficiency-induced premenopausal osteoporosis. Cream: Prevention of nosebleeds.*

PRECAUTIONS

CONTRAINDICATIONS: Known or suspected breast cancer (except select pts with metastasis), estrogen-dependent neoplasia; undiagnosed abnormal genital bleeding; active thrombophlebitis or thromboembolic disorders; history of thrombophlebitis, thrombosis, or thromboembolic disorders with previous estrogen use, hypersensitivity to estrogen. *CAUTIONS:* Conditions that may be aggravated by fluid retention: cardiac, renal, or hepatic dysfunction, epilepsy, migraine, mental depression, metabolic bone disease with potential hypercalcemia, history of jaundice during pregnancy, strong family history of breast cancer, fibrocystic disease or breast nodules, children in whom bone growth is not complete.

▷*LIFESPAN CONSIDERATIONS:* **Pregnancy/Lactation:** Distributed in breast milk. May be harmful to fetus. Not for use during lactation. **Pregnancy Category X. Children:** Safety and efficacy not established. **Elderly:** No age related precautions noted.

INTERACTIONS

DRUG: May interfere with effects of **bromocriptine.** May increase concentration of **cyclosporine,** increase hepatic, nephrotoxicity. **Hepatotoxic medications** may increase hepatotoxicity. *HERBAL:* None known. *FOOD:* None known. *LAB VALUES:* May affect metapyrone, thyroid function tests. May decrease cholesterol, LDH. May increase calcium, glucose, HDL, triglycerides.

AVAILABILITY (Rx)

TABLETS: 0.3 mg, 0.625 mg, 0.9 mg, 1.25 mg, 2.5 mg. ***INJECTION:*** 25 mg. ***VAGINAL CREAM.***

ADMINISTRATION/HANDLING

PO:

• Administer at the same time each day. • Give with milk or food if nausea occurs.

IV

Storage:

• Refrigerate vials for IV use. • Reconstituted solution stable for 60 days refrigerated. • Do not use if solution darkens or precipitate forms.

Reconstitution:

• Reconstitute with 5 ml Sterile Water for Injection containing benzyl alcohol (diluent provided). • Slowly add diluent, shaking gently. Avoid vigorous shaking.

Rate of administration:

• Give slowly to prevent flushing reaction.

IV INCOMPATIBILITY ⊘

No information available via Y-site administration.

INDICATIONS/ROUTES/DOSAGE

Vasomotor symptoms associated with menopause, atrophic vaginitis, kraurosis vulvae:

***PO:* Adults, elderly:** 0.3–1.25 mg/day cyclically (21 days on; 7 days off or continuously).

***INTRAVAGINAL:* Adults, elderly:** 2–4 g/day cyclically.

Female hypogonadism:

***PO:* Adults:** 2.5–7.5 mg/day in divided doses for 20 days; rest 10 days.

Female castration, primary ovarian failure:

***PO:* Adults:** Initially, 1.25 mg/day cyclically.

Osteoporosis:

***PO:* Adults, elderly:** 0.3–0.625 mg/day, cyclically.

Breast cancer:

***PO:* Adults, elderly:** 10 mg 3 times/day for at least 3 mos.

Prostate cancer:

***PO:* Adults, elderly:** 1.25–2.5 mg 3 times/day.

Abnormal uterine bleeding:

***IM/IV:* Adults:** 25 mg, may repeat once in 6–12 hrs.

SIDE EFFECTS

FREQUENT: Change in vaginal bleeding (spotting, breakthrough), breast pain/tenderness, gynecomastia. ***OCCASIONAL:*** Headache, increased B/P, intolerance to contact lenses. ***High-dose therapy:*** Anorexia, nausea. ***RARE:*** Loss of scalp hair, clinical depression.

ADVERSE REACTIONS/TOXIC EFFECTS

Prolonged administration may increase risk of gallbladder, thromboembolic disease, and breast, cervical, vaginal, endometrial, and liver carcinoma.

NURSING IMPLICATIONS

BASELINE ASSESSMENT:

Question hypersensitivity to estrogen, previous jaundice, or thromboembolic disorders associated with pregnancy or estrogen therapy.

INTERVENTION/EVALUATION:

Assess B/P periodically. Check for swelling; weigh daily. Monitor blood glucose 4 times/day for pts with diabetes. Promptly report signs and symptoms of thromboembolic or thrombotic disorders: sudden severe headache, shortness of breath, vision or speech disturbance, weakness or numbness of an extremity, loss of coordination, pain in chest, groin, or leg.

PATIENT/FAMILY TEACHING:

Avoid smoking due to increased risk of heart attack or blood clots. Explain importance of diet and exercise when taken to retard osteoporosis. Teach how to perform Homan's test, signs and symptoms of blood clots (report these to physician immediately). Notify physician of abnormal vaginal bleeding, depression. Teach female pts to perform breast self-exam. Report weekly gain of >5 lbs. Stop taking medication and contact physician if pregnancy is suspected.

corticotropin injection

kore-tih-koe-**troe**-pin
(ACTH, Acthar)

corticotropin repository

(Cortigel, Cortrophin-Gel, Acthar Gel)

▶CLASSIFICATION

PHARMACOTHERAPEUTIC: Adrenocortical steroid. *CLINICAL:* Corticotropin

ACTION/*THERAPEUTIC EFFECT*

Stimulates adrenal cortex to secrete cortisol, corticosterone, aldosterone and androgenic substances. Acts to stimulate synthesis of adrenocortical hormones. *Suppresses immune response, inflammation.*

USES

Diagnostic testing of adrenocortical function. Limited therapeutic value in conditions responsive to corticosteroid therapy. May be used in hypercalcemia of cancer, acute exacerbations of multiple sclerosis, nonsuppurative thyroiditis.

PRECAUTIONS

CONTRAINDICATIONS: Hypersensitivity to any corticosteroid or porcine proteins, systemic fungal infection, peptic ulcers (except life-threatening situations), scleroderma, primary adrenocortical insufficiency. Avoid live virus vaccine; long-term therapy in children. *CAUTIONS:* Thromboembolic disorders, history of tuberculosis (may reactivate disease), hypothyroidism, cirrhosis, nonspecific ulcerative colitis, CHF, hypertension, psychosis, renal insufficiency, seizures. Prolonged therapy should be discontinued slowly.

INTERACTIONS

DRUG: **Amphotericin** may increase hypokalemia. May decrease effect of **oral hypoglycemics, insulin, diuretics, potassium supplements.** May increase **digoxin** toxicity (due to hypokalemia). **Hepatic enzyme inducers** may decrease effect. **Live virus vaccines** may potentiate virus replication, increase vaccine side effects, decrease pt's antibody response to vaccine. *HERBAL:* None known. *FOOD:* None known. *LAB VALUES:* May decrease calcium, potassium, thyroxine. May increase cholesterol, lipids, glucose, sodium, amylase.

AVAILABILITY (Rx)

POWDER FOR INJECTION: 25

units, 40 units. **REPOSITORY FOR INJECTION:** 40 units/ml, 80 units/ml.

INDICATIONS/ROUTES/DOSAGE

Note: May give IM, SubQ. Use IV only for corticotropin injection; IM only for corticotropin zinc hydroxide.

Diagnostic testing:
IV: **Adults:** 10–25 units in 500 ml D_5W infused over 8 hrs.
IM/SubQ: **Adults:** 20 units 4 times/day.

Acute exacerbation of multiple sclerosis:
IM: **Adults:** 80–120 units/day for 2–3 wks.

Infantile spasms:
IM: **Infants:** 20–40 units/day or 80 units every other day for 3 mos (or 1 mo after cessation of seizures).

Usual repository injection dosage:
IM/SubQ: **Adults:** 40–80 units q24–72h.

SIDE EFFECTS

FREQUENT: Insomnia, heartburn, nervousness, abdominal distention, increased sweating, acne, mood swings, increased appetite, facial flushing, delayed wound healing, increased susceptibility to infection, diarrhea/constipation. ***OCCASIONAL:*** Headache, edema, change in skin color, frequent urination. ***RARE:*** Tachycardia, allergic reaction (rash, hives), pain, redness, swelling at injection site, psychic changes, hallucinations, depression.

ADVERSE REACTIONS/TOXIC EFFECTS

Long-term therapy: Hypocalcemia, hypokalemia, muscle wasting (esp. arms, legs), osteoporosis, spontaneous fractures, amenorrhea, cataracts, glaucoma, peptic ulcer, CHF. *Abrupt withdrawal following long-term therapy:* Anorexia, nausea, fever, headache, joint pain, rebound inflammation, fatigue, weakness, lethargy, dizziness, orthostatic hypertension.

NURSING IMPLICATIONS

BASELINE ASSESSMENT:

Question for hypersensitivity to any of the corticosteroids. Obtain baseline values for weight, B/P, glucose, cholesterol, electrolytes.

INTERVENTION/EVALUATION:

Be alert to infection (reduced immune response): sore throat, fever, or vague symptoms. For those on long-term therapy, watch for hypocalcemia (muscle twitching, cramps, positive Trousseau's or Chvostek's signs) or hypokalemia (weakness and muscle cramps, numbness/tingling esp. lower extremities, nausea and vomiting, irritability, EKG changes). Assess emotional status, ability to sleep.

PATIENT/FAMILY TEACHING:

Do not change dose/schedule or stop taking drug; *must* taper off under medical supervision. Notify physician of fever, sore throat, muscle aches, sudden weight gain/swelling. Inform dentist or other physicians of cortisone therapy now or within past 12 mos.

cortisone acetate

kore-tih-zone
(Cortone✚, Cortone Acetate)

C

▶CLASSIFICATION

PHARMACOTHERAPEUTIC: Adrenocortical steroid. **CLINICAL:** Glucocorticoid (see p. 78C)

ACTION/*THERAPEUTIC EFFECT*

Inhibits accumulation of inflammatory cells at inflammation sites, phagocytosis, lysosomal enzyme release and synthesis and/or release of mediators of inflammation. *Prevents/suppresses cell-mediated immune reactions. Decreases/prevents tissue response to inflammatory process.*

USES

Management of adrenocortical insufficiency.

PRECAUTIONS

CONTRAINDICATIONS: Hypersensitivity to any corticosteroid, systemic fungal infection, peptic ulcers (except life-threatening situations). Avoid live virus vaccine. **CAUTIONS:** Thromboembolic disorders, history of tuberculosis (may reactivate disease), hypothyroidism, cirrhosis, nonspecific ulcerative colitis, CHF, hypertension, psychosis, renal insufficiency, seizure disorders. Prolonged therapy should be discontinued slowly.

INTERACTIONS

DRUG: Amphotericin may increase hypokalemia. May decrease effect of **oral hypoglycemics, insulin, diuretics, potassium supplements.** May increase **digoxin** toxicity (due to hypokalemia). **Hepatic enzyme inducers** may decrease effect. **Live virus vaccines** may potentiate virus replication, increase vaccine side effects, decrease pt's antibody response to vaccine. **HERBAL:** None known. **FOOD:** None known. **LAB VALUES:** May decrease calcium, potassium, thyroxine. May increase cholesterol, lipids, glucose, sodium, amylase.

AVAILABILITY (Rx)

TABLETS: 5 mg, 10 mg, 25 mg.

INDICATIONS/ROUTES/DOSAGE

Usual adult dosage:

PO: Adults: Initially, 25–300 mg/day. **Maintenance:** Lowest dosage that maintains adequate clinical response.

Usual elderly dosage:

PO: Use lowest effective dosage.

SIDE EFFECTS

FREQUENT: Insomnia, heartburn, nervousness, abdominal distention, increased sweating, acne, mood swings, increased appetite, facial flushing, delayed wound healing, increased susceptibility to infection, diarrhea/constipation. **OCCASIONAL:** Headache, edema, change in skin color, frequent urination. **RARE:** Tachycardia, allergic reaction (rash, hives), psychic changes, hallucinations, depression.

ADVERSE REACTIONS/TOXIC EFFECTS

Long-term therapy: Hypocalcemia, hypokalemia, muscle wasting (esp. arms, legs), osteoporosis, spontaneous fractures, amenorrhea, cataracts, glaucoma, peptic ulcer, CHF. **Abrupt withdrawal following long-term therapy:** Anorexia, nausea, fever, headache, joint pain, rebound inflammation, fatigue, weakness, lethargy, dizziness, orthostatic hypertension.

BASELINE ASSESSMENT:

Question for hypersensitivity to any of the corticosteroids. Obtain baseline values for weight, B/P, glucose, cholesterol, electrolytes.

INTERVENTION/EVALUATION:

Be alert to infection (reduced immune response): sore throat, fever, or vague symptoms. For those on long-term therapy, watch for hypocalcemia (muscle twitching, cramps, positive Trousseau's or Chvostek's signs) or hypokalemia (weakness and muscle cramps, numbness/tingling esp. lower extremities, nausea and vomiting, irritability, EKG changes). Assess emotional status, ability to sleep.

PATIENT/FAMILY TEACHING:

Do not change dose/schedule or stop taking drug; *must* taper off under medical supervision. Notify physician of fever, sore throat, muscle aches, sudden weight gain/swelling. Inform dentist or other physicians of cortisone therapy now or within past 12 mos.

cosyntropin

koe-syn-**troe**-pin
(Cortrosyn)

▶CLASSIFICATION

PHARMACOTHERAPEUTIC:
Adrenocortical steroid. ***CLINI-CAL:*** Glucocorticoid

ACTION/*THERAPEUTIC EFFECT*

Stimulates initial reaction in synthesis of adrenal steroids from cholesterol, *increasing endogenous corticoid synthesis.*

USES

Diagnostic testing of adrenocortical function.

PRECAUTIONS

CONTRAINDICATIONS: Hypersensitivity to cosyntropin or corticotropin. ***CAUTIONS:*** Short duration for diagnostic use does not produce effects of long-term corticotropin therapy.

INTERACTIONS

DRUG: None significant. ***HERBAL:*** None known. ***FOOD:*** None known. ***LAB VALUES:*** None significant.

AVAILABILITY (Rx)

POWDER FOR INJECTION: 0.25 mg.

INDICATIONS/ROUTES/DOSAGE

Screening test for adrenal function:

IM: **Adults:** 0.25–0.75 mg one time. **Children (<2 yrs):** 0.125 mg one time. **Neonates:** 0.015 mg/kg/dose.

IV INFUSION: **Adults:** 0.25 mg in D_5W or 0.9% NaCl, infuse over 4–8 hrs.

SIDE EFFECTS

OCCASIONAL: Nausea, vomiting. ***RARE:*** Hypersensitivity reaction (fever, pruritus).

ADVERSE REACTIONS/TOXIC EFFECTS

None significant.

NURSING IMPLICATIONS

BASELINE ASSESSMENT:

Hold cortisone, hydrocortisone, or spironolactone on the test day. Assure that baseline plasma cortisol concentration has been drawn prior to start of test, or 24 hr urine for 17-KS or 17-OHCS is initiated.

INTERVENTION/EVALUATION:

Adhere to time frame for blood draws; monitor collection of urine if indicated.

PATIENT/FAMILY TEACHING:

Explain procedure and purpose of the test.

co-trimoxazole (sulfamethoxazole-trimethoprim)

koe-try-mox-oh-zole
(Apo-Sulfatrim✤, Bactrim, Cotrim, Novotrimel✤, Septra, Sulfamethoprim)

FIXED-COMBINATION(S)

With sulfamethoxazole, a sulfonamide and trimethoprim, a folate antagonist. With phenazopyridine, an analgesic **(Zotrim)**

▶CLASSIFICATION

PHARMACOTHERAPEUTIC:
Sulfonamide/folate antagonist.
CLINICAL: Anti-infective

ACTION/*THERAPEUTIC EFFECT*

Blocks bacterial synthesis of essential nucleic acids, *producing bactericidal action in susceptible microorganisms.*

PHARMACOKINETICS

Rapidly, well absorbed from GI tract. Widely distributed. Protein binding: 45–60%. Metabolized in liver. Excreted in urine. Minimally removed by hemodialysis. Half-life: 6–12 hrs (trimethoprim 8–10 hrs). Half-life increased with impaired renal function.

USES/*UNLABELED*

Acute/complicated and recurrent/chronic urinary tract infection, *Pneumocystis carinii* pneumonia, shigellosis, enteritis, otitis media, chronic bronchitis, traveler's diarrhea. Prophylaxis of *Pneumocystis carinii* pneumonia. *Treatment of biliary tract, bone/joint, chancroid, bacterial endocarditis, chlamydial infection, gonorrhea, intra-abdominal, meningitis, sinusitis, septicemia, skin/soft tissue.*

PRECAUTIONS

CONTRAINDICATIONS: Hypersensitivity to trimethoprim or any sulfonamides, megaloblastic anemia due to folate deficiency, infants <2 mos. Not for treatment of streptococcal pharyngitis. ***CAUTIONS:*** Elderly, impaired renal or hepatic function, history of severe allergy or bronchial asthma (allergic reaction to metabisulfite in injection more likely), AIDS (higher incidence of adverse reactions).
▷***LIFESPAN CONSIDERATIONS:***
Pregnancy/Lactation: Contraindicated during pregnancy at term and lactation. Readily crosses placenta; distributed in breast milk. May produce kernicterus in newborns. **Pregnancy Category C. Children:** Contraindicated in those <2 mos, may increase risk of kernicterus in newborn. **Elderly:** Increased risk for severe skin reaction, bone

marrow depression, or decreased platelet count.

INTERACTIONS

DRUG: May increase, prolong effects, increase toxicity with **warfarin, hydantoin anticonvulsants, oral hypoglycemics.** May increase risk of toxicity with other **hemolytics. Hepatotoxic medications** may increase risk of hepatotoxicity. **Methenamine** may form precipitate. May increase effect of **methotrexate.** ***HERBAL:*** None known. ***FOOD:*** None known. ***LAB VALUES:*** May increase SGOT (AST), SGPT (ALT), alkaline phosphatase, BUN, creatinine, potassium.

AVAILABILITY (Rx)

TABLETS: 80 mg trimethoprim/ 400 mg sulfamethoxazole; 160 mg/800 mg. ***ORAL SUSPENSION:*** 40 mg/200 mg. ***INJECTION:*** 80 mg/400 mg per 5 ml.

ADMINISTRATION/HANDLING

Note: Space doses evenly around the clock.

PO:

• Store tablets, suspension at room temperature. • Administer on empty stomach with 8 oz water. • Give several extra glasses of water/day.

IV

Storage:

• IV infusion (piggyback) stable for 2–6 hrs (use immediately). • Discard if cloudy or precipitate forms.

Reconstitution:

• For IV infusion (piggyback), dilute each 5 ml with 75–125 ml D_5W. • Do not mix with other drugs or solutions.

Rate of administration:

• Infuse over 60–90 min. Must avoid bolus or rapid infusion. • Do not give IM. • Assure adequate hydration.

IV INCOMPATIBILITIES ⊘

Fluconazole (Diflucan), foscarnet (Foscavir), midazolam (Versed), vinorelbine (Navelbine).

IV COMPATIBILITIES

Diltiazem (Cardizem), lorazepam (Ativan), magnesium.

INDICATIONS/ROUTES/DOSAGE

Note: Potency expressed in terms of trimethoprim content.

UTI, enteritis, acute otitis media:
***PO:* Adults, elderly:** 160 mg q12h for 7–14 days. **Children >2 mos:** 7.5–8 mg/kg/day q12h for 5–10 days.

Severe UTI, enteritis:
***IV:* Adults, elderly, children >2 mos:** 8–10 mg/kg/day in 2–4 equally divided doses q6–12h for 5–14 days. **Maximum:** 960 mg/day.

Pneumocystis carinii pneumonia:
***PO:* Adults, elderly, children >2 mos:** 20 mg/kg/day in 4 divided doses q6h.
***IV:* Adults, elderly, children >2 mos:** 15–20 mg/kg/day in 3–4 divided doses q6–8h.

Prevention of Pneumocystis carinii pneumonia:
***PO:* Adults:** One double-strength tablet/day. **Children:** 150 mg/m²/ day on 3 consecutive days/wk.

Traveler's diarrhea:
***PO:* Adults, elderly:** One double-strength tablet q12h for 5 days.

C

Acute exacerbation of chronic bronchitis:

PO: Adults, elderly: One double-strength tablet q12h for 14 days.

Dosage in renal impairment:

The dose and/or frequency is modified based on severity of infection, degree of renal impairment, and serum concentration of drug. For those with creatinine clearance of 15–30 ml/min, a reduction in dose of 50% is recommended.

SIDE EFFECTS

FREQUENT: Anorexia, nausea, vomiting, rash (generally 7–14 days after therapy begins), urticaria. ***OCCASIONAL:*** Diarrhea, abdominal pain, local pain/irritation at IV site. ***RARE:*** Headache, vertigo, insomnia, seizures, hallucinations, depression.

ADVERSE REACTIONS/TOXIC EFFECTS

Rash, fever, sore throat, pallor, purpura, cough, shortness of breath may be early signs of serious adverse reactions. Fatalities are rare but have occurred in sulfonamide therapy following Stevens-Johnson syndrome, toxic epidermal necrolysis, fulminant hepatic necrosis, agranulocytosis, aplastic anemia, other blood dyscrasias. Elderly are at increased risk of adverse reactions: bone marrow suppression, decreased platelets, severe dermatologic reactions.

NURSING IMPLICATIONS

BASELINE ASSESSMENT:

Obtain history for hypersensitivity to trimethoprim or any sulfonamide, sulfite sensitivity, severe allergy or bronchial asthma. Determine renal, hepatic, hematologic baselines.

INTERVENTION/EVALUATION:

Evaluate food tolerance. Determine pattern of bowel activity. Assess skin for rash, pallor, purpura. Check IV site, flow rate. Monitor renal, hepatic, hematology reports. Assess I&O. Check for CNS symptoms: headache, vertigo, insomnia, hallucinations. Monitor vital signs at least twice a day. Monitor for cough or shortness of breath. Assess for overt bleeding, bruising, or swelling.

PATIENT/FAMILY TEACHING:

Continue medication for full length of therapy. Space doses evenly around the clock. Take oral doses with 8 oz water and drink several extra glasses of water daily. Notify physician of new symptoms immediately, esp. rash or other skin changes, bleeding or bruising, fever, sore throat.

---

cromolyn sodium

krom-oh-lin
(Apo-Cromolyn✦, Crolom, Gastrocom, Intal, Nasalcrom, Opticrom)

▶CLASSIFICATION

PHARMACOTHERAPEUTIC: Mast cell stabilizer. ***CLINICAL:*** Antiasthmatic, antiallergic (see p. 64C)

ACTION/*THERAPEUTIC EFFECT*

Possesses no direct antihistaminic, anti-inflammatory properties. *Prevents release of mast cells (e.g., histamine) after exposure to allergens that produce allergic reaction.*

PHARMACOKINETICS

Minimal absorption following PO,

inhalation, or nasal administration. Absorbed portion excreted in urine or via biliary elimination.

USES

Oral inhalation and nebulization: Prophylactic management of severe bronchial asthma, exercise-induced bronchospasm. ***Intranasal:*** Perennial or seasonal allergic rhinitis. ***Systemic:*** Symptomatic treatment of systemic mastocytosis, food allergy, treatment of inflammatory bowel disease (IBD). ***Ophthalmic:*** Conjunctivitis.

PRECAUTIONS

CONTRAINDICATIONS: None significant. ***CAUTIONS:*** Impaired renal or hepatic function.

▷***LIFESPAN CONSIDERATIONS:*** **Pregnancy/Lactation:** Unknown if drug crosses placenta or is distributed in breast milk. **Pregnancy Category B. Children:** No age-related precautions noted. **Elderly:** Age-related renal/liver impairment may require dosage adjustment.

INTERACTIONS

DRUG: None significant. ***HERBAL:*** None known. ***FOOD:*** None known. ***LAB VALUES:*** None significant.

AVAILABILITY (Rx)

ORAL CONCENTRATE: 100 mg/5 ml. ***SOLUTION FOR NEBULIZATION:*** 20 mg amp. ***AEROSOL SPRAY:*** 800 mcg/spray. ***NASAL SPRAY (OTC):*** 40 mg/ml ***OPHTHALMIC SOLUTION:*** 4%.

ADMINISTRATION/HANDLING

Inhalation:

• Shake container well; exhale completely; place mouthpiece fully into mouth and inhale deeply and slowly while depressing the cannister and hold breath as long as possible before exhaling. • Wait 1–10 min before inhaling 2nd dose (allows for deeper bronchial penetration). • Rinse mouth with water immediately after inhalation (prevents mouth/throat dryness). • **Nebulization, inhalation capsules:** Inhalation capsules are not to be swallowed; instruct patient on use of Spinhaler.

Ophthalmic:

• Place finger on lower eyelid and pull out until pocket is formed between eye and lower lid. Hold dropper above pocket and place prescribed number of drops in pocket. Instruct pt to close eyes gently so medication will not be squeezed out of sac. • Apply gentle finger pressure to the lacrimal sac at inner canthus for 1 min following installation (lessens risk of systemic absorption).

PO:

• Give at least 30 min before meals. • Pour contents of capsule in hot water, stirring until completely dissolved; add equal amount cold water while stirring. • Do not mix with fruit juice, milk, or food.

Nasal:

• Nasal passages should be clear (may require nasal decongestant). • Inhale through nose.

INDICATIONS/ROUTES/DOSAGE

Asthma:

INHALATION (nebulization): **Adults, elderly, children >2 yrs:** 20 mg 3–4 times/day.

AEROSOL SPRAY: **Adults, elderly, children ≥12 yrs:** Initially, 2 sprays 4 times/day. **Maintenance:** 2–4 sprays 3–4 times/day. **Children (5–12 yrs):** Initially, 2 sprays

4 times/day, then 1–2 sprays 3–4 times/day.

Prevention of bronchospasm:

INHALATION (nebulization): **Adults, elderly, children >2 yrs:** 20 mg not longer than 1 hr prior to exercise or allergic exposure.

AEROSOL SPRAY: **Adults, elderly, children >5 yrs:** 2 sprays not longer than 1 hr prior to exercise or allergic exposure.

Food allergy, IBD:

PO: **Adults, elderly, children >12 yrs:** 200–400 mg 4 times/day. **Children (2–12 yrs):** 100–200 mg 4 times/day. **Maximum:** 40 mg/kg/day.

Allergic rhinitis:

INTRANASAL: **Adults, elderly, children >6 yrs:** 1 spray each nostril 3–4 times/day. May increase up to 6 times/day.

Systemic mastocytosis:

PO: **Adults, elderly, children >12 yrs:** 200 mg 4 times/day. **Children 2–12 yrs:** 100 mg 4 times/day. **Maximum:** 40 mg/kg/day. **Children <2 yrs:** 20 mg/kg/day in 4 divided doses. **Maximum** *(children 6 mos–2 yrs):* 30 mg/kg/day.

Usual ophthalmic dose:

OPHTHALMIC: **Adults, elderly, children >4 yrs:** 1–2 drops in both eyes 4–6 times/day.

SIDE EFFECTS

FREQUENT: Inhalation: Cough, dry mouth/throat, stuffy nose, throat irritation, unpleasant taste. **Nasal:** Burning, stinging, irritation of nose, increased sneezing. **Ophthalmic:** Burning, stinging of eye. **PO:** Headache, diarrhea. **OCCASIONAL: Inhalation:** Bronchospasm, hoarseness, watering eyes. **Nasal:** Cough, headache, unpleasant taste, postnasal drip.

Ophthalmic: Increased watering/itching of eye. **PO:** Skin rash, abdominal pain, joint pain, nausea, insomnia. **RARE: Inhalation:** Dizziness, painful urination, muscle/joint pain, skin rash. **Nasal:** Nosebleeds, skin rash. **Ophthalmic:** Chemosis (edema of conjunctiva), eye irritation.

ADVERSE REACTIONS/TOXIC EFFECTS

Nasal, PO, inhalation: Anaphylaxis occurs rarely.

NURSING IMPLICATIONS

INTERVENTION/EVALUATION:

Monitor rate, depth, rhythm, type of respiration; quality and rate of pulse. Assess lung sounds for rhonchi, wheezing, rales. Observe lips, fingernails for blue or dusky color in light-skinned patients; gray in dark-skinned patients.

PATIENT/FAMILY TEACHING:

Increase fluid intake (decreases lung secretion viscosity). Rinsing mouth with water immediately after inhalation may prevent mouth/throat dryness. Effect of therapy dependent on administration at regular intervals.

cyanocobalamin (vitamin B$_{12}$)

sye-ah-no-koe-**bal**-a-min (Rubramin ♣, Rubramin PC, Crysti-12, Cyanoject, Cyomin, Nascobal)

hydroxocobalamin (vitamin B$_{12}$)

(Hydrobexan, Hydro-Cobex)

FIXED-COMBINATION(S)

With liver extract, 10 mcg/ml (liver injection); with liver excrete crude, 2 mcg/ml; vitamin B$_{12}$ with intrinsic factor **(Ciopar Forte).**

▶CLASSIFICATION

PHARMACOTHERAPEUTIC: Coenzyme. ***CLINICAL:*** Vitamin, antianemic (see p. 128C)

ACTION/*THERAPEUTIC EFFECT*

Coenzyme for metabolic functions (fat, carbohydrate metabolism, protein synthesis). *Necessary for growth, cell replication, hematopoiesis, and myelin synthesis.*

PHARMACOKINETICS

Absorbed in lower half of ileum in presence of calcium. Initially bound to intrinsic factor; this complex passes down intestine, binding to receptor sites on ileal mucosa. In presence of calcium, absorbed systemically. Protein binding: High. Metabolized in liver. Eliminated via biliary excretion. Half-life: 6 days.

USES

Prophylaxis, treatment of pernicious anemia, vitamin B$_{12}$ deficiency due to inadequate diet or intestinal malabsorption, hemolytic anemia, hyperthyroidism, malignancy of pancreas, bowel, gastrectomy, GI lesions, neurologic damage, malabsorption syndrome, vegetarians, breast-fed infants, metabolic disorders, prolonged stress, chronic fever, renal disease. Deficiency generally occurs concurrently with other B-vitamin deficiencies.

PRECAUTIONS

CONTRAINDICATIONS: History of allergy to cobalamin, folate deficient anemia, hereditary optic nerve atrophy. ***CAUTIONS:*** None significant.

▷***LIFESPAN CONSIDERATIONS:*** **Pregnancy/Lactation:** Crosses placenta; excreted in breast milk. **Pregnancy Category A. Category C** if used at doses greater than RDA). **Children/Elderly:** No age-related precautions noted.

INTERACTIONS

DRUG:* Alcohol, colchicine** may decrease absorption. **Ascorbic acid** may destroy vitamin B$_{12}$. **Folic acid** (large doses) may decrease concentration. ***HERBAL: None known. ***FOOD:*** None known. ***LAB VALUES:*** None significant.

AVAILABILITY (Rx)

TABLETS: 25 mcg, 50 mcg, 100 mcg, 250 mcg, 500 mcg, 1,000 mcg. ***INJECTION:*** 100 mcg/ml, 1,000 mcg/ml. ***NASAL GEL:*** 500 mcg/spray.

ADMINISTRATION/HANDLING

PO:

• Give with meals (increases absorption).

INDICATIONS/ROUTES/DOSAGE

Deficiency:

S$_{UB}$Q/IM: **Adults, elderly:** Initially, 100 mcg/day for 6–7 days, then every other day for 7 doses, then q3–4days for 2–3 wks. **Maintenance:** 100–200 mcg every month. **Children:** Initially, 30–50 mcg/day for at least 2 wks. **Maintenance:** 100 mcg every month.

Usual nasal dosage:

Adults, elderly: 500 mcg (1 spray) every week (after deficiency corrected).

Supplement:

PO: **Adults, elderly:** 2–6 mcg/day. **Children:** 0.3–2 mcg/day.

SIDE EFFECTS

OCCASIONAL: Diarrhea, itching.

ADVERSE REACTIONS/TOXIC EFFECTS

Rare allergic reaction generally due to impurities in preparation. May produce peripheral vascular thrombosis, pulmonary edema, hypokalemia, CHF.

NURSING IMPLICATIONS

INTERVENTION/EVALUATION:

Assess for CHF, pulmonary edema, hypokalemia in cardiac pts receiving SubQ/IM therapy. Monitor potassium levels (3.5–5 mEq/L), serum B_{12} (200–800 pg/ml), rise in reticulocyte count (peaks in 5–8 days). Assess for reversal of deficiency symptoms: hyporeflexia, loss of positional sense, ataxia, fatigue, irritability, insomnia, anorexia, pallor, palpitation on exertion. Therapeutic response to treatment usually dramatic within 48 hrs.

PATIENT/FAMILY TEACHING:

Lifetime treatment may be necessary with pernicious anemia. Report symptoms of infection. Foods rich in vitamin B_{12} include organ meats, clams, oysters, herring, red snapper, muscle meats, fermented cheese, dairy products, egg yolks.

cyclobenzaprine hydrochloride

cy-klow-**benz**-ah-preen
(Flexeril, Novo-Cycloprine✤)

▶CLASSIFICATION

CLINICAL: Skeletal muscle relaxant

ACTION/*THERAPEUTIC EFFECT*

Acts within CNS at brain stem, *relieving local skeletal muscle spasm.*

PHARMACOKINETICS

	Onset	Peak	Duration
PO	1 hr	3–4 hrs	12–24 hrs

Well (but slowly) absorbed from GI tract. Protein binding: 93%. Metabolized in GI tract, liver. Primarily excreted in urine. Half-life: 1–3 days.

USES/*UNLABELED*

Short-term (2–3 wks) use as adjunct to rest, physical therapy, other measures for relief of discomfort due to acute, painful musculoskeletal conditions. *Treatment of fibromyalgia.*

PRECAUTIONS

CONTRAINDICATIONS: Concurrent use of MAO inhibitors or within 14 days after their discontinuation, acute recovery phase of MI, those with arrhythmias, heart blocks or conduction disturbances, CHF, hyperthyroidism. *CAUTIONS:* Impaired renal or hepatic function, history of urinary retention, angle-closure glaucoma, increased intraocular pressure.

▷*LIFESPAN CONSIDERATIONS:* **Pregnancy/Lactation:** Unknown if drug crosses placenta or is distributed in breast milk. **Pregnancy Category B. Children:** Safety and efficacy not established. **Elderly:** Increased sensitivity to anticholinergic effects (e.g., confusion, urinary retention).

INTERACTIONS

DRUG:* Tricyclic antidepressants, CNS depression-producing medications** may increase CNS depression. **MAO inhibitors** may increase risk of hypertensive crisis, severe seizures. ***HERBAL: None known. ***FOOD:*** None known. ***LAB VALUES:*** None significant.

AVAILABILITY (Rx)

TABLETS: 10 mg.

ADMINISTRATION/HANDLING

PO:

• Give without regard to food.

INDICATIONS/ROUTES/DOSAGE

Note: Do not use longer than 2–3 wks.

Acute, painful musculoskeletal conditions:

***PO:* Adults, elderly:** 10 mg 3 times/day. **Range:** 20–40 mg/day in 2–4 divided doses. **Maximum:** 60 mg/day.

SIDE EFFECTS

FREQUENT: Drowsiness (39%), dry mouth (27%), dizziness (11%). ***RARE*** (1–3%): Fatigue, tiredness, asthenia, blurred vision, headache, nervousness, confusion, nausea, constipation, dyspepsia, unpleasant taste.

ADVERSE REACTIONS/TOXIC EFFECTS

Overdosage may result in visual hallucinations, hyperactive reflexes, muscle rigidity, vomiting, hyperpyrexia.

NURSING IMPLICATIONS

BASELINE ASSESSMENT:

Record onset, type, location, and duration of muscular spasm. Check for immobility, stiffness, swelling.

INTERVENTION/EVALUATION:

Assist with ambulation at all times. Evaluate for therapeutic response: decreased intensity of skeletal muscle pain/tenderness, improved mobility, decrease in stiffness.

PATIENT/FAMILY TEACHING:

Drowsiness usually diminishes with continued therapy. Avoid tasks that require alertness, motor skills until response to drug is established. Avoid alcohol or other depressants while taking medication. Avoid sudden changes in posture. Sugarless gum, sips of water may relieve dry mouth.

cyclophosphamide

sigh-klo-**phos**-fah-mide
(Cytoxan, Neosar, Procytox✢)

▶CLASSIFICATION

PHARMACOTHERAPEUTIC: Alkylating agent. ***CLINICAL:*** Antineoplastic (see p. 69C)

ACTION/*THERAPEUTIC EFFECT*

Inhibits DNA, RNA protein synthesis by cross-linking with DNA, RNA strands, *inhibiting protein synthesis, preventing cell growth.* Potent immunosuppressant.

PHARMACOKINETICS

Well absorbed from GI tract. Crosses blood-brain barrier. Pro-

C

tein binding: Low. Metabolized in liver to active metabolites. Primarily excreted in urine. Removed by hemodialysis. Half-life: 3–12 hrs.

USES/*UNLABELED*

Treatment of Hodgkin's disease, non-Hodgkin's lymphomas, multiple myeloma, leukemia (acute lymphoblastic, acute myelogenous, acute monocytic, chronic granulocytic, chronic lymphocytic), mycosis fungoides, disseminated neuroblastoma, adenocarcinoma of ovary, retinoblastoma, carcinoma of breast. Biopsy-proven "minimal change" nephrotic syndrome in children. *Treatment of carcinoma of lung, cervix, endometrium, bladder, prostate, testicles, osteosarcoma, germ cell ovarian tumors, rheumatoid arthritis, systemic lupus erythematosus.*

PRECAUTIONS

CONTRAINDICATIONS: None significant. ***CAUTIONS:*** Severe leukopenia, thrombocytopenia, tumor infiltration of bone marrow, previous therapy with other antineoplastic agents, radiation.
▷***LIFESPAN CONSIDERATIONS:***
Pregnancy/Lactation: If possible, avoid use during pregnancy. May cause malformations (limb abnormalities, cardiac anomalies, hernias). Distributed in breast milk. Breast feeding not recommended. **Pregnancy Category D. Children:** No age-related precautions noted. **Elderly:** Age-related renal impairment may require caution.

INTERACTIONS

DRUG: May decrease effect of **antigout medications. Allopurinol, bone marrow depressants** may increase bone marrow depression. **Cytarabine** may in-

crease cardiomyopathy. Immunosuppressants may increase risk of infection, development of neoplasms. **Live virus vaccines** may potentiate virus replication, increase vaccine side effects, decrease pt's antibody response to vaccine. ***HERBAL:*** None known. ***FOOD:*** None known. ***LAB VALUES:*** May increase uric acid.

AVAILABILITY (Rx)

TABLETS: 25 mg, 50 mg. ***POWDER FOR INJECTION:*** 100 mg, 200 mg, 500 mg, 1 g, 2 g.

ADMINISTRATION/HANDLING

Note: May be carcinogenic, mutagenic, or teratogenic. Handle with extreme care during preparation/administration.

PO:
• Give on an empty stomach. If GI upset occurs, give with food.

IV 🔢

Storage:
• Reconstituted solution is stable for 24 hrs at room temperature or up to 6 days if refrigerated.

Reconstitution:
• For IV push, reconstitute each 100 mg with 5 ml Sterile Water for Injection or Bacteriostatic Water for Injection to provide concentration of 20 mg/ml. • Shake to dissolve. Allow to stand until clear.

Rate of administration:
• May give by IV push or further dilute with 250 ml D_5W, 0.9% NaCl, 0.45% NaCl, lactated Ringer's solution (LR) or D_5W/LR. • Infuse each 100 mg or fraction thereof over 15 min or longer. • IV may produce faintness, facial flushing, diaphoresis, oropharyngeal sensation.

IV INCOMPATIBILITIES ⊘

Amphotericin B complex (Abelcet, Ambisome, Amphotec).

IV COMPATIBILITIES

Cisplatin (Platinol), diphenhydramine (Benadryl), ondansetron (Zofran).

INDICATIONS/ROUTES/DOSAGE

Note: Dosage individualized based on clinical response, tolerance to adverse effects. When used in combination therapy, consult specific protocols for optimum dosage, sequence of drug administration.

Malignant diseases:

PO: Adults: 1–5 mg/kg/day. **Children:** Initially, 2–8 mg/kg/day. **Maintenance:** 2–5 mg/kg 2 times/wk.

IV: Adults: 40–50 mg/kg in divided doses over 2–5 days; or 10–15 mg/kg q7–10 days or 3–5 mg/kg 2 times/wk. **Children:** Initially, 40–50 mg/kg in divided doses over 2–5 days. **Maintenance:** 10–15 mg/kg q7–10 days or 3–5 mg/kg 2 times/wk.

Biopsy-proven "minimal change" nephrotic syndrome:

PO: Children: 2.5–3 mg/kg/day for 60–90 days.

SIDE EFFECTS

EXPECTED: Marked leukopenia 8–15 days after initial therapy. **FREQUENT:** Nausea, vomiting begins about 6 hrs after administration and lasts about 4 hrs; alopecia (33%). **OCCASIONAL:** Diarrhea, darkening of skin/fingernails, stomatitis (may include oral ulceration), headache, diaphoresis. **RARE:** Pain/redness at injection site.

ADVERSE REACTIONS/TOXIC EFFECTS

Major toxic effect is bone marrow depression resulting in blood dyscrasias (leukopenia, anemia, thrombocytopenia, hypoprothrombinemia). Thrombocytopenia may occur 10–15 days after drug initiation. Anemia generally occurs after large doses or prolonged therapy. Hemorrhagic cystitis occurs commonly in long-term therapy (esp. in children). Pulmonary fibrosis, cardiotoxicity noted with high doses. Amenorrhea, azoospermia, hyperkalemia may also occur.

NURSING IMPLICATIONS

BASELINE ASSESSMENT:

Obtain WBC count weekly during therapy or until maintenance dose is established, then at intervals of 2–3 wks.

INTERVENTION/EVALUATION:

Monitor CBC, serum uric acid concentration, blood chemistries. Monitor WBC closely during initial therapy. Monitor for hematologic toxicity (fever, sore throat, signs of local infection, easy bruising or unusual bleeding from any site), symptoms of anemia (excessive tiredness, weakness). Recovery from marked leukopenia due to bone marrow depression can be expected in 17–28 days.

PATIENT/FAMILY TEACHING:

Encourage copious fluid intake and frequent voiding (assists in preventing cystitis) at least 24 hrs before, during, after therapy. Do not have immunizations without physician's approval (drug lowers body's resistance). Avoid contact with those who have recently received live virus vaccine. Promptly report fever, sore throat, signs of local infection, easy bruising, or unusual bleeding from any site. Alopecia is reversible, but new hair growth may have different color or texture.

cyclosporine

sigh-klo-**spore**-in
(Neoral, Restasis, Sandimmune, Sang Cya)

▶ CLASSIFICATION

PHARMACOTHERAPEUTIC:
Cyclic polypeptide. **CLINICAL:**
Immunosuppressant

ACTION/*THERAPEUTIC EFFECT*

Inhibits interleukin-2, a proliferative factor needed for T cell activity. *Inhibits both cellular and humoral immune responses.*

PHARMACOKINETICS

Variably absorbed from GI tract. Widely distributed. Protein binding: 90%. Metabolized in liver. Eliminated primarily by biliary/fecal excretion. Not removed by hemodialysis. Half-life: adults 10–27 hrs, children 7–19 hrs.

USES/*UNLABELED*

Prevents rejection of kidney, liver, heart in combination with steroid therapy. Treatment of chronic allograft rejection in those previously treated with other immunosuppressives. **Capsules/solution:** Treatment of severe, active rheumatoid arthritis, psoriasis. *Treatment of alopecia areata, aplastic anemia, atopic dermatitis, Behçet's disease,* *biliary cirrhosis, corneal transplantation.*

PRECAUTIONS

CONTRAINDICATIONS: History of hypersensitivity to cyclosporine or polyoxyethylated castor oil. **CAUTIONS:** Impaired hepatic, renal, cardiac function, malabsorption syndrome, pregnancy, chickenpox, herpes zoster, infection, hypokalemia.

▷**LIFESPAN CONSIDERATIONS:**
Pregnancy/Lactation: Readily crosses placenta, distributed in breast milk. Avoid nursing. **Pregnancy Category C. Children:** No age-related precautions noted in transplant patients. **Elderly:** Increased risk of hypertension, increased serum creatinine.

INTERACTIONS

DRUG: Cimetidine, danazol, diltiazem, erythromycin, ketoconazole may increase concentration, risk of hepatotoxicity, nephrotoxicity; **ACE inhibitors, potassium-sparing diuretics, potassium supplements** may cause hyperkalemia. **Immunosuppressants** may increase risk of infection, lymphoproliferative disorders. **Lovastatin** may increase risk of rhabdomyolysis, acute renal failure. **Live virus vaccines** may potentiate virus replication, increase vaccine side effects, decrease pt's antibody response to vaccine. **HERBAL: St. John's wort** may alter absorption. **FOOD: Grapefruit/grapefruit juice** may increase absorption, risk of toxicity. **LAB VALUES:** May increase BUN, creatinine, SGOT (AST), SGPT (ALT), alkaline phosphatase, amylase, bilirubin, uric acid, potassium. May decrease magnesium. Therapeutic blood serum level: Peak: 50–300 ng/ml; toxic blood serum level: >400 ng/ml.

AVAILABILITY (Rx)

CAPSULES: 25 mg, 50 mg, 100 mg. **ORAL SOLUTION:** 100 mg/ml (in 50 ml calibrated liquid measuring device). **IV SOLUTION:** 50 mg/ml (5 ml amps).

ADMINISTRATION/HANDLING

Note: Oral solution available in bottle form with calibrated liquid measuring device. Oral form should replace IV administration as soon as possible.

PO:

• Oral solution may be mixed in glass container with milk, chocolate milk, or orange juice (preferably at room temperature). Stir well. Drink immediately. • Add more diluent to glass container and mix with remaining solution to ensure total amount is given. • Dry outside of calibrated liquid measuring device before replacing in cover. Do not rinse with water. • Avoid refrigeration of oral solution (separation of solution may occur). Discard oral solution after 2 mos once bottle is opened.

IV 🔟

Storage:

• Store parenteral form at room temperature. • Protect IV solution from light. • After diluted, stable for 24 hrs.

Reconstitution:

• Dilute each ml concentrate with 20–100 ml 0.9% NaCl or D_5W.

Rate of administration:

• Infuse over 2–6 hrs. • Monitor pt continuously for first 30 min after instituting infusion and frequently thereafter for hypersensitivity reaction (facial flushing, dyspnea).

IV INCOMPATIBILITIES 🚫

Amphotericin B complex (Ambisome, Amphotec, Abelcet).

IV COMPATIBILITY

Propofol (Diprivan).

INDICATIONS/ROUTES/DOSAGE

Note: May be given with adrenal corticosteroids, but not with other immunosuppressive agents (increases susceptibility to infection, development of lymphoma).

Prevention of allograft rejection:

PO: Adults, elderly, children: Initially, 15 mg/kg as single dose 4–12 hrs prior to transplantation, continue daily dose of 10–14 mg/kg/day for 1–2 wks. Taper dose by 5%/wk over 6–8 wks. **Maintenance:** 5–10 mg/kg/day.

IV: Adults, elderly, children: Give about one-third of oral dose: 5–6 mg/kg as single dose 4–12 hrs prior to transplantation, continue this daily single dose until pt is able to take oral medication.

Psoriasis, rheumatoid arthritis:

PO: Adults: 2.5 mg/kg daily in 2 divided doses.

SIDE EFFECTS

FREQUENT: Mild to moderate hypertension (26%), increased hair growth [hirsutism] (21%), tremor (12%). **OCCASIONAL** (2–4%): Acne, cramping, gingival hyperplasia (bleeding, tender gums), paresthesia, diarrhea, nausea, vomiting, headache. **RARE** (<1%): Hypersensitivity reaction, abdominal discomfort, gynecomastia, sinusitis.

ADVERSE REACTIONS/TOXIC EFFECTS

Mild nephrotoxicity occurs in 25% of renal transplants after transplan-

---

tation, 38% in cardiac transplants, and 37% of liver transplants, respectively. Hepatotoxicity occurs in 4% of renal, 7% of cardiac, and 4% of liver transplants, respectively. Both toxicities usually responsive to dosage reduction. Severe hyperkalemia, hyperuricemia occur occasionally.

NURSING IMPLICATIONS

BASELINE ASSESSMENT:
Note that if nephrotoxicity occurs, mild toxicity is generally noted 2–3 mos after transplantation; more severe toxicity noted early after transplantation; hepatotoxicity may be noted during first month after transplantation.

INTERVENTION/EVALUATION:
Diligently monitor BUN, creatinine, bilirubin, SGOT (AST), SGPT (ALT), LDH blood serum levels for evidence of hepatotoxicity or nephrotoxicity (mild toxicity noted by slow rise in serum levels; more overt toxicity noted by rapid rise in levels; hematuria also noted). Assess potassium level for evidence of hyperkalemia. Encourage diligent oral hygiene (gum hyperplasia). Monitor B/P for evidence of hypertension. Therapeutic blood serum level: Peak: 50–300 ng/ml; toxic blood serum level: >400 ng/ml.

PATIENT/FAMILY TEACHING:
Essential to repeat blood testing on a routine basis while receiving medication. Headache, tremor may occur as a response to medication. Avoid grapefruit, grapefruit juice (increases concentration, side effects).

cyproheptadine hydrochloride

C

sigh-pro-**hep**-tah-deen
(Periactin)

▶CLASSIFICATION
PHARMACOTHERAPEUTIC:
Phenothiazine. **CLINICAL:** Antihistamine (see p. 48C)

ACTION/*THERAPEUTIC EFFECT*
Competes with histamine at histaminic receptor sites, *relieving allergic conditions (urticaria, pruritus).* Anticholinergic effects cause drying of nasal mucosa.

USES/*UNLABELED*
Relief of nasal allergies, allergic dermatitis, cold urticaria, hypersensitivity reactions. *Stimulates appetite in underweight pts, those with anorexia nervosa. Treatment of vascular cluster headaches.*

PRECAUTIONS
CONTRAINDICATIONS: Acute asthmatic attack, pts receiving MAO inhibitors. **CAUTIONS:** Narrow-angle glaucoma, peptic ulcer, prostatic hypertrophy, pyloroduodenal or bladder neck obstruction, asthma, COPD, increased intraocular pressure, cardiovascular disease, hyperthyroidism, hypertension, seizure disorders.

INTERACTIONS
DRUG: Alcohol, CNS depressants may increase CNS depressant effects. **MAO inhibitors** may increase anticholinergic, CNS depressant effects. **HERBAL:** None known. **FOOD:** None known. **LAB VALUES:** May suppress wheal,

---

flare reactions to antigen skin testing, unless antihistamines discontinued 4 days prior to testing.

AVAILABILITY (Rx)

TABLETS: 4 mg. **SYRUP:** 2 mg/5 ml.

ADMINISTRATION/HANDLING

PO:

• Give without regard to meals. • Scored tablets may be crushed.

INDICATIONS/ROUTES/DOSAGE

Allergic condition:

PO: Adults, children >15 yrs: 4 mg 3 times/day. May increase dose but do not exceed 0.5 mg/kg/day. **Children 7–14 yrs:** 4 mg 2–3 times/day, or 0.25 mg/kg daily in divided doses. **Children 2–6 yrs:** 2 mg 2–3 times/day, or 0.25 mg/kg daily in divided doses.

Usual elderly dosage:

PO: Initially, 4 mg 2 times/day.

Note: Reduce dosage in pts with severe liver impairment.

SIDE EFFECTS

FREQUENT: Drowsiness, dizziness, muscular weakness, dry mouth/nose/throat/lips, urinary retention, thickening of bronchial secretions. Sedation, dizziness, hypotension more likely noted in elderly. **OCCASIONAL:** Epigastric distress, flushing, visual disturbances, hearing disturbances, paresthesia, sweating, chills.

ADVERSE REACTIONS/TOXIC EFFECTS

Children may experience dominant paradoxical reaction (restlessness, insomnia, euphoria, nervousness, tremors). Overdosage in children may result in hallucinations, convulsions, death. Hypersensitivity reaction (eczema, pruritus, rash, cardiac disturbances, angioedema, photosensitivity) may occur. Overdosage may vary from CNS depression (sedation, apnea, cardiovascular collapse, death) to severe paradoxical reaction (hallucinations, tremor, seizures).

NURSING IMPLICATIONS

BASELINE ASSESSMENT:

If pt is undergoing allergic reaction, obtain history of recently ingested foods, drugs, environmental exposure, recent emotional stress.

INTERVENTION/EVALUATION:

Monitor B/P, esp. in elderly (increased risk of hypotension). Monitor children closely for paradoxical reaction.

PATIENT/FAMILY TEACHING:

Tolerance to antihistaminic effect generally does not occur; tolerance to sedative effect may occur. Avoid tasks that require alertness, motor skills until response to drug is established. Dry mouth, drowsiness, dizziness may be an expected response of drug. Avoid alcoholic beverages during antihistamine therapy.

---

cytarabine

sigh-**tar**-ah-bean
(Ara-C, Cytosar✤, Cytosar-U, DepoCyt)

▶CLASSIFICATION

PHARMACOTHERAPEUTIC: Antimetabolite. **CLINICAL:** Antineoplastic (see p. 69C)

C

ACTION/*THERAPEUTIC EFFECT*

Converted intracellularly to nucleotide; *appears to inhibit DNA synthesis.* Cell cycle-specific for S phase of cell division. Potent immunosuppressive activity.

PHARMACOKINETICS

Widely distributed; moderate amount crosses blood-brain barrier. Protein binding: 15%. Primarily excreted in urine. Half-life: 1–3 hrs.

USES/*UNLABELED*

Treatment of acute and chronic myelocytic leukemia, acute lymphocytic leukemia, meningeal leukemia, non-Hodgkin's lymphoma in children. *DepoCyt:* Intrathecal treatment of lymphomatous meningitis. *Treatment of Hodgkin's lymphoma, myelodysplastic syndrome.*

PRECAUTIONS

CONTRAINDICATIONS: None significant. ***CAUTIONS:*** Impaired hepatic function.

▷*LIFESPAN CONSIDERATIONS:* **Pregnancy/Lactation:** If possible, avoid use during pregnancy. May cause malformations. Unknown if distributed in breast milk. Breast feeding not recommended. **Pregnancy Category D. Children:** No age-related precautions noted. **Elderly:** Age-related renal impairment may require dosage adjustment.

INTERACTIONS

DRUG: May decrease effect of **antigout medications. Bone marrow depressants** may increase bone marrow depression. **Cyclophosphamide** may increase cardiomyopathy risk. **Live virus vaccines** may potentiate virus replication, increase vaccine side effects, decrease pt's antibody response to vaccine. ***HERBAL:*** None known. ***FOOD:*** None known. ***LAB VALUES:*** May increase SGOT (AST), bilirubin, alkaline phosphatase, uric acid.

AVAILABILITY (Rx)

POWDER FOR INJECTION: 100 mg, 500 mg, 1 g, 2 g. ***INJECTABLE SUSTAINED-RELEASE FORMULATION:*** 10 mg/ml.

ADMINISTRATION/HANDLING

Note: May give by SubQ, IV push, IV infusion, or intrathecally. May be carcinogenic, mutagenic, or teratogenic (embryonic deformity). Handle with extreme care during preparation/administration.

SubQ, IV, intrathecal:

Storage:
• Reconstituted solution is stable for 48 hrs at room temperature. • IV infusion solutions at concentration up to 0.5 mg/ml is stable for 7 days at room temperature. • Discard if slight haze develops.

Reconstitution:
• Reconstitute 100 mg vial with 5 ml Bacteriostatic Water for Injection with benzyl alcohol (10 ml for 500 mg vial) to provide concentration of 20 mg/ml and 50 mg/ml, respectively. • Dose may be further diluted with up to 1,000 ml D_5W or 0.9% NaCl for IV infusion. • For intrathecal use, reconstitute vial with preservative-free 0.9% NaCl or pt's spinal fluid. Dose usually administered in 5–15 ml of solution, after equivalent volume of CSF removed.

Rate of administration:
• For IV push, give over 1–3 min. • For IV infusion, give over 30 min to 24 hrs.

IV INCOMPATIBILITIES ⊘

Amphotericin B complex (Ambisome, Amphotec, Abelcet), ganciclovir (Cytovene).

IV COMPATIBILITIES

Diphenhydramine (Benadryl), dexamethasone (Decadron), granisetron (Kytril), ondansetron (Zofran).

INDICATIONS/ROUTES/DOSAGE

Note: Dosage individualized based on clinical response, tolerance to adverse effects. When used in combination therapy, consult specific protocols for optimum dosage, sequence of drug administration. Modify dose when serious hematologic depression occurs.

Acute nonlymphocytic leukemia:

IV INFUSION: **Adults, children** (Combination): 100 mg/m²/day, days 1–7.

IV: **Adults:** 100 mg/m² q12h, days 1–7.

Acute lymphocytic leukemia:

Refer to specific protocol.

SIDE EFFECTS

FREQUENT: SubQ, IV (16–33%): Asthenia, fever, pain, change in taste/smell, nausea, vomiting (risk of nausea and vomiting greater with IV push than with continuous IV infusion). **Intrathecal** (11–28%): Headache, asthenia, change in taste/smell, confusion, somnolence, nausea, vomiting. ***OCCASIONAL: SubQ, IV*** (7–11%): Abnormal gait, somnolence, constipation, back pain, urinary incontinence, peripheral edema, headache, confusion. **Intrathecal** (3–7%): Peripheral edema, back pain, constipation, abnormal gait, urinary incontinence.

ADVERSE REACTIONS/TOXIC EFFECTS

Major toxic effect is bone marrow depression resulting in blood dyscrasias (leukopenia, anemia, thrombocytopenia, megaloblastosis, reticulocytopenia), occurring minimally after single IV dose, but leukopenia, anemia, thrombocytopenia should be expected with daily or continuous IV. Cytarabine syndrome (fever, myalgia, rash, conjunctivitis, malaise, chest pain), hyperuricemia may be noted. High-dose therapy may produce severe CNS, GI, pulmonary toxicity.

NURSING IMPLICATIONS

BASELINE ASSESSMENT:
Leukocyte count decreases within 24 hrs after initial dose, continues to decrease for 7–9 days followed by brief rise at 12 days, then decreases again at 15–24 days, then rises rapidly for next 10 days. Platelet count decreases 5 days after drug initiation to low count at 12–15 days, then rises rapidly for next 10 days.

INTERVENTION/EVALUATION:
Monitor CBC for evidence of bone marrow depression. Monitor for blood dyscrasias (fever, sore throat, signs of local infection, easy bruising, or unusual bleeding from any site), symptoms of anemia (excessive tiredness, weakness). Monitor for signs of neuropathy (gait disturbances, handwriting difficulties, numbness).

PATIENT/FAMILY TEACHING:
Increase fluid intake (may protect against hyperuricemia). Do not have immunizations without physician's approval (drug lowers body's resistance). Avoid contact with those who have recently received live virus vaccine. Promptly report fever, sore throat, signs of local infection, easy bruising or unusual bleeding from any site.

dacarbazine

day-**car**-bah-zeen
(DTIC-Dome)
Do not confuse with Dicarbosil.

▶CLASSIFICATION

PHARMACOTHERAPEUTIC:
Alkaylating agent. ***CLINICAL:***
Antineoplastic (see p. 69C).

ACTION/*THERAPEUTIC EFFECT*

Cell cycle-phase nonspecific.
Some activity and toxicity results
from activation of drug by hepatic
enzymes. Forms carbonium ions,
inhibiting DNA, RNA synthesis.

PHARMACOKINETICS

Minimally crosses blood-brain barrier. Protein binding: Low. Metabolized in liver. Excreted in urine.
Half-life: 5 hrs (half-life increased
with impaired renal function).

USES/*UNLABELED*

Treatment of metastatic malignant
melanoma, second-line therapy of
Hodgkin's disease. *Treatment of
soft tissue sarcoma.*

PRECAUTIONS

CONTRAINDICATIONS: Demonstrated hypersensitivity to drug.
CAUTIONS: Impaired hepatic
function.

▷*LIFESPAN CONSIDERATIONS:*
Pregnancy/Lactation: If possible, avoid use during pregnancy,
esp. first trimester. Breast feeding
not recommended. **Pregnancy
Category C. Children:** Safety and
efficacy not established. **Elderly:**
Age-related renal impairment
may require dosage adjustment.

INTERACTIONS

DRUG: **Bone marrow depressants** may enhance myelosuppression. **Live virus vaccines**
may potentiate virus replication,
increase vaccine side effects, decrease pt's antibody response to
vaccine. ***HERBAL:*** None known.
FOOD: None known. ***LAB VALUES:***
May increase SGOT (AST), SGPT
(ALT), alkaline phosphatase, BUN.

AVAILABILITY (Rx)

POWDER FOR INJECTION: 10
mg/ml.

ADMINISTRATION/HANDLING

Note: May give by IV push or IV
infusion. May be carcinogenic,
mutagenic, or teratogenic. Handle
with extreme care during prepa-
ration/administration.

IV

Storage:

• Protect from light; refrigerate
vials. • Color change from ivory to
pink indicates decomposition; discard. • Solution containing 10 mg/
ml is stable for 8 hrs at room temperature or 72 hrs if refrigerated. •
Solution diluted with up to 500 ml
D_5W or 0.9% NaCl is stable for at
least 8 hrs at room temperature or
24 hrs if refrigerated.

Reconstitution:

• Reconstitute 100 mg vial with 9.9
ml Sterile Water for Injection (19.7
ml for 200 mg vial) to provide
concentration of 10 mg/ml.

Rate of administration:

• Give IV push over 1–2 min. • For
IV infusion, further dilute with up
to 250 ml D_5W or 0.9% NaCl. Infuse over 15–30 min. • Apply hot
packs if local pain, burning sensation, irritation at injection site occurs. • Avoid extravasation (stinging, swelling, coolness, slight or no
blood return at injection site).

IV INCOMPATIBILITIES ⊘

Allopurinol (Aloprim), cefepime (Maxipime), heparin, piperacillin/tazobactam (Zosyn).

IV COMPATIBILITIES

Etoposide (Vepesed), granisetron (Kytril), ondansetron (Zofran), paclitaxel (Taxol).

INDICATIONS/ROUTES/DOSAGE

Note: Dosage individualized based on clinical response, tolerance to adverse effects. When used in combination therapy, consult specific protocols for optimum dosage, sequence of drug administration.

Malignant melanoma:

IV: Adults, elderly: 2–4.5 mg/kg/day for 10 days, repeated at 4 wk intervals, or 250 mg/m^2 daily for 5 days, repeated q3wks.

Hodgkin's disease:

IV: Adults, elderly: Combination therapy: 150 mg/m^2 daily for 5 days, repeated q4wks, or 375 mg/m^2 once, repeated q15days. **Children:** 375 mg/m^2 on days 1 and 15; repeat q28days.

Solid tumors:

IV: Children: 200–470 mg/m^2/day over 5 days q21–28days.

Neuroblastoma:

IV: Children: 800–900 mg/m^2 as single dose on day 1 of therapy q3–4wks in combination therapy.

SIDE EFFECTS

FREQUENT (90%): Nausea, vomiting, anorexia (occurs within 1 hr of initial dose, may last up to 12 hrs). **OCCASIONAL:** Facial flushing, paresthesia, alopecia, flulike syndrome (fever, myalgia, malaise), dermatologic reactions, CNS symptoms (confusion, blurred vision, headache, lethargy). **RARE:** Diarrhea, stomatitis (redness/burning of oral mucous membranes, gum/tongue inflammation), photosensitivity.

ADVERSE REACTIONS/TOXIC EFFECTS

Bone marrow depression resulting in blood dyscrasias (leukopenia, thrombocytopenia) generally appears 2–4 wks after last drug dose. Hepatotoxicity occurs rarely.

NURSING IMPLICATIONS

BASELINE ASSESSMENT:

Some clinicians recommend food/fluids be restricted 4–6 hrs before treatment; other clinicians believe good hydration to within 1 hr of treatment will avoid dehydration due to vomiting. Conflicting reports of effectiveness of administering antiemetics for nausea, vomiting.

INTERVENTION/EVALUATION:

Monitor leukocyte, erythrocyte, platelet counts for evidence of bone marrow depression. Monitor for hematologic toxicity (fever, sore throat, signs of local infection, easy bruising, unusual bleeding from any site).

PATIENT/FAMILY TEACHING:

Tolerance to GI effects occurs rapidly (generally after 1–2 days treatment). Do not have immunizations without physician's approval (drug lowers body's resistance). Avoid contact with those who have recently received live virus vaccine. Promptly report fever, sore throat, signs of local infection, easy bruising, unusual bleeding from any site. Contact physician if nausea/vomiting continues at home.

daclizumab

day-**cly**-zu-mab
(Zenapax)

▶CLASSIFICATION

PHARMACOTHERAPEUTIC:
Monoclonal antibody. ***CLINI-CAL:*** Immunosuppressive

ACTION/*THERAPEUTIC EFFECT*

Binds to and inhibits interleukin-2 mediated lymphocyte activation (critical pathway in cellular immune response involved in allograft rejection), *preventing organ rejection.*

USES

Prophylaxis of acute organ rejection in pts receiving renal transplants.

PRECAUTIONS

CONTRAINDICATIONS: None significant. ***CAUTIONS:*** Infection, history of malignancy.
▷***LIFESPAN CONSIDERATIONS:***
Pregnancy/Lactation: Unknown if crosses placenta, distributed in breast milk. **Pregnancy Category C. Children/Elderly:** No age-related precautions noted.

INTERACTIONS

DRUG: None significant. ***HERBAL:*** None known. ***FOOD:*** None known. ***LAB VALUES:*** None known.

AVAILABILITY (Rx)

INJECTION: 25 mg/5 ml.

ADMINISTRATION/HANDLING

IV 🔲

Storage:

• Protect from light; refrigerate vials.• Once reconstituted, stable for 4 hrs at room temperature, 24 hrs if refrigerated.

Reconstitution:
• Dilute in 50 ml 0.9% NaCl. • Invert gently. • Avoid shaking.

Rate of administration:
• Infuse over 15 min.

IV INCOMPATIBILITY ⊘

Do not mix with any other medication.

INDICATIONS/ROUTES/DOSAGE

***IV:* Adults, children:** 1 mg/kg over 15 min. First dose no more than 24 hrs before transplantation, then q14 days for total of 5 doses. **Maximum:** 100 mg.

SIDE EFFECTS

OCCASIONAL (>2%): Constipation, nausea, diarrhea, vomiting, abdominal pain, edema, headache, dizziness, fever, pain, fatigue, insomnia, weakness, arthralgia, myalgia, increased sweating.

ADVERSE REACTIONS/TOXIC EFFECTS

None significant.

NURSING IMPLICATIONS

BASELINE ASSESSMENT:

Obtain baseline blood serum levels and vital signs, particularly B/P, pulse rate.

INTERVENTION/EVALUATION:

Diligently monitor all blood serum levels. Assess B/P for hypertension/hypotension; pulse for evidence of tachycardia. Question for GI disturbances, urinary changes. Monitor for presence of wound infection, CBC, signs of infection (fever, sore throat), unusual bleeding/bruising.

PATIENT/FAMILY TEACHING:
Report difficulty in breathing or swallowing, rapid heartbeat, rash, or itching, swelling of lower extremities and weakness. Avoid pregnancy.

---

dactinomycin

dak-tin-oh-**my**-sin
(Cosmegen)

▶CLASSIFICATION
PHARMACOTHERAPEUTIC:
Antibiotic. ***CLINICAL:*** Antineoplastic (see p. 69C)

ACTION/*THERAPEUTIC EFFECT*
Forms DNA complex, *inhibiting DNA-dependent RNA synthesis.* Actively growing cells are most sensitive to drug's action. Cell cycle-phase nonspecific.

USES/*UNLABELED*
Treatment of Wilms' tumor, rhabdomyosarcoma, Ewing's sarcoma, advanced nonseminomatous testicular carcinoma, sarcoma botryoides, metastatic and nonmetastatic choriocarcinoma. *Treatment of ovarian cancer, Kaposi's sarcoma, osteosarcoma, malignant melanoma.*

PRECAUTIONS
CONTRAINDICATIONS: Those with chickenpox or herpes zoster. ***CAUTIONS:*** Within first 2 mos of radiation therapy.

INTERACTIONS
DRUG: May decrease effect of **antigout medications. Bone marrow depressants** may enhance myelosuppression. **Live virus vaccines** may potentiate virus replication, increase vaccine side effects, decrease pt's antibody response to vaccine. ***HERBAL:*** None known. ***FOOD:*** None known. ***LAB VALUES:*** May increase uric acid.

AVAILABILITY (Rx)
POWDER FOR INJECTION: 0.5 mg.

ADMINISTRATION/HANDLING
IV 💉
Note: Give by IV push or IV infusion. Wear protective gloves when handling drug. May be carcinogenic, mutagenic, or teratogenic. Handle with extreme care during preparation/administration.

Storage:
• Prepare solution immediately before use. • Discard unused portion. • Solution should be clear, gold color.

Reconstitution:
• Reconstitute 500 mcg vial with 1.1 ml Sterile Water for Injection without preservative (avoids precipitate) to provide concentration of 500 mcg/ml.

Rate of administration:
• For IV push, administer over 1–3 min into tubing of running IV. Withdraw dose from vial with one needle, use 2nd needle for injection. • For IV infusion, add up to 50 ml D₅W or 0.9% NaCl and infuse over 20–30 min. • Extravasation usually produces immediate pain, severe local tissue damage. Aspirate as much infiltrated drug as possible; then infiltrate area with hydrocortisone, sodium succinate injection (50–100 mg hydrocortisone), and/or isotonic sodium thiosulfate injection or ascorbic acid injection (1 ml of 5% injection). Apply cold compresses.

IV INCOMPATIBILITY ⊘
Filgrastim (Neupogen).

IV COMPATIBILITIES
Allopurinol (Aloprim), etoposide (Vepesed), granisetron (Kytril), ondansetron (Zofran).

INDICATIONS/ROUTES/DOSAGE
Note: Dosage is individualized based on clinical response and tolerance to adverse effects. When used in combination therapy, consult specific protocols for optimum dosage and sequence of drug administration. Do not exceed 15 mcg/kg or 400–600 mcg/m²/day. Dosage for obese or edematous pts based on surface area. Repeat dosage at least at 3 wk intervals, provided all signs of toxicity have disappeared.

Usual dosage:

***IV:* Adults, elderly, children:** 15 mcg/kg/day (up to maximum of 500 mcg/day) for 5 days, or total dosage of 2.5 mg/m² in divided doses over 1 wk.

***ISOLATION PERFUSION:* Adults, elderly:** 50 mcg/kg for lower extremity or pelvis; 35 mcg/kg for upper extremity.

SIDE EFFECTS
FREQUENT: Nausea, vomiting, buccal/pharangeal/skin erythema, rash (particularly when combined with radiation). ***OCCASIONAL:*** Anorexia, alopecia, abdominal distress.

ADVERSE REACTIONS/TOXIC EFFECTS
Bone marrow depression resulting in hematologic toxicity (leukopenia, thrombocytopenia, and to lesser extent, anemia, pancytopenia, reticulopenia, agranulocytosis, aplastic anemia). GI and oral mucosal toxicity may result in diarrhea, oral/GI ulceration, stomatitis, glossitis, esophagitis, pharyngitis.

NURSING IMPLICATIONS

BASELINE ASSESSMENT:
Obtain baseline hematologic results. Nausea/vomiting occurs a few hrs after dosing, can last up to 24 hrs. Decrease in platelet count generally appears 1–7 days after last drug dose, reaches lowest count at 14–21 days, returns to normal within 21–25 days.

INTERVENTION/EVALUATION:
Monitor hematologic status, renal/hepatic function studies, serum uric acid level. Assess pattern of daily bowel activity and stool consistency. Monitor for hematologic toxicity (fever, sore throat, signs of local infection, easy bruising, or unusual bleeding from any site), symptoms of anemia (excessive tiredness, weakness). Assess skin for dermatologic effects.

PATIENT/FAMILY TEACHING:
Alopecia is reversible, but new hair growth may have different color or texture. Pain, redness may occur at injection site. Do not have immunizations without physician's approval (drug lowers body's resistance). Avoid contact with those who have recently received live virus vaccine. Promptly report fever, sore throat, signs of local infection, easy bruising, unusual bleeding from any site. Increase fluid intake. Contact physician if nausea/vomiting continues at home.

dalteparin sodium

dawl-teh-pear-in
(Fragmin)

▶CLASSIFICATION

PHARMACOTHERAPEUTIC:
Low molecular weight heparin.
CLINICAL: Anticoagulant (see
p. 28C)

ACTION/THERAPEUTIC EFFECT

Antithrombin; in presence of low
molecular weight heparin, *produces anticoagulation* by inhibition
of factor Xa and thrombin by antithrombin. Only slightly influences
platelet aggregation, prothrombin
time (PT), activated partial thromboplastin time (APTT).

PHARMACOKINETICS

	Onset	Peak	Duration
SubQ	—	4 hrs	—

Protein binding: <10%. Terminal
half-life following SubQ administration: 3–5 hrs.

USES

Treatment of unstable angina and
non Q-wave myocardial infarction
(MI) to prevent ischemic events.
Prevention of deep vein thrombosis (DVT) in pts undergoing hip
replacement or abdominal surgery who are at risk of thromboembolic complications. Those at
risk are >40 yrs, obese, undergoing surgery under general anesthesia lasting >30 min, malignancy or history of DVT or
pulmonary embolism.

PRECAUTIONS

CONTRAINDICATIONS: Active
major bleeding, concurrent heparin therapy, thrombocytopenia
associated with positive in vitro
test for antiplatelet antibody, hypersensitivity to dalteparin, heparin, or pork products. **CAUTIONS:** Conditions with increased
risk of hemorrhage, bacterial endocarditis, history of heparin-induced thrombocytopenia, impaired renal or hepatic function,
uncontrolled arterial hypertension, history of recent GI ulceration and hemorrhage, hypertensive or diabetic retinopathy.

▷**LIFESPAN CONSIDERATIONS:**
Pregnancy/Lactation: Use with
caution, particularly during last
trimester, immediate postpartum
period (increased risk of maternal
hemorrhage). Unknown if distributed in breast milk. **Pregnancy
Category B. Children:** Safety and
efficacy not established. **Elderly:**
No age-related precautions noted.

INTERACTIONS

**DRUG: Anticoagulants, platelet
inhibitors** may increase bleeding.
HERBAL: None known. **FOOD:**
None known. **LAB VALUES:** Reversible increases in SGOT (AST),
SGPT (ALT), alkaline phosphatase,
lactate dehydrogenase (LDH).

AVAILABILITY (Rx)

SOLUTION: 2,500 anti-Factor Xa IU
per 0.2 ml. **SINGLE-DOSE SYRINGE:**
5,000 IU. **MULTIDOSE VIAL:** 95,000
IU.

ADMINISTRATION/HANDLING
SubQ:

• Store at room temperature. • Instruct pt to sit or lie down before administering by deep SubQ injection. • Inject in U-shaped area
around the navel, upper outer side
of thigh, or upper outer quadrangle
of buttock. • Use a fine needle
(25–26 gauge) to minimize tissue

trauma. • Introduce entire length of needle (½ inch) into skin fold held between thumb and forefinger, holding skin fold during injection at a 45° to 90° angle. • Do not rub injection site after administration (prevents bruising). • Alternate the administration site with each injection.

INDICATIONS/ROUTES/DOSAGE

Prevention of deep vein thrombosis:

SUBQ: **Adults:** 2,500–5,000 IU each day, starting 1–2 hrs before surgery. Repeat once daily for 5–10 days postoperatively.

Prevention of ischemic events in unstable angina, non Q-wave MI:

SUBQ: **Adults, elderly:** 120 IU/kg q12h (with concurrent aspirin). **Maximum:** 10,000 IU.

SIDE EFFECTS

OCCASIONAL (3–7%): Hematoma at injection site. ***RARE*** (<1%): Hypersensitivity reaction (chills, fever, pruritus, urticaria, asthma, rhinitis, lacrimation, headache), mild, local skin irritation.

ADVERSE REACTIONS/TOXIC EFFECTS

Accidental overdosage may lead to bleeding complications ranging from local ecchymoses to major hemorrhage. Thrombocytopenia occurs rarely.

NURSING IMPLICATIONS

BASELINE ASSESSMENT:

Assess CBC, including platelet count. Determine initial B/P.

INTERVENTION/EVALUATION:

Periodically monitor CBC, platelet count, stool for occult blood (no need for daily monitoring in pts with normal presurgical coagulation parameters). Assess for any sign of bleeding: bleeding at surgical site, hematuria, blood in stool, bleeding from gums, petechiae, bruising, bleeding from injection sites.

PATIENT/FAMILY TEACHING:

Usual length of therapy is 5–10 days. Report any sign of bleeding. Do not take any OTC medication (esp. aspirin) without consulting physician. Report bleeding, bruising, dizziness or lightheadedness, rash, itching, fever, swelling, breathing difficulty. Rotate injection sites daily. Teach proper injection technique. Excessive bruising at injection site may be lessened by ice massage prior to injection.

danaparoid

dan-ah-**pear**-oid
(Orgaran k)

▶CLASSIFICATION

PHARMACOTHERAPEUTIC: Low molecular weight heparin. ***CLINICAL:*** Antithrombotic (see p. 28C)

ACTION/*THERAPEUTIC EFFECT*

Inhibits thrombin formation through factor anti-Xa and anti II-A effects, *producing anthrombotic activity, anticoagulation.* Does not significantly influence bleeding time, prothrombin time (PT), activated partial thromboplastin time (APTT), platelet function. Possesses greater antithrombotic activity than anticoagulant activity.

PHARMACOKINETICS

	Onset	Peak	Duration
PO	—	2–5 hrs	—

Well absorbed following SubQ administration. Eliminated primarily in the urine. Half-life: 24 hrs (half-life prolonged in those with severely impaired renal function).

USES/*UNLABELED*

Prophylaxis of postop deep vein thrombosis (DVT) following elective hip replacement surgery. *Treatment of thromboembolism, to produce anticoagulation during hemodialysis, hemofiltration during cardiovascular operation, pregnant pts at increased risk of thrombosis.*

PRECAUTIONS

CONTRAINDICATIONS: Severe hemorrhagic diathesis (hemophilia, idiopathic thrombocytopenic purpura), active major bleeding state, including hemorrhagic stroke in the acute phase, type II phase thrombocytopenia associated with positive in vitro test for antiplatelet antibody in presence of danaparoid, hypersensitivity to pork products, danaparoid. ***CAUTIONS:*** Conditions with increased risk of hemorrhage, acute bacterial endocarditis, congenital or acquired bleeding disorders, active ulcerative and angiodysplastic GI disease, nonhemorrhagic stroke, shortly after brain, spinal, or ophthalmologic surgery, postop indwelling epidural catheter use, severe uncontrolled hypertension, renal/hepatic function impairment, those with sulfite sensitivity (more frequently seen in asthmatics).

▷*LIFESPAN CONSIDERATIONS:*
Pregnancy/Lactation: Unknown if distributed in breast milk. **Pregnancy Category B. Children:** Safety and efficacy not established. **Elderly:** No age-related precautions noted.

INTERACTIONS

DRUG: **Anticoagulants, platelet inhibitors** may increase bleeding (use with care). ***HERBAL:*** None known. ***FOOD:*** None known. ***LAB VALUES:*** None significant.

AVAILABILITY (Rx)

INJECTION: 750 anti-Xa units/0.6 ml.

ADMINISTRATION/HANDLING

SubQ:

• Instruct pt to sit or lie down before administering by deep SubQ injection. • Inject between left and right anterolateral and left and right posterolateral abdominal wall (avoid navel area). • Use a fine needle (25–26 gauge) to minimize tissue trauma. • Introduce entire length of needle into skin fold held between thumb and forefinger, holding skin fold during injection at a 45° to 90° angle. • Do not pinch or rub injection site after administration (prevents bruising). • Alternate the administration site with each injection.

INDICATIONS/ROUTES/DOSAGE

Note: Give initial dose as soon as possible after surgery but not more than 24 hrs after surgery.

Prevention of deep vein thrombosis:

SubQ: **Adults, elderly:** 750 anti-Xa units twice daily beginning 1–4 hrs preoperatively, and then not sooner than 2 hrs after surgery. Continue treatment throughout postop care until risk of DVT has diminished (average duration 7–14 days).

SIDE EFFECTS

FREQUENT (13%): Injection site pain. **OCCASIONAL** (4–9%): Fever, pain, nausea, urinary tract infection, constipation. **RARE** (≤2%): Rash, pruritus, infection.

ADVERSE REACTIONS/TOXIC EFFECTS

Accidental overdosage may lead to bleeding complications ranging from minor ecchymosis to major hemorrhage. A unexplained fall in hematocrit or fall in B/P should lead to consideration of a hemorrhagic event. **Antidote:** Protamine sulfate only partially neutralizes danaparoid activity and is incapable of reducing severe nonsurgical bleeding during treatment. If serious bleeding occurs, discontinue danaparoid, give blood or blood product transfusions.

NURSING IMPLICATIONS

BASELINE ASSESSMENT:

Assess CBC, including platelet count.

INTERVENTION/EVALUATION:

Periodically monitor CBC, platelet count, stool for occult blood. Assess for any sign of bleeding: bleeding at surgical site, hematuria, blood in stool, bleeding from gums, petechiae, bruising, bleeding from injection sites. A unexplained fall in hematocrit or fall in B/P should lead to consideration of a hemorrhagic event. In those with renal function impairment, monitor those with serum creatinine ≥2 mg/dl.

PATIENT/FAMILY TEACHING:

Usual length of therapy is 7–14 days. Report any sign of bleeding. Do not take any OTC medication (esp. aspirin) without consulting physician.

danazol ✳ D

dan-ah-zole
(Cyclomen ♣, Danocrine)

▶**CLASSIFICATION**

PHARMACOTHERAPEUTIC: Testosterone derivative. **CLINICAL:** Androgen, hormone

ACTION/*THERAPEUTIC EFFECT*

Suppresses the pituitary-ovarian axis by inhibiting the output of pituitary gonadotropins. In endometriosis, causes atrophy of both normal and ectopic endometrial tissue, *producing anovulation and amenorrhea.* For fibrocystic breast disease, follicle-stimulating hormone (FSH) and luteinizing hormone (LH) are depressed, *reducing the production of estrogen;* inhibits steroid synthesis and binding of steroids to their receptors in breast tissue. Increases serum levels of esterase inhibitor, *correcting biochemical deficiency as seen in hereditary angioedema.*

USES/*UNLABELED*

Palliative treatment of endometriosis, fibrocystic breast disease; prophylactic treatment of hereditary angioedema. *Treatment of gynecomastia, menorrhagia, precocious puberty.*

PRECAUTIONS

CONTRAINDICATIONS: Severe cardiac function impairment, liver function impairment, renal function impairment. Active or history of thromboembolic disease, androgen tumor, abnormal vaginal

---

bleeding. ***CAUTIONS:*** Renal function impairment, cardiac impairment, epilepsy, migraine headaches, diabetes.

INTERACTIONS

DRUG: May enhance effects of **anticoagulants.** May increase nephrotoxicity with **cyclosporine** and **tacrolimus.** ***HERBAL:*** None significant. ***FOOD:*** None significant. ***LAB VALUES:*** May increase liver function tests.

AVAILABILITY (Rx)

CAPSULES: 20 mg, 100 mg, 200 mg.

INDICATIONS/ROUTES/DOSAGE

Note: Initiate therapy during menstruation or when pt is not pregnant.

Endometriosis:

PO: **Adults:** 200–800 mg/day in 2 divided doses for 3–9 mos.

Fibrocystic breast disease:

PO: **Adults:** 100–400 mg/day in 2 divided doses.

Hereditary angioedema:

PO: **Adults:** Initially, 200 mg 2–3 times/day. Decrease dose by 50% or less at 1–3 mo intervals. If attack occurs, increase dose by up to 200 mg/day.

SIDE EFFECTS

FREQUENT: **Females:** Amenorrhea, breakthrough bleeding/spotting, decreased breast size, increased weight, irregular menstrual period. ***OCCASIONAL:*** **Males/females:** Edema, rhabdomyolysis (muscle cramps, unusual fatigue), virilism (acne, oily skin), flushed skin, altered moods. ***RARE:*** **Males/females:** Hematuria, gingivitis, carpal tunnel syndrome, cataracts, severe headache, vomiting, rash, photosensitivity.

Females: Enlarged clitoris, hoarseness, deepening voice, hair growth, monilial vaginitis. **Males:** Decreased testicle size.

ADVERSE REACTIONS/TOXIC EFFECTS

Jaundice may occur in those receiving 400 mg/day or more. Liver dysfunction, eosinophilia, thrombocytopenia, pancreatitis occur rarely.

NURSING IMPLICATIONS

BASELINE ASSESSMENT:

Inquire about menstrual cycle: Therapy should begin during menstruation. Establish baseline weight, B/P.

INTERVENTION/EVALUATION:

Weigh 2–3 times/week; report >5 lbs/wk gain or swelling of fingers or feet. Monitor B/P periodically. Check for jaundice (yellow eyes or skin, dark urine, claycolored stools).

PATIENT/FAMILY TEACHING:

Patient should use nonhormonal contraceptive during therapy. Do not take drug, check with physician if suspect pregnancy (risk to fetus). Importance of full length of therapy, regular visits to physician's office (hepatic function tests, etc.). Notify physician promptly of masculinizing effects (may not be reversible), weight gain, muscle cramps, or fatigue. Spotting or bleeding may occur in first mos of therapy for endometriosis (does not mean lack of efficacy). In fibrocystic breast disease, irregular menstrual periods and amenorrhea may occur with or without ovulation.

dantrolene sodium

dan-trow-lean
(Dantrium)
Do not confuse with Daraprim.

▶CLASSIFICATION

CLINICAL: Skeletal muscle relaxant

ACTION/*THERAPEUTIC EFFECT*

Reduces muscle contraction by interfering with release of calcium ion, *dissociating excitation-contraction coupling*. Reduced calcium ion concentration, *interfering with catabolic process associated with malignant hyperthermic crisis*.

PHARMACOKINETICS

Poorly absorbed from GI tract. Protein binding: High. Metabolized in liver. Primarily excreted in urine. Half-life: IV: 4–8 hrs; PO: 8.7 hrs.

USES/*UNLABELED*

PO: Relief of signs and symptoms of spasticity due to spiral cord injuries, stroke, cerebral palsy, multiple sclerosis, esp. flexor spasms, concomitant pain, clonus, and muscular rigidity. **Parenteral:** Management of fulminant hypermetabolism of skeletal muscle due to malignant hyperthermia crisis. *Treatment of neuroleptic malignant syndrome, relief of exercise-induced pain in pts with muscular dystrophy, treatment of flexor spasms.*

PRECAUTIONS

CONTRAINDICATIONS: PO: Active liver disease (i.e., hepatitis, cirrhosis), when spasticity is needed to maintain upright posture and balance when walking or to achieve or support increased function, severely impaired cardiac function, previous liver disease/dysfunction. **CAUTIONS:** Females, those >35 yrs of age, impaired liver, or pulmonary function.

▷*LIFESPAN CONSIDERATIONS:* **Pregnancy/Lactation:** Readily crosses placenta; do not use in breast-feeding mothers. **Pregnancy Category C. Children:** No age-related precautions noted in those >5 yrs. **Elderly:** No information available.

INTERACTIONS

DRUG: CNS depressants may increase CNS depression (short-term use). **Hepatotoxic medications** may increase risk of hepatotoxicity (chronic use). **HERBAL:** None known. **FOOD:** None known. **LAB VALUES:** May alter liver function tests.

AVAILABILITY (Rx)

CAPSULES: 25 mg, 50 mg, 100 mg. **POWDER FOR INJECTION:** 20 mg vial.

ADMINISTRATION/HANDLING
PO:
• Give without regard to meals.
IV
Storage:
• Store at room temperature. • Use within 6 hrs after reconstitution. Solution is clear, colorless. Discard if cloudy, precipitate formed.

Reconstitution:
• Reconstitute 20 mg vial with 60 ml Sterile Water for Injection to provide concentration of 0.33 mg/ml.

Rate of administration:
• For IV infusion, administer over 1 hr. • Diligently monitor for extravasation (high pH of IV prepara-

tion). May produce severe complications.

IV INCOMPATIBILITY ⊘

None known.

INDICATIONS/ROUTES/DOSAGE

Spasticity:

Note: Best to begin with low-dose therapy, then increase gradually at 4–7 day intervals (reduces incidence of side effects).

PO: **Adults, elderly:** Initially, 25 mg/day. Increase to 25 mg 2–4 times/day, then by 25 mg increments up to 100 mg 2–4 times/day. **Children >5 yrs:** Initially, 0.5 mg/kg 2 times/day. Increase to 0.5 mg/kg 3–4 times/day, then increase by 0.5 mg/kg/day up to 3 mg/kg 2–4 times/day. **Maximum:** 400 mg/day.

Prevention of malignant hyperthermia crisis:

PO: **Adults, elderly, children:** 4–8 mg/kg/day in 3–4 divided doses 1–2 days prior to surgery (give last dose 3–4 hrs prior to surgery).

IV INFUSION: **Adults, elderly, children:** 2.5 mg/kg about 1.25 hrs prior to surgery.

Management of hyperthermia crisis:

IV: **Adults, elderly, children:** Initially (minimum), 1 mg/kg rapid IV; may repeat up to total maximum dose of 10 mg/kg. May follow with 4–8 mg/kg/day orally in 4 divided doses up to 3 days after crisis.

SIDE EFFECTS

Note: Effects are generally transient.

FREQUENT: Drowsiness, dizziness, weakness, general malaise, diarrhea (may be severe). *OCCASIONAL:* Confusion, headache, insomnia, constipation, urinary frequency. *RARE:* Paradoxical CNS excitement/restlessness, paresthesia, tinnitus, slurred speech, tremor, blurred vision, dry mouth, diarrhea, nocturia, impotence.

ADVERSE REACTIONS/TOXIC EFFECTS

Risk of hepatotoxicity, most notably in females, those >35 yrs of age, those taking other medications concurrently. Overt hepatitis noted most frequently between 3rd and 12th mo of therapy. Overdosage results in vomiting, muscular hypotonia, muscle twitching, respiratory depression, seizures.

NURSING IMPLICATIONS

BASELINE ASSESSMENT:

Obtain baseline liver function tests (SGOT [AST], SGPT [ALT], alkaline phosphatase, total bilirubin). Record onset, type, location, and duration of muscular spasm. Check for immobility, stiffness, swelling.

INTERVENTION/EVALUATION:

Assist with ambulation. For those on long-term therapy, liver/renal function tests, blood counts should be performed periodically. Evaluate for therapeutic response: decreased intensity of skeletal muscle pain.

PATIENT/FAMILY TEACHING:

Drowsiness usually diminishes with continued therapy. Avoid tasks that require alertness, motor skills until response to drug is established. Avoid alcohol or other depressants while taking medication. Report continued weakness, fatigue, nausea or diarrhea, skin rash, itching, bloody/black stools.

✐ - see color pill atlas

darbepoetin alfa

dar-bee-eh-poe-**ee**-tin alfa
(Aranesp)

▶CLASSIFICATION

PHARMACOTHERAPEUTIC:
Glycoprotein. **CLINICAL:** Hematopoietic

ACTION/*THERAPEUTIC EFFECT*

Stimulates formation of red blood cells in bone marrow; increases serum half-life of epoetin, *induces erythropoiesis, release of reticulocytes from marrow.*

PHARMACOKINETICS

Well absorbed following SubQ administration. Half-life: 48.5 hrs.

USES/*UNLABELED*

Treatment of anemia associated with chronic renal failure, including pts on dialysis and those not on dialysis. *Treatment of chemotherapy-induced anemia.*

PRECAUTIONS

CONTRAINDICATIONS: Uncontrolled hypertension, history of sensitivity to mammalian cell-derived products or human albumin. **CAUTIONS:** Pts with known porphyria (impairment of erythrocyte formation in bone marrow or responsible for liver impairment), hemolytic anemia, sickle cell anemia, thalassemia.
▷*LIFESPAN CONSIDERATIONS:*
Pregnancy/Lactation: Unknown if drug crosses placenta or is distributed in breast milk. **Pregnancy Category C**. **Children:** Safety and efficacy not established. **Elderly:** No age-related precautions noted.

INTERACTIONS

DRUG: None significant. **HERBAL:** None significant. **FOOD:** None significant. **LAB VALUES:** May decrease bleeding time, iron concentration, serum ferritin. May increase BUN, creatinine, phosphorus, potassium, sodium, uric acid.

AVAILABILITY (Rx)

INJECTION: 225 mcg/ml, 40 mcg/ml, 60 mcg/ml, 100 mcg/ml, 200 mcg/ml.

ADMINISTRATION/HANDLING

Note: Avoid excessive agitation of vial; do not shake (foaming).

SubQ:

• Use 1 dose per vial; do not re-enter vial. Discard unused portion. May be mixed in a syringe with Bacteriostatic 0.9% NaCl with Benzyl Alcohol 0.9% (Bacteriostatic Saline) at a 1:1 ratio (benzyl alcohol acts as a local anesthetic; may reduce injection site discomfort).

IV

Storage:

• Refrigerate vials. Vigorous shaking may denature medication, rendering it inactive.

IV reconstitution:

• No reconstitution necessary.

Rate of IV administration:

• May be given as an IV bolus.

IV INCOMPATIBILITY ⊘

Do not mix with any other medications.

INDICATIONS/ROUTES/DOSAGE

Anemia in chronic renal failure pts:
SuBQ/IV BOLUS: **Adults, elderly:** Initially, 0.45 mcg/kg once weekly. Adjust dosage to achieve and maintain a target hemoglobin not to exceed 12 g/dL. Do not in-

---

crease dose more frequently than once moly.

SIDE EFFECTS

FREQUENT: Myalgia, hypertension or hypotension, headache, diarrhea. ***OCCASIONAL:*** Fatigue, edema, vomiting, reaction at administration site, asthenia, dizziness.

ADVERSE REACTIONS/TOXIC EFFECTS

Vascular access thrombosis, CHF, sepsis, arrhythmias, anaphylactic reaction occurs rarely.

NURSING IMPLICATIONS

BASELINE ASSESSMENT:

Assess B/P before drug initiation (80% of pts with chronic renal failure have history of hypertension). B/P often rises during early therapy in those with history of hypertension. Consider that all pts will eventually need supplemental iron therapy. Assess serum iron (transferrin saturation: should be >20%) and serum ferritin (>100 ng/ml) prior to and during therapy. Establish baseline CBC (esp. note Hct). Monitor B/P aggressively for increase (25% of those on medication require antihypertension therapy, dietary restrictions).

INTERVENTION/EVALUATION:

Monitor Hct level diligently (if level increases >4 points in 2 wk period, dosage should be reduced); assess CBC routinely. Monitor BUN, uric acid, creatinine, phosphorus, potassium.

PATIENT/FAMILY TEACHING:

Compliance with dietary guidelines and frequency of dialysis is essential in chronic renal failure pts.

daunorubicin

dawn-oh-**rue**-bih-sin
(Cerubidine, DaunoXome)
Do not confuse with Doxorubicin.

▶CLASSIFICATION

PHARMACOTHERAPEUTIC:
Anthracycline antibiotic. ***CLINICAL:*** Antineoplastic (see p. 69C)

ACTION/*THERAPEUTIC EFFECT*

Cell cycle-phase nonspecific. Most active in S phase of cell division. Appears to bind to DNA, *inhibiting DNA, DNA-dependent RNA synthesis.*

PHARMACOKINETICS

Widely distributed. Does not cross blood-brain barrier. Protein binding: High. Metabolized in liver to active metabolite. Excreted in urine, eliminated by biliary excretion. Half-life: 18.5 hrs; metabolite: 55 hrs.

USES/*UNLABELED*

Remission induction in acute non-lymphocytic leukemia (myelogenous, monocytic, erythroid) of adults; acute lymphocytic leukemia of both children and adults. DaunoXome: Advanced HIV-related Kaposi's sarcoma. *Treatment of neuroblastoma, non-Hodgkin's lymphoma, Ewing's sarcoma, Wilms' tumor, chronic myelocytic leukemia.*

PRECAUTIONS

CONTRAINDICATIONS: None significant. ***CAUTIONS:*** Preexisting bone marrow depression.

▷***LIFESPAN CONSIDERATIONS:***
Pregnancy/Lactation: If possible, avoid use during pregnancy, esp. first trimester. May cause fetal harm. Breast feeding not recommended.

Pregnancy Category D. Children: Safety and efficacy not established. **Elderly:** Cardiotoxicity may be more frequent, reduced bone marrow reserves requires caution. Age-related renal impairment may require dosage adjustment.

INTERACTIONS

DRUG: May decrease effect of **antigout medications. Bone marrow depressants** may enhance myelosuppression. **Live virus vaccines** may potentiate virus replication, increase vaccine side effects, decrease pt's antibody response to vaccine. **HERBAL:** None known. **FOOD:** None known. **LAB VALUES:** May increase serum bilirubin, SGOT (AST), and alkaline phosphatase levels. May raise blood uric acid level.

AVAILABILITY (Rx)

INJECTION: 2 mg/ml.

ADMINISTRATION/HANDLING

IV 💊

Note: Give by IV push or IV infusion. IV infusion not recommended due to vein irritation, risk of thrombophlebitis. Avoid small veins, swollen or edematous extremities, areas overlying joints and tendons. May be carcinogenic, mutagenic, or teratogenic. Handle with extreme care during preparation/administration.

Storage:

• Reconstituted solution is stable for 24 hrs at room temperature and 48 hrs if refrigerated. • Color change from red to blue-purple indicates decomposition; discard.

DaunoXome:

• Refrigerate unopened vials. • Reconstituted solution is stable for 6 hrs refrigerated. • Do not use if opaque.

Reconstitution:

• Reconstitute each 20 mg vial with 4 ml Sterile Water for Injection to provide concentration of 5 mg/ml. • Gently agitate vial until completely dissolved.

DaunoXome:

• Must dilute with equal part D_5W to provide concentration of 1 mg/ml. • Do not use any other diluent.

Rate of administration:

• For IV push, withdraw desired dose into syringe containing 10–15 ml 0.9% NaCl. Inject over 2–3 min into tubing of running IV solution of D_5W or 0.9% NaCl. • For IV infusion, further dilute with 100 ml D_5W or 0.9% NaCl. Infuse over 30–45 min. • Extravasation produces immediate pain, severe local tissue damage. Aspirate as much infiltrated drug as possible, then infiltrate area with hydrocortisone sodium succinate injection (50–100 mg hydrocortisone) and/or isotonic sodium thiosulfate injection or ascorbic acid injection (1 ml of 5% injection). Apply cold compresses.

DaunoXome:

• Infuse over 60 min.

IV INCOMPATIBILITIES ⊘

Allopurinal (Aloprim), aztreonam (Azactam), cefepime (Maxipime), fludarabine (Fludara), piperacillin/tazobactam (Zosyn). **DaunoXome:** Do not mix with any other solution esp. NaCl or bacteriostatic agents (e.g., benzyl alcohol).

IV COMPATIBILITIES

Etoposide (Vepesed), granisetron (Kytril), ondansetron (Zofran).

INDICATIONS/ROUTES/DOSAGE

Note: Dosage individualized based on clinical response, tolerance to ad-

---

verse effects. When used in combination therapy, consult specific protocols for optimum dosage, sequence of drug administration. Do not exceed total dosage of 500–600 mg/m^2 in adults, 400–450 mg/m^2 in those who received irradiation of cardiac region, 300 mg/m^2 in children >2 yrs, 10 mg/kg in children <2 yrs (increases risk of cardiotoxicity). Reduce dosage in those with liver and/or renal impairment. Use body weight to calculate dose in children <2 yrs or surface area <0.5 m^2.

Acute nonlymphocytic leukemia (induction remission):

IV: Adults <60 yrs: Combined with cytosine: 45 mg/m^2/day for 3 successive days for first course of induction therapy. Give 45 mg/m^2/day for 2 successive days on subsequent courses. **Adults >60 yrs:** 30 mg/m^2/day following same dosage regimen as above.

Acute lymphocytic leukemia (induction remission):

IV: Adults, elderly: Combination therapy: 45 mg/m^2/day first 3 days of induction therapy. **Children:** 25 mg/m^2 on day 1 once a wk for 4 wks.

Kaposi's sarcoma (DaunoXome):

IV: Adults: 40 mg/m^2 over 1 hr. Repeat q2wks.

SIDE EFFECTS

FREQUENT: Complete alopecia (scalp, axillary, pubic hair), nausea, vomiting begins a few hrs after administration, lasts 24–48 hrs. ***DaunoXome:*** Mild to moderate nausea, fatigue, fever. ***OCCASIONAL:*** Diarrhea, abdominal pain, esophagitis, stomatitis (redness/burning of oral mucous membranes, inflammation of gums/tongue), transverse pigmentation of fingernails/toenails. ***RARE:*** Transient fever, chills.

ADVERSE REACTIONS/TOXIC EFFECTS

Bone marrow depression manifested as hematologic toxicity (generally severe leukopenia, anemia, thrombocytopenia). Decrease in platelet count, WBC occurs in 10–14 days, returns to normal level by third week. Cardiotoxicity noted as either acute, transient, abnormal EKG findings and/or cardiomyopathy manifested as CHF (risk increases when cumulative dose exceeds 550 mg/m^2 in adults and 300 mg/m^2 in children >2 yrs, or total dosage more than 10 mg/kg in children <2 yrs).

NURSING IMPLICATIONS

BASELINE ASSESSMENT:

Obtain WBC, platelet, erythrocyte counts prior to and at frequent intervals during therapy. EKG should be obtained prior to therapy. Antiemetics may be effective in preventing, treating nausea.

INTERVENTION/EVALUATION:

Monitor for stomatitis (burning, erythema of oral mucosa). May lead to ulceration within 2–3 days. Assess skin, nailbeds for hyperpigmentation. Monitor hematologic status, renal/hepatic function studies, serum uric acid level. Assess pattern of daily bowel activity and stool consistency. Monitor for hematologic toxicity (fever, sore throat, signs of local infection, easy bruising, or unusual bleeding from any site), symptoms of anemia (excessive tiredness, weakness).

PATIENT/FAMILY TEACHING:

Urine may turn reddish color for 1–2 days after beginning therapy. Alopecia is reversible, but new hair growth may have different color or texture. New hair growth resumes about 5 wks after last therapy dose. Maintain fastidious oral hygiene. Do not have immunizations without physician's approval (drug lowers body's resistance). Avoid contact with those who have recently received live virus vaccine. Promptly report fever, sore throat, signs of local infection, easy bruising, or unusual bleeding from any site. Increase fluid intake (may protect against hyperuricemia). Contact physician if nausea/vomiting continues at home.

deferoxamine mesylate

deaf-er-**ox**-ah-meen
(Desferal)
Do not confuse with
cefuroxime, Disaphrol.

▶CLASSIFICATION
CLINICAL: Antidote

ACTION/*THERAPEUTIC EFFECT*

Binds with iron to form complex, *promoting urine excretion of acute iron poisoning.*

USES/*UNLABELED*

Treatment of acute iron toxicity, chronic iron toxicity secondary to multiple transfusions associated with some chronic anemia (e.g., thalassemia). *Treatment/diagnosis of aluminum toxicity.*

PRECAUTIONS

CONTRAINDICATIONS: Severe renal disease, anuria, primary hemochromatosis. *CAUTIONS:* None significant.

INTERACTIONS

DRUG: **Vitamin C** may increase effect. *HERBAL:* None known. *FOOD:* None known. *LAB VALUES:* May cause a falsely high total iron-binding capacity (TIBC).

AVAILABILITY (Rx)

INJECTION: 500 mg.

ADMINISTRATION/HANDLING

Note: Reconstitute each 500 mg vial with 2 ml Sterile Water for Injection to provide a concentration of 250 mg/ml.

SubQ:

• Administer SubQ very slowly; may give undiluted.

IM:

• Inject deeply into upper outer quadrant of buttock.; may give undiluted.

IV 🔊

• For IV infusion, further dilute with 0.9% NaCl, D_5W, and administer at maximum rate of 15 mg/kg/hr. • A too-rapid IV administration may produce skin flushing, urticaria, hypotension, shock.

IV INCOMPATIBILITY ⊘

Do not mix with any other IV medications.

INDICATIONS/ROUTES/DOSAGE

Acute iron intoxication:

IM: **Adults:** Initially, 1 g, then 0.5 g q4h for 2 doses; may give additional doses of 0.5 g q4–12h. **Maximum:** 6 g/day. **Children:** 50 mg/kg/dose q6h.

IV: **Adults:** 15 mg/kg/hr. **Maximum:** 6 g/day. **Children:** 15 mg/kg/hr.

Chronic iron overload:

SubQ: **Adults:** 1–2 g/day over 8–24

hrs. **Children:** 20–50 mg/kg/day over 8–12 hrs. **Maximum:** 2 g/day. **IM: Adults:** 0.5–1 g/day. **IV:** 15 mg/kg/hr. **Maximum:** 12 g/day.

SIDE EFFECTS

FREQUENT: Pain, induration at injection site, urine color change (to orange-rose). **OCCASIONAL:** Abdominal discomfort, diarrhea, leg cramps, impaired vision.

ADVERSE REACTIONS/TOXIC EFFECTS

Neurotoxicity, including high-frequency hearing loss, has been noted.

NURSING IMPLICATIONS

BASELINE ASSESSMENT:

Inform pt injection may produce discomfort at IM or SubQ injection site. Assess serum iron levels, iron binding capacity before and during therapy.

INTERVENTION/EVALUATION:

Question pt for evidence of hearing loss (neurotoxicity). Periodic slit-lamp ophthalmic exams should be obtained in those treated for chronic iron overload. If using SubQ technique, monitor for pruritus, erythema, skin irritation, and swelling.

PATIENT/FAMILY TEACHING:

Urine will appear reddish. Discomfort may occur at site of injection.

delavirdine mesylate

dell-ah-**veer**-deen
(Rescriptor)

CLASSIFICATION

PHARMACOTHERAPEUTIC: Non-nucleoside reverse transcriptase inhibitor. **CLINICAL:** Antiretroviral (see pp. 58C, 95C)

ACTION/THERAPEUTIC EFFECT

Inhibits catalytic reaction of HIV reverse transcriptase that is independent of nucleoside binding, *nterrupting HIV replication, slowing progression of HIV infection.*

PHARMACOKINETICS

Rapidly absorbed following PO administration. Primarily distributed in blood plasma. Protein binding: 98%. Metabolized in the liver. Eliminated in feces and urine. Half-life: 2–11 hrs.

USES

Treatment of HIV infection (in combination with other antivirals).

PRECAUTIONS

CONTRAINDICATIONS: None significant. **CAUTIONS:** Liver impairment.

▷**LIFESPAN CONSIDERATIONS:** **Pregnancy/Lactation:** Unknown if drug crosses placenta or distributed in breast milk. **Pregnancy Category C. Children:** Safe and efficacy not established in those <16 yrs of age. **Elderly:** Safety and efficacy not established.

INTERACTIONS:

DRUG: Benzodiazepines, calcium channel blockers may cause life-threatening adverse effects. **Carbamazepine, phenobarbital, phenytoin** may decrease concentrations. **H_2 blockers** may decrease absorption. **Rifampin** may decrease concentrations. **HERBAL:** None known. **FOOD:** None known. **LAB VALUES:** May increase SGOT (AST), SGPT (ALT); may decrease neutrophil count.

AVAILABILITY (Rx)
TABLETS: 100 mg, 200 mg.

ADMINISTRATION/HANDLING
PO:
• May disperse in water prior to consumption. • May give with or without food. • Patients with achlorhydria should take with orange juice or cranberry juice.

INDICATIONS/ROUTES/DOSAGE
HIV infection:
PO: Adults: 400 mg 3 times/day on empty stomach.

SIDE EFFECTS
FREQUENT (18%): Rash, pruritus. ***OCCASIONAL*** (>2%): Headache, nausea, diarrhea, fatigue, anorexia.

ADVERSE REACTIONS/TOXIC EFFECTS
None significant.

NURSING IMPLICATIONS

BASELINE ASSESSMENT:
Obtain baseline laboratory testing, esp. liver function tests, before beginning therapy and at periodic intervals during therapy. Offer emotional support.

INTERVENTION/EVALUATION:
Assess skin for evidence of rash. Question if nausea is noted. Determine pattern of bowel activity and stool consistency. Assess eating pattern; monitor for weight loss. Monitor lab values carefully, particularly liver function.

PATIENT/FAMILY TEACHING:
Do not take any medications, including OTC drugs without con-

sulting physician. Small, frequent meals may offset anorexia, nausea. Delavirdine is not a cure for HIV infection, nor does it reduce risk of transmission to others.

D

demecarium

(Humorsol)
See Classification section under: Antiglaucoma agents

demeclocycline hydrochloride

deh-meh-clo-**sigh**-clean
(Declomycin)

▶CLASSIFICATION
PHARMACOTHERAPEUTIC: Tetracycline. ***CLINICAL:*** Antibiotic

ACTION/*THERAPEUTIC EFFECT*
Bacteriostatic due to binding to ribosomes, *inhibiting protein synthesis.* Inhibits ADH-induced water reabsorption, *producing water diuresis.*

USES
Treatment of respiratory and urinary tract infections, uncomplicated gonorrhea, brucellosis, rheumatic fever prophylaxis, trachoma, Rocky Mountain spotted fever, typhus, Q fever, rickettsialpox, psittacosis, ornithosis, granuloma inguinale, lymphogranuloma venereum. Treatment of syndrome of inappropriate ADH secretion (SIADH).

PRECAUTIONS

CONTRAINDICATIONS: Last half of pregnancy, infants–8 yrs. **CAUTIONS:** Renal impairment, sun or ultraviolet exposure (severe photosensitivity reaction).

INTERACTIONS

DRUG: Antacids containing aluminum/calcium/magnesium, **laxatives** containing magnesium, oral iron preparations, **dairy products** impair absorption of tetracyclines (give 1–2 hrs before or after tetracyclines). **Cholestyramine, colestipol** may decrease absorption. May decrease effect of **oral contraceptives**. **HERBAL:** None known. **FOOD: Milk, dairy products** may decrease absorption. **LAB VALUES:** May increase BUN, SGOT (AST), SGPT (ALT), alkaline phosphatase, amylase, bilirubin concentrations.

AVAILABILITY (Rx)

CAPSULES: 150 mg. **TABLETS:** 150 mg, 300 mg.

INDICATIONS/ROUTES/DOSAGE

Note: Space doses evenly around the clock.

Mild to moderate infections:

PO: Adults, elderly: 600 mg/day in 2–4 divided doses. **Children >8 yrs:** 6–12 mg/kg/day in 2–4 divided doses.

Uncomplicated gonorrhea:

PO: Adults: Initially, 600 mg, then 300 mg q12h for 4 days for total of 3 g.

Chronic form of SIADH:

PO: Adults, elderly: 600 mg–1.2 g/day in 3–4 divided doses, or 3.25–3.75 mg/kg q6h.

SIDE EFFECTS

FREQUENT: Anorexia, nausea, vomiting, diarrhea, dysphagia, exaggerated sunburn reaction with moderate to high dosage. **OCCASIONAL:** Urticaria, rash. Long-term therapy may result in diabetes insipidus syndrome: polydipsia, polyuria, weakness.

ADVERSE REACTIONS/TOXIC EFFECTS

Superinfection (esp. fungal), anaphylaxis, increased intracranial pressure occur rarely. Bulging fontanelles occur rarely in infants.

NURSING IMPLICATIONS

BASELINE ASSESSMENT:
Question for history of allergies, esp. to tetracyclines.

INTERVENTION/EVALUATION:
Determine pattern of bowel activity and stool consistency. Check food intake, tolerance. Monitor I&O, renal function test results. Assess for rash. Be alert to superinfection: diarrhea, ulceration or changes of oral mucosa, tongue, anal/genital pruritus. Monitor B/P and LOC because of potential for increased intracranial pressure.

PATIENT/FAMILY TEACHING:
Continue antibiotic for full length of treatment. Space doses evenly. Take oral doses on empty stomach with full glass of water. Avoid sun/ultraviolet light exposure.

denileukin diftitox

den-ee-**lew**-kin
(Ontak)

▶CLASSIFICATION

PHARMACOTHERAPEUTIC:
Biologic response modifier.
CLINICAL: Antineoplastic (see p. 69C)

ACTION/*THERAPEUTIC EFFECT*

A cytotoxic fusion protein that targets cells expressing interleukin-2 (IL-2) receptors. After binding to IL-2 receptor, directs cytocidal action to malignant cutaneous T-cell lymphoma (CTCL) cells, *causing inhibition of protein synthesis and cell death.*

USES

Treatment of persistent or recurrent T-cell lymphoma whose malignant cells express the CD25 component of the IL-2 receptor.

PRECAUTIONS

CONTRAINDICATIONS: Diphtheria toxin, interleukin-2. ***CAUTIONS:*** None significant.

INTERACTIONS

DRUG: None significant. ***HERBAL:*** None known. ***FOOD:*** None known. ***LAB VALUES:*** May decrease serum albumin, calcium, potassium, WBC count, hemoglobin, hematocrit. Increases transaminase level.

AVAILABILITY [Rx]

SOLUTION FOR INJECTION: 150 mcg/ml.

ADMINISTRATION/HANDLING
IV 🔳

Storage:
• Store frozen. • Solutions for IV infusion stable for 6 hrs.

Reconstitution:
• Thaw in refrigerator for up to 24 hrs or at room temperature for 1–2 hrs. • Inject calculated dose into empty infusion bag. No more than 9 ml 0.9% NaCl to be added to each ml denileuklin.

Rate of administration:
• Infuse over 15 min.

IV INCOMPATIBILITY ⊘

Do not mix with any other IV medications.

INDICATIONS/ROUTES/DOSAGE
CTCL:

IV INFUSION: **Adults:** 9 or 18 mcg/kg/day for 5 consecutive days q21days. Infuse over at least 15 min.

SIDE EFFECTS

Two distinct syndromes occur very commonly: A hypersensitivity reaction (69%), consisting of at least more than one of the following: hypotension, back pain, dyspnea, vasodilation, vascular leak syndrome characterized by hypotension, edema, hypoalbuminemia, rash, chest tightness, tachycardia, dysphagia, sycope. Also, a flulike symptom complex (91%), consisting of at least more than one of the following: fever, chills, nausea, vomiting, diarrhea, myalgia, arthralgia. ***OCCASIONAL*** (10–25%): Dizziness, chest pain, vasodilation, decreased weight, rhinitis, pruritus.

ADVERSE REACTIONS/TOXIC EFFECTS

Pancreatitis, acute renal insufficiency, hematuria, hypothyroidism or hyperthyroidism occur rarely.

NURSING IMPLICATIONS

BASELINE ASSESSMENT:

CBC, blood chemistries including renal and hepatic function tests, chest x-ray should be performed before therapy begins and weekly thereafter. Assess serum albumin level before initiation of each treatment (should be ≥3 g/dl).

INTERVENTION/EVALUATION:

Monitor serum albumin for hypoalbuminemia (generally occurs 1–2 wks after administration). Monitor for evidence of infection (strong potential due to lowered immune response).

PATIENT/FAMILY TEACHING:

At home, increase fluid intake (protects against renal impairment). Do not have immunizations without physician's approval (drug lowers body resistance); avoid contact with those who have recently taken live virus vaccine.

---

desipramine hydrochloride

deh-**sip**-rah-meen
(Norpramin)
Do not confuse with
disopyramide, imipramine.

▶**CLASSIFICATION**

PHARMACOTHERAPEUTIC:
Tricyclic. **CLINICAL:** Antidepressant (see p. 34C)

ACTION/THERAPEUTIC EFFECT

Increases synaptic concentration of norepinephrine and/or serotonin (inhibits reuptake by presynaptic membrane), *producing antidepressant effect.* Strong anticholinergic activity.

PHARMACOKINETICS

Rapidly, well absorbed from GI tract. Protein binding: 90%. Metabolized in liver. Primarily excreted in urine. Minimally removed by hemodialysis. Half-life: 12–27 hrs.

USES/UNLABELED

Treatment of various forms of depression, often in conjunction with psychotherapy. *Treatment of panic disorder, neurogenic pain, attention deficit hyperactivity disorder, narcolepsy/cataplexy, bulimia nervosa, cocaine withdrawal.*

PRECAUTIONS

CONTRAINDICATIONS: Acute recovery period following MI, within 14 days of MAO inhibitor ingestion. **CAUTIONS:** Prostatic hypertrophy, history of urinary retention or obstruction, glaucoma, diabetes mellitus, history of seizures, hyperthyroidism, cardiac/hepatic/renal disease, schizophrenia, increased intraocular pressure, hiatal hernia.
▷**LIFESPAN CONSIDERATIONS:**
Pregnancy/Lactation: Crosses placenta; minimally distributed in breast milk. **Pregnancy Category C. Children:** Not recommended in those <6 yrs of age. **Elderly:** Use lower doses (higher doses not tolerated, increases risk of toxicity).

INTERACTIONS

DRUG: Alcohol, CNS depressants may increase CNS, respiratory depression, hypotensive effects. **Antithyroid agents** may increase risk of agranulocytosis. **Phenothiazines** may increase sedative, anticholinergic effects. **Cimetidine** may increase concentration, toxicity. May decrease effects of **clonidine, guanadrel.** May increase cardiac effects with **sympathomimetics.** May increase risk of hypertensive crisis, hyperpyrexia, convulsions with **MAO inhibitors. Phenytoin** may decrease desipramine concentration. ***HERBAL:*** St. John's wort may have additivie effects. ***FOOD:*** None known. ***LAB VALUES:*** May alter EKG readings, glucose serum level. Therapeutic blood serum level: 115–300 ng/ml; toxic blood serum level: >400 ng/ml.

AVAILABILITY (Rx)

TABLETS: 10 mg, 25 mg, 50 mg, 75 mg, 100 mg, 150 mg. ***CAPSULES:*** 25 mg, 50 mg.

ADMINISTRATION/HANDLING
PO:
• Give with food or milk if GI distress occurs.

INDICATIONS/ROUTES/DOSAGE
Depression:
PO: Adults: Initially, 75–150 mg daily as single daily dose, or in divided doses. Gradually increase to lowest effective therapeutic level. Do not exceed 300 mg daily.

Usual dose for children:
PO: Children 6–12 yrs: 1–3 mg/kg/day. **Maximum:** 5 mg/kg/day. **Adolescents:** 25–50 mg/day. **Maximum:** 150 mg/day.

Usual elderly dosage:
PO: 25–100 mg/day. **Maximum:** 150 mg/day.

SIDE EFFECTS

FREQUENT: Drowsiness, fatigue, dry mouth, blurred vision, constipation, delayed micturition, postural hypotension, excessive sweating, disturbed concentration, increased appetite, urinary retention. ***OCCASIONAL:*** GI disturbances (nausea, GI distress, metallic taste sensation). ***RARE:*** Paradoxical reaction (agitation, restlessness, nightmares, insomnia), extrapyramidal symptoms (particularly fine hand tremor).

ADVERSE REACTIONS/TOXIC EFFECTS

High dosage may produce confusion, seizures, severe drowsiness, fast/slowith irregular heartbeat, fever, hallucinations, agitation, shortness of breath, vomiting, unusual tiredness/weakness. Abrupt withdrawal from prolonged therapy may produce severe headache, malaise, nausea, vomiting, vivid dreams.

NURSING IMPLICATIONS

BASELINE ASSESSMENT:

For those on long-term therapy, liver/renal function tests, blood counts should be performed periodically.

INTERVENTION/EVALUATION:

Supervise suicidal risk pt closely during early therapy (as depression lessens, energy level improves, increasing suicide potential). Assess appearance, behavior, speech pattern, level of interest, mood. Therapeutic blood serum level: 115–300 ng/ml; toxic blood serum level: >400 ng/ml.

PATIENT/FAMILY TEACHING:

Change positions slowly to avoid hypotensive effect. Tolerance to postural hypotension, sedative, and anticholinergic effects usually develops during early therapy. Maximum therapeutic effect may be noted in 2–4 wks. Do not abruptly discontinue medication.

desloratidine

(Clarinex)
See New Drug Supplement.

desmopressin

des-moe-**press**-in
(DDAVP, Octostim✦, Stimate)

▶CLASSIFICATION

PHARMACOTHERAPEUTIC:
Synthetic pituitary hormone.
CLINICAL: Antidiuretic

ACTION/*THERAPEUTIC EFFECT*
Increases reabsorption of water
by increasing permeability of collecting ducts of the kidneys, *decreasing urinary output.* Increases
plasma factor VIII (antihemophilic
factor), plasminogen activator.

PHARMACOKINETICS

Onset	Peak	Duration
PO		
1 hr	4–7 hrs	—
Intranasal		
15 min–1 hr	1–5 hrs	5–21 hrs
IV		
15–30 min	1.5–3 hrs	—

Absorption 10–20% with nasal administration. Metabolized renally.
Half-life: 75 min.

USES

DDAVP intranasal: Primary nocturnal enuresis, central cranial diabetes insipidus. **Parenteral:** Central cranial diabetes insipidus,
hemophilia A, von Willebrand's
disease (type I). *Stimate intranasal:* Hemophilia A, von Willebrand's disease (type I).

PO: Central cranial diabetes insipidus.

PRECAUTIONS
CONTRAINDICATIONS: Type IIB
or platelet-type von Willebrand's
disease; nasal scarring, blockage,
or other impairment with intranasal
administration. Intranasal administration with impaired LOC. **CAU-
TIONS:** Coronary artery insufficiency, hypertensive cardiovascular
disease, infants, and children <6 yrs.
▷*LIFESPAN CONSIDERATIONS:*
**Pregnancy/Lactation: Pregnancy
Category B. Children:** Caution in
neonates, those <3 mos (increased
risk fluid balance problems). Careful
fluid restrictions recommended in infants. **Elderly:** Increased risk of hyponatremia and water intoxication.

INTERACTIONS
**DRUG: Carbamazepine, chlor-
propamide, clofibrate** may increase effect. **Demeclocycline,
lithium, norepinephrine** may decrease effect. **HERBAL:** None
known. **FOOD:** None known. **LAB
VALUES:** None significant.

AVAILABILITY (Rx)
TABLETS: 0.1 mg, 0.2 mg. **NASAL
SOLUTION:** 0.1 mg/ml, 1.5 mg/
ml. **NASAL SPRAY. INJECTION:** 4
mcg/ml.

ADMINISTRATION/HANDLING
Intranasal:

• Refrigerate. • Nasal solution is
stable for up to 3 wks at room temperature. Store nasal spray at room
temperature. • A calibrated catheter (rhinyle) is used to draw up a
measured quantity of desmo-
pressin; with one end inserted in
the nose, the pt blows on the other
end to deposit the solution deep in
the nasal cavity. • For infants, young

children, obtunded pts, an air-filled syringe may be attached to the catheter to deposit the solution.

SubQ:

• Evening dosage should consider satisfactory sleep response.
• Morning and evening doses should be adjusted separately.

IV 💊

Storage:

• Refrigerate.

Reconstitution:

• For IV infusion, dilute in 10–50 ml 0.9% NaCl.

Rate of administration:

• Infuse over 15–30 min. • For preop use, administer 30 min before procedure. • Monitor B/P and pulse during IV infusion. • IV dose = 1/10 intranasal dose.

IV INCOMPATIBILITY ⊘
Information not available.

INDICATIONS/ROUTES/DOSAGE
Primary nocturnal enuresis:

INTRANASAL: **Children ≥6 yrs:** Initially, 20 mcg (0.2 ml) at bedtime (½ dose each nostril). Adjust up to 40 mcg.

PO: **Children >12 yrs:** 0.2–0.4 mg once before bedtime.

Central cranial diabetes insipidus:

PO: **Adults, elderly:** Initially, 0.05 mg 2 times/day. **Range:** 0.1–1.2 mg/day in 2–3 divided doses. **Children:** 0.05 mg initially, then 2 times/day. **Range:** 0.1–0.8 mg daily.

INTRANASAL: **Adults, elderly:** 0.1–0.4 ml/day as single or 2–3 divided doses. **Children (3 mos–12 yrs):** 0.05–0.3 ml/day as single or 2 divided doses.

SubQ/IV: **Adults, elderly:** 0.5–1 ml/day in 2 divided doses.

Hemophilia A, von Willebrand's disease (type I):

IV INFUSION: **Adults, elderly, children >10 kg:** 0.3 mcg/kg diluted in 50 ml 0.9% NaCl. **Children <10 kg:** 0.3 mcg/kg diluted in 10 ml 0.9% NaCl.

INTRANASAL: **Adults, elderly, children >12 yrs, >50 kg:** 300 mcg (1 spray each nostril). **Adults, elderly, children >12 yrs, <50 kg:** 150 mcg as single spray.

SIDE EFFECTS
OCCASIONAL: IV: Pain/redness/swelling at injection site, headache, abdominal cramps, vulval pain, flushed skin; mild elevation of B/P; nausea with high doses. ***Nasal:*** Runny/stuffy nose; slight elevation of B/P.

ADVERSE REACTIONS/TOXIC EFFECTS
Water intoxication or hyponatremia (coma, confusion, drowsiness, headache, decreased urination, seizures, rapid weight gain) may occur in overhydration. Elderly, infants, children are esp. at risk.

NURSING IMPLICATIONS

BASELINE ASSESSMENT:
Establish baselines for B/P, pulse, weight, electrolytes, urine specific gravity. Check lab values for factor VIII coagulant concentration for hemophilia A and von Willebrand's disease; bleeding times.

INTERVENTION/EVALUATION:
Monitor I&O closely, restrict intake as necessary to prevent water intoxication (early signs of water intoxication: drowsiness, listlessness, headache). Check B/P and pulse q15min during IV administration, 2 times/day for

other routes. Evaluate parenteral injection site for erythema, pain.

PATIENT/FAMILY TEACHING:

Teach pt/family proper technique for intranasal administration. Report headache, nausea, shortness of breath, or other symptoms promptly.

desonide

(Otic Tridesilon, Tridesilon)

See Classification section under: Corticosteroids: topical (p. 81C)

desoximetasone

(Topicort)

See Classification section under: Corticosteroids: topical (p. 81C)

dexamethasone

dex-a-**meth**-a-sone
(Delalone, Decadron, Dexasone, Diodex✿, Hexadrol✿, Maxidex)
Do not confuse with desoximetasone, Maxzide.

FIXED-COMBINATION(S)

With neomycin and polymyxin, anti-infectives **(Maxitrol, Dexacidin)**

▶CLASSIFICATION

PHARMACOTHERAPEUTIC:
Long-acting glucocorticoid.
CLINICAL: Corticosteroid (see pp. 79C, 81C)

ACTION/*THERAPEUTIC EFFECT*

Inhibits accumulation of inflammatory cells at inflammation sites, phagocytosis, lysosomal enzyme release and synthesis and/or release of mediators of inflammation. *Prevents/suppresses cell and tissue immune reactions, inflammatory process.*

PHARMACOKINETICS

Rapidly, completely absorbed from GI tract after IM administration. Widely distributed. Protein binding: High. Metabolized in liver. Primarily excreted in urine. Minimally removed by hemodialysis. Half-life: 3–4.5 hrs.

USES

Treatment of chronic inflammations; allergic, neoplastic, and autoimmune diseases; management of cerebral edema, septic shock; adjuvant antiemetic in treatment of chemotherapy-induced emesis.

PRECAUTIONS

CONTRAINDICATIONS: Hypersensitivity to any corticosteroid, systemic fungal infection, peptic ulcers (except life-threatening situations). Avoid live virus vaccine such as smallpox. **Topical:** Marked circulation impairment. Do not instill ocular solutions when topical corticosteroids are being used on eyelids or surrounding skin. **CAUTIONS:** Thromboembolic disorders, history of tuberculosis (may reactivate disease), hypothyroidism, cirrhosis, nonspecific ulcerative colitis, CHF, hypertension, psychosis, renal insufficiency, seizure disorders. Prolonged therapy should be discontinued slowly. **Topical:** Do not apply to extensive areas.
▷**LIFESPAN CONSIDERATIONS:**
Pregnancy/Lactation: Crosses

placenta, distributed in breast milk. **Pregnancy Category C. Children:** Prolonged treatment of high-dose therapy may decrease short-term growth rate, cortisol secretion. **Elderly:** More likely to develop hypertension or osteoporosis.

INTERACTIONS

DRUG: Amphotericin may increase hypokalemia. May decrease effect of **oral hypoglycemics, insulin, diuretics, potassium supplements.** May increase **digoxin** toxicity (due to hypokalemia). **Hepatic enzyme inducers** may decrease effect. **Live virus vaccines** may potentiate virus replication, increase vaccine side effects, decrease pt's antibody response to vaccine. **HERBAL:** None known. **FOOD:** None known. **LAB VALUES:** May decrease calcium, potassium, thyroxine. Increases cholesterol, glucose, lipids, sodium, amylase serum levels.

AVAILABILITY (Rx)

TABLETS: 0.25 mg, 0.5 mg, 0.75 mg, 1 mg, 1.5 mg, 2 mg, 4 mg, 6 mg. **ELIXIR:** 0.5 mg/5 ml. **ORAL SOLUTION:** 0.5 mg/5 ml, 0.5 mg/0.5 ml. **INJECTION:** 4 mg/ml, 8 mg/ml (suspension), 10 mg/ml, 16 mg/ml (suspension), 20 mg/ml, 24 mg/ml. **INHALANT, INTRANASAL, OPHTHALMIC:** Solution, suspension, ointment. **TOPICAL:** Aerosol, cream.

ADMINISTRATION/HANDLING

PO:
• Give with milk or food.

IM:
• Give deep IM, preferably in gluteus maximus.

IV
Note: Dexamethasone sodium

phosphate may be given by IV push or IV infusion.
• For IV push, give over 1 min. • For IV infusion, mix with 0.9% NaCl or D₅W. • For neonate, solution must be preservative free. • IV solution must be used within 24 hrs.

Ophthalmic:
• Place finger on lower eyelid and pull out until a pocket is formed between eye and lower lid. Hold dropper above pocket and place correct number of drops (1/4–1/2 inch ointment) into pocket. Close eye gently. **Solution:** Apply digital pressure to lacrimal sac for 1–2 min (minimizes drainage into nose and throat, reducing risk of systemic effects). **Ointment:** Close eye for 1–2 min, rolling eyeball (increases contact area of drug to eye). Remove excess solution or ointment around eye with tissue. • Ointment may be used at night to reduce frequency of solution administration. • As with other corticosteroids, taper dosage slowly when discontinuing.

Topical:
• Gently cleanse area prior to application. • Use occlusive dressings only as ordered. • Apply sparingly and rub into area thoroughly.

IV INCOMPATIBILITIES
Ciprofloxacin (Cipro), idarubicin (Idamycin), midazolam (Versed).

IV COMPATIBILITIES
Cisplatin (Platinol), cyclophosphamide (Cytoxan), cytarabine (ARA-C), docetaxel (Taxotere), doxorubicin (Adriamycin), etoposide (Vepesid), paclitaxel (Taxol), propofol (Diprivan).

INDICATIONS/ROUTES/DOSAGE
Anti-inflammatory:
PO/IM/IV: Adults, elderly: 0.75–9

mg/day in divided doses q6–12h. **Children:** 0.08–0.3 mg/kg/day in divided doses q6–12h.

Cerebral edema:

IV: **Adults, elderly:** Initially, 10 mg, then 4 mg (IM/IV) q6h.

PO/IM/IV: **Children:** Loading dose of 1–2 mg/kg, then 1–1.5 mg/kg/day in divided doses q4–6h.

Chemotherapy antiemetic:

IV: **Adults, elderly:** 8–20 mg once, then (PO) 4 mg q4–6h or 8 mg q8h. **Children:** 10 mg/m^2/dose (maximum: 20 mg), then 5 mg/m^2/dose q6h.

Physiologic replacement:

PO/IM/IV: **Adults, elderly:** 0.03–0.15 mg/kg/day in divided doses q6–12h.

Usual ophthalmic dosage:

Adults, elderly, children: *Ointment:* Thin coating 3–4 times/day. *Suspension:* Initially, 2 drops q1h while awake and q2h at night; then reduce to 3–4 times/day.

SIDE EFFECTS

FREQUENT: Inhalation: Cough, dry mouth, hoarseness, throat irritation. **Intranasal:** Burning, dryness inside nose. **Ophthalmic:** Blurred vision. **Systemic:** Insomnia, facial swelling ("moon face"), moderate abdominal distention, indigestion, increased appetite, nervousness, facial flushing, increased sweating. **OCCASIONAL: Inhalation:** Localized fungal infection (thrush). **Intranasal:** Crusting inside nose, nosebleed, sore throat, ulceration of nasal mucosa. **Ophthalmic:** Decreased vision, watering of eyes, eye pain, nausea, vomiting, burning, stinging, redness of eyes. **Systemic:** Dizziness, decreased/blurred vision. **Topical:** Allergic contact dermatitis, purpura (blood-containing blisters), thinning of skin with easy bruising, telangiectasis (raised dark red spots on skin). **RARE: Inhalation:** Increased bronchospasm, esophageal candidiasis. **Intranasal:** Nasal/pharyngeal candidiasis, eye pain. **Systemic:** General allergic reaction (rash, hives), pain, redness, swelling at injection site, psychic changes, false sense of well-being, hallucinations, depression.

ADVERSE REACTIONS/TOXIC EFFECTS

Long-term therapy: Muscle wasting (esp. arms, legs), osteoporosis, spontaneous fractures, amenorrhea, cataracts, glaucoma, peptic ulcer, CHF. **Abrupt withdrawal following long-term therapy:** Severe joint pain, severe headache, anorexia, nausea, fever, rebound inflammation, fatigue, weakness, lethargy, dizziness, orthostatic hypotension. *Ophthalmic:* Glaucoma, ocular hypertension, cataracts.

NURSING IMPLICATIONS

BASELINE ASSESSMENT:

Question for hypersensitivity to any of the corticosteroids. Obtain baselines for height, weight, B/P, glucose, electrolytes.

INTERVENTION/EVALUATION:

Monitor I&O, daily weight: Assess for edema. Evaluate food tolerance and bowel activity: report hyperacidity promptly. Check vitals at least 2 times/day. Be alert to infection: sore throat, fever, or vague symptoms. Monitor electrolytes. Watch for hypercalcemia (muscle twitching, cramps), hypokalemia (weakness and muscle cramps, numbness/tingling esp. lower extremities, nausea and vomiting, irritability). Assess emotional status, ability to sleep.

PATIENT/FAMILY TEACHING:

Do not change dose/schedule or stop taking drug. *Must* taper off gradually under medical supervision. Notify physician of fever, sore throat, muscle aches, sudden weight gain/swelling. Severe stress (serious infection, surgery, or trauma) may require increased dosage. Inform dentist or other physicians of dexamethasone therapy now or within past 12 mos. *Topical:* Apply after shower or bath for best absorption.

dexmedetomidine hydrochloride

decks-meh-deh-**tome**-ih-deen (Precedex)

▶CLASSIFICATION

PHARMACOTHERAPEUTIC: Alpha₂ agonist. ***CLINICAL:*** Non-barbiturate sedative, hypnotic

ACTION/*THERAPEUTIC EFFECT*

Selective alpha₂ adrenoceptor agonist with sedative properties. Alpha₂ activity seen following slow IV infusion of low to medium doses, alpha₁ observed following slow IV infusion of high doses or rapid IV administration. Half-life: 8 min.

USES

Sedation of initially intubated and mechanically ventilated adults during treatment in intensive care setting.

PRECAUTIONS

CONTRAINDICATIONS: None

significant. ***CAUTIONS:*** Hepatic function impairment, those >65 yrs, dysrhythmias.

INTERACTIONS

DRUG: Concurrent administration with **anesthetics, sedatives, hypnotics, opioids** may enhance effects. ***HERBAL:*** None known. ***FOOD:*** None known. ***LAB VALUES:*** May increase AST (SGOT), ALT (SGPT), potassium alkaline phosphatase.

AVAILABILITY (Rx)

INJECTION: 100 mcg/ml.

ADMINISTRATION/HANDLING

IV ▧

Storage:
• Store at room temperature.

Reconstitution:
• Dilute 2 ml of dexmedetomidine with 48 ml 0.9 NaCl.

Rate of administration:
• Give as maintenance infusion.

IV INCOMPATIBILITY ⊘

Do not mix with any other medications.

INDICATIONS/ROUTES/DOSAGE

Note: Must be diluted with 48 ml 0.9% NaCl prior to use.

Sedation:

IV INFUSION: **Adults:** Loading dose of 1 mcg/kg over 10 min followed by maintenance dose of 0.2–0.7 mcg/kg/hr. Can be continuously infused in mechanically ventilated pt before, during, after extubation.

SIDE EFFECTS

FREQUENT: Hypotension (30%), nausea (11%). ***OCCASIONAL*** (2–3%): Pain, fever, oliguria, thirst.

ADVERSE REACTIONS/TOXIC EFFECTS

Bradycardia, atrial fibrillation, hypoxia, anemia, pain, pleural effusion may occur if IV is infused too rapidly.

NURSING IMPLICATIONS

INTERVENTION/EVALUATION:

Monitor EKG for atrial fibrillation, pulse for bradycardia, B/P for hypotension. Assess respiratory rate, rhythm.

dexmethylphenidate

(Focalin)
See New Drug Supplement.

dexrazoxane

dex-rah-**zox**-ann
(Zinecard)

▶CLASSIFICATION

PHARMACOTHERAPEUTIC: Cytoprotective agent. **CLINICAL:** Antineoplastic adjunct

ACTION/*THERAPEUTIC EFFECT*

Readily penetrates cell membranes converting intracellularly to a chelating agent, *binding iron and preventing free radical formation by anthracycline, protecting against anthracycline-induced cardiomyopathy.*

PHARMACOKINETICS

Rapidly distributed following IV administration. Not bound to plasma proteins. Primarily excreted in urine. Elimination half-life: 2.1–2.5 hrs.

USES

Reduction of incidence and severity of cardiomyopathy associated with doxorubicin therapy in women with metastatic breast cancer. Not recommended with initiation of doxorubicin therapy.

PRECAUTIONS

CONTRAINDICATIONS: Chemotherapy regimens that do not contain an anthracycline. **CAUTIONS:** Chemotherapeutic agents that are additive to myelosuppression, concurrent FAC therapy (fluorouracil, doxorubicin, cyclophosphamide).

▷**LIFESPAN CONSIDERATIONS:** **Pregnancy/Lactation:** May be embryotoxic, tetragenic. Unknown if distributed in breast milk. Recommended not to breast-feed during therapy. **Pregnancy Category C. Children:** Safety and efficacy not established. **Elderly:** Information not available.

INTERACTIONS

DRUG: Concurrent FAC therapy (**fluorouracil, doxorubicin, cyclophosphamide**) may produce severe blood dyscrasias. **HERBAL:** None known. **FOOD:** None known. **LAB VALUES:** Concurrent FAC (fluorouracil, doxorubicin, cyclophosphamide) therapy may produce abnormal hepatic or renal function tests.

AVAILABILITY (Rx)

POWDER FOR INJECTION: 250 mg (10 mg/ml reconstituted in 25 ml single-use vial), 500 mg (10 mg/ml reconstituted in 50 ml single-use vial).

ADMINISTRATION/HANDLING

Note: Do not mix with other drugs. Use caution in handling and preparation of reconstituted solution (glove use recommended).

IV ⚕

Storage:

• Store vials at room temperature.
• Reconstituted solution is stable for 6 hrs at room temperature or if refrigerated. Discard unused solution.

Reconstitution:

• Reconstitute with 0.167 molar (M/6) sodium lactate injection to give concentration of 10 mg dexrazoxane for each ml of sodium lactate. • May further dilute with 0.9% NaCl or D_5W. Concentration should range from 1.3–5 mg/ml.

Rate of administration:

• Give reconstituted solution by slow IV push or rapid drip IV infusion from a bag. • After infusion is completed, and before a total elapsed time of 30 min from beginning of dexrazoxane infusion, give IV injection of doxorubicin.

IV INCOMPATIBILITY ⊘

Do not mix with other medications.

INDICATIONS/ROUTES/DOSAGE

Note: Dexrazoxane should only be used in those who have received a cumulative doxorubicin dose of 300 mg/m² and are continuing with doxorubicin therapy. The reconstituted dexrazoxane solution may be diluted with 0.9% NaCl injection or D_5W to a concentration range of 1.3 to 5 mg/ml in IV infusion bags.

Cardioprotective:

IV: **Adults, children:** Recommended dosage ratio of dexrazoxane:doxorubicin is 10:1 (e.g., 500 mg/m² dexrazoxane: 50 mg/m² doxorubicin).

SIDE EFFECTS

FREQUENT: Alopecia, nausea, vomiting, fatigue, malaise, anorexia, stomatitis, fever, infection, diarrhea. **OCCASIONAL:** Pain with injection, neurotoxicity, phlebitis, dysphagia, streaking/erythema. **RARE:** Urticaria, skin reaction.

ADVERSE REACTIONS/TOXIC EFFECTS

FAC therapy with dexrazoxane may produce more severe leukopenia, granulocytopenia, and thrombocytopenia than those receiving FAC without dexrazoxane. Overdosage can be removed with peritoneal or hemodialysis.

NURSING IMPLICATIONS

BASELINE ASSESSMENT:

Use gloves when preparing solution. If powder or solution comes in contact with skin, wash immediately with soap and water. Antiemetics may be effective in preventing, treating nausea.

INTERVENTION/EVALUATION:

Frequently monitor blood counts for evidence of blood dyscrasias. Monitor for stomatitis (burning/erythema of oral mucosa at inner margin of lips, sore throat, difficulty swallowing). Monitor hematologic status, renal/hepatic function studies, cardiac function. Assess pattern of daily bowel activity, stool consistency. Monitor for hematologic toxicity (fever, signs of local infection, easy bruising, unusual bleeding from any site).

PATIENT/FAMILY TEACHING:

Alopecia is reversible, but new hair growth may have different color or texture. New hair growth resumes 2–3 mos after last therapy dose. Maintain fastidious oral hygiene. Promptly report fever, sore throat, signs of local infection. Contact physician if nausea/vomiting continues at home.

dextran, low molecular weight (dextran 40)

dex-tran
(Gentran, Hyskon✦, Rheomacrodex)

dextran, high molecular weight (dextran 75)

(Macrodex)

▶CLASSIFICATION

PHARMACOTHERAPEUTIC: Branched polysaccharide. **CLINICAL:** Plasma volume expander

ACTION/*THERAPEUTIC EFFECT*

Draws fluid from interstitial to intravascular space (colloidal osmotic effect) *resulting in increased central venous pressure, cardiac output, stroke volume, B/P, urine output, capillary perfusion, pulse pressure, and decreased heart rate, peripheral resistance, blood viscosity.* Reduces aggregation of erythrocytes. Enhances blood flow *(corrects hypovolemia, improves circulation).*

PHARMACOKINETICS

Evenly distributed in vascular circulation. Enzymatically degraded to glucose. Excreted in urine, feces.

USES

Fluid replacement and blood volume expander in treatment of hypovolemia, shock, or impending shock.

PRECAUTIONS

CONTRAINDICATIONS: Marked hemostatic defects, including drug-induced, marked cardiac decompensation, renal disease with severe oliguria or anuria, hypervolemic conditions, severe bleeding disorders, when use of sodium or chloride could be detrimental. **CAUTIONS:** Those with thrombocytopenia, CHF, pulmonary edema, severe renal insufficiency, those on corticosteroids or corticotropin, presence of edema with sodium retention, impaired renal clearance, chronic liver disease, pathologic abdominal conditions, those undergoing bowel surgery.

▷**LIFESPAN CONSIDERATIONS:**
Pregnancy/Lactation: Unknown if drug crosses placenta or is distributed in breast milk. **Pregnancy Category C. Children/ Elderly:** No age-related precautions noted.

INTERACTIONS

DRUG: None significant. **HERBAL:** None known. **FOOD:** None known. **LAB VALUES:** Prolongs bleeding time, increases bleeding tendency, depresses platelet count. Decreases factor VIII, factor V, factor IX.

AVAILABILITY (Rx)

INJECTION: 10% dextran 40 in NaCl or D_5W, 6% dextran 75 in NaCl or D_5W.

ADMINISTRATION/HANDLING

Note: Use caution in handling and preparation of reconstituted solution (glove use recommended).

IV ⓦ

Storage:

• Store at room temperature. • Use only clear solutions. • Discard partially used containers.

Rate of administration:

• Give by IV infusion only. • Monitor pt closely during first mins of infusion for anaphylactoid reaction. Monitor vital signs q5min. • Monitor urine flow rates during administration (if oliguria or anuria occurs, dextran 40 should be discontinued and osmotic diuretic given (minimizes vascular overloading). • Monitor central venous pressure (CVP) when given by rapid infusion. If there is a precipitous rise in CVP, immediately discontinue drug (overexpansion of blood volume). • Monitor B/P diligently during infusion; if marked hypotension occurs, stop infusion immediately (imminent anaphylactoid reaction). • If evidence of blood volume overexpansion occurs, discontinue IV until blood volume adjusts via urine output.

IV INCOMPATIBILITY ⊘

Do not add any medications to dextran solution.

INDICATIONS/ROUTES/DOSAGE

Volume expansion/shock:

IV: **Adults, elderly:** 500–1,000 ml at rate of 20–40 ml/min. **Maximum dose:** 20 ml/kg first 24 hrs, 10 ml/kg thereafter. **Children:** Total dose not to exceed 20 ml/kg day 1, 10 ml/kg/day thereafter.

Note: Therapy should not continue >5 days.

SIDE EFFECTS

OCCASIONAL: Mild hypersensitivity reaction (urticaria, nasal congestion, wheezing).

ADVERSE REACTIONS/TOXIC EFFECTS

Severe or fatal anaphylaxis (marked hypotension, cardiac/respiratory arrest) may occur, noted early during IV infusion, generally in those not previously exposed to IV dextran.

NURSING IMPLICATIONS

INTERVENTION/EVALUATION:

Monitor urine output closely (increase in output generally occurs in oliguric pts after dextran administration). If no increase is observed after 500 ml dextran is infused, discontinue drug until diuresis occurs. Monitor for fluid overload (peripheral and/or pulmonary edema, impending CHF symptoms). Assess lung sounds for rales. Monitor central venous pressure (detects overexpansion of blood volume). Observe closely for allergic reaction. Assess for bleeding esp. following surgery or those on anticoagulant therapy (overt bleeding esp. at surgical site and bruising, petechiae development).

dextroamphetamine sulfate ✳

dex-tro-am-**fet**-ah-meen
(Dexedrine)
Do not confuse with Dextran, Excedrin.

▶CLASSIFICATION

PHARMACOTHERAPEUTIC:
Amphetamine **(Schedule II).**
CLINICAL: CNS stimulant

ACTION/*THERAPEUTIC EFFECT*

Enhances release, action of catecholamine (dopamine, norepinephrine) by blocking reuptake, inhibiting MAO. *Increases motor activity, mental alertness, decreases drowsiness, fatigue.*

USES

Treatment of narcolepsy; treatment of attention deficit disorder in hyperactive children; short-term treatment to assist caloric restriction in exogenous obesity.

PRECAUTIONS

CONTRAINDICATIONS: Hyperthyroidism, advanced arteriosclerosis, agitated states, moderate to severe hypertension, symptomatic cardiovascular disease, history of drug abuse, glaucoma, history of hypersensitivity to sympathomimetic amines, within 14 days of MAO inhibitor ingestion. **CAUTIONS:** Elderly, debilitated, tartrazine-sensitive pts.

INTERACTIONS

DRUG: Tricyclic antidepressants may increase cardiovascular effects. Beta-blockers may increase risk of hypertension, bradycardia, heart block. CNS stimulants may increase effects. May increase risk of arrhythmias with digoxin. Meperidine may increase risk of hypotension, respiratory depression, convulsions, vascular collapse. MAO inhibitors may prolong, intensify effects. May increase effects of thyroid hormone. Thyroid hormones may increase effects. **HERBAL:** None known. **FOOD:** None known. **LAB VALUES:** May increase plasma corticosteroid concentrations.

AVAILABILITY (Rx)

TABLETS: 5 mg, 10 mg. **CAP-** **SULES (sustained-release):** 5 mg, 10 mg, 15 mg.

INDICATIONS/ROUTES/DOSAGE

Narcolepsy:

PO: Adults, children >12 yrs: Initially, 10 mg/day. Increase by 10 mg at weekly intervals until therapeutic response achieved. **Children 6–12 yrs:** Initially, 5 mg/day. Increase by 5 mg/day at weekly intervals until therapeutic response achieved. **Maximum:** 60 mg/day.

Attention deficit disorder:

PO: Children >6 yrs: Initially, 5 mg 1–2 times/day. Increase by 5 mg/day at weekly intervals until therapeutic response achieved. **Children 3–5 yrs:** Initially, 2.5 mg/day. Increase by 2.5 mg/day at weekly intervals until therapeutic response achieved. **Maximum:** 40 mg/day.

Appetite suppressant:

PO: Adults: 5–30 mg daily in divided doses of 5–10 mg each dose, given 30–60 min before meals. **EXTENDED-RELEASE:** 1 capsule in morning.

SIDE EFFECTS

FREQUENT: Irregular heartbeat, CNS stimulation, false sense of well-being, nervousness, insomnia. Increased motor activity, talkativeness, nervousness, mild euphoria, insomnia. **OCCASIONAL:** Headache, chilliness, dry mouth, GI distress, increased depression in depressed pts, tachycardia, palpitations, chest pain.

ADVERSE REACTIONS/TOXIC EFFECTS

Overdose may produce pallor or flushing, cardiac irregularities, psychotic syndrome. Abrupt withdrawal following prolonged administration of high dosage may produce lethargy (may last for wks). Prolonged administration to children with ADD may produce a temporary suppression of weight and/or height patterns.

NURSING IMPLICATIONS

PATIENT/FAMILY TEACHING:

Normal dosage levels may produce tolerance to drug's anorexic mood-elevating effects within a few wks. Avoid tasks that require alertness, motor skills until response to drug is established. Dry mouth may be relieved by sugarless gum, sips of tepid water. Take early in day. May mask extreme fatigue. Report pronounced nervousness, dizziness, decreased appetite, dry mouth.

DHEA

Also known as prasterone

▶CLASSIFICATION

HERBAL

ACTION/EFFECT

Produced in adrenal glands and liver, metabolized to androstenedione, major precursor to androgens and estrogens. Also produced in the CNS and concentrated in the limbic regions; may function as an excitatory neuroregulator. *Androgen or estrogen-like effects may be responsible for DHEA benefits.*

USES

Used for increasing strength, energy, muscle mass, stimulation of immunity, improvement of cogni-tive function and memory, improvement of depressed mood/fatigue in HIV pts. Treatment of atherosclerosis, hyperglycemia, cancer, prevention of osteoporosis and to increase bone mineral density.

PRECAUTIONS

CONTRAINDICATIONS: None significant. ***CAUTIONS:*** May increase risk of prostate, breast, and hormone-sensitive cancers. Avoid use during pregnancy/lactation. Avoid use in those with breast, uterine, ovarian cancer, endometriosis, uterine fibroids, diabetes (can increase insulin resistance/sensitivity), depression (may increase risk of adverse psychiatric effects).
▷***LIFESPAN CONSIDERATIONS:***
Pregnancy/Lactation: May adversely effect pregnancy by increasing androgen levels. **Children:** Safety and efficacy not established. **Elderly:** Age-related liver impairment may require caution.

INTERACTIONS

DRUG: Can increase **triazolam** concentration, inhibit **triazolam** metabolism. May interfere with **estrogen/androgen** therapy. ***HERBAL:*** None significant. ***FOOD:*** None significant. ***LAB VALUES:*** None significant.

AVAILABILITY (OTC)

CAPSULES: 25 mg. ***TABLETS:*** 25 mg

INDICATIONS/ROUTES/DOSAGE

Depression:
PO: **Adults, elderly:** 30–90 mg/day.
Usual adult dosage:
PO: **Adults, elderly:** 25–50 mg/day.

SIDE EFFECTS

Acne, hair loss, hirsutism, voice deepening, insulin resistance, altered menstrual pattern, hypertension, abdominal pain, fatigue, headache, nasal congestion.

ADVERSE REACTIONS/TOXIC EFFECTS

None significant.

NURSING IMPLICATIONS

BASELINE ASSESSMENT:

Assess for hormone-sensitive tumors (may stimulate growth). Use of hormone replacement therapy (avoid).

INTERVENTION/EVALUATION:

Assess changes in mood, sleep disturbances. Monitor changes in aggressiveness, irritability, restlessness.

PATIENT/FAMILY TEACHING:

Avoid use in pregnancy/lactation. Lower dosage if acne develops.

diazepam

dye-**az**-eh-pam
(Apo-Diazepam✤, Diastat, Diazemuls✤, Dizac, Valium, Valrelease, Vivol✤)
Do not confuse with diazoxide, Ditropan, Valcyte.

▶**CLASSIFICATION**

PHARMACOTHERAPEUTIC:
Benzodiazepine **(Schedule IV).**
CLINICAL: Antianxiety, skeletal muscle relaxant, anticonvulsant (see pp. 11C, 32C)

ACTION/*THERAPEUTIC EFFECT*

Enhances action of neurotransmitter gamma-aminobutyric acid (GABA) neurotransmission at CNS, *producing anxiolytic effect.* Enhances presynaptic inhibition, *elevating seizure threshold* in response to electrical/chemical stimulation. Inhibits spinal afferent pathways, *producing skeletal muscle relaxation.*

PHARMACOKINETICS

Onset	Peak	Duration
PO		
30 min	1–2 hrs	2–3 hrs
IM		
15 min	30–90 min	30–90 min
IV		
1–5 min	15 min	15–60 min

Well absorbed from GI tract. Widely distributed. Protein binding: 98%. Metabolized in liver to active metabolite. Excreted in urine. Minimally removed by hemodialysis. Half-life: 20–70 hrs (half-life increased in elderly, liver dysfunction).

USES/*UNLABELED*

Short-term relief of anxiety symptoms, preanesthetic medication, relief of acute alcohol withdrawal. Adjunct for relief of acute musculoskeletal conditions, treatment of seizures (IV route used for termination of status epilepticus). **Gel:** Control of increased seizure activity in refractory epilepsy in those on stable regimens. *Treatment of panic disorders, tension headache, tremors.*

PRECAUTIONS

CONTRAINDICATIONS: Acute narrow-angle glaucoma, acute alcohol intoxication. ***CAUTIONS:*** Impaired kidney/liver function.
▷***LIFESPAN CONSIDERATIONS:***
Pregnancy/Lactation: Crosses placenta; distributed in breast milk. May increase risk of fetal abnormalities if administered dur-

ing first trimester of pregnancy. Chronic ingestion during pregnancy may produce withdrawal symptoms, CNS depression in neonates. **Pregnancy Category D. Children/Elderly:** Use small initial doses with gradual increases to avoid ataxia or excessive sedation.

INTERACTIONS

DRUG: Alcohol, CNS depressants may increase CNS depressant effect. **HERBAL: Kava kava, valerian** may increase CNS depressant effects. **FOOD:** None known. **LAB VALUES:** May produce abnormal renal function tests, elevate SGOT (AST), SGPT (ALT), LDH, alkaline phosphatase, serum bilirubin. Therapeutic blood serum level: 0.5–2 mcg/ml; toxic blood serum level: >3 mcg/ml.

AVAILABILITY (Rx)

TABLETS: 2 mg, 5 mg, 10 mg. **CAPSULES (sustained-release):** 15 mg. **ORAL SOLUTION:** 5 mg/5 ml. **INJECTION:** 5 mg/ml. **INJECTABLE EMULSION:** 5 mg/ml. **RECTAL GEL:** 2.5 mg, 10 mg, 15 mg, 20 mg.

ADMINISTRATION/HANDLING

PO:

• Give without regard to meals. • Dilute oral concentrate with water, juice, carbonated beverages; may also be mixed in semisolid food (applesauce, pudding). • Tablets may be crushed. • Do not crush or break capsule.

IM:

• Injection may be painful. Inject deeply into deltoid muscle.

IV

Storage:

• Store at room temperature.

Rate of administration:

• Give by IV push. • Administer directly into a large vein (reduces risk of thrombosis/phlebitis). If not possible, administer into tubing of a flowing IV solution as close to the vein insertion point as possible. Do not use small veins (e.g., wrist/dorsum of hand). • Administer IV rate not exceeding 5 mg/min. For children, give over a 3 min period (a too rapid IV may result in hypotension, respiratory depression). • Monitor respirations q5–15min for 2h. May produce arrhythmias when used prior to cardioversion.

IV INCOMPATIBILITIES ⊘

Amphotericin B complex (Ambisome, Amphotec, Abelcet), cefepime (Maxipime), diltiazem (Cardizem), fluconazole (Diflucan), foscarnet (Foscavir), heparin, hydrocortisone (Solu-Cortef), hydromorphone, meropenem (Merrem IV), potassium chloride, propofol (Diprivan), vitamins.

IV COMPATIBILITY

Dobutamine (Dobutrex).

INDICATIONS/ROUTES/DOSAGE

Anxiety/skeletal muscle relaxant:

PO: Adults: 2–10 mg 2–4 times/day. **Elderly:** 2.5 mg 2 times/day. **Children:** 0.12–0.8 mg/kg/day in divided doses q6–8h.

IM/IV: Adults: 2–10 mg; repeat in 3–4 hrs. **Children:** 0.04–0.3 mg/kg/dose q2–4h. **Maximum:** 0.5 mg/kg in an 8 hr period.

Preanesthesia:

IV: Adults, elderly: 5–15 mg 5–10 min prior to procedure. **Children:** 0.2–0.3 mg/kg. **Maximum:** 10 mg.

Alcohol withdrawal:

PO: Adults, elderly: 10 mg 3–4

times during first 24 hrs, then reduce to 5–10 mg 3–4 times/day as needed.

IM/IV: Adults, elderly: Initially, 10 mg, followed by 5–10 mg q3–4h.

Status epilepticus:

IV: Adults, elderly: 5–10 mg q10–15 min up to 30 mg/8 hrs. **Children ≥5 yrs:** 0.05–0.3 mg/kg/dose q15–30min. **Maximum total dose:** 10 mg. **Children >1 mo to ≤5 yrs:** 0.05–0.3 mg/kg/dose q15–30min. **Maximum total dose:** 5 mg.

RECTAL GEL: Adults, children ≥12 yrs: 0.2 mg/kg. **Children 6–11 yrs:** 0.3 mg/kg. **Children 2–5 yrs:** 0.5 mg/kg. Dose may be repeated in 4–12 hrs.

Note: Do not use more than 5 times/ mo or more than once q5days.

SIDE EFFECTS

FREQUENT: Pain with IM injection, drowsiness, fatigue, ataxia (muscular incoordination). **OCCASIONAL:** Slurred speech, orthostatic hypotension, headache, hypoactivity, constipation, nausea, blurred vision. **RARE:** Paradoxical CNS hyperactivity/nervousness in children, excitement/restlessness in elderly/debilitated (generally noted during first 2 wks of therapy, particularly noted in presence of uncontrolled pain).

ADVERSE REACTIONS/TOXIC EFFECTS

IV route may produce pain, swelling, thrombophlebitis, carpal tunnel syndrome. Abrupt or too rapid withdrawal may result in pronounced restlessness, irritability, insomnia, hand tremors, abdominal/muscle cramps, sweating, vomiting, seizures. Abrupt withdrawal in pts with epilepsy may produce increase in frequency and/or severity of seizures. Overdosage results in somnolence, confusion, diminished reflexes, coma.

NURSING IMPLICATIONS

BASELINE ASSESSMENT:

Assess B/P, pulse, respirations immediately before administration. Pt must remain recumbent for up to 3 hrs (individualized) after parenteral administration to reduce hypotensive effect. **Anxiety:** Assess autonomic response (cold, clammy hands, sweating) and motor response (agitation, trembling, tension). **Musculoskeletal spasm:** Record onset, type, location, duration of pain. Check for immobility, stiffness, swelling. **Seizures:** Review history of seizure disorder (length, intensity, frequency, duration, LOC). Observe frequently for recurrence of seizure activity. Initiate seizure precautions.

INTERVENTION/EVALUATION:

Assess children, elderly for paradoxical reaction, particularly during early therapy. Evaluate for therapeutic response: a decrease in intensity/frequency of seizures; a calm, facial expression, decreased restlessness; decreased intensity of skeletal muscle pain. Therapeutic blood serum level: 0.5–2 mcg/ml; toxic blood serum level: >3 mcg/ml.

PATIENT/FAMILY TEACHING:

Discomfort may occur with IM injection. Drowsiness usually diminishes with continued therapy. Smoking reduces drug effectiveness. Do not abruptly withdraw medication after long-term therapy. Strict maintenance of drug therapy is essential for seizure control. Avoid alcohol.

---

diazoxide

dye-ah-**zocks**-eyd
(Hyperstat, Proglycem)
Do not confuse with diazepam,
Dyazide.

▶CLASSIFICATION

PHARMACOTHERAPEUTIC:
Vasodilator. *CLINICAL:* Antihypertensive, antihypoglycemic

ACTION/THERAPEUTIC EFFECT

Directly relaxes smooth muscle in
peripheral arterioles, *reducing
peripheral vascular resistance, B/P.*
Inhibits insulin release from pancreas, *increasing blood glucose.*

USES

Emergency lowering of B/P in
adults with severe, nonmalignant
and malignant hypertension; children with acute severe hypertension. Management of hypoglycemia caused by hyperinsulinism
associated with islet cell adenoma, carcinoma, or extrapancre-
atic malignancy.

PRECAUTIONS

CONTRAINDICATIONS: History
of hypersensitivity to thiazide derivatives. *IV:* Hypertension associated with aortic coarctation, arteriovenous shunt. *PO:* Management
of functional hypoglycemia. *CAU-
TIONS:* Impaired renal function,
cardiac reserve; caution when reducing severely elevated B/P.

INTERACTIONS

DRUG: **Beta-blockers, vasodilators, hypotension-producing medications** may increase hypotensive
effect. *PO:* May decrease effect of
phenytoin. *HERBAL:* None known.
FOOD: None known. *LAB VALUES:*
May increase SGOT (AST), alkaline
phosphatase, free fatty acids,
sodium, uric acid, glucose, BUN.
May decrease hemoglobin, hematocrit, creatinine clearance.

AVAILABILITY (Rx)

CAPSULES: 50 mg. *ORAL SUS-
PENSION:* 50 mg/ml. *INJECTION:*
15 mg/ml.

ADMINISTRATION/HANDLING

IV

Storage:
• Store at room temperature.

Rate of administration:
• Administer undiluted over ≤30 sec.

IV INCOMPATIBILITY ⊘

Do not mix with any other medications.

INDICATIONS/ROUTES/DOSAGE

Note: Administer only in a peripheral vein.

Severe hypertension:

IV: **Adults, elderly, children:** 1–3
mg/kg (up to maximum of 150 mg).
Repeat q5–15min until adequate
decrease in B/P occurs. Thereafter,
give at intervals of 4–24 hrs.

Hypoglycemia:

PO: **Adults, elderly, children:** Initially, 3 mg/kg/day in 3 divided
doses q8h. **Maintenance:** 3–8
mg/kg/day in 2–3 divided doses at
12 or 8 hr intervals. **Maximum:**
Up to 15 mg/kg/day. **Infants, neonates:** Initially, 10 mg/kg/day in 3
divided doses q8h. **Maintenance:**
8–15 mg/kg/day in 2–3 divided
doses at 12 or 8 hr intervals.

SIDE EFFECTS

FREQUENT: Edema (increased
weight, swelling of feet). *OCCA-
SIONAL:* Tachycardia, altered

taste, constipation, anorexia, nausea, vomiting, abdominal pain. **Parenteral:** Back pain, tinnitus, facial flushing, headache, pain/warmth along injection site. **RARE: IV/PO:** Sensitivity reaction (rash, fever), confusion, paresthesia, orthostatic hypotension.

ADVERSE REACTIONS/TOXIC EFFECTS

Overdose may cause hyperglycemia/ketoacidosis (increased urination, thirst, fruitlike breath). Angina, myocardial infarction, thrombocytopenia occur rarely.

NURSING IMPLICATIONS

BASELINE ASSESSMENT:

Establish baseline B/P, blood glucose. When administering IV, achieve desired B/P over as long a period of time as possible.

INTERVENTION/EVALUATION:

If excessive reduction in B/P occurs, place pt in Trendelenburg position. If parenteral form leaks in SubQ tissue, apply warm compresses to decrease pain sensation. Monitor for development of hyperglycemia, particularly in those with renal or liver disease, diabetes mellitus.

PATIENT/FAMILY TEACHING:

Blood glucose or daily urine testing should be attained in those on chronic oral therapy.

dibucaine

(Nupercainal)

See Classification section under: Anesthetics: local

diclofenac

dye-**klo**-feh-nak
(Cataflam, Diclotek♣, Novo-Difenac♣, Solaraze, Voltaren, Voltaren XR)
Do not confuse with Diflucan, Duphalac, Verelan.

FIXED-COMBINATION(S)

With misoprostil, an antisecretory gastric protectant **(Arthrotec)**

▶CLASSIFICATION

PHARMACOTHERAPEUTIC: Nonsteroidal anti-inflammatory. **CLINICAL:** Analgesic, anti-inflammatory (see p. 106C)

ACTION/*THERAPEUTIC EFFECT*

Inhibits prostaglandin synthesis, reducing inflammatory response and intensity of pain stimulus reaching sensory nerve endings, *producing analgesic and anti-inflammatory effect.* Constricts iris sphincter, *preventing miosis during cataract surgery.*

PHARMACOKINETICS

	Onset	Peak	Duration
PO	—	2–3 hrs	—

Completely absorbed from GI tract, penetrates cornea after ophthalmic administration (may be systemically absorbed). Widely distributed. Protein binding: >99%. Metabolized in liver. Primarily excreted in urine. Minimally removed by hemodialysis. Half-life: 1.2–2 hrs.

USES/*UNLABELED*

Symptomatic treatment of acute and/or chronic rheumatoid arthritis, osteoarthritis, ankylosing spondylitis; postop inflammation of cataract extraction; analgesic, primary dysmenorrhea. Treatment of photophobia, relief of pain in incisional refractive surgery. *Solaraze:* Treatment of actinic keratoses. *Ophthalmic: Reduces occurrence/severity of cystoid macular edema post cataract surgery. PO: Treatment of vascular headaches.*

PRECAUTIONS

CONTRAINDICATIONS: History of severe reaction induced by aspirin, other NSAIDs, nasal polyps associated with bronchospasm, bone marrow depression, blood dyscrasias. **CAUTIONS:** History of inflammatory or ulcerative disease of GI tract (e.g., peptic ulcer, Crohn's disease), hemophilia or other bleeding problem. Impaired renal or liver function. Stomatitis.
▷**LIFESPAN CONSIDERATIONS:**
Pregnancy/Lactation: Crosses placenta, unknown if distributed in breast milk. Avoid use during last trimester (may adversely affect fetal cardiovascular system: premature closure of ductus arteriosus). **Pregnancy Category B (Category D** if used in third trimester or near delivery). **Children:** Safety and efficacy not established. **Elderly:** GI bleeding or ulceration more likely to cause serious adverse effects. Age-related renal impairment may increase risk of liver or renal toxicity; reduced dosage recommended.

INTERACTIONS

DRUG: May increase effects of **oral anticoagulants, heparin, thrombolytics.** May decrease effect of **antihypertensives, diuretics. Salicylates, aspirin** may increase risk of GI side effects, bleeding. **Bone marrow depressants** may increase risk of hemato-

logic reactions. May increase concentration, toxicity of **lithium.** May increase **methotrexate** toxicity. **Probenecid** may increase concentration. *Ophthalmic:* May decrease effect of **acetylcholine, carbachol.** May decrease antiglaucoma effect of **epinephrine, other antiglaucoma medications. HERBAL: Ginkgo biloba** may increase risk of bleeding. **FOOD:** None known. **LAB VALUES:** May increase alkaline phosphatase, LDH, serum transaminase, potassium urine protein, BUN, serum creatinine. May decrease uric acid.

AVAILABILITY (Rx)

GEL: 3%. **TABLETS:** 50 mg (Cataflam). **TABLETS (delayed-release):** 25 mg, 50 mg, 75 mg. **TABLETS (extended-release):** 100 mg. **OPHTHALMIC SOLUTION:** 0.1%.

ADMINISTRATION/HANDLING

PO:

* Do not crush or break enteric-coated form. * May give with food, milk, or antacids if GI distress occurs.

Ophthalmic:

* Place finger on lower eyelid and pull out until pocket is formed between eye and lower lid. Hold dropper above pocket and place prescribed number of drops in pocket. * Close eye gently. Apply digital pressure to lacrimal sac for 1–2 min (minimized drainage into nose and throat, reducing risk of systemic effects). * Remove excess solution with tissue.

INDICATIONS/ROUTES/DOSAGE

Osteoarthritis:

PO: Adults, elderly: 100–150 mg/day in 2–3 divided doses. **Extended-release:** 100 mg/day as single dose.

Rheumatoid arthritis:

PO: **Adults, elderly:** 150–200 mg/day in 2–4 divided doses. *Extended-release:* 100 mg/day.

Ankylosing spondylitis:

PO: **Adults, elderly:** 100–125 mg/day in 4–5 divided doses.

Analgesic, primary dysmenorrhea:

PO: **Adults:** 150 mg/day in 3 divided doses.

Usual ophthalmic dosage:

Adults, elderly: Apply 1 drop to eye 4 times/day commencing 24 hrs after cataract surgery. Continue for 2 wks after surgery.

Actinic keratoses:

TOPICAL: **Adults, adolescents:** Apply 2 times/day to lesion for 60–90 days.

Usual pediatric dosage:

PO: 2–3 mg/kg/day in divided doses 2–4 times/day.

Photophobia:

Adults, elderly: 1 drop to affected eye 1 hr preop, within 15 min postop, then 4 times/day for 3 days.

SIDE EFFECTS

FREQUENT (3–9%): *PO:* Headache, abdominal cramping, constipation, diarrhea, nausea, dyspepsia. *Ophthalmic:* Burning, stinging on instillation, ocular discomfort. *OCCASIONAL* (1–3%): *PO:* Flatulence, dizziness, epigastric pain. *Ophthalmic:* Itching, tearing. *RARE* (<1%): *PO:* Rash, peripheral edema/fluid retention, visual disturbances, vomiting, drowsiness.

ADVERSE REACTIONS/TOXIC EFFECTS

Overdosage may result in acute renal failure. In those treated chronically, peptic ulcer, GI bleeding, gastritis, severe hepatic reaction (jaundice), nephrotoxicity (hematuria, dysuria, proteinuria), severe hypersensitivity reaction (bronchospasm, angiofacial edema) occur rarely.

NURSING IMPLICATIONS

BASELINE ASSESSMENT:

Anti-inflammatory: Assess onset, type, location, and duration of pain or inflammation. Inspect appearance of affected joints for immobility, deformities, and skin condition.

INTERVENTION/EVALUATION:

Monitor for headache, dyspepsia. Monitor pattern of daily bowel activity and stool consistency. Evaluate for therapeutic response: relief of pain, stiffness, swelling, increase in joint mobility, reduced joint tenderness, improved grip strength.

PATIENT/FAMILY TEACHING:

Swallow tablet whole; do not crush or chew. Avoid aspirin, alcohol during therapy (increases risk of GI bleeding). If GI upset occurs, take with food, milk. Report skin rash, itching, weight gain, changes in vision, black stools, persistent headache.

dicloxacillin sodium

Dynapen, Dycill, Pathocil

See Classification section under: Antibiotic: Penicillins (p. 26C)

---

dicyclomine hydrochloride

dye-**sigh**-clo-meen
(Antispaz, Bentyl, Bentylol♣,
Dibent, Di-Spaz, Formulex♣,
Lomine♣, Neoquess, OrTyl,
Spasmoject)
Do not confuse with Aventyl,
Benedryl, doxycycline, dyclonine.

▶CLASSIFICATION

CLINICAL: GI antispasmodic,
anticholinergic (see p. 27C)

ACTION/THERAPEUTIC EFFECT

Direct relaxant action on smooth
muscle, *reducing tone, motility of
GI tract.*

PHARMACOKINETICS

Readily absorbed from GI tract.
Widely distributed. Metabolized
in liver. Half-life: 9–10 hrs.

USES

Treatment of functional disturbances of GI motility (i.e., irritable
bowel syndrome).

PRECAUTIONS

CONTRAINDICATIONS: Narrow-
angle glaucoma, severe ulcerative
colitis, toxic megacolon, obstructive disease of GI tract, paralytic
ileus, intestinal atony, bladder
neck obstruction due to prostatic
hypertrophy, myasthenia gravis in
those not treated with neostigmine, tachycardia secondary to
cardiac insufficiency or thyrotoxicosis, cardiospasm, unstable cardiovascular status in acute hemorrhage. **EXTREME CAUTION:**
Autonomic neuropathy, known or
suspected GI infections, diarrhea,
mild to moderate ulcerative colitis.
CAUTIONS: Hyperthyroidism, hepatic or renal disease, hypertension, tachyarrhythmias, CHF, coronary artery disease, gastric ulcer,
esophageal reflux or hiatal hernia
associated with reflux esophagitis,
infants, elderly, COPD.

▷**LIFESPAN CONSIDERATIONS:**
Pregnancy/Lactation: Unknown
if drug crosses placenta or is distributed in breast milk. **Pregnancy Category B. Children:** Infants, young children more
susceptible to toxic effects. **Elderly:** May cause excitement, agitation, drowsiness or confusion.

INTERACTIONS

DRUG: Antacids, antidiarrheals
may decrease absorption. **Anticholinergics** may increase effects. May decrease absorption of
ketoconazole. May increase
severity of GI lesions with **KCl
(wax matrix). HERBAL:** None
known. **FOOD:** None known. **LAB
VALUES:** None significant.

AVAILABILITY (Rx)

CAPSULES: 10 mg, 20 mg. **TAB-
LETS:** 20 mg. **SYRUP:** 10 mg/5 ml.
INJECTION: 10 mg/ml.

ADMINISTRATION/HANDLING

• Store capsules, tablets, syrup,
parenteral form at room temperature.

PO:

• Dilute oral solution with equal
volume of water just before administration. • May give without
regard to meals (food may slightly
decrease absorption).

IM:

• Injection should appear colorless. • Do not administer IV or
SubQ. • Inject deep into large
muscle mass. • Do not give longer
than 2 days.

INDICATIONS/ROUTES/DOSAGE
Functional disturbances of GI motility:

PO: Adults: 10–20 mg 3–4 times/day up to 40 mg 4 times/day. **Children 6 mos–2 yrs:** 5 mg 3–4 times/day. **Children >2 yrs:** 10 mg 3–4 times/day.

IM: Adults: 20 mg q4–6h.

Usual elderly dosage:

PO: 10–20 mg 4 times/day. May increase up to 160 mg/day.

SIDE EFFECTS
FREQUENT: Dry mouth (sometimes severe), constipation, decreased sweating. ***OCCASIONAL:*** Blurred vision, intolerance to light, urinary hesitancy, drowsiness (with high dosage), agitation/excitement/drowsiness noted in elderly (even with low doses). IM may produce transient lightheadedness, irritation at injection site. ***RARE:*** Confusion, hypersensitivity reaction, increased intraocular pressure, nausea, vomiting, unusual tiredness.

ADVERSE REACTIONS/TOXIC EFFECTS
Overdosage may produce temporary paralysis of ciliary muscle, pupillary dilation, tachycardia, palpitation, hot/dry/flushed skin, absence of bowel sounds, hyperthermia, increased respiratory rate, EKG abnormalities, nausea, vomiting, rash over face/upper trunk, CNS stimulation, psychosis (agitation, restlessness, rambling speech, visual hallucination, paranoid behavior, delusions), followed by depression.

NURSING IMPLICATIONS

BASELINE ASSESSMENT:
Before giving medication, instruct pt to void (reduces risk of urinary retention).

INTERVENTION/EVALUATION:
Monitor daily bowel activity and stool consistency. Assess for urinary retention. Monitor changes in B/P, temperature. Assess skin turgor, mucous membranes to evaluate hydration status (encourage adequate fluid intake), bowel sounds for peristalsis. Be alert for fever (increased risk of hyperthermia).

PATIENT/FAMILY TEACHING:
Do not become overheated during exercise in hot weather (may result in heat stroke). Avoid hot baths, saunas. Avoid tasks that require alertness, motor skills until response to drug is established. Do not take antacids or medicine for diarrhea within 1 hr of taking this medication (decreased effectiveness).

didanosine

dye-**dan**-oh-sin
(Videx, Videx-EC)

▶CLASSIFICATION
PHARMACOTHERAPEUTIC: Purine nucleoside analogue. ***CLINICAL:*** Antiviral (see pp. 58C, 94C)

ACTION/*THERAPEUTIC EFFECT*
Intracellularly converted into a triphosphate, interfering with RNA-directed DNA polymerase (reverse transcriptase). *Virustatic,* inhibiting replication of retroviruses, including human immunodeficiency virus (HIV).

PHARMACOKINETICS

Variably absorbed from GI tract. Protein binding: <5%. Rapidly metabolized intracellularly to active form. Primarily excreted in urine. Partially (20%) removed by hemodialysis. Half-life: 1.5 hrs; metabolite: 8–24 hrs.

USES

Management (not cure) of advanced HIV disease in pts who cannot tolerate zidovudine or who have had clinically or immunologically significant deterioration during zidovudine therapy. Initial therapy in AIDS.

PRECAUTIONS

CONTRAINDICATIONS: Hypersensitivity to drug or any component of preparation. **CAUTIONS:** Renal or hepatic dysfunction, alcoholism, elevated triglycerides, T cell counts <100 cells/mm^3; extreme caution with history of pancreatitis. Phenylketonuria and sodium-restricted diets due to phenylalanine and sodium content of preparations.

▷**LIFESPAN CONSIDERATIONS:** **Pregnancy/Lactation:** Use during pregnancy only if clearly needed. Discontinue nursing during didanosine therapy. **Pregnancy Category B. Children:** Well tolerated in children >3 mos of age. **Elderly:** Age-related renal impairment may require dosage adjustment.

INTERACTIONS

DRUG: May increase risk of pancreatitis, peripheral neuropathy with medications producing pancreatitis, peripheral neuropathy, respectively. May decrease absorption of **dapsone, itraconazole, ketoconazole, tetracyclines, fluoroquinolones. Stavudine** may increase risk of fatal lactic acidosis in pregnant women. **HERBAL:** None known. **FOOD:** Decreases absorption. **LAB VALUES:** May increase alkaline phosphatase, SGOT (AST), SGPT (ALT), bilirubin, amylase, lipase, triglycerides, uric acid. May decrease potassium.

AVAILABILITY (Rx)

TABLETS (chewable): 25 mg, 50 mg, 100 mg, 150 mg, 200 mg. **CAPSULES (delayed-release):** 125 mg, 200 mg, 250 mg, 400 mg. **POWDER FOR ORAL SOLUTION (single-dose packet):** 100 mg, 167 mg, 250 mg. **PEDIATRIC SOLUTION:** 10 mg/ml.

ADMINISTRATION/HANDLING
PO:

• Store at room temperature. • If tablets are dispersed in water, is stable for 1 hr at room temperature; after reconstitution of buffered powder, oral solution is stable for 4 hrs at room temperature. • Pediatric powder for oral solution after reconstitution as directed, stable for 30 days refrigerated. • Give 1 hr before or 2 hrs after meals (food decreases rate and extent of absorption). • *Chewable tablets:* Thoroughly crush and disperse in at least 30 ml water before swallowing. Mixture should be stirred well (2–3 min) and swallowed immediately. • *Buffered powder for oral solution:* Reconstitute prior to administration by pouring contents of packet into about 4 oz water; stir until completely dissolved (up to 2–3 min). Do not mix with fruit juice or other acidic liquid because didanosine is unstable at acidic pH. • *Unbuffered pediatric powder:* Add 100–200 ml water to 2 or 4 g, respectively, to provide concentration of 20 mg/ml. Immediately mix with equal amount of antacid to provide concentration of 10 mg/ml. Shake thoroughly prior to removing each dose. • *Enteric-coated capsules:* Swallow whole, take on empty stomach.

INDICATIONS/ROUTES/DOSAGE

HIV:

Adults, children (≥13 yrs, ≥60 kg): 200 mg q12h or 400 mg once daily. *Oral solution:* 250 mg q12h. *Delayed-release capsules:* 400 mg once daily. **Adults (≥13 yrs, ≤60 kg):** 125 mg q12h or 250 mg once daily. *Oral solution:* 167 mg q12h. *Delayed-release capsules:* 250 mg once daily. **Children (3 mos–<13 yrs):** 180–300 mg/m^2/day in divided doses q12h. **Children <3 mos:** 50 mg/m^2/day in divided doses q12h.

Dosage in renal impairment:

Pts <60 kg:

Creatinine Clearance (ml/min)	Tablets	Oral Solution	Delayed-Release Capsules
30–59	75 mg 2 times/day	100 mg 2 times/day	125 mg once daily
10–29	100 mg once daily	100 mg once daily	125 mg once daily
<10	75 mg once daily	100 mg once daily	—

Pts >60 kg:

Creatinine Clearance (ml/min)	Tablets	Oral Solution	Delayed-Release Capsules
30–59	100 mg 2 times/day	100 mg 2 times/day	200 mg once daily
10–29	150 mg once daily	167 mg once daily	125 mg once daily
<10	100 mg once daily	100 mg once daily	125 mg once daily

SIDE EFFECTS

FREQUENT: Adults (>10%): Diarrhea, neuropathy, chills/fever. **Children** (>25%): Chills, fever, decreased appetite, pain, malaise, nausea, diarrhea, vomiting, abdominal pain, headache, nervousness, cough, rhinitis, dyspnea, asthenia, rash, itching. **OCCASIONAL: Adults** (2–9%): Rash, itching, headache, abdominal pain, nausea, vomiting, pneumonia, myopathy, decreased appetite, dry mouth, dyspnea. **Children** (10–25%): Failure to thrive, decreased weight, stomatitis, oral thrush, ecchymosis, arthritis, myalgia, insomnia, epistaxis, pharyngitis.

ADVERSE REACTIONS/TOXIC EFFECTS

Pneumonia, opportunistic infection occur occasionally. Peripheral neuropathy, potentially fatal pancreatitis are the major toxicities.

NURSING IMPLICATIONS

BASELINE ASSESSMENT:

Obtain baseline values for CBC, renal and hepatic function tests, vital signs, weight.

INTERVENTION/EVALUATION:

In event of abdominal pain and nausea, vomiting, or elevated serum amylase, triglycerides, contact physician before administering medication (potential pancreatitis). Be alert to burning feet, "restless leg syndrome" (unable to find comfortable position for legs and feet), lack of coordination and other signs of peripheral neuropathy. Monitor consistency and frequency of stools. Check skin for rash, eruptions. Assess for opportunistic infections: onset of fever, oral mucosa changes, cough, or other respiratory symptoms. Assess children for epistaxis or other bleeding, petechiae. Check weight at least twice a week. Assess for visual or hearing difficulty; provide protection from light if photophobia develops.

PATIENT/FAMILY TEACHING:

Explain correct administration of medication. Eat small, frequent meals to offset anorexia, vomiting.

dienestrol

dye-en-**ess**-troll
(Ortho Dienestrol)

▶CLASSIFICATION

PHARMACOTHERAPEUTIC: Hormone. **CLINICAL:** Estrogen

ACTION/*THERAPEUTIC EFFECT*

Increases synthesis of DNA, RNA, and various proteins in responsive tissues, *alleviating signs and symptoms of vulvovaginal epithelial atrophy (atrophic vaginitis), kraurosis vulvae associated with menopause.*

USES

Treatment of atrophic vaginitis, kraurosis vulvae.

PRECAUTIONS

CONTRAINDICATIONS: Known or suspected breast cancer, estrogen-dependent neoplasia; undiagnosed abnormal genital bleeding; active thrombophlebitis or thromboembolic disorders; history of thrombophlebitis, thrombosis, or thromboembolic disorders with previous estrogen use, hypersensitivity to estrogen or ingredients of cream. **CAUTIONS:** Mental depression, hypercal-

cemia, history of jaundice during pregnancy, or strong family history of breast cancer, fibrocystic disease, or breast nodules. Also, cautions in conditions that may be aggravated by fluid retention: cardiac, renal, or hepatic dysfunction, epilepsy, migraine.

INTERACTIONS

DRUG: May interfere with effects of bromocriptine. May increase concentration cyclosporine, increase hepatic, nephrotoxicity. Hepatotoxic medications may increase hepatotoxicity. **HERBAL:** None known. **FOOD:** None known. **LAB VALUES:** May affect metapyrone, thyroid function tests. May decrease cholesterol, LDH. May increase calcium, glucose, HDL, triglycerides.

AVAILABILITY (Rx)

VAGINAL CREAM: 0.01%.

INDICATIONS/ROUTES/DOSAGE

Atrophic vaginitis, kraurosis vulvae:
INTRAVAGINAL: Adults, elderly: Initially, 1–2 applicatorsful/day for 7–14 days. Reduce dose by ½ for additional 1–2 wks. **Maintenance:** 1 applicatorful 1–3 times/wk.

SIDE EFFECTS

FREQUENT: Breast pain/tenderness, enlarged breasts, edema (swelling of feet, increased weight), decreased appetite, abdominal cramping. **OCCASIONAL:** Diarrhea, dizziness, headache, increased libido, abnormal vaginal bleeding (amenorrhea, breakthrough bleeding, spotting, menorrhagia), breast tumors, gallbladder obstructions. Local irritation (itching, redness, swelling).

ADVERSE REACTIONS/TOXIC EFFECTS

Prolonged administration increases risk of gallbladder, thromboembolic disease, and breast, cervical, vaginal, endometrial, and liver carcinoma.

NURSING IMPLICATIONS

BASELINE ASSESSMENT:

Question hypersensitivity to estrogen or ingredients of cream, previous jaundice or thromboembolic disorders associated with pregnancy or estrogen therapy.

INTERVENTION/EVALUATION:

Monitor blood glucose 4 times/day for pts with diabetes. Assess for vaginal discharge, local irritation.

PATIENT/FAMILY TEACHING:

With systemic absorption, smoking may increase risk of heart attack or blood clots. Notify physician of abnormal vaginal bleeding pain or numbness of an extremity. Remain recumbent at least 30 min after application and do not use tampons. Stop using dienestrol, contact physician at once if suspect pregnancy.

diflunisal

dye-**flew**-neh-sol
(Apo-Diflunisal✤, Dolobid, Novo-Diflunisal✤)
Do not confuse with Slo-bid.

▶CLASSIFICATION

PHARMACOTHERAPEUTIC:
Nonsteroidal anti-inflammatory.
CLINICAL: Antirheumatic, analgesic, vascular headache suppressant (see p. 106C)

ACTION/*THERAPEUTIC EFFECT*

Inhibits prostaglandin synthesis, reducing inflammatory response and intensity of pain stimulus reaching sensory nerve endings, *producing analgesic and anti-inflammatory effect.*

PHARMACOKINETICS

	Onset	Peak	Duration
PO	1 hr	2–3 hrs	—

Completely absorbed from GI tract. Widely distributed. Protein binding: >99%. Metabolized in liver. Primarily excreted in urine. Not removed by hemodialysis. Half-life: 8–12 hrs.

USES/*UNLABELED*

Treatment of acute or long-term mild to moderate pain associated with acute and/or chronic rheumatoid arthritis, osteoarthritis. *Treatment of psoriatic arthritis, vascular headache.*

PRECAUTIONS

CONTRAINDICATIONS: History of severe allergic reaction induced by aspirin, other NSAIDs, nasal polyps associated with bronchospasm, bone marrow depression, blood dyscrasias. **CAUTIONS:** History of inflammatory or ulcerative disease of GI tract (e.g., peptic ulcer, Crohn's disease), hemophilia or other bleeding problem. Impaired renal or liver function. Stomatitis.

▷**LIFESPAN CONSIDERATIONS:**
Pregnancy/Lactation: Crosses placenta; distributed in breast milk. Avoid use during last trimester (may adversely affect fetal cardiovascular system: premature closure of ductus arteriosus). **Pregnancy Category C (Category D** if used in third trimester or near

delivery). **Children:** Safety and efficacy not established. **Elderly:** GI bleeding or ulceration more likely to cause serious adverse effects. Age-related renal impairment may increase risk liver or renal toxicity; decreased dosage recommended.

INTERACTIONS

DRUG: May increase effects of **oral anticoagulants, heparin, thrombolytics.** May decrease effect of **antihypertensives, diuretics. Salicylates, aspirin** may increase risk of GI side effects, bleeding. **Bone marrow depressants** may increase risk of hematologic reactions. May increase concentration, toxicity of **lithium.** May increase **methotrexate** toxicity. **Probenecid** may increase concentration. **HERBAL: Gingko biloba** may increase risk of bleeding. **FOOD:** None known. **LAB VALUES:** May increase serum transaminase activity. May decrease uric acid.

AVAILABILITY (Rx)
TABLETS: 250 mg, 500 mg.

ADMINISTRATION/HANDLING
PO:

• May give with water, milk, or meals. • Do not crush or break film-coated tablets.

INDICATIONS/ROUTES/DOSAGE
Mild to moderate pain:

PO: Adults, elderly: Initially, 0.5–1 g, then 250–500 mg q8–12h.

Rheumatoid arthritis, osteoarthritis:

PO: Adults, elderly: 0.5–1 g/day in 2 divided doses.

SIDE EFFECTS

Side effects appear less frequently with short-term treatment. **OCCA-SIONAL** (3–9%): Nausea, dyspepsia (heartburn, indigestion, epigastric pain), diarrhea, headache, rash. **RARE** (1–3%): Vomiting, constipation, flatulence, dizziness, insomnolence, insomnia, fatigue, tinnitus.

ADVERSE REACTIONS/TOXIC EFFECTS

Overdosage may produce drowsiness, vomiting, nausea, diarrhea, hyperventilation, tachycardia, sweating, stupor, coma. Peptic ulcer, GI bleeding, gastritis, severe hepatic reaction (cholestasis, jaundice) occur rarely. Nephrotoxicity (dysuria, hematuria, proteinuria, nephrotic syndrome) and severe hypersensitivity reaction (bronchospasm, angiofacial edema) occur rarely.

NURSING IMPLICATIONS

BASELINE ASSESSMENT:
Assess onset, type, location, and duration of pain or inflammation. Inspect appearance of affected joints for immobility, deformities, and skin condition.

INTERVENTION/EVALUATION:
Monitor for nausea, dyspepsia. Assess skin for evidence of rash. Monitor pattern of daily bowel activity and stool consistency. Evaluate for therapeutic response: relief of pain, stiffness, swelling, increase in joint mobility, reduced joint tenderness, improved grip strength.

PATIENT/FAMILY TEACHING:
Swallow tablet whole; do not crush or chew. If GI upset occurs, take with food, milk. Report GI distress, headache, rash.

digoxin 🖋

di-**jox**-in
(Lanoxin, Lanoxicaps)
Do not confuse with Desoxyn,
doxepin, Levsinex, Lonox.

▶CLASSIFICATION

PHARMACOTHERAPEUTIC:
Cardiac glycoside. **CLINICAL:**
Antiarrhythmic, cardiotonic (see
p. 76C)

ACTION/THERAPEUTIC EFFECT

Direct action on cardiac muscle,
conduction system. Decreases
conduction rate through SA, AV
node. *Increases force, velocity of
myocardial contraction.*

PHARMACOKINETICS

Readily absorbed from GI tract.
Widely distributed. Protein binding: 30%. Partially metabolized in
liver. Primarily excreted in urine.
Minimally removed by hemodialysis. Half-life: 36–48 hrs (half-life increased with impaired renal function, elderly).

USES

Prophylactic management and
treatment of CHF; control of ventricular rate in pts with atrial fibrillation. Treatment and prevention of
recurrent paroxysmal atrial tachycardia.

PRECAUTIONS

CONTRAINDICATIONS: Ventricular fibrillation, ventricular tachycardia unrelated to CHF. **CAUTIONS:**
Impaired renal function, impaired
hepatic function, hypokalemia, advanced cardiac disease, acute myocardial infarction, incomplete AV
block, cor pulmonale, hypothyroidism, pulmonary disease.

▷**LIFESPAN CONSIDERATIONS:**
Pregnancy/Lactation: Crosses
placenta; distributed in breast
milk. **Pregnancy Category C.**
Children: Premature infants more
susceptible to toxicity. **Elderly:**
Age-related liver or renal function
impairment may require adjusted
dosage. Increased risk of loss of
appetite.

INTERACTIONS

**DRUG: Glucocorticoids, ampho-
tericin, potassium-depleting diuretics** may increase toxicity (due
to hypokalemia). **Amiodarone** may
increase concentration, toxicity; additive effect on SA, AV nodes. **Antiarrhythmics, parenteral calcium, sympathomimetics** may
increase risk of arrhythmias. **Antidiarrheals, cholestyramine,
colestipol, sucralfate** may decrease absorption. **Diltiazem, verapamil, fluoxetine, quinidine**
may increase concentration. **Parenteral magnesium** may cause
conduction changes, heart block.
HERBAL: Siberian gingseng may
increase serum levels. **FOOD:**
None known. **LAB VALUES:** None
significant. Therapeutic blood
serum level: 0.8–2 ng/ml; toxic
blood serum level: >2 ng/ml.

AVAILABILITY (Rx)

TABLETS: 0.125 mg, 0.25 mg, 0.5
mg. **CAPSULES:** 0.05 mg, 0.1 mg,
0.2 mg. **ELIXIR:** 0.05 mg/ml. **IN-
JECTION:** 0.25 mg/ml, 0.1 mg/ml.

ADMINISTRATION/HANDLING

Note: IM rarely used (produces
severe local irritation, erratic absorption). If no other route possible, give deep into muscle followed by massage. Give no more
than 2 ml at any one site.

PO:

• May give without regard to meals. • Tablets may be crushed.

IV ▨

• May give undiluted or dilute with at least a 4-fold volume of Sterile Water for Injection, or D₅W (less than this may cause a precipitate). Use immediately. • Give IV slowly over at least 5 min.

IV INCOMPATIBILITIES ⊘

Amphotericin B complex (Abelcet, Amphotec, Ambisome), fluconazole (Diflucan), foscarnet (Foscavir), propofol (Diprivan).

IV COMPATIBILITIES

Diltiazem (Cardizem), midazolam (Versed), milrinone (Primacor), potassium chloride.

INDICATIONS/ROUTES/DOSAGE

Note: Adjust dose in elderly, pts with renal dysfunction. Larger doses often required for adequate control of ventricular rate in pts with atrial fibrillation or flutter. Administer loading dosage in several doses at 4–8 hr intervals.

Usual Dosage for Adults:

Rapid loading dosage:

IV: **Adults, elderly:** 0.6–1 mg.

PO: **Adults, elderly:** Initially, 0.5–0.75 mg, additional doses of 0.125–0.375 mg at 6–8 hr intervals. **Range:** 0.75–1.25 mg.

Maintenance dosage:

PO/IV: **Adults, elderly:** 0.125–0.375 mg/day.

Usual Dosage for Children:

Rapid loading dosage:

IV: **Children (>10 yrs):** 8–12 mcg/kg; **(5–10 yrs):** 15–30 mcg/kg; **(2–5 yrs):** 25–35 mcg/kg; **(1–24 mos):** 30–50 mcg/kg; **(Full term):** 20–30 mcg/kg; **(Premature):** 15–25 mcg/kg.

PO: **Children (>10 yrs):** 10–15 mcg/kg; **(5–10 yrs):** 20–35 mcg/kg; **(2–5 yrs):** 30–40 mcg/kg; **(1–24 mos):** 35–60 mcg/kg; **(Full term):** 25–35 mcg/kg; **(Premature):** 20–30 mcg/kg.

Maintenance dosage:

PO/IV: **Children:** 25–35% loading dose (20–30% for premature).

SIDE EFFECTS

None significant; however, there is a very narrow margin of safety between a therapeutic and toxic result. Chronic therapy may produce mammary gland enlargement in women but is reversible when drug is withdrawn.

ADVERSE REACTIONS/TOXIC EFFECTS

The most common early manifestations of toxicity are GI disturbances (anorexia, nausea, vomiting) and neurologic abnormalities (fatigue, headache, depression, weakness, drowsiness, confusion, nightmares). Facial pain, personality change, ocular disturbances (photophobia, light flashes, halos around bright objects, yellow or green color perception) may be noted.

NURSING IMPLICATIONS

BASELINE ASSESSMENT:

Assess apical radial pulse for 60 sec (30 sec if on maintenance therapy). If pulse is 60/min or below (70/min or below for children), withhold drug and contact physician. Blood samples are best taken 6–8 hrs after dose or just prior to next dose.

INTERVENTION/EVALUATION:

Monitor pulse for bradycardia, EKG for arrhythmias for 1–2 hrs after administration (excessive slowing of pulse may be a first clinical sign of toxicity). Assess for GI disturbances, neurologic abnormalities (signs of toxicity) q2–4h during digitalization (daily during maintenance). Monitor serum potassium, magnesium levels. Therapeutic blood serum level: 0.8–2 ng/ml; toxic blood serum level: >2 ng/ml.

PATIENT/FAMILY TEACHING:

Importance of follow-up visits, tests. Teach pt to take pulse correctly and to report pulse below 60/min (or as indicated by physician). Assure pt understands signs of toxicity and need to notify physician if any occur. Wear/carry identification of digoxin therapy and inform dentist or other physician of taking digoxin. Do not increase or skip doses. Do not take OTC medications without consulting physician. Report nausea, vomiting, extremely slow pulse.

digoxin immune FAB

(Digibind, DigiFab)

▶**CLASSIFICATION**
CLINICAL: Antidote

ACTION/*THERAPEUTIC EFFECT*

Acts in extracellular space. Binds molecules of digoxin, *making digoxin unavailable for binding at its site of action on cells in the body.*

PHARMACOKINETICS

	Onset	Peak	Duration
IV	30 min	—	3–4 days

Widely distributed into extracellular space. Excreted in urine. Half-life: 15–20 hrs.

USES

Treatment of potentially life-threatening digoxin intoxication.

PRECAUTIONS

CONTRAINDICATIONS: None significant. **CAUTIONS:** Impaired cardiac, renal function.
▷**LIFESPAN CONSIDERATIONS:** **Pregnancy/Lactation:** Unknown if drug crosses placenta or is distributed in breast milk. **Pregnancy Category C. Children:** No age-related precautions noted. **Elderly:** Age-related renal impairment may require caution.

INTERACTIONS

DRUG: None significant. **HERBAL:** None known. **FOOD:** None known. **LAB VALUES:** May alter potassium concentration. Serum digoxin concentration may increase precipitously and persist for up to 1 wk (until FAB/digoxin complex is eliminated from body).

AVAILABILITY (Rx)

POWDER FOR INJECTION: 38 mg vial.

ADMINISTRATION/HANDLING
IV 💉

Storage:

• Refrigerate vials. • After reconstitution, is stable for 4 hrs if refrigerated. • Use immediately after reconstitution.

Reconstitution:

• Reconstitute each 38 mg vial with 4 ml Sterile Water for Injection to provide a concentration of 9.5 mg/ml. • Further dilute with 50 ml 0.9% NaCl.

Rate of administration:

• Infuse over 30 min (recommended that solution be infused through a 0.22 micron filter). • If cardiac arrest imminent, may give IV push.

IV INCOMPATIBILITY ⊘

None known.

INDICATIONS/ROUTES/DOSAGE

Dosage varies according to amount of digoxin to be neutralized. Refer to manufacturer's dosing guidelines.

SIDE EFFECTS

None significant.

ADVERSE REACTIONS/TOXIC EFFECTS

As result of digitalis intoxication, hyperkalemia may present (diarrhea, paresthesia of extremities, heaviness of legs, decreased B/P, cold skin, grayish pallor, hypotension, mental confusion, irritability, flaccid paralysis, tented T waves, widening QRS, ST depression). When effect of digitalis is reversed, hypokalemia may develop rapidly (muscle cramping, nausea, vomiting, hypoactive bowel sounds, abdominal distention, difficulty breathing, postural hypotension). Rarely, low cardiac output, CHF may occur.

NURSING IMPLICATIONS

BASELINE ASSESSMENT:

Obtain serum digoxin level before administering drug. If drawn <6 hrs before last digoxin ,dose, serum digoxin level may be unreliable. Those with impaired renal function may require >1 wk before serum digoxin assay is reliable. Assess muscle strength, mental status.

INTERVENTION/EVALUATION:

Closely monitor temperature, B/P, EKG, and potassium serum level during and after drug is administered. Watch for changes from initial assessment (hypokalemia may result in muscle strength changes, tremor, muscle cramps, change in mental status, cardiac arrhythmias; hyponatremia may result in confusion, thirst, cold/clammy skin).

---

dihydroergotamine

See ergotamine

---

dihydrotachysterol

See vitamin D

---

diltiazem hydrochloride 🖊

dill-**tie**-ah-zem
(Apo-Diltiaz❧, Cardizem, Cardizem CD, Dilacor XR, Novo-Diltiazem❧, Tiazac)
Do not confuse with Cardene, Ziac.

FIXED-COMBINATION(S)

With enalapril, an ACE inhibitor **(Teczem)**

▶CLASSIFICATION

PHARMACOTHERAPEUTIC: Calcium channel blocker. ***CLINICAL:*** Antianginal, antihypertensive, antiarrhythmic (see pp. 14C, 65C)

ACTION/*THERAPEUTIC EFFECT*

Inhibits calcium movement across cell membranes of cardiac and vascular smooth muscle (dilates coronary arteries, peripheral arteries/arterioles); *decreases heart rate, myocardial contractility, slows SA and AV conduction. Decreases total peripheral vascular resistance by vasodilation.*

PHARMACOKINETICS

	Onset	Peak	Duration
PO	30–60 min	—	—

Well absorbed from GI tract. Protein binding: 70–80%. Undergoes first-pass metabolism in liver. Metabolized in liver to active metabolite. Primarily excreted in urine. Not removed by hemodialysis. Half-life: 3–8 hrs.

USES

PO: Treatment of angina due to coronary artery spasm (Prinzmetal's variant angina), chronic stable angina (effort-associated angina). **Extended-release:** Treatment of essential hypertension, angina. **Parenteral:** Temporary control of rapid ventricular rate in atrial fibrillation/flutter. Rapid conversion of PSVT to normal sinus rhythm.

PRECAUTIONS

CONTRAINDICATIONS: Sick sinus syndrome/second- or third-degree AV block (except in presence of pacemaker), severe hypotension (<90 mm Hg, systolic), acute MI, pulmonary congestion. **CAUTIONS:** Impaired renal/hepatic function, CHF.
▷**LIFESPAN CONSIDERATIONS:** **Pregnancy/Lactation:** Distributed in breast milk. **Pregnancy Category C. Children:** No age-related precautions noted. **El-**

derly: Age-related renal impairment may require caution.

INTERACTIONS

DRUG: Beta-blockers may have additive effect. May increase **digoxin** concentration. **Procainamide, quinidine** may increase risk of QT interval prolongation. **Carbamazepine, quinidine, theophylline** may increase concentration, toxicity. **HERBAL:** None known. **FOOD:** None known. **LAB VALUES:** PR interval may be increased.

AVAILABILITY (Rx)

TABLETS: 30 mg, 60 mg, 90 mg, 120 mg. **CAPSULES (sustained-release):** 60 mg, 90 mg, 120 mg, 180 mg, 240 mg, 300 mg, 360 mg, 420 mg. **INJECTION:** 5 mg/ml vials.

ADMINISTRATION/HANDLING

PO:

• Give before meals and at bedtime. • Tablets may be crushed. • Do not crush sustained-release capsules.

IV 🔟

Storage:

• Refrigerate vials. • After dilution, stable for 24 hrs.

Reconstitution:

• Add 125 mg to 100 ml D_5W, 0.9% NaCl, or D_5W/0.45% NaCl to provide a concentration of 1 mg/ml. Add 250 mg to 250 or 500 ml diluent to provide a concentration of 0.83 mg/ml or 0.45 mg/ml, respectively. Maximum concentration: 1.25 g/250 ml (5 mg/ml).

Rate of administration:

• Infuse per dilution/rate chart provided by manufacturer.

IV INCOMPATIBILITIES ⊘

Acetazolamide (Diamox), acyclovir (Zovirax), aminophyllin, ampicillin, ampicillin/sulbactam (Unasyn), cefoperazone (Cefobid), diazepam (Valium), furosemide (Lasix), heparin, insulin, nafcillin, phenytoin (Dilantin), rifampin (Rifampin), sodium bicarbonate.

IV COMPATIBILITIES

Bumetanide (Bumex), cefazolin (Ancef), ceftriaxone (Rocephin), ciprofloxacin (Cipro), clindamycin (Cleocin), dobutamine (Dobutrex), dopamine (Intropin), fluconazole (Diflucan), gentamicin (Garamycin), labetalol (Normodyne, Trandate), lidocaine, lorazepam (Ativan), metoclopramide (Reglan), metronidazole (Flagyl), midazolam (Versed), multivitamins, nitroglycerin, norepinephrine (Levophed), potassium chloride, tobramycin (Nebcin), vancomycin (Vancocin).

INDICATIONS/ROUTES/DOSAGE

Angina:

PO: **Adults, elderly:** Initially, 30 mg 4 times/day. Increase up to 180–360 mg/day in 3–4 divided doses at 1–2 day intervals.

(CD capsules): **Adults, elderly:** Initially, 120–180 mg/day; titrate over 7–14 days. **Range:** Up to 480 mg/day.

Essential hypertension:

PO (extended-release): **Adults, elderly:** Initially, 60–120 mg 2 times/day.

(CD capsules): **Adults, elderly:** Initially, 180–240 mg/day. **Range:** 240–360 mg in 2 divided doses.

(Dilacor XR): **Adults, elderly:** Initially, 180–240 mg/day. **Range:** 180–480 mg/day.

Usual parenteral dosage:

IV PUSH: **Adults, elderly:** Initially, 0.25 mg/kg actual body weight over 2 min. May repeat in 15 min at dose of 0.35 mg/kg actual body weight. Subsequent doses individualized.

IV INFUSION: **Adults, elderly:** After initial bolus injection, 5–10 mg/hr, may increase at 5 mg/hr up to 15 mg/hr. Maintain over 24 hrs. **Note:** Refer to manufacturer's information for dose concentration/infusion rates.

SIDE EFFECTS

FREQUENT (5–10%): Peripheral edema, dizziness, lightheadedness, headache, bradycardia, asthenia (loss of strength, weakness). *OCCASIONAL* (2–5%): Nausea, constipation, flushing, altered EKG. *RARE* (<2%): Rash, micturition disorder (polyuria, nocturia, dysuria, frequency of urination), abdominal discomfort, somnolence.

ADVERSE REACTIONS/TOXIC EFFECTS

Abrupt withdrawal may increase frequency/duration of angina. CHF, second- and third-degree AV block occur rarely. Overdosage produces nausea, drowsiness, confusion, slurred speech, profound bradycardia.

NURSING IMPLICATIONS

BASELINE ASSESSMENT:

Concurrent therapy of sublingual nitroglycerin may be used for relief of anginal pain. Record onset, type (sharp, dull, squeezing), radiation, location, intensity, and duration of anginal pain, and precipitating factors (exertion, emotional stress). Assess baseline renal/liver function tests. Assess B/P, apical pulse immediately before drug is administered.

INTERVENTION/EVALUATION:

Assist with ambulation if dizziness occurs. Assess for peripheral edema behind medial malleolus (sacral area in bedridden pts). Monitor pulse rate for bradycardia. Question for asthenia, headache.

PATIENT/FAMILY TEACHING:

Do not abruptly discontinue medication. Compliance with therapy regimen is essential to control anginal pain. To avoid hypotensive effect rise slowly from lying to sitting position, wait momentarily before standing. Avoid tasks that require alertness, motor skills until response to drug is established. Contact physician/nurse if irregular heartbeat, shortness of breath, pronounced dizziness, nausea, or constipation occurs.

dimenhydrinate

(Dramamine)
See Classification section under: Antihistamines

dinoprostone

dye-noe-**pros**-tone
(Cervidil, Prepidil Gel, Prostaglandin E₂, Prostin E₂)

▶CLASSIFICATION

PHARMACOTHERAPEUTIC: Prostaglandin. **CLINICAL:** Oxytoxic, abortifacient, antihemorrhagic

ACTION/*THERAPEUTIC EFFECT*

Direct action on myometrium. Direct softening, dilation effect on cervix. *Stimulates myometrial contractions in gravid uterus.*

PHARMACOKINETICS

Undergoes rapid enzymatic deactivation primarily in maternal lungs. Protein binding: 73%. Primarily excreted in urine.

USES/*UNLABELED*

Suppository: To induce abortion from the 12th wk of pregnancy through the second trimester; to evacuate uterine contents in missed abortion or intrauterine fetal death up to 28 wks gestational age (as calculated from the first day of the last normal menstrual period), benign hydatidiform mole. **Gel:** Ripening unfavorable cervix in pregnant women at or near term with medical or obstetrical need for labor induction. **Suppository:** Treatment of postpartum/postabortion hemorrhage, induction labor at or near term. **Gel:** Induction labor at or near term.

PRECAUTIONS

CONTRAINDICATIONS: Hypersensitivity to dinoprostone or other prostaglandins; acute pelvic inflammatory disease; active cardiac, renal, hepatic, or pulmonary disease; fetal malpresentation or significant cephalopelvic disproportion. **CAUTIONS:** Cervicitis, infected endocervical lesions or acute vaginitis, history of asthma, hypo/hypertension, anemia, jaundice, diabetes, epilepsy, uterine fibroids, compromised (scarred) uterus, cardiovascular, renal, or hepatic disease.

▷*LIFESPAN CONSIDERATIONS:*
Pregnancy/Lactation: *Suppository:*

Teratogenic; therefore abortion must be complete. *Gel:* Sustained uterine hyperstimulation may affect fetus (e.g., abnormal heart rate). **Pregnancy Category C. Children/Elderly:** Not used in these pt populations.

INTERACTIONS

DRUG: **Oxytocics** may cause uterine hypertonus, possibly causing uterine rupture or cervical laceration. *HERBAL:* None known. *FOOD:* None known. *LAB VALUES:* None significant.

AVAILABILITY (Rx)

VAGINAL SUPPOSITORY: 20 mg. *VAGINAL GEL:* 0.5 mg (Prepidil). *VAGINAL INSERTS:* 10 mg (Cervidil).

ADMINISTRATION/HANDLING

Suppository:

• Keep frozen (<4°F); bring to room temperature just prior to use. • Administer only in hospital setting with emergency equipment available. • Warm suppository to room temperature before removing foil wrapper. • Avoid skin contact because of risk of absorption. • Insert high in vagina. • Pt should remain supine for 10 min after administration.

Gel:

• Refrigerate. • Use caution in handling, prevent skin contact. Wash hands thoroughly with soap and water after administration. • Bring to room temperature just before use (avoid forcing the warming process). • Assemble dosing apparatus as described in manufacturer insert. • Have pt in dorsal position with cervix visualized using a speculum. • Introduce gel into cervical canal just below level of internal os. • Have pt remain in supine position at least 15–30 min (minimizes leakage from cervical canal).

INDICATIONS/ROUTES/DOSAGE

Abortifacient:

INTRAVAGINAL: **Adults:** 20 mg (one suppository) high into vagina. May repeat at 3–5 hr intervals until abortion occurs. Do not administer >2 days.

Ripening unfavorable cervix:

INTRACERVICAL: (Prepidil): **Adults:** Initially, 0.5 mg (2.5 ml); if no cervical/uterine response, may repeat 0.5 mg dose in 6 hrs. **Maximum:** 1.5 mg (7.5 ml) for a 24 hr period. *(Cervidil):* **Adults:** 10 mg over 12 hr period. Remove upon onset of active labor or 12 hrs after insertion.

SIDE EFFECTS

FREQUENT: Vomiting (66%), diarrhea (40%), nausea (33%). *OCCASIONAL:* Headache (10%), chills/shivering (10%), hives, bradycardia, increased uterine pain accompanying abortion, peripheral vasoconstriction. *RARE:* Flushing, vulvae edema.

ADVERSE REACTIONS/TOXIC EFFECTS

Excessive dosage may cause uterine hypertonicity with spasm and tetanic contraction, leading to cervical laceration/perforation, uterine rupture or hemorrhage.

NURSING IMPLICATIONS

BASELINE ASSESSMENT:

Offer emotional support. *Suppository:* Obtain orders for antiemetics and antidiarrheals, meperidine or other pain medication for abdominal cramps. Assess any uterine activity or vaginal bleeding. *Gel:* Assess Bishop score. Assess degree of effacement (determines size of shielded endocervical catheter).

INTERVENTION/EVALUATION:

Suppository: Check strength, duration, and frequency of contractions and monitor vital signs q15min until stable, then hrly until abortion complete. Check resting uterine tone. Administer medications for relief of GI effects if indicated, abdominal cramps. **Gel:** Monitor uterine activity (onset of uterine contractions), fetal status (heart rate), character of cervix (dilation, effacement). Have pt remain recumbent 12 hrs after application with continuous electronic monitoring of fetal heart rate and uterine activity. Record maternal vital signs at least hrly in presence of uterine activity. Reassess Bishop score.

PATIENT/FAMILY TEACHING:

Suppository: Report fever, chills, foul-smelling/increased vaginal discharge, uterine cramps, or pain promptly.

diphenhydramine hydrochloride

dye-phen-**high**-dra-meen
(Allerdryl✤, Benadryl, Nytol✤)
Do not confuse with benazepril, Bentyl, Benylin, calamine, dimenhydrinate.

FIXED-COMBINATION(S)

With calamine, an astringent, and camphor, a counterirritant **(Caladryl)**

▶CLASSIFICATION

PHARMACOTHERAPEUTIC:
Ethanolamine. **CLINICAL:** Antihistamine, anticholinergic, antipruritic, antitussive, antiemetic, antidyskinetic (see p. 48C)

ACTION/THERAPEUTIC EFFECT

Competes with histamine at histaminic receptor sites, *resulting in anticholinergic, antipruritic, antitussive, antiemetic effects.* Inhibits central acetylcholine, *producing antidyskinetic, sedative effect.*

PHARMACOKINETICS

Onset	Peak	Duration
PO		
15–30 min	1–4 hrs	4–6 hrs
IM/IV		
<15 min	1–4 hrs	4–6 hrs

Well absorbed following oral, parenteral administration. Widely distributed. Protein binding: 98–99%. Metabolized in liver. Primarily excreted in urine. Half-life: 1–4 hrs.

USES

Treatment of allergic reactions, parkinsonism, prevention and treatment of nausea, vomiting, vertigo due to motion sickness; antitussive, short-term management of insomnia. Topical form used for relief of pruritus, insect bites, skin irritations.

PRECAUTIONS

CONTRAINDICATIONS: Acute asthmatic attack, those receiving MAO inhibitors. **CAUTIONS:** Narrow-angle glaucoma, peptic ulcer, prostatic hypertrophy, pyloro-duodenal or bladder neck obstruction, asthma, COPD, increased intraocular pressure, cardiovascular disease, hyperthyroidism, hypertension, seizure disorders.

▷**LIFESPAN CONSIDERATIONS:**
Pregnancy/Lactation: Crosses placenta; detected in breast milk (may produce irritability in nursing infants). Increased risk of seizures in neonates, premature infants if used during third trimester of

pregnancy. May prohibit lactation. **Pregnancy Category B. Children:** Not recommended in newborns or premature infants (increased risk of anticholinergic effects). Paradoxical excitement may occur. **Elderly:** Increased risk for dizziness, sedation, confusion, hypotension, hyperexcitability.

INTERACTIONS

DRUG: **Alcohol, CNS depressants** may increase CNS depressant effects. **MAO inhibitors** may increase anticholinergic, CNS depressant effects. **Anticholinergics** may increase anticholinergic effects. *HERBAL:* None known. *FOOD:* None known. *LAB VALUES:* May suppress wheal and flare reactions to antigen skin testing unless antihistamines are discontinued 4 days prior to testing.

AVAILABILITY (OTC)

CAPSULES: 25 mg, 50 mg. *TABLETS:* 25 mg, 50 mg. *TABLETS (chewable):* 12.5 mg. *SYRUP:* 12.5 mg/5 ml. *ELIXIR:* 12.5 mg/5 ml. *INJECTION (Rx):* 50 mg/ml.

ADMINISTRATION/HANDLING

PO:
• Give without regard to meals. • Scored tablets may be crushed. • Do not crush capsules or film-coated tablets.

IM:
• Give deep IM into large muscle mass.

IV 🏥
• May be given undiluted. • Give IV injection over at least 1 min.

IV INCOMPATIBILITIES ⊘

Allopurinol (Aloprim), amphotericin B complex (Abelcet, Ambisome, Amphotec), cefepime (Maxipime), foscarnet (Foscavir).

IV COMPATIBILITIES

Cisplatin (Platinol), cyclophosphamide (Cytoxan), cytarabine (ARA-C), heparin, hydrocortisone (Solu-Cortef), potassium chloride, propofol (Diprivan).

INDICATIONS/ROUTES/DOSAGE

Moderate to severe allergic reaction, dystonic reaction:
PO/IM/IV: **Adults, elderly:** 25–50 mg q4h. **Maximum:** 400 mg/day. **Children:** 5 mg/kd/day in divided doses q6–8h. **Maximum:** 300 mg/day.

Motion sickness, minor allergic rhinitis:
PO/IM/IV: **Adults, elderly, children ≥12 yrs:** 25–50 mg q4–6h. **Maximum:** 300 mg/day. **Children (6–12 yrs):** 12.5–25 mg q4–6h. **Maximum:** 150 mg/day. **Children 2–6 yrs:** 6.25 mg q4–6h. **Maximum:** 37.5 mg/day.

Antitussive:
PO: **Adults, elderly, children ≥12 yrs:** 25 mg q4h. **Maximum:** 150 mg/day. **Children (6–12 yrs):** 12.5 mg q4h. **Maximum:** 75 mg/day. **Children (2–6 yrs):** 6.25 mg q4h. **Maximum:** 37.5 mg/day.

Nighttime sleep aid:
PO: **Adults, elderly, children ≥12 yrs:** 50 mg qh. **Children (2–12 yrs):** 1 mg/kg/dose. **Maximum:** 50 mg.

Pruritus relief:
TOPICAL: **Adults, elderly, children ≥12 yrs:** *1% or 2% strength:* Apply 3–4 times/day. **Children (2–12 yrs):** *1% strength:* Apply 3–4 times/day.

SIDE EFFECTS

FREQUENT: Drowsiness, dizziness, muscular weakness, hypotension, dry mouth/nose/throat/lips, urinary retention, thickening of bronchial secretions. Sedation, dizziness, hypotension more likely noted in elderly. **OCCASIONAL:** Epigastric distress, flushing, visual disturbances, hearing disturbances, paresthesia, sweating, chills.

ADVERSE REACTIONS/TOXIC EFFECTS

Children may experience dominant paradoxical reactions (restlessness, insomnia, euphoria, nervousness, tremors). Overdosage in children may result in hallucinations, convulsions, death. Hypersensitivity reaction (eczema, pruritus, rash, cardiac disturbances, photosensitivity) may occur. Overdosage may vary from CNS depression (sedation, apnea, cardiovascular collapse, death) to severe paradoxical reaction (hallucinations, tremor, seizures).

NURSING IMPLICATIONS

BASELINE ASSESSMENT:

If pt is undergoing allergic reaction, obtain history of recently ingested foods, drugs, environmental exposure, recent emotional stress. Monitor rate, depth, rhythm, type of respiration, and quality and rate of pulse. Assess lung sounds for rhonchi, wheezing, rales.

INTERVENTION/EVALUATION:

Monitor B/P, esp. in elderly (increased risk of hypotension). Monitor children closely for paradoxical reaction.

PATIENT/FAMILY TEACHING:

Tolerance to antihistaminic effect generally does not occur; tolerance to sedative effect may occur. Avoid tasks that require alertness, motor skills until response to drug is established. Dry mouth, drowsiness, dizziness may be an expected response of drug. Avoid alcoholic beverages during antihistamine therapy.

diphenoxylate hydrochloride with atropine sulfate

dye-pen-**ox**-e-late
(Lonox, Lomotil)
Do not confuse with Lamictal, Lanoxin, Loprox.

▶CLASSIFICATION

PHARMACOTHERAPEUTIC: Meperidine derivative. **CLINICAL:** Antidiarrheal (see p. 41C)

ACTION/*THERAPEUTIC EFFECT*

Acts locally, centrally *to reduce intestinal motility.*

PHARMACOKINETICS

Well absorbed from GI tract. Metabolized in liver to active metabolite. Primarily eliminated in feces. Halflife: 2.5 hrs; metabolite: 12–24 hrs.

USES

Adjunctive treatment of acute, chronic diarrhea.

PRECAUTIONS

CONTRAINDICATIONS: Obstructive jaundice, diarrhea associated with pseudomembranous entero-

---

colitis due to broad-spectrum antibiotics or with organisms that invade intestinal mucosa *(E. coli, Shigella, Salmonella)*, acute ulcerative colitis (may produce toxic megacolon). ***CAUTIONS:*** Advanced hepatorenal disease, abnormal liver function.

▷ *LIFESPAN CONSIDERATIONS:*
Pregnancy/Lactation: Unknown if drug crosses placenta or is distributed in breast milk. **Pregnancy Category C. Children:** Not recommended (increased susceptibility to toxicity including respiratory depression). **Elderly:** More susceptible to anticholinergic effects, confusion, respiratory depression.

INTERACTIONS
DRUG:* Alcohol, CNS depressants** may increase effect. **Anticholinergics** may increase effect of atropine. **MAO inhibitors** may precipitate hypertensive crisis. ***HERBAL: None known. ***FOOD:*** None known. ***LAB VALUES:*** May increase amylase.

AVAILABILITY (Rx)
TABLETS: 2.5 mg. ***LIQUID:*** 2.5 mg/5 ml.

ADMINISTRATION/HANDLING
PO:
• Give without regard to meals. If GI irritation occurs, give with food or meals. • Use liquid for children under 12 yrs (use dropper for administration of liquids).

INDICATIONS/ROUTES/DOSAGE
Antidiarrheal:

***PO:* Adults, elderly:** Initially, 15–20 mg/day in 3–4 divided doses, then 5–15 mg/day in 2–3 divided doses. **Children 8–12 yrs:** 2 mg 5 times/day; **5–8 yrs:** 2 mg 4 times/day; **2–5 yrs:** 2 mg 3 times/day.

SIDE EFFECTS
FREQUENT: Drowsiness, lightheadedness, dizziness, nausea. ***OCCASIONAL:*** Headache, dry mouth. ***RARE:*** Flushing, tachycardia, urinary retention, constipation, paradoxical reaction (restlessness, agitation), blurred vision.

ADVERSE REACTIONS/TOXIC EFFECTS
Dehydration may predispose to toxicity. Paralytic ileus, toxic megacolon (constipation, decreased appetite, stomach pain with nausea/vomiting) occurs rarely. Severe anticholinergic effects (severe drowsiness, hypotonic reflexes, hyperthermia) may result in severe respiratory depression, coma.

NURSING IMPLICATIONS

BASELINE ASSESSMENT:
Check baseline hydration status: skin turgor, mucous membranes for dryness, urinary status.

INTERVENTION/EVALUATION:
Encourage adequate fluid intake. Assess bowel sounds for peristalsis. Monitor daily bowel activity, stool consistency (watery loose, soft, semisolid, solid) and record time of evacuation. Assess for abdominal disturbances. Discontinue medication if abdominal distention occurs.

PATIENT/FAMILY TEACHING:
Avoid tasks that require alertness, motor skills until response to drug is established. Do not ingest alcohol or barbiturates. Contact physician if fever, palpitations occur or diarrhea persists. Report abdominal distention.

---

dipivefrin

(Propine)

See Classification section under: Antiglaucoma agents (p. 45C)

dipyridamole

die-pie-**rid**-ah-mole
(Apo-Dipyridamole✦, Novodipiradol✦, Persantine)
Do not confuse with Aggrastat, disopyramide, Periactin.

FIXED-COMBINATION(S)

With aspirin, an antiplatelet **(Aggrenox)**

▶CLASSIFICATION

PHARMACOTHERAPEUTIC: Blood modifier, anticoagulant. *CLINICAL:* Antiplatelet, antianginal, diagnostic agent (see p. 29C)

ACTION/*THERAPEUTIC EFFECT*

Direct action on small vessels of coronary vascular bed, *increasing coronary blood flow, coronary sinus O_2 saturation.*

PHARMACOKINETICS

Slowly, variably absorbed from GI tract. Widely distributed. Protein binding: 91–99%. Metabolized in liver. Primarily eliminated via biliary excretion. Half-life: 10–15 hrs.

USES/*UNLABELED*

Adjunct to coumarin anticoagulant in prevention of postop thromboembolic complications of cardiac valve replacement. *IV:* Alternative to exercise in thallium myocardial perfusion imaging for evaluation of coronary artery disease. *Prophylaxis of myocardial reinfarction, treatment of transient ischemic attacks (TIAs).*

PRECAUTIONS

CONTRAINDICATIONS: None significant. *CAUTIONS:* Hypotension.

▷*LIFESPAN CONSIDERATIONS:* **Pregnancy/Lactation:** Distributed in breast milk. **Pregnancy Category C. Children:** Safety and efficacy not established. **Elderly:** No age-related precautions noted.

INTERACTIONS

DRUG: May increase risk of bleeding with **anticoagulants, heparin, thrombolytics, aspirin, salicylates.** *HERBAL:* None known. *FOOD:* None known. *LAB VALUES:* None significant.

AVAILABILITY (Rx)

TABLETS: 25 mg, 50 mg, 75 mg. *INJECTION:* 10 mg.

ADMINISTRATION/HANDLING

PO:

• Best taken on empty stomach with full glass of water.

IV ▩

• Dilute to at least 1:2 ratio with 0.9% NaCl or D_5W for total volume of 20–50 ml (undiluted may cause irritation). • Infuse over 4 min. • Inject thallium within 5 min after dipyridamole infusion.

IV INCOMPATIBILITY ⊘

No information available via Y-site administration.

INDICATIONS/ROUTES/DOSAGE

Prevention of thromboembolic disorders:

PO: Adults, elderly: 75–100 mg 4 times/day in combination with other medications. **Children:** 3–6 mg/kg/day in 3 divided doses.

Diagnostic:

IV: **Adults, elderly (based on weight):** 0.142 mg/kg/min infused over 4 min; doses >60 mg not needed for any pt.

SIDE EFFECTS

FREQUENT (14%): Dizziness. *OCCASIONAL* (2–6%): Abdominal distress, headache, rash. *RARE* (<2%): Diarrhea, vomiting, flushing, pruritis.

ADVERSE REACTIONS/TOXIC EFFECTS

Overdosage produces peripheral vasodilation, resulting in hypotension.

NURSING IMPLICATIONS

BASELINE ASSESSMENT:
Assess chest pain, B/P, pulse. When used as antiplatelet, check hematologic levels.

INTERVENTION/EVALUATION:
Assist with ambulation if dizziness occurs. Monitor heart sounds by auscultation. Assess B/P for hypotension. Assess skin for flushing, rash.

PATIENT/FAMILY TEACHING:
If nausea occurs, cola, unsalted crackers, or dry toast may relieve effect. Therapeutic response may not be achieved before 2–3 mos of continuous therapy. Use caution when getting up suddenly from lying or sitting position.

dirithromycin

dih-**rith**-row-my-sin
(Dynabac)
Do not confuse with Dynacin, DynaCirc.

▶CLASSIFICATION

PHARMACOTHERAPEUTIC: Macrolide. *CLINICAL:* Antibiotic (see p. 23C)

ACTION/THERAPEUTIC EFFECT

Binds to ribosomal receptor sites of susceptible organisms, *inhibiting protein synthesis.*

PHARMACOKINETICS

Rapidly absorbed from GI tract. Widely distributed into tissues and within cells. Protein binding: 15–30%. Eliminated primarily unchanged via biliary excretion. Not removed by hemodialysis. Half-life: 30–44 hrs.

USES

Treatment of mild to moderate infections of upper respiratory tract (pharyngitis, tonsillitis), acute bronchitis, chronic bronchitis, uncomplicated skin/skin structure infections, community-acquired pneumonia.

PRECAUTIONS

CONTRAINDICATIONS: Hypersensitivity to dirithromycin, erythromycins, any macrolide antibiotic, concurrent terfenadine therapy, electrolyte disturbances (may cause cardiac dysrhythmias), bacteremia. *CAUTIONS:* Hepatic/renal dysfunction.

▷*LIFESPAN CONSIDERATIONS:*
Pregnancy/Lactation: Unknown if distributed in breast milk. **Pregnancy Category C. Children:** Safety and efficacy not established in those <12 yrs of age. **Elderly:** No age-related precautions noted.

INTERACTIONS

DRUG: **H₂ antagonists** increase dirithromycin absorption. **Aluminum/magnesium-containing antacids** may decrease concentra-

---

tion (give 1 hr before or 2 hrs after antacid). **HERBAL:** None known. **FOOD:** None known. **LAB VALUES:** May increase platelet count, potassium CPK, eosinophils, neutrophils. Decreases bicarbonate level.

AVAILABILITY (Rx)

TABLETS (enteric-coated): 250 mg.

ADMINISTRATION/HANDLING
PO:

• Administer with food or within an hr of having eaten (food increases absorption). • Swallow whole (tablets not to be cut, crushed, or chewed).

INDICATIONS/ROUTES/DOSAGE
Pharyngitis/tonsillitis:

PO: Adults, elderly, children ≥12 yrs: 500 mg once daily for 10 days.

Acute bronchitis, chronic bronchitis:

PO: Adults, elderly, children ≥12 yrs: 500 mg once daily for 7 days.

Community-acquired pneumonia:

PO: Adults, elderly, children ≥12 yrs: 500 mg once daily for 14 days.

Skin, skin structure infections:

PO: Adults, elderly, children ≥12 yrs: 500 mg once daily for 7 days.

SIDE EFFECTS

FREQUENT (8–10%): Abdominal pain, headache, nausea, diarrhea. **OCCASIONAL** (2–3%): Vomiting, dyspepsia, dizziness, nonspecific pain, asthenia. **RARE** (<2%): Increased cough, flatulence, rash, dyspnea, pruritus/urticaria, insomnia.

ADVERSE REACTIONS/TOXIC EFFECTS

Superinfections, esp. antibiotic-associated colitis (abdominal cramps, watery severe diarrhea, fever) may result from altered bacterial balance.

NURSING IMPLICATIONS

BASELINE ASSESSMENT:
Question pt for history of allergies to dirithromycin, erythromycins.

INTERVENTION/EVALUATION:
Check for GI discomfort, nausea, headache, diarrhea. Determine pattern of bowel activity and stool consistency. Evaluate for superinfection: genital/anal pruritus, sore mouth or tongue, moderate to severe diarrhea.

PATIENT/FAMILY TEACHING:
Continue therapy for full length of treatment. Doses should be evenly spaced. Take medication with food or within an hr of having eaten.

disopyramide phosphate ✳

dye-so-**peer**-ah-myd
(Norpace, Rythmodan✶)
Do not confuse with desipramine, dipyridamole, Rhythmol.

▶**CLASSIFICATION**
PHARMACOTHERAPEUTIC: Non-nitrate. **CLINICAL:** Antiarrhythmic (see p. 12C)

ACTION/THERAPEUTIC EFFECT
Prolongs refractory period by direct effect, decreasing myocardial excitability and conduction velocity. *Depresses myocardial contrac-*

tility. Has anticholinergic, negative inotropic effects.

USES/*UNLABELED*

Suppression and prevention of unifocal/multifocal premature ventricular contractions (ectopic), paired ventricular contractions (couplets), episodes of ventricular tachycardia. *Prophylaxis/treatment of supraventricular tachycardia.*

PRECAUTIONS

CONTRAINDICATIONS: Preexisting urinary retention, preexisting second- or third-degree AV block, cardiogenic shock, narrow-angle glaucoma, unless pt is undergoing cholinergic therapy. ***CAUTIONS:*** CHF, myasthenia gravis, narrow-angle glaucoma, prostatic hypertrophy, sick-sinus syndrome (bradycardia/tachycardia), Wolff-Parkinson-White syndrome, bundle-branch block, impaired renal/hepatic function.

INTERACTIONS

DRUG: Other antiarrhythmics (e.g., **propranolol, diltiazem, verapamil**) may prolong conduction, decrease cardiac output. **Pimozide** may increase cardiac arrhythmias. ***HERBAL:*** None known. ***FOOD:*** None known. ***LAB VALUES:*** May decrease glucose. May cause EKG changes. Therapeutic blood serum level: 2–8 mcg/ml; toxic blood serum level: >8 mcg/ml.

AVAILABILITY (Rx)

CAPSULES: 100 mg, 150 mg. ***CAPSULES (extended-release):*** 100 mg, 150 mg.

INDICATIONS/ROUTES/DOSAGE

Usual dosage:

PO: **Adults, elderly >50 kg:** 150 mg q6h (300 mg q12h with extended-release). **Adults, elderly <50 kg:** 100 mg q6h (200 mg q12h with extended-release). **Children 12–18 yrs:** 6–15 mg/kg/day in divided doses q6h. **Children 4–12 yrs:** 10–15 mg/kg/day in divided doses q6h. **Children 1–4 yrs:** 10–20 mg/kg/day in divided doses q6h. **Children <1 yr:** 10–30 mg/kg/day in divided doses q6h.

Rapid control of arrhythmias:

Note: Do not use extended-release capsules.

PO: **Adults, elderly >50 kg:** Initially, 300 mg, then 150 mg q6h.

Adults, elderly <50 kg: Initially, 200 mg, then 100 mg q6h.

Severe refractory arrhythmias:

PO: **Adults, elderly:** Up to 400 mg q6h.

Dosage in renal impairment:

With or without loading dose of 150 mg:

Creatinine Clearance	Dosage
>40 ml/min	100 mg q6h (extended-release 200 mg q12h)
30–40 ml/min	100 mg q8h
15–30 ml/min	100 mg q12h
<15 ml/min	100 mg q24h

Dosage in hepatic impairment:

100 mg q6h (200 mg q12h with extended-release).

Dosage in cardiomyopathy, decompensated myocardium:

No loading dose; 100 mg q6–8h with gradual dosage adjustments.

SIDE EFFECTS

FREQUENT (>9%): Dry mouth (32%), urinary hesitancy, constipation. ***OCCASIONAL*** (3–9%): Blurred vision, dry eyes, nose, or throat, urinary retention, headache, dizziness, fatigue, nausea. ***RARE*** (<1%): Impotence, hypotension, edema, weight gain, shortness of breath, syncope, chest pain, nervousness, diarrhea, vomiting, decreased appetite, rash, itching.

ADVERSE REACTIONS/TOXIC EFFECTS

May produce or aggravate CHF. May produce severe hypotension, compounded with shortness of breath, chest pain, syncope (esp. in those with primary cardiomyopathy or in inadequately compensated CHF). Hepatic toxicity occurs rarely.

NURSING IMPLICATIONS

BASELINE ASSESSMENT:
Before giving medication, instruct pt to void (reduces risk of urinary retention).

INTERVENTION/EVALUATION:
Monitor EKG for cardiac changes, particularly widening of QRS complex, prolongation of PR and QT intervals. Assess pattern of daily bowel activity, stool consistency. Monitor I&O (be alert to urinary retention). Assess for evidence of CHF (cough, dyspnea [particularly on exertion], rales at base of lungs, fatigue). Assist with ambulation if dizziness occurs. Therapeutic blood serum level: 2–8 mcg/ml; toxic blood serum level: >8 mcg/ml.

PATIENT/FAMILY TEACHING:
Report shortness of breath, productive cough. Compliance with therapy regimen is essential to control cardiac dysrhythmias. Do not use nasal decongestants, OTC cold preparations (stimulants) without physician approval. Restrict salt, alcohol intake.

disulfiram

dye-**sul**-fi-ram
(Antabuse)
Do not confuse with Anturane, Diflucan.

▶**CLASSIFICATION**
CLINICAL: Alcohol abuse deterrent

ACTION/*THERAPEUTIC EFFECT*

Inhibits enzyme aldehyde dehydrogenase, responsible for breakdown of ethanol metabolite acetaldehyde. Increased acetaldehyde responsible for *disulfiram reaction after alcohol ingestion.*

PHARMACOKINETICS

Slowly absorbed from GI tract. Metabolized in liver. Primarily excreted in urine. Up to 20% of dose remains in body for at least 1 wk.

USES

Adjunct in management of selected chronic alcoholic pts who want to remain in state of enforced sobriety.

PRECAUTIONS

CONTRAINDICATIONS: Severe heart disease, psychosis. *CAUTIONS:* Alcoholic disease.
▷*LIFESPAN CONSIDERATIONS:*
Pregnancy/Lactation: Safety during pregnancy not established. **Pregnancy Category C. Children:** Safety and efficacy not established. **Elderly:** Age-related renal impairment may require caution.

INTERACTIONS

DRUG: **Alcohol** within 14 days results in disulfiram/alcohol reaction. **Oral anticoagulant** effect may be increased. May increase concentration, toxicity of **phenytoin. Isoniazid** may increase CNS effects. **Metronidazole** may increase toxicity. **HERBAL:** None known. **FOOD:** None known. **LAB VALUES:** May increase cholesterol concentrations. May decrease VMA concentrations.

AVAILABILITY (Rx)
TABLETS: 250 mg, 500 mg.

ADMINISTRATION/HANDLING
PO:

• Scored tablets may be crushed.
• Give without regard to meals.

INDICATIONS/ROUTES/DOSAGE
Note: Pts must abstain from alcohol for at least 12 hrs before initial dose is administered.

PO: Adults, elderly: Initially, administer maximum of 500 mg daily given as a single dose for 1–2 wks. **Maintenance:** 250 mg daily (normal range: 125–500 mg). Do not exceed maximum daily dose of 500 mg.

SIDE EFFECTS
FREQUENT: Drowsiness. **OCCASIONAL:** Headache, restlessness, optic neuritis (impaired color perception, altered vision), peripheral neuropathy, metallic or garlic taste, rash.

ADVERSE REACTIONS/TOXIC EFFECTS
Disulfiram-alcohol reaction to ingestion of alcohol in any form: flushing/throbbing in head and neck, throbbing headache, nausea, copious vomiting, diaphoresis, dyspnea, hyperventilation, tachycardia, hypotension, marked uneasiness, vertigo, blurred vision, confusion. Can produce death.

NURSING IMPLICATIONS

INTERVENTION/EVALUATION:
Do not give without pt's knowledge. Fully inform pt of consequences of alcohol ingestion. Therapy cannot be started until a minimum of 12 hrs has elapsed since pt's last ingestion of alcohol.

PATIENT/FAMILY TEACHING:
Avoid cough syrups, vinegars, fluid extracts, elixirs because of their alcohol content. Even external application of liniments, shaving or body lotion may precipitate a crisis. Effects of medication may occur several days after discontinuance. Avoid alcohol in all forms, including beverages, vinegar, liquid medications, colognes, etc. Use caution driving, performing tasks requiring alertness.

dobutamine hydrochloride

do-**byew**-ta-meen
(Dobutrex)
Do not confuse with Dopamine.

▶CLASSIFICATION

PHARMACOTHERAPEUTIC: Sympathomimetic. **CLINICAL:** Cardiac stimulant (see p. 125C)

ACTION/THERAPEUTIC EFFECT
Direct-acting inotropic agent acting primarily on beta$_1$-adrenergic receptors, *enhancing myocardial contractility, stroke volume, cardiac output.* Decreases preload, afterload. Excessive doses *increase heart rate. Improves renal blood flow, urine output.*

PHARMACOKINETICS

	Onset	Peak	Duration
IV			
	1–2 min	10 min	Length of infusion

Metabolized in liver. Primarily excreted in urine. Not removed by hemodialysis. Half-life: 2 min.

USES

Prophylaxis/treatment of acute hypotension, shock (associated with myocardial infarction, trauma, renal failure, cardiac decompensation, open heart surgery), treatment of low cardiac output, CHF.

PRECAUTIONS

CONTRAINDICATIONS: Idiopathic hypertrophic subaortic stenosis, hypovolemic pts, sulfite sensitivity. ***CAUTIONS:*** Atrial fibrillation, hypertension. Safety in children not established.

▷***LIFESPAN CONSIDERATIONS:*** **Pregnancy/Lactation:** Unknown if drug crosses placenta or is distributed in breast milk. Has not been administered to pregnant women. **Pregnancy Category C. Children/Elderly:** No age-related precautions noted.

INTERACTIONS

DRUG: **Tricyclic antidepressants, MAO inhibitors, oxytocics** may increase effect (arrhythmias, hypertension), **beta-blockers** may antagonize effects, **digoxin** may increase risk of arrhythmias, additional inotropic effect. ***HERBAL:*** None known. ***FOOD:*** None known. ***LAB VALUES:*** Decreases potassium serum levels.

AVAILABILITY (Rx)

INJECTION: 250 mg vial. ***INFUSION:*** 500 mg/250 ml solution.

ADMINISTRATION/HANDLING

Note: Correct hypovolemia with volume expanders before dobutamine infusion. Those with atrial fibrillation should be digitalized prior to infusion. Administer by IV infusion only.

IV

Storage:
• Store at room temperature. Freezing produces crystallization. • Pink discoloration of solution (due to oxidation) does not indicate loss of potency if used within recommended time period. • Reconstituted, concentrated solution maintains potency for 6 hrs at room temperature, 48 hrs if refrigerated. • Further diluted solution for infusion must be used within 24 hrs.

Reconstitution:
• Dilute 250 mg ampule with 10 ml Sterile Water for Injection or D_5W for injection. Resulting solution: 25 mg/ml. Add additional 10 ml of diluent if not completely dissolved (resulting solution: 12.5 mg/ml). • Dilute further to at least 50 ml with D_5W, 0.9% NaCl, or sodium lactate injection before administration. Maximum concentration: 3.125 g/250 ml (12.5 mg/ml).

Rate of administration:
• Use infusion pump to control flow rate. • Titrate dosage to individual response.

IV INCOMPATIBILITIES ⊘

Acyclovir (Zovirax), alteplase (Activase), amphotericin B complex (Abelcet, Ambisome, Amphotec), cefepime (Maxipime), foscarnet (Foscavir), furosemide (Lasix), heparin, piperacillin/tazobactam (Zosyn).

IV COMPATIBILITIES

Amiodarone (Cordarone), calcium gluconate, diltiazem (Cardizem), dopamine (Intropin), enalapril (Vasotec), insulin, labetalol (Normodyne, Trandate), lidocaine, lorazepam (Ativan), magnesium, milrinone (Primacor), nitroglycerin, norepinephrine (Levophed), potassium chloride, propofol (Diprivan), verapamil (Calan).

INDICATIONS/ROUTES/DOSAGE
Note: Dosage determined by pt response.
IV INFUSION: **Adults, elderly, children:** 2.5–15 mcg/kg/min. Rarely, infusion rate up to 40 mcg/kg/min to increase cardiac output.

SIDE EFFECTS
FREQUENT (5%): Increased heart rate, blood pressure. ***OCCASIONAL*** (3–5%): Pain at injection site. ***RARE*** (1–3%): Nausea, headache, anginal pain, shortness of breath, fever.

ADVERSE REACTIONS/TOXIC EFFECTS
Overdosage may produce marked increase in heart rate (30 beats/min or greater), marked increase in systolic B/P (50 mm Hg or greater), anginal pain, premature ventricular beats.

NURSING IMPLICATIONS

BASELINE ASSESSMENT:
Pt must be on continuous cardiac monitoring. Determine weight (for dosage calculation). Obtain initial B/P, heart rate, and respirations.

INTERVENTION/EVALUATION:
Continuously monitor for cardiac rate, arrhythmias. With physician, establish parameters for adjusting rate or stopping infusion.

Maintain accurate I&O; measure urine output frequently. Assess potassium levels and dobutamine plasma level (therapeutic range = 40–190 ng/ml). Check cardiac output. Monitor B/P continuously (hypertension greater risk in pts with preexisting hypertension) and pulmonary wedge pressure or central venous pressure frequently. Immediately notify physician of decreased urine output, cardiac arrhythmias, significant increase in B/P or heart rate, and less commonly hypotension.

docetaxel

dox-eh-**tax**-el
(Taxotere)
Do not confuse with Taxol.

▶CLASSIFICATION
PHARMACOTHERAPEUTIC: Antimitotic agent, taxoid. ***CLINICAL:*** Antineoplastic (see p. 69C)

ACTION/*THERAPEUTIC EFFECT*
Disrupts the microtubular cell network, essential for cellular function, *inhibiting cell mitosis.*

PHARMACOKINETICS
Distributed into peripheral compartments. 94% protein bound. Extensively metabolized. Excreted primarily in feces with lesser amount in urine.

USES/*UNLABELED*
Treatment of locally advanced or metastatic breast carcinoma after the failure of any prior chemotherapy. Treatment of metastatic non-small lung cancer. *Treatment*

of small-cell lung, ovarian, head and neck, prostate, bladder cancer.

PRECAUTIONS

CONTRAINDICATIONS: Neutrophil count <1,500 cells/mm^3, history of severe hypersensitivity to docetaxel or other drugs formulated with polysorbate 80. **CAUTIONS:** Abnormal liver function, those receiving higher doses than normal (increased risk of mortality).

▷**LIFESPAN CONSIDERATIONS:**
Pregnancy/Lactation: May cause fetal harm. Unknown if distributed in breast milk; do not breast-feed. **Pregnancy Category D. Children:** Safety and efficacy not established in those <16 yrs of age. **Elderly:** No age-related precautions noted.

INTERACTIONS

DRUG: Cyclosporine, ketoconazole, erythromycin may significantly modify docetaxel metabolism. **HERBAL:** None known. **FOOD:** None known.. **LAB VALUES:** May significantly increase bilirubin, BUN, serum creatinine, transaminase, alkaline phosphatase. Reduces neutrophils, thrombocytes, WBC count.

AVAILABILITY (Rx)

INJECTION: 20 mg in 0.5 ml with diluent, 80 mg in 2 ml with diluent.

ADMINISTRATION/HANDLING

Note: Dilution is required before administration. Pt should be premedicated with oral corticosteroids (dexamethasone 16 mg/day for 5 days beginning day 1 before docetaxel therapy; reduces severity of fluid retention, hypersensitivity reaction).

IV 💊

Storage:
• Refrigerate vial. Freezing does not adversely affect drug. • Protect from bright light. • Stand vial at room temperature for 5 min before administering (do not store in PVC bags). • Premixed solution is stable for 8 hrs either at room temperature or if refrigerated.

Reconstitution:
• Withdraw contents of diluent (provided by manufacturer) and add to vial of docetaxel. • Gently rotate to ensure thorough mixing. This provides a solution of 10 mg/ml. • Withdraw dose and add to 250 ml 0.9% NaCl injection or D$_5$W glass or polyolefin container. This provides a final concentration of 0.3–0.9 mg/ml.

Rate of administration:
• Administer as a 1 hr infusion. • Monitor closely for hypersensitivity reaction, i.e., flushing, localized skin reaction, bronchospasm (may occur within a few mins after infusion).

IV INCOMPATIBILITIES ⊘

Amphotericin (Fungizone), doxorubicin liposome (DaunoXome), methylprednisolone (Solu-Medrol), nalbuphine (Nubain).

IV COMPATIBILITIES

Granisetron (Kytril), lorazepam (Ativan), ondansetron (Zofran).

INDICATIONS/ROUTES/DOSAGE
Breast carcinoma:

IV INFUSION: Adults: 60–100 mg/m^2 given over 1 hr q3wks. Those dosed initially at 100 mg/m^2 who experience febrile neutropenia, neutrophils <500 cells/mm^3 for >1 wk, severe or cumulative cutaneous reactions, or severe peripheral neuropathy during therapy should have dose adjusted from 100 to 75 mg/m^2. If reaction continues, lower dose from 75 to 55 mg/m^2 or stop therapy. Those dosed at 60 mg/m^2 and do not experience above symptoms may tolerate increased dose.

Non–small-cell lung carcinoma:

IV INFUSION: **Adults:** 75 mg/m^2 q3wks.

SIDE EFFECTS

FREQUENT: Alopecia (80%), asthenia, i.e., loss of strength (62%), hypersensitivity reaction, i.e., dermatitis (59%). Hypersensitivity reaction decreases to 16% in those treated with premedicated oral corticosteroids. Fluid retention (49%), stomatitis (redness/burning of oral mucous membranes, gum/tongue inflammation) (43%), nausea, diarrhea (40%), fever (30%), nail changes (28%), vomiting (24%), myalgia (19%). *OCCASIONAL:* Hypotension, edema, anorexia, headache, weight gain, infection (urinary tract, injection site, catheter tip), dizziness. *RARE:* Dry skin, sensory disorders (vision, speech, taste), dermatitis, arthralgia, myalgia, weight loss, conjunctivitis, hematuria, proteinuria.

ADVERSE REACTIONS/TOXIC EFFECTS

In those with normal liver function tests, neutropenia (<2,000 cells/mm^3) and leukopenia (<4,000 cells/mm^3) occurs in 96% of pts. Anemia (<11 g/dl) occurs in 90%. Thrombocytopenia (<100,000 cells/mm^3) occurs in 8%. Infection occurs in 28%. Neurosensory, neuromotor (distal extremity weakness) occur in 54% and 13%, respectively.

NURSING IMPLICATIONS

BASELINE ASSESSMENT:

Offer emotional support to pt and family. Antiemetics may be effective in preventing, treating nausea, vomiting. Pt should be pre-treated with corticosteroids before therapy to reduce fluid retention, hypersensitivity reaction.

INTERVENTION/EVALUATION:

Frequent monitoring of blood counts is essential, particularly neutrophil count (<1,500 cells/mm^3 requires discontinuation of therapy), renal, hepatic function studies, serum uric acid levels. Monitor for cutaneous reactions characterized by rash with eruptions, mainly on hands or feet. Assess for extravascular fluid accumulation: rales in lungs, edema in dependent areas, dyspnea at rest, pronounced abdominal distention (due to ascites).

PATIENT/FAMILY TEACHING:

Alopecia is reversible, but new hair growth may have different color or texture. New hair growth resumes 2–3 mos after last therapy dose. Maintain fastidious oral hygiene. Do not have immunizations without physician approval (drug lowers body's resistance). Avoid those who have recently taken live virus vaccine.

docosanol

dough-**coe**-san-all
(Abreva)

▶CLASSIFICATION

PHARMACOTHERAPEUTIC: Anti-infective. *CLINICAL:* Topical antiviral

ACTION/*THERAPEUTIC EFFECT*

Interferes with one or more of the common pathways for viral entry into target cell and subsequent migration to the cell nucleus. Inhibits the fusion between the plasma membrane and the herpes simplex virus (HSV) envelope, *reducing the duration of symptoms attributed to cold sores and fever blisters.*

USES
Treatment of cold sores or fever blisters due to either herpes simplex virus type 1 or type 2.

AVAILABILITY (OTC)
CREAM: 10%.

INDICATIONS/ROUTES/DOSAGE
Cold sores, fever blisters:
TOPICAL: Adults, elderly: Apply to lesions 5 times/day beginning at the onset of symptoms, continuing until the lesions are healed, up to a maximum of 10 days.

PRECAUTIONS
CONTRAINDICATIONS: None significant. **CAUTIONS:** None significant.

INTERACTIONS
DRUG: None significant. **HERBAL:** None significant. **FOOD:** None significant. **LAB VALUES:** None significant.

SIDE EFFECTS
RARE (1–5%): Headache, mild erythema.

ADVERSE REACTIONS/TOXIC EFFECTS
None significant.

NURSING IMPLICATIONS

BASELINE ASSESSMENT:
Use only on lips or face. Do not apply to oral mucous membranes. Avoid application in or near eyes (produces irritation).

PATIENT/FAMILY TEACHING:
Avoid exposure of cold sores to direct sunlight.

docusate calcium

dock-cue-sate
(Pro-Cal-Sof, Surfak)

docusate potassium
(Dialose, Diocto-K, Kasof)

docusate sodium
(Colace, Doxinate, Modane Soft)

FIXED-COMBINATION(S)
With casanthranol, a stimulant laxative **(Peri-colace)**; with phenolphthalein, a laxative **(Correctol, Doxidan)**

▶CLASSIFICATION
PHARMACOTHERAPEUTIC: Bulk-producing laxative. **CLINICAL:** Stool softener (see p. 100C)

ACTION/THERAPEUTIC EFFECT
Decreases surface film tension by mixing liquid and bowel contents, *increasing infiltration of liquid to form a softer stool.*

PHARMACOKINETICS
Minimal absorption from GI tract. Acts in small/large intestine. Results occur 1–2 days after first dose (may take 3–5 days).

USES
Prophylaxis/treatment of constipation.

PRECAUTIONS
CONTRAINDICATIONS: Abdominal pain, nausea, vomiting, appendicitis. **CAUTIONS:** None significant.

D

▷**LIFESPAN CONSIDERATIONS:**
Pregnancy/Lactation: Unknown if drug is distributed in breast milk. **Pregnancy Category C. Children:** Not recommended in children <6 yrs of age. **Elderly:** No age-related precautions noted.

INTERACTIONS

DRUG: May increase absorption of **mineral oil, danthron, phenolphthalein. HERBAL:** None known. **FOOD:** None known. **LAB VALUES:** None significant.

AVAILABILITY (OTC)

Calcium: CAPSULES: 50 mg, 240 mg.
Potassium: CAPSULES: 100 mg, 240 mg.
Sodium: TABLETS: 100 mg. *CAPSULES:* 50 mg, 100 mg, 240 mg, 250 mg. *SYRUP:* 60 mg/15 ml, 50 mg/15 ml. *LIQUID:* 150 mg/15 ml. *SOLUTION:* 50 mg/ml.

ADMINISTRATION/HANDLING

• Drink 6–8 glasses of water/day (aids stool softening). • Give each dose with full glass of water or fruit juice.

INDICATIONS/ROUTES/DOSAGE

STOOL SOFTENER:

Calcium docusate:

PO: Adults, elderly: 240 mg/day until evacuation. **Children >6 yrs:** 50–150 mg/day.

Potassium docusate:

PO: Adults, elderly: 100–300 mg/day until evacuation. **Children >6 yrs:** 100 mg at bedtime.

Sodium docusate:

PO: Adults, elderly: 50–500 mg/day. **Children 6–12 yrs:** 40–120 mg/day. **Children 3–6 yrs:** 20–60 mg/day. **Children <3 yrs:** 10–40 mg/day.

SIDE EFFECTS

OCCASIONAL: Mild GI cramping, throat irritation (liquid preparation). **RARE:** Rash.

ADVERSE REACTIONS/TOXIC EFFECTS

None significant.

NURSING IMPLICATIONS

INTERVENTION/EVALUATION:

Encourage adequate fluid intake. Assess bowel sounds for peristalsis. Monitor daily bowel activity and stool consistency (watery, loose, soft, semisolid, solid) and record time of evacuation.

PATIENT/FAMILY TEACHING:

Institute measures to promote defecation: increase fluid intake, exercise, high-fiber diet.

dofetilide

doe-**fet**-ill-ide
(Tikosyn)

▶CLASSIFICATION

PHARMACOTHERAPEUTIC: Potassium channel blocker. **CLINICAL:** Antiarrhythmic: Class III (see p. 14C)

ACTION/THERAPEUTIC EFFECT

A selective potassium channel blocker; prolongs repolarization without affecting conduction velocity by blocking one or more time-dependent potassium currents. No effect on sodium channels, adrenergic alpha, beta receptors. *Terminates reentrant tachyarrhythmias, preventing reinduction.*

USES

Maintenance of normal sinus rhythm (NSR) in pts with atrial fibrillation/atrial flutter of >1 wk duration who have been converted to NSR.

PRECAUTIONS

CONTRAINDICATIONS: Congenital or acquired QT syndromes, severe renal impairment (Ccr <20 ml/min), concurrent use of verapamil, cimetidine, trimethoprim, ketakonazole, prochlorperazine, megestrol, QT interval of >440 msec. **CAUTIONS:** Renal or hepatic function impairment, fertility impairment.

INTERACTIONS

DRUG: Amiloride, metformin, megestrol, prochlorperaine, triamterine increases dofetilide serum levels. **Bepredil, cisapride, phenothiazines, tricyclic antidepressants** may increase QT interval. **Cimetidine, verapamil** increases dofetilide serum plasma levels. **Ketoconazole, trimethoprim** increases maximum plasma concentration. **HERBAL:** None known. **FOOD:** None known. **LAB VALUES:** None significant.

AVAILABILITY (Rx)

CAPSULES: 125 mcg, 250 mcg, 500 mcg.

INDICATIONS/ROUTES/DOSAGE

Antiarrhythmias:

PO: Adults, elderly: Individualized using a seven-step dosing algorithm dependent upon calculated creatinine clearance and QT measurements.

SIDE EFFECTS

OCCASIONAL (<5%): Headache, chest pain, dizziness, dyspnea, nausea, insomnia, back/abdominal pain, diarrhea, rash.

ADVERSE REACTIONS/TOXIC EFFECTS

Angioedema, bradycardia, cerebral ischemia, facial paralysis, serious arrhythmias (ventricular, various forms of block) may be noted.

NURSING IMPLICATIONS

BASELINE ASSESSMENT:

Have cardiac monitoring equipment and personnel for constant cardiac and B/P monitoring. Anticipate proarrhythmic events.

INTERVENTION/EVALUATION:

Assess for conversion of ventricular arrhythmias and absence of new arrhythmias. Constantly monitor EKG. Provide emotional support to pt and family. Monitor for electrolyte imbalance (prolonged or excessive diarrhea, sweating, vomiting, thirst).

PATIENT/FAMILY TEACHING:

Instruct pt on need for compliance and requirement for periodic monitoring.

dolasetron

dole-**ah**-seh-tron
(Anzemet)
Do not confuse with Aldomet.

▶CLASSIFICATION

PHARMACOTHERAPEUTIC: Selective receptor antagonist. **CLINICAL:** Antiemetic

ACTION/*THERAPEUTIC EFFECT*

Exhibits selective 5-HT$_3$ receptor antagonism for *preventing nausea/vomiting associated with can-*

cer chemotherapy. Action may be central (CTZ) or peripheral (vagus nerve terminal).

PHARMACOKINETICS

Oral form readily absorbed from GI tract. Protein binding: 69–77%. Metabolized in liver. Primarily excreted in urine. Unknown if removed by hemodialysis. Half-life: 7.5 hrs.

USES/UNLABELED

Prevention of nausea/vomiting associated with cancer chemotherapy, including high-dose cisplatin; prevention of postop nausea/vomiting. **Injection:** Treatment of postop nausea/vomiting. Radiation therapy–induced nausea and vomiting.

PRECAUTIONS

CONTRAINDICATIONS: None significant. **CAUTIONS:** Those who have or may have prolongation of cardiac conduction intervals, hypokalemia, hypomagnesemia, those taking diuretics with potential for inducing electrolyte disturbances, congenital QT syndrome, those taking antiarrhythmics that may lead to QT prolongation and cumulative high-dose anthracycline therapy.

▷**LIFESPAN CONSIDERATIONS:**
Pregnancy/Lactation: Unknown if distributed in breast milk. **Pregnancy Category B. Children:** Safety and efficacy not established in those <2 yrs of age. **Elderly:** No age-related precautions noted.

INTERACTIONS

DRUG: None significant. **HERBAL:** None known. **FOOD:** None known. **LAB VALUES:** May alter liver function tests.

AVAILABILITY (Rx)

TABLETS: 50 mg, 100 mg. **INJECTION:** 20 mg/ml.

ADMINISTRATION/HANDLING

PO:
• Do not cut, break, or chew film-coated tablets. • For children 2–16 yrs, injection form may be mixed in apple or apple-grape juice for oral dosing at 1.8 mg/kg up to a maximum of 100 mg.

IV

Storage:
• Store vials at room temperature. • After dilution, solution is stable for 24 hrs or 48 hrs if refrigerated.

Reconstitution:
• May dilute in 0.9% NaCl, D_5W, D_5W with 0.45% NaCl, D_5W with lactated Ringer's, lactated Ringer's, or 10% mannitol injection to 50 ml.

Rate of administration:
• Can be given as IV push as rapidly as 100 mg/30 sec. • Intermittent IV infusion (piggyback) may be infused over 15 min.

IV INCOMPATIBILITY ⊘

No information available via Y-site administration.

INDICATIONS/ROUTES/DOSAGE

Prevention of chemotherapy-induced nausea/vomiting:

IV: Adults/children (1–16 yrs): 1.8 mg/kg as a single dose 30 min before chemotherapy. **Maximum:** 100 mg for children.

PO: Adults: 100 mg within 1 hr of chemotherapy. **Children 2–16 yrs:** 1.8 mg/kg within 1 hr of chemotherapy. **Maximum:** 100 mg.

Treatment/prevention of postop nausea/vomiting:

IV: Adults: 12.5 mg. **Children 2–16 yrs:** 0.35 mg/kg. **Maximum:**

12.5 mg. Give approximately 15 min before cessation of anesthesia or as soon as nausea presents.

PO: **Adults:** 100 mg. **Children 2–16 yrs:** 1.2 mg/kg. **Maximum:** 100 mg within 2 hrs of surgery.

SIDE EFFECTS

FREQUENT (5–10%): Headache, diarrhea, fatigue. *OCCASIONAL* (1–5%): Fever, dizziness, tachycardia, dyspepsia.

ADVERSE REACTIONS/TOXIC EFFECTS

Overdose may produce combination of CNS stimulation and depressant effects.

NURSING IMPLICATIONS

BASELINE ASSESSMENT:

Assess for dehydration if excessive vomiting occurs (poor skin turgor, dry mucous membranes, longitudinal furrows in tongue). Provide emotional support.

INTERVENTION/EVALUATION:

Monitor for therapeutic relief from nausea/vomiting. Maintain quiet, supportive atmosphere.

donepezil hydrochloride

doh-**neh**-peh-zil
(Aricept)
Do not confuse with Aciphex, Ascriptin.

▶CLASSIFICATION

PHARMACOTHERAPEUTIC: Cholinesterase inhibitor. *CLINICAL:* Cholinergic

ACTION/*THERAPEUTIC EFFECT*

Enhances cholinergic function by increasing the concentration of acetylcholine through inhibition of the hydrolysis of acetylcholine by the enzyme acetycholinesterase, *slowing the progression of Alzheimer's disease*.

PHARMACOKINETICS

Well absorbed following PO administration. Protein binding: 96%. Extensively metabolized. Eliminated in urine and feces. Half-life: 70 hrs.

USES

Treatment of mild to moderate dementia of Alzheimer's disease.

PRECAUTIONS

CONTRAINDICATIONS: History of hypersensitivity to donepezil or piperidine derivatives. *CAUTIONS:* Asthma, COPD, bladder outflow obstruction, history of ulcer disease, those on concurrent NSAIDs, "sick-sinus syndrome" or other supraventricular cardiac conduction conditions, seizures.

▷*LIFESPAN CONSIDERATIONS:* **Pregnancy/Lactation:** Unknown if distributed in breast milk. **Pregnancy Category C. Children:** Safety and efficacy not established. **Elderly:** No age-related precautions noted.

INTERACTIONS

DRUG: **Ketoconazole, quinidine** inhibit metabolism of donepezil. Decreases effect of **anticholinergics.** Increases gastric acid secretion of **NSAIDs,** synergistic effects of **succinylcholine, neuromuscular blocking agents, cholinergic agonists. Paroxetine** may decrease metabolism, increase concentration. *HERBAL:* None known. *FOOD:* None known.. *LAB VALUES:* May decrease potassium, increase creatine kinase, blood sugar, lactate dehydrogenase.

AVAILABILITY (Rx)

TABLETS: 5 mg, 10 mg.

ADMINISTRATION/HANDLING

PO:

• May be given without regard to meals or time of administration (morning vs. evening dose), although it is suggested dose be given in the evening, just prior to bedtime.

INDICATIONS/ROUTES/DOSAGE

Alzheimer's disease:

PO: Adults, elderly: 5–10 mg/day as a single dose. If initial dose is 5 mg, do not increase to 10 mg for 4–6 wks.

SIDE EFFECTS

FREQUENT (8–11%): Nausea, diarrhea, headache, insomnia, pain in various locations, dizziness. **OCCASIONAL** (3–6%): Mild muscle cramps, fatigue, vomiting, anorexia, ecchymosis. **RARE** (2–3%): Depression, abnormal dreams, weight decrease, arthritis, somnolence, syncope, frequent urination.

ADVERSE REACTIONS/TOXIC EFFECTS

Overdosage may result in cholinergic crisis characterized by severe nausea, increased salivation/sweating, bradycardia, hypotension, flushed skin, stomach pain, respiratory depression, seizures, collapse. Increasing muscle weakness may occur, resulting in death if respiratory muscles are involved. **Antidote:** 1–2 mg IV atropine sulfate with subsequent doses based on therapeutic response.

NURSING IMPLICATIONS

BASELINE ASSESSMENT:

Obtain baseline vital signs. Obtain history of peptic ulcer, urinary obstruction, asthma, COPD.

INTERVENTION/EVALUATION:

Monitor for cholinergic reaction: GI discomfort/cramping, feeling of facial warmth, excessive salivation and sweating, lacrimation, pallor, urinary urgency, dizziness. Assess eyes for pupillary contraction. Monitor for nausea, diarrhea, headache, insomnia.

PATIENT/FAMILY TEACHING:

Report nausea, vomiting, diarrhea, sweating, increased salivary secretions, severe abdominal pain, dizziness.

dong quai

Also known as Chinese angelica, dang gui, tang kuei, toki

▶CLASSIFICATION

HERBAL

ACTION/EFFECT

Competitively inhibits estradiol binding to estrogen receptors. Has vasodilation, antispasmodic, and CNS stimulant activity. *Reduces symptoms of menopause.*

USES

Gynecological ailments including menstrual cramps, menopause symptoms, uterine stimulant. Also used to control hypertension and as anti-inflammatory, vasodilator, immunosuppressant, analgesic, and antipyretic.

PRECAUTIONS

CONTRAINDICATIONS: Pregnancy due to uterine stimulant effect, bleeding disorders, excessive menstrual flow. **CAUTIONS:** Lactation, breast, ovarian, uterine cancer.
▷**LIFESPAN CONSIDERATIONS:**
Pregnancy/Lactation: Contraindicated. **Children:** Safety and efficacy not established. **Elderly:** No age-related precautions noted.

INTERACTIONS

DRUG: Increases anticoagulant effect, risk of bleeding with **warfarin. HERBAL: Feverfew, garlic, ginger, ginkgo, ginseng** may increase risk of bleeding. **FOOD:** None significant. **LAB VALUES:** May increase prothrombin time/INR.

AVAILABILITY

(DONG QUAI SOFTGEL): 200 mg, 530 mg, 565 mg.

INDICATIONS/ROUTES/DOSAGE

Gynecological ailments, other purported uses:
PO: Adults, elderly: 3–4 g/day in divided doses with meals.

SIDE EFFECTS

Diarrhea, photosensitivity, nausea, vomiting, anorexia, increased menstrual flow.

ADVERSE REACTIONS/TOXIC EFFECTS

None significant.

NURSING IMPLICATIONS

BASELINE ASSESSMENT:

Assess if pt is pregnant/breast-feeding, taking other medica-

tions, esp. those that increase risk of bleeding.

INTERVENTION/EVALUATION:

Assess for hypersensitivity reaction.

PATIENT/FAMILY TEACHING:

Inform physician if pregnant or planning to become pregnant, breast-feeding: do not use. May cause photosensitivity reaction—sunscreen or protective clothing should be worn.

dopamine hydrochloride

dope-a-meen
(Intropin, Dopastat)
Do not confuse with
dobutamine, Dopram, Isoptin.

▶CLASSIFICATION

PHARMACOTHERAPEUTIC: Sympathomimetic (adrenergic agonist). **CLINICAL:** Cardiac stimulant, vasopressor (see p. 125C)

ACTION/THERAPEUTIC EFFECT

Stimulates adrenergic receptors; effects are dose dependent. **Low doses (1–5 mcg/kg/min):** Stimulates dopaminergic receptors causing renal vasodilation (*increases renal blood flow, urine flow, sodium excretion*). **Low to moderate doses (5–15 mcg/kg/min):** Positive inotropic effect by direct action, release of norepinephrine (*increases myocardial contractility, stroke volume, cardiac output*). **High doses (>15 mcg/kg/min):** Stimulates alpha receptors (*increased peripheral resistance,* *renal vasoconstriction, increases systolic and diastolic B/P).*

PHARMACOKINETICS

	Onset	Peak	Duration
IV	1–2 min	<5 min	<10 min

Widely distributed. Does not cross blood-brain barrier. Metabolized in liver, kidney, plasma. Primarily excreted in urine. Not removed by hemodialysis. Half-life: 2 min.

USES

Prophylaxis/treatment of acute hypotension, shock (associated with myocardial infarction, trauma, renal failure, cardiac decompensation, open heart surgery), treatment of low cardiac output, CHF.

PRECAUTIONS

CONTRAINDICATIONS: Pheochromocytoma, uncorrected tachyarrhythmias, ventricular fibrillation, sulfite sensitivity. ***CAUTIONS:*** Ischemic heart disease, occlusive vascular disease. Safety and efficacy for use in children has not been established.
▷***LIFESPAN CONSIDERATIONS:***
Pregnancy/Lactation: Unknown if drug crosses placenta or is distributed in breast milk. **Pregnancy Category C. Children:** Recommended close hemodynamic monitoring (gangrene due to extravasation reported). **Elderly:** No age-related precautions noted.

INTERACTIONS

DRUG:* Tricyclic antidepressants** may increase cardiovascular effects. **Beta-blockers** may decrease effects. May increase risk of arrhythmias with **digoxin. Ergot alkaloids** may increase vasoconstriction. **MAO inhibitors** may increase cardiac stimulation, vasopressor effects. ***HERBAL: None known. ***FOOD:*** None known. ***LAB VALUES:*** Increases urea nitrogen in blood.

AVAILABILITY (Rx)

INJECTION: 40 mg/ml, 80 mg/ml, 160 mg/ml. ***INJECTION (with Dextrose):*** 80 mg/100 ml, 160 mg/100 ml, 320 mg/100 ml.

ADMINISTRATION/HANDLING

Note: Blood volume depletion must be corrected before administering dopamine (may be used concurrently with fluid replacement).

IV

Storage:
• Do not use solutions darker than slightly yellow or discolored to yellow, brown, or pink to purple (indicates decomposition of drug). • Stable for 24 hrs following dilution.

Reconstitution:
• Available prediluted in 250 or 500 ml D₅W or dilute each 5 ml (200 mg) ampule in 250–500 ml 0.9% NaCl, D₅W/0.45 NaCl, D₅W/0.45 NaCl, D₅W/lactated Ringer's or lactated Ringer's (concentration is dependent on dosage and fluid requirement of pt); 250 ml solution yields 800 mcg/ml; 500 ml solution yields 400 mcg/ml. Maximum concentration: 3.2 g/250 ml (12.8 mg/ml).

Rate of administration:
• Administer into large vein (antecubital fossa or central line) to prevent extravasation. • Use infusion pump to control rate of flow. • Titrate each pt to the desired hemodynamic or renal response (optimum urine flow determines dosage).

IV INCOMPATIBILITIES ⊘

Acyclovir (Zovirax), amphotericin B complex (Abelcet, Ambisome, Amphotec), cefepime (Maxipime), furosemide (Lasix), insulin.

IV COMPATIBILITIES

Amiodarone (Cordarone), ciprofloxacin (Cipro), diltiazem (Cardizem), dobutamine (Dobutrex), enalapril (Vasotec), heparin, labetalol (Normodyne, Trandate), lidocaine, lorazepam (Ativan), methylprednisolone (Solu-Medrol), midazolam (Versed), milrinone (Primacor), nitroglycerin, potassium chloride.

INDICATIONS/ROUTES/DOSAGE

***IV:* Adults, elderly:** 1 mcg/kg/min up to 50 mcg/kg/min titrated to desired response. **Children:** 1–20 mcg/kg/min. **Maximum:** 50 mcg/kg/min. **Neonates:** 1–20 mcg/kg/min.

SIDE EFFECTS

FREQUENT: Headache, ectopic beats, tachycardia, anginal pain, palpitations, vasoconstriction, hypotension, nausea, vomiting, dyspnea. ***OCCASIONAL:*** Piloerection (goose bumps), bradycardia, widening of QRS complex.

ADVERSE REACTIONS/TOXIC EFFECTS

High doses may produce ventricular arrhythmias. Pts with occlusive vascular disease are high-risk candidates for further compromise of circulation to extremities, which may result in gangrene. Extravasation resulting in tissue necrosis with sloughing may occur with IV administration.

NURSING IMPLICATIONS

BASELINE ASSESSMENT:

Check for MAO inhibitor therapy within last 2–3 wks (requires dosage reduction). Pt must be on continuous cardiac monitoring. Determine weight (for dosage calculation). Obtain initial B/P, heart rate, and respirations.

INTERVENTION/EVALUATION:

Continuously monitor for cardiac arrhythmias. Measure urine output frequently. If extravasation occurs, immediately infiltrate the affected tissue with 10–15 ml 0.9% NaCl solution containing 5–10 mg phentolamine mesylate. Monitor B/P, heart rate, and respirations q15min during administration (or more often if indicated). Assess cardiac output, pulmonary wedge pressure or central venous pressure frequently. Assess peripheral circulation (palpate pulses, note color and temperature of extremities). Immediately notify physician of decreased urine output, cardiac arrhythmias, significant changes in B/P or heart rate (or failure to respond to increase/decrease in infusion rate), decreased peripheral circulation (cold, pale, or mottled extremities). Taper dosage before discontinuing because abrupt cessation of therapy may result in marked hypotension. Be alert to excessive vasoconstriction (as evidenced by decreased urine output, increased heart rate or arrhythmias, and a disproportionate increase in diastolic B/P and decrease in pulse pressure); slow or temporarily stop the infusion and notify physician.

---

dornase alfa

door-naze **al**-fah
(Pulmozyme)

▶CLASSIFICATION

PHARMACOTHERAPEUTIC:
Respiratory inhalant. ***CLINI-CAL:*** Cystic fibrosis therapy
adjunct

ACTION/*THERAPEUTIC EFFECT*

Selectively splits, hydrolyzes DNA
in sputum, *reducing sputum viscid
elasticity.*

USES

Management (with standard therapy) of cystic fibrosis pts (including pts with advanced disease) to
reduce frequency of respiratory
infections, improve pulmonary
function.

PRECAUTIONS

CONTRAINDICATIONS: None
significant. ***CAUTIONS:*** None significant.

INTERACTIONS

DRUG: None significant. ***HERBAL:***
None known. ***FOOD:*** None known.
LAB VALUES: None significant.

AVAILABILITY (Rx)

SOLUTION FOR INHALATION:
1 mg/ml.

INDICATIONS/ROUTES/DOSAGE

**Management of pulmonary
function:**

NEBULIZATION: **Adults, children >5 yrs:** 2.5 mg (1 ampule)
once daily via recommended
nebulizer. (Twice daily dosing
may be beneficial for some pts.)

SIDE EFFECTS

FREQUENT: Pharyngitis (36%),
chest pain or discomfort (18%),
sore throat, changes in voice
(12%). ***OCCASIONAL*** (3–10%):
Conjunctivitis, hoarseness, skin
rash.

ADVERSE REACTIONS/TOXIC
EFFECTS

None significant.

NURSING IMPLICATIONS

BASELINE ASSESSMENT:

Assess arterial blood gases,
lung sounds, dyspnea and fatigue, pulmonary secretions
(amount, color, viscosity).

INTERVENTION/EVALUATION:

Provide emotional support to pt,
family, parents. Assess for relief
of dyspnea, fatigue. Observe for
decreased viscosity of pulmonary secretions. Encourage
fluid intake.

PATIENT/FAMILY TEACHING:

Refrigerate. Do not dilute/mix
with other medications. May
have hoarseness or other upper
airway irritation.

dorzolamide

(Trusopt)

**See Classification section
under: Antiglaucoma agents
(p. 46C)**

doxacurium chloride

(Nuromax)

**See Classification section
under: Neuromuscular
blockers (p. 102C)**

doxazosin mesylate

docks-ah-**zoe**-sin
(<u>Cardura</u>)
Do not confuse with doxapram,
doxepin, doxorubicin, Cardene,
Cordarone, Coumadin, K-Dur,
Ridaura.

▶CLASSIFICATION

PHARMACOTHERAPEUTIC:
Alpha-adrenergic blocker. **CLINI-CAL:** Antihypertensive (see p. 52C)

ACTION/*THERAPEUTIC EFFECT*

Selectively blocks alpha₁ adrenergic receptors, decreasing peripheral vascular resistance. Resulting
peripheral vasodilation *lowers B/P,
relaxes smooth muscle of blad-
der/prostate.*

PHARMACOKINETICS

	Onset	Peak	Duration
PO	—	2–6 hrs	—

Well absorbed from GI tract. Protein binding: 98–99%. Metabolized in liver. Primarily eliminated
in feces. Not removed by hemodialysis. Half-life: 19–22 hrs.

USES

Treatment of mild to moderate hypertension. Used alone or in combination
with other antihypertensives. Treatment of benign prostatic hyperplasia.

PRECAUTIONS

CONTRAINDICATIONS: None
significant. **CAUTIONS:** Chronic
renal failure, impaired hepatic
function.

▷*LIFESPAN CONSIDERATIONS:*
Pregnancy/Lactation: Unknown
if drug crosses placenta or is distributed in breast milk. **Preg-**

nancy Category B. Children:
Safety and efficacy not established. **Elderly:** May be more sensitive to hypotensive effects.

INTERACTIONS

DRUG: NSAIDs, estrogen may
decrease effect. **Hypotension-
producing medications** may increase effect. **HERBAL:** None
known. **FOOD:** None known. **LAB
VALUES:** None significant.

AVAILABILITY (Rx)

TABLETS: 1 mg, 2 mg, 4 mg, 8 mg.

ADMINISTRATION/HANDLING

PO:
• Give without regard to food.

INDICATIONS/ROUTES/DOSAGE
Hypertension:

PO: Adults: Initially, 1 mg/day.
May increase to 2, 4, 8, and 16 mg
if necessary. **Elderly:** Initially, 0.5
mg/day.

Note: Doses >4 mg increase potential postural effects.

Benign prostatic hyperplasia:
PO: Adults, elderly: 2–16 mg/day.

SIDE EFFECTS

FREQUENT (10–20%): Dizziness,
asthenia, headache, edema. **OC-
CASIONAL** (3–9%): Nausea, pharyngitis, rhinitis, pain in extremities, somnolence. **RARE** (1–3%):
Palpitations, diarrhea, constipation,
dyspnea, muscle pain, altered vision, dizziness, nervousness.

ADVERSE REACTIONS/TOXIC
EFFECTS

First-dose syncope (hypotension
with sudden loss of consciousness) generally occurs 30–90 min
after giving initial dose of 2 mg or
greater, a too rapid increase in

dose, or addition of another hypotensive agent to therapy. May be preceded by tachycardia (120–160 beats/min).

BASELINE ASSESSMENT:

Give first dose at bedtime. If initial dose is given during daytime, pt must remain recumbent for 3–4 hrs. Assess B/P, pulse immediately before each dose, and q15–30min until stabilized (be alert to B/P fluctuations).

INTERVENTION/EVALUATION:

Monitor pulse diligently (first-dose syncope may be preceded by tachycardia). Assess for edema, headache. Assist with ambulation if dizziness, lightheadedness occurs.

PATIENT/FAMILY TEACHING:

Full therapeutic effect may not occur for 3–4 wks. May cause syncope (fainting). Avoid driving for 12–24 hrs after first dose or increase in dosage. Use caution driving or operating machinery, or when rising from sitting or lying position.

doxepin hydrochloride

dox-eh-pin
(Novo-Doxepin✦, Prudoxin, Sinequan, Zonalon)
Do not confuse with doxapram, doxazosin, Doxidan, saquinavir.

▶**CLASSIFICATION**

PHARMACOTHERAPEUTIC: Tricyclic. **CLINICAL:** Antidepressant, antianxiety, antineuralgic, antiulcer, antipruritic (see p. 35C)

ACTION/*THERAPEUTIC EFFECT*

Increases synaptic concentration of norepinephrine and/or serotonin (inhibits reuptake by presynaptic membrane), *producing antidepressant, anxiolytic effect.* Strong anticholinergic activity. Topical may produce antihistamine/sedative effect.

PHARMACOKINETICS

Rapidly, well absorbed from GI tract. Protein binding: >90%. Metabolized in liver to active metabolite. Primarily excreted in urine. Not removed by hemodialysis. Half-life: 11–23 hrs. **Topical:** Absorbed through skin, distributed to body tissues, metabolized to active metabolite, eliminated renally.

USES/*UNLABELED*

Treatment of various forms of depression, often in conjunction with psychotherapy. Treatment of anxiety. **Topical:** Treatment of pruritus associated with eczema. *Treatment of panic disorder, neurogenic pain, prophylaxis vascular headache, pruritus in idiopathic cold urticaria.*

PRECAUTIONS

CONTRAINDICATIONS: Acute recovery period following MI, within 14 days of MAO inhibitor ingestion. ***CAUTIONS:*** Prostatic hypertrophy, history of urinary retention/obstruction, glaucoma, diabetes mellitus, history of seizures, hyperthyroidism, cardiac/hepatic/renal disease, schizophrenia, increased intraocular pressure, hiatal hernia.

▷***LIFESPAN CONSIDERATIONS:***
Pregnancy/Lactation: Crosses placenta; distributed in breast milk. **Pregnancy Category C.**

Topical: **Pregnancy Category B. Children:** Safety and efficacy not established. **Elderly:** Increased risk of toxicity (lower doses recommended).

INTERACTIONS

DRUG: **Alcohol, CNS depressants** may increase CNS, respiratory depression, hypotensive effects. **Antithyroid agents** may increase risk of agranulocytosis. **Phenothiazines** may increase sedative, anticholinergic effects. **Cimetidine** may increase concentration, toxicity. May decrease effects of clonidine, guanadrel. May increase cardiac effects with **sympathomimetics.** May increase risk of hypertensive crisis, hyperpyretic, convulsions with **MAO inhibitors. HERBAL:** None known. **FOOD:** None known. **LAB VALUES:** May alter EKG readings, glucose. Therapeutic blood serum level: 110–250 ng/ml; toxic blood serum level: >300 ng/ml.

AVAILABILITY (Rx)

CAPSULES: 10 mg, 25 mg, 50 mg, 75 mg, 100 mg, 150 mg. **ORAL CONCENTRATE:** 10 mg/ml. **CREAM:** 5%.

ADMINISTRATION/HANDLING
PO:

• Give with food or milk if GI distress occurs. • Dilute concentrate in 8 oz glass of water, milk, orange, grapefruit, tomato, prune, pineapple juice. Incompatible with carbonated drinks.

INDICATIONS/ROUTES/DOSAGE
Depression/anxiety:

PO: Adults: 30–150 mg/day at bedtime or in 2–3 divided doses. May increase to 300 mg/day. **Adolescents:** Initially, 25–50 mg/day as single or divided doses. May increase to 100 mg/day. **Children <12 yrs:** 1–3 mg/kg/day.

Usual elderly dosage:

PO: Initially, 10–25 mg at bedtime. May increase by 10–25 mg/day q3–7days. **Maximum:** 75 mg/day.

Usual topical dosage:

TOPICAL: Adults, elderly: Apply thin film 4 times/day.

SIDE EFFECTS

FREQUENT: PO: Orthostatic hypotension, drowsiness, dry mouth, headache, increased appetite/weight, nausea, unusual tiredness, unpleasant taste. **Topical:** Edema at application site, increased itching/eczema, burning, stinging of skin, altered taste, dizziness, drowsiness, dry skin, dry mouth, fatigue, headache, thirst. **OCCASIONAL: PO:** Blurred vision, confusion, constipation, hallucinations, difficult urination, eye pain, irregular heartbeat, fine muscle tremors, nervousness, impaired sexual function, diarrhea, increased sweating, heartburn, insomnia. **Topical:** Anxiety, skin irritation/cracking, nausea. **RARE:** Allergic reaction, alopecia, tinnitus, breast enlargement. **Topical:** Fever.

ADVERSE REACTIONS/TOXIC EFFECTS

High dosage may produce confusion, seizures, severe drowsiness, fast/slowith irregular heartbeat, fever, hallucinations, agitation, shortness of breath, vomiting, unusual tiredness/weakness. Abrupt withdrawal from prolonged therapy may produce headache, malaise, nausea, vomiting, vivid dreams.

NURSING IMPLICATIONS

INTERVENTION/EVALUATION:

Supervise suicidal risk pt closely during early therapy (as depression lessens, energy level improves, increasing suicide potential). Assess appearance, behavior, speech pattern, level of interest, mood. Therapeutic blood serum level: 110–250 ng/ml; toxic blood serum level: >300 ng/ml.

PATIENT/FAMILY TEACHING:

Change positions slowly to avoid hypotensive effect. Tolerance to postural hypotension, sedative and anticholinergic effects usually develops during early therapy. Therapeutic effect may be noted within 2–5 days, maximum effect within 2–3 wks. Avoid tasks that require alertness, motor skills until response to drug is established.

doxercalciferol

(Hectorol)
See vitamin D

doxorubicin

dox-o-**roo**-bi-sin
(Adriamycin, Doxil, Rubex)
Do not confuse with
Daunorubicin, Idamycin, Idarubicin.

▶CLASSIFICATION

PHARMACOTHERAPEUTIC:
Anthracycline antibiotic. **CLINICAL:** Antineoplastic (see p. 70C)

ACTION/*THERAPEUTIC EFFECT*

Inhibits DNA, DNA-dependent RNA synthesis by binding with DNA strands, *preventing cellular division.* Cell cycle-specific for S phase of cell division.

PHARMACOKINETICS

Widely distributed. Does not cross blood-brain barrier. Protein binding: 74–76%. Metabolized rapidly in liver to active metabolite. Primarily eliminated via biliary system. Not removed by hemodialysis. Half-life: 16 hrs; metabolite: 32 hrs.

USES/*UNLABELED*

Produces regression in breast, ovarian, thyroid, transitional cell bladder, bronchogenic, gastric carcinoma; soft tissue and bone sarcomas, neuroblastoma, Wilms' tumor, lymphomas of Hodgkin's and non-Hodgkin's type, acute lymphoblastic and myeloblastic leukemia. **Doxil:** Treatment of AIDS-related Kaposi's sarcoma, metastatic ovarian cancer. *Treatment of head/neck, cervical, liver, pancreatic, prostatic, testicular, endometrial carcinoma; treatment of germ cell tumors, multiple myeloma.*

PRECAUTIONS

CONTRAINDICATIONS: Preexisting myelosuppression, impaired cardiac function, previous treatment with complete cumulative doses of doxorubicin and/or daunorubicin. **CAUTIONS:** Impaired hepatic, renal function. Children at increased risk of cardiotoxicity.
▷*LIFESPAN CONSIDERATIONS:*
Pregnancy/Lactation: If possible, avoid use during pregnancy, esp. first trimester. Breast feeding not recommended. **Pregnancy**

Category D. Children/Elderly: Cardiotoxicity may be more frequent in those <2 yrs or >70 yrs.

INTERACTIONS

DRUG: May decrease effect of **antigout medication. Bone marrow depressants** may increase bone marrow depression. May increase cardiotoxicity with **daunorubicin. Live virus vaccines** may potentiate virus replication, increase vaccine side effects, decrease pt's antibody response to vaccine. **HERBAL:** None known. **FOOD:** None known. **LAB VALUES:** May cause EKG changes. May increase uric acid. **Doxil:** May reduce neutrophil, RBC count.

AVAILABILITY (Rx)

POWDER FOR INJECTION: 10 mg, 20 mg, 50 mg, 100 mg, 150 mg. **LIPID COMPLEX (Doxil):** 20 mg.

ADMINISTRATION/HANDLING

Note: Wear gloves. If powder or solution comes in contact with skin, wash thoroughly. Avoid small veins, swollen or edematous extremities, and areas overlying joints, tendons. **Doxil:** Do not use with in-line filter or mix with any diluent except D_5W. May be carcinogenic, mutagenic, or teratogenic. Handle with extreme care during preparation/administration.

IV 💊

Storage:

• Refrigerate unopened vials. • Reconstituted solution is stable for 24 hrs at room temperature or 48 hrs if refrigerated. • Protect from prolonged exposure to sunlight; discard unused solution.

DOXIL:

• Refrigerate unopened vials. •

After solution is diluted, use within 24 hrs.

Reconstitution:

• Reconstitute each 10 mg vial with 5 ml preservative-free 0.9% NaCl (10 ml for 20 mg; 25 ml for 50 mg) to provide concentration of 2 mg/ml. • Shake vial; allow contents to dissolve. • Withdraw appropriate volume of air from vial during reconstitution (avoids excessive pressure buildup). • May be further diluted with 50 ml D_5W or 0.9% NaCl and give as a continuous infusion through a central venous line.

DOXIL:

• Dilute each dose in 250 ml D_5W.

Rate of administration:

• For IV push, administer into tubing of freely running IV infusion of D_5W or 0.9% NaCl, preferably via butterfly needle, at rate no faster than 3–5 min (avoids local erythematous streaking along vein and facial flushing). • Must test for flashback q30sec to be certain needle remains in vein during injection. • Extravasation produces immediate pain, severe local tissue damage. Terminate immediately; withdraw as much medication as possible, obtain extravasation kit, follow protocol.

DOXIL:

• Give as infusion over >30 min. • Do not use in-line filters.

IV INCOMPATIBILITIES ⊘

Doxorubicin: Allopurinol (Aloprim), amphotericin B complex (Abelcet, Ambisome, Amphotec), cefepime (Maxipime), furosemide (Lasix), ganciclovir (Cytovene), heparin, piperacillin/tazobactam (Zosyn), propofol (Diprivan). **Doxil:** Do not mix with any other medications.

IV COMPATIBILITIES

Dexamethasone (Decadron), diphenhydramine (Benadryl), granisetron (Kytril), lorazepam (Ativan), ondansetron (Zofran).

INDICATIONS/ROUTES/DOSAGE

Note: Dosage individualized based on clinical response, tolerance to adverse effects. When used in combination therapy, consult specific protocols for optimum dosage, sequence of drug administration.

Usual dose:

IV: **Adults:** 60–75 mg/m^2 single dose q21days, 20 mg/m^2 once weekly, or 25–30 mg/m^2 daily on 2–3 successive days q4wks. Due to cardiotoxicity, do not exceed cumulative dose of 550 mg/m^2 (400–450 mg/m^2 for those whose previous therapy included related compounds or irradiation of cardiac region). **Children:** 25–40 mg/m^2 or per individual protocol.

Kaposi's sarcoma: (Doxil)

IV INFUSION: **Adults:** 20 mg/m^2 q3wks (infuse over 30 min).

Ovarian cancer: (Doxil)

IV INFUSION: **Adults:** 50 mg/m^2 q4wks.

Dosage in hepatic impairment:

Serum Bilirubin Concentration	Dosage
1.2–3 mg/dl	50% usual dose
>3 mg/dl	25% usual dose

SIDE EFFECTS

FREQUENT: Complete alopecia (scalp, axillary, pubic hair), nausea, vomiting, stomatitis, esophagitis (esp. if drug given daily on several successive days), reddish urine. **Doxil:** Nausea. **OCCASIONAL:** Anorexia, diarrhea, hyperpigmentation of nailbeds, phalangeal and dermal creases. **RARE:** Fever, chills, conjunctivitis, lacrimation.

ADVERSE REACTIONS/TOXIC EFFECTS

Bone marrow depression manifested as hematologic toxicity (principally leukopenia and, to lesser extent, anemia, thrombocytopenia). Generally occurs within 10–15 days, returns to normal levels by third week. Cardiotoxicity noted as either acute, transient abnormal EKG findings and/or cardiomyopathy manifested as CHF.

NURSING IMPLICATIONS

BASELINE ASSESSMENT:

Obtain WBC, platelet, erythrocyte counts before and at frequent intervals during therapy. Obtain EKG prior to therapy, liver function studies prior to each dose. Antiemetics may be effective in preventing, treating nausea.

INTERVENTION/EVALUATION:

Monitor for stomatitis (burning/erythema of oral mucosa at inner margin of lips, difficulty swallowing). May lead to ulceration of mucous membranes within 2–3 days. Assess skin, nailbeds for hyperpigmentation. Monitor hematologic status, renal/hepatic function studies, serum uric acid levels. Assess pattern of daily bowel activity, stool consistency. Monitor for hematologic toxicity (fever, sore throat, signs of local infection, easy bruising, unusual bleeding from any site), symptoms of anemia (excessive tiredness, weakness).

PATIENT/FAMILY TEACHING:

Alopecia is reversible, but new hair growth may have different color or texture. New hair growth resumes 2–3 mos after last therapy dose. Maintain fastidious oral hygiene. Do not have immunizations without physician's approval (drug lowers body's resistance). Avoid contact with those who have recently received live virus vaccine. Promptly report fever, sore throat, signs of local infection, easy bruising, or unusual bleeding from any site. Contact physician if nausea/vomiting continues at home. Avoid alcohol.

doxycycline

dock-see-**sigh**-clean
(Adoxa, Apo-Doxy♣, Doryx, Doxycin♣, Periostat, Vibra-Tabs, Vibramycin, Vibramycin Calcium syrup)
Do not confuse with Dicyclomine, doxylamine.

▶CLASSIFICATION

PHARMACOTHERAPEUTIC: Tetracycline. **CLINICAL:** Antibiotic

ACTION/*THERAPEUTIC EFFECT*

Inhibits protein synthesis by binding to ribosomes, *preventing bacterial cell growth.*

USES/*UNLABELED*

Treatment of periodontitis, respiratory, skin/soft tissue, urinary tract infections, syphilis, uncomplicated gonorrhea, pelvic inflammatory disease, rheumatic fever prophylaxis, brucellosis, trachoma, Rocky Mountain spotted fever, typhus, Q fever, rickettsia, smallpox, psittacosis, ornithosis, granuloma inguinale, lymphogranuloma venereum, adjunctive treatment of intestinal amebiasis.

Adoxa: Treatment of severe acne. *Treatment of gonorrhea, malaria, atypical mycobacterial infections, prophylaxis/treatment of traveler's diarrhea, rheumatoid arthritis, prevention of Lyme disease.*

PRECAUTIONS

CONTRAINDICATIONS: Hypersensitivity to tetracyclines, sulfite, last half of pregnancy, children <8 yrs. **CAUTIONS:** Sun/ultraviolet light exposure (severe photosensitivity reaction).

INTERACTIONS

DRUG: Antacids containing aluminum/calcium/magnesium, **laxatives** containing magnesium. **Oral iron preparations** impair absorption of tetracyclines (give 1–2 hrs before or after tetracyclines). **Barbiturates, phenytoin, carbamazepine** may decrease doxycycline concentrations. **Cholestyramine, colestipol** may decrease absorption. May decrease effect of **oral contraceptives. Carbamazepine, phenytoin** may decrease concentrations. **HERBAL:** None known. **FOOD:** None known. **LAB VALUES:** May increase SGOT (AST), SGPT (ALT), alkaline phosphatase, amylase, bilirubin concentrations; alter CBC.

AVAILABILITY (Rx)

CAPSULES: 20 mg, 50 mg, 100 mg. **TABLETS:** 50 mg, 100 mg. **POWDER FOR ORAL SUSPENSION:** 25 mg/5 ml, 50 mg/5 ml. **SYRUP:** 50 mg/5 ml. **POWDER FOR INJECTION:** 100 mg, 200 mg.

ADMINISTRATION/HANDLING

Note: Do not administer IM or SubQ. Space doses evenly around clock.

PO:

• Store capsules, tablets at room temperature. • Oral suspension is stable for 2 wks at room temperature. Give with full glass of fluid. • May take with food or milk.

IV 🔟

Storage:

• After reconstitution, IV infusion (piggyback) is stable for 12 hrs at room temperature, 72 hrs if refrigerated. • Protect from direct sunlight. Discard if precipitate forms.

Reconstitution:

• Reconstitute each 100 mg vial with 10 ml Sterile Water for Injection for concentration of 10 mg/ml. • Further dilute each 100 mg with at least 100 ml D_5W, 0.9% NaCl, lactated Ringer's.

Rate of administration:

• Give by intermittent IV infusion (piggyback). • Infuse >1–4 hrs.

IV INCOMPATIBILITIES ⊘

Allopurinol (Aloprim), heparin, piperacillin/tazobactam (Zosyn).

IV COMPATIBILITY

Magnesium.

INDICATIONS/ROUTES/DOSAGE

Usual dosage:

PO: **Adults, elderly:** Initially, 200 mg (100 mg q12h), then 100 mg/day as single dose or in 2 divided doses (100 mg q12h in severe infections). **Children >8 yrs, >45 kg:** 2–4 mg/kg/day divided q12–24h. **Maximum:** 200 mg/day.

IV: **Adults, elderly:** Initially, 200 mg as 1–2 infusions; then 100–200 mg/day (200 mg as 12 infusions). **Children:** 2–4 mg/kg/day divided q12–24h. **Maximum:** 200 mg/day.

Acute gonococcal infections:

PO: **Adults:** Initially, 200 mg, then 100 mg at bedtime on first day; then 100 mg 2 times/day for 3 days.

Syphilis:

PO/IV: **Adults:** 300 mg/day in divided doses for 10 days.

Traveler's diarrhea:

PO: **Adults, elderly:** 100 mg daily during a period of risk (up to 14 days) and for 2 days after returning home.

Periodonitis:

PO: **Adults:** 20 mg 2 times/day.

SIDE EFFECTS

FREQUENT: Anorexia, nausea, vomiting, diarrhea, dysphagia, photosensitivity (may be severe). **OCCASIONAL:** Rash, urticaria.

ADVERSE REACTIONS/TOXIC EFFECTS

Superinfection (esp. fungal), benign intracranial hypertension (headache, visual changes). Liver toxicity, fatty degeneration of liver, pancreatitis occur rarely.

NURSING IMPLICATIONS

BASELINE ASSESSMENT:

Question for history of allergies esp. to tetracyclines, sulfite.

INTERVENTION/EVALUATION:

Determine pattern of bowel activity, stool consistency. Assess skin for rash. Monitor LOC due to potential for increased intracranial pressure. Be alert for superinfection: diarrhea, ulceration or changes of oral mucosa, anal/genital pruritus.

PATIENT/FAMILY TEACHING:

Continue antibiotic for full length of treatment. Space doses evenly. May take with food or milk. Protect skin from sun/ultraviolet light exposure.

dronabinol

drow-**nab**-in-all
(Marinol)
Do not confuse with droperidol.

▶CLASSIFICATION

PHARMACOTHERAPEUTIC:
Controlled substance **(Schedule III). CLINICAL:** Antinausea, antiemetic, appetite stimulant

ACTION/*THERAPEUTIC EFFECT*

Inhibit vomiting control mechanisms in medulla oblongata. *Dose-related reversible effects on appetite, mood, cognition, memory, perception.*

USES

Prevention, treatment of nausea, vomiting due to cancer chemotherapy; appetite stimulant in AIDS, cancer pts.

PRECAUTIONS

CONTRAINDICATIONS: Nausea, vomiting other than due to chemotherapy. **CAUTIONS:** Hypertension, heart disease; manic, depressive, or schizophrenic pts. Not recommended in children.

INTERACTIONS

DRUG: CNS depressants may enhance sedative effects. **HERBAL:** None known. **FOOD:** None known. **LAB VALUES:** None significant.

AVAILABILITY (Rx)

CAPSULES, GELATIN: 2.5 mg, 5 mg, 10 mg.

INDICATIONS/ROUTES/DOSAGE
Nausea, vomiting:

PO: Adults, children: Initially, 5 mg/m^2, 1–3 hrs before chemother-

apy, then q2–4h after chemotherapy for total of 4–6 doses/day. May increase by 2.5 mg/m^2 up to 15 mg/m^2 dose.

Appetite stimulant:

PO: Adults: Initially, 2.5 mg 2 times/day (before lunch, dinner). **Range:** 2.5–20 mg/day.

SIDE EFFECTS

FREQUENT (3–24%): Euphoria, dizziness, paranoid reaction, somnolence. **OCCASIONAL** (1–3%): Asthenia, ataxia, confusion, abnormal thinking, depersonalization. **RARE** (<1%): Diarrhea, depression, nightmares, speech difficulties, headache, anxiety, ringing in ears, flushed skin.

ADVERSE REACTIONS/TOXIC EFFECTS

Mild intoxication may produce increased sensory awareness (e.g., taste, smell, sound), altered time perception, reddened conjunctiva, dry mouth, tachycardia. Moderate intoxication may produce memory impairment, urinary retention. Severe intoxication may produce lethargy, decrease motor coordination, slurred speech, postural hypotension.

NURSING IMPLICATIONS

BASELINE ASSESSMENT:

Assess for dehydration if excessive vomiting occurs (poor skin turgor, dry mucous membranes, decreased urine output).

INTERVENTION/EVALUATION:

Supervise closely for serious mood and behavior responses.

PATIENT/FAMILY TEACHING:

Report visual disturbances. Relief from nausea/vomiting generally occurs within 15 min of drug administration. Avoid alcohol, barbiturates. Avoid tasks that require alertness, motor skills until response to drug is established. For appetite stimulation take before lunch and dinner.

droperidol

droe-**pear**-ih-dall
(Inapsine)

FIXED-COMBINATION(S)
With fentanyl, a narcotic **(Innovar)**
Do not confuse with Indinavir.

▶**CLASSIFICATION**

PHARMACOTHERAPEUTIC:
General anesthetic. *CLINICAL:*
Anesthesia adjunct, antiemetic

ACTION/*THERAPEUTIC EFFECT*
Antagonizes dopamine neurotransmission at synapses by blocking postsynaptic dopamine receptor sites; partially blocks adrenergic receptor binding sites, *producing tranquilization, antiemetic effect.*

PHARMACOKINETICS

	Onset	Peak	Duration
IM	3–10 min	30 min	2–4 hrs
IV	3–10 min	30 min	2–4 hrs

Well absorbed after IM administration. Crosses blood-brain barrier. Metabolized in liver. Primarily excreted in urine.

USES
Tranquilization, control of nausea/vomiting during surgical, diagnostic procedures. Used preoperatively with opiate analgesics during general anesthesia as anxiolytic, to increase analgesic effect of opiate.

PRECAUTIONS

CONTRAINDICATIONS: None significant. *CAUTIONS:* Impaired hepatic/renal/cardiac function (may cause cardiac arrhythmias during administration).

▷*LIFESPAN CONSIDERATIONS:*
Pregnancy/Lactation: Crosses placenta; unknown if drug is distributed in breast milk. **Pregnancy Category C. Children:** Dystonias more likely. **Elderly:** May be more sensitive to sedative, hypotensive effects.

INTERACTIONS

DRUG: **CNS depressants** may increase CNS depressant effect. **Hypotensives** may increase hypotension. *HERBAL:* None known. *FOOD:* None known. *LAB VALUES:* None significant.

AVAILABILITY (Rx)
INJECTION: 2.5 mg/ml.

ADMINISTRATION/HANDLING
Note: Pt must remain recumbent for 30–60 min in head-low position with legs raised, to minimize hypotensive effect.

Storage:
• Store parenteral form at room temperature.

IM:
• Inject slowly, deep IM into upper outer quadrant of gluteus maximus.

IV
• May give undiluted as IV push at a rate of 10 mg or less over 1 min.
• Dose for high-risk pts should be added to D_5W or lactated Ringer's injection to a concentration of 1 mg/50 ml and given as an IV infusion.

IV INCOMPATIBILITIES ⊘

Allopurinol (Aloprim), amphotericin B complex (Abelcet, Ambisome, Amphotic), cefepime (Maxipime), foscarnet (Foscavir), heparin, methotrexate, piperacillin/tazobactam (Zosyn).

IV COMPATIBILITIES

Metoclopramide (Reglan), potassium chloride.

INDICATIONS/ROUTES/DOSAGE

Preop:

IM/IV: **Adults, elderly:** 2.5–10 mg 30–60 min before induction of general anesthesia. **Children 2–12 yrs:** 0.088–0.165 mg/kg.

Adjunct for induction of general anesthesia:

IV: **Adults, elderly:** 0.22–0.275 mg/kg. **Children 2–12 yrs:** 0.088–0.165 mg/kg.

Adjunct for maintenance of general anesthesia:

IV: **Adults, elderly:** 1.25–2.5 mg.

Diagnostic procedures without general anesthesia:

IM: **Adults, elderly:** 2.5–10 mg 30–60 min before procedure. If needed, may give additional doses of 1.25–2.5 mg (usually by IV injection).

Adjunct to regional anesthesia:

IM/IV: **Adults, elderly:** 2.5–5 mg.

Nausea/vomiting:

IM/IV: **Adults, elderly:** 2.5–5 mg/ dose q3–4h as needed. **Children 2–12 yrs:** 0.05–0.06 mg/kg/dose q4–6h as needed.

SIDE EFFECTS

FREQUENT: Mild to moderate hypotension. **OCCASIONAL:** Tachycardia, postop drowsiness, dizziness, chills, shivering. **RARE:** Postop nightmares, facial sweating, bronchospasm.

ADVERSE REACTIONS/TOXIC EFFECTS

May produce cardiac arrhythmias. Extrapyramidal symptoms may appear as akathisia (motor restlessness) and dystonias: torticollis (neck muscle spasm), opisthotonos (rigidity of back muscles), and oculogyric crisis (rolling back of eyes).

NURSING IMPLICATIONS

BASELINE ASSESSMENT:

Assess vital signs. Have pt void. Raise side rails. Instruct to remain recumbent.

INTERVENTION/EVALUATION:

Monitor B/P and pulse diligently for hypotensive reaction during and after procedure. Assess pulse for tachycardia. Monitor for extrapyramidal symptoms. Evaluate for therapeutic response from anxiety: a calm facial expression, decreased restlessness.

drotrecogin

(Xigris)

See New Drug Supplement.

echinacea

Also known as black susans, comb flower, red sunflower, scurvy root

▶CLASSIFICATION
HERBAL

ACTION/EFFECT

Possesses antiviral/immune stimulatory effects. Increases phagocytosis and lymphocyte activity (possibly by releasing tumor necrosis factor, interleukin-1, and interferon), *preventing/reducing symptoms associated with influenza-like upper respiratory infection.*

USES

Immune system stimulant used for treatment/prevention of the common cold and other upper respiratory infections. Also used for urinary tract infections, vaginal candidiasis.

PRECAUTIONS

CONTRAINDICATIONS: Pregnancy/lactation, children <2 yrs, those with autoimmune disease (e.g., multiple sclerosis, SLE, HIV/AIDS), tuberculosis, history of allergic conditions. **CAUTIONS:** Diabetes (may alter control of blood sugar). Do not use longer than 8 wks (may decrease effectiveness).

▷**LIFESPAN CONSIDERATIONS:**
Pregnancy/Lactation: Contraindicated. **Children:** Safety and efficacy not established in those <2 yrs. **Elderly:** No age-related precautions noted.

INTERACTIONS

DRUG: May interfere with immunosuppressant therapy (e.g., **corticosteroids, cyclosporine, mycophenolate**). Topical **econazole** may reduce recurring vaginal candida infections. **HERBAL:** None significant. **FOOD:** None significant. **LAB VALUES:** None significant.

AVAILABILITY (OTC)

CAPSULES: 200 mg, 380 mg, 400 mg, 500 mg. **POWDER:** 25 g, 100 g, 500 g. **LIQUID.**

INDICATIONS/ROUTES/DOSAGE
Usual adult dosage:

PO: Adults, elderly: 6–9 ml herbal juice for up to a maximum of 8 wks.

Note: A wide variety of doses have been used depending upon the preparation.

SIDE EFFECTS

Well tolerated. May cause allergic reaction (urticaria, acute asthma/dyspnea, angioedema), fever, nausea, vomiting, diarrhea, unpleasant taste, abdominal pain, dizziness.

ADVERSE REACTIONS/TOXIC EFFECTS

None significant.

NURSING IMPLICATIONS

BASELINE ASSESSMENT:

Assess if pregnant/breast-feeding, history of autoimmune disease, receiving immunosuppressant therapy.

INTERVENTION/EVALUATION:

Assess for hypersensitivity reaction, improvement in infection.

PATIENT/FAMILY TEACHING:

Do not use during pregnancy/lactation, children <2 yrs. Do not use longer than 8 wks without at least 1 wk rest.

---

echothiophate

(Phospholine Iodide)

See Classification section under: Antiglaucoma agents (p. 44C)

---

edetate calcium

See Appendix A: Antidotes

---

efavirenz

eh-fah-**vir**-enz
(Sustiva)

▶CLASSIFICATION

PHARMACOTHERAPEUTIC:
Non-nucleoside reverse tran-
scriptase inhibitors. **CLINICAL:**
Antiretroviral (see pp. 58C, 95C)

ACTION/*THERAPEUTIC EFFECT*

Inhibits activity of HIV reverse transcriptase (RT) of human immunodeficiency virus type 1 (HIV-1), *interrupting HIV replication, slowing
progression of HIV infection.*

PHARMACOKINETICS

Rapidly absorbed following PO
administration. Protein binding:
99%. Metabolized to major isoen-
zymes in liver. Eliminated in urine
and feces. Half-life: 40–55 hrs.

USES

Treatment of HIV infection in combination with other appropriate
antiretroviral agents.

PRECAUTIONS

CONTRAINDICATIONS: History
of hypersensitivity to efavirenz,
monotherapy, concurrent administration with midazolam, triazolam,
ergot derivatives. **CAUTIONS:**
History of mental illness or substance abuse, liver impairment.
▷**LIFESPAN CONSIDERATIONS:**
Pregnancy/Lactation: Breast
feeding not recommended. **Pre-
gancy Category C. Children:**
Safety and efficacy not established
in those <3 yrs of age. May have increased incidence of rash. **Elderly:**
No age-related precautions noted.

INTERACTIONS

**DRUG:Midazolam, triazolam, ergot
derivatives** may create serious or life-
threatening events (cardiac arrhythmias, prolonged sedation, respiratory
depression). **Alcohol, psychoactive
drugs** may produce additive CNS effects. **Phenobarbital, rifampin, rifabutin** lowers efavirenz plasma concentration. Decreases **clarithromycin**
plasma levels. Decreases **indinavir,
saquinavir** plasma concentrations, increases **nelfinavir, ritonavir** plasma
concentrations, alters **warfarin** plasma
concentrations. **HERBAL:** None
known. **FOOD:** None known. **LAB
VALUES:** May produce false-positive
urine cannabinoid test results, increase total cholesterol, triglycerides,
increase SGOT (AST), SGPT (ALT)
liver enzymes.

AVAILABILITY (Rx)

CAPSULES: 50 mg, 100 mg, 200 mg.

ADMINISTRATION/HANDLING

PO:

• Give without regard to meals. •
High-fat meal may increase absorption and should be avoided.

INDICATIONS/ROUTES/DOSAGE

HIV infection:

PO: Adults, elderly: 600 mg once
daily in combination. Bedtime dosing is recommended during first
2–4 wks (due to temporary nervous system side effects). **Children >3 yrs, 88 lbs:** 600 mg once
daily. **71.5–88 lbs:** 400 mg once
daily. **55–71.5 lbs:** 350 mg once
daily. **44–55 lbs:** 300 mg once daily.
33–44 lbs: 250 mg once daily.
22–33 lbs: 200 mg once daily.

SIDE EFFECTS

FREQUENT (52%, mild to severe
symptoms): Dizziness, abnormal
dreaming, insomnia, confusion, abnormal thinking, impaired concen-

tration, amnesia, agitation, depersonalization, hallucinations, euphoria. **_OCCASIONAL_** (27%): Maculopapular rash, mild to moderate degree; (<26%): Nausea, fatigue, headache, diarrhea, fever, cough.

ADVERSE REACTIONS/TOXIC EFFECTS

None significant.

NURSING IMPLICATIONS

BASELINE ASSESSMENT:

Offer emotional support to pt and family. Obtain baseline SGOT (AST), SGPT (ALT) in pts with history of hepatitis B or C, cholesterol, triglycerides prior to initiating therapy and at intervals during therapy. Obtain history of all prescription and nonprescription medication (high level of drug interaction).

INTERVENTION/EVALUATION:

Monitor for CNS psychiatric symptoms: severe acute depression, including suicidal ideation/attempts, dizziness, impaired concentration, somnolence, abnormal dreams, insomnia (begins during first or second day of therapy, generally resolves in 2–4 wks). Assess for evidence of rash (common side effect). Monitor liver enzyme studies for abnormalities. Assess for headache, nausea, diarrhea.

PATIENT/FAMILY TEACHING:

Avoid high-fat meals during therapy. If rash appears, contact physician immediately. CNS symptoms occur in over half the pts and may cause dizziness, impaired concentration, delusions, depression. Take medication every day as prescribed. Do not alter dose or discontinue medication without informing physician. Avoid tasks that require alertness, motor skills until response to drug is established. Drug is not a cure for HIV infection, nor does it reduce risk of transmission to others.

E

eflornithine hydrochloride

eh-**floor**-nigh-theen
(Vaniqa)
Do not confuse with Viagra.

▶CLASSIFICATION

PHARMACOTHERAPEUTIC: Topical anti-infective. **_CLINICAL:_** Antiprotozoal

ACTION/_THERAPEUTIC EFFECT_

Inhibits ornithine deczarboxylase cell division and synthetic function in the skin, _affecting rate of hair growth_

USES

For reduction of unwanted facial hair in women.

PRECAUTIONS

CONTRAINDICATIONS: None significant. **_CAUTIONS:_** None significant.

INTERACTIONS

DRUG: None significant. **_HERBAL:_** None significant. **_FOOD:_** None significant. **_LAB VALUES:_** May elevate serum transaminase.

AVAILABILITY (Rx)

CREAM: 30 g tube.

ADMINISTRATION/HANDLING

• Continue to use hair-removal techniques in conjunction with eflornithine. • Apply eflornithine

≥5 min after hair removal. • Avoid application on abraded or broken skin. • Cosmetics or sunscreen may be applied over treated areas after cream has dried.

INDICATIONS/ROUTES/DOSAGE

TOPICAL: Adults, elderly: Apply thin layer to affected area of face and adjacent involved areas under chin; rub in thoroughly. Use twice daily ≥8 hrs apart. Do not wash area for ≥4 hrs.

SIDE EFFECTS

FREQUENT (10%): Acne. **OCCASIONAL** (3–5%): Headache, stinging/burning skin, dry skin, pruritus, erythema. **RARE** (1–2%): Tingling skin, rash, dyspepsia (heartburn, GI distress).

ADVERSE REACTIONS/TOXIC EFFECTS

None significant.

NURSING IMPLICATIONS

INTERVENTION/EVALUATION:
Assess skin for rash, erythema, acne. Therapeutic improvement noted in 4–8 wks. Condition may return to pretreatment levels 8 wks after discontinuing treatment.

PATIENT/FAMILY TEACHING:
Continue therapy for full length of treatment. Notify physician in event rash, skin irritation, or intolerance develops. Transient stinging or burning may occur when applied to broken or abraded skin.

emedastine difumarate

em-eh-**das**-teen
(Emadine)

► CLASSIFICATION

PHARMACOTHERAPEUTIC: Ophthalmic H$_1$-receptor antagonist. **CLINICAL:** Antiallergic, antihistamine

ACTION/THERAPEUTIC EFFECT

Inhibits histamine-stimulated vascular permeability in the conjunctiva, *relieving ocular itching associated with allergic conjunctivitis.*

USES

Treatment of signs/symptoms of allergic conjunctivitis.

PRECAUTIONS

CONTRAINDICATIONS: None significant. **CAUTIONS:** None significant.

INTERACTIONS

DRUG: None significant. **HERBAL:** None known. **FOOD:** None known. **LAB VALUES:** None significant.

AVAILABILITY (Rx)

SOLUTION: 0.05%.

INDICATIONS/ROUTES/DOSAGE
Usual ophthalmic dosage:
Adults: 1–2 drops 2 times/day.

SIDE EFFECTS

FREQUENT (11%): Headache. **OCCASIONAL** (<5%): Abnormal dreams, asthenia (loss of strength, energy), bad taste, blurred vision, burning or stinging, dry eyes, foreign body sensation, tearing.

ADVERSE REACTIONS/TOXIC EFFECTS

Somnolence, malaise occurs rarely.

NURSING IMPLICATIONS

INTERVENTIONS/EVALUATION:
Monitor for headache, abnormal

dreams, loss of strength/energy, bad taste, blurred vision, burning or stinging, dry eyes, foreign body sensation, tearing.

PATIENT/FAMILY TEACHING:

Do not touch eyelids or surrounding area with dropper tip of the bottle. Do not apply medication while wearing soft contact lenses (absorbs drug preservative). Reinsert lenses ≥10 min after drug is administered.

enalapril maleate

en-**al**-ah-prill
(Vasotec)
Do not confuse with Anafranil, Eldepryl, ramipril.

FIXED-COMBINATION(S)

With hydrochlorothiazide, a diuretic **(Vaseretic)**; with diltrazem, a calcium channel blocker **(Teczem);** with felodipine, a calcium channel blocker **(Lexxel)**

▶**CLASSIFICATION**

PHARMACOTHERAPEUTIC:
Angiotensin-converting enzyme (ACE) inhibitor. ***CLINICAL:*** Antihypertensive, vasodilator (see p. 6C)

ACTION/THERAPEUTIC EFFECT

Suppresses renin-angiotensin-aldosterone system (prevents conversion of angiotensin I to angiotensin II, a potent vasoconstrictor; may inhibit angiotensin II at local vascular, renal sites). Decreases plasma angiotensin II, increases plasma renin activity, decreases aldosterone secretion. *In hypertension, reduces peripheral arterial resistance. In CHF, increases cardiac output, decreases peripheral vascular resistance, B/P, pulmonary capillary wedge pressure, heart size.*

PHARMACOKINETICS

	Onset	Peak	Duration
PO	1 hr	4–6 hrs	24 hrs
IV	15 min	1–4 hrs	6 hrs

Readily absorbed from GI tract (not affected by food). Protein binding: 50–60%. Converted to active metabolite. Primarily excreted in urine. Removed by hemodialysis. Half-life: 11 hrs (half-life increased with impaired renal function).

USES/*UNLABELED*

Treatment of hypertension alone or in combination with other antihypertensives. Adjunctive therapy for CHF (in combination with cardiac glycosides, diuretics). *Treatment of diabetic nephropathy, hypertension, or renal crisis in scleroderma.*

PRECAUTIONS

CONTRAINDICATIONS: History of angioedema with previous treatment with ACE inhibitors. ***CAUTIONS:*** Renal impairment, those with sodium depletion or on diuretic therapy, dialysis, hypovolemia, coronary/cerebrovascular insufficiency.

▷***LIFESPAN CONSIDERATIONS:***
Pregnancy/Lactation: Crosses placenta; distributed in breast milk. May cause fetal/neonatal mortality/morbidity. **Pregnancy Category D. Children:** Safety and efficacy not established. **Elderly:** May be more susceptible to hypotensive effects.

INTERACTIONS

***DRUG:* Alcohol, diuretics, hypotensive agents** may increase effects. **HERBAL:** None known. **FOOD:** None known. **LAB VALUES:** May increase potassium, SGOT (AST), SGPT (ALT), alkaline phosphatase, bilirubin, BUN, creatinine. May decrease sodium. May cause positive ANA titer.

AVAILABILITY (Rx)

TABLETS: 2.5 mg, 5 mg, 10 mg, 20 mg. **INJECTION:** 1.25 mg/ml.

ADMINISTRATION/HANDLING
PO

• Give without regard to food. • Tablets may be crushed.

IV 💊

Storage:

• Store parenteral form at room temperature. • Use only clear, colorless solution. • Diluted IV solution is stable for 24 hrs at room temperature.

Reconstitution:

• May give undiluted or dilute with D_5W or 0.9% NaCl.

Rate of administration:

• For IV push, give undiluted over 5 min. • For IV piggyback, infuse over 10–15 min.

IV INCOMPATIBILITIES ⊘

Amphotericin (Fungizone), amphotericin B complex (Abelcet, Ambisome, Amphotec), cefefime (Maxipime), phenytoin (Dilantin).

IV COMPATIBILITIES

Calcium gluconate, dobutamine (Dobutrex), heparin, lidocaine, magnesium, potassium chloride, potassium phosphate.

INDICATIONS/ROUTES/DOSAGE
Hypertension:

PO: Adults, elderly: Initially, 2.5–5 mg/day. **Range:** 10–40 mg/day in 1–2 divided doses.

IV: Adults, elderly: 0.625–1.25 mg q6h up to 5 mg q6h.

CHF:

PO: Adults, elderly: Initially, 2.5–5 mg/day. **Range:** 5–20 mg/day in 2 divided doses.

Usual pediatric dose:

PO: Children: 0.1 mg/kg/day in 1–2 divided doses. **Maximum:** 0.5 mg/kg/day. **Neonates:** 0.1 mg/kg/day q24h.

IV: Children, neonates: 5–10 mcg/kg/dose q8–24h.

Dosage in renal impairment:

Creatinine Clearance	% Usual Dose
10–50 ml/min	75–100
<10 ml/min	50

SIDE EFFECTS

FREQUENT (5–7%): Postural hypotension, headache, dizziness. **OCCASIONAL** (2–3%): Orthostatic hypotension, fatigue, diarrhea, cough, syncope. **RARE** (<2%): Angina, abdominal pain, vomiting, nausea, rash, asthenia (loss of strength/energy), fainting.

ADVERSE REACTIONS/TOXIC EFFECTS

Excessive hypotension ("first-dose syncope") may occur in those with CHF, severely salt/volume depleted. Angioedema (swelling of face, lips), hyperkalemia occur rarely. Agranulocytosis, neutropenia may be noted in pts with impaired renal function or collagen vascular disease (systemic lupus erythematosus, scleroderma). Nephrotic syndrome may be noted in those with history of renal disease.

NURSING IMPLICATIONS:

BASELINE ASSESSMENT:
Obtain B/P immediately before

each dose (be alert to fluctuations). In pts with renal impairment, autoimmune disease, or taking drugs that affect leukocytes or immune response, CBC should be performed before therapy begins and q2wks for 3 mo, then periodically thereafter.

INTERVENTION/EVALUATION:

Assist with ambulation if dizziness occurs. Monitor serum potassium, BUN, serum creatinine levels. Monitor pattern of daily bowel activity, stool consistency.

PATIENT/FAMILY TEACHING:

To reduce hypotensive effect, rise slowly from lying to sitting position and permit legs to dangle from bed momentarily before standing. Several weeks may be needed for full therapeutic effect of B/P reduction. Skipping doses or voluntarily discontinuing drug may produce severe, rebound hypertension.

enoxacin

(Penetrex)
See Classification section under: Antibiotic: fluoroquinolone (p. 22C)

enoxaparin sodium

en-**ox**-ah-pear-in
(Lovenox)
Do not confuse with Lotronex.

▶CLASSIFICATION

PHARMACOTHERAPEUTIC:
Low molecular weight heparin.
CLINICAL: Anticoagulant (see p. 29C)

ACTION/*THERAPEUTIC EFFECT*

Antithrombin; in presence of low molecular weight heparin, *produces anticoagulation* by inhibition of factor Xa. Enoxaparin causes less inactivation of thrombin, inhibition of platelets, and bleeding than standard heparin. Does not significantly influence bleeding time, prothrombin time (PT), activated partial thromboplastin time (APTT).

PHARMACOKINETICS

	Onset	Peak	Duration
SubQ	—	3–5 hrs	12 hrs

Well absorbed after SubQ administration. Eliminated primarily in urine. Not removed by hemodialysis. Half-life: 4.5 hrs.

USES/*UNLABELED*

Prevention of postop deep vein thrombosis (DVT) following hip or knee replacement surgery, abdominal surgery. Long-term DVT prevention following hip replacement surgery, nonsurgical acute illness. Treatment of unstable angina, non-Q-wave myocardial infarction, acute DVT (with warfarin). *Prevents DVT following general surgical procedures.*

PRECAUTIONS

CONTRAINDICATIONS: Active major bleeding, concurrent heparin therapy, thrombocytopenia associated with positive in vitro test for antiplatelet antibody, hypersensitivity to heparin or pork products. ***CAUTIONS:*** Conditions with increased risk of hemorrhage, history of heparin-induced thrombocytopenia, impaired renal function, elderly, uncontrolled arterial hypertension, history of recent GI ulceration and hemorrhage.

▷*LIFESPAN CONSIDERATIONS:*
Pregnancy/Lactation: Use with caution, particularly during last trimester, immediate postpartum period (increased risk of maternal hemorrhage). Unknown if excreted in breast milk. **Pregnancy Category B. Children:** Safety and efficacy not established. **Elderly:** May be more susceptible to bleeding.

INTERACTIONS

DRUG: **Anticoagulants, platelet inhibitors** may increase bleeding. *HERBAL:* None known. *FOOD:* None known. *LAB VALUES:* Reversible increases in SGOT (AST), SGPT (ALT), alkaline phosphatase, lactic dehydrogenase (LDH).

AVAILABILITY (Rx)

INJECTION: 30 mg/0.3 ml, 40 mg/0.4 ml, 60 mg/0.6 ml, 80 mg/0.8 ml, 100 mg/1 ml, prefilled syringes.

ADMINISTRATION/HANDLING

Note: Do not mix with other injections or infusions. Do not give IM.

SubQ:

• Parenteral form appears clear and colorless to pale yellow. • Store at room temperature. • Instruct pt to lie down before administering by deep SubQ injection. • Inject between left and right anterolateral and left and right posterolateral abdominal wall. • Introduce entire length of needle (½ inch) into skin fold held between thumb and forefinger, holding skin fold during injection.

INDICATIONS/ROUTES/DOSAGE

Note: Give initial dose as soon as possible after surgery but not more than 24 hrs after surgery.

Prevention of deep vein thrombosis (hip, knee surgery):
SubQ: **Adults, elderly:** 30 mg twice daily, generally for 7–10 days.

Prevention of DVT abdominal surgery:
SubQ: **Adults, elderly:** 40 mg daily for 7–10 days.

Prevention of long-term DVT, nonsurgical acute illness:
SubQ: **Adults, elderly:** 40 mg once daily for 3 wks.

Angina, myocardial infarction:
SubQ: **Adults, elderly:** 1 mg/kg q12h (treatment).

Acute DVT:
SubQ: **Adults, elderly:** 1 mg/kg q12h or 1.5 mg/kg once daily.

Usual dosage for children:
SubQ: 0.5 mg/kg q12h (prophylaxis); 1 mg/kg q12h (treatment).

Dosage in renal impairment:
Clearance decreased when creatinine clearance <30 ml/min. Monitor, adjust dosage.

SIDE EFFECTS

OCCASIONAL (1–4%): Injection site hematoma, nausea, peripheral edema.

ADVERSE REACTIONS/TOXIC EFFECTS

Accidental overdosage may lead to bleeding complications ranging from local ecchymoses to major hemorrhage. *Antidote:* Protamine sulfate (1% solution) should be equal to the dose of enoxaparin injected. One mg protamine sulfate neutralizes 1 mg enoxaparin. A second dose of 0.5 mg/mg protamine sulfate may be given if APTT tested 2–4 hrs after the first infusion remains prolonged.

NURSING IMPLICATIONS

BASELINE ASSESSMENT:
Assess CBC, including platelet count.

INTERVENTION/EVALUATION:

Periodically monitor CBC, platelet count, stool for occult blood (no need for daily monitoring in pts with normal presurgical coagulation parameters). Assess for any sign of bleeding: bleeding at surgical site, hematuria, blood in stool, bleeding from gums, petechiae, bruising, bleeding from injection sites.

PATIENT/FAMILY TEACHING:

Usual length of therapy is 7–10 days. Do not take any OTC medication (esp. aspirin) without consulting physician.

entacapone

en-tah-cah-**pone**
(Comtan)

▶CLASSIFICATION

PHARMACOTHERAPEUTIC:
Enzyme inhibitor. ***CLINICAL:***
Antiparkinson agent

ACTION/THERAPEUTIC EFFECT

Inhibits the enzyme, catechol-O-methyltransferase (COMT), potentiating dopamine activity and increasing the duration of action of levodopa, *decreasing signs and symptoms of Parkinson's disease.*

PHARMACOKINETICS

Rapidly absorbed following PO administration. Protein binding: 98%. Metabolized in the liver. Primarily eliminated via bile. Not removed by hemodialysis.

USES

In conjunction with levodopa/carbidopa, improves quality of life in pts with Parkinson's disease.

PRECAUTIONS

CONTRAINDICATIONS: Hypersensitivity, concomitant use of MAOIs (see interactions). ***CAUTIONS:*** Rapid withdrawal or abrupt reduction in dosage could lead to emergence of signs/symptoms of Parkinson's disease, may lead to hyperpyrexia and confusion. Liver impairment. May increase occurrence of orthostatic hypotension, hallucinations, dyskinesias.

▷*LIFESPAN CONSIDERATIONS:*
Pregnancy/Lactation: Unknown if distributed in breast milk. **Pregnancy Category C. Children:** N/A. **Elderly:** No age-related precautions noted.

INTERACTIONS

DRUG: Other **CNS depressants** may have additive effect. Nonselective MAOIs (e.g., **phenelzine)** may result in inhibiting pathway for normal catecholamine metabolism. **Probencid, cholestyramine, erythromycin, ampicillin** may decrease excretion of **entacapone. Isoproterenol, epinephrine, norepinephrine, dopamine, dobutamine, methyldopa, isoetharine, bitolterol** may increase risk of arrhythmias, changes in blood pressure. ***HERBAL:*** None known. ***FOOD:*** None known. ***LAB VALUES:*** None significant.

AVAILABILITY (Rx)
TABLETS: 200 mg.

ADMINISTRATION/HANDLING
PO:
• Give without regard to food.

INDICATIONS/ROUTES/DOSAGE
Note: Always administer with levodopa/carbidopa.

Parkinson's disease:
PO: Adults, elderly: 200 mg con-

comitantly with each dose of levodopa/carbidopa to maximum of 8 times/daily (1,600 mg).

SIDE EFFECTS

FREQUENT (>10%): Dyskinesia (uncontrolled body movements), nausea, urine discoloration (dark yellow or orange), diarrhea. **OCCASIONAL** (3–9%): Abdominal pain, vomiting, constipation, dry mouth, fatigue, back pain. **RARE** (<2%): Anxiety, somnolence, agitation, dyspepsia, flatulence, increased sweating, asthenia, dyspnea.

ADVERSE REACTIONS/TOXIC EFFECTS

None significant.

NURSING IMPLICATIONS

INTERVENTION/EVALUATION:

Monitor for evidence of dyskinesia (difficulty with movement). Assess for clinical reversal of symptoms (improvement of tremor of head/hands at rest, masklike facial expression, shuffling gait, muscular rigidity).

PATIENT/FAMILY TEACHING:

Avoid tasks that require alertness, motor skills until response to drug is established. May cause color change in urine/sweat (dark yellow or orange). Report any uncontrolled movement of face, eyelids, mouth, tongue, arms, hands, legs.

ephedra

Also known as ma huang, sea grape, teamsters tea, yellow horse

▶CLASSIFICATION
HERBAL/CNS STIMULANT

ACTION/EFFECT

A nonselective alpha and beta receptor agonist that stimulates the sympathetic nervous system. *Increases blood pressure, heart rate, causes peripheral vasoconstriction, bronchodilation.*

USES

Weight loss, cardiovascular and CNS stimulant. Also used for allergic disorders, nasal congestion, bronchospasm, asthma, bronchitis.

PRECAUTIONS

CONTRAINDICATIONS: Angina, anorexia, bulimia, cerebral insufficiency. Heart disease (may cause tachycardia, arrhythmias), hyperthyroidism, uncontrolled hypertension, pregnancy/lactation. **CAUTIONS:** Anxiety, benign prostate hypertrophy (BPH), diabetes, glaucoma, those with urinary retention.

▷**LIFESPAN CONSIDERATIONS:**
Pregnancy/Lactation: Contraindicated. **Children:** Safety and efficacy not established; avoid use. **Elderly:** Safety and efficacy not established.

INTERACTIONS

DRUG: May decrease effects of **beta blockers.** May increase toxicity with **MAOIs, theophylline, decongestants. HERBAL: Caffeine** can increase risk of side effects. **FOOD: Coffee, tea** can increase risk of stimulatory effects. **LAB VALUES:** May increase blood glucose.

AVAILABILITY

TABLETS: 25 mg. **TEA, TINCTURE, EXTRACT.**

INDICATIONS/ROUTES/DOSAGE
Usual adult dosage:
PO: **Adults, elderly:** 25 mg 3 times/day.

Note: Doses as low as 12–36 mg/day associated with severe adverse effects. Probably unsafe when used orally.

SIDE EFFECTS

Most common include dizziness, restlessness, anxiety, insomnia, headache, anorexia, nausea, vomiting, flushing, tingling, tachycardia, increased blood pressure.

ADVERSE REACTIONS/TOXIC EFFECTS

Psychosis, myalgia, cardiomyopathy, rhabdomyolysis, myocardial infarction, stroke have been reported.

NURSING IMPLICATIONS

BASELINE ASSESSMENT:

Assess all medications (esp. decongestants, theophylline, MAOIs, beta blockers). Assess if pregnant/breast-feeding (contraindicated), history of cardiovascular disease, glaucoma, seizures, hyperthyroidism, hypertension, psychosis.

INTERVENTION/EVALUATION:

Assess for hypersensitivity reactions, dermatitis, increase in cardiovascular side effects (e.g., hypertension, palpitations, chest pain), CNS stimulation (e.g., insomnia, anxiety, nervousness, tremors, hallucinations).

PATIENT/FAMILY TEACHING:

Do not use if pregnant/breast-feeding, history of cardiovascular disease, diabetes, hypertension, glaucoma, thyroid disorders.

Avoid use longer than 1 wk. Avoid use in combination with other stimulants such as caffeine.

epinephrine   ✳   E

eh-pih-**nef**-rin
(Adrenalin, AsthmaHaler, Bronitin, Bronkaid, EpiPen, MedihalerEpi, Primatene, Sus-Phrine, Vaponefrin ♣)

▶CLASSIFICATION

PHARMACOTHERAPEUTIC:
Sympathomimetic (adrenergic agonist). ***CLINICAL:*** Antiglaucoma, bronchodilator, cardiac stimulant, antiallergic, antihemorrhagic, priapism reversal agent (see pp. 45C, 125C)

ACTION/*THERAPEUTIC EFFECT*

Stimulates alpha-adrenergic receptors (vasoconstriction, pressor effects), beta$_1$-adrenergic receptors (cardiac stimulation), and beta$_2$-adrenergic receptors (bronchial dilation, vasodilation), *resulting in relaxation of smooth muscle of bronchial tree, peripheral vasculature.* **Ophthalmic:** Increases outflow of aqueous humor from anterior eye chamber, *dilates pupils (constricts conjunctival blood vessels).*

PHARMACOKINETICS

Onset	Peak	Duration
SubQ		
5–10 min	20 min	1–4 hrs
IM		
5–10 min	20 min	1–4 hrs
Inhalation		
3–5 min	20 min	1–3 hrs
Ophthalmic		
1 hr	4–8 hrs	12–24 hrs

Minimal absorption after inhalation, well absorbed after parenteral administration. Metabolized in liver, other tissues, sympathetic nerve endings. Excreted in urine. **Ophthalmic:** May have systemic absorption from drainage into nasal pharyngeal passages. Mydriasis occurs within several mins, persists several hrs; vasoconstriction occurs within 5 min, lasts <1 hr.

USES/*UNLABELED*

Treatment of acute bronchial asthma attacks, reversible bronchospasm in pts with chronic bronchitis, emphysema, hypersensitivity reactions. Restores cardiac rhythm in cardiac arrest. **Ophthalmic:** *Management of chronic open-angle glaucoma.* **Systemic:** *Treatment of gingival/pulpal hemorrhage; priapism.* **Ophthalmic:** *Treatment of conjunctival congestion during surgery; secondary glaucoma.*

PRECAUTIONS

CONTRAINDICATIONS: Hypertension, hyperthyroidism, ischemic heart disease, cardiac arrhythmias, cerebrovascular insufficiency, narrow-angle glaucoma, shock. **CAUTIONS:** Elderly, diabetes mellitus, angina pectoris, tachycardia, MI, severe renal/hepatic impairment, psychoneurotic disorders, hypoxia.

▷*LIFESPAN CONSIDERATIONS:* **Pregnancy/Lactation:** Crosses placenta; distributed in breast milk. **Pregnancy Category C. Children/Elderly:** No age-related precautions noted.

INTERACTIONS

DRUG: **Tricyclic antidepressants** may increase cardiovascular effects. May decrease effects of **beta-blockers. Ergonovine, methergine, oxytocin** may increase vasoconstriction. **Digoxin, sympathomimetics** may increase risk of arrhythmias. **HERBAL:** None known. **FOOD:** None known. **LAB VALUES:** May decrease serum potassium levels.

AVAILABILITY (Rx)

SOLUTION FOR INHALATION: 2%, 2.25%. **AEROSOL:** 0.2 mg/spray, 0.25 mg/spray, 0.3 mg/spray. **INJECTION:** 1 mg/ml, 0.1 mg/ml, 0.01 mg/ml. **INJECTION (suspension):** 5 mg/ml. **OPHTHALMIC SOLUTION:** 0.1%, 0.5%, 1%, 2%.

ADMINISTRATION/HANDLING
SubQ:

• Shake ampule thoroughly. • Use tuberculin syringe for SubQ into lateral deltoid region. • Massage rejection site (minimizes vasoconstriction effect).

IV 🔆

Storage:

• Store parenteral forms at room temperature. • Do not use if solution appears discolored or contains a precipitate.

Reconstitution:

• For injection, dilute each 1 mg of 1:1,000 solution with 10 ml 0.9 NaCl to provide 1:10,000 solution and inject each 1 mg or fraction thereof >1 min. • For infusion, further dilute with 250–500 D_5W. Maximum concentration: 64 mg/250 ml.

Rate of administration:

• For IV infusion, give at 1–10 mcg/min (titrate to desired response).

IV INCOMPATIBILITY ⃠

Ampicillin (Omnipen, Polycillin).

IV COMPATIBILITIES

Diltiazem (Cardizem), dobutamine (Dobutrex), dopamine (Intropin), heparin, lorazepam (Ativan), midazolam (Versed), milrinone (Primacor), nitroglycerin, norepinephrine (Levophed), potassium chloride, propofol (Diprivan).

INDICATIONS/ROUTES/DOSAGE

Cardiac arrest:

IV: **Adults, elderly:** 0.1–1 mg (1–10 ml of 1:10,000 concentration). May repeat q5min (or may be followed by 0.3 mg SubQ or IV infusion initially at 1 mcg/min up to 4 mcg/min).

Children: 0.01 mg/kg (0.1 ml/kg of 1:10,000 concentration). May repeat q5min (or may give IV infusion initially at 0.1 mcg/kg/min increased at 0.1 mcg/kg/min increments up to maximum of 1 mcg/kg/min). **Neonates:** 0.01–0.03 mg/kg (0.1–0.3 ml/kg of 1:10,000 concentration). May repeat q5min.

INTRACARDIAC: **Adults, elderly:** 0.1–1 mg (1–10 ml of 1:10,000 concentration). **Children:** 0.005–0.01 mg/kg (0.05–0.1 ml/kg of 1:10,000 concentration).

Severe anaphylaxis or asthma:

SubQ/IM: **Adults, elderly:** 0.1–0.5 mg (0.1–0.5 ml of 1:1,000 concentration). May repeat at 10–15 min intervals for anaphylaxis; 20 min–4 hrs for asthma.

SubQ: **Children:** 0.01 mg/kg (0.01 ml/kg of 1:1,000 concentration). **Maximum single dose:** 0.5 mg. May repeat at 20 min–4 hr intervals.

Asthma (prolonged effect):

SubQ: **Adults, elderly:** Initially, 0.5 mg (0.1 ml of 1:200 concentration). May repeat with 0.5–1.5 mg no sooner than 6 hrs from previous dose. **Children:** 0.02–0.025 mg/kg (0.004–0.005 ml/kg of 1:200 concentration). **Maximum single dose:** 0.75 mg. May repeat no sooner than 6 hrs from previous dose.

Severe anaphylactic shock:

IV: **Adults, elderly:** 0.1–0.25 mg (1–2.5 ml of 1:10,000 concentration) over 5–10 min. May repeat q5–15min, or continuous IV infusion initially at 1 mcg/min up to 4 mcg/min. **Children:** 0.1 mg (10 ml of 1:100,000 concentration) over 5–10 min followed with IV infusion of 0.1 mcg/kg/min up to 1.5 mcg/kg/min.

Usual inhalation dosage:

INHALATION: **Adults, elderly, children >4 yrs:** 1 inhalation, may repeat in at least 1 min; subsequent doses no sooner than 3 hrs.
NEBULIZER: **Adults, elderly, children >4 yrs:** 1–3 deep inhalations; subsequent doses no sooner than 3 hrs.

Glaucoma:

OPHTHALMIC: **Adults, elderly:** 1–2 drops 1–2 times/day.

SIDE EFFECTS

FREQUENT: Systemic: Fast/pounding heartbeat, nervousness. *Ophthalmic:* Headache/brow ache, stinging, burning, other eye irritation, watering of eyes. *OCCASIONAL: Systemic:* Dizziness, lightheadedness, facial flushing, headache, diaphoresis, increased B/P, nausea, trembling, insomnia, vomiting, weakness. *Ophthalmic:* Blurred/decreased vision, eye pain. *RARE: Systemic:* Chest discomfort/pain, irregular heartbeats, bronchospasm, dry mouth/throat.

ADVERSE REACTIONS/TOXIC EFFECTS

Excessive doses may cause acute hypertension, arrhythmias. Prolonged or excessive use may result in metabolic acidosis (due to increased serum lactic acid concentrations). Observe for disorientation, weakness, hyperventilation, headache, nausea, vomiting, diarrhea.

NURSING IMPLICATIONS

INTERVENTION/EVALUATION:

Monitor for vital sign changes. Assess lung sounds for rhonchi, wheezing, rales. Monitor arterial blood gases. In cardiac arrest, monitor EKG, B/P, pulse.

PATIENT/FAMILY TEACHING:

Avoid excessive use of caffeine derivatives (chocolate, coffee, tea, cola, cocoa). *Ophthalmic:* Slight burning, stinging may occur on initial instillation. Report any new symptoms (rapid pulse, shortness of breath, or dizziness) immediately: may be systemic effects.

epirubicin

eh-pea-**rew**-bih-sin
(Ellence)

►CLASSIFICATION

PHARMACOTHERAPEUTIC:
Anthracycline antibiotic. *CLINICAL:* Antineoplastic (see p. 70C)

ACTION/*THERAPEUTIC EFFECT*

Exact mechanism unknown but may include formation of a complex with DNA by intercalation of its planar rings with consequent inhibition of DNA, RNA, protein synthesis. Inhibits DNA helicase activity, preventing enzymatic separation of double-stranded DNA and interfering with replication and transcription, producing *antiproliferative and cytotoxic activity.*

PHARMACOKINETICS

Widely distributed into tissues. Protein binding: 77%. Metabolized in liver, red blood cells. Primarily eliminated through biliary excretion. Not removed by hemodialysis. Half-life: 33 hrs.

USES/*UNLABELED*

Component of adjuvant therapy in pts with evidence of axillary node tumor involvement following resection of primary breast cancer. *Lung, ovarian carcinoma, non-Hodgkin's lymphoma, sarcomas.*

PRECAUTIONS

CONTRAINDICATIONS: Baseline neutrophil count <1,500 cells/mm³. Severe myocardial insufficiency, recent myocardial infarction. Previous treatment with anthracyclines up to maximum cumulative dose. Hypersensitivity to epirubicin. Severe liver impairment. *CAUTIONS:* Liver function impairment, renal function impairment.

▷*LIFESPAN CONSIDERATIONS:*
Pregnancy/Lactation: May cause fetal harm, unknown if distributed in breast milk. **Pregnancy Category D. Children:** Safety and efficacy not established. **Elderly:** No age-related precautions noted but monitor for toxicity.

INTERACTIONS

DRUG: **Cimetidine** may increase serum concentrations. *HERBAL:* None known. *FOOD:* None known. *LAB VALUES:* None significant.

AVAILABILITY (Rx)

INJECTION: 2 mg/ml single-use vial.

ADMINISTRATION/HANDLING

Note: Exclude pregnant staff from working with epirubicin; wear protective clothing; treat accidental contact with skin/eyes immediately with copious lavage with water.

IV 🔳

Storage:

• Refrigerate vial. • Protect from light. • Use within 24 hrs of first penetration of rubber stopper. • Discard unused portion.

Reconstitution:

• Ready-to-use vials require no re-constitution.

Rate of administration:

• Infuse medication into tubing of free-flowing IV of 0.9% NaCl or D_5W over 3–5 min.

IV INCOMPATIBILITIES ⊘

Heparin, 5-fluorouracil. Do not mix with other medications in same syringe.

INDICATIONS/ROUTES/DOSAGE

Breast cancer:

IV INFUSION: **Adults:** (in combination with 5-FU and Cytoxan). Initially, 100–120 mg/m² in repeated cycles of 3–4 wks. Total dose may be given day 1 of each cycle or divided equally on days 1 and 8 of each cycle.

Note: Dosage adjustment for pts with bone marrow, liver dysfunction, and hematologic toxicities, severe renal impairment.

SIDE EFFECTS

Note: Venous sclerosis may result if infused into a small vein. *FRE-QUENT* (70–83%): Nausea, vomiting alopecia, amenorrhea. *OCCA-SIONAL* (5–9%): Stomatitis (burning/erythema of oral mucosa, oral ulceration of mucous membranes, difficulty swallowing), diarrhea, hot flashes. *RARE* (1–2%): Rash, pruritus, fever, lethargy, conjunctivitis.

ADVERSE REACTIONS/TOXIC EFFECTS

Cardiotoxicity noted as either acute, transient abnormal EKG findings and/or cardiomyopathy manifested as CHF. Risk increased with total cumulative dose in excess of 900 mg/m². Severe local tissue necrosis will occur if extravasation occurs during administration. Bone marrow depression manifested as hematologic toxicity (principally leukopenia and, to lesser extent, anemia, thrombocytopenia).

NURSING IMPLICATIONS

BASELINE ASSESSMENT:

Obtain WBC, platelet, erythrocyte counts before and at frequent intervals during therapy. Obtain EKG prior to therapy, liver function studies prior to each dose. Antiemetics may be effective in preventing, treating nausea.

INTERVENTION/EVALUATION:

Monitor for stomatitis (may lead to ulceration of mucous membranes within 2–3 days). Monitor blood counts for evidence of myelosuppression, renal/hepatic function studies, cardiac function. Assess pattern of daily bowel activity, stool consistency. Monitor for hematologic toxicity (fever, sore throat, signs of local infection, easy bruising, unusual bleeding from any site), symptoms of anemia (excessive tiredness, weakness).

PATIENT/FAMILY TEACHING:

Alopecia is reversible, but new hair growth may have different color or texture. New hair growth resumes 2–3 mos after last therapy dose. Maintain fastidious oral hygiene. Do not have immunizations without physician's approval (drug lowers body's resistance). Avoid contact with those who have recently received live virus vaccine. Promptly report fever, sore throat, signs of local infection, easy bruising, or unusual bleeding from any site.

epoetin alfa

eh-po-**ee**-tin
(Epogen, Eprex✦, Procrit)
Do not confuse with Neupogen.

▶CLASSIFICATION

PHARMACOTHERAPEUTIC:
Glycoprotein. **CLINICAL:** Erythropoietin

ACTION/*THERAPEUTIC EFFECT*

Stimulates division, differentiation of erythroid progenitor cells in bone marrow, *inducing erythropoiesis, release of reticulocytes from marrow.*

PHARMACOKINETICS

Well absorbed following SubQ administration. After administration, an increase in reticulocyte count seen within 10 days, increases in Hgb, Hct, and RBC count within 2–6 wks. Half-life: 4–13 hrs.

USES/*UNLABELED*

Treatment of anemia in pts receiving or who have received chemotherapy, those associated with chronic renal failure, HIV-infected pts on zidovudine (AZT) therapy, those scheduled for elective nonvascular surgery, reducing need for allogenic blood transfusions. *Prevents anemia in pts donating blood prior to elective surgery, autologous transfusion; treatment of anemia associated with neoplastic diseases.*

AVAILABILITY (Rx)

INJECTION: 2,000 units, 3,000 units, 4,000 units, 10,000 units.

ADMINISTRATION/HANDLING

Note: Avoid excessive agitation of vial; do not shake (foaming).

SubQ

• Use 1 dose per vial; do not re-enter vial. Discard unused portion. May be mixed in a syringe with Bacteriostatic 0.9% NaCl with benzyl alcohol 0.9% (Bacteriostatic Saline) at a 1:1 ratio (benzyl alcohol acts as a local anesthetic; may reduce injection site discomfort).

IV 🗓

Storage:

• Refrigerate vials. Vigorous shaking may denature medication, rendering it inactive.

IV reconstitution:

• No reconstitution necessary.

Rate of IV administration:

• May be given as an IV bolus.

IV INCOMPATIBILITY ⊘

Do not mix with any other medications.

INDICATIONS/ROUTES/DOSAGE

Chemotherapy pts:

SubQ: **Adults, elderly:** Initially, 150 units/kg 3 times/wk up to 300 units/kg 3 times/wk.

Reduction of allogenic blood transfusions:

SubQ: **Adults, elderly:** 300 units/kg/day 10 days prior to, on day of, and 4 days after surgery.

Chronic renal failure:

SubQ/IV BOLUS: **Adults, elderly:** Initially, 50–100 units/kg 3 times/wk. **Target Hct Range** 30–36%. Dosage adjustments not earlier than 1 mo intervals unless clinically indicated. ***Decrease dose:*** Hct increasing and approaching 36% (temporarily hold doses if Hct continues to rise, reinstate lower dose when Hct begins to decrease); Hct increases by >4 points in 2 wk period (monitor Hct 2 times/wk for 2–6 wks). ***Increase dose:*** Hct does not increase 5–6 points after 8 wks (with iron stores adequate) and Hct below target range. **Maintenance:** *(Dialysis):* 75 units/kg 3 times/wk. **Range:** 12.5–525 units/kg. *(Nondialysis):* 75–150 units/kg/wk.

AZT-treated, HIV-infected pts:

Note: Pts receiving AZT with serum erythropoietin levels >500 milliunits likely not to respond to therapy.

SubQ/IV: **Adults:** Initially, 100 units/kg 3 times/wk for 8 wks; may increase by 50–100 units/kg 3 times/wk. Evaluate response q4–8 wks thereafter; adjust dose by 50–100 units/kg 3 times/wk. If doses >300 units/kg 3 times/wk are not eliciting response, unlikely pt will respond. **Maintenance:** Titrate to maintain desired Hct.

PRECAUTIONS

CONTRAINDICATIONS: Uncontrolled hypertension, history of sensitivity to mammalian cell-derived products or human albumin. ***CAUTIONS:*** Pts with known porphyria (impairment of erythrocyte formation in bone marrow or responsible for liver impairment).

▷***LIFESPAN CONSIDERATIONS:***
Pregnancy/Lactation: Unknown if drug crosses placenta or is distributed in breast milk. **Pregnancy Category C**. **Children:** Safety and efficacy not established in those <12 yrs. **Elderly:** No age-related precautions noted.

INTERACTIONS

DRUG: May need to increase **he-parin** (increase in RBC volume may enhance blood clotting). ***HERBAL:*** None significant. ***FOOD:*** None significant. ***LAB VALUES:*** May decrease bleeding time, iron concentration, serum ferritin. May increase BUN, creatinine, phosphorus, potassium, sodium, uric acid.

SIDE EFFECTS

Cancer pts on chemotherapy: ***FREQUENT*** (17–20%): Fever, diarrhea, nausea, vomiting, edema. ***OCCASIONAL*** (11–13%): Asthenia (loss of strength, energy), shortness of breath, paresthesia. ***RARE:*** (3–5%): Dizziness, trunk pain. ***Chronic renal failure pts:*** ***FREQUENT*** (11–24%): Hypertension, headache, nausea, arthralgia. ***OCCASIONAL*** (7–9%): Fatigue, edema, diarrhea, vomiting, chest pain, reactions at administration site, asthenia, dizziness. ***AZT-treated HIV-infected pts:*** ***FREQUENT*** (15–38%): Fever, fatigue, headache, cough, diarrhea, rash, nausea. ***OCCASIONAL*** (9–14%): Shortness of breath, asthenia (loss of strength, weakness), skin reaction at injection site, dizziness.

ADVERSE REACTIONS/TOXIC EFFECTS

Hypertensive encephalopathy, thrombosis, cerebrovascular accident, MI, seizures have occurred rarely. Hyperkalemia occurs occasionally in pts with chronic renal failure, usually in those who do not conform to medication compliance, dietary guidelines, frequency of dialysis.

NURSING IMPLICATIONS

BASELINE ASSESSMENT:

Assess B/P before drug initiation (80% of pts with chronic renal failure have history of hypertension). B/P often rises during early therapy in pts with history of hypertension. Consider that all pts will eventually need supplemental iron therapy. Assess serum iron (transferrin saturation: should be >20%) and serum ferritin (>100 ng/ml) prior to and during therapy. Establish baseline CBC (esp. note Hct). Monitor aggressively for increased B/P (25% of pts on medication require antihypertension therapy, dietary restrictions).

INTERVENTION/EVALUATION:

Monitor Hct level diligently (if level increases >4 points in 2 wk period, dosage should be reduced); assess CBC routinely. Monitor temperature, esp. in cancer pts on chemotherapy and zidovudine-treated HIV pts, and BUN, uric acid, creatinine, phosphorus, potassium, esp. in chronic renal failure pts.

PATIENT/FAMILY TEACHING:

Compliance with dietary guidelines and frequency of dialysis is essential in chronic renal failure pts. Evidence of response to epoetin alfa may be seen in increased reticulocyte count within 10 days;

---

epoprostenol sodium, PG₂, PGX, prostacyclin

ep-oh-**pros**-ten-awl
(Flolan)

▶CLASSIFICATION

PHARMACOTHERAPEUTIC:
Vasodilator. ***CLINICAL:*** Antihypertensive

ACTION/*THERAPEUTIC EFFECT*

Directly vasodilates pulmonary and systemic arterial vascular beds and inhibits platelet aggregation. *Reduces right and left ventricular afterload, increases cardiac output, stroke volume.*

USES/*UNLABELED*

Long-term treatment of primary pulmonary hypertension in class III and class IV pts (New York Heart Association). *Pulmonary hypertension associated with adult respiratory syndrome, systemic lupus erythematosus, or congenital heart disease; neonatal pulmonary hypertension, cardiopulmonary bypass surgery, hemodialysis, refractory CHF, severe community-acquired pneumonia.*

PRECAUTIONS

CONTRAINDICATIONS: Chronic use in those with CHF (severe ventricular systolic dysfunction). ***CAUTIONS:*** Elderly.

INTERACTIONS

DRUG: Hypotensive effects may be increased by other **vasodilators** or using acetate in dialysis fluids. **Anticoagulants, antiplatelets** may increase risk of bleeding. **Vasoconstrictors** may decrease effect. ***HERBAL:*** None known. ***FOOD:*** None known. ***LAB VALUES:*** None significant.

AVAILABILITY (Rx)

POWDER FOR RECONSTITUTION: 0.5 mg, 1.5 mg.

ADMINISTRATION/HANDLING

IV 🔟

Storage:

• Store unopened vial at room temperature. • Do not freeze. •

Reconstituted solutions may be refrigerated for no more than 48 hrs.

Reconstitution:
• Must use diluent provided by manufacturer. • Follow instructions of manufacturer for dilution to specific concentrations.

Rate of administration:
• Give as IV infusion via pump as continuous infusion.

IV INCOMPATIBILITY ⃠

Do not mix with any other medications.

INDICATIONS/ROUTES/DOSAGE
Pulmonary hypertension:

Note: Infused continuously through permanent indwelling central venous catheter using an ambulatory infusion pump. May give through peripheral vein on temporary basis.
IV INFUSION: Adults, elderly: *(Acute dose-ranging procedure):* Initially, 2 ng/kg/min increased in increments of 2 ng/kg/min q15min until dose-limiting adverse effects occur. *(Chronic infusion):* Start at 4 ng/kg/min less than the maximum dose rate tolerated during acute dose ranging (or ½ maximum rate if rate was below 5 ng/kg/min).

SIDE EFFECTS

FREQUENT: Acute phase: Flushing (58%), headache (49%), nausea (32%), vomiting (32%), hypotension (16%), anxiety (11%), chest pain (11%), dizziness (8%). **OCCASIONAL** (2–5%): Bradycardia, abdominal pain, muscle pain, dyspnea, back pain. **RARE** (<2%): Diaphoresis, dyspepsia, paresthesia, tachycardia. **Chronic phase: FREQUENT** (>20%): Dyspnea, asthenia, dizziness, headache, chest pain, nausea, vomiting, palpitations, edema, jaw pain, tachycardia, flushing, myalgia, nonspecific muscle pain, paresthesia, diarrhea, anxiety, chills/fever/flulike symptoms. **OCCASIONAL** (10–20%): Rash, depression, hypotension, pallor, syncope, bradycardia, ascites.

ADVERSE REACTIONS/TOXIC EFFECTS

Overdose may cause hyperglycemia/ketoacidosis (increased urination, thirst, fruitlike breath). Angina, myocardial infarction, thrombocytopenia occur rarely. Abrupt withdrawal (including large reduction in dosage, interruption in drug delivery) may produce rebound pulmonary hypertension (dyspnea, dizziness, asthenia).

E

NURSING IMPLICATIONS

INTERVENTION/EVALUATION:
Monitor standing/supine B/P with any dosage adjustment for several hrs after adjustment. Assess for therapeutic response: improvement in pulmonary function, decreased dyspnea on exertion (DOE), fatigue, syncope, chest pain, pulmonary vascular resistance, pulmonary arterial pressure.

PATIENT/FAMILY TEACHING:
Instruct pt on drug reconstitution, drug administration, care of the permanent central venous catheter. Brief interruptions in drug delivery may result in rapid, deteriorating symptoms. Drug therapy will be necessary for a prolonged period, possibly yrs.

eprosartan

eh-pro-**sar**-tan
(Teveten)

►CLASSIFICATION

PHARMACOTHERAPEUTIC:
Angiotensin II receptor antagonist.
CLINICAL: Antihypertensive
(see p. 7C)

ACTION/*THERAPEUTIC EFFECT*

Potent vasodilator. Blocks vasoconstrictor and aldosterone-secreting effects of angiotensin II, inhibiting the binding of angiotensin
II to the ATI receptors, *causing vasodilation, decreased peripheral
resistance, decrease in B/P.*

PHARMACOKINETICS

Rapidly absorbed following PO
administration. Protein binding:
98%. Undergoes first-pass metabolism in liver to active metabolites.
Excreted in urine and biliary system. Minimally removed by hemodialysis. Half-life: 5–9 hrs.

USES

Treatment of hypertension.

PRECAUTIONS

CONTRAINDICATIONS: None
significant. **CAUTIONS:** Renal/he-
patic function impairment, renal
arterial stenosis.
▷**LIFESPAN CONSIDERATIONS:**
Pregnancy/Lactation: Has caused
fetal/neonatal morbidity, mortality.
Potential for adverse effects on nursing infant. Do not breast-feed. **Pregnancy Category C (first trimester);
Category D (second and third
trimesters). Children:** Safety and
efficacy not established. **Elderly:** No
age-related precautions noted.

INTERACTIONS

DRUG: None significant. **HERBAL:**
None known. **FOOD:** None known.
LAB VALUES: May increase BUN,
serum creatinine, SGOT (AST),
SGPT (ALT), alkaline phosphatase,
bilirubin. May decrease hemoglobin, hematocrit.

AVAILABILITY (Rx)

TABLETS: 400 mg, 600 mg.

ADMINISTRATION/HANDLING
PO:

• Give without regard to food. •
Do not crush or break tablets.

INDICATIONS/ROUTES/DOSAGE
Hypertension:

PO: Adults, elderly: Initially, 600
mg/day. **Range:** 400–800 mg/day.

SIDE EFFECTS

OCCASIONAL (2–5%): Headache,
cough, dizziness. **RARE** (<2%): Muscle pain, fatigue, diarrhea, upper respiratory infection, dyspepsia.

ADVERSE REACTIONS/TOXIC
EFFECTS

Overdosage may manifest as hypotension and tachycardia; bradycardia occurs less often.

NURSING IMPLICATIONS

BASELINE ASSESSMENT:

Obtain B/P and apical pulse immediately before each dose, in
addition to regular monitoring
(be alert to fluctuations). Question possibility of pregnancy
(see Pregnancy Category). Assess medication history (esp. diuretic). Question for history of
hepatic/renal impairment, renal
artery stenosis.

INTERVENTION/EVALUATION:

If excessive reduction in B/P occurs, place pt in supine position,
feet slightly elevated. Assist with
ambulation if dizziness occurs.

PATIENT/FAMILY TEACHING:

Inform female pt regarding consequences of second and third

𝒷 - see color pill atlas   <u>underscored</u> - top 100 prescribed drug trimester exposure to medication. Avoid tasks that require alertness, motor skills (possible dizziness effect). Restrict sodium and alcohol intake. Follow diet and control weight. Do not stop taking medication. Need for lifelong control. Caution against exercising during hot weather (risk of dehydration, hypotension).

eptifibatide

ep-tih-**fye**-bah-tide
(Integrilin)

▶CLASSIFICATION

PHARMACOTHERAPEUTIC: Glycoprotein IIb/IIIa inhibitor. ***CLINICAL:*** Antiplatelet, antithrombotic (see p. 30C)

ACTION/*THERAPEUTIC EFFECT*

Produces rapid inhibition of platelet aggregation by preventing binding of fibrinogen to receptor sites on platelets. *Prevents closure of treated coronary arteries. Prevents acute cardiac ischemic complications.*

USES

Treatment of pts with acute coronary syndrome (ACS), including those managed medically and those undergoing percutaneous coronary intervention (PCI).

PRECAUTIONS

CONTRAINDICATIONS: Active internal bleeding, recent (within 6 wks) GI or GU bleeding, history of CVA <2 yrs or CVA with residual neurologic defect, oral anticoagulants <7 days unless prothrombin time <1.22 × control, thrombocytopenia (<100,000 cells/mcl), recent surgery or trauma (within 6

wks), intracranial neoplasm, arteriovenous malformation or aneurysm, severe uncontrolled hypertension, history of vasculitis, prior IV dextran use before or during PTCA. ***CAUTIONS:*** Pts who weigh <75 kg, those >65 yrs, those with history of GI disease, those receiving thrombolytics, heparin, aspirin, PTCA <12 hrs of onset of symptoms for acute MI, prolonged PTCA (>70 min), failed PTCA.

▷***LIFESPAN CONSIDERATIONS:***
Pregnancy/Lactation: Unknown if drug causes fetal harm or can affect reproduction capacity. Unknown if distributed in breast milk. **Pregnancy Category C. Children:** Safety and efficacy not established. **Elderly:** Major bleeding risk increased.

INTERACTIONS

DRUG:* Anticoagulants, heparin** may increase risk of hemorrhage. **Platelet aggregation inhibitors (e.g., aspirin, dextran, thrombolytic agents)** may increase risk of bleeding. ***HERBAL: None known. ***FOOD:*** None known. ***LAB VALUES:*** Increases clotting time (ACT), prothrombin time (PT), activated partial thromboplastin time (APTT); decreases platelet count.

ADMINISTRATION/HANDLING
IV 💉

Storage:
• Store vials in refrigerator. Solution appears clear, colorless. Do not shake. Discard any unused portion left in vial or if preparation contains *any* opaque particles.

Reconstitution:
• Withdraw bolus dose from 10 ml vial; for IV infusion withdraw from 100 ml vial. • IV push and infusion administration may be given undiluted.

Rate of administration:
• Give IV push over 1–2 min.

IV INCOMPATIBILITY ⊘

Administer in separate line; no other medication should be added to infusion solution.

AVAILABILITY (Rx)

INJECTION: 0.75 mg/ml, 2 mg/ml.

INDICATIONS/ROUTES/DOSAGE

Adjunct percutaneous coronary intervention (PCI):

IV BOLUS/IV INFUSION: **Adults, elderly:** 180 mcg/kg before PCI initiation, then continuous drip of 2 mcg/kg/min and a second 180 mcg/kg bolus 10 min after the first.

ACS:

IV BOLUS/IV INFUSION: **Adults, elderly:** 180 mcg/kg bolus then 2 mcg/kg/min until discharge or CABG, up to 72 hrs.

SIDE EFFECTS

OCCASIONAL (7%): Hypotension.

ADVERSE REACTIONS/TOXIC EFFECTS

Minor to major bleeding complications may occur, most commonly at arterial access site for cardiac catherization.

| NURSING IMPLICATIONS |

BASELINE ASSESSMENT:

Assess platelet count, hemoglobin, hematocrit prior to treatment. If platelet count <90,000/mm³, additional platelet counts should be obtained routinely to avoid thrombocytopenia.

INTERVENTION/EVALUATION:

Diligently monitor for potential bleeding, particularly at other arterial and venous puncture sites. If possible, urinary catheters, NG tubes should be avoided.

ergoloid mesylates

ur-go-loyd mess-**ah**-lates
(Gerimal, Hydergine)

▶CLASSIFICATION

PHARMACOTHERAPEUTIC: Ergot alkaloid. *CLINICAL:* Psychotherapeutic

ACTION/*THERAPEUTIC EFFECT*

Central action decreases vascular tone, slows heart rate. Peripheral action blocks alpha adrenergic receptors. *Improves O_2 uptake, improves cerebral metabolism.*

USES

Treatment of age-related (those >60 yrs) mental capacity decline (cognitive and interpersonal skills, mood, self-care, apparent motivation).

PRECAUTIONS

CONTRAINDICATIONS: Acute or chronic psychosis, regardless of etiology. *CAUTIONS:* None significant.

INTERACTIONS

DRUG: None significant. *HERBAL:* None known. *FOOD:* None known. *LAB VALUES:* None significant.

AVAILABILITY (Rx)

TABLETS (sublingual): 0.5 mg, 1 mg. *TABLETS (oral):* 0.5 mg, 1 mg. *CAPSULES:* 1 mg. *LIQUID:* 1 mg/ml.

INDICATIONS/ROUTES/DOSAGE

Age-related decline in mental capacity:

PO/SUBLINGUAL: **Adults, elderly:**

Initially, 1 mg 3 times/day. **Range:** 1.5–12 mg/day.

SIDE EFFECTS

OCCASIONAL: GI distress, transient nausea, sublingual irritation.

ADVERSE REACTIONS/TOXIC EFFECTS

Overdose may produce blurred vision, dizziness, syncope, headache, flushed face, nausea, vomiting, decreased appetite, stomach cramps, stuffy nose.

NURSING IMPLICATIONS

BASELINE ASSESSMENT:

Exclude possibility that pt's signs and symptoms arise from a possibly reversible and treatable condition secondary to systemic disease, neurologic disease, or primary disturbance of mood before administering medication.

PATIENT/FAMILY TEACHING:

Elimination of symptoms appears gradual; results may not be noted for 3–4 wks. May cause nausea, GI upset. Allow sublingual tablets to dissolve completely under tongue.

ergotamine tartrate

er-**got**-a-meen
(Ergostar Medihaler Ergotamine)

dihydroergotamine

(D.H.E., Ergomar ♣, Migranal)

FIXED-COMBINATION(S)

With caffeine, a stimulant **(Cafergot, Wigraine)**. With belladonna, an anticholinergic, and phenobarbital, a sedative-hypnotic **(Bellergal-S)**

▶CLASSIFICATION

PHARMACOTHERAPEUTIC:
Ergotamine derivative. **CLINICAL:** Antimigraine

ACTION/*THERAPEUTIC EFFECT*

May have agonist/antagonist actions with alpha adrenergic, serotonergic, dopaminergic receptors. Directly stimulates vascular smooth muscle, *constricting arteries and veins*. May inhibit reuptake of norepinephrine.

PHARMACOKINETICS

Slow, incomplete absorption from GI tract; rapid, extensive absorption rectally. Protein binding: >90%. Undergoes extensive first-pass metabolism in liver. Metabolized to active metabolite. Eliminated in feces via biliary system. Half-life: 21 hrs.

USES

Ergotamine: Prevents or aborts vascular headaches (e.g., migraine, cluster headaches). **Dihydroergotamine:** Treatment of migraine headache with or without aura; injection also used to treat cluster headache.

PRECAUTIONS

CONTRAINDICATIONS: Peripheral vascular disease (thromboangitis obliterans, syphilitic arteritis, severe arteriosclerosis, thrombophlebitis, Raynaud's disease), impaired renal/hepatic function, severe pruritus, coronary artery disease, hypertension, sepsis, malnutrition. **CAUTIONS:** None significant.

▷*LIFESPAN CONSIDERATIONS:*
Pregnancy/Lactation: Contraindicated in pregnancy (produces uterine stimulant action, resulting in possible fetal death or retarded

fetal growth); increases vasoconstriction of placental vascular bed. Drug distributed in breast milk. May produce diarrhea, vomiting in neonate. May prohibit lactation. **Pregnancy Category D. Children:** No precautions in those >6 yrs of age, but only use when unresponsive to other medication. **Elderly:** Age-related occlusive peripheral vascular disease increases risk of peripheral vasoconstriction. Age-related renal impairment may require caution.

INTERACTIONS

DRUG: **Beta-blockers, erythromycin** may increase risk of vasospasm. May decrease effect of **nitroglycerin. Ergot alkaloids, systemic vasoconstrictors** may increase pressor effect. *HERBAL:* None known. *FOOD:* None known. *LAB VALUES:* None significant.

AVAILABILITY (Rx)

TABLETS (sublingual): 2 mg. *INJECTION:* 1 mg/ml. *NASAL SPRAY:* 0.5 mg/spray. *SUPPOSITORY:* 2 mg (with 100 mg caffeine).

ADMINISTRATION/HANDLING

Sublingual:
• Place under tongue; do not swallow.

INDICATIONS/ROUTES/DOSAGE

VASCULAR HEADACHES:

Ergotamine:

PO: **Adults, elderly:** *Cafergot:* 2 mg at onset of attack, then 1–2 mg q30min. **Maximum:** 6 mg/attack; 10 mg/wk.

SUBLINGUAL: **Adults, elderly:** *Ergomar:* 1 tablet at onset of attack, then 1 tablet q30min. **Maximum:** 3 tablets/24 hrs; 5 tabs/wk.

PO/SUBLINGUAL: **Children:** 1 mg at onset of attack, then 1 mg q30min. **Maximum:** 3 mg/attack.

RECTAL: **Adults, elderly:** 1 suppository at onset of attack, then second dose in 1 hr. **Maximum:** 2/attack; 5/wk.

Dihydroergotamine:

IM/SUBQ: **Adults, elderly:** 1 mg at onset of attack; repeat hourly. **Maximum:** 3 mg/day; 6 mg/wk.

IV: **Adults, elderly:** 1 mg at onset of attack; repeat hourly. **Maximum:** 2 mg/day; 6 mg/wk.

INTRANASAL: **Adults, elderly:** 1 spray (0.5 mg) into each nostril; repeat in 15 min. **Maximum:** 4 sprays/day; 8 sprays/wk.

SIDE EFFECTS

OCCASIONAL (2–5%): Cough, dizziness. *RARE* (<2%): Muscle pain, fatigue, diarrhea, upper respiratory infection, dyspepsia.

ADVERSE REACTIONS/TOXIC EFFECTS

Prolonged administration or excessive dosage may produce ergotamine poisoning: nausea, vomiting, weakness of legs, pain in limb muscles, numbness and tingling of fingers/toes, precordial pain, tachycardia or bradycardia, hyper/hypotension. Localized edema, itching due to vasoconstriction of peripheral arteries and arterioles. Feet, hands will become cold, pale, numb. Muscle pain occurs when walking and later, even at rest. Gangrene may occur. Occasionally confusion, depression, drowsiness, convulsions appear.

NURSING IMPLICATIONS

BASELINE ASSESSMENT:
Question pt regarding history of peripheral vascular disease, renal/hepatic impairment, or pos-

sibility of pregnancy. Question pt regarding onset, location, and duration of migraine and possible precipitating symptoms.

INTERVENTION/EVALUATION:

Monitor closely for evidence of ergotamine overdosage as result of prolonged administration or excessive dosage (see Adverse Reactions/Toxic Effects).

PATIENT/FAMILY TEACHING:

Initiate therapy at first sign of migraine attack. Report if there is need to progressively increase dose to relieve vascular headaches or if irregular heartbeat, nausea, vomiting, numbness/tingling of fingers/toes, or pain or weakness of extremities is noted. Discuss contraception with physician; report suspected pregnancy immediately.

ertapenem

(Invanz)
See New Drug Supplement.

erythromycin base 🖊

eh-rith-row-**my**-sin
(E-Mycin, Erybid✤, Eryc, Erytab, Erythromid✤, Ilotycin, Novoryihro✤, PCE✤, PCE Dispertab)

erythromycin estolate

(Ilosone)

erythromycin ethylsuccinate

(EES, EryPed, Pediamycin)

erythromycin lactobionate

(Erythrocin)

erythromycin stearate

(Erythrocin, Wyamycin)

erythromycin topical

(Akne-mycin, Eryderm, Erymax)

FIXED-COMBINATION(S)

Erythromycin ethylsuccinate combined with sulfisoxazole, a sulfonamide **(Pediazole)**

▶**CLASSIFICATION**

PHARMACOTHERAPEUTIC: Macrolide. ***CLINICAL:*** Antibiotic, antiacne (see p. 24C)

ACTION/*THERAPEUTIC EFFECT*

Bacteriostatic. Penetrates bacterial cell membrane and reversibly binds to bacterial ribosomes, *inhibiting protein synthesis.*

PHARMACOKINETICS

Variably absorbed from GI tract (affected by dosage form used). Widely distributed. Protein binding: 70–90%. Metabolized in liver. Primarily eliminated in feces via bile. Not removed by hemodialysis. Half-life: 1.4–2 hrs (half-life increased with impaired renal function).

USES/*UNLABELED*

Respiratory infections, otitis media, pertussis, inflammatory acne vulgaris, diphtheria (adjunctive therapy), Legionnaires' disease, intestinal amebiasis, preop intestinal antisepsis. Prophylaxis for rheumatic fever, bacterial endocarditis, respiratory tract surgery/invasive procedures, gonococcal ophthalmia neonatorum; if penicillin, tetracycline is contraindicated: gonorrheal pelvic inflammatory disease, coexisting chlamydial infections, uncomplicated urogenital infections, Lyme disease (<9 yrs). **Topical:** Treatment of acne vulgaris. **Ophthalmic:** Treatment of ocular infections, prophylaxis of neonatal conjunctivitis, ophthalmia neonatorum. **Systemic:** Treatment of acne vulgaris, chancroid, Campylobacter enteritis, gastroparesis, Lyme disease. **Topical:** Treatment of minor skin bacterial infections. **Ophthalmic:** *Treatment of blepharitis, conjunctivitis, chlamydia, keratitis, trachoma.*

PRECAUTIONS

CONTRAINDICATIONS: Hypersensitivity to erythromycins, preexisting liver disease, history of hepatitis due to erythromycins. Do not administer Pediazole to infants <2 mos. **CAUTIONS:** Hepatic dysfunction. If combination used (Pediazole), consider precautions of sulfonamides. IV may cause increased HR, prolonged QT interval.

▷**LIFESPAN CONSIDERATIONS:**
Pregnancy/Lactation: Crosses placenta, distributed in breast milk. Erythromycin estolate may increase liver function test results in pregnant women. **Pregnancy Category B. Children/Elderly:** No age-related precautions noted. High dose in those with decreased liver or renal function increases risk of hearing loss.

INTERACTIONS

DRUG: May inhibit metabolism of **carbamazepine.** May decrease effects of **chloramphenicol, clindamycin.** May increase concentration, toxicity of **buspirone, cyclosporine, felodipine, lovastatin, simvastatin. Hepatotoxic medications** may increase hepa-

totoxicity. May increase risk of toxicity with **theophylline.** May increase effect of **warfarin. HERBAL:** None known. **FOOD:** None known. **LAB VALUES:** May increase SGOT (AST), SGPT (ALT), alkaline, phosphatase, bilirubin.

AVAILABILITY (Rx)

POWDER FOR INJECTION: 500 mg, 1 g.

Base: TABLETS: 250 mg, 333 mg, 500 mg. **TABLETS (delayed-release):** 333 mg. **CAPSULES (delayed-release):** 250 mg.

Estolate: TABLETS: 500 mg. **CAPSULES:** 250 mg. **ORAL SUSPENSION:** 125 mg/5 ml, 250 mg/5 ml.

Ethylsuccinate: TABLETS (chewable): 200 mg. **TABLETS:** 400 mg. **ORAL SUSPENSION:** 200 mg/5 ml, 400 mg/5 ml. **ORAL DROPS:** 100 mg/2.5 ml.

Stearate: TABLETS: 250 mg, 500 mg.

OPHTHALMIC OINTMENT: 5 mg/g. **TOPICAL SOLUTION:** 1.5%, 2%. **TOPICAL GEL:** 2%. **TOPICAL OINTMENT:** 2%.

ADMINISTRATION/HANDLING
PO:

• Store capsules, tablets at room temperature. • Oral suspension is stable for 14 days at room temperature. • Administer erythromycin base, stearate 1 hr before or 2 hrs after food. Erythromycin estolate, ethylsuccinate may be given without regard to meals, but optimal absorption occurs when given on empty stomach. • Give with 8 oz water. • If swallowing difficulties exist, sprinkle capsule contents on teaspoon of applesauce, follow with water. • Do not swallow chewable tablets whole.

IV 🏵

Storage:

• Store parenteral form at room

temperature. • Initial reconstituted solution in vial is stable for 2 wks refrigerated or 24 hrs at room temperature. • Diluted IV solutions stable for 8 hrs at room temperature, 24 hrs if refrigerated. • Discard if precipitate forms.

Reconstitution:

• Reconstitute each 500 mg with 10 ml Sterile Water for Injection without preservative to provide a concentration of 50 mg/ml. • Further dilute with 100–250 ml D_5W or 0.9% NaCl.

Rate of administration:

• For intermittent IV infusion (piggyback), infuse over 20–60 min. • For continuous infusion, infuse over 6–24 hrs.

Ophthalmic:

• Place finger on lower eyelid and pull out until a pocket is formed between eye and lower lid. Place $1/4$–$1/2$ inch ointment into pocket. • Have pt close eye gently for 1–2 min, rolling eyeball (increases contact area of drug to eye). • Remove excess ointment around eye with tissue.

IV INCOMPATIBILITY ⊘

Fluconazole (Diflucan).

IV COMPATIBILITIES

Diltiazem (Cardizem), heparin, lorazepam (Ativan), magnesium, midazolam (Versed), multivitamins.

INDICATIONS/ROUTES/DOSAGE

Usual parenteral dosage:

IV: Adults, elderly, children: 15–20 mg/kg/day in divided doses. **Maximum:** 4 g/day.

Usual oral dosage:

PO: Adults, elderly: 250 mg q6h; 500 mg q12h; or 333 mg q8h. Increase up to 4 g/day. **Children:** 30–50 mg/kg/day in divided doses

up to 60–100 mg/kg/day for severe infections. **Neonates:** 20–40 mg/kg/day in divided doses q6–12h.

Preop intestinal antisepsis:

PO: Adults, elderly: Give 1 g at 1, 2, and 11 PM on day prior to surgery (with neomycin). **Children:** 20 mg/kg; same regimen as above.

Acne vulgaris:

TOPICAL: Adults: Apply to skin 2 times/day.

Gonococcal ophthalmia neonatorum:

OPHTHALMIC: Neonates: 0.5–2 cm no later than 1 hr after delivery.

SIDE EFFECTS

FREQUENT: Abdominal discomfort/cramping, phlebitis/thrombophlebitis with IV administration. **Topical:** Dry skin (50%). **OCCASIONAL:** Nausea, vomiting, diarrhea, rash, urticaria. **RARE: Ophthalmic:** Sensitivity reaction with increased irritation, burning, itching, inflammation. **Topical:** Urticaria.

ADVERSE REACTIONS/TOXIC EFFECTS

Superinfections, esp. antibiotic-associated colitis (genital/anal pruritus, sore mouth or tongue, moderate to severe diarrhea), reversible cholestatic hepatitis may occur. High dosage in renal impairment may lead to reversible hearing loss. Anaphylaxis occurs rarely.

NURSING IMPLICATIONS

BASELINE ASSESSMENT:

Question pt for history of allergies (particularly erythromycins), hepatitis.

INTERVENTION/EVALUATION:
Determine pattern of bowel activity, stool consistency. Assess skin for rash. Assess for hepatotoxicity: malaise, fever, abdominal pain, GI disturbances. Evaluate for superinfection. Check for phlebitis (heat, pain, red streaking over vein).

PATIENT/FAMILY TEACHING:
Continue therapy for full length of treatment. Doses should be evenly spaced. Do *not* swallow chewable tablets whole. Take medication with 8 oz water 1 hr before or 2 hrs after food/beverage. *Ophthalmic:* Report burning, itching, or inflammation: *Topical:* Report excessive dryness, itching, burning. Improvement of acne may not occur for 1–2 mos; maximum benefit may take 3 mos; therapy may last mos or yrs. Use caution in use of other topical acne preparations containing peeling or abrasive agents, medicated or abrasive soaps, cosmetics containing alcohol (e.g., astringents, aftershave lotion).

esmolol hydrochloride

ez-moe-lol
(Brevibloc)

▶CLASSIFICATION

PHARMACOTHERAPEUTIC:
Beta₁-adrenergic blocker. **CLINICAL:** Antiarrhythmic (see pp. 13C, 61C)

ACTION/*THERAPEUTIC EFFECT*
Selectively blocks $beta_1$-adrenergic receptors, *slowing sinus heart rate, decreasing cardiac output, decreasing B/P.* Antiarrhythmic activity due to blocking stimulation of cardiac pacemaker potentials.

USES
Rapid, short-term control of ventricular rate in those with supraventricular arrhythmias, sinus tachycardia. Intra/postop control of tachycardia/hypertension.

PRECAUTIONS
CONTRAINDICATIONS: Overt cardiac failure, cardiogenic shock, heart block greater than first degree, sinus bradycardia. **CAUTIONS:** History of allergy, bronchial asthma, emphysema, bronchitis, CHF, diabetes, impaired renal function.

INTERACTIONS
DRUG: Sympathomimetics, xanthines may mutually inhibit effects. May mask symptoms of hypoglycemia, prolong hypoglycemic effect of **insulin, oral hypoglycemics. MAO inhibitors** may cause significant hypertension. **HERBAL:** None known. **FOOD:** None known. **LAB VALUES:** None significant.

AVAILABILITY (Rx)
INJECTION: 10 mg/ml, 250 mg/ml.

ADMINISTRATION/HANDLING
Note: Give by IV infusion. Avoid butterfly needles, very small veins.
IV ▨
Storage:
• Use only clear and colorless to light yellow solution. • Alter dilution, solution is stable for 24 hrs. • Discard solution if it is discolored or if precipitate forms.

Reconstitution:
• Must be diluted to concentration of 10 mg/ml (prevents vein irritation). • For IV infusion, remove

20 ml from 500 ml container of D_5W, D_5W/Ringer's, D_5W/lactated Ringer's, D_5W/0.9% NaCl, D_5W/ 0.45% NaCl, 0.9% NaCl, lactated Ringer's or 0.45% NaCl and dilute 5 g vial esmolol to remaining 480 ml of solution to provide concentration of 10 mg/ml. Maximum concentration: 10 g/250 ml (40 mg/ml).

Rate of administration:

• Administer by controlled infusion device set at rate judged by tolerance and response. • Hypotension (systolic B/P below 90 mm Hg) is greatest during first 30 min of IV infusion.

IV INCOMPATIBILITIES ⊘

Amphotericin B complex (Abelcet, Ambisome, Amphotec), furosemide (Lasix).

IV COMPATIBILITIES

Amiodarone (Cordarone), diltiazem (Cardizem), dopamine (Intropin), heparin, magnesium, midazolam (Versed), potassium chloride, propofol (Diprivan).

INDICATIONS/ROUTES/DOSAGE

IV: **Adults, elderly:** Initially, loading dose of 500 mcg/kg/min for 1 min, followed by 50 mcg/kg/min for 4 min. If optimum response is not attained in 5 min, give second loading dose of 500 mcg/kg/min for 1 min, followed by infusion of 100 mcg/kg/min for 4 min. Additional loading doses can be given and infusion increased by 50 mcg/kg/min (up to 200 mcg/kg/min) for 4 min. Once desired response is attained, cease loading dose and increase infusion by no more than 25 mcg/kg/min. Interval between doses may be increased to 10 min. Infusion usually administered over 24–48 hrs in most pts.

SIDE EFFECTS

Generally well tolerated, with transient and mild side effects. ***FREQUENT:*** Hypotension (systolic B/P below 90 mm Hg) manifested as dizziness, nausea, diaphoresis, headache, cold extremities, fatigue. ***OCCASIONAL:*** Anxiety, drowsiness, flushed skin, vomiting, confusion, inflammation at injection site, fever.

ADVERSE REACTIONS/TOXIC EFFECTS

Excessive dosage may produce profound hypotension, bradycardia, dizziness, syncope, drowsiness, breathing difficulty, bluish fingernails/palms of hands, seizures. May potentiate insulin-reduced hypoglycemia in diabetic pts.

NURSING IMPLICATIONS

BASELINE ASSESSMENT:

Assess B/P, apical pulse immediately before drug is administered (if pulse is 60/min or below, or systolic B/P is below 90 mm Hg, withhold medication, contact physician).

INTERVENTION/EVALUATION:

Monitor B/P for hypotension, development of diaphoresis or dizziness (usually first sign of impending hypotension). Assess pulse for strength/weakness, irregular rate, bradycardia. Assess extremities for coldness. Assist with ambulation if dizziness occurs. Assess for nausea, diaphoresis, headache, fatigue.

esomeprazole

es-oh-**mep**-rah-zole
(Nexium)

▶CLASSIFICATION

PHARMACOTHERAPEUTIC: Benzimidazole. **CLINICAL:** Proton pump inhibitor (see p. 122C).

ACTION/*THERAPEUTIC EFFECT*

Converted to active metabolites that irreversibly bind to and inhibit H+/K+ ATPase (an enzyme on surface of gastric parietal cells). Inhibits hydrogen ion transport into gastric lumen, *increasing gastric pH, reducing gastric acid production.*

PHARMACOKINETICS

Primarily distributed into gastric parietal cells. Metabolized slowly, leading to slower systemic clearance and achieving greater and longer inhibition of gastric acid secretion than other proton pump inhibitors. Therapeutic intragastric pH is maintained 2–6 hrs longer than omeprazole.

USES

Short-term treatment (4–8 wks) of erosive esophagitis (diagnosed by endoscopy); symptomatic gastroesophageal reflux disease (GERD). Used in triple therapy with amoxicillin and clarithromycin for treatment of *H. pylori* infection in pts with duodenal ulcer.

PRECAUTIONS

CONTRAINDICATIONS: None significant. **CAUTIONS:** None significant.

▷*LIFESPAN CONSIDERATIONS:* **Pregnancy/Lactation:** Unknown if drug crosses placenta or is distributed in breast milk. **Pregnancy Category B**. **Children:** Safety and efficacy not established. **Elderly:** No age-related precautions noted.

INTERACTIONS

DRUG: May decrease concentration of **ketoconazole, iron, digoxin. HERBAL:** None significant. **FOOD:** None significant. **LAB VALUES:** None significant.

AVAILABILITY (Rx)

CAPSULES (delayed-release): 20 mg, 40 mg.

ADMINISTRATION/HANDLING

PO:

• Give ≥1 hr before eating. • Do not crush or chew capsule; swallow whole. For those with difficulty swallowing capsules, open capsule and mix pellets with 1 tbs applesauce. Swallow spoonful without chewing.

INDICATIONS/ROUTES/DOSAGE

Erosive esophagitis:

PO: **Adults, elderly:** 20–40 mg once daily for 4–8 wks.

Maintenance healing of erosive esophagitis:

PO: **Adults, elderly:** 20 mg/day.

GERD:

PO: **Adults, elderly:** 20 mg once daily for 4 wks.

***H. pylori* duodenal ulcer:**

PO: **Adults, elderly:** Esomeprazole: 40 mg once daily, with amoxicillin 1,000 mg and clarithromycin 500 mg twice daily for 10 days.

SIDE EFFECTS

FREQUENT (7%): Headache. **OCCASIONAL** (2–3%): Diarrhea, abdominal pain, nausea. **RARE** (<2%): Dizziness, asthenia (loss of strength), vomiting, constipation, rash, cough.

ADVERSE REACTIONS/TOXIC EFFECTS

None significant.

NURSING IMPLICATIONS

INTERVENTION/EVALUATION:

Evaluate for therapeutic response, i.e., relief of GI symptoms. Question if GI discomfort, nausea, diarrhea occur.

PATIENT/FAMILY TEACHING:

Report headache. Take ≥1 hr before eating. For pts with difficulty swallowing capsules, open capsule and mix pellets with 1 tbs applesauce. Swallow spoonful without chewing.

---

estazolam

es-**tay**-zoe-lam
(ProSom)
Do not confuse with Proscar, Prozac, Psorcon.

▶CLASSIFICATION

PHARMACOTHERAPEUTIC:
Benzodiazepine **(Schedule IV).**
CLINICAL: Sedative-hypnotic
(see p. 123C)

ACTION/*THERAPEUTIC EFFECT*

Enhances action of inhibitory neurotransmitter gamma-aminobutyric acid (GABA). *Depressant effects occur at all levels of CNS.*

USES

Short-term treatment of insomnia (up to 6 wks). Reduces sleep induction time, number of nocturnal awakenings; increases length of sleep.

PRECAUTIONS

CONTRAINDICATIONS: Sensitivity to other benzodiazepines, pregnancy (Pregnancy Category X). ***CAUTIONS:*** Impaired renal/hepatic function.

INTERACTIONS

DRUG: **Alcohol, CNS depressants** may increase CNS depressant effect. ***HERBAL:*** **Kava kava, valerian** may increase CNS depression. ***FOOD:*** None known. ***LAB VALUES:*** None significant.

AVAILABILITY (Rx)

TABLETS: 1 mg, 2 mg.

INDICATIONS/ROUTES/DOSAGE

Note: Use smallest effective dose in those with liver disease, low serum albumin.

Insomnia:
***PO:* Adults >18 yrs:** 1–2 mg at bedtime. **Elderly/debilitated:** 0.5–1 mg at bedtime.

SIDE EFFECTS

FREQUENT: Drowsiness, sedation, rebound insomnia (may occur for 1–2 nights after drug is discontinued), dizziness, confusion, euphoria. ***OCCASIONAL:*** Weakness, anorexia, diarrhea. ***RARE:*** Paradoxical CNS excitement, restlessness (particularly noted in elderly/debilitated).

ADVERSE REACTIONS/TOXIC EFFECTS

Overdosage results in somnolence, confusion, diminished reflexes, coma.

NURSING IMPLICATIONS

BASELINE ASSESSMENT:

Raise bed rails. Provide environment conductive to sleep (backrub, quiet environment, low lighting). Question possibility of pregnancy (Pregnancy Category X),

INTERVENTION/EVALUATION:

Assess sleep pattern of pt. Assess elderly/debilitated for para-

---

doxical reaction, particularly during early therapy. Evaluate for therapeutic response: decrease in number of nocturnal awakenings, increase in length of sleep.

PATIENT/FAMILY TEACHING:

Smoking reduces drug effectiveness. Rebound insomnia may occur when drug is discontinued after short-term therapy. Do not use during pregnancy. Avoid alcohol.

estradiol

ess-tra-**dye**-ole
(Estrace)

estradiol cypionate

(Depo Estradiol, Depogen)

estradiol valerate

(Delestrogen, Valogen)

estradiol transdermal

(Alora, Climara, Esclim, Estraderm, Vivelle, Vivelle Dot)
Do not confuse with Testoderm.

FIXED-COMBINATION(S)

With medroxyprogesterone, a progestin **(Lunelle);** with norethindrone, a progestogen **(Femhrt 1/5) (CombiPatch);** with norgestimate, a progestogen **(Ortho-Prefest);** estradiol cypionate with testosterone cypionate, an androgen **(DepoTestadiol);** estradiol valerate with testosterone enanthate, an androgen **(Deladumone, Estra-Testrin);** ethinyl estradiol with fluoxymesterone, an androgen **(Halodrin);** esterified estrogens with methyltestosterone, an androgen **(Estratest)**

▶**CLASSIFICATION**

PHARMACOTHERAPEUTIC: Estrogen. ***CLINICAL:*** Estrogen antineoplastic

ACTION/*THERAPEUTIC EFFECT*

Increases synthesis of DNA, RNA, and various proteins in responsive tissues. Reduces release of gonadotropin-releasing hormone, reducing follicle-stimulating hormone (FSH) and luteinizing hormone (LH). *Promotes normal growth, development of female sex organs, maintaining GU function, vasomotor stability. Prevents accelerated bone loss by inhibiting bone resorption, restoring balance of bone resorption and formation.* Inhibits LH, decreases serum concentration of testosterone.

PHARMACOKINETICS

Well absorbed from GI tract. Widely distributed. Protein binding: 50–80%. Metabolized in liver. Primarily excreted in urine. Half-life: 50–60 min.

USES/*UNLABELED*

Management of moderate to severe vasomotor symptoms associated with menopause, female hypogonadism. Palliative treatment of advanced, inoperable metastatic carcinoma of the breast in postmenopausal women (estradiol, ethinyl estradiol), prostate in men (estradiol, estradiol valerate, ethinyl estradiol). Prevention of postpartum breast engorgement (estradiol valerate). Treatment of atrophic vaginitis, kraurosis vulvae (estradiol, estradiol valerate). Treatment of postmenopausal osteoporosis (estradiol transdermal system). Prevention of osteoporosis. *Treatment of Turner's syndrome.*

PRECAUTIONS

CONTRAINDICATIONS: Known or suspected breast cancer (except select pts with metastasis), estrogen-dependent neoplasia; undiagnosed abnormal genital bleeding; active thrombophlebitis or thromboembolic disorders; history of thrombophlebitis, thrombosis or thromboembolic disorders with previous estrogen use. **CAUTIONS:** Conditions that may be aggravated by fluid retention: cardiac, renal/hepatic dysfunction, epilepsy, migraine. Mental depression, metabolic bone disease with potential hypercalcemia, history of jaundice during pregnancy or strong family history of breast cancer, fibrocystic disease, or breast nodules, children in whom bone growth is not complete.

▷**LIFESPAN CONSIDERATIONS:**
Pregnancy/Lactation: Distributed in breast milk. May be harmful to offspring. Not for use during lactation. **Pregnancy Category X. Children:** Caution in those whom bone growth not complete (may accelerate epiphyseal closure). **Elderly:** No age-related precautions noted.

INTERACTIONS

DRUG: May interfere with effects of **bromocriptine.** May increase concentration of **cyclosporine**, increase hepatic, nephrotoxicity. **Hepatotoxic medications** may increase hepatotoxicity. **HERBAL: Saw palmetto** effects increased. **FOOD:** None known. **LAB VALUES:** May affect metapyrone, thyroid function tests. May decrease cholesterol, LDH. May increase calcium, glucose, HDL, triglycerides.

AVAILABILITY (Rx)

TABLETS: (Estrace): 0.5 mg, 1 mg, 2 mg. **INJECTION: (Cypionate):** 5 mg/ml; **(Valerate):** 20 mg/ml, 40 mg/ml. **VAGINAL TABLETS:** 25 mcg. **TRANSDERMAL:** 0.025 mg, 0.0375 mg, 0.05 mg, 0.075 mg, 0.1 mg. **VAGINAL CREAM:** 100 mcg/g.

Note: Climara is administered once weekly; others are twice weekly.

ADMINISTRATION/HANDLING
PO:
• Administer at the same time each day.

IM:
• Rotate vial to disperse drug in solution. • Inject deep IM in gluteus maximus.

Vaginal:
• Apply at bedtime for best absorption. • Insert end of filled applicator into vagina, directed slightly toward sacrum; push plunger down completely. • Avoid skin contact with cream (prevents skin absorption).

Transdermal:
• Remove old patch; select new site (buttocks an alternative application site). • Peel off protective strip to expose adhesive surface. • Apply to clean, dry, intact skin on the trunk of the body (area with as little hair as possible). • Press in place for at least 10 sec (do not apply to the breasts or waistline).

INDICATIONS/ROUTES/DOSAGE
Female hypogonadism:

IM (Cypionate): 1.5–2 mg/mo.
(Valerate): 10–20 mg/mo.

PO: 0.5–2 mg/day cyclically (3 wks on, 1 wk off).

TRANSDERMAL: Once weekly **(Climara):** 0.025–0.05 mg. Twice weekly: 0.05 mg 2 times/wk cyclically in pts with intact uterus, continuous in those without a uterus.

Vaginal/vulvae atrophy:

INTRAVAGINAL: Initially, 200–400 mcg/day (2–4 g of cream) estradiol daily for 1–2 wks; then 100–200 mcg (1–2 g) daily for 1–2 wks. **Maintenance:** After vaginal mucosa restored: 100 mcg 1–3 times/wk for 3 wks, off 1 wk per cycle.

Menopausal symptoms:

IM (Cypionate): 1–5 mg/day cyclically (3 wks on, 1 wk off). **(Valerate):** 10–20 mg q4wks.

PO: 0.5–2 mg/day cyclically or continuously.

TRANSDERMAL: 25–50 mcg 1–2 times/wk depending on product used.

Breast cancer:

PO: 10 mg 3 times/day for at least 3 mos.

Prostate cancer:

PO: 1–2 mg 3 times/day.

IM (Valerate): 30 mg q1–2wks.

Prevention of postmenopausal osteoporosis:

PO: 0.5 mg/day, cyclically (23 days on, 5 days off).

TRANSDERMAL (Climara, Vivelle): 25–100 mcg/day.

SIDE EFFECTS

FREQUENT: Anorexia, nausea, swelling of breasts, peripheral edema evidenced by swollen ankles, feet. **Transdermal route:** Skin irritation, redness. **OCCASIONAL:** Vomiting (esp. with high dosages), headache (may be severe), intolerance to contact lenses, increased B/P, glucose intolerance, brown spots on exposed skin. **Vaginal route:** Local irritation, vaginal discharge, changes in vaginal bleeding (spotting, breakthrough or prolonged bleeding). **RARE:** Chorea (involuntary movements), hirsutism (abnormal hairiness), loss of scalp hair, depression.

ADVERSE REACTIONS/TOXIC EFFECTS

Prolonged administration increases risk of gallbladder, thromboembolic disease, and breast, cervical, vaginal, endometrial, and liver carcinoma. Cholestatic jaundice occurs rarely.

NURSING IMPLICATIONS

BASELINE ASSESSMENT:

Question hypersensitivity to estrogen, previous jaundice or thromboembolic disorders associated with pregnancy or estrogen therapy. Question possibility of pregnancy (Pregnancy Category X).

INTERVENTION/EVALUATION:

Promptly report signs and symptoms of thromboembolic or thrombotic disorders: sudden severe headache, shortness of breath, vision or speech disturbance, numbness of an extremity.

PATIENT/FAMILY TEACHING:

Avoid smoking due to increased risk of heart attack or blood clots. Notify physician of abnormal vaginal bleeding, depression. With vaginal application, remain recumbent at least 30 min after application and do not use tampons. Stop taking the medication and contact physician at once if pregnancy is suspected.

estramustine phosphate sodium

es-trah-**mew**-steen
(Emcyt)

▶CLASSIFICATION

PHARMACOTHERAPEUTIC:
Alkylating agent, estrogen/nitrogen mustard. **CLINICAL:** Antineoplastic (see p. 70C)

ACTION/*THERAPEUTIC EFFECT*

Action may be due to direct effect of estrogen component or antimitotic activity. *Reduces serum testosterone concentration.*

PHARMACOKINETICS

Well absorbed from GI tract. Highly localized in prostatic tissue. Rapidly dephosphorylated during absorption into peripheral circulation. Metabolized in liver. Primarily eliminated in feces via biliary system. Half-life: 20 hrs.

USES

Treatment of metastatic or progressive carcinoma of prostate gland.

PRECAUTIONS

CONTRAINDICATIONS: Hypersensitivity to estradiol or nitrogen mustard, active thrombophlebitis or thrombolic disorders unless tumor is cause for thrombolic disorders and benefits outweigh risk. **CAUTIONS:** History of thrombophlebitis, thrombosis, or thromboembolic disorders, cerebrovascular or coronary artery disease, impaired hepatic function, metabolic bone disease in those with hypercalcemia or renal insufficiency.

▷*LIFESPAN CONSIDERATIONS:*
Pregnancy/Lactation and **Children:** Not used in these populations. **Elderly:** Age-related renal impairment and/or peripheral vascular disease may require caution.

INTERACTIONS

DRUG: Hepatotoxic drugs may increase risk of hepatotoxicity. **HERBAL:** None known. **FOOD:** None known. **LAB VALUES:** May increase SGOT (AST), LDH, bilirubin, cortisol, glucose, phospholipids, prolactin, prothrombin, sodium, triglycerides. May decrease antithrombin 3, folate, pregnanediol excretion, phosphate. May alter thyroid function tests.

AVAILABILITY (Rx)

CAPSULES: 140 mg.

ADMINISTRATION/HANDLING

PO:
• Refrigerate capsules (may remain at room temperature for 24–48 hrs without loss of potency).
• Give with water 1 hr before or 2 hrs after meals.

INDICATIONS/ROUTES/DOSAGE

Prostatic carcinoma:
PO: Adults, elderly: 10–16 mg/kg/day (140 mg for each 10 kg weight) in 3–4 doses/day.

SIDE EFFECTS

FREQUENT: Peripheral edema of lower extremities, breast tenderness or enlargement, diarrhea, flatulence, nausea. **OCCASIONAL:** Increase in B/P, thirst, dry skin, easy bruising, flushing, thinning hair, night sweats. **RARE:** Headache, rash, fatigue, insomnia, vomiting.

E

✤ - Canadian trade name   ✳ - see also www.wbsaunders.com/SIMON/SaundersNDH

ADVERSE REACTIONS/TOXIC EFFECTS

May exacerbate CHF, pulmonary emboli, thrombophlebitis, cerebrovascular accident.

NURSING IMPLICATIONS

INTERVENTION/EVALUATION:
Monitor B/P periodically.

PATIENT/FAMILY TEACHING:
Do not take with milk, milk products or calcium-rich food, calcium-containing antacids. Use contraceptive measures during therapy. If headache (migraine or severe), vomiting, disturbed speech or vision, dizziness, numbness, shortness of breath, calf pain, heaviness in chest, unexplained cough occurs, contact physician.

estropipate

ess-troe-**pie**-pate
(Ogen)

▶CLASSIFICATION

PHARMACOTHERAPEUTIC:
Estrogen. **CLINICAL:** Hormone

ACTION/THERAPEUTIC EFFECT

Increases synthesis of DNA, RNA, and various proteins in responsive tissues. Reduces release of gonadotropin-releasing hormone, reducing follicle-stimulating hormone (FSH) and luteinizing hormone (LH). *Promotes normal growth, development of female sex organs, maintaining GU function, vasomotor stability. Prevents accelerated bone loss by inhibiting bone resorption, restoring balance of bone resorption and formation.*

USES

Management of moderate to severe vasomotor symptoms associated with menopause. Treatment of atrophic vaginitis, kraurosis vulvae, female hypogonadism and castration, primary ovarian failure. Prevention of osteoporosis.

PRECAUTIONS

CONTRAINDICATIONS: Known or suspected breast cancer, estrogen-dependent neoplasia; undiagnosed abnormal genital bleeding; active thrombophlebitis or thromboembolic disorders; history of thrombophlebitis, thrombosis, or thromboembolic disorders with previous estrogen use, hypersensitivity to estrogen. **CAUTIONS:** Conditions that may be aggravated by fluid retention: cardiac, renal, or hepatic dysfunction, epilepsy, migraine. Mental depression, hypercalcemia, history of jaundice during pregnancy or strong family history of breast cancer, fibrocystic disease, or breast nodules, children in whom bone growth is not complete.

INTERACTIONS

DRUG: May interfere with effects of **bromocriptine.** May increase concentration of **cyclosporine**, increase hepatic, nephrotoxicity. **Hepatotoxic medications** may increase hepatotoxicity. **HERBAL: Saw palmetto** effects increased. **FOOD:** None known. **LAB VALUES:** May affect metapyrone, thyroid function tests. May decrease cholesterol, LDL. May increase calcium, glucose, HDL, triglycerides.

AVAILABILITY (Rx)

TABLETS: 0.625 mg, 1.25 mg, 2.5 mg. **VAGINAL CREAM:** 1.5 mg/g.

INDICATIONS/ROUTES/DOSAGE

Vasomotor symptoms, atrophic vaginitis, kraurosis vulvae:

PO: Adults, elderly: 0.625–5 mg/day cyclically.

Atrophic vaginitis, kraurosis vulvae:

INTRAVAGINAL: Adults, elderly: 2–4 g/day cyclically.

Female hypogonadism, castration, primary ovarian failure:

PO: Adults, elderly: 1.25–7.5 mg/day for 21 days; off 8–10 days. Repeat if bleeding does not occur by end of rest period.

Osteoporosis prevention:

PO: Adults, elderly: 0.625 mg/day (25 days of 31 day cycle/month).

SIDE EFFECTS

FREQUENT: Anorexia, nausea, swelling of breasts, peripheral edema evidenced by swollen ankles, feet. **OCCASIONAL:** Vomiting (esp. with high dosages), headache (may be severe), intolerance to contact lenses, increased B/P, glucose intolerance, brown spots on exposed skin. **Vaginal route:** Local irritation, vaginal discharge, changes in vaginal bleeding (spotting, breakthrough or prolonged bleeding). **RARE:** Chorea (involuntary movements), hirsutism (abnormal hairiness), loss of scalp hair, depression.

ADVERSE REACTIONS/TOXIC EFFECTS

Prolonged administration increases risk of gallbladder, thromboembolic disease, and breast, cervical, vaginal, endometrial, and liver carcinoma. Cholestatic jaundice occurs rarely.

NURSING IMPLICATIONS

BASELINE ASSESSMENT:

Question hypersensitivity to estrogen, previous jaundice or thromboembolic disorders associated with pregnancy or estrogen therapy. Question possibility of pregnancy (Pregnancy Category X).

INTERVENTION/EVALUATION:

Promptly report signs and symptoms of thromboembolic or thrombotic disorders: sudden severe headache, shortness of breath, vision or speech disturbance, numbness of an extremity.

PATIENT/FAMILY TEACHING:

Avoid smoking due to increased risk of heart attack or blood clots. Notify physician of abnormal vaginal bleeding, depression. With vaginal application, remain recumbent at least 30 min after application and do not use tampons. Stop taking the medication and contact physician at once if pregnancy is suspected.

etanercept

ee-**tan**-er-cept
(Enbrel)

▶CLASSIFICATION

PHARMACOTHERAPEUTIC: Protein. **CLINICAL:** Antiarthritic

ACTION

Binds to tumor necrosis factor (TNF), blocking its interaction with cell surface receptors (TNF is involved in inflammatory and immune responses; elevated TNF is found in synovial fluid of rheumatoid arthritis pts, *reducing rheumatoid arthritis effects.*

PHARMACOKINETICS

Well absorbed following SubQ administration. Blocks interactions with cell surface tumor necrosis factor receptors (TNFR). Half-life: 115 hrs.

USES

Reduces signs and symptoms of moderately to severely active rheumatoid arthritis (RA). Treatment of active juvenile rheumatoid arthritis.

PRECAUTIONS

CONTRAINDICATIONS: Sepsis. ***CAUTIONS:*** Avoid use in pts with infections (etanercept may cause serious infections), including tuberculosis.

▷*LIFESPAN CONSIDERATIONS:*
Pregnancy/Lactation: Unknown if excreted in breast milk. **Pregnancy Category B. Children:** No age-related precautions noted in those >4 yrs of age. **Elderly:** No age-related precautions noted.

INTERACTIONS

DRUG: None significant. ***HERBAL:*** None known. ***FOOD:*** None known. ***LAB VALUES:*** None significant.

AVAILABILITY (Rx)

POWDER FOR INJECTION: 25 mg.

ADMINISTRATION/HANDLING

Note: Do not add other medications to solution. Do not use filter during reconstitution or administration.

SubQ:

• Reconstitute with 1 ml of sterile Bacteriostatic Water for Injection (0.9% benzyl alcohol). Do not reconstitute with other diluents. • Slowly inject the diluent into the vial. Some foaming will occur. To avoid excessive foaming, do not shake or agitate vigorously, but slowly swirl contents until powder is dissolved (<5 min). • Visually inspect solution for particles or discoloration. Reconstituted solution should appear clear and colorless. If discolored, cloudy, or particles remain, discard solution; do not use. • Withdraw all the solution into syringe. Final volume should be approximately 1 ml. • Inject into thigh, abdomen, or upper arm. Rotate injection sites. • Give new injection at least 1 inch from an old site and never into area when skin is tender, bruised, red, or hard. • Refrigerate. Once reconstituted, may be stored under refrigeration for up to 6 hrs.

INDICATIONS/ROUTES/DOSAGE

Rheumatoid arthritis:

SubQ: **Adults, elderly:** 25 mg twice weekly given 72–96 hrs apart. **Children (4–17 yrs):** 0.4 mg/kg (maximum 25 mg dose) twice weekly given 72–96 hrs apart.

SIDE EFFECTS

FREQUENT (37%): Injection site reaction (erythema, itching, pain, swelling). Incidence of abdominal pain, vomiting is higher in children than adults. ***OCCASIONAL*** (4–16%): Headache, rhinitis, dizziness, pharyngitis, cough, asthenia, abdominal pain, dyspepsia. ***RARE*** (<3%): Sinusitis, allergic reaction.

ADVERSE REACTIONS/TOXIC EFFECTS

Infection (pyelonephritis, cellulitis, osteomyelitis, wound infection, leg ulcer, septic arthritis, diarrhea), upper respiratory tract infection (bronchitis, pneumonia) occurs frequently (29–38%): Formation of autoimmune antibodies may occur. Serious adverse effects occur rarely (heart failure, hypertension, hypotension, pancreatitis, GI hemorrhage, dyspnea).

NURSING IMPLICATIONS

BASELINE ASSESSMENT:

Assess onset, type, location, duration of pain/inflammation. The needle cover of the diluent syringe contains latex and should not be handled by those sensitive to this substance. If pt is to self-administer, instruct in SubQ injection technique, including areas of the body acceptable as injection sites. If a significant exposure to varicella virus has occurred during treatment, therapy should be temporarily discontinued and treatment with varicella zoster immune globulin be considered.

INTERVENTION/EVALUATION:

Assess for therapeutic response (relief from pain, improved mobility).

PATIENT/FAMILY TEACHING:

Injection site reaction generally occurs in first mo of treatment and decreases in frequency during continued therapy. Do not receive live vaccines during treatment.

ethacrynic acid ✳

eth-ah-**krin**-ick
(Edecrin)
Do not confuse with Ecotrin.

▶CLASSIFICATION

PHARMACOTHERAPEUTIC:
Diuretic. ***CLINICAL:*** Loop (see p. 84C)

ACTION/*THERAPEUTIC EFFECT*

Enhances excretion of sodium, chloride, potassium at ascending limb of loop of Henle and distal renal tubule *producing diuretic effect.*

USES/*UNLABELED*

Treatment of edema associated with CHF, severe renal impairment, nephrotic syndrome, hepatic cirrhosis; short-term management of ascites, children with CHF. *Treatment of hypertension, hypercalcemia.*

PRECAUTIONS

CONTRAINDICATIONS: Anuria, severe renal impairment. ***CAUTIONS:*** Hepatic cirrhosis, ascites, history of gout, pancreatitis, systemic lupus erythematosus, diabetes mellitus, elderly, debilitated.

INTERACTIONS

DRUG: **Amphotericin, ototoxic and nephrotoxic agents** may increase toxicity. May decrease effect of **anticoagulants, heparin.** Hypokalemia-causing agents may increase risk of hypokalemia. May increase risk of lithium toxicity. ***HERBAL:*** None known. ***FOOD:*** None known. ***LAB VALUES:*** May increase glucose, BUN, uric acid, urinary phosphate. May decrease calcium, chloride, magnesium, potassium, sodium.

ADMINISTRATION/HANDLING

PO:

• Give with food to avoid GI upset, preferably with breakfast (may prevent nocturia).

IV 🏺

Storage:

• Store vials at room temperature.
• Discard if parenteral form appears hazy or opalescent. • Dis-

E

card unused reconstituted solution after 24 hrs.

Reconstitution:

• For IV infusion, reconstitute each 50 mg ethacrynate sodium with 50 ml D_5W or 0.9% NaCl.

Rate of administration:

• For IV push, administer slowly over several mins. • For IV infusion, infuse over 20–30 min.

IV INCOMPATIBILITY ⊘

No information available via Y-site administration.

IV COMPATIBILITIES

Heparin, potassium chloride.

AVAILABILITY (Rx)

TABLETS: 25 mg, 50 mg. **POWDER FOR INJECTION:** 50 mg.

INDICATIONS/ROUTES/DOSAGE

Edema:

PO: Adults, elderly: 25–400 mg/day in 1–2 divided doses. **Children:** 1 mg/kg/dose once daily. May increase at 2–3 day intervals. **Maximum:** 3 mg/kg/day.

IV: Adults, elderly: 0.5–1 mg/kg/dose. **Maximum:** 100 mg/dose. **Children:** 1 mg/kg/dose.

SIDE EFFECTS

FREQUENT: Expected: Increase in urine frequency/volume. **OCCASIONAL:** Nausea, gastric upset with cramping, diarrhea, headache, fatigue, apprehension. **RARE:** Severe, watery diarrhea.

ADVERSE REACTIONS/TOXIC EFFECTS

Vigorous diuresis may lead to profound water loss and electrolyte depletion, resulting in hypokalemia, hyponatremia, dehydration, coma, circulatory collapse. Acute hypotensive episodes may also occur, sometimes several days after beginning of therapy. Ototoxicity may occur, esp. in those with severe renal impairment. Can exacerbate diabetes, systemic lupus erythematosus, gout, pancreatitis. Blood dyscrasias have been reported.

NURSING IMPLICATIONS

BASELINE ASSESSMENT:

Check B/P for hypotension prior to administration. Obtain baseline electrolytes (particularly check for low potassium). Assess for edema, skin turgor, mucous membranes for hydration status. Initiate I&O.

INTERVENTION/EVALUATION:

Monitor B/P, vital signs, electrolytes, I&O, weight. Note extent of diuresis. Watch for changes from initial assessment (hypokalemia may result in muscle strength changes, tremor, muscle cramps, change in mental status, cardiac arrhythmias; hyponatremia may result in confusion, thirst, cold/clammy skin).

PATIENT/FAMILY TEACHING:

Expect increased frequency and volume of urination. Eat foods high in potassium such as whole grains (cereals), legumes, meat, bananas, apricots, orange juice, potatoes (white, sweet), raisins.

ethambutol

eth-**am**-byoo-toll
(Etibi✚, Myambutol)
Do not confuse with Nembutal.

►CLASSIFICATION

PHARMACOTHERAPEUTIC:
Isonicotinic acid derivative.
CLINICAL: Antitubercular

ACTION/*THERAPEUTIC EFFECT*

Interferes with cell metabolism and multiplication by inhibiting one or more metabolites in susceptible bacteria. Active only during cell division. *Bacteriostatic.*

PHARMACOKINETICS

Rapidly, well absorbed from GI tract. Widely distributed. Protein binding: 20–30%. Metabolized in liver. Primarily excreted in urine. Removed by hemodialysis. Half-life: 3–4 hrs (half-life increased with impaired renal function).

USES/*UNLABELED*

In conjunction with at least one other antitubercular agent for initial treatment and retreatment of clinical tuberculosis. *Treatment of atypical mycobacterial infections.*

PRECAUTIONS

CONTRAINDICATIONS: Optic neuritis. ***CAUTIONS:*** Renal dysfunction, gout, ocular defects: diabetic retinopathy, cataracts, recurrent ocular inflammatory conditions. Not recommended for children under 13 yrs of age.

▷***LIFESPAN CONSIDERATIONS:***
Pregnancy/Lactation: Crosses placenta; excreted in breast milk. **Pregnancy Category B. Children:** Safety and efficacy not performed in those <13 yrs of age. **Elderly:** Age-related renal impairment may require dosage adjustment.

INTERACTIONS

DRUG: **Neurotoxic medications** may increase risk of neurotoxicity. ***HERBAL:*** None known. ***FOOD:***

None known. ***LAB VALUES:*** May increase uric acid.

AVAILABILITY (Rx)
TABLETS: 100 mg, 400 mg.

ADMINISTRATION/HANDLING
PO:
• Give with food (decreases GI upset).

INDICATIONS/ROUTES/DOSAGE
Tuberculosis:
***PO:* Adults, elderly, children:** 15–25 mg/kg/day as single dose or 50 mg/kg 2 times/wk. **Maximum:** 2.5 g/dose.

Nontuberculosis mycobacterium:
***PO:* Adults, elderly, children:** 15 mg/kg/day. **Maximum:** 1 g/day.

Dosage in renal impairment:

Creatinine Clearance	Dosage Interval
10–50 ml/min	q24–36h
<10 ml/min	q48h

SIDE EFFECTS

OCCASIONAL: Acute gouty arthritis (chills, pain, swelling of joints with hot skin), confusion, abdominal pain, nausea, vomiting, anorexia, headache. ***RARE:*** Rash, fever, blurred vision, eye pain, red-green color blindness.

ADVERSE REACTIONS/TOXIC EFFECTS

Optic neuritis (occurs more often with high dosage, long-term therapy), peripheral neuritis, thrombocytopenia, anaphylactoid reaction occur rarely.

NURSING IMPLICATIONS

BASELINE ASSESSMENT:
Evaluate initial CBC, renal and hepatic test results.

INTERVENTION/EVALUATION:

Assess for vision changes (altered color perception, decreased visual acuity may be first signs): Discontinue drug and notify physician immediately. Give with food if GI distress occurs. Monitor serum uric acid and assess for hot/painful/swollen joints, esp. big toe, ankle, or knee (gout). Report numbness, tingling, burning of extremities (peripheral neuritis).

PATIENT/FAMILY TEACHING:

Do not skip doses; take for full length of therapy (may take mos, yrs). Notify physician immediately of any visual problem (visual effects generally reversible with discontinuation of ethambutol, but in rare cases may take up to a yr to disappear or may be permanent); promptly report swelling and pain of joints, numbness/tingling/burning of hands or feet.

---

ethosuximide

(Zarontin)
See Classification section under: Anticonvulsants

---

etidronate disodium

eh-**tye**-droe-nate
(Didronel)
Do not confuse with etidocaine, etomidate.

▶**CLASSIFICATION**

PHARMACOTHERAPEUTIC: Bisphosphonate. **CLINICAL:** Calcium regulator

ACTION/*THERAPEUTIC EFFECT*

Binds to calcium phosphate surface of calcium crystals, *retarding bone resorption, bone formation. May also retard accelerated rate of bone turnover in Paget's disease.*

USES

PO: Treatment of symptomatic Paget's disease of the bone, prevention and treatment of heterotopic ossification following hip replacement or due to spinal injury. **IV:** Treatment of hypercalcemia associated with malignant neoplasms inadequately managed by dietary modification or oral hydration; treatment of hypercalcemia of malignancy persisting after adequate hydration has been restored.

PRECAUTIONS

CONTRAINDICATIONS: Children, severe renal function. **CAUTIONS:** Enterocolitis, renal impairment, pts unable to maintain adequate intake of vitamin D or calcium.

INTERACTIONS

DRUG: Antacids with **calcium, magnesium, aluminum,** foods with **calcium, mineral supplements** may decrease absorption. **HERBAL:** None known. **FOOD:** None known. **LAB VALUES:** None significant.

AVAILABILITY (Rx)

TABLETS: 200 mg, 400 mg. **INJECTION:** 300 mg amps.

ADMINISTRATION/HANDLING
IV 🏥

Storage:
• Store at room temperature.

Reconstitution:
- Must dilute with at least 250 ml 0.9% NaCl or D₅W.

Rate of administration:
- Infuse over at least 2 hrs.

IV INCOMPATIBILITY ⊘
Do not mix with other medications.

INDICATIONS/ROUTES/DOSAGE
Paget's disease:

PO: **Adults, elderly:** Initially, 5–10 mg/kg/day not to exceed 6 mos or 11–20 mg/kg/day not to exceed 3 mos. Repeat only after drug-free period of at least 90 days.

Heterotopic ossification (due to spinal cord injury):

PO: **Adults, elderly:** 20 mg/kg/day for 2 wks; then 10 mg/kg/day for 10 wks.

Heterotopic ossification (complicating total hip replacement):

PO: **Adults, elderly:** 20 mg/kg/day for 1 mo preop; follow with 20 mg/kg/day for 3 mos postop.

Hypercalcemia associated with malignancy:

IV: **Adults, elderly:** 7.5 mg/kg/day for 3 days; retreatment no sooner than 7 day intervals between courses. Follow with oral therapy on day after last infusion (20 mg/kg/day for 30 days; may extend up to 90 days).

SIDE EFFECTS
FREQUENT: Nausea, increased diarrhea, continuing or more frequent bone pain in those with Paget's disease. **OCCASIONAL:** Bone fractures (esp. femur). **Parenteral:** Metallic, altered, or loss of taste. **RARE:** Hypersensitivity reaction.

ADVERSE REACTIONS/TOXIC EFFECTS
Nephrotoxicity (hematuria, dysuria, proteinuria) noted with parenteral route.

NURSING IMPLICATIONS

BASELINE ASSESSMENT:
Obtain lab baselines, esp. electrolytes, renal function.

INTERVENTION/EVALUATION:
Assess for diarrhea. Monitor electrolytes. Check I&O, BUN, creatinine in pts with impaired renal function. Evaluate pain in pts with Paget's disease.

PATIENT/FAMILY TEACHING:
May take up to 3 mos for therapeutic response. Assure milk, dairy products in diet for calcium, vitamin D. Take medication on empty stomach, 2 hrs from food, vitamins, antacids.

etodolac

eh-**toe**-doe-lack
(Apo-Etodolac✤, Lodine, Lodine XL, Ultradol✤)

▶CLASSIFICATION
PHARMACOTHERAPEUTIC: NSAID. **CLINICAL:** Nonsteroidal anti-inflammatory analgesic (see p. 106C)

ACTION/THERAPEUTIC EFFECT
Produces analgesic and anti-inflammatory effect by inhibiting prostaglandin synthesis, *reducing*

inflammatory response and intensity of pain stimulus reaching sensory nerve endings.

PHARMACOKINETICS

Onset	Peak	Duration
PO analgesic		
30 min	—	4–12 hrs

Completely absorbed from GI tract. Widely distributed. Protein binding: >99%. Metabolized in liver. Primarily excreted in urine. Not removed by hemodialysis. Half-life: 6–7 hrs.

USES/*UNLABELED*

Acute and long-term treatment of osteoarthritis, management of pain, treatment of rheumatoid arthritis. *Treatment of acute gouty arthritis, vascular headache.*

PRECAUTIONS

CONTRAINDICATIONS: Active peptic ulcer, GI ulceration, chronic inflammation of GI tract, GI bleeding disorders, history of hypersensitivity to aspirin or NSAIDs. **CAUTIONS:** Impaired renal/hepatic function, history of GI tract disease, predisposition to fluid retention.

▷*LIFESPAN CONSIDERATIONS:*
Pregnancy/Lactation: Unknown if drug crosses placenta or is distributed in breast milk. Avoid use during last trimester (may adversely affect fetal cardiovascular system: premature closure of ductus arteriosus). **Pregnancy Category C. Children:** Safety and efficacy not established. **Elderly:** GI bleeding and ulceration more likely to cause serious adverse effects. Age-related renal impairment may increase risk of liver or renal toxicity; decreased dosage recommended.

INTERACTIONS

DRUG: May increase effects of **oral anticoagulants, heparin, thrombolytics.** May decrease effect of **antihypertensives, diuretics. Salicylates, aspirin** may increase risk of GI side effects, bleeding. **Bone marrow depressants** may increase risk of hematologic reactions. May increase concentration, toxicity of **lithium.** May increase **methotrexate** toxicity. **Probenecid** may increase concentration. **HERBAL: Feverfew, gingko biloba** may increase risk of bleeding. **FOOD:** None known. **LAB VALUES:** May increase bleeding time, creatinine, liver function tests. May decrease uric acid.

AVAILABILITY (Rx)

CAPSULES: 200 mg, 300 mg, 400 mg, 500 mg. **CAPSULES (extended-release):** 400 mg, 500 mg, 600 mg, 1,200 mg.

ADMINISTRATION/HANDLING

PO:
• Do not crush or break capsules, extended-release capsules. • May give with food, milk, or antacids if GI distress occurs.

INDICATIONS/ROUTES/DOSAGE

Note: Reduce dosage in elderly; maximum dose for pts weighing <60 kg: 20 mg/kg.

Osteoarthritis:

PO: Adults, elderly: Initially, 800–1,200 mg/day in 2–4 divided doses. **Maintenance:** 600–1,200 mg/day.

Rheumatoid arthritis:

PO: Adults, elderly: Initially, 300 mg 2–3 times/day or 400–500 mg 2 times/day. **Maintenance:** 600–1,200 mg/day.

Analgesia:

***PO:* Adults, elderly:** 200–400 mg q6–8h as needed. **Maximum:** 1,200 mg/day.

SIDE EFFECTS

OCCASIONAL (3–9%): Dizziness, headache, abdominal pain or cramps, bloated feeling, diarrhea, nausea, indigestion. ***RARE*** (1–3%): Constipation, rash, itching, visual changes, ringing in ears.

ADVERSE REACTIONS/TOXIC EFFECTS

Overdosage may result in acute renal failure. In those treated chronically, peptic ulcer, GI bleeding, gastritis, severe hepatic reaction (jaundice), nephrotoxicity (hematuria, dysuria, proteinuria), severe hypersensitivity reaction (bronchospasm, angiofacial edema) occur rarely.

NURSING IMPLICATIONS

BASELINE ASSESSMENT:

Assess onset, type, location, duration of pain or inflammation. Inspect appearance of affected joints for immobility, deformities, skin condition.

INTERVENTION/EVALUATION:

Evaluate for therapeutic response: relief of pain, stiffness, swelling, increase in joint mobility, reduced joint tenderness, improved grip strength.

PATIENT/FAMILY TEACHING:

Swallow capsule whole; do not crush or chew. Avoid aspirin, alcohol during therapy (increases risk of GI bleeding). Report GI distress, visual disturbances, rash, edema, headache.

etoposide, VP-16

eh-**toe**-poe-side
(Etopophos, VePesid)
Do not confuse with Versed.

▶ CLASSIFICATION

E

PHARMACOTHERAPEUTIC: Epipodophyllotoxin. ***CLINICAL:*** Antineoplastic (see p. 70C)

ACTION/*THERAPEUTIC EFFECT*

Induces single- and double-stranded breaks in DNA, *inhibiting or altering DNA synthesis.* Cell cycle-dependent and phase specific with maximum effect on S, G_2 phase of cell division.

PHARMACOKINETICS

Variably absorbed from GI tract. Rapidly distributed. Low concentrations in CSF. Protein binding: 97%. Metabolized in liver. Primarily excreted in urine. Not removed by hemodialysis. Half-life: 3–12 hrs.

USES/*UNLABELED*

Treatment of refractory testicular tumors, small cell lung carcinoma. *Treatment of bladder carcinoma, Hodgkin's, non-Hodgkin's lymphoma, acute myelocytic leukemia, Ewing's sarcoma, AIDS-associated Kaposi's sarcoma.*

PRECAUTIONS

CONTRAINDICATIONS: None significant. ***CAUTIONS:*** Impaired hepatic function.
▷*LIFESPAN CONSIDERATIONS:*
Pregnancy/Lactation: If possible, avoid use during pregnancy, esp. first trimester. May cause fetal harm. Breast feeding not recommended. **Pregnancy Category D. Children:** Safety and efficacy not

established. **Elderly:** Age-related renal impairment may require dosage adjustment.

INTERACTIONS

DRUG: Bone marrow depressants may increase bone marrow depression. **Live virus vaccines** may potentiate virus replication, increase vaccine side effects, decrease pt's antibody response to vaccine. **HERBAL:** None known. **FOOD:** None known. **LAB VALUES:** None significant.

AVAILABILITY (Rx)

CAPSULES: 50 mg. **INJECTION:** 20 mg/ml. **INJECTION (water soluble). Etopophos:** 20 mg/ml.

ADMINISTRATION/HANDLING

Note: Administer by slow IV infusion. Wear gloves when preparing solution. If powder or solution comes in contact with skin, wash immediately and thoroughly with soap, water. May be carcinogenic, mutagenic, or teratogenic. Handle with extreme care during preparation/administration.

IV 🖤

Storage:
• Refrigerate gelatin capsules.

VePesid:
• Store injection at room temperature before dilution. • Concentrate for injection is clear, yellow. • Diluted solution is stable at room temperature for 96 hrs at 0.2 mg/ml, 48 hrs at 0.4 mg/ml. • Discard if crystallization occurs.

Etopophos:
• Refrigerate vials. • Stable for 24 hrs after reconstitution.

Reconstitution:

VePesid:
• Dilute each 100 mg (5 ml) with at least 250 ml D_5W or 0.9% NaCl to provide concentration of 0.4 mg/ml (500 ml for concentration of 0.2 mg/ml).

Etopophos:
• Reconstitute each 100 mg with 5–10 ml Sterile Water for Injection, D_5W, or 0.9% NaCl to provide concentration of 20 mg/ml or 10 mg/ml, respectively. • May give without further dilution or further dilute to concentration as low as 0.1 mg/ml with 0.9% NaCl or D_5W.

Rate of administration:

VePesid:
• Infuse slowly, over 30–60 min (rapid IV may produce marked hypotension). • Monitor for anaphylactic reaction during infusion (chills, fever, dyspnea, sweating, lacrimation, sneezing, throat/back/chest pain).

Etopophos:
• May give over as little as 5 min up to 210 min.

IV INCOMPATIBILITIES ⊘

Cefepime (Maxipime), filgrastim (Neupogen), idarubicin (Idamycin). *Etopophos:* amphotericin (Fungizone), cefepime (Maxipime), chlorpromazine (Thorazine), methylprednisolone (Solu-Medrol), prochlorperazine (Compazine).

IV COMPATIBILITIES

Dexamethasone (Decadron), diphenhydramine (Benadryl), granisetron (Kytril), ondansetron (Zofran).

INDICATIONS/ROUTES/DOSAGE

Note: Dosage individualized based on clinical response, tolerance to adverse effects. Treatment repeated at 3–4 wk intervals.

Refractory testicular tumors:

IV: **Adults:** Combination therapy: 50–100 mg/m^2/day on days 1 to 5 or 100 mg/m^2/day on days 1, 3, 5.

Small cell lung carcinoma:

PO: **Adults:** 2 times IV dose rounded to nearest 50 mg.

IV: **Adults:** *Combination therapy:* 35 mg/m^2 daily for 4 consecutive days up to 50 mg/m^2 daily for 5 consecutive days.

Usual dose for children:

IV: 60–150 mg/m^2/day for 2–5 days q3–6wks.

SIDE EFFECTS

FREQUENT (43–66%): Mild to moderate nausea and vomiting, alopecia. ***OCCASIONAL*** (6–13%): Diarrhea, anorexia, stomatitis (redness/burning of oral mucous membranes, gum/tongue inflammation). ***RARE*** (≤2%): Hypotension, peripheral neuropathy.

ADVERSE REACTIONS/TOXIC EFFECTS

Bone marrow depression manifested as hematologic toxicity (principally leukopenia, thrombocytopenia, anemia, and, to lesser extent, pancytopenia). Leukopenia occurs within 7–14 days after drug administration, thrombocytopenia occurs within 9–16 days after administration. Bone marrow recovery occurs by day 20. Hepatotoxicity occurs occasionally.

NURSING IMPLICATIONS

BASELINE ASSESSMENT:

Obtain hematology tests prior to and at frequent intervals during therapy. Antiemetics readily control nausea, vomiting.

INTERVENTION/EVALUATION:

Monitor hemoglobin, hematocrit, WBC, platelet count. Assess pattern of daily bowel activity and stool consistency. Monitor for hematologic toxicity (fever, sore throat, signs of local infection, easy bruising, unusual bleeding from any site), symptoms of anemia (excessive tiredness, weakness). Assess for paresthesias (peripheral neuropathy). Monitor for stomatitis (redness/burning of oral mucous membranes, gum/tongue inflammation).

PATIENT/FAMILY TEACHING:

Alopecia is reversible, but new hair growth may have different color or texture. Do not have immunizations without physician's approval (drug lowers body's resistance). Avoid contact with those who have recently received live virus vaccine. Promptly report fever, sore throat, signs of local infection, easy bruising, or unusual bleeding from any site.

exemestane

x-eh-**mess**-tane
(Aromasin)

▶CLASSIFICATION

PHARMACOTHERAPEUTIC: Hormone. ***CLINICAL:*** Antineoplastic (see p. 70C)

ACTION/*THERAPEUTIC EFFECT*

An irreversible, steroidal aromatase inactivator (aromatase is the principal enzyme that converts androgens to estrogens in both pre- and postmenopausal women); acts as false substrate for aromatase enzyme; binds irreversibly to active site of enzyme, causing its inactivation. *Significantly lowers circulating estrogen concentration in postmenopausal women.*

PHARMACOKINETICS

Rapidly absorbed following PO administration. Distributed extensively into tissues. Protein binding: 90%. Metabolized in liver; eliminated in urine and feces. Half-life: 24 hrs.

USES/*UNLABELED*

Treatment of advanced breast cancer in postmenopausal women whose disease has progressed following tamoxifen therapy. *Prevention of prostate cancer.*

PRECAUTIONS

CONTRAINDICATIONS: Hypersensitivity to exemestane. ***CAUTIONS:*** None known. Do not give to premenopausal women.

▷***LIFESPAN CONSIDERATIONS:*** **Pregnancy/Lactation:** Indicated for postmenopausal women. **Pregnancy Category D. Children:** Not applicable. **Elderly:** No age-related precautions noted.

INTERACTIONS

DRUG: None significant. ***HERBAL:*** None known. ***FOOD:*** None known. ***LAB VALUES:*** May increase AST, ALT, alkaline phosphatase.

AVAILABILITY (Rx)

TABLETS: 25 mg.

ADMINISTRATION/HANDLING

PO:

• Give after a meal.

INDICATIONS/ROUTES/DOSAGE

Breast cancer:

PO: Adults, elderly: 25 mg once daily after a meal.

SIDE EFFECTS

FREQUENT (10–22%): Fatigue, nausea, depression, hot flashes, pain, insomnia, anxiety, dyspnea. ***OCCASIONAL*** (5–8%): Headache, dizziness, vomiting, edema (peripheral, leg), abdominal pain, anorexia, flulike symptoms, increased sweating, constipation, hypertension. ***RARE*** (3–4%): Diarrhea, increased sweating.

ADVERSE REACTIONS/TOXIC EFFECTS

None significant.

NURSING IMPLICATIONS

INTERVENTION/EVALUATION:

Monitor for onset of depression. Assess sleep pattern. Monitor for and assist with ambulation if dizziness occurs. Assess for headache. Offer antiemetic for nausea/vomiting.

PATIENT/FAMILY TEACHING:

Notify physician if nausea, hot flashes become unmanageable.

factor IX complex (human)

(Benefix, Heat-treated Propex T, Immunine VH✦, Konyne, Profilnine)

▶CLASSIFICATION

PHARMACOTHERAPEUTIC: Blood modifier. ***CLINICAL:*** Antihemophilic

ACTION/*THERAPEUTIC EFFECT*

Raises plasma levels of factor IX, restores hemostasis in pts with factor IX deficiency. *Increases blood clotting factors II, VII, IX, and X.*

USES

Note: Only Propex T controls bleeding in pts with factor VII deficiency. Treatment of bleeding caused by hemophilia B (deficiency of factor IX is demonstrated). Treatment of bleeding in pts with hemophilia A who have factor VIII inhibitors. Reversal of anticoagulant effect of coumarin anticoagulants.

PRECAUTIONS

CONTRAINDICATIONS: Sensitivity to mouse protein. ***CAUTIONS:*** Sensitivity to factor IX, liver impairment, recent surgery.

INTERACTIONS

DRUG: **Aminocaproic acid** may increase risk of thrombosis. ***HERBAL:*** None known. ***FOOD:*** None known. ***LAB VALUES:*** None significant.

AVAILABILITY (Rx)

INJECTION: Number of units indicated on each vial.

ADMINISTRATION/HANDLING

IV 💉

Storage:

• Store in refrigerator. • Reconstituted solution is stable for 12 hrs at room temperature. • Begin administration within 3 hrs. • Do not refrigerate reconstituted solutions.

Reconstitution:

• Before reconstitution, warm diluent to room temperature. • Gently agitate vial until powder is completely dissolved (prevents removal of active components during administration through filter).

Rate of administration:

• Administer by slow IV push or IV infusion. • Filter before administration. • Infuse slowly, not to exceed 3 ml/min. A too rapid IV may produce headache, flushing, change in B/P and pulse rate, tingling sensation. Discontinuing infusion will eliminate effects immediately. Resume IV at slower rate. • If evidence of disseminated intravascular coagulation (DIC) occurs (change in B/P and pulse rate, respiratory distress, chest pain, cough), stop infusion immediately.

IV INCOMPATIBILITY ⊘

Do not mix with any other medications.

INDICATIONS/ROUTES/DOSAGE

Note: Amount of factor IX required is individualized. Dosage depends on degree of deficiency, level of each factor desired, weight of pt, severity of bleeding. Give sufficient drug to achieve/maintain plasma level at least 20% of normal until hemostasis achieved.

SIDE EFFECTS

RARE: Mild hypersensitivity reaction (fever, chills, change in B/P and pulse rate, rash, urticaria [hives]).

ADVERSE REACTIONS/TOXIC EFFECTS

High risk of venous thrombosis during postop period. Acute hypersensitivity reaction, anaphylactoid reaction may occur. ***Antidote:*** Epinephrine 1:1,000. High dosage may produce DIC, MI, thrombosis,

---

pulmonary embolism. There is a risk of transmitting viral hepatitis, other viral diseases.

NURSING IMPLICATIONS

BASELINE ASSESSMENT:

When monitoring B/P, avoid overinflation of cuff. Remove adhesive tape from any pressure dressing very carefully and slowly. Assess results of coagulation studies and extent of existing bleeding (overt bleeding, bruising, joint pain, and swelling).

INTERVENTION/EVALUATION:

Monitor vital signs, I&O. Assess for hypersensitivity reaction (slow infusion and notify physician). Monitor results of coagulation studies closely. Avoid IM or SubQ injections or rectal temperatures. After IV administration, apply direct pressure to venipuncture site for a full 5 min or longer to assure bleeding has stopped. Monitor IV site for oozing q5–15min for 1–2 hrs after administration. Report any evidence of hematuria or change in vital signs immediately. Assess for decrease in B/P, increase in pulse rate, complaint of abdominal/back pain, severe headache (may be evidence of hemorrhage). Question for increase in amount of discharge during menses. Assess peripheral pulses; skin for bruises, petechiae. Check for excessive bleeding from minor cuts, scratches. Assess gums for erythema, gingival bleeding. Evaluate for therapeutic relief of pain, reduction of swelling, and restricted joint movement.

PATIENT/FAMILY TEACHING:

Use electric razor, soft toothbrush to prevent bleeding. Report any sign of red/dark urine, black/red stool, coffee-ground vomitus, red-speckled mucus from cough. Do not use OTC medication without physician approval (may interfere with platelet aggregation). Carry identification that indicates disease.

famciclovir

fam-**sigh**-klo-vir
(Famvir)

▶CLASSIFICATION

PHARMACOTHERAPEUTIC: Synthetic nucleoside. ***CLINICAL:*** Antiviral (see p. 58C)

ACTION/*THERAPEUTIC EFFECT*

Inhibits viral DNA synthesis, *suppressing herpes simplex virus and varicella zoster virus replication.*

PHARMACOKINETICS

Rapidly, extensively absorbed following PO administration. Protein binding: 20–25%. Rapidly metabolized to penciclovir by enzymes in gut wall, plasma, and liver. Eliminated unchanged in urine. Removed by hemodialysis. Half-life: 2 hrs.

USES

Management of acute herpes zoster (shingles), treatment or suppression of recurrent genital herpes; treatment of recurrent mucocutaneous herpes simplex in HIV pts.

PRECAUTIONS

CONTRAINDICATIONS: None significant. ***CAUTIONS:*** Renal function impairment.
▷***LIFESPAN CONSIDERATIONS:***
Pregnancy/Lactation: Increase in mammary adenocarcinoma in animals. Unknown if excreted in breast milk. **Pregnancy Category B. Children:** Safety and efficacy not established. **Elderly:** Age-related renal function impairment may require dosage adjustment.

INTERACTIONS

DRUG: None significant. ***HERBAL:*** None known. ***FOOD:*** None known. ***LAB VALUES:*** None significant.

AVAILABILITY (Rx)

TABLETS: 125 mg, 250 mg, 500 mg.

ADMINISTRATION/HANDLING

PO:

• Give without regard to meals.

INDICATIONS/ROUTES/DOSAGE

Herpes zoster:

PO: Adults: 500 mg q8h for 7 days.

Recurrent genital herpes:

PO: Adults: 125 mg twice daily for 5 days.

Suppression of recurrent genital herpes:

PO: Adults: 250 mg twice daily for up to 1 yr.

Recurrent herpes simplex:

PO: Adults: 500 mg twice daily for 7 days.

Dosage in renal impairment:

Dosage based upon creatinine clearance (ml/min):

Creatinine Clearance	Herpes Zoster	Genital Herpes
40–59	500 mg q12h	125 mg q12h
20–39	500 mg q24h	125 mg q24h
<20	250 mg q24h	125 mg q24h

Hemodialysis pts:

PO: Adults: 250 mg (herpes zoster) or 125 mg (genital herpes) following each dialysis treatment.

SIDE EFFECTS

FREQUENT: Headache (23%), nausea (12%). ***OCCASIONAL*** (2–10%): Dizziness, somnolence, numbness of feet, diarrhea, vomiting, constipation, decreased appetite, fatigue, fever, pharyngitis, sinusitis, pruritus. ***RARE*** (<2%): Inability to sleep, abdominal pain, dyspepsia, flatulence, back pain, arthralgia.

ADVERSE REACTIONS/TOXIC EFFECTS

None significant.

NURSING IMPLICATIONS

INTERVENTION/EVALUATION:

Evaluate cutaneous lesions. Be alert to neurologic effects: headache, dizziness. Provide analgesics and comfort measures; esp. exhausting to elderly.

PATIENT/FAMILY TEACHING:

Drink adequate fluids. Fingernails should be kept short, hands clean. Do not touch lesions with fingers to avoid spreading infection to new site. **Genital herpes:** Continue therapy for full length of treatment. Space doses evenly. Use finger cot or rubber glove to apply topical ointment. Avoid sexual intercourse during duration of lesions to prevent infecting partner. Notify physician if lesions do not improve or recur.

famotidine

fah-**mow**-tih-deen
(Maalox H₂ Acid Controller❖, Mylanta AR, Novo-Famotidine❖, <u>Pepcid</u>, Pepcid AC, Pepcid RPD, Ulcidine❖)

FIXED-COMBINATION(S)

With calcium carbonate and magnesium hydroxide, antacids **(Pepcid Complete)**

▶CLASSIFICATION

PHARMACOTHERAPEUTIC: H₂ receptor antagonist. ***CLINICAL:*** Antiulcer, gastric acid secretion inhibitor (see p. 88C)

ACTION/*THERAPEUTIC EFFECT*

Inhibits histamine action at H₂ receptors of parietal cells, *inhibiting gastric acid secretion (fasting, nocturnal, or when stimulated by food, caffeine, insulin).*

PHARMACOKINETICS

Rapidly, incompletely absorbed from GI tract. Protein binding: 15–20%. Partially metabolized in liver. Primarily excreted in urine. Not removed by hemodialysis. Half-life: 2.5–3.5 hrs (half-life increased with impaired renal function).

USES/*UNLABELED*

Short-term treatment of active duodenal ulcer. Prevention of duodenal ulcer recurrence. Treatment of active benign gastric ulcer, pathologic GI hypersecretory conditions. Short-term treatment of gastroesophageal reflux disease including erosive esophagitis. OTC formulation for relief of heartburn, acid indigestion, sour stomach. *Prophylaxis vs. aspiration pneumonitis. Autism.*

PRECAUTIONS

CONTRAINDICATIONS: None significant. ***CAUTIONS:*** Impaired renal/hepatic function.
▷***LIFESPAN CONSIDERATIONS:*** **Pregnancy/Lactation:** Unknown if drug crosses placenta or is distributed in breast milk. **Pregnancy Category B. Children:** No age-related precautions noted. **Elderly:** Confusion more likely to occur esp. in those with impaired renal or liver function.

INTERACTIONS

DRUG: **Antacids** may decrease absorption (do not give within ½–1 hr). May decrease absorption of **ketoconazole** (give at least 2 hrs after). ***HERBAL:*** None known. ***FOOD:*** None known. ***LAB VALUES:*** Interferes with skin tests using allergen extracts. May increase liver function tests.

AVAILABILITY (Rx)

CAPSULES: 10 mg (OTC). ***TABLETS:*** 20 mg, 40 mg. ***CHEWABLE TABLETS:*** 10 mg. ***POWDER FOR ORAL SUSPENSION:*** 40 mg/5 ml. ***INJECTION:*** 10 mg/ml, 20 mg/50 ml NaCl infusion.

ADMINISTRATION/HANDLING
PO:

• Store tablets, suspension at room temperature. • Give without regard to meals or antacids. Best given after meals or at bedtime. • Shake suspension well before use. • Pepcid RPD dissolves under tongue; does not require water for dosing.

IV ▥

Storage:

• After reconstitution, oral suspension is stable for 30 days at room temperature. • Refrigerate unreconstituted vials. • IV solution appears clear, colorless. • After dilution, IV solution is stable for 48 hrs at room temperature.

Reconstitution:

• For IV push, dilute 20 mg with 5–10 ml 0.9% NaCl, D_5W, $D_{10}W$, lactated Ringer's, or 5% sodium bicarbonate. • For intermittent IV infusion (piggyback), dilute with 100 ml D_5W, $D_{10}W$, 0.9% NaCl, or lactated Ringer's.

Rate of administration:

• IV push given over at least 2 min. • Infuse piggyback over 15–30 min.

IV INCOMPATIBILITIES ⊘

Amphotericin B complex (Abelcet, Amphotec, Ambisome), cefepime (Maxipime), furosemide (Lasix), piperacillin/tazobactam (Zosyn).

IV COMPATIBILITIES

Calcium gluconate, heparin, magnesium, potassium chloride.

INDICATIONS/ROUTES/DOSAGE
Acute therapy—duodenal ulcer:
PO: **Adults, elderly:** 40 mg at bedtime or 20 mg q12h. **Maintenance:** 20 mg at bedtime. **Children 1–6 yrs:** 0.5 mg/kg/day. **Maximum:** 40 mg.

Acute therapy—benign gastric ulcer:
PO: **Adults, elderly:** 40 mg at bedtime.

Gastroesophageal reflux disease:
PO: **Adults, elderly:** 20 mg 2 times/day up to 6 wks; 20–40 mg 2 times/day up to 12 wks in pts with esophagitis (including erosions, ulcerations). **Children 1–16 yrs:** 1 mg/kg/day in 2 divided doses. **Maximum:** 80 mg/day.

Pathologic hypersecretory conditions:
PO: **Adults, elderly:** Initially, 20 mg q6h up to 160 mg q6h.

Acid indigestion, heartburn, sour stomach:
PO: **Adults, elderly:** 10 mg 15–60 min before eating. **Maximum:** 2 tablets/day.

Usual parenteral dosage:
IV: **Adults, elderly:** 20 mg q12h. **Children:** 0.25 mg/kg q12h. **Maximum:** 40 mg/day.

Dosage in renal impairment:

Creatinine Clearance (ml/min)	Dosing Frequency
10–50	q24h
<10	q36–48h

SIDE EFFECTS

OCCASIONAL (5%): Headache. ***RARE*** (≤2%): Constipation, diarrhea, dizziness.

ADVERSE REACTIONS/TOXIC EFFECTS

None significant.

NURSING IMPLICATIONS

INTERVENTION/EVALUATION:
Monitor daily bowel activity and stool consistency. Monitor for diarrhea/constipation, headache.

PATIENT/FAMILY TEACHING:
May take without regard to meals or antacids. Report headache. Avoid tasks that require alertness, motor skills until drug response is established.

felodipine

feh-**low**-dih-peen
(Plendil, Renedil✦)
Do not confuse with pindolol, Pletal, Prinivil.

FIXED-COMBINATION(S)
With enalapril, an ACE inhibitor **(Lexxel)**

▶ CLASSIFICATION

PHARMACOTHERAPEUTIC: Calcium channel blocker. ***CLINICAL:*** Antihypertensive, antianginal (see p. 65C)

ACTION/*THERAPEUTIC EFFECT*

Inhibits calcium movement across cardiac, vascular smooth muscle. Potent peripheral vasodilator (does not depress SA, AV nodes). *Increases myocardial contractility, heart rate, cardiac output; decreases peripheral vascular resistance.*

PHARMACOKINETICS

	Onset	Peak	Duration
PO	2–5 hrs	—	—

Rapidly, completely absorbed from GI tract. Protein binding: >99%. Undergoes first-pass metabolism in liver. Metabolized in liver. Primarily excreted in urine. Not removed by hemodialysis. Half-life: 11–16 hrs.

USES/*UNLABELED*

Management of hypertension. May be used alone or with other antihypertensives. *Treatment of chronic angina pectoris, Raynaud's phenomena.*

PRECAUTIONS

CONTRAINDICATIONS: Sick-sinus syndrome/second- or third-degree AV block (except in presence of pacemaker). Severe hypotension, extreme bradycardia, CHF. ***CAUTIONS:*** Impaired renal/hepatic function, CHF. Grapefruit juice may increase concentration of felodipine.

▷ *LIFESPAN CONSIDERATIONS:* **Pregnancy/Lactation:** Unknown if drug crosses placenta or is distributed in breast milk. **Pregnancy Category C. Children:** Safety and efficacy not established. **Elderly:** Age-related renal impairment may require caution.

INTERACTIONS

DRUG: **Beta-blockers** may have additive effect. May increase **digoxin** concentration. **Procainamide, quinidine** may increase risk of QT interval prolongation. **Erythromycin** may increase concentration/toxicity. **Hypokalemia-producing agents** may increase risk of arrhythmias. ***HERBAL:*** **DHEA** may increase concentrations. ***FOOD:*** **Grapefruit/grapefruit juice** may increase absorption, concentrations. ***LAB VALUES:*** None significant.

AVAILABILITY (Rx)

TABLETS (extended-release): 2.5 mg, 5 mg, 10 mg

✐ - see color pill atlas

ADMINISTRATION/HANDLING

PO:

• Give without regard to food. • Do not crush or break tablets.

INDICATIONS/ROUTES/DOSAGE

Hypertension:

PO: Adults: Initially, 5 mg/day as single dose. **Elderly, pts with impaired liver function:** Initially, 2.5 mg/day. Adjust dosage at no less than 2 wk intervals. **Maintenance:** 2.5–10 mg/day.

SIDE EFFECTS

FREQUENT (18–22%): Headache, peripheral edema. **OCCASIONAL** (4–6%): Flushing, respiratory infection, dizziness, lightheadedness, asthenia (loss of strength, weakness). **RARE** (<3%): Paresthesia, abdominal discomfort, nervousness, muscle cramping, cough, diarrhea, constipation.

ADVERSE REACTIONS/TOXIC EFFECTS

Overdosage produces nausea, drowsiness, confusion, slurred speech.

NURSING IMPLICATIONS

BASELINE ASSESSMENT:

Assess B/P, apical pulse immediately before drug is administered (if pulse is 60/min or below, or systolic B/P is below 90 mm Hg, withhold medication, contact physician).

INTERVENTION/EVALUATION:

Assist with ambulation if lightheadedness, dizziness occur. Assess for peripheral edema behind media/malleolus (sacral area in bedridden pts). Monitor pulse rate for bradycardia. Assess skin for flushing. Monitor

liver enzyme tests. Question for headache, asthenia.

PATIENT/FAMILY TEACHING:

Do not abruptly discontinue medication. Compliance with therapy regimen is essential to control hypertension. To avoid hypotensive effect, rise slowly from lying to sitting position. Wait momentarily before standing. Avoid tasks that require alertness, motor skills until response to drug is established. Contact physician/nurse if irregular heartbeat, shortness of breath, pronounced dizziness, or nausea occurs. Swallow whole; do not crush or chew. Avoid grapefruit juice.

fenofibrate

fen-oh-**figh**-brate
(Apo-Fenofibrate, Tricor)

▶**CLASSIFICATION**

CLINICAL: Antihyperlipidemic (see p. 50C)

ACTION/*THERAPEUTIC EFFECT*

Reduces very low-density lipoprotein (VLDL) and stimulates the catabolism of triglyceride-rich lipoprotein (VLDL), *decreasing plasma triglycerides, cholesterol. Reduces serum uric acid levels* by increasing urinary excretion of uric acid.

PHARMACOKINETICS

Well absorbed from GI tract. Absorption increased when given with food. Protein binding: 99%. Rapidly metabolized in liver to active metabolite. Binds to plasma proteins. Excreted primarily in urine, lesser amount in feces. Not removed by hemodialysis. Half-life: 20 hrs.

USES

Adjunct to diet therapy in adult pts with very high elevations of serum triglyceride levels who are at risk of pancreatitis and who do not respond adequately to a determined dietary effort to control triglyceride levels. Increases HDL.

PRECAUTIONS

CONTRAINDICATIONS: Hypersensitivity to fenofibrate, severe renal or hepatic dysfunction including primary biliary cirrhosis, unexplained persistent liver function abnormality, gallbladder disease. **CAUTIONS:** Anticoagulant therapy, history of liver disease, substantial alcohol consumption.

▷**LIFESPAN CONSIDERATIONS:** **Pregnancy/Lactation:** Safety in pregnancy not established. Avoid use in nursing mothers. **Pregnancy Category C. Children:** Safety and efficacy not established. **Elderly:** No age-related precautions noted.

INTERACTIONS

DRUG: Potentiates effects of **anticoagulants.** Concurrent administration with **cyclosporine** increases risk of nephrotoxicity. Increased risk of severe myopathy, rhabdomyolysis, acute renal failure may occur with **HMG-CoA reductase inhibitors. Bile acid sequestrants** impede fenofibrate absorption (give fenofibrate 1 hr before or 4–6 hrs after bile acid sequestrant administration). **HERBAL:** None known. **FOOD:** Food increases drug absorption. **LAB VALUES:** May increase serum transaminase (AST, ALT), creatinine kinase (CK), blood urea lev-

els. May decrease hemoglobin, hematocrit, WBC, uric acid.

AVAILABILITY (Rx)

CAPSULES: 67 mg.

ADMINISTRATION/HANDLING

PO:

• Give with meals.

INDICATIONS/ROUTES/DOSAGE

Hyperlipidemia:

PO: Adults, renal function impairment (Ccr <50 ml/min): Initially, 67 mg/day given with meals. **Maximum:** 3 capsules/day (201 mg). **Elderly:** Initially, 67 mg/day.

SIDE EFFECTS

FREQUENT (4–8%): Pain, rash, headache, asthenia/fatigue, flu syndrome, dyspepsia, nausea/vomiting, rhinitis. **OCCASIONAL** (2–3%): Diarrhea, abdominal pain, constipation, flatulence, arthralgia, decreased libido, dizziness, pruritus. **RARE** (<2%): Increased appetite, insomnia, polyuria, cough, blurred vision, eye floaters, earache.

ADVERSE REACTIONS/TOXIC EFFECTS

May increase cholesterol excretion into the bile, leading to cholelithiasis. Pancreatitis, hepatitis, thrombocytopenia, agranulocytosis occur rarely.

NURSING IMPLICATIONS

BASELINE ASSESSMENT:

Obtain lipid cholesterol, triglycerides, liver function tests, including serum ALT, and blood counts during initial therapy and periodically during treatment. Treatment should be discontinued if liver enzyme levels persist >3 times normal limit.

INTERVENTION/EVALUATION:

For those on concurrent therapy with HMG-CoA reductase inhibitors, monitor for complaints of myopathy (muscle pain, weakness), including serum creatinine kinase levels. Monitor cholesterol and triglyceride concentrations for therapeutic response.

PATIENT/FAMILY TEACHING:

Periodic lab tests are essential part of therapy. Do not stop medication without consulting physician.

fenoldopam

phen-**ole**-doe-pam
(Corlopam)

▶CLASSIFICATION

PHARMACOTHERAPEUTIC:
Vasodilator (dopamine receptor agonist). **CLINICAL:** Antihypertensive

ACTION/*THERAPEUTIC EFFECT*

Rapid-acting vasodilator. An agonist for D_1-like dopamine receptor, produces vasodilation in coronary, renal, mesenteric and peripheral arteries, *reducing systolic and diastolic B/P, increase in heart rate.*

PHARMACOKINETICS

Following IV administration, metabolized in the liver. Primarily excreted in urine. Unknown if removed by hemodialysis. Half-life: Approximately 5 min.

USES

Short-term (≤48 hrs) management of severe hypertension when rapid, but quickly reversible, emergency reduction of B/P is clinically indicated, including malignant hypertension with deteriorating end-organ function.

PRECAUTIONS

CONTRAINDICATIONS: None significant. **CAUTIONS:** Glaucoma, intraocular hypertension, tachycardia, hypotension, hypokalemia, sulfite sensitivity.
▷**LIFESPAN CONSIDERATIONS:**
Pregnancy/Lactation: Unknown if distributed in breast milk. **Pregnancy Category B. Children:** Safety and efficacy not established. **Elderly:** No age-related precautions noted.

INTERACTIONS

DRUG: Concurrent use of **beta-blockers** may produce excessive hypotension. **HERBAL:** None known. **FOOD:** None known. **LAB VALUES:** May elevate BUN, glucose, transaminase, LDH. May decrease potassium.

AVAILABILITY (Rx)
INJECTION: 10 mg/ml.

ADMINISTRATION/HANDLING

Note: Must give by continuous IV infusion, not as a bolus injection.

IV ▥
Storage:
• Store ampules at room temperature. • Diluted solution is stable for 24 hrs. Discard any solution not used within 24 hrs.

Reconstitution:
• Each 10 mg (1 ml) must be diluted with 250 ml 0.9% NaCl or

D_5W to provide a concentration of 40 mcg/ml.

Rate of administration:

• Administer as IV infusion at initial rate of 0.1 mcg/kg/min. • Use infusion pump.

IV INCOMPATIBILITIES ⊘

Do not mix with any other medication. Specific IV incompatibilities not available.

INDICATIONS/ROUTES/DOSAGE
Hypertension:

IV INFUSION (continuous): **Adults:** Initially, 0.1 mcg/kg/min. **Maximum:** 1.7 mcg/kg/min. Titrate dose up or down in increments of 0.05 to 0.1 mcg/kg/min no more frequently than q15min. May discontinue gradually or abruptly.

SIDE EFFECTS

Note: Avoid beta-blockers (may cause unexpected hypotension).

OCCASIONAL: Headache (7%), flushing (3%), nausea (4%), hypotension (2%). *RARE* (≤2%): Nervousness/anxiety, vomiting, constipation, nasal congestion, diaphoresis, back pain.

ADVERSE REACTIONS/TOXIC EFFECTS

Excessive hypotension occurs occasionally; B/P must be monitored diligently during infusion. Substantial tachycardia may lead to ischemic cardiac events or worsened heart failure. Allergic-type reactions, including anaphylaxis and life-threatening asthmatic attack, in those with sulfite sensitivity.

NURSING IMPLICATIONS

BASELINE ASSESSMENT:

Determine initial B/P and apical pulse. It is essential to diligently monitor B/P and EKG during infusion to avoid hypotension and too

rapid decrease of B/P. Assess medication history (esp. beta-blockers). Obtain baseline serum electrolytes, particularly potassium, and periodically thereafter during infusion. Question asthmatic pts for history of sulfite sensitivity. Check with physician for desired B/P level.

INTERVENTION/EVALUATION:

Monitor rate of infusion frequently. Monitor B/P for tachycardia (may lead to ischemic heart disease, MI, angina, extrasystoles, worsening heart failure). Monitor closely for symptomatic hypotension.

fenoprofen calcium

fen-oh-**pro**-fen
(Nalfon)
Do not confuse with Naldecon.

▶CLASSIFICATION

PHARMACOTHERAPEUTIC: NSAID. *CLINICAL:* Nonsteroidal anti-inflammatory, analgesic, anti-gout, vascular headache prophylactic/suppressant (see p. 106C)

ACTION/*THERAPEUTIC EFFECT*

Produces analgesic and anti-inflammatory effect by inhibiting prostaglandin synthesis, *reducing inflammatory response and intensity of pain stimulus reaching sensory nerve endings.*

USES/*UNLABELED*

Treatment of acute or long-term mild to moderate pain, symptomatic treatment of acute and/or chronic rheumatoid arthritis, osteoarthritis. *Treatment of vascular headaches, ankylosing spondylitis, psoriatic arthritis.*

PRECAUTIONS

CONTRAINDICATIONS: Active peptic ulcer, GI ulceration, chronic inflammation of GI tract, GI bleeding disorders, history of hypersensitivity to aspirin/NSAIDs, history of significantly impaired renal function. ***CAUTIONS:*** Impaired renal/hepatic function, history of GI tract diseases, predisposition to fluid retention.

INTERACTIONS

DRUG: May increase effects of **oral anticoagulants, heparin, thrombolytics.** May decrease effect of **antihypertensives, diuretics. Salicylates, aspirin** may increase risk of GI side effects, bleeding. **Bone marrow depressants** may increase risk of hematologic reactions. May increase concentration, toxicity of **lithium.** May increase **methotrexate** toxicity. Probenecid may increase concentrations. ***HERBAL:*** None known. ***FOOD:*** None known. ***LAB VALUES:*** May increase serum transaminase, LDH, alkaline phosphatase, BUN, creatinine, potassium, glucose, protein, bleeding time.

AVAILABILITY (Rx)

CAPSULES: 200 mg, 300 mg. ***TABLETS:*** 600 mg.

INDICATIONS/ROUTES/DOSAGE

Note: Do not exceed 3.2 g/day.

Mild to moderate pain:

PO: Adults, elderly: 200 mg q4–6h as needed.

Rheumatoid arthritis, osteoarthritis:

PO: Adults, elderly: 300–600 mg 3–4 times/day.

SIDE EFFECTS

FREQUENT (3–9%): Headache, somnolence/drowsiness, dyspepsia (heartburn, indigestion, epigastric pain), nausea, vomiting, constipation. ***OCCASIONAL*** (1–2%): Dizziness, pruritus, nervousness, asthenia (loss of strength), diarrhea, abdominal cramps, flatulence, tinnitus, blurred vision, peripheral edema/fluid retention.

ADVERSE REACTIONS/TOXIC EFFECTS

Overdosage may result in acute hypotension, tachycardia. Peptic ulcer, GI bleeding, nephrotoxicity (dysuria, cystitis, hematuria, proteinuria, nephrotic syndrome), gastritis, severe hepatic reaction (cholestasis, jaundice), severe hypersensitivity reaction (bronchospasm, angiofacial edema) occur rarely.

NURSING IMPLICATIONS

BASELINE ASSESSMENT:

Assess onset, type, location, duration of pain or inflammation. Inspect appearance of affected joints for immobility, deformities, skin condition.

INTERVENTION/EVALUATION:

Assist with ambulation if somnolence/drowsiness/dizziness occurs. Monitor for evidence of dyspepsia. Monitor pattern of daily bowel activity, stool consistency. Check behind medial malleolus for fluid retention (usually first area noted). Evaluate for therapeutic response: relief of pain, stiffness, swelling, increase in joint mobility, reduced joint tenderness, improved grip strength.

PATIENT/FAMILY TEACHING:

Swallow capsule whole; do not crush or chew. Avoid tasks that require alertness, motor skills

F

until response to drug is established. If GI upset occurs, take with food, milk. Avoid aspirin, alcohol during therapy (increases risk of GI bleeding).

fentanyl

fen-**tah**-nil
(Actig, Duragesic)
Do not confuse with alfentanil.

fentanyl citrate

(Fentanyl Oralet, Sublimaze)

FIXED-COMBINATION(S)

With droperidol, an antianxiety, antiemetic **(Innovar)**

▶CLASSIFICATION

PHARMACOTHERAPEUTIC: Opioid, narcotic agonist **(Schedule II).** *CLINICAL:* Analgesic (see p. 116C)

ACTION/*THERAPEUTIC EFFECT*

Binds at opiate receptor sites within CNS, reducing stimuli from sensory nerve endings, *affecting pain perception, emotional response to pain.*

PHARMACOKINETICS

Onset	Peak	Duration
IM		
7–15 min	20–30 min	1–2 hrs
IV		
1–2 min	3–5 min	0.5–1 hr

Well absorbed after topical, IM administration. Transmucosal absorbed through mucosal tissue of mouth, GI tract. Protein binding: 80–85%. Metabolized in liver. Primarily eliminated via biliary system. Half-life: 3.6 hrs (half-life increased in elderly).

USES

For sedation; relief of pain, preop medication, adjunct to general or regional anesthesia. Management of chronic pain *(transdermal).* *Actig:* Treatment breakthrough for pain in chronic cancer or AIDS-related pain.

PRECAUTIONS

CONTRAINDICATIONS: Transdermal: Diarrhea, acute respiratory depression. *EXTREME CAUTION:* Bradyarrhythmias, severe CNS depression, anoxia, hypercapnia, respiratory depression, seizures, acute alcoholism, shock, untreated myxedema, respiratory dysfunction. *CAUTIONS: Transdermal:* Acute asthma attack, chronic respiratory disease, severe inflammatory bowel disease, impaired liver/renal function, increased intracranial pressure, head injury.

▷*LIFESPAN CONSIDERATIONS:* **Pregnancy/Lactation:** Readily crosses placenta; unknown if distributed in breast milk. May prolong labor if administered in latent phase of first stage of labor, or before cervical dilation of 4–5 cm has occurred. Respiratory depression may occur in neonate if mother received opiates during labor. **Pregnancy Category B** (Category D if used for prolonged periods or in high doses at term). **Children: Patch:** Safety and efficacy not established in those <12 yrs of age. Neonates more susceptible to respiratory depressant effects. **Elderly:** May be more susceptible to respiratory depressant effects. Age-related renal impairment may require dosage adjustment.

INTERACTIONS

DRUG: Benzodiazepines may increase risk of hypotension, respiratory depression. **Buprenorphine** may decrease effect. **CNS depressants** may increase CNS, respiratory depression, hypotension. **_HERBAL:_** None known. **_FOOD:_** None known. **_LAB VALUES:_** May increase amylase, lipase plasma concentrations.

AVAILABILITY (Rx)

INJECTION: 0.05 mg/ml. **_TRANSDERMAL PATCH:_** 25 mcg/hr, 50 mcg/hr, 75 mcg/hr, 100 mcg/hr. **_LOZENGES:_** 200 mcg, 300 mcg, 400 mcg.

ADMINISTRATION/HANDLING

IV

Storage:
• Store parenteral form at room temperature.

Rate of administration:
• For initial anesthesia induction dosage, give small amount, via tuberculin syringe. • Give by slow IV injection (over 1–2 min). • Too rapid IV increases risk of severe adverse reactions (skeletal and thoracic muscle rigidity resulting in apnea, laryngospasm, bronchospasm, peripheral circulatory collapse, anaphylactoid effects, cardiac arrest). • Opiate antagonist (naloxone) should be readily available.

Transdermal:
• Apply to nonhairy area of intact skin of upper torso. • Use flat, nonirritated site. • Firmly press evenly for 10–20 sec assuring adhesion is in full contact with skin and edges are completely sealed. • Use only water to cleanse site prior to application (soaps, oils, etc., may irritate skin). • Rotate sites of application. • Used patches are carefully folded so system adheres to itself; discard in toilet.

Transmucosal:
• Suck lozenge vigorously.

IV INCOMPATIBILITY ⊘

None significant.

IV COMPATIBILITIES

Diltiazem (Cardizem), dobutamine (Dobutrex), dopamine (Intropin), heparin, lorazepam (Ativan), midazolam (Versed), milrinone (Primacor), nitroglycerin, norepinephrine (Levophed), potassium chloride, propofol (Diprivan).

INDICATIONS/ROUTES/DOSAGE

Sedation (minor procedures/analgesia):
IM: Adults, elderly, children >12 yrs: 0.5–1 mcg/kg/dose; may repeat after 30–60 min. **Children (1–12 yrs):** 1–2 mcg/kg/dose. **Children <1 yr:** 1–4 mcg/kg/dose.

**Preop sedation,
adjunct regional anesthesia,
postop pain:**
IM/IV: Adults, elderly, children >12 yrs: 50–100 mcg/dose.

Adjunct to general anesthesia:
IV: Adults, elderly, children >12 yrs: 2–50 mcg/kg.

Transdermal dose:
Adults, elderly, children >12 yrs: Initially, 25 mcg/hr system. May increase after 3 days.

Transmucosal dose:
Adults, children: 200–400 mcg for breakthrough cancer pain.

Usual epidural dose:
Note: May be combined with local anesthetic (e.g., bupivacaine).

Adults, elderly: Bolus of 100 mcg, then continuous infusion rate of 4–12 ml/hr of a 10 mcg/ml concentration.

Usual PCA dosage:

Adults, elderly: Loading dose: 25–75 mcg; intermittent bolus dose: 15–50 mcg; lockout interval: 3–10 min; continuous infusion: 20–100 mcg/hr; 4 hr lockout: 200–400 mcg.

Usual transmucosal dosage:

TRANSMUCOSAL: **Adults, children:** 200–400 mcg for breakthrough cancer pain.

SIDE EFFECTS

FREQUENT: Transdermal (3–10%): Headache, itching skin, nausea, vomiting, sweating, difficulty breathing, confusion, dizziness, drowsiness, diarrhea, constipation, decreased appetite. *IV:* Postop drowsiness, nausea, vomiting. *OCCASIONAL: Transdermal* (1–3%): Chest pain, irregular heartbeat, redness, itching, swelling of skin, fainting, agitation, tingling/burning of skin. *IV:* Postop confusion, blurred vision, chills, orthostatic hypotension, constipation, difficulty urinating.

ADVERSE REACTIONS/TOXIC EFFECTS

Overdosage or too rapid IV results in severe respiratory depression, skeletal and thoracic muscle rigidity resulting in apnea, laryngospasm, bronchospasm, cold and clammy skin, cyanosis, coma. Tolerance to analgesic effect may occur with repeated use.

NURSING IMPLICATIONS

BASELINE ASSESSMENT:

Resuscitative equipment and opiate antagonist (naloxone, 0.5 mcg/kg) must be available. Establish baseline B/P and respirations. Assess type, location, intensity, and duration of pain.

INTERVENTION/EVALUATION:

Monitor B/P and respirations closely. Assist with ambulation. Encourage pt to turn, cough, and deep breathe q2h. Check for constipation; increase fluids, bulk, and exercise as appropriate. Assess for relief of pain.

PATIENT/FAMILY TEACHING:

Avoid alcohol; do not take other medications without consulting physician. Do not drive or perform other activities requiring alertness, coordination. Teach pt proper application of transdermal. Use as directed to avoid overdosage; potential for physical dependence with prolonged use. After long-term use, must be discontinued slowly.

ferrous fumarate

fair-us **fume**-ah-rate
(Feostat, Palafer✦)

ferrous gluconate

fair-us **glue**-kuh-nate
(Apo-Ferrous Gluconate✦, Fergon, Ferralet, Simron)

ferrous sulfate

fair-us **sul**-fate
(Apo-Ferrous Sulfate✦, Feosol, Fer-In-Sol✦, Slow-Fe)

FIXED-COMBINATION(S)

With docusate sodium, a stool softener **(Ferro-Sequels)**; with aluminum and magnesium hydroxide, antacids **(Fermalox)**

▶CLASSIFICATION

PHARMACOTHERAPEUTIC: Enzymatic mineral. *CLINICAL:* Iron preparation (see p. 89C).

ACTION/*THERAPEUTIC EFFECT*

Essential component in formation of hemoglobin, myoglobin, and enzymes, *necessary for effective erythropoiesis and for transport and utilization of O_2.*

PHARMACOKINETICS

Absorption increased when iron stores depleted. Primarily absorbed in duodenum, proximal jejunum and stored in hepatocytes and reticuloendothelial system. Protein binding: >90%. No physiologic system of elimination (small amounts lost daily in shedding skin, hair, nails). Not removed by hemodialysis. Half-life: 6 hrs.

USES

Prevention and treatment of iron deficiency anemia due to inadequate diet, malabsorption, pregnancy, and/or blood loss.

PRECAUTIONS

CONTRAINDICATIONS: Hemochromatosis, hemosiderosis, hemolytic anemias, peptic ulcer, regional enteritis, or ulcerative colitis. ***CAUTIONS:*** Bronchial asthma, iron hypersensitivity.
▷***LIFESPAN CONSIDERATIONS:***
Pregnancy/Lactation: Crosses placenta; excreted in breast milk. **Pregnancy Category A. Children/Elderly:** No age-related precautions noted.

INTERACTIONS

DRUG: **Antacids, calcium supplements, pancreatin, pancrelipase** may decrease absorption. May decrease absorption of **quinolones, etidronate, tetracyclines. *HERBAL:*** None known. ***FOOD:*** None known. ***LAB VALUES:*** May increase bilirubin. May decrease calcium. May obscure occult blood in stools.

AVAILABILITY (OTC)

Ferrous Fumarate: TABLETS: 63 mg, 195 mg, 200 mg, 324 mg, 350 mg. ***TABLETS (chewable):*** 100 mg. ***CAPSULES (controlled-release):*** 325 mg. ***SUSPENSION:*** 100 mg/5 ml. ***ORAL DROPS:*** 45 mg/0.6 ml.
Ferrous Gluconate: TABLETS: 300 mg, 320 mg. ***TABLETS (sustained-release):*** 320 mg.
Ferrous Sulfate: TABLETS: 195 mg, 300 mg, 324 mg. ***CAPSULES:*** 250 mg. ***TABLETS (timed-release):*** 525 mg. ***SYRUP:*** 90 mg/5 ml. ***ELIXIR:*** 220 mg/5 ml. ***ORAL DROPS:*** 125 mg/ml.
Ferrous Sulfate (exsiccated): TABLETS: 200 mg. ***CAPSULES:*** 190 mg. ***CAPSULES (timed-release):*** 159 mg, 250 mg. ***TABLETS (slow-release):*** 160 mg.

ADMINISTRATION/HANDLING

PO:

• Store all forms (tablets, capsules, suspension, drops) at room temperature. • Ideally, give between meals with water but may give with meals if GI discomfort occurs. • Transient staining of mucous membranes and teeth will occur with liquid iron preparation. Place liquid on back of tongue with dropper or straw. • Avoid simultaneous administration of antacids or tetracycline. • Do not crush sustained-release preparations.

INDICATIONS/ROUTES/DOSAGE

Note: Dosage expressed in terms of elemental iron. Elemental iron content: ferrous fumarate: 33% (99 mg iron/300 mg tablet); ferrous gluconate: 11.6% (35 mg iron/300 mg tablet); ferrous sulfate: 20% (60 mg iron/300 mg tablet).

Deficiency:

PO: Adults, elderly: 2–3 mg/kg/day in 3 divided doses. **Children 2–12 yrs:** 1–1.5 mg/kg/day in 3–4 divided doses. **Children 6 mos–2 yrs:** Up to 6 mg/kg/day in 3–4 divided doses. **Infants:** 10–25 mg/day in 3–4 divided doses.

SIDE EFFECTS

OCCASIONAL: Mild, transient nausea. ***RARE:*** Heartburn, anorexia, constipation, or diarrhea.

ADVERSE REACTIONS/TOXIC EFFECTS

Large doses may aggravate existing GI tract disease (peptic ulcer, regional enteritis, ulcerative colitis). Severe iron poisoning occurs mostly in children and is manifested as vomiting, severe abdominal pain, diarrhea, dehydration, followed by hyperventilation, pallor or cyanosis, cardiovascular collapse.

NURSING IMPLICATIONS

BASELINE ASSESSMENT:

To prevent mucous membrane and teeth staining with liquid preparation, use dropper or straw and allow solution to drop on back of tongue. Eggs, milk inhibit absorption.

INTERVENTION/EVALUATION:

Those with normal iron balance should not take iron preparation routinely. Monitor daily pattern of bowel activity and stool consistency. Assess for clinical improvement and record relief of iron deficiency symptoms (fatigue, irritability, pallor, paresthesia of extremities, headache).

PATIENT/FAMILY TEACHING:

Expect stools to darken in color. If GI discomfort occurs, take after meals or with food. Do not take within 2 hrs of antacids (prevents absorption).

feverfew

Also known as bachelor's button, featherfew, midsummer daisy, Santa Maria

▶**CLASSIFICATION**
HERBAL

ACTION/*EFFECT*

Exact mechanism unknown. May inhibit platelet aggregation and serotonin release from platelets and leukocytes. Also inhibits/blocks prostaglandin synthesis, *reducing pain intensity, vomiting, noise sensitivity with severe migraine headaches.*

USES

Fever, headache, prevention of migraine and menstrual irregularities. Also used for arthritis, psoriasis, allergies, asthma, and vertigo

PRECAUTIONS

CONTRAINDICATIONS: Pregnancy/lactation (may cause uterine contraction/abortion). Allergies to ragweed, chrysanthemums, marigolds, daisies. ***CAUTIONS:*** None significant.

▷***LIFESPAN CONSIDERATIONS:*** **Pregnancy/Lactation:** Contraindicated. **Children:** Safety and efficacy not established; avoid use. **Elderly:** No age-related precautions noted.

INTERACTIONS

DRUG: May increase risk of bleeding with **anticoagulants, antiplatelets. NSAIDs** may decrease effectiveness of feverfew. **HERBAL:** Garlic, ginger, ginkgo may increase risk of bleeding. **FOOD:** None significant. **LAB VALUES:** None significant.

AVAILABILITY

CAPSULES: 100 mg. **FEVERFEW LEAF:** 380 mg.

INDICATIONS/ROUTES/DOSAGE

Migraine headache:
PO: Adults, elderly: 50–100 mg extract/day. **LEAF:** 50–125 mg/day.

SIDE EFFECTS

Oral: Abdominal pain, muscle stiffness, pain, indigestion, diarrhea, flatulence, nausea, vomiting. **Chewing leaf:** Mouth ulceration, inflammation of oral mucosa and tongue, swelling of lips, loss of taste.

ADVERSE REACTIONS/TOXIC EFFECTS

Hypersensitivity reaction.

NURSING IMPLICATIONS

BASELINE ASSESSMENT:
Assess if pregnant/breast-feeding (contraindicated).

INTERVENTION/EVALUATION:
Assess for hypersensitivity reaction. Assess for mouth ulcers and muscle/joint pain.

PATIENT/FAMILY TEACHING:
Do not use during pregnancy/lactation. Avoid use in children.

fexofenadine hydrochloride

fecks-**oh**-fen-ah-deen
(Allegra)

FIXED-COMBINATION(S)
With pseudoephedrine, a sympathomimetic (**Allegra-D**)

▶**CLASSIFICATION**

PHARMACOTHERAPEUTIC: Piperidine. **CLINICAL:** Antihistamine (see p. 48C)

ACTION/THERAPEUTIC EFFECT

Prevents, antagonizes most histamine effects (e.g., urticaria, pruritus). *Relieves allergic rhinitis symptoms.*

PHARMACOKINETICS

Rapidly absorbed following PO administration. Does not cross blood-brain barrier. Protein binding: 20–30%. Minimally metabolized. Eliminated in feces, excreted in urine. Not removed by hemodialysis. Half-life: 14.4 hrs (half-life increased with impaired renal function).

USES

Relief of symptoms associated with seasonal allergic rhinitis (sneezing, rhinorrhea, itching of throat/eyes) in adults, children >12 yrs.

PRECAUTIONS

CONTRAINDICATIONS: None significant. **CAUTIONS:** Severe renal impairment.

▷*LIFESPAN CONSIDERATIONS:*
Pregnancy/Lactation: Unknown if drug crosses placenta or is distributed in breast milk. **Pregnancy Category C. Children:** Safety and efficacy not established in those <12 yrs of age. **Elderly:** No age-related precautions noted.

INTERACTIONS

DRUG: None significant. *HERBAL:* None known. *FOOD:* None known. *LAB VALUES:* May suppress wheal and flare reactions to antigen skin testing. Discontinue at least 4 days before testing.

AVAILABILITY (Rx)

CAPSULES: 30 mg, 60 mg, 180 mg.

ADMINISTRATION/HANDLING

PO:

• Give without regard to food.

INDICATIONS/ROUTES/DOSAGE

Allergic rhinitis:

PO: **Adults, elderly, children >12 yrs:** 60 mg 2 times/day.

Dosage in renal impairment:

PO: **Adults, elderly, children >12 yrs:** 60 mg once daily.

SIDE EFFECTS

RARE (<2%): Drowsiness, headache, fatigue, nausea, vomiting, abdominal distress, dysmenorrhea.

ADVERSE REACTIONS/TOXIC EFFECTS

None significant.

NURSING IMPLICATIONS

BASELINE ASSESSMENT:

If pt is undergoing allergic reaction, obtain history of recently ingested foods, drugs, environmental exposure, recent emotional stress. Monitor rate, depth, rhythm, type of respiration; quality and rate of pulse. Assess lung sounds for rhonchi, wheezing, rales.

INTERVENTION/EVALUATION:

Assess for therapeutic response from allergy: itching, red, watery eyes, relief from rhinorrhea, sneezing.

PATIENT/FAMILY TEACHING:

Avoid tasks that require alertness, motor skills until response to drug is established. Avoid alcoholic beverages during antihistamine therapy. Coffee or tea may help reduce drowsiness.

filgrastim

fill-**grass**-tim
(Neupogen, G-CSF)
Do not confuse with Epogen, Nutramigin.

▶CLASSIFICATION

PHARMACOTHERAPEUTIC: Biologic modifier. *CLINICAL:* Granulocyte colony stimulating factor (GCSF)

ACTION/*THERAPEUTIC EFFECT*

Regulates production of neutrophils within bone marrow. A glycoprotein, primarily affects neutrophil progenitor proliferation, differentiation, and selected end-cell functional activation *(e.g., increased phagocytic ability, antibody-dependent killing).*

PHARMACOKINETICS

Readily absorbed after SubQ administration. Not removed by hemodialysis. Half-life: 3.5 hrs.

USES/*UNLABELED*

Decrease infection incidence in pt

with nonmyeloid malignancies receiving myelosuppressive therapy associated with severe neutropenia, fever. Reduce neutropenia duration (and sequelae) in pt with nonmyeloid malignancies having myeloablative therapy followed by bone marrow transplant (BMT). Mobilization of hematopoietic progenitor cells into peripheral blood for collection by leukapheresis. Improve neutrophil recovery, reduce fever duration following chemotherapy for acute myeloid leukemia (AML). *Treatment of AIDS-related neutropenia; chronic, severe neutropenia, drug-induced neutropenia; myelodysplastic syndrome.*

PRECAUTIONS

CONTRAINDICATIONS: Hypersensitivity to *Escherichia coli*–derived proteins, 24 hrs before or after cytotoxic chemotherapy, use with other drugs that may result in lowered platelet count. ***CAUTIONS:*** Concurrent use with mycoloid properties.
▷***LIFESPAN CONSIDERATIONS:***
Pregnancy/Lactation: Unknown if drug crosses placenta or is distributed in breast milk. **Pregnancy Category C. Children/Elderly:** No age-related precautions noted.

INTERACTIONS

DRUG: None significant. ***HERBAL:*** None known. ***FOOD:*** None known. ***LAB VALUES:*** May increase alkaline phosphatase, LDH, uric acid, leukocyte (LAP) scores.

AVAILABILITY (Rx)

INJECTION: 300 mcg/ml.

ADMINISTRATION/HANDLING

Note: May be given by SubQ

bolus injection or short IV infusion (15–30 min) or by continuous SubQ or IV infusion.

SubQ:
Storage:
• Store in refrigerator, but remove before use and allow to warm to room temperature. • Aspirate syringe before injection (avoid intra-arterial administration).

IV
Storage:
• Refrigerate vials. • Stable for up to 24 hrs at room temperature (provided vial contents are clear, contain no particulate matter). Remains stable if accidentally exposed to freezing temperature.

Reconstitution:
• Use single-dose vial, do not reenter vial. Do not shake. • Dilute with 10–50 ml D_5W to concentration of 15 mcg/ml or greater. For concentration from 5–15 mcg/ml, add 2 ml of 5% albumin to each 50 ml D_5W to provide a final concentration of 2 mg/ml. Do not dilute to a final concentration of <5 mcg/ml.

Rate of administration:
• For intermittent infusion (piggyback), infuse over 15–30 min. • For continuous infusion, give single dose over 4–24 hrs. • In all situations, flush IV line with D_5W before and after administration.

IV INCOMPATIBILITIES ⊘

Amphotericin (Fungizone), cefepime (Maxipime), cefotaxime (Claforan), cefoxitin (Mefoxin), ceftizoxime (Cefizox), ceftriaxone (Rocephin), cefuroxime (Zinacef), clindamycin (Cleocin), dactinomycin (Cosmegen), etoposide (Vepesid), fluorouracil, furosemide (Lasix), heparin, mannitol, methylprednisolone (Solu-Medrol), mito-

mycin (Mutamycin), prochlorperazine (Compazine).

IV COMPATIBILITIES

Bumetanide (Bumex), calcium gluconate, lorazepam (Ativan), potassium chloride.

INDICATIONS/ROUTES/DOSAGE

Note: Begin at least 24 hrs after
last dose of chemotherapy; discontinue at least 24 hrs prior to
next dose of chemotherapy.

Myelosuppressive:

SubQ/IV or SubQ INFUSION:
Adults, elderly: Initially, 5 mcg/kg/
day. May increase by 5 mcg/kg for
each chemotherapy cycle based
on duration/severity of absolute
neutrophil count (ANC) nadir.

Note: Begin at least 24 hrs after
last dose of chemotherapy and at
least 24 hrs after bone marrow infusion.

BMT:

IV or SubQ INFUSION: **Adults, elderly:** 5–10 mcg/kg/day. Adjust
dose daily during period of neutrophil recovery based on neutrophil response.

Mobilize progenitor cells:

IV/SubQ: **Adults:** 10 mcg/kg/day
beginning at least 4 days before
first leukapheresis and continuing
until last leukapheresis.

SIDE EFFECTS

FREQUENT (57%): Nausea/vomit-
ing (57%), bone pain (22%), mild
to severe (occurs more frequently
in those receiving high dose via
IV form, less frequently in low-
dose, SubQ form), alopecia
(18%), diarrhea (14%), fever
(12%), fatigue (11%). *OCCA-
SIONAL* (5–9%): Anorexia, dyspnea, headache, cough, skin rash.
RARE (<5%): Psoriasis, hema-
turia/proteinuria, osteoporosis.

ADVERSE REACTIONS/TOXIC EFFECTS

Chronic administration occasionally produces chronic neutropenia, splenomegaly. Thrombocytopenia, MI arrhythmias occur
rarely. Adult respiratory distress
syndrome may occur in septic pts.

NURSING IMPLICATIONS

BASELINE ASSESSMENT:

A CBC, platelet count (differential) should be obtained before
initiation of therapy and twice
weekly thereafter.

INTERVENTION/EVALUATION:

In septic pts, be alert to adult
respiratory distress syndrome.
Closely monitor those with preexisting cardiac conditions.
Monitor B/P (transient decrease
in B/P may occur).

finasteride

fin-**ah**-stir-eyd
(Propecia, Proscar)
Do not confuse with Posicor,
ProSom, Prozac, Psorcon.

▶CLASSIFICATION

PHARMACOTHERAPEUTIC:
Androgen hormone inhibitor.
CLINICAL: Benign prostatic hy-
perplasia agent

ACTION/*THERAPEUTIC EFFECT*

Inhibits steroid 5-alpha reductase,
an intracellular enzyme that converts testosterone into dihydrotestosterone (DHT) in the
prostate gland, providing a reduction in serum DHT, *regressing the
enlarged prostate gland.*

PHARMACOKINETICS

	Onset	Peak	Duration
PO	24 hrs	1–2 days	5–7 days

Protein binding: 90%. Rapidly absorbed from GI tract. Widely distributed. Metabolized in liver. Half-life: 6–8 hrs.

USES

Reduce risk of acute urinary retention, need for surgery in symptomatic benign prostatic hypertrophy (BPH). Most improvement noted in hesitancy, feeling of incomplete bladder emptying, interruption of urinary stream, difficulty initiating flow, dysuria, impaired size and force of urinary stream. Treatment for hair loss.

PRECAUTIONS

CONTRAINDICATIONS: Physical handling of tablet in those who may become, or are, pregnant, exposure to semen in those who may become pregnant. ***CAUTIONS:*** Liver function abnormalities.
▷***LIFESPAN CONSIDERATIONS:*** **Pregnancy/Lactation:** Physical handling of tablet in those who may become, or are, pregnant. May produce abnormalities of external genitalia of male fetus. **Pregnancy Category X. Children:** Not indicated in children. **Elderly:** No age-related precautions noted.

INTERACTIONS

DRUG: None significant. ***HERBAL:*** None known. ***FOOD:*** None known. ***LAB VALUES:*** Produces decrease in serum prostate-specific antigen (PSA) levels (even in presence of prostate cancer).

AVAILABILITY (Rx)

TABLETS: 1 mg, 5 mg.

ADMINISTRATION/HANDLING

PO:
• Do not break or crush film-coated tablets. • Give without regard to meals.

INDICATIONS/ROUTES/DOSAGE

Benign prostatic hypertrophy:
PO: Adults, elderly: 5 mg once daily (minimum 6 mos).

Hair loss:
PO: Adults: 1 mg daily.

SIDE EFFECTS

OCCASIONAL (2–4%): Impotence, decreased libido, gynecomastia, decreased volume of ejaculate.

ADVERSE REACTIONS/TOXIC EFFECTS

None significant.

NURSING IMPLICATIONS

BASELINE ASSESSMENT:

Digital rectal exam, serum PSA determination should be performed in those with benign prostatic hypertrophy before initiating therapy and periodically thereafter.

INTERVENTION/EVALUATION:

Diligent monitoring of I&O, esp. in those with large residual urinary volume or severely diminished urinary flow for obstructive uropathy.

PATIENT/FAMILY TEACHING:

Pt should be aware of potential impotence. May not notice improved urinary flow even if prostate gland shrinks, need to take medication >6 mos, and it is unknown if medication decreases need for surgery. Because of potential risk to male fetus, a woman who is or may become pregnant should not handle tablets or be exposed to pt's semen. Volume of ejaculate may be decreased during treatment.

flavoxate

flay-**vocks**-ate
(Urispas)
Do not confuse with Urised.

▶CLASSIFICATION

PHARMACOTHERAPEUTIC: Anticholinergic. **CLINICAL:** Antispasmodic

ACTION/THERAPEUTIC EFFECT

Relaxes detrusor and other smooth muscle by cholinergic blockade, counteracting muscle spasm of urinary tract. *Produces anticholinergic, local anesthetic, analgesic effect, relieving urinary symptoms.*

USES

Symptomatic relief of dysuria, urgency, nocturia, frequency, incontinence associated with cystitis, prostatitis, urethritis, urethrocystitis, or urethrotrigonitis.

PRECAUTIONS

CONTRAINDICATIONS: GI tract obstructive disease, GI hemorrhage, paralytic ileus, obstructive uropathy. **CAUTIONS:** None significant.

INTERACTIONS

DRUG: None significant. **HERBAL:** None known. **FOOD:** None known. **LAB VALUES:** None significant.

AVAILABILITY (Rx)

TABLETS: 100 mg.

INDICATIONS/ROUTES/DOSAGE

Urinary antispasmodic:
PO: Adults, elderly, adolescents: 100–200 mg 3–4 times/day.

SIDE EFFECTS

Generally well tolerated. Side effects usually mild and transient. **FREQUENT:** Drowsiness, dry mouth, throat. **OCCASIONAL:** Constipation, difficult urination, blurred vision, dizziness, headache, increased light sensitivity, nausea, vomiting, stomach pain. **RARE:** Confusion (primarily in elderly), hypersensitivity, increase intraocular pressure, leukopenia.

ADVERSE REACTIONS/TOXIC EFFECTS

Anticholinergic effect with overdose (unsteadiness, severe dizziness, drowsiness, fever, flushed face, shortness of breath, nervousness, irritability).

NURSING IMPLICATIONS

BASELINE ASSESSMENT:
Assess dysuria, urgency, frequency, incontinence, or suprapubic pain.

INTERVENTION/EVALUATION:
Monitor for symptomatic relief. Observe elderly esp. for mental confusion.

PATIENT/FAMILY TEACHING:
Avoid driving or other tasks requiring alertness, coordination, or manual dexterity (blurred vision, drowsiness).

flecainide

(Tambocor)

See Classification section under: Antiarrhythmics (p. 13C)

floxuridine

flocks-**your**-ih-deen
(FUDR)
Do not confuse with Fludara.

▶**CLASSIFICATION**

PHARMACOTHERAPEUTIC: Antimetabolite. **CLINICAL:** Antineoplastic (see p. 70C)

ACTION/THERAPEUTIC EFFECT

Inhibits action of thymidylate synthetase, an essential component of DNA, RNA synthesis, *inducing cell death.* Cell cycle-specific for S phase cell division.

USES/UNLABELED

Palliative management of GI adenocarcinoma metastatic to liver. *Treatment of breast, cervical, ovarian, bladder, renal, prostate carcinoma.*

PRECAUTIONS

CONTRAINDICATIONS: Poor nutritional state, depressed bone marrow function (WBC <5,000/mm³ and/or platelet count <100,000/mm³), serious infection. **EXTREME CAUTION:** Previous high-dose pelvic irradiation therapy or alkylating agents, impaired liver, kidney function.

INTERACTIONS

DRUG: Bone marrow depressants may increase bone marrow depression. **Live virus vaccines** may potentiate virus replication, increase vaccine side effects, decrease pt's antibody response to vaccine. **HERBAL:** None known. **FOOD:** None known. **LAB VALUES:** May increase SGOT (AST), SGPT (ALT), alkaline phosphatase, LDH, bilirubin. Interferes with bromosulfophthalein (BSP) test, prothrombin, sedimentation rate assays.

ADMINISTRATION/HANDLING

Note: Give by continuous intraarterial infusion via catheter inserted into arterial blood supply of tumor.

• Reconstitute each 500 mg vial with 5 ml Sterile Water for Injection to provide concentration of 100 mg/ml. • Further dilute with D_5W or 0.9% NaCl to volume appropriate for specific infusion apparatus used.

IV INCOMPATIBILITY ⊘

Allopurinol (Aloprim).

IV COMPATIBILITIES

Granisetron (Kytril), ondansetron (Zofran).

AVAILABILITY (Rx)

POWDER FOR INJECTION: 500 mg.

INDICATIONS/ROUTES/DOSAGE

Note: Dosage individualized based on clinical response, tolerance to adverse effects. When used in combination therapy, consult specific protocols for optimum dosage, sequence of drug administration.

INTRA-ARTERIAL INFUSION:
Adults: 0.1–0.6 mg/kg/day (0.4–0.6 mg/kg/day for hepatic artery infusion). Continue therapy until toxicity or as long as response continues.

SIDE EFFECTS

FREQUENT: Nausea, vomiting, diarrhea, anorexia, abdominal cramping, rash, pruritus. ***OCCA-SIONAL:*** Duodenal ulcer, gastritis, glossitis, pharyngitis, ataxia, blurred vision, vertigo, weakness, mental depression, lethargy.

ADVERSE REACTIONS/TOXIC EFFECTS

Toxicity manifested as stomatitis, enteritis. Hepatic arterial infusion associated with sclerosis of bile ducts, cirrhosis of liver.

NURSING IMPLICATIONS

BASELINE ASSESSMENT:

Notify physician if intractable vomiting, diarrhea, severe stomatitis, GI bleeding occurs (drug may need to be discontinued).

INTERVENTION/EVALUATION:

Monitor blood counts diligently. Check for stomatitis (burning/erythema of oral mucosa at inner margin of lips, sore throat, difficulty swallowing). May lead to ulceration within 2–3 days. Assess intra-arterial site for signs of bleeding, infection, or catheter displacement.

PATIENT/FAMILY TEACHING:

Maintain fastidious but gentle oral hygiene. Promptly report fever, sore throat, signs of local infection, easy bruising, unusual bleeding from any site. Increase fluids.

fluconazole

flu-**con**-ah-zole
(Diflucan)
Do not confuse with diclofenac.

▶**CLASSIFICATION**
CLINICAL: Antifungal

ACTION/*THERAPEUTIC EFFECT*

Interferes with cytochrome (necessary for ergosterol formation). Fungistatic. *Directly damages fungal membrane, altering membrane function.*

PHARMACOKINETICS

Well absorbed from GI tract. Widely distributed (including CSF). Protein binding: 11%. Partially metabolized in liver. Primarily excreted unchanged in urine. Partially removed by hemodialysis. Half-life: 20–50 hrs (half-life increased with impaired renal function).

USES/*UNLABELED*

Treatment of oropharyngeal, esophageal, vaginal candidiasis, serious systemic candidal infections (e.g., urinary tract infections, peritonitis, pneumonia), *Cryptococcus neoformans* meningitis. Prevention of candidiasis in bone marrow transplants. *Treatment of coccidiomycosis, cryptococcosis, onychomycosis, fungal pneumonia/septicemia, ringworm of the hand.*

PRECAUTIONS

CONTRAINDICATIONS: None significant. ***CAUTIONS:*** Hepatic impairment, hypersensitivity to other triazoles (e.g., itraconazole, terconazole) or imidazoles (butoconazole, ketoconazole, etc.).

▷***LIFESPAN CONSIDERATIONS:***
Pregnancy/Lactation: Unknown if excreted in breast milk. **Pregnancy Category C. Children:** No age-related precautions noted. **Elderly:** Age-related renal impairment may require dosage adjustment.

INTERACTIONS

DRUG: May increase concentration,

effects of **oral hypoglycemics.** High doses increase **cyclosporine** concentration. May decrease metabolism of **phenytoin, warfarin. Rifampin** may increase metabolism. **HERBAL:** None known. **FOOD:** None known. **LAB VALUES:** May increase SGOT (AST), SGPT (ALT), alkaline phosphatase, bilirubin.

AVAILABILITY (Rx)

TABLETS: 50 mg, 100 mg, 150 mg, 200 mg. **POWDER FOR ORAL SUSPENSION:** 10 mg/ml, 40 mg/ml. **INJECTION:** 2 mg/ml (in 100 or 200 ml containers).

ADMINISTRATION/HANDLING
PO:

• Give without regard to meals. • PO and IV therapy equally effective; IV therapy for pt intolerant of the drug or unable to take orally.

IV

Storage:

• Store at room temperature. • Do not remove from outer wrap until ready to use. • Squeeze inner bag to check for min leaks. • Do not use parenteral form if solution is cloudy, precipitate forms, seal is not intact, or it is discolored. • Do not add supplementary medication.

Rate of administration:

• Do not exceed maximum flow rate 200 mg/hr.

IV INCOMPATIBILITIES ⊘

Amphotericin (Fungizone), amphotericin B complex (Abelcet, Amphotec, Ambisome), ampicillin (Polycillin), calcium gluconate, cefotaxime (Claforan), ceftazidime (Fortaz), ceftriaxone (Rocephin), cefuroxime (Zinacef), chloramphenicol (Chloromycetin), clindamycin (Cleocin), diazepam

(Valium), digoxin (Lanoxin), erythromycin (Erythrocin), furosemide (Lasix), haloperidol (Haldol), hydroxyzine (Vistaril), imipenem/cilastatin (Primaxin), sulfamethoxazole-trimethoprim (Bactrim).

IV COMPATIBILITIES

Diltiazem (Cardizem), dobutamine (Dobutrex), dopamine (Intropin), heparin, lorazepam (Ativan), midazolam (Versed), propofol (Diprivan).

INDICATIONS/ROUTES/DOSAGE
Oropharyngeal candidiasis:

PO/IV: Adults, elderly: Initially, 200 mg once, then 100 mg/day for at least 14 days. **Children:** Initially, 6 mg/kg/day once, then 3 mg/kg/day.

Esophageal candidiasis:

PO/IV: Adults, elderly: 200 mg once, then 100 mg/day (up to 400 mg/day) for 21 days and at least 14 days following resolution of symptoms. **Children:** 6 mg/kg/day once, then 3 mg/kg/day (up to 12 mg/kg/day).

Vaginal candidiasis:

PO: Adults: 150 mg once.

Candidiasis prevention:

PO: Adults: 400 mg/day.

Systemic candidiasis:

PO/IV: Adults, elderly: Initially, 400 mg once, then 200 mg/day (up to 400 mg/day) for at least 28 days and at least 14 days following resolution of symptoms. **Children:** 6–12 mg/kg/day.

Cryptococcal meningitis:

PO/IV: Adults, elderly: Initially, 400 mg once, then 200 mg/day (up to 400 mg/day). Continue for 10–12 wks after CSF becomes negative (200 mg/day for suppression of relapse in pts with

AIDS). **Children:** 12 mg/kg/day once, then 6–12 mg/kg/day; 6 mg/kg/day for suppression.

Onychomycosis:

PO: **Adults:** 150 mg weekly.

Dosage in renal impairment:

After loading dose of 400 mg, daily dose based on creatinine clearance:

Creatinine Clearance	% of Recommended Dose
>50	100
21–50	50
11–20	25
Dialysis	Dose after dialysis

SIDE EFFECTS

OCCASIONAL (1–4%): Hypersensitivity reaction (fever, chills, rash, pruritus), dizziness, drowsiness, headache, constipation, diarrhea, nausea, vomiting, abdominal pain.

ADVERSE REACTIONS/TOXIC EFFECTS

Exfoliative skin disorders, serious hepatic effects, blood dyscrasias (eosinophilia, thrombocytopenia, anemia, leukopenia) have been reported rarely.

NURSING IMPLICATIONS

BASELINE ASSESSMENT:

Establish baselines for CBC, potassium, hepatic function studies.

INTERVENTION/EVALUATION:

Assess for hypersensitivity reaction (chills, fever). Monitor hepatic function tests; be alert for hepatotoxicity. Report rash, itching promptly. Monitor temperature at least daily. Determine pattern of bowel activity, stool consistency. Assess for dizziness and provide assistance as needed.

PATIENT/FAMILY TEACHING:

Do not drive car or use machinery if dizziness, drowsiness occur. Notify physician of dark urine, pale stool, yellow skin/ eyes or rash with or without itching. Pts with oropharyngeal infections should be taught good oral hygiene. Consult physician before taking any other medication.

fludarabine phosphate

flew-**dare**-ah-bean
(Fludara)
Do not confuse with FUDR.

▶CLASSIFICATION

PHARMACOTHERAPEUTIC: Antimetabolite. *CLINICAL:* Antineoplastic (see p. 70C)

ACTION/*THERAPEUTIC EFFECT*

Interferes with DNA polymerase alpha, ribonucleotide reductase, and DNA primase, *inhibiting DNA synthesis, inducing cell death.*

PHARMACOKINETICS

Rapidly dephosphorylated in serum, then phosphorylated intracellularly to active triphosphate. Primarily excreted in urine. Half-life: 10 hrs.

USES

Treatment of chronic lymphocytic leukemia in those who have not responded to or have progressed with another standard alkylating agent.

PRECAUTIONS

CONTRAINDICATIONS: None significant. *CAUTIONS:* Impaired renal function.

F

▷*LIFESPAN CONSIDERATIONS:*
Pregnancy/Lactation: If possible, avoid use during pregnancy, esp. first trimester. May cause fetal harm. Not known whether distributed in breast milk. Breast feeding not recommended. **Pregnancy Category D. Children:** Safety and efficacy not established. **Elderly:** Age-related renal impairment may require dosage adjustment.

INTERACTIONS

DRUG: May decrease effect of **antigout** medications. **Bone marrow depressants** may increase risk of bone marrow depression. **Live virus vaccines** may potentiate virus replication, increase vaccine side effects, decrease pt's antibody response to vaccine. **HERBAL:** None known. **FOOD:** None known. **LAB VALUES:** May increase uric acid, alkaline phosphatase, SGOT (AST).

AVAILABILITY (Rx)

INJECTION: 50 mg.

ADMINISTRATION/HANDLING

Note: Give by IV infusion. Do not add to other IV infusions. Avoid small veins, swollen or edematous extremities, areas overlying joints, tendons.

IV 🏥

Storage:
• Store in refrigerator. • Handle with extreme care during preparation and administration. If contact with skin or mucous membranes, wash thoroughly with soap and water; rinse eyes profusely with plain water. • After reconstitution, use within 8 hrs; discard unused portion.

Reconstitution:
• Reconstitute 50 mg vial with 2 ml Sterile Water for Injection to provide a concentration of 25 mg/ml. • Further dilute with 100–125 ml 0.9% NaCl or D₅W.

Rate of administration:
• Infuse over 30 min.

IV INCOMPATIBILITIES ⊘

Acyclovir (Zovirax), amphotericin (Fungizone), hydroxyzine (Vistaril), prochlorperazine (Compazine).

IV COMPATIBILITIES

Heparin, lorazepam (Ativan), magnesium, multivitamins, potassium chloride.

INDICATIONS/ROUTES/DOSAGE

Note: Dosage is individualized on basis of clinical response and tolerance to adverse effects. When used in combination therapy, consult specific protocols for optimum dosage, sequence of drug administration. Dosage based on pt's actual weight. Use ideal body weight in obese or edematous pts.

Chronic lymphocytic leukemia:

IV: Adults: 25 mg/m² daily for 5 consecutive days. Continue up to 3 additional cycles. Begin each course of treatment q28days.

Acute leukemia:

IV: Children: 10 mg/m² bolus (over 15 min), then IV infusion of 30.5 mg/m²/day.

Solid tumors:

IV: Children: 9 mg/m² bolus, then 27 mg/m²/day for 5 days as continuous infusion.

SIDE EFFECTS

FREQUENT: Fever (60%), nausea/vomiting (36%), chills (11%). **OCCASIONAL** (10–20%): Fatigue, generalized pain, rash, diarrhea, cough, weakness, stomatitis (burning/erythema of oral mucosa, sore throat, difficulty swallowing), dyspnea, weakness, peripheral edema. **RARE** (3–7%): Anorexia, sinusitis, dysuria, myalgia, paresthesia, headaches, visual disturbances.

ADVERSE REACTIONS/TOXIC EFFECTS

Pneumonia occurs frequently. Severe bone marrow toxicity (anemia, thrombocytopenia, neutropenia) may occur. Tumor lysis syndrome may occur with onset of flank pain, hematuria. This syndrome may include hypercalcemia, hyperphosphatemia, hyperuricemia and result in renal failure. GI bleeding may occur. High dosage may produce acute leukemia, blindness, coma.

NURSING IMPLICATIONS

BASELINE ASSESSMENT:

Assess baseline CBC, platelet, serum creatinine. Drug should be discontinued if intractable vomiting, diarrhea, stomatitis, GI bleeding occurs.

INTERVENTION/EVALUATION:

Assess for weakness, visual disturbances, peripheral edema. Assess for onset of pneumonia. Monitor for dyspnea, cough, rapidly falling WBC and/or intractable diarrhea, GI bleeding (bright red or tarry stool). Assess oral mucosa for mucosal erythema, ulceration at inner margin of lips, sore throat, difficulty swallowing (stomatitis). Assess skin for rash. Be alert to possible tumor lysis syndrome (onset with flank pain and hematuria).

PATIENT/FAMILY TEACHING:

Avoid crowds and exposure to infection. Maintain fastidious oral hygiene. Promptly report fever, sore throat, signs of local infection, easy bruising, unusual bleeding from any site. Contact physician if nausea/vomiting continues at home.

fludrocortisone

floo-droe-**kor**-tih-sone
(Florinef)
Do not confuse with Fiorinal.

▶CLASSIFICATION

PHARMACOTHERAPEUTIC: Mineralocorticoid. ***CLINICAL:*** Glucocorticosteroid (see p. 79C)

ACTION/*THERAPEUTIC EFFECT*

Acts at distal tubules to *increase potassium, hydrogen ion excretion, sodium reabsorption, and water retention.*

PHARMACOKINETICS

Well absorbed from GI tract. Widely distributed. Metabolized in liver, kidney. Primarily excreted in urine. Half-life: 3.5 hrs.

USES/*UNLABELED*

Partial replacement therapy for primary and secondary adrenocortical insufficiency in Addison's disease. Adjunctive treatment of salt-losing forms of congenital adrenogenital syndrome. *Treatment of idiopathic orthostatic hypotension, acidosis in renal tubular disorders.*

PRECAUTIONS

CONTRAINDICATIONS: Any condition except those requiring high mineralocorticoid activity. ***CAUTIONS:*** CHF, hypertension, renal insufficiency. Prolonged therapy should be discontinued slowly.

▷**LIFESPAN CONSIDERATIONS:**
Pregnancy/Lactation: Not known whether drug crosses placenta or is distributed in breast milk. **Pregnancy Category C. Children:** May cause growth suppression and inhibition of endogenous steroid production. **Elderly:** Studies in elderly not performed.

INTERACTIONS

DRUG: May increase **digoxin** toxicity (hypokalemia). **Hepatic enzyme inducers (e.g., phenytoin)** may increase metabolism. **Hypokalemia-causing medications** may increase effect. **Sodium-containing medication** may increase sodium, edema, B/P. **HERBAL:** None known. **FOOD:** None known. **LAB VALUES:** May increase sodium. May decrease potassium, hematocrit.

AVAILABILITY (Rx)
TABLETS: 0.1 mg.

ADMINISTRATION/HANDLING
PO:
• Give with food or milk.

INDICATIONS/ROUTES/DOSAGE
Addison's disease:
PO: Adults, elderly: 0.05–0.1 mg/day. **Range:** 0.1 mg 3 times/wk–0.2 mg/day. Administration with cortisone/hydrocortisone preferred.

Salt-losing adrenogenital syndrome:
PO: Adults, elderly: 0.1–0.2 mg/day.

Usual pediatric dosage:
PO: 0.05–0.1 mg/day.

SIDE EFFECTS
FREQUENT: Increased appetite, exaggerated sense of well-being, abdominal distention, weight gain, insomnia, mood swings. *High-dose, prolonged therapy, too rapid withdrawal:* Increased susceptibility to infection (signs/symptoms masked); delayed wound healing, hypokalemia, hypocalcemia, GI distress, diarrhea or constipation, hypertension. **OCCASIONAL:** Headache (frontal or occipital), dizziness, menstrual difficulty or amenorrhea, ulcer development. **RARE:** Hypersensitivity reaction.

ADVERSE REACTIONS/TOXIC EFFECTS

Long-term therapy: Muscle wasting (esp. arms, legs), osteoporosis, spontaneous fractures, amenorrhea, cataracts, glaucoma, peptic ulcer, CHF. **Abrupt withdrawal following long-term therapy:** Anorexia, nausea, fever, headache, joint pain, rebound inflammation, fatigue, weakness, lethargy, dizziness, orthostatic hypotension.

NURSING IMPLICATIONS

BASELINE ASSESSMENT:
Obtain baselines for weight, B/P, blood glucose, electrolytes, chest x-ray, EKG.

INTERVENTION/EVALUATION:
Monitor I&O, daily weight. Check B/P, pulse at least 2 times/day. Assess for signs of edema. Monitor blood glucose and electrolytes. Be alert to signs/symptoms of hypokalemia (weakness and muscle cramps, numbness/tingling, esp. lower extremities, nausea and vomiting, irritability, EKG changes). Evaluate food tolerance and bowel activity; report hyperacidity promptly. Assess emotional status, ability to sleep. Assess for

infection: fever, sore throat, vague symptoms.

PATIENT/FAMILY TEACHING:
Do not change dose/schedule or stop taking drug; must taper off gradually. Report fever, sore throat, muscle aches, sudden weight gain/swelling, continuing headaches. Maintain careful personal hygiene, avoid exposure to disease or trauma. Severe stress (serious infection, surgery, or trauma) may require increased dosage.

flumazenil

flew-**maz**-ah-nil
(Anexate ✤, Romazicon)

▶CLASSIFICATION
PHARMACOTHERAPEUTIC:
Benzodiazepine receptor antagonist. ***CLINICAL:*** Antidote

ACTION/*THERAPEUTIC EFFECT*
Antagonizes sedation, impairment of recall and psychomotor impairment due to benzodiazepine activity on CNS.

PHARMACOKINETICS

	Onset	Peak	Duration
IV	1–2 min	6–10 min	—

Duration, degree of benzodiazepine reversal related to dosage, plasma concentration. Protein binding: 50%. Metabolized by liver; excreted in urine.

USES
Complete or partial reversal of sedative effects of benzodiazepines when general anesthesia has been induced and/or maintained with benzodiazepines, when sedation has been produced with benzodiazepines for diagnostic and therapeutic procedures, management of benzodiazepine overdosage.

PRECAUTIONS
CONTRAINDICATIONS: History of hypersensitivity to benzodiazepines, in those who have been given a benzodiazepine for control of a potentially life-threatening condition (control of intracranial pressure, status epilepticus), those showing signs of serious cyclic antidepressant overdose manifested by motor abnormalities, dysrhythmias, anticholinergic signs, cardiovascular collapse.
CAUTIONS: Head injury, impaired hepatic function, alcoholism, drug dependency.

▷*LIFESPAN CONSIDERATIONS:*
Pregnancy/Lactation: Not known whether drug crosses placenta or is distributed in breast milk. Not recommended during labor, delivery. **Pregnancy Category C. Children:** Not approved for neonates/infants. **Elderly:** Benzodiazepine-induced sedation tends to be deeper and more prolonged requiring careful monitoring.

INTERACTIONS
DRUG: **Seizure-induced medications** may increase risk of seizures. ***HERBAL:*** None knonw. ***FOOD:*** None known. ***LAB VALUES:*** None significant.

AVAILABILITY (Rx)
INJECTION: 0.1 mg/ml.

ADMINISTRATION/HANDLING

Note: Compatible with D$_5$W, lactated Ringer's, 0.9% NaCl.

IV ⚠

Storage:

• Store parenteral form at room temperature. • Discard after 24 hrs once medication is drawn into syringe, is mixed with any solutions, or if particulate or discoloration is noted. • Rinse spilled medication from skin with cool water.

Rate of administration:

• *Reverse conscious sedation or general anesthesia:* Give over 15 sec. • *Benzodiazepine overdose:* Give over 30 sec. • Administer through freely running IV infusion into large vein (local injection produces pain, inflammation at injection site).

IV INCOMPATIBILITY ⊘

No information available via Y-site administration.

INDICATIONS/ROUTES/DOSAGE

Reversal of conscious sedation, in general anesthesia:

***IV:* Adults, elderly:** Initially, 0.2 mg (2 ml) over 15 sec; may repeat 0.2 mg dose in 45 sec; then at 60 sec intervals. **Maximum:** 1 mg (10 ml total dose).

Note: If resedation occurs, repeat dose at 20 min intervals. **Maximum:** 1 mg (given as 0.2 mg/min) at any one time, 3 mg in any 1 hr.

Benzodiazepine overdose:

***IV:* Adults, elderly:** Initially, 0.2 mg (2 ml) over 30 sec; may repeat after 30 sec with 0.3 mg (3 ml) over 30 sec if desired LOC not achieved. Further doses of 0.5 mg (5 ml) over 30 sec may be administered at 60 sec intervals. **Maximum:** 3 mg (30 ml) total dose.

Note: If resedation occurs, repeat dose at 20 min intervals. **Maximum:** 1 mg (given as 0.5 mg/min) at any one time, 3 mg in any 1 hr.

Usual dosage for children:

IV: Initially, 0.01 mg/kg (**Maximum:** 2 mg). May repeat in 45 seconds, then at 60 second intervals. **Maximum cumulative dose:** 1 mg.

SIDE EFFECTS

FREQUENT (3–11%): Agitation, anxiety, dry mouth, dyspnea, insomnia, palpitations, tremors, headache, blurred vision, dizziness, ataxia, nausea, vomiting, pain at injection site, increased sweating. ***OCCASIONAL*** (1–3%): Fatigue, flushing, hearing disturbances, thrombophlebitis, skin rash. ***RARE*** (<1%): Hives, itching, hallucinations.

ADVERSE REACTIONS/TOXIC EFFECTS

May produce onset of seizures (particularly those on long-term benzodiazepine use), overdosage, concurrent sedative-hypnotic drug withdrawal, recent therapy with repeated doses of parenteral benzodiazepine, myoclonic jerking, concurrent cyclic antidepressant poisoning. May provoke panic attack in those with history of panic disorder.

NURSING IMPLICATIONS

BASELINE ASSESSMENT:

Arterial blood gases should be obtained before and at 30 min intervals during IV administration. Prepare to intervene in reestablishing airway, assisting ventilation (drug may not fully reverse ventilatory insufficiency induced by benzodiazepines). Note that effects of flumazenil may wear off before effects of benzodiazepines.

INTERVENTION/EVALUATION:

Properly manage airway, assisted breathing, circulatory access and support, internal decontamination by lavage and charcoal, adequate clinical evaluation. Monitor for reversal of benzodiazepine effect. Assess for possible resedation, respiratory depression, hypoventilation. Assess closely for return of unconsciousness (narcosis) for at least 1 hr after pt is fully alert.

PATIENT/FAMILY TEACHING:

Avoid tasks that require alertness, motor skills, ingestion of alcohol, or taking nonprescription drugs until at least 18–24 hrs after discharge.

---

flunisolide

flew-**nis**-oh-lide
(AeroBid, Bronalide aerosol✸,
Nasalide, Nasarel, Rhinalar✸)
Do not confuse with
fluocinonide, Nasalcrom.

▶**CLASSIFICATION**

PHARMACOTHERAPEUTIC:
Adrenocorticosteroid. ***CLINI-CAL:*** Antiasthmatic, anti-inflammatory (see pp. 64C, 79C)

ACTION/*THERAPEUTIC EFFECT*

Decreases number, activity of anti-inflammatory cells. *Inhibits bronchoconstriction, produces smooth muscle relaxation. Decreases immediate and late-phase allergic reactions.*

USES/*UNLABELED*

Inhalation: Control of bronchial asthma in those requiring chronic steroid therapy. ***Intranasal:*** Relief of symptoms of seasonal/perennial rhinitis. *Prevent recurrence of postsurgical nasal polyps.*

PRECAUTIONS

CONTRAINDICATIONS: Hypersensitivity to any corticosteroid, primary treatment of status asthmaticus, systemic fungal infections, persistently positive sputum cultures for *Candida albicans*. ***CAUTIONS:*** Adrenal insufficiency.

INTERACTIONS

DRUG: None significant. ***HERBAL:*** None known. ***FOOD:*** None known. ***LAB VALUES:*** None significant.

AVAILABILITY (Rx)

AEROSOL: 250 mcg/activation. ***NASAL SPRAY:*** 25 mcg/activation.

ADMINISTRATION/HANDLING
Inhalation:

• Shake container well; exhale as completely as possible. • Place mouthpiece fully into mouth, holding inhaler upright, inhale deeply and slowly while pressing the top of the cannister and hold breath as long as possible before exhaling; then exhale slowly. • Wait 1 min between inhalations when multiple inhalations ordered (allows for deeper bronchial penetration). • Rinse mouth with water immediately after inhalation (prevents mouth/throat dryness).

Intranasal:

• Clear nasal passages before use (topical nasal decongestants may be needed 5–15 min before use). • Tilt head slightly forward. • In-

---

sert spray tip up in 1 nostril, pointing toward inflamed nasal turbinates, away from nasal septum. • Pump medication into 1 nostril while holding other nostril closed and concurrently inspire through nose. • Discard used nasal solution after 3 mos.

INDICATIONS/ROUTES/DOSAGE

Usual inhalation dosage:

INHALATION: **Adults, elderly:** 2 inhalations 2 times/day, morning and evening. **Maximum:** 4 inhalations 2 times/day. **Children (6–15 yrs):** 2 inhalations 2 times/day.

Usual intranasal dosage:

Note: Improvement seen within few days; may take 3 wks. Do not continue beyond 3 wks if no significant improvement occurs.

INTRANASAL: **Adults, elderly:** Initially, 2 sprays each nostril 2 times/day, may increase to 2 sprays 3 times/day. **Maximum:** 8 sprays each nostril/day. **Children (6–14 yrs):** Initially, 1 spray 3 times/day or 2 sprays 2 times/day. **Maximum:** 4 sprays each nostril/day. **Maintenance:** Smallest amount to control symptoms.

SIDE EFFECTS

FREQUENT: Inhalation (10–25%): Unpleasant taste, nausea, vomiting, sore throat, diarrhea, upset stomach, cold symptoms, nasal congestion. ***OCCASIONAL: Inhalation*** (3–9%): Dizziness, irritability, nervousness, shakiness, abdominal pain, heartburn, fungal infection in mouth, pharynx, larynx, edema. ***Intranasal:*** Mild nasopharyngeal irritation, dryness, rebound congestion, bronchial asthma, rhinorrhea, loss of sense of taste.

ADVERSE REACTIONS/TOXIC EFFECTS

Acute hypersensitivity reaction (urticaria, angioedema, severe bronchospasm) occurs rarely. Transfer from systemic to local steroid therapy may unmask previously suppressed bronchial asthma condition.

F

NURSING IMPLICATIONS

BASELINE ASSESSMENT:

Establish baseline assessment of asthma, rhinitis.

INTERVENTION/EVALUATION:

In those receiving bronchodilators by inhalation concomitantly with steroid inhalation therapy, advise pts to use bronchodilator several mins before corticosteroid aerosol (enhances penetration of steroid into bronchial tree). Monitor rate, depth, rhythm, type of respiration; quality and rate of pulse. Assess lung sounds for rhonchi, wheezing, rales. Monitor arterial blood gases.

PATIENT/FAMILY TEACHING:

Do not change dose schedule or stop taking drug; must taper off gradually under medical supervision. Maintain careful mouth hygiene. Rinse mouth with water immediately after inhalation (prevents mouth/throat dryness, fungal infection of mouth). Increase fluid intake (decreases lung secretion viscosity). ***Intranasal:*** Teach proper use of nasal spray. Clear nasal passages prior to use. Contact physician if no improvement in symptoms, sneezing or nasal irritation occur. Improvement noted in several days.

fluocinolone acetonide

(Flurosyn, Synalar, Synemol)

fluocinonide

(Lidex, Vasoderm)

See Classification section under: Corticosteroids: topical (p. 81C)

fluoride

flur-eyd
(Fluor-A-Day✦, Fluoritab, Fluotic✦, Luride)

▶CLASSIFICATION

PHARMACOTHERAPEUTIC:
Trace element. *CLINICAL:* Dietary supplement

ACTION/*THERAPEUTIC EFFECT*

Increases tooth resistance to acid dissolution by *promoting remineralization of decalcified enamel, inhibiting dental plaque bacteria, increasing resistance to development of caries.* Maintains bone strength.

USES

Dietary supplement for prevention of dental caries in children.

PRECAUTIONS

CONTRAINDICATIONS: Arthralgia, GI ulceration, severe renal insufficiency. *CAUTIONS:* None significant.

INTERACTIONS

DRUG: **Aluminum hydroxide, calcium** may decrease absorption. *HERBAL:* None known. *FOOD:* None known. *LAB VALUES:*

May increase SGOT (AST), alkaline phosphatase.

AVAILABILITY (Rx)

TABLETS (chewable): 0.25 mg, 0.5 mg, 1 mg. *TABLETS:* 1 mg. *DROPS:* 0.125 mg/drop; 0.25 mg/drop; 0.5 mg/ml.

INDICATIONS/ROUTES/DOSAGE

Dietary supplement:

Water Fluoride	Age	mg/Day
<0.3 ppm	<2 yrs	0.25 mg/day
	2–3 yrs	0.5 mg/day
	3–13 yrs	1 mg/day
0.3–0.7 ppm	<2 yrs	None
	2–3 yrs	0.25 mg/day
	3–13 yrs	0.5 mg/day
>0.7 ppm	None	None

SIDE EFFECTS

RARE: Oral mucous membrane ulceration.

ADVERSE REACTIONS/TOXIC EFFECTS

Hypocalcemia, tetany, bone pain (esp. ankles, feet), electrolyte disturbances, arrhythmias occur rarely. May cause skeletal fluorosis, osteomalacia, osteosclerosis.

NURSING IMPLICATIONS

PATIENT/FAMILY TEACHING:

Do not take with milk or other dairy products (decreases absorption). Rinses and gels should be used at bedtime after brushing or flossing. Expectorate excess—do not swallow. Do not eat, drink, or rinse mouth after application.

fluorouracil

phlur-oh-**your**-ah-sill
(Adrucil, Efudex, Fluoroplex)
Do not confuse with Efidac.

▶CLASSIFICATION

PHARMACOTHERAPEUTIC:
Antimetabolite. ***CLINICAL:*** Antineoplastic (see p. 70C)

ACTION/*THERAPEUTIC EFFECT*

Blocks formation of thymidylic acid, *inhibiting DNA, RNA synthesis. Topical:* Destroys rapidly proliferating cells. Cell cycle-specific for S phase of cell division.

PHARMACOKINETICS

Crosses blood-brain barrier. Widely distributed. Rapidly metabolized in tissues to active metabolite, which is localized intracellularly. Primarily excreted via lungs as CO_2. Removed by hemodialysis. Half-life: 20 hrs.

USES/*UNLABELED*

Parenteral: Treatment of carcinoma of colon, rectum, breast, stomach, pancreas. Used in combination with levamisole after surgical resection in pts with Duke's stage C colon cancer. ***Topical:*** Treatment of multiple actinic or solar keratoses, superficial basal cell carcinomas. ***Parenteral:*** *Treatment of bladder, prostate, ovarian, cervical, endometrial, lung, liver, head/neck carcinomas; treatment of pericardial, peritoneal, pleural effusions.* ***Topical:*** *Treatment of actinic cheilitis, radiodermatitis.*

PRECAUTIONS

CONTRAINDICATIONS: Poor nutritional status, depressed bone marrow function, potentially serious infections, major surgery within previous mo. ***CAUTIONS:*** History of high-dose pelvic irradiation, metastatic cell infiltration of bone marrow, impaired hepatic, renal function.

▷*LIFESPAN CONSIDERATIONS:*
Pregnancy/Lactation: If possible, avoid use during pregnancy, esp. first trimester. May cause fetal harm. Not known whether distributed in breast milk. Breast feeding not recommended. **Pregnancy Category D. Children:** No age-related precautions noted. **Elderly:** Age-related renal impairment may require dosage adjustment.

INTERACTIONS

DRUG: **Bone marrow depressant** may increase risk of bone marrow depression. **Live virus vaccines** may potentiate virus replication, increase vaccine side effects, decrease pt's antibody response to vaccine. ***HERBAL:*** None known. ***FOOD:*** None known. ***LAB VALUES:*** May decrease albumin. May increase excretion of 5-HIAA in urine. ***Topical:*** May cause eosinophilia, leukocytosis, thrombocytopenia, toxic granulation.

AVAILABILITY (Rx)

INJECTION: 50 mg/ml. ***CREAM:*** 1%, 5%. ***TOPICAL SOLUTION:*** 1%, 2%, 5%.

ADMINISTRATION/HANDLING

Note: Give by IV injection or IV infusion. Do not add to other IV infusions. Avoid small veins, swollen or edematous extremities, areas overlying joints, tendons. May be carcinogenic, mutagenic, or teratogenic. Handle with extreme care during preparation/administration.

IV 💊

Storage:

• Solution appears colorless to faint yellow. Slight discoloration does not adversely affect potency or safety. • If precipitate forms, redissolve by heating, shaking vigorously; allow to cool to body temperature.

Reconstitution:

• IV push does not need to be diluted or reconstituted. Inject through Y-tube or 3-way stopcock of free-flowing solution. • For IV infusion, further dilute with D_5W or 0.9% NaCl.

Rate of administration:

• Give IV push slowly over 1–2 min. • IV infusion is administered over 30 min–24 hrs. • Extravasation produces immediate pain, severe local tissue damage. Follow protocol.

IV INCOMPATIBILITIES ⊘

Amphotericin B complex (Abelcet, Amphotec, Ambisome), droperidol (Inapsine), filgrastim (Neupogen), ondansetron (Zofran), vinorelbine (Navelbine).

IV COMPATIBILITIES

Granisetron (Kytril), potassium chloride, propofol (Diprivan).

INDICATIONS/ROUTES/DOSAGE

Note: Dosage is individualized on basis of clinical response and tolerance to adverse effects. When used in combination therapy, consult specific protocols for optimum dosage, sequence of drug administration. Dosage based on pt's actual weight. Use ideal body weight in obese or edematous pts.

Initial course:

IV: Adults, elderly, children: Initially, 12 mg/kg/day for 4–5 days. **Maximum:** 800 mg/day. **Maintenance:** 6 mg/kg every other day for 4 doses. Repeat in 4 wks or 15 mg/kg as a single bolus dose. **Maintenance:** 5–15 mg/kg/wk as a single dose, not to exceed 1 g.

Usual topical dosage:

Adults: Apply 2 times/day to cover lesions.

SIDE EFFECTS

OCCASIONAL: Anorexia, diarrhea, minimal alopecia, fever, dry skin, fissuring, scaling, erythema. **Topical:** pain, pruritus, hyperpigmentation, irritation, inflammation, burning at application site. **RARE:** Nausea, vomiting, anemia, esophagitis, proctitis, GI ulcer, confusion, headache, lacrimation, visual disturbances, angina, allergic reactions.

ADVERSE REACTIONS/TOXIC EFFECTS

Earliest sign of toxicity (4–8 days after beginning of therapy) is stomatitis (dry mouth, burning sensation, mucosal erythema, ulceration at inner margin of lips). Most common dermatologic toxicity is pruritic rash (generally appears on extremities, less frequently on trunk). Leukopenia generally occurs within 9–14 days after drug administration (may occur as late as 25th day). Thrombocytopenia occasionally occurs within 7–17 days after administration. Hematologic toxicity may also manifest itself as pancytopenia, agranulocytosis.

NURSING IMPLICATIONS

BASELINE ASSESSMENT:

Monitor hematology test results. Drug should be discontinued if intractable diarrhea, stomatitis, GI bleeding occurs.

INTERVENTION/EVALUATION:

Monitor for rapidly falling WBC and/or intractable diarrhea, GI bleeding (bright red or tarry stool). Assess oral mucosa for mucosal erythema, ulceration of inner margin of lips, sore throat, difficulty swallowing (stomatitis). Assess skin for rash.

PATIENT/FAMILY TEACHING:

Contraceptive measures should be used during therapy. Maintain fastidious oral hygiene. Promptly report fever, sore throat, signs of local infection, easy bruising, unusual bleeding from any site. Avoid ultraviolet rays with topical or parenteral therapy. *Topical:* Apply only to affected area. Do not use occlusive coverings. Be careful near eyes, nose, and mouth. Wash hands thoroughly after application. Treated areas may be unsightly for several wks after therapy.

fluoxetine hydrochloride 🖉

flew-**ox**-eh-teen
(Novo-Fluoxetine ♣, <u>Prozac</u>, Prozac Weekly, Sarafen)
Do not confuse with fluvastatin, Prilosec, Proscar, ProSom, Serophene.

▶**CLASSIFICATION**

PHARMACOTHERAPEUTIC:
Psychotherapeutic. ***CLINICAL:*** Antidepressant, antiobsessional agent, antibulimic (see p. 35C)

ACTION/*THERAPEUTIC EFFECT*

Selectively inhibits serotonin uptake in CNS, enhancing serotonergic function. *Resulting enhancement of synaptic activity produces antidepressant, antiobsessional, antibulimic effect.*

PHARMACOKINETICS

Well absorbed from GI tract. Crosses blood-brain barrier. Protein binding: 94%. Metabolized in liver to active metabolite. Primarily excreted in urine. Not removed by hemodialysis. Half-life: 2–3 days; metabolite: 7–9 days.

USES/*UNLABELED*

Outpatient treatment of major depression exhibited as persistent, prominent dysphoria (occurring nearly every day for at least 2 wks) manifested by 4 of 8 symptoms: change in appetite, change in sleep pattern, increased fatigue, impaired concentration, feelings of guilt or worthlessness, loss of interest in usual activities, psychomotor agitation or retardation, or suicidal tendencies. Treatment of obsessive-compulsive disorder (OCD). Treatment of panic disorder, premenstrual dyphoric disorder, bulimia. *Decreases hot flashes.*

PRECAUTIONS

CONTRAINDICATIONS: Within 14 days of MAO inhibitor ingestion. ***CAUTIONS:*** Impaired renal or hepatic function.
▷***LIFESPAN CONSIDERATIONS:***
Pregnancy/Lactation: Unknown whether drug crosses placenta or is distributed in breast milk. **Pregnancy Category B. Children:** May be more sensitive to behavioral side effects (e.g., insomnia, restlessness). **Elderly:** No age-related precautions noted.

INTERACTIONS

DRUG: Alcohol, CNS depressants antagonize CNS depressant effect. May displace **highly protein-bound medications** from protein-binding sites (e.g., **oral anticoagulants). MAO inhibitors** may produce serotonin syndrome. May increase phenytoin concentration, toxicity. **HERBAL: St. John's wort** may have additive effect. **FOOD:** None known. **LAB VALUES:** None significant.

AVAILABILITY (Rx)

CAPSULES: 10 mg, 20 mg, 90 mg. **LIQUID:** 20 mg/5 ml. **TABLETS:** 10 mg.

ADMINISTRATION/HANDLING
PO:

• Give with food or milk if GI distress occurs.

INDICATIONS/ROUTES/DOSAGE

Note: Use lower or less frequent doses in those with renal, hepatic impairment, elderly, those with concurrent disease or on multiple medications.

Depression, OCD:

PO: Adults: Initially, 20 mg each morning. If therapeutic improvement does not occur after 2 wks, gradually increase dose to maximum 80 mg/day in 2 equally divided doses in morning, noon. **Elderly:** Initially, 10 mg/day. May increase by 10–20 mg q2wks. Avoid administration at night. **Children:** Initially, 5–10 mg/day. Titrate upward as needed (20 mg/day usual dosage).

Prozac Weekly: Adults: 90 mg/wk begin 7 days after last dose of 20 mg.

Bulimia:

PO: Adults: 60 mg once daily in morning.

Premenstrual dyphoric disorder:
PO: Adults: 20 mg/day.

SIDE EFFECTS

FREQUENT (>10%): Headache, asthenia (loss of strength), inability to sleep, anxiety, nervousness, drowsiness, nausea, diarrhea, decreased appetite. **OCCASIONAL** (2–9%): Dizziness, tremor, fatigue, vomiting, constipation, dry mouth, abdominal pain, nasal congestion, increased sweating. **RARE** (<2%): Flushed skin, lightheadedness, decreased ability to concentrate.

ADVERSE REACTIONS/TOXIC EFFECTS

Overdosage may produce seizures, nausea, vomiting, excessive agitation, restlessness.

NURSING IMPLICATIONS

BASELINE ASSESSMENT:

For those on long-term therapy, liver/renal function tests, blood counts should be performed periodically.

INTERVENTION/EVALUATION:

Supervise suicidal risk pt closely during early therapy (as energy level improves, suicide potential increases). Assess appearance, behavior, speech pattern, level of interest, mood. Monitor stool frequency and consistency. Assess skin for appearance of rash.

PATIENT/FAMILY TEACHING:

Maximum therapeutic response may require 4 or more wks of therapy. Do not abruptly discontinue medication. Avoid tasks that require alertness, motor skills until response to drug is established.

fluoxymesterone

floo-ox-ih-**mes**-teh-rone
(Android-F, Halotestin)
Do not confuse with Halotex, halothane.

FIXED-COMBINATION(S)

With ethinyl estradiol, an estrogen **(Halodrin)**

▶CLASSIFICATION

PHARMACOTHERAPEUTIC: Androgen. **CLINICAL:** Sex hormone, antineoplastic

ACTION/THERAPEUTIC EFFECT

Suppresses gonadotropin-releasing hormone, LH, and FSH. *Stimulates spermatogenesis, development of male secondary sex characteristics, sexual maturation at puberty.* Stimulates production of RBCs.

USES/UNLABELED

Replacement of endogenous testicular hormone, palliative treatment of breast cancer in women, postpartum breast engorgement. *Treatment of anemia.*

PRECAUTIONS

CONTRAINDICATIONS: Serious cardiac, renal, or hepatic dysfunction. Do not use for men with carcinomas of the breast or prostate. **CAUTIONS:** Decreased renal or liver function, benign prostate hypertrophy, hypercalcemia (may be aggravated in pts with metastatic breast cancer), history of myocardial infarction, diabetes mellitus.

INTERACTIONS

DRUG: May increase effect of **oral anticoagulants.** Hepatotoxic medications may increase hepatotoxicity. **HERBAL:** None known. **FOOD:** None known. **LAB VALUES:** May increase alkaline phosphatase, SGOT (AST), bilirubin, calcium, potassium, sodium, hemoglobin, hematocrit, LDL. May decrease HDL.

AVAILABILITY (Rx)

TABLETS: 2 mg, 5 mg, 10 mg.

INDICATIONS/ROUTES/DOSAGE

Males (hypogonadism):
PO: Adults: 5–20 mg/day.

Males (delayed puberty):
PO: Adults: 2.5–20 mg/day for 4–6 mos.

Females (inoperable breast cancer):
PO: Adults: 10–40 mg/day in divided doses for 1–3 mos.

Females (prevent postpartum breast pain/engorgement):
PO: Adults: Initially, 2.5 mg shortly after delivery, then 5–10 mg/day in divided doses for 4–5 days.

SIDE EFFECTS

FREQUENT: Females: Amenorrhea, virilism (e.g., acne, decreased breast size, enlarged clitoris, male pattern baldness), deepening voice. **Males:** UTI, breast soreness, gynecomastia, priapism, virilism (e.g., acne, early pubic hair growth). **OCCASIONAL:** Edema, nausea, vomiting, mild acne, diarrhea, stomach pain. **Males:** Impotence, testicular atrophy.

ADVERSE REACTIONS/TOXIC EFFECTS

Peliosis hepatitis (liver, spleen replaced with blood-filled cysts), hepatic neoplasms, and hepatocellular carcinoma have been associated with prolonged high dosage.

NURSING IMPLICATIONS

BASELINE ASSESSMENT:

Establish baseline weight, B/P, hemoglobin, hematocrit. Check liver function test results, electrolytes, and cholesterol if ordered. Wrist x-rays may be ordered to determine bone maturation in children.

INTERVENTION/EVALUATION:

Assess electrolytes, cholesterol, hemoglobin, hematocrit (periodically for high dosage), liver function test results. With breast cancer or immobility, check for hypercalcemia (lethargy, muscle weakness, confusion, irritability). Be alert to signs of virilization. Monitor sleep patterns.

PATIENT/FAMILY TEACHING:

Weigh daily, report weekly gain of 5 lbs or more. Notify physician if jaundice, nausea, vomiting, acne, ankle swelling occur. *Female:* Promptly report menstrual irregularities, hoarseness, deepening of voice. *Male:* Report frequent erections, difficulty urinating, gynecomastia.

fluphenazine

flew-**phen**-ah-zeen
(Apo-Fluphenazine✿,
Moditen✿, Permitil, Prolixin)

▶**CLASSIFICATION**

PHARMACOTHERAPEUTIC:
Phenothiazine. **CLINICAL:** Antipsychotic (see p. 55C)

ACTION/*THERAPEUTIC EFFECT*

Antagonizes dopamine neurotransmission at synapses by blocking postsynaptic dopaminergic receptors in brain, *decreasing psychotic behavior*. Produces weak anticholinergic, sedative, antiemetic effects, strong extrapyramidal activity.

USES/*UNLABELED*

Management of psychotic disturbances (schizophrenia, delusions, hallucinations). *Treatment of neurogenic pain (adjunct to tricyclic antidepressants).*

PRECAUTIONS

CONTRAINDICATIONS: Severe CNS depression, comatose states, severe cardiovascular disease, bone marrow depression, subcortical brain damage. **CAUTIONS:** Impaired respiratory/hepatic/renal/cardiac function, alcohol withdrawal, history of seizures, urinary retention, glaucoma, prostatic hypertrophy, hypocalcemia (increased susceptibility to dystonias).

INTERACTIONS

DRUG: Alcohol, CNS depressants may increase CNS, respiratory depression, hypotensive effects. **Tricyclic antidepressants, MAO inhibitors** may increase sedative, anticholinergic effects. **Antithyroid agents** may increase risk of agranulocytosis. Extrapyramidal symptoms (EPS) may increase with **EPS-producing medications. Hypotensives** may increase hypotension. May decrease **levodopa** effects. **Lithium** may decrease absorption, produce adverse neurologic effects. **HERBAL:** None known. **FOOD:** None known. **LAB VALUES:** May produce false-positive pregnancy test, PKU. EKG changes may occur, including Q and T wave disturbances.

AVAILABILITY (Rx)

TABLETS: 1 mg, 2.5 mg, 5 mg, 10 mg. **ELIXIR:** 2.5 mg/5 ml. **CONCENTRATE:** 5 mg/ml. **INJECTION:** 2.5 mg/ml, 25 mg/ml.

INDICATIONS/ROUTES/DOSAGE

PSYCHOTIC DISORDERS:

PO: Adults: Initially, 2.5–10 mg/day in divided doses q6–8h. **Maintenance:** 1–5 mg/day. **Elderly:** 1–2.5 mg/day; increase gradually as needed. **Children:** 0.25–0.75 mg 1–4 times/day.

Decanoate:

IM/SUBQ: Adults: 12.5–25 mg, may repeat q1–3wks. **Maintenance:** Up to 50 mg q1–4wks. **Maximum:** 100 mg/dose. **Children >12 yrs:** 6.25–18.75 mg/wk, may increase to 12.5–25 mg q1–3wks. **Children 5–12 yrs:** 3.125–12.5 mg, may repeat q1–3wks.

Enanthate:

IM/SUBQ: Adults, children >12 yrs: Initially, 25 mg q2wks. **Maximum:** 100 mg/dose.

SIDE EFFECTS

FREQUENT: Hypotension, dizziness, and fainting occur frequently after first injection, occasionally after subsequent injections, and rarely with oral dosage. **OCCASIONAL:** Drowsiness during early therapy, dry mouth, blurred vision, lethargy, constipation or diarrhea, nasal congestion, peripheral edema, urinary retention. **RARE:** Ocular changes, skin pigmentation (those on high doses for prolonged periods).

ADVERSE REACTIONS/TOXIC EFFECTS

Extrapyramidal symptoms appear dose related (particularly high dosage), divided into 3 categories: akathisia (inability to sit still, tapping of feet, urge to move around); parkinsonian symptoms (masklike face, tremors, shuffling gait, hypersalivation); and acute dystonias: torticollis (neck muscle spasm), opisthotonos (rigidity of back muscles), and oculogyric crisis (rolling back of eyes). Dystonic reaction may also produce profuse sweating, pallor. Tardive dyskinesia (protrusion of tongue, puffing of cheeks, chewing/puckering of the mouth) occurs rarely (may be irreversible). Abrupt withdrawal after long-term therapy may precipitate nausea, vomiting, gastritis, dizziness, tremors. Blood dyscrasias, particularly agranulocytosis, mild leukopenia (sore mouth/gums/throat) may occur. May lower seizure threshold.

NURSING IMPLICATIONS

BASELINE ASSESSMENT:

Avoid skin contact with solution (contact dermatitis). Assess behavior, appearance, emotional status, response to environment, speech pattern, thought content.

INTERVENTION/EVALUATION:

Monitor B/P for hypotension. Monitor CBC for blood dyscrasias. Monitor for fine tongue movement (may be early sign of tardive dyskinesia). Supervise suicidal risk pt closely during early therapy (as depression lessens, energy level improves, increasing suicide potential). Assess for therapeutic response (interest in surroundings, improvement in self-care, increased ability to concentrate, relaxed facial expression).

PATIENT/FAMILY TEACHING:

Full therapeutic effect may take up to 6 wks. Urine may darken. Do not abruptly withdraw from long-term drug therapy. Drowsiness generally subsides during continued therapy. Avoid tasks that require alertness, motor skills until response to drug is established.

flurandrenolide

(Cordran)

See Classification section under: Corticosteroids: topical

flurazepam hydrochloride

flur-**ah**-zah-pam
(Apo-Flurazepam❖, Dalmane)
Do not confuse with Dialume.

▶CLASSIFICATION

PHARMACOTHERAPEUTIC: Benzodiazepine **(Schedule IV).** ***CLINICAL:*** Sedative-hypnotic (see p. 123C)

ACTION/*THERAPEUTIC EFFECT*

Enhances action of inhibitory neurotransmitter gamma-aminobutyric acid (GABA), *producing hypnotic effect due to CNS depression.*

𝒮 - see color pill atlas

PHARMACOKINETICS

	Onset	Peak	Duration
PO	15–45 min	—	7–8 hrs

Well absorbed from GI tract. Protein binding: 97%. Crosses blood-brain barrier. Widely distributed. Metabolized in liver to active metabolite. Primarily excreted in urine. Not removed by hemodialysis. Half-life: 2.3 hrs; metabolite: 40–114 hrs.

USES

Short-term treatment of insomnia (up to 4 wks). Reduces sleep-induction time, number of nocturnal awakenings; increases length of sleep.

PRECAUTIONS

CONTRAINDICATIONS: Acute narrow-angle glaucoma, acute alcohol intoxication. ***CAUTIONS:*** Impaired renal/hepatic function.

▷*LIFESPAN CONSIDERATIONS:* **Pregnancy/Lactation:** Crosses placenta; may be distributed in breast milk. Chronic ingestion during pregnancy may produce withdrawal symptoms, CNS depression in neonates. **Pregnancy Category X. Children:** Safety and efficacy not established in those <15 yrs of age. **Elderly:** Use small initial doses with gradual dose increases to avoid ataxia or excessive sedation.

INTERACTIONS

DRUG:* Alcohol, CNS depressants** may increase CNS depressant effect. ***HERBAL:* Kava kava, valerian** may have additive CNS depression. ***FOOD: None known. ***LAB VALUES:*** None significant.

AVAILABILITY (Rx)

CAPSULES: 15 mg, 30 mg.

ADMINISTRATION/HANDLING

PO:

• Give without regard to meals. • Capsules may be emptied and mixed with food.

INDICATIONS/ROUTES/DOSAGE

Insomnia:

***PO:* Adults:** 15–30 mg at bedtime. **Elderly/debilitated/liver disease/low serum albumin, children >15 yrs:** 15 mg at bedtime.

SIDE EFFECTS

FREQUENT: Drowsiness, dizziness, ataxia, sedation. Morning drowsiness may occur initially. ***OCCASIONAL:*** GI disturbances, nervousness, blurred vision, dry mouth, headache, confusion, skin rash, irritability, slurred speech. ***RARE:*** Paradoxical CNS excitement/restlessness (particularly noted in elderly/debilitated).

ADVERSE REACTIONS/TOXIC EFFECTS

Abrupt or too rapid withdrawal following long-term use may result in pronounced restlessness and irritability, insomnia, hand tremors, abdominal/muscle cramps, sweating, vomiting, seizures. Overdosage results in somnolence, confusion, diminished reflexes, coma.

NURSING IMPLICATIONS

BASELINE ASSESSMENT:

Assess B/P, pulse, respirations immediately before administration. Raise bed rails. Provide environment conducive to sleep (back rub, quiet environment, low lighting).

INTERVENTION/EVALUATION:

Assess for paradoxical reaction, particularly during early therapy.

Evaluate for therapeutic response: decrease in number of nocturnal awakenings, increase in length of sleep duration.

PATIENT/FAMILY TEACHING:

Smoking reduces drug effectiveness. Do not abruptly withdraw medication after long-term use. May have disturbed sleep 1–2 nights after discontinuing. Notify physician if pregnant or planning to become pregnant (Pregnancy Category X).

flurbiprofen

fleur-bih-pro-fen
(Ansaid, Froben✦)

flurbiprofen sodium

(Ocufen)

▶CLASSIFICATION

PHARMACOTHERAPEUTIC: Phenylalkanoic acid. ***CLINICAL:*** Nonsteroidal anti-inflammatory, antidysmenorrheal (see p. 106C)

ACTION/*THERAPEUTIC EFFECT*

Produces analgesic and anti-inflammatory effect by inhibiting prostaglandin synthesis, *reducing inflammatory response and intensity of pain stimulus reaching sensory nerve endings.* Prevents, reduces miosis by relaxing iris sphincter.

PHARMACOKINETICS

Well absorbed from GI tract, penetrates cornea after ophthalmic administration (may be systemically absorbed). Widely distributed. Protein binding: 99%. Metabolized in liver. Primarily excreted in urine. Half-life: 3–4 hrs.

USES

Symptomatic treatment of acute and/or chronic rheumatoid arthritis, osteoarthritis, dysmenorrhea, pain; inhibits intraoperative miosis.

PRECAUTIONS

CONTRAINDICATIONS: Active peptic ulcer, GI ulceration, chronic inflammation of GI tract, GI bleeding disorders, history of hypersensitivity to aspirin or NSAIDs. ***CAUTIONS:*** Impaired renal/hepatic function, history of GI tract disease, predisposition to fluid retention, those wearing soft contact lenses, surgical pts with bleeding tendencies.

▷***LIFESPAN CONSIDERATIONS:***
Pregnancy/Lactation: Crosses placenta; not known whether distributed in breast milk. Avoid use during last trimester (may adversely affect fetal cardiovascular system: premature closure of ductus arteriosus). **Pregnancy Category B.** (Category D if used in third trimester or near delivery). *Ophthalmic:* **Pregnancy Category C. Children:** *Safety and efficacy not established.* **Elderly:** *GI bleeding or ulceration more likely to cause serious adverse effects. Age-related renal impairment may increase risk of liver or renal toxicity, decreased dossage recommended.*

INTERACTIONS

DRUG: May increase effects of **oral anticoagulants, heparin, thrombolytics.** May decrease effect of **antihypertensives, diuretics. Salicylates, aspirin** may increase risk of GI side effects, bleeding. **Bone marrow depressants** may increase risk of hematologic reactions. May increase concentration, toxicity of **lithium.** May increase **methotrexate** toxicity. **Probenecid** may increase concentration. *Ophthalmic:* May decrease effect of **acetylcholine, carbachol.** May decrease antiglaucoma effect of **epinephrine, other antiglaucoma medications. *HERBAL:*** **Feverfew** may have decreased effect. **Ginkgo biloba** may increase risk of bleeding. ***FOOD:*** None known. ***LAB VALUES:*** May increase serum transaminase, alkaline phosphatase, LDH, bleeding time.

AVAILABILITY (Rx)

TABLETS: 50 mg, 100 mg. ***OPHTHALMIC SOLUTION:*** 0.03%.

ADMINISTRATION/HANDLING
PO:

• Do not crush or break enteric-coated form. • May give with food, milk, or antacids if GI distress occurs.

Ophthalmic:

• Place finger on lower eyelid and pull out until pocket is formed between eye and lower lid. • Hold dropper above pocket and place prescribed number of drops into pocket. Close eye gently. • Apply digital pressure to lacrimal sac for 1–2 min (minimizes drainage into nose and throat, reducing risk of systemic effects). • Remove excess solution with tissue.

INDICATIONS/ROUTES/DOSAGE
Rheumatoid arthritis, osteoarthritis:

PO: **Adults, elderly:** 200–300 mg/day in 2–4 divided doses. Do not give >100 mg/dose or 300 mg/day.

Usual ophthalmic dosage:

OPHTHALMIC: **Adults, elderly, children:** 1 drop q30 min starting 2 hrs before surgery for total of 4 doses.

SIDE EFFECTS

OCCASIONAL: PO (3–9%): Headache, abdominal pain, diarrhea, indigestion, nausea, fluid retention. ***Ophthalmic:*** Burning, stinging on instillation, keratitis, elevated intraocular pressure. ***RARE*** (<3%): Blurred vision, flushed skin, dizziness, drowsiness, nervousness, insomnia, unusual weakness, constipation, decreased appetite, vomiting, confusion.

ADVERSE REACTIONS/TOXIC EFFECTS

Overdosage may result in acute renal failure. In those treated chronically, peptic ulcer, GI bleeding, gastritis, severe hepatic reaction (jaundice), nephrotoxicity (hematuria, dysuria, proteinuria), severe hypersensitivity reaction (bronchospasm, angiofacial edema), cardiac arrhythmias occur rarely.

NURSING IMPLICATIONS

BASELINE ASSESSMENT:

Anti-inflammatory: Assess onset, type, location, and duration of pain or inflammation. Inspect appearance of affected joints for immobility, deformities, and skin condition.

INTERVENTION/EVALUATION:

Monitor for headache, dyspepsia, dizziness. Monitor pattern of daily bowel activity and stool consistency. ***Anti-inflammatory:*** Evaluate for therapeutic response: relief of pain, stiffness, swelling, increase in joint mobility, reduced joint tenderness, improved grip strength.

PATIENT/FAMILY TEACHING:

Swallow tablet whole; do not crush or chew. Avoid aspirin, alcohol during therapy (increases risk of GI bleeding). If GI upset occurs, take with food, milk. Report GI distress, visual disturbances, rash, edema, headache. ***Ophthalmic:*** Eye burning may occur with instillation.

flutamide

flew-tah-myd
(Euflex✤, Eulexin, Novo-Flutamide✤)
Do not confuse with Flumadine.

▶**CLASSIFICATION**

PHARMACOTHERAPEUTIC: Antiandrogen, hormone. ***CLINICAL:*** Antineoplastic (see p. 70C)

ACTION/*THERAPEUTIC EFFECT*

Inhibits androgen uptake and/or binding of androgen in tissues. Interferes with testosterone at cellular level (complements leuprolide, *suppressing testicular androgen production* by inhibiting LH secretion).

PHARMACOKINETICS

Completely absorbed from GI tract. Protein binding: 94–96%. Metabolized in liver to active metabolite. Primarily excreted in urine. Not removed by hemodialysis. Half-life: 6 hrs (half-life increased in elderly).

USES

Treatment of metastatic carcinoma of prostate (in combination with LHRH analogues, i.e., leuprolide). Management of locally confined stage B_2-C and stage D_2.

PRECAUTIONS

CONTRAINDICATIONS: None significant. ***CAUTIONS:*** None significant.

▷**LIFESPAN CONSIDERATIONS:**
Pregnancy/Lactation: Not used in this pt population. **Children:** Not used in children. **Elderly:** No age-related precautions noted.

INTERACTIONS

DRUG: None significant. **HERBAL:** None known. **FOOD:** None known. **LAB VALUES:** May increase estradiol, testosterone, SGOT (AST), SGPT (ALT), bilirubin, creatinine, glucose.

AVAILABILITY (Rx)
CAPSULES: 125 mg.

ADMINISTRATION/HANDLING
PO:
• Give without regard to food.

INDICATIONS/ROUTES/DOSAGE
Prostatic carcinoma:
PO: Adults, elderly: 250 mg q8h.

SIDE EFFECTS

FREQUENT: Hot flashes (50%), loss of libido, impotence, diarrhea (24%), generalized pain (23%), asthenia (loss of strength, energy) (17%), constipation (12%), nausea, nocturia (11%). **OCCASIONAL** (6–8%): Dizziness, paresthesia, insomnia, impotence, peripheral edema, gynecomastia. **RARE** (4–5%): Rash, sweating, hypertension, sweating, hematuria, vomiting, urinary incontinence, headache, flu syndrome, photosensitivity.

ADVERSE REACTIONS/TOXIC EFFECTS

Hepatotoxicity including hepatic encephalopathy, hemolytic anemia may be noted.

NURSING IMPLICATIONS

INTERVENTION/EVALUATION:

Periodically monitor hepatic function tests in long-term therapy. Assess bowel activity and stool consistency. Nausea may be controlled with use of antiemetics.

PATIENT/FAMILY TEACHING:

Do not stop taking medication (both drugs must be continued). Urine color may change to an amber or yellow-green appearance. Avoid prolonged exposure to the sun or tanning beds. Wear protective clothing from ultraviolet exposure until tolerance is determined.

fluticasone propionate

flew-**tih**-cah-sewn
(Flonase, Cutivate, Flovent)

FIXED-COMBINATION(S)

With salmeterol, a bronchodilator **(Advair)**

▶**CLASSIFICATION**

PHARMACOTHERAPEUTIC: Corticosteroid. **CLINICAL:** Antiinflammatory, antipruritic (see pp. 64C, 79C, 81C)

ACTION/THERAPEUTIC EFFECT

Nasal: Inhibits early activation of inflammatory cells, release of inflammatory mediators, generally on late-phase allergic reactions, *decreasing response to seasonal and perennial rhinitis.* **Topical:** Stimulates protein synthesis of inhibitory enzymes responsible for anti-inflammatory effects. **Inhala-**

tion: Inhibits inflammatory cascade reducing airway hyper-responsiveness. *Decreases bronchial reactivity inhibiting early/late bronchoconstriction* occurring when exposed to inhaled allergens.

PHARMACOKINETICS

Inhalation/intranasal: Protein binding: 91%. Undergoes extensive first-pass metabolism in liver. Excreted in urine. Half-life: 3–7.8 hrs. *Topical:* Amount absorbed dependent on drug, area, skin condition (absorption increased with elevated skin temperature, hydration, inflamed/denuded skin).

USES

Nasal: Relief of seasonal/perennial allergic rhinitis. *Topical:* Relief of inflammation/pruritus associated with steroid-responsive disorders (e.g., contact dermatitis, eczema). *Inhalation:* Maintenance treatment of asthma for those requiring oral corticosteroid therapy for asthma. *Powder:* Maintenance of asthma treatment in children 4 yrs and older.

PRECAUTIONS

CONTRAINDICATIONS: Untreated localized infection of nasal mucosa. *Inhalation:* Primary treatment of status asthmaticus or other acute asthma episodes. ***CAUTIONS:*** Active or quiescent tuberculosis, untreated fungal, bacterial, or systemic viral infection of ocular herpes simplex.

▷*LIFESPAN CONSIDERATIONS:* **Pregnancy/Lactation:** Unknown if drug crosses placenta or is distributed in breast milk. **Pregnancy Category C. Children:** Safety and efficacy not established in those <4 yrs of age. Children >4 yrs may experience growth suppression with prolonged or high doses. **Elderly:** No age-related precautions noted.

INTERACTIONS

DRUG: None significant. ***HERBAL:*** None known. ***FOOD:*** None known. ***LAB VALUES:*** None significant.

AVAILABILITY (Rx)

CREAM: 0.05%. ***OINTMENT:*** 0.005%. ***INTRANASAL:*** 50 mcg/actuation. ***INHALATION:*** 44 mcg/actuation, 110 mcg/actuation, 220 mcg/actuation. ***POWDER FOR INHALATION (Diskus, Rotadisk):*** 50 mcg, 100 mcg, 250 mcg.

ADMINISTRATION/HANDLING

Inhalation:

• Shake container well; exhale as completely as possible. • Place mouthpiece fully into mouth, holding inhaler upright, inhale deeply and slowly while pressing the top of the cannister and hold breath as long as possible before exhaling; then exhale slowly. • Wait 1 min between inhalations when multiple inhalations ordered (allows for deeper bronchial penetration). • Rinse mouth with water immediately after inhalation (prevents mouth/throat dryness).

Intranasal:

• Clear nasal passages before use (topical nasal decongestants may be needed 5–15 min before use). • Tilt head slightly forward. • Insert spray tip up in 1 nostril, pointing toward inflamed nasal turbinates, away from nasal septum. • Pump medication into 1 nostril while holding other nostril closed and concurrently inspire through nose.

INDICATIONS/ROUTES/DOSAGE

Allergic rhinitis:

INTRANASAL: Adults, elderly: Initially, 200 mcg (2 sprays each nostril once daily or 1 spray each nostril q12h). **Maintenance:** 1 spray each nostril once daily. **Maximum:** 200 mcg/day. **Children >4 yrs:** Initially, 100 mcg (1 spray each nostril once daily). **Maximum:** 200 mcg/day.

Usual topical dosage:

TOPICAL: Adults, elderly, children >3 mos: Apply sparingly to affected area 1–2 times/day.

Usual inhalation dosage (dry powder formulation):

INHALATION: Children (4–11 yrs): 50–100 mcg twice daily.

Previous treatment: bronchodilators:

INHALATION: Adults, elderly, children >12 yrs: Initially, 100 mcg q12h. **Maximum:** 500 mcg/day.

Previous treatment: inhaled steroids:

INHALATION: Adults, elderly, children >12 yrs: Initially, 100–250 mcg q12h. **Maximum:** 500 mcg q12h.

Previous treatment: oral steroids:

INHALATION: Adults, elderly, children >12 yrs: *DISKUS:* 500–1,000 mcg 2 times/day. *ROTA-DISK:* 1,000 mcg 2 times/day.

SIDE EFFECTS

FREQUENT: Inhalation: Throat irritation, hoarseness, dry mouth, coughing, temporary wheezing, localized fungal infection in mouth, pharynx, larynx (particularly if mouth is not rinsed with water after each administration). **Intranasal:** Mild nasopharyngeal irritation; nasal irritation, burning, stinging, dryness, rebound congestion, rhinorrhea, loss of sense of taste. **OCCASIONAL: Intranasal:** Nasal/pharyngeal candidiasis, headache. **Inhalation:** Oral candidiasis. **Topical:** Burning/itching of skin.

ADVERSE REACTIONS/TOXIC EFFECTS

None significant.

NURSING IMPLICATIONS

BASELINE ASSESSMENT:

Establish baseline history of skin disorder, asthma, or rhinitis.

INTERVENTION/EVALUATION:

In those receiving bronchodilators by inhalation concomitantly with steroid inhalation therapy, advise pts to use bronchodilator several mins before corticosteroid aerosol (enhances penetration of steroid into bronchial tree). Monitor rate, depth, rhythm, type of respiration; quality and rate of pulse. Assess lung sounds for rhonchi, wheezing, rales. Monitor arterial blood gases. **Topical:** Assess involved area for therapeutic response to irritation.

PATIENT/FAMILY TEACHING:

Do not change dose schedule or stop taking drug; must taper off gradually under medical supervision. Maintain careful mouth hygiene. Rinse mouth with water immediately after inhalation (prevents mouth/throat dryness, fungal infection of mouth). Increase fluid intake (decreases lung secretion viscosity). **Intranasal:** Teach proper use of nasal spray. Clear nasal passages prior to use. Contact physician if no improvement in symptoms, sneezing or nasal irritation occur. Improvement noted in several days. **Topical:** Rub thin film gently into affected area. Use only for prescribed area and no longer than ordered. Avoid contact with eyes.

fluvastatin

flu-vah-**stah**-tin
(Lescol)
Do not confuse with fluoxetine.

▶**CLASSIFICATION**

PHARMACOTHERAPEUTIC: HMG-CoA reductase inhibitor. ***CLINICAL:*** Antihyperlipidemic (see p. 50C)

ACTION/*THERAPEUTIC EFFECT*

Inhibits HMG-CoA reductase, the enzyme that catalyzes the early step in cholesterol synthesis. *Decreases LDL cholesterol, VLDL, plasma triglycerides.* Increases HDL cholesterol concentration slightly.

PHARMACOKINETICS

Well absorbed from GI tract (unaffected by food). Does not cross blood-brain barrier. Protein binding: >98%. Primarily eliminated in feces.

USES

Adjunct to diet therapy to decrease elevated total and LDL cholesterol concentrations in those with primary hypercholesterolemia (types IIa and IIb) and in those with combined hypercholesterolemia, hypertriglyceridemia. Treatment of elevated triglycerides and apolipoprotein.

PRECAUTIONS

CONTRAINDICATIONS: Active liver disease, unexplained increased serum transaminase. ***CAUTIONS:*** Anticoagulant therapy, history of liver disease, substantial alcohol consumption. Withholding/ discontinuing fluvastatin may be necessary when pt at risk for renal failure (secondary to rhabdomyolysis); major surgery, severe acute infection, trauma, hypotension, severe metabolic, endocrine, or electrolyte disorders, or uncontrolled seizures.

▷***LIFESPAN CONSIDERATIONS:***
Pregnancy/Lactation: Contraindicated in pregnancy (suppression of cholesterol biosynthesis may cause fetal toxicity) and lactation. Unknown whether drug is distributed in breast milk. **Pregnancy Category X. Children:** Safety and efficacy not established. **Elderly:** No age-related precautions noted.

INTERACTIONS

DRUG: Increased risk of rhabdomyolysis, acute renal failure with **cyclosporine, erythromycin, gemfibrozil, niacin, other immunosuppressants. HERBAL:** None known. **FOOD:** None known. **LAB VALUES:** May increase creatinine kinase (CK), serum transaminase concentrations.

AVAILABILITY (Rx)

CAPSULES: 20 mg, 40 mg. ***EXTENDED-RELEASE TABLETS:*** 80 mg.

ADMINISTRATION/HANDLING
PO:
• Give without regard to food.

INDICATIONS/ROUTES/DOSAGE
Hyperlipoproteinemia:
PO: Adults, elderly: Initially, 20

mg/day in the evening. May increase up to 40 mg/day. **Maintenance:** 20–40 mg/day in single or divided doses.

SIDE EFFECTS

FREQUENT (5–8%): Headache, dyspepsia, back pain, myalgia, arthralgia, diarrhea, abdominal cramping, rhinitis. *OCCASIONAL* (2–4%): Nausea, vomiting, insomnia, constipation, flatulence, rash, fatigue, cough, dizziness.

ADVERSE REACTIONS/TOXIC EFFECTS

Myositis (inflammation of voluntary muscle), with or without increased CK, muscle weakness, occurs rarely. May progress to frank rhabdomyolysis and renal impairment.

NURSING IMPLICATIONS

BASELINE ASSESSMENT:

Question for possibility of pregnancy before initiating therapy (Pregnancy Category X). Assess baseline lab results: cholesterol, triglycerides, liver function tests.

INTERVENTION/EVALUATION:

Determine pattern of bowel activity. Check for headache, dizziness, blurred vision. Assess for rash, pruritus. Monitor cholesterol and triglyceride lab results for therapeutic response. Be alert for malaise, muscle cramping or weakness.

PATIENT/FAMILY TEACHING:

Follow special diet (important part of treatment). Periodic lab tests are essential part of therapy. Report promptly any muscle pain or weakness, esp. if accompanied by fever or malaise.

fluvoxamine maleate

flew-**vox**-ah-meen
(Luvox)
Do not confuse with Lasix.

▶CLASSIFICATION

PHARMACOTHERAPEUTIC: Serotonin reuptake inhibitor. *CLINICAL:* Antidepressant, antiobsessional (see p. 35C)

ACTION/*THERAPEUTIC EFFECT*

Selectively inhibits serotonin neuronal uptake in CNS, *producing antidepressant, antiobsessive effects.*

USES/*UNLABELED*

Treatment of obsessive-compulsive disorder (OCD). *Treatment of depression.*

PRECAUTIONS

CONTRAINDICATIONS: Within 14 days of MAO inhibitor ingestion, concurrent astemizole or terfenadine therapy. *CAUTIONS:* Impaired renal or hepatic function, elderly.

INTERACTIONS

DRUG: **MAO inhibitors** may produce serious reactions (hyperthermia, rigidity, myoclonus). **Tryptophan, lithium** may enhance serotonergic effects. **Tricyclic antidepressants** may increase concentration. Fluvoxamine may increase concentration/toxicity of **benzodiazepines, carbamazepine, clozapine, theophylline.** May increase effects of **warfarin.** *HERBAL:* **St. John's wort** may have additive effect. *FOOD:* None known. *LAB VALUES:* None significant.

AVAILABILITY (Rx)

TABLETS: 50 mg, 100 mg.

INDICATIONS/ROUTES/DOSAGE

Note: Use lower or less frequent dosing in impaired hepatic function, elderly.

Obsessive-compulsive disorder:

***PO:* Adults:** 50 mg at bedtime; increase by 50 mg q4–7days. Doses >100 mg/day in 2 divided doses. **Maximum:** 300 mg/day. **Children 8–17 yrs:** 25 mg at bedtime; increase by 25 mg q4–7 days. Doses >50 mg/day in 2 divided doses. **Maximum:** 200 mg/day.

SIDE EFFECTS

FREQUENT: Nausea (40%), headache, somnolence, insomnia (21–22%). ***OCCASIONAL*** (8–14%): Nervousness, dizziness, diarrhea/loose stools, dry mouth, asthenia (loss of strength, weakness), dyspepsia, constipation, abnormal ejaculation. ***RARE*** (3–6%): Anorexia, anxiety, tremor, vomiting, flatulence, urinary frequency, sexual dysfunction, taste change.

ADVERSE REACTIONS/TOXIC EFFECTS

Overdosage may produce seizures, nausea, vomiting, excessive agitation, extreme restlessness.

NURSING IMPLICATIONS

INTERVENTION/EVALUATION:

Supervise suicidal risk pt closely during early therapy (as energy level improves, suicide potential increases). Assess appearance, behavior, speech pattern, level of interest, mood. Assist with ambulation if dizziness, somnolence occurs. Monitor stool frequency and consistency.

PATIENT/FAMILY TEACHING:

Maximum therapeutic response may require 4 or more wks of therapy. Dry mouth may be relieved by sugarless gum, sips of tepid water. Do not abruptly discontinue medication. Avoid tasks that require alertness, motor skills until response to drug is established.

F

folic acid (vitamin B$_9$)

foe-lick
(Apo-Folic✦, Folvite)
Do not confuse with Florvite.

sodium folate

(Folvite-parenteral)

▶CLASSIFICATION

PHARMACOTHERAPEUTIC:
Coenzyme. ***CLINICAL:*** Nutritional supplement

ACTION/*THERAPEUTIC EFFECT*

Stimulates production of red and white blood cells and platelets, *essential for nucleoprotein synthesis, maintenance of normal erythropoiesis.*

PHARMACOKINETICS

Oral form almost completely absorbed from GI tract (upper duodenum). Protein binding: High. Metabolized in liver, plasma to active form. Excreted in urine. Removed by hemodialysis.

USES/*UNLABELED*

Treatment of megaloblastic, macrocytic anemia associated with pregnancy, infancy, childhood, inadequate dietary intake. *Decreases risk of colon cancer.*

PRECAUTIONS
CONTRAINDICATIONS: Anemias (pernicious, aplastic, normocytic, refractory). ***CAUTIONS:*** None significant.

▷***LIFESPAN CONSIDERATIONS:***
Pregnancy/Lactation: Distributed in breast milk. **Pregnancy Category A.** If more than RDA: **Pregnancy Category C. Children/Elderly:** No age-related precautions noted.

INTERACTIONS
DRUG: May decrease effects of **hydantoin anticonvulsants. Analgesics, anticonvulsants, carbamazepine, estrogens** may increase folic acid requirements. **Antacids, cholestyramine** may decrease absorption. **Methotrexate, triamterene, trimethoprim** may antagonize effects. ***HERBAL:*** None known. ***FOOD:*** None known. ***LAB VALUES:*** May decrease vitamin B_{12} concentration.

AVAILABILITY (Rx)
TABLETS: 0.4 mg, 0.8 mg ***(OTC)***, 1 mg ***(Rx)***. ***INJECTION (Rx):*** 5 mg/ml.

ADMINISTRATION/HANDLING
Note: Parenteral form used in acutely ill, parenteral or enteral alimentation, those unresponsive to oral route in GI malabsorption syndrome. Dosage >0.1 mg daily may conceal pernicious anemia.

INDICATIONS/ROUTES/DOSAGE
Deficiency:
PO/IM/IV: **Adults, children:** Up to 1 mg/day. **Infants:** 50 mcg/day.

Supplement:
PO/IM/IV/SubQ: **Adults, elderly, children >4 yrs:** 0.4 mg/day. **Children <4 yrs:** 0.3 mg/day. **Children**

<1 yr: 0.1 mg/day. **Pregnancy:** 0.8 mg/day.

SIDE EFFECTS
None significant.

ADVERSE REACTIONS/TOXIC EFFECTS
Allergic hypersensitivity occurs rarely with parenteral form. Oral folic acid is nontoxic.

NURSING IMPLICATIONS

BASELINE ASSESSMENT:
Pernicious anemia should be ruled out by Schilling test and vitamin B_{12} blood level before therapy is initiated (may produce irreversible neurologic damage). Resistance to treatment may occur if decreased hematopoiesis, alcoholism, antimetabolic drugs, or deficiency of vitamin B_6, B_{12}, C, or E is evident.

INTERVENTION/EVALUATION:
Assess for therapeutic improvement: improved sense of well-being, relief from iron deficiency symptoms (fatigue, shortness of breath, sore tongue, headache, pallor).

PATIENT/FAMILY TEACHING:
Eat foods rich in folic acid including fruits, vegetables, and organ meats.

follitropin alpha

(Gonal-F)

See Classification section under: Fertility agents (p. 86C)

fomepizole

(Antizol)
See Appendix A: Antidotes

fomvirsen sodium

foam-ih-**vir**-sen
(Vitravene)

▶CLASSIFICATION

PHARMACOTHERAPEUTIC:
Antiviral. ***CLINICAL:*** Antiretinitis
(see p. 56C)

ACTION/*THERAPEUTIC EFFECT*

Inhibits protein synthesis by binding to target mRNA transcripts, *preventing human cytomegalovirus (CMV) replication.*

USES

Treatment of cytomegalovirus (CMV) retinitis in pts with acquired immunodeficiency syndrome (AIDS).

AVAILABILITY (Rx)

INJECTION: 6.6 mg/ml.

INDICATIONS/ROUTES/DOSAGE

Cytomegalovirus (CMV) retinitis:

INTRAVITREAL (ophthalmic): **Adults, elderly:** 330 mcg (0.05 ml/eye) as a single intravitreal injection every other week for 2 doses. **Maintenance:** 330 mcg (0.05 ml/eye) once q4wks.

SIDE EFFECTS

FREQUENT (25%): Ocular inflammation (uveitis), including iritis and vitritis. ***OCCASIONAL*** (5–20%): Blurred vision, decreased visual acuity, eye pain, floaters, photophobia, abdominal pain, asthenia, diarrhea, fever, headache, nausea, rash, sinusitis, vomiting, increased intraocular pressure (IOP), retinal pigment changes. ***RARE*** (2–5%): Conjunctivitis, decreased peripheral vision, eye irritation, application site reaction.

ADVERSE REACTIONS/TOXIC EFFECTS

Cataracts, conjunctival bleeding, retinal detachment, retinal edema, abnormal liver function may occur.

NURSING IMPLICATIONS

PATIENT/FAMILY TEACHING:
Regular ophthalmic follow-up exams are required.

formoterol fumarate

four-**moh**-tur-all
(Foradil Aerolizer)

▶CLASSIFICATION

PHARMACOTHERAPEUTIC:
Sympathomimetic (beta$_2$-adrenergic agonist). ***CLINICAL:*** Bronchodilator (see p. 63C)

ACTION/*THERAPEUTIC EFFECT*

Long-acting bronchodilator. Stimulates beta$_2$-adrenergic receptors in the lungs resulting in relaxation of bronchial smooth muscle. Also inhibits release of mediators from various cells in the lungs, including mast cells. *Relieves bronchospasm, reduces airway resistance. Produces better bronchodilation than albuterol, better nighttime asthma control, better peak flow rates*

PHARMACOKINETICS

	Onset	Peak	Duration
Inhalation	<5 min	—	12 hrs

Absorbed from bronchi following inhalation. Metabolized in liver. Primarily excreted in urine. Unknown if removed by hemodialysis.

USES

For long-term maintenance treatment of asthma, prevention of exercise-induced bronchospasm, treatment of bronchoconstriction in pts with COPD. Can be used concomitantly with short-acting beta agonists, inhaled or systemic corticosteroids, theophylline therapy.

PRECAUTIONS

CONTRAINDICATIONS: None significant. ***CAUTIONS:*** Hypertension, cardiovascular disease.
▷***LIFESPAN CONSIDERATIONS:***
Pregnancy/Lactation: Unknown if drug crosses placenta or is distributed in breast milk. **Pregnancy Category C**. **Children:** Safety and efficacy not established in children <5 yrs. **Elderly:** May be more sensitive to tremor or tachycardia due to age-related increased sympathetic sensitivity.

INTERACTIONS

DRUG: **Beta-adrenergic blocking agents (beta blockers)** can antagonize bronchodilating effects. May potentiate cardiovascular effects with **MAO inhibitors, tricyclic antidepressants,** drugs that can prolong QT interval **(erythromycin, thioridazine, quinidine).** Diuretics, xanthine derivatives, steroids can increase risk of hypokalemia. ***HERBAL:*** None significant. ***FOOD:*** None significant. ***LAB VALUES:*** May reduce serum potassium level, increase blood glucose level.

AVAILABILITY (Rx)

INHALATION POWDER IN CAPSULES: 12 mcg.

ADMINISTRATION/HANDLING

Storage:
• Maintain capsules in individual blister pack until immediately before use. Do not swallow capsules. Do not use with a spacer.

Inhalation:
• Pull off *Aerolizer Inhaler* cover, twisting mouthpiece in direction of the arrow to open. • Place capsule in chamber. Capsule is pierced by pressing and releasing buttons on the side of the *Aerolizer*, once only. • Exhale completely; place mouthpiece into mouth and close lips. • Inhale quickly and deeply through mouth (this causes capsule to spin, dispensing the drug). Hold breath as long as possible before exhaling slowly. • Check capsule to make sure all the powder is gone. If not, inhale again to receive rest of the dose. Rinse mouth with water immediately after inhalation (prevents mouth/throat dryness).

INDICATIONS/ROUTES/DOSAGE

Maintenance treatment of asthma:

INHALATION: Adults, elderly, children >5 yrs: Inhale contents of 1 capsule every 12 hrs.

Exercise-induced asthma:

INHALATION: Adults, elderly, children >12 yrs: Inhale contents of 1 capsule at least 15 min before exercise.

SIDE EFFECTS

OCCASIONAL: Tremor, cramps,

tachycardia, insomnia, headache, irritability, irritation of mouth or throat.

ADVERSE REACTIONS/TOXIC EFFECTS

Excessive sympathomimetic stimulation may produce palpitations, extrasystoles, chest pain.

NURSING IMPLICATIONS

INTERVENTION/EVALUATION:

Monitor rate, depth, rhythm, type of respiration; quality and rate of pulse, EKG, serum potassium, arterial blood gases (ABGs) determinations. Assess lung sounds for wheezing (bronchoconstriction) and rales.

PATIENT/FAMILY TEACHING:

Instruct on proper use of inhaler. Increase fluid intake (decreases lung secretion viscosity). Rinsing mouth with water immediately after inhalation may prevent mouth/throat irritation. Avoid excessive use of caffeine derivatives (chocolate, coffee, tea, cola).

foscarnet sodium

fos-**car**-net
(Foscavir)

▶CLASSIFICATION

CLINICAL: Antiviral (see p. 58C).

ACTION/THERAPEUTIC EFFECT

Provides selective inhibition at binding site on virus-specific DNA polymerases and reverse transcriptases, *inhibiting replication of herpes virus.*

PHARMACOKINETICS

Sequestered into bone, cartilage. Protein binding: 14–17%. Primarily excreted unchanged in urine. Removed by hemodialysis. Half-life: 3.3–6.8 hrs (half-life increased with impaired renal function).

USES/*UNLABELED*

Treatment of CMV retinitis in pts with AIDS; in combination with ganciclovir for relapsed AIDS-related CMV retinitis; acyclovir-resistant herpes simplex virus (HSV) in immunocompromised pts. *Treatment of CMV disease, herpes simplex, varicella zoster.*

PRECAUTIONS

CONTRAINDICATIONS: None significant. **CAUTIONS:** Neurologic or cardiac abnormalities, history of renal impairment, altered calcium or other electrolyte levels.
▷**LIFESPAN CONSIDERATIONS:**
Pregnancy/Lactation: Unknown if distributed in breast milk. **Pregnancy Category C. Children:** Safety and efficacy not established. **Elderly:** Age-related renal impairment may require dosage adjustment.

INTERACTIONS

DRUG: Nephrotoxic medications may increase risk of renal toxicity. **Pentamidine (IV)** may cause reversible hypocalcemia, hypomagnesemia, nephrotoxicity. **Zidovudine** may increase anemia. **HERBAL:** None known. **FOOD:** None known. **LAB VALUES:** May increase SGOT (AST), SGPT (ALT), alkaline phosphatase, bilirubin, creatinine. May decrease magnesium, potassium. May alter calcium, phosphate concentrations.

AVAILABILITY (Rx)

INJECTION: 24 mg/ml.

✤ - Canadian trade name   ✳ - see also www.wbsaunders.com/SIMON/SaundersNDH

ADMINISTRATION/HANDLING
IV 💊

Storage:
• Store parenteral vials at room temperature. • After dilution, stable for 24 hrs at room temperature. • Do not use if solution is discolored or contains particulate material.

Reconstitution:
• The standard 24 mg/ml solution may be used without dilution when central venous catheter is used for infusion; 24 mg/ml solution *must* be diluted to 12 mg/ml when peripheral vein catheter is being used. • Only D_5W or 0.9% NaCl solution for injection should be used for dilution.

Rate of administration:
• Since dosage is calculated on body weight, unneeded quantity may be removed before start of infusion to avoid overdosage. Aseptic technique must be used and solution administered within 24 hrs of first entry into sealed bottle. • Do not give IV injection or rapid infusion (increases toxicity). • Administer only by IV infusion over a minimum of 1 hr (no more than 1 mg/kg/min). • To minimize toxicity and phlebitis, use central venous lines or veins with adequate blood to permit rapid dilution and dissemination of foscarnet. • Use IV infusion pump to prevent accidental overdose.

IV INCOMPATIBILITIES ⊘
Acyclovir (Zovirax), amphotericin (Fungizone), diazepam (Valium), digoxin (Lanoxin), diphenhydramine (Benadryl), dobutamine (Dobutrex), droperidol (Inapsine), ganciclovir (Cytovene), haloperidol (Haldol), leucovorin, midazolam (Versed), pentamidine (Pentam IV), prochlorperazine (Compazine), sulfamethoxazole-trimethoprim (Bactrim), vancomycin (Vancocin).

IV COMPATIBILITY
Heparin.

INDICATIONS/ROUTES/DOSAGE
CMV retinitis:
IV: Adults: Initially, 60 mg/kg q8h for 2–3 wks. **Maintenance:** 90 mg/kg/day; may increase up to 120 mg/kg/day if retinitis progresses.

Herpes simplex:
IV: Adults: 40 mg/kg q8–12h for 2–3 wks or until healed.

Dosage in renal impairment:
Dosage individualized according to pt's creatinine clearance. Refer to dosing guide provided by manufacturer.

SIDE EFFECTS
FREQUENT: Fever (65%), nausea (47%), vomiting, diarrhea (30%). **OCCASIONAL** (≥5%): Anorexia, pain and inflammation at injection site, fever, rigors, malaise, hyper/hypotension, headache, paresthesia, dizziness, rash, increased sweating, nausea, vomiting, abdominal pain. **RARE** (1–5%): Back/chest pain, edema, hyper/hypotension, flushing, pruritus, constipation, dry mouth.

ADVERSE REACTIONS/TOXIC EFFECTS
Renal impairment is a major toxicity that occurs to some extent in most pts. Seizures and mineral/electrolyte imbalances may be life threatening.

BASELINE ASSESSMENT:
Obtain baseline mineral and electrolyte levels, vital signs, CBC values, renal functioning. Risk of renal impairment can be reduced by sufficient fluid intake to assure diuresis before and during dosing.

INTERVENTION/EVALUATION:
Assess for signs of electrolyte imbalance, esp. hypocalcemia (perioral tingling, numbness/paresthesia of extremities) or hypokalemia (weakness, muscle cramps, numbness/tingling of extremities, irritability). Monitor renal function tests. Assess for tremors; provide safety measures for potential seizures. Assess for bleeding, anemia, or developing superinfections.

PATIENT/FAMILY TEACHING:
Important to report perioral tingling, numbness in the extremities, or paresthesias during or after infusion (may indicate electrolyte abnormalities). Tremors should be reported promptly due to potential for seizures.

fosfomycin tromethamine

foss-foe-**my**-sin
(Monurol)
Do not confuse with Monopril.

▶CLASSIFICATION
PHARMACOTHERAPEUTIC: Antibiotic. **CLINICAL:** Urinary tract infection agent

ACTION/*THERAPEUTIC EFFECT*
Inhibits synthesis of peptidoglycan, the initial step in *preventing bacterial cell wall synthesis. Bactericidal.*

USES
Single-dose treatment for uncomplicated urinary tract infections (UTI) in women.

PRECAUTIONS
CONTRAINDICATIONS: None significant. **CAUTIONS:** None significant.

INTERACTIONS
DRUG: Metoclopramide lowers serum concentration, urinary excretion of fosfomycin. **HERBAL:** None known. **FOOD:** None known. **LAB VALUES:** May increase eosinophil count, bilirubin, SGOT, SGPT, alkaline phosphatase. May alter WBC, platelet count. May decrease hematocrit, hemoglobin.

AVAILABILITY (Rx)
POWDER: 3 g.

ADMINISTRATION/HANDLING
• Give without regard to food.

INDICATIONS/ROUTES/DOSAGE
UTI:
PO: Adults, elderly: 3 g mixed in water as a single dose.

SIDE EFFECTS
OCCASIONAL (3–9%): Diarrhea, nausea, headache, back pain. **RARE** (<2%): Dysmenorrhea, pharyngitis, abdominal pain, rash.

ADVERSE REACTIONS/TOXIC EFFECTS
None significant.

PATIENT/FAMILY TEACHING:
Symptoms should improve in
2–3 days. Always mix medication with water before taking.

fosinopril

foh-**sin**-oh-prill
(Monopril)
Do not confuse with Monurol.

▶CLASSIFICATION

PHARMACOTHERAPEUTIC:
Angiotensin-converting enzyme
(ACE) inhibitor. **CLINICAL:** Antihypertensive (see p. 6C).

ACTION/THERAPEUTIC EFFECT

Suppresses renin-angiotensin-aldosterone system (prevents
conversion of angiotensin I to angiotensin II, a potent vasoconstrictor; may also inhibit angiotensin II
at local vascular and renal sites).
Decreases plasma angiotensin II,
increases plasma renin activity,
decreases aldosterone secretion.
*Reduces peripheral arterial resistance, pulmonary capillary wedge
pressure, improves cardiac output,
exercise tolerance.*

PHARMACOKINETICS

	Onset	Peak	Duration
PO	1 hr	2–6 hrs	24 hrs

Slowly absorbed from GI tract.
Protein binding: 97–98%. Metabolized in liver, GI mucosa to active
metabolite. Primarily excreted in
urine. Minimal removal by hemodialysis. Half-life: 11.5 hrs.

USES/*UNLABELED*
Treatment of hypertension. Used
alone or in combination with other
antihypertensives. Treatment of
heart failure. *Treatment of renal
crisis in scleroderma.*

PRECAUTIONS

CONTRAINDICATIONS: History
of angioedema with previous
treatment with ACE inhibitors.
CAUTIONS: Renal impairment,
those with sodium depletion or on
diuretic therapy, dialysis, hypovolemia, coronary or cerebrovascular insufficiency.
▷**LIFESPAN CONSIDERATIONS:**
Pregnancy/Lactation: Crosses
placenta; distributed in breast
milk. May cause fetal/neonatal
mortality/morbidity. **Pregnancy
Category D. Children:** Safety and
efficacy not established. Neonates
and infants may be at increased
risk for oliguria and neurologic
abnormalities. **Elderly:** May be
more sensitive to hypotensive effects.

INTERACTIONS

DRUG: Alcohol, diuretics, hypotensive agents may increase
effects. **NSAIDs** may decrease effect. **Potassium-sparing diuretics, potassium supplements** may
cause hyperkalemia. May increase **lithium** concentration, toxicity. **HERBAL:** None known.
FOOD: None known. **LAB VALUES:**
May increase potassium, SGOT
(AST), SGPT (ALT), alkaline phosphatase, bilirubin, BUN, creatinine.
May decrease sodium. May cause
positive ANA titer.

AVAILABILITY (Rx)
TABLETS: 10 mg, 20 mg.

ADMINISTRATION/HANDLING

PO:

• Give without regard to food. •
Tablets may be crushed.

INDICATIONS/ROUTES/DOSAGE

Hypertension (used alone):

PO: **Adults, elderly:** Initially, 10
mg/day. **Maintenance:** 20–40
mg/day. **Maximum:** 80 mg/day.

Hypertension (with diuretic):

Note: Discontinue diuretic 2–3
days before initiation of fosinopril
therapy.

PO: **Adults, elderly:** Initially, 10
mg/day titrated to pt's needs.

Heart failure:

PO: **Adults, elderly:** Initially, 5–10
mg. **Maintenance:** 20–40 mg/day.

SIDE EFFECTS

FREQUENT (9–12%): Dizziness,
cough. *OCCASIONAL* (2–4%): Hypotension, nausea, vomiting,
upper respiratory infection.

ADVERSE REACTIONS/TOXIC EFFECTS

Excessive hypotension ("first-dose
syncope") may occur in pts with
CHF, severely salt/volume depleted.
Angioedema (swelling of face/lips),
hyperkalemia occur rarely. Agranulocytosis, neutropenia may be
noted in those with impaired renal
function or collagen vascular disease (systemic lupus erythematosus, scleroderma). Nephrotic syndrome may be noted in those with
history of renal disease.

NURSING IMPLICATIONS

BASELINE ASSESSMENT:

Obtain B/P immediately before
each dose, in addition to regular
monitoring (be alert to fluctuations). Renal function tests
should be performed before
therapy begins. In pts with renal
impairment, autoimmune disease, or taking drugs that affect
leukocytes or immune response,
CBC and differential count
should be performed before
therapy begins and q2wks for 3
mos, then periodically thereafter.

INTERVENTION/EVALUATION:

If excessive reduction in B/P occurs, place pt in supine position
with legs elevated. Assist with
ambulation if dizziness occurs.
Assess for urinary frequency.
Auscultate lung sounds for rales,
wheezing in those with CHF.
Monitor urinalysis for proteinuria. Monitor serum potassium
levels in those on concurrent diuretic therapy.

PATIENT/FAMILY TEACHING:

Report any sign of infection (sore
throat, fever). Several wks may be
needed for full therapeutic effect
of B/P reduction. Skipping doses
or voluntarily discontinuing drug
may produce severe, rebound
hypertension. To reduce hypotensive effect, rise slowly from
lying to sitting position and permit legs to dangle from bed momentarily before standing.

fosphenytoin

fos-**phen**-ih-twon
(Cerebyx)
Do not confuse with Celebrex.

▶CLASSIFICATION

PHARMACOTHERAPEUTIC:
Hydantoin. *CLINICAL:* Anticonvulsant (see p. 32C)

ACTION/*THERAPEUTIC EFFECT*

Stabilizes neuronal membranes, limits spread of seizure activity. Decreases sodium, calcium, ion influx in neurons. Decreases post-tetanic potentiation and repetitive afterdischarge. *Decreases seizure activity.*

PHARMACOKINETICS

Completely absorbed following IM administration. Protein binding: 95–99%. After IM or IV administration, rapidly/completely hydrolyzed to phenytoin. Half-life for conversion to phenytoin: 8–15 min.

USES

Acute treatment, control of generalized convulsive status epilepticus, prevention, treatment of seizures occurring during neurosurgery, short-term substitution of oral phenytoin.

PRECAUTIONS

CONTRAINDICATIONS: Hypersensitivity to fosphenytoin, phenytoin, severe bradycardia, SA block, second- or third-degree AV block, Adams-Stokes syndrome. **CAUTIONS:** Porphyria, hypotension, severe myocardial insufficiency, renal/hepatic disease, hypoalbuminemia.

▷*LIFESPAN CONSIDERATIONS:* **Pregnancy/Lactation:** May increase frequency of seizures during pregnancy. Increased risk of congenital malformations. Unknown if excreted in breast milk. **Pregnancy Category D. Children:** Safety not established. **Elderly:** Lower dosage recommended.

INTERACTIONS

DRUG: May decrease effect of **glucocorticoids. Alcohol, CNS depressants** may increase CNS depression. **Antacids** may decrease absorption. **Amiodarone, anticoagulants, cimetidine, disulfiram, fluoxetine, isoniazid, sulfonamides** may increase fosphenytoin concentration, effects, toxicity. **Fluconazole, ketoconazole, miconazole** may increase concentration. **Lidocaine, propranolol** may increase cardiac depressant effects. **Valproic acid** may increase concentration, decrease metabolism. May increase **xanthine** metabolism. *HERBAL:* None known. *FOOD:* None known. *LAB VALUES:* May increase alkaline phosphatase, GGT, glucose.

AVAILABILITY (Rx)

INJECTION: 75 mg/ml (50 mg phenytoin sodium).

ADMINISTRATION/HANDLING

IV 🍴

• Refrigerate. Do not store at room temperature >48 hrs. • After dilution, solution is stable for 8 hrs at room temperature or 24 hrs if refrigerated.

Reconstitution:

• Dilute in D_5W or 0.9% NaCl to a concentration ranging from 1.5 to 25 mg PE/ml (PE: phenytoin equivalent).

Rate of administration:

• Administer at rate of ≤150 mg PE/min (decreases risk of hypotension).

IV INCOMPATIBILITY ⊘

Do not mix with any other medications.

IV COMPATIBILITY

Potassium chloride.

INDICATIONS/ROUTES/DOSAGE

Note: 150 mg fosphenytoin yields 100 mg phenytoin. Dose, concentration solution, infusion rate of fosphenytoin expressed in terms of phenytoin equivalents (PE). Lower, less frequent dosing in elderly may be required. Not approved for pediatric use.

Status epilepticus:

IV: **Adults: Loading dose:** 15–20 mg PE/kg infused at rate of 100–150 mg PE/min.

Nonemergent seizures:

IV: **Adults: Loading dose:** 10–20 mg PE/kg. **Maintenance:** 4–6 mg PE/kg/day.

SIDE EFFECTS

FREQUENT: Dizziness, paresthesia, tinnitus, pruritus, headache, somnolence. *OCCASIONAL:* Morbilliform rash.

ADVERSE REACTIONS/TOXIC EFFECTS

A too high fosphenytoin blood concentration may produce ataxia (muscular incoordination), nystagmus (rhythmic oscillation of eyes), double vision, lethargy, slurred speech, nausea, vomiting, hypotension. As level increases, extreme lethargy to comatose states occur.

NURSING IMPLICATIONS

BASELINE ASSESSMENT:

Review history of seizure disorder (intensity, frequency, duration, LOC). Initiate seizure precautions. Obtain vital signs, medication history (esp. use of phenytoin or other anticonvulsants). Observe clinically.

INTERVENTION/EVALUATION:

Measure cardiac function, EKG, determination of respiratory function, B/P during and immediately after infusion (10–20 min). Discontinue if skin rash appears. Interrupt or decrease rate if hypotension or arrhythmias are detected. Assess pt postinfusion (may feel dizzy, ataxic, or drowsy). Assess blood levels of fosphenytoin (2 hrs post IV infusion or 4 hrs post IM injection).

PATIENT/FAMILY TEACHING:

Teach pts about their seizure condition and role in its management. If noncompliance is an issue in causing acute seizures, discuss reasons for noncompliance and address them.

F

frovatriptan

(Frovar)
See New Drug Supplement.

furosemide 🖊

feur-**oh**-sah-mide
(Apo-Furosemide ♣, Lasix)
Do not confuse with Torsemide.

▶ CLASSIFICATION

PHARMACOTHERAPEUTIC:
Loop. ***CLINICAL:*** Diuretic (see p. 84C)

ACTION/THERAPEUTIC EFFECT

Enhances excretion of sodium, chloride, potassium by direct action at ascending limb of loop of Henle, *producing diuretic effect.*

PHARMACOKINETICS

Onset	Peak	Duration
PO		
30–60 min	1–2 hrs	6–8 hrs
IM		
—	30 min	—
IV		
5 min	20–60 min	2 hrs

Well absorbed from GI tract. Protein binding: 91–97%. Partially metabolized in liver. Primarily excreted in urine (in severe renal impairment, nonrenal clearance increases). Not removed by hemodialysis. Half-life: 30–90 min (half-life increased with impaired renal, liver function and in neonates).

USES/UNLABELED

Treatment of edema associated with CHF, chronic renal failure including nephrotic syndrome, hepatic cirrhosis, acute pulmonary edema. Treats hypertension, either alone or in combination with other antihypertensives. *Treatment of hypercalcemia.*

PRECAUTIONS

CONTRAINDICATIONS: Anuria, hepatic coma, severe electrolyte depletion. **CAUTIONS:** Acute MI, oliguria, hepatic cirrhosis, history of gout, diabetes, systemic lupus erythematosus, pancreatitis.

▷**LIFESPAN CONSIDERATIONS:** **Pregnancy/Lactation:** Crosses placenta; distributed in breast milk. **Pregnancy Category C. Children:** Half-life increased in neonates; may require increasing dosage interval. **Elderly:** May be more sensitive to hypotensive or electrolyte effects, developing circulatory collapse, or thromboembolic effect. Age-related renal function impairment may require dosage adjustment.

INTERACTIONS

DRUG: Amphotericin, ototoxic, nephrotoxic agents may increase toxicity. May decrease effect of **anticoagulants, heparin. Hypokalemia-causing agents** may increase risk of hypokalemia. May increase risk of **lithium** toxicity. **Probenecid** may increase concentrations. **HERB-**

AL: None known. **FOOD:** None known. **LAB VALUES:** May increase glucose, BUN, uric acid. May decrease calcium, chloride, magnesium, potassium, sodium.

AVAILABILITY (Rx)

TABLETS: 20 mg, 40 mg, 80 mg. **ORAL SOLUTION:** 10 mg/ml, 40 mg/5 ml. **INJECTION:** 10 mg/ml.

ADMINISTRATION/HANDLING
PO:

• Give with food to avoid GI upset, preferably with breakfast (may prevent nocturia).

IM:

• Temporary pain at injection site may be noted.

IV ▥

Storage:

• Solution appears clear, colorless. • Discard yellow injections.

Rate of administration:

• May give undiluted but is compatible with D_5W, 0.9% NS, or lactated Ringer's solutions. • Administer each 40 mg or fraction by IV push over 1–2 min. Do not exceed administration rate of 4 mg/min in those with renal impairment.

IV INCOMPATIBILITIES ⊘

Ciprofloxacin (Cipro), diltiazem (Cardizem), dobutamine (Dobutrex), dopamine (Intropin), doxorubicin (Adriamycin), droperidol (Inapsine), esmolol (Brevibloc), famotidine (Pepcid), filgrastim (Neupogen), fluconazole (Diflucan), gemcitabine (Gemzar), gentamicin (Garamycin), idarubicin (Idamycin), labetolol (Trandate), meperidine, mctoclopramide (Reglan), midazolam (Versed), milrinone (Primacor), nicardipen (Cardene), ondansetron (Zofran), quinidine, thiopental (Pentothal), vecuronium (Norcuron), vinblastine (Velban), vincristine (Oncovin), vinorelbine (Navelbine).

IV COMPATIBILITIES

Heparin, lorazepam (Ativan), potassium chloride.

INDICATIONS/ROUTES/DOSAGE

Edema/hypertension:

PO: **Adults, elderly:** Initially, 20–80 mg/dose; may increase by 20–40 mg/dose at 6–8 hr intervals. **Children:** 1–6 mg/kg/day in divided doses q6–12h.

IM/IV: **Adults, elderly:** 20–40 mg/dose; may repeat in 1–2 hrs and increase by 20 mg/dose. **Children:** 1–2 mg/kg/dose q6–12h. **Neonates:** 1–2 mg/kg/dose q12–24h.

IV INFUSION: **Adults, elderly:** Bolus of 0.1 mg/kg, then 0.1 mg/kg/hr; may double q2h. **Maximum:** 0.4 mg/kg/hr. **Children:** 0.05 mg/kg/hr; titrate to desired effect.

SIDE EFFECTS

EXPECTED: Increase in urinary frequency/volume. ***FREQUENT:*** Nausea, gastric upset with cramping, diarrhea, or constipation, electrolyte disturbances. ***OCCASIONAL:*** Dizziness, lightheadedness, headache, blurred vision, paresthesia, photosensitivity, rash, weakness, urinary frequency/bladder spasm, restlessness, diaphoresis. ***RARE:*** Flank pain, loin pain.

ADVERSE REACTIONS/TOXIC EFFECTS

Vigorous diuresis may lead to profound water loss and electrolyte depletion, resulting in hypokalemia, hyponatremia, dehydration. Sudden volume depletion may result in increased risk of thrombosis, circulatory collapse, sudden death. Acute hypotensive episodes may also occur, sometimes several days after beginning of therapy. Ototoxicity manifested as deafness, vertigo, tinnitus (ringing/roaring in ears) may occur, esp. in those with severe renal impairment. Can exacerbate diabetes mellitus, systemic lupus erythematosus, gout, pancreatitis. Blood dyscrasias have been reported.

F

NURSING IMPLICATIONS

BASELINE ASSESSMENT:

Check vital signs, esp. B/P for hypotension before administration. Assess baseline electrolytes, particularly check for low potassium. Assess edema, skin turgor, mucous membranes for hydration status. Assess muscle strength, mental status. Note skin temperature, moisture. Obtain baseline weight. Initiate I&O monitoring.

INTERVENTION/EVALUATION:

Monitor B/P, vital signs, electrolytes, I&O, weight. Note extent of diuresis. Watch for changes from initial assessment (hypokalemia may result in changes in muscle strength, tremor, muscle cramps, change in mental status, cardiac arrhythmias). Hyponatremia may result in confusion, thirst, cold/clammy skin.

PATIENT/FAMILY TEACHING:

Expect increased frequency and volume of urination. Report irregular heartbeat, signs of electrolyte imbalances (noted above), hearing abnormalities (such as sense of fullness in ears, ringing/roaring in ears). Eat foods high in potassium such as whole grains (cereals), legumes, meat, bananas, apricots, orange juice, potatoes (white, sweet), raisins. Avoid sun/sunlamps.

gabapentin

gah-bah-**pen**-tin
(<u>Neurontin</u>)
Do not confuse with Noroxin.

▶CLASSIFICATION

CLINICAL: Anticonvulsant, anti-neuralgic (see p. 33C)

ACTION/*THERAPEUTIC EFFECT*

Exact mechanism unknown. May be due to increased gamma-aminobutyric acid (GABA) synthesis rate, increased GABA accumulation, or binding to as yet undefined receptor sites in brain tissue *to produce anticonvulsant activity, reduce neuropathic pain.*

PHARMACOKINETICS

Well absorbed from GI tract (not affected by food). Protein binding: <5%. Widely distributed. Crosses blood-brain barrier. Primarily excreted unchanged in urine. Removed by hemodialysis. Half-life: 5–7 hrs (half-life increased with impaired renal function, elderly).

USES

Adjunctive therapy in treatment of partial seizures and partial seizures with secondary generalization in adults. Treatment of migraines, essential tremors, hot flashes, neuropathic pain, psychiatric disorders.

PRECAUTIONS

CONTRAINDICATIONS: None significant. **CAUTIONS:** Renal impairment. Discontinue/add anticonvulsant therapy gradually (reduces loss of seizure control). Children <18 yrs of age.

▷**LIFESPAN CONSIDERATIONS:**
Pregnancy/Lactation: Unknown whether it is distributed in breast milk. **Pregnancy Category C. Children:** Safety and efficacy not established in those <12 yrs of age. **Elderly:** Age-related renal impairment may require dosage adjustment.

INTERACTIONS

DRUG: None significant. **HERBAL:** None known. **FOOD:** None known. **LAB VALUES:** May decrease WBCs.

AVAILABILITY (Rx)

CAPSULES: 100 mg, 300 mg, 400 mg. **ORAL SOLUTION:** 250 mg/5 ml. **TABLETS:** 600 mg, 800 mg.

ADMINISTRATION/HANDLING
PO:

• Give without regard to meals; may give with food to avoid or reduce GI upset. • If treatment is discontinued or anticonvulsant therapy is added, do so gradually over at least 1 wk (reduces risk of loss of seizure control).

INDICATIONS/ROUTES/DOSAGE
Seizure control:

Note: Maximum time between doses should not exceed 12 hrs.

PO: Adults >18 yrs, elderly: 900–1,800 mg/day given in divided doses q8h. May titrate to effective dose rapidly: *Day 1:* 300 mg (give at bedtime). *Day 2:* 300 mg q12h. *Day 3:* 300 mg q8h. **Maximum:** 3,600 mg/day. **Children 3–12 yrs:** Initially, 10–15 mg/kg/day. Titrate upward over 3 days up to 25–40 mg/kg/day in 3 divided doses.

Renal function impairment:

Based on creatinine clearance:

Creatinine Clearance	Dosage
>60 ml/min	400 mg q8h
30–60 ml/min	300 mg q12h
15–30 ml/min	300 mg daily
<15 ml/min	300 mg every other day
Hemodialysis	200–300 mg after each 4 hr hemodialysis

SIDE EFFECTS

FREQUENT (11–19%): Fatigue, somnolence, dizziness, ataxia. **OCCASIONAL** (3–8%): Nystagmus (rolling eye movements), tremor, diplopia (double vision), rhinitis, weight gain. **RARE** (<2%): Nervousness, dysarthria (speech difficulty), memory loss, dyspepsia, pharyngitis, myalgia.

ADVERSE REACTIONS/TOXIC EFFECTS

Abrupt withdrawal may increase seizure frequency. Overdosage may result in double vision, slurred speech, drowsiness, lethargy, diarrhea.

NURSING IMPLICATIONS

BASELINE ASSESSMENT:

Review history of seizure disorder (type, onset, intensity, frequency, duration, LOC). Routine laboratory monitoring of blood serum levels unnecessary for safe use.

INTERVENTION/EVALUATION:

Provide safety measures as needed. Assess for seizure activity.

PATIENT/FAMILY TEACHING:

Take gabapentin only as prescribed; do not abruptly stop taking drug because seizure frequency may be increased. Do not drive, operate machinery, or perform activities requiring mental acuity due to potential dizziness, somnolence. Avoid alcohol. Carry identification card/bracelet to note anticonvulsant therapy. If noncompliance is an issue in causing acute seizures, discuss reasons for noncompliance and address them.

G

galantamine

gal-**an**-tah-mine
(Reminyl)

▶CLASSIFICATION

PHARMACOTHERAPEUTIC: Cholinesterase inhibitor. **CLINICAL:** Antidementia

ACTION/THERAPEUTIC EFFECT

Elevates acetylcholine concentrations in cerebral cortex by slowing degeneration of acetylcholine released by still intact cholinergic neurons (Alzheimer's disease involves degeneration of cholinergic neuronal pathways). *Resultant effect slows progression of Alzheimer's disease.*

PHARMACOKINETICS

Rapidly absorbed from GI tract. Protein binding: 18%. Distributed to blood cells; binds to plasma proteins, mainly albumin. Metabolized in the liver. Excreted in the urine. Plasma concentration increases in pts with moderate-to-severe hepatic impairment. Half-life: 7 hrs.

USES

Treatment of mild-to-moderate dementia of Alzheimer's type.

PRECAUTIONS

CONTRAINDICATIONS: Severe hepatic or renal impairment. ***CAUTIONS:*** Moderately impaired renal/hepatic function, history of ulcer disease, those on concurrent NSAIDs, asthma, COPD, bladder outflow obstruction, supraventricular cardiac conduction conditions. ▷***LIFESPAN CONSIDERATIONS:*** **Pregnancy/Lactation:** Unknown if drug crosses placenta or is distributed in breast milk. **Pregnancy Category B. Children:** Not prescribed for this pt population. **Elderly:** No age-related precautions noted but use is not recommended in those with severe hepatic or renal impairment (creatinine clearance <9 ml/min).

INTERACTIONS

DRUG: **Cimetidine, ketoconazole, paroxetine, erythromycin** may increase galantamine concentration; may interfere with **succinylcholine, bethanechol** effects. ***HERBAL:*** None significant. ***FOOD:*** None significant. ***LAB VALUES:*** None significant.

AVAILABILITY (Rx)

TABLETS: 4 mg, 8 mg, 12 mg. ***ORAL SOLUTION:*** 4 mg/ml.

ADMINISTRATION/HANDLING
PO:
• Give with morning and evening meals.

INDICATIONS/ROUTES/DOSAGE
Alzheimer's disease:

PO: Adults, elderly: Initially, 4 mg twice daily (8 mg/day). If well tolerated and after a minimum of 4 wks, may increase to 8 mg twice daily (16 mg/day). After a minimum of 4 wks, may increase to 12 mg twice daily (24 mg/day). Do not exceed 16 mg/day in pts with moderate renal impairment.

Note: If therapy is interrupted for several days or longer, must retitrate as noted above.

SIDE EFFECTS

FREQUENT (5–17%): Nausea, vomiting, diarrhea, anorexia, weight decrease. ***OCCASIONAL*** (4–9%): Abdominal pain, insomnia, depression, headache, dizziness, fatigue, rhinitis. ***RARE*** (<3%): Tremors, constipation, confusion, cough, anxiety, urinary incontinence.

ADVERSE REACTIONS/TOXIC EFFECTS

Overdose can cause cholinergic crises (increased salivation, lacrimation, urination, defecation, bradycardia, hypotension, increased muscle weakness). Treatment aimed at general supportive measures, use of anticholinergics (e.g., atropine).

NURSING IMPLICATIONS

BASELINE ASSESSMENT:

Assess cognitive, behavioral, and functional deficits of pt. Assess liver, renal function.

INTERVENTION/EVALUATION:

Monitor cognitive, behavioral, and functional status of pt. Evaluate EKG, periodic rhythm strips in pts with underlying arrhythmias. Monitor for symptoms of ulcer, GI bleeding.

PATIENT/FAMILY TEACHING:

Take with morning and evening meals (reduces risk of nausea).

Do not reduce or stop medication; do not increase dosage without physician direction. Ensure adequate fluid intake. If therapy is interrupted for several days, restart at lowest dose and titrate to current dose at 4 wk intervals. Inform family of local chapter of Alzheimer's Disease Association (provides a guide to services for these pts).

ganciclovir sodium

gan-**sye**-klo-vir
(Cytovene, Vitrasert)
Do not confuse with Cytosar.

▶CLASSIFICATION

PHARMACOTHERAPEUTIC: Synthetic nucleoside. ***CLINICAL:*** Antiviral (see p. 58C)

ACTION/*THERAPEUTIC EFFECT*

Converted intracellularly, competes with viral DNA polymerases and direct incorporation into growing viral DNA chains, *interfering with DNA synthesis and viral replication.* Congener of acyclovir.

PHARMACOKINETICS

Widely distributed. Protein binding: 1–2%. Undergoes minimal metabolism. Primarily excreted unchanged in urine. Removed by hemodialysis. Half-life: 2.5–3.6 hrs (half-life increased with impaired renal function).

USES/*UNLABELED*

Treatment of cytomegalovirus (CMV) retinitis in immunocompromised pts (e.g., AIDS, bone marrow recipients); CMV, GI infections, pneumonitis. Possesses antiviral activity against herpes simplex. Prevention of CMV in transplant pts. ***PO:*** Maintenance treatment of CMV. *Vitrasert: Intraocular implant:* Treatment of CMV in pts with AIDS. ***IV:*** *Treatment of other CMV infections (e.g., pneumonitis, gastroenteritis, hepatitis).*

PRECAUTIONS

CONTRAINDICATIONS: Hypersensitivity to ganciclovir or acyclovir. Not for use in immunocompetent persons or those with congenital or neonatal CMV disease. ***CAUTIONS:*** Extreme caution in children because of long-term carcinogenicity, reproductive toxicity. Renal impairment, preexisting cytopenias or history of cytopenic reactions to other drugs, elderly (at greater risk of renal impairment).

▷*LIFESPAN CONSIDERATIONS:*
Pregnancy/Lactation: Effective contraception should be used during therapy; ganciclovir should not be used during pregnancy. Nursing should be discontinued; may be resumed no sooner than 72 hrs after the last dose of ganciclovir. **Pregnancy Category C. Children:** Safety and efficacy not established in those <12 yrs of age. **Elderly:** Age-related renal impairment may require dosage adjustment.

INTERACTIONS

DRUG: **Bone marrow depressants** may increase bone marrow depression. May increase risk of seizures with **imipenem-cilastatin.** May increase hematologic toxicity with **zidovudine. *HERBAL:*** None known. ***FOOD:*** None known. ***LAB VALUES:*** May increase SGOT (AST), SGPT (ALT), alkaline phosphatase, bilirubin.

G

AVAILABILITY (Rx)

CAPSULES: 250 mg, 500 mg. ***POWDER FOR INJECTION:*** 500 mg. ***IMPLANT.***

ADMINISTRATION/HANDLING

PO:

* Give with food.

IV 🍽

Storage:

* Store vials at room temperature. Do not refrigerate. * Reconstituted solution in vial is stable for 12 hrs at room temperature. * After dilution, refrigerate, use within 24 hrs. * Discard if precipitate forms, discoloration occurs. * Avoid exposure to skin, eyes, mucous membranes. * Latex gloves and safety glasses should be used during preparation and handling of solution. * Avoid inhalation. * If solution contacts skin or mucous membranes, wash carefully with soap and water; rinse eyes thoroughly with plain water).

Reconstitution:

* Reconstitute 500 mg vial with 10 ml Sterile Water for Injection to provide a concentration of 50 mg/ml; do *not* use Bacteriostatic Water (contains parabens, which is incompatible with ganciclovir). * Further dilute with 100 ml D_5W, 0.9% NaCl, lactated Ringer's, or any combination thereof to provide a concentration of 5 mg/ml.

Rate of administration:

* Administer only by IV infusion over 1 hr. * Do not give by IV push or rapid IV infusion (increases risk of toxicity; protect from infiltration (high pH causes severe tissue irritation). * Use veins with adequate blood to permit rapid dilution and dissemination of ganciclovir (minimize phlebitis); central venous catheters tunneled under SubQ tissue may reduce catheter-associated infection.

IV INCOMPATIBILITIES 🚫

Aldesleukin (Proleukin), amifostine (Ethyol), aztreonam (Azactam), cefepime (Maxipime), cytarabine (ARA-C), doxorubicin (Adriamycin), fludarabine (Fludara), foscarnet (Foscavir), gemcitabine (Gemzar), ondansetron (Zofran), piperacillin/tazobactam (Zosyn), sargramostim (Leukine), vinorelbine (Navelbine).

IV COMPATIBILITIES

Cisatracurium (Nimbex), propofol (Diprivan).

INDICATIONS/ROUTES/DOSAGE

Retinitis:

IV: **Adults, children >3 mos:** 10 mg/kg/day in divided doses q12h for 14–21 days, then 5 mg/kg/day as a single daily dose.

Prevention of CMV in transplant pts:

IV: **Adults, children:** 10 mg/kg/day in divided doses q12h for 7–14 days, then 5 mg/kg/day as a single daily dose.

Other CMV infections:

IV: **Adults, children:** Initially, 10 mg/kg/day in divided doses q12h for 14–21 days, then 5 mg/kg/day as a single daily dose.

Maintenance:

PO: **Adults:** 1,000 mg 3 times/day or 500 mg q3h (6 times/day). **Children:** 30 mg/kg/dose q8h.

Intravitreal implant:

Adults: 1 implant q6–9mos plus ganciclovir orally. **Children >9 yrs:** 1 implant q6–9mos plus ganciclovir orally (30 mg/dose q8h).

Adult dosage in renal impairment:

Creatinine Clearance (ml/min)	IV Indications	IV Maintenance	Oral
50–69	2.5 mg/kg q12h	2.5 mg/kg q24h	1,500 mg/day
25–49	2.5 mg/kg q24h	1.25 mg/kg q24h	1,000 mg/day
10–24	1.25 mg/kg q24h	0.625 mg/kg q24h	500 mg/day
<10	1.25 mg/kg 3 times/wk	0.625 mg 3 times/wk	500 mg 3 times/wk

SIDE EFFECTS

FREQUENT: Diarrhea (41%), fever (40%), nausea (25%), abdominal pain (17%), vomiting (13%). **OCCASIONAL** (6–11%): Sweating, infection, paresthesia, flatulence, pruritus. **RARE** (2–4%): Headache, stomatitis, dyspepsia, vomiting, phlebitis.

ADVERSE REACTIONS/TOXIC EFFECTS

Hematologic toxicity occurs commonly: leukopenia (29–41%), anemia (19–25%). Intraocular insert produces visual acuity loss, vitreous hemorrhage, retinal detachment occasionally. GI hemorrhage occurs rarely.

NURSING IMPLICATIONS

BASELINE ASSESSMENT:

Evaluate hematologic baseline. Obtain specimens for support of differential diagnosis (urine, feces, blood, throat) because usually retinal infection is due to hematogenous dissemination.

INTERVENTION/EVALUATION:

Monitor I&O and assure adequate hydration (minimum 1,500 ml/24 hrs). Diligently evaluate hematology reports, neutropenia, thrombocytopenia, decreased platelets. Question pt regarding vision, therapeutic improvement, or complications. Assess for rash, pruritus.

PATIENT/FAMILY TEACHING:

Ganciclovir provides suppression, not cure of CMV retinitis. Frequent blood tests and eye exams are necessary during therapy because of toxic nature of drug. It is essential to report any new symptom promptly. May temporarily or permanently inhibit sperm production in men, suppress fertility in women. Barrier contraception should be used during and for 90 days after therapy because of mutagenic potential.

ganirelix

(Antagon)

See Classification section under: Fertility agents (p. 86C)

garlic

Also known as ail, allium, nectar of the gods, poor man's treacle, stinking rose

▶CLASSIFICATION
HERBAL

ACTION/EFFECT

Possesses antithrombotic properties, can increase fibrinolytic activity, decrease platelet aggregation, increase prothrombin time. Acts as an HMG-CoA reductase inhibitor (statins), *lowering cholesterol levels.* Causes smooth muscle relaxation/vasodilation, *reducing blood pressure*. Reduces oxidative stress and LDL oxidation, *preventing age-related vascular changes and atherosclerosis*. Prevents endothelial cell depletion, *producing antioxidant effect.*

USES

Treatment of hypertension, hyperlipidemia; prevention of coronary artery disease, age-related vascular changes, atherosclerosis.

PRECAUTIONS

CONTRAINDICATIONS: Pts with bleeding disorders. ***CAUTIONS:*** Diabetes (may decrease blood sugar levels), inflammatory GI conditions (may irritate the GI tract). Hypothyroidism (may reduce iodine uptake). May prolong bleeding time (discontinue 1–2 wks prior to surgery).

▷***LIFESPAN CONSIDERATIONS:*** **Pregnancy/Lactation:** Caution: may stimulate labor and cause colic in infants. **Children:** Safety and efficacy not established (may be beneficial in children with hypercholesterolemia). **Elderly:** No age-related precautions noted.

INTERACTIONS

DRUG: May increase hypoglycemic effect of **insulin, oral antidiabetic agents.** May enhance effects of **anticoagulants/antiplatelets (e.g., warfarin, aspirin, clopidogrel, enoxaparin).** May decrease effect of **cyclosporine, oral contraceptive.** May decrease concentration/effects of **saquinavir, other HIV antiretrovirals. HERBAL:** Feverfew, **ginger, ginkgo, ginseng** may increase risk of bleeding. ***FOOD:*** None significant. ***LAB VALUES:*** May decrease blood glucose, cholesterol, increase INR.

AVAILABILITY (OTC)

CAPSULES: 100 mg, 300 mg, 500 mg, 1,000 mg, 1.5 g. ***TABLETS:*** 400 mg, 1,250 mg. ***TEA. EXTRACT. OIL. POWDER.***

INDICATIONS/ROUTES/DOSAGE

Hyperlipidemia, hypertension:

PO: Adults, elderly: (Capsules, powder, tea): 600–1,200 mg/day in divided doses 3 times/day.

Note: Appropriate doses for other conditions vary depending on the preparation used.

SIDE EFFECTS

Breath/body odor, mouth/GI burning, heartburn, nausea, vomiting, diarrhea, allergic reactions (e.g., rhinitis, urticaria, angioedema).

ADVERSE REACTIONS/TOXIC EFFECTS

None significant.

NURSING IMPLICATIONS

BASELINE ASSESSMENT:

Assess lipid levels, determine if pt is taking anticoagulants/antiplatelets. Assess if diabetic, taking insulin or oral hypoglycemic agents.

INTERVENTION/EVALUATION:

Monitor CBC, coagulation studies, lipid levels, glucose levels. Assess for hypersensitivity reaction and contact dermatitis.

PATIENT/FAMILY TEACHING:

Avoid use in pregnancy/breastfeeding. Inform all health care providers of garlic usage. Discontinue 1–2 wks prior to any procedure in which bleeding may occur.

gatifloxacin

gat-ih-**flocks**-ah-sin
(Tequin)

▶CLASSIFICATION

PHARMACOTHERAPEUTIC:
Fluorouinolone. **CLINICAL:** Antibacterial (see p. 22C)

ACTION/*THERAPEUTIC EFFECT*

Inhibits two enzymes, topoisomerase II and IV, in susceptible microorganisms, *interfering with bacterial DNA replication.* Prevents or delays resistance emergence. Bactericidal.

PHARMACOKINETICS

Well absorbed from GI tract following PO administration. Protein binding: 20%. Widely distributed. Metabolized in liver. Primarily excreted in urine. Half-life: 7–14 hrs.

USES

Treatment of infections due to acute bacterial exacerbation of chronic bronchitis, acute sinusitis, community-acquired pneumonia, cystitis, complicated urinary tract infections, pyelonephritis, urethral gonorrhea in men/women, endocervical and rectal gonorrhea in women.

PRECAUTIONS

CONTRAINDICATIONS: Hypersensitivity to quinolones. ***CAUTIONS:*** Renal/hepatic impairment, CNS disorders, cerebral anthrosclerosis, seizures, those with prolonged QT interval, uncorrected hypokalemia, those receiving quinidine, procainamide, amiodarone, sotalol.

▷*LIFESPAN CONSIDERATIONS:*
Pregnancy/Lactation: Unknown if distributed in breast milk. **Pregnancy Category C. Children:** Safety and efficacy not established. **Elderly:** Age-related renal impairment may require dosage adjustment.

INTERACTIONS

DRUG: **Probenecid** may increase plasma concentration, half-life of gatifloxacin. **Antacids, iron preparations, digoxin** may decrease plasma concentration, half-life. ***HERBAL:*** None known. ***FOOD:*** None known. ***LAB VALUES:*** None significant.

AVAILABILITY (Rx)

TABLETS: 200 mg, 400 mg. ***INJECTION:*** 200 mg, 400 mg vials.

ADMINISTRATION/HANDLING
PO:

• Give without regard to meals. • Oral gatifloxacin should be administered 4 hrs before giving antacids, multivitamins, ferrous sulfate, or buffered tablets or solutions.

Note: Do not give by rapid or bolus IV.

IV 🎖

Storage:

• Available prediluted and ready for use. • Also available in 20 ml and 40 ml vials, which must be diluted in 100–200 ml D_5W, 0.9% NaCl, lactated Ringer's, Plasma Lyte 56/D_5W, M/6 sodium lactate or Sterile Water for Injection. Also compatible with KCl.

Rate of administration:

• Infuse over 60 min.

IV INCOMPATIBILITY ⊘

Do not mix with any other medications.

INDICATIONS/ROUTES/DOSAGE

Chronic bronchitis, complicated urinary tract infections, pyelonephritis:

PO/IV: Adults >18 yrs, elderly: 400 mg/day for 7–10 days (5 days for chronic bronchitis).

Sinusitis:

PO/IV: Adults >18 yrs, elderly: 400 mg/day for 10 days.

Pneumonia:

PO/IV: Adults >18 yrs, elderly: 400 mg/day for 7–14 days.

Cystitis:

PO/IV: Adults >18 yrs, elderly: 400 mg as a single dose or 200 mg/day for 3 days.

Urethral gonorrhea in men/women, endocervical and rectal gonorrhea in women:

PO/IV: Adults >18 yrs, elderly: 400 mg as a single dose.

Dosage in renal impairment:

Creatinine Clearance	Dosage
40 ml/min	400 mg/day
<40 ml/min	Initially, 400 mg/day then 200 mg/day
Hemodialysis	Initially, 400 mg/day then 200 mg/day
Peritoneal dialysis	Initially, 400 mg/day then 200 mg/day

SIDE EFFECTS

OCCASIONAL (3–8%): Nausea, vaginitis, diarrhea, headache, dizziness. ***RARE*** (0.1–3%): Abdominal pain, constipation, dyspepsia, stomatitis, edema, insomnia, abnormal dreams, sweating, change in taste, rash.

ADVERSE REACTIONS/TOXIC EFFECTS

Pseudomembranous colitis (severe abdominal pain/cramps, severe watery diarrhea, fever) may occur. Superinfection (genital-anal pruritus, ulceration or changes in oral mucosa, moderate to severe diarrhea) may occur.

NURSING IMPLICATIONS

BASELINE ASSESSMENT:

Question for history of hypersensitivity to gatifloxacin, quinolones.

INTERVENTION/EVALUATION:

Determine pattern of bowel activity. Assist with ambulation if dizziness occurs. Assess for headache, nausea, vaginitis.

PATIENT/FAMILY TEACHING:

Do not skip dose; take full course of therapy. Take with 8 oz water; drink several glasses of water between meals. Do not take antacids within 4 hrs of medication (reduces/destroys effectiveness).

gemcitabine hydrochloride

gem-**cih**-tah-bean
(Gemzar)

▶CLASSIFICATION

PHARMACOTHERAPEUTIC: Antimetabolite. ***CLINICAL:*** Antineoplastic (see p. 71C)

ACTION/*THERAPEUTIC EFFECT*

Inhibits ribonucleotide reductase, the enzyme necessary for catalyzing DNA synthesis, thereby *producing cell death in those cells undergoing DNA synthesis.*

PHARMACOKINETICS

Following IV infusion, not extensively distributed (increased with length of infusion). Protein binding: <10%. Excreted primarily in urine as metabolite. Half-life: 42–94 min (influenced by gender/duration of infusion).

USES

Treatment of locally advanced (stage II or stage III) or metastatic (stage IV) adenocarcinoma of pancreas. Indicated for pts previously treated with 5-fluorouracil. Monotherapy or in combination with cisplatin for treatment for locally advanced/metastatic non small cell lung cancer.

PRECAUTIONS

CONTRAINDICATIONS: None significant. ***CAUTIONS:*** Impaired renal function, hepatic insufficiency. ▷***LIFESPAN CONSIDERATIONS:*** **Pregnancy/Lactation:** If possible, avoid use during pregnancy, esp. first trimester. May cause fetal harm. Unknown if distributed in breast milk. Breast feeding not recommended. **Pregnancy Category D. Children:** Safety and efficacy not established. **Elderly:** Increased risk of hematologic toxicity.

INTERACTIONS

DRUG: **Bone marrow depressants** may increase risk of bone marrow depression. **Live virus vaccines** may potentiate virus replication, increase vaccine side effects, decrease pt's antibody response to vaccine. ***HERBAL:*** None known. ***FOOD:*** None known. ***LAB VALUES:*** May increase SGOT (AST), SGPT (ALT), alkaline phosphatase, bilirubin, creatinine, BUN.

AVAILABILITY (Rx)

POWDER FOR RECONSTITUTION: 200 mg, 1 g vial.

ADMINISTRATION/HANDLING

IV 〽

Storage:

• Store at room temperature (refrigeration may cause crystallization). • Reconstituted solution is stable for 24 hrs at room temperature.

Reconstitution:

• Use gloves when handling/preparing gemcitabine. • Reconstitute 200 mg or 1 g vial with 0.9% NaCl injection without preservative (5 ml or 25 ml, respectively) to provide a concentration of 40 mg/ml. • Shake to dissolve.

Rate of administration:

• May give without further dilution. • May be further diluted with 0.9% NaCl to a concentration as low as 0.1 mg/ml. • Infuse over 30 min (do not exceed rate over 1 hr—increases toxicity).

IV INCOMPATIBILITIES ⊘

Acyclovir (Zovirax), amphotericin (Fungizone), cefoperazone (Cefobid), fuosemide (Lasix), ganciclivir (Cytovene), imipenem-cilastatin (Primaxin), irinotecan (Camptosar), methotrexate, methylprednisolone (Solu-Medrol), mitomycin (Mutamycin), piperacillin/tazobactam (Zosyn), prochlorperazine (Compazine).

IV COMPATIBILITIES

Bumetanide (Bumex), calcium gluconate, dexamethasone (Decadron), diphenhydramine (Benadryl), dobutamine (Dobutrex), dopamine (Intropin), granisetron (Kytril), heparin, hydrocortisone (Solu-Cortef), lorazepam (Ativan), ondansetron (Zofran), potassium.

INDICATIONS/ROUTES/DOSAGE

Note: Dosage is individualized on basis of clinical response and tolerance to adverse effects. When used in combination therapy, consult specific protocols for optimum dosage, sequence of drug administration.

Pancreatic cancer:

***IV INFUSION:* Adults:** 1,000 mg/m^2 once weekly for up to 7 wks (or until toxicity necessitates decreasing/holding the dose), followed by 1 wk of rest. Subsequent cycles should consist of once weekly for 3 consecutive wks out of every 4 wks. Pts completing cycles at 1,000 mg/m^2 may increase dose to 1,250 mg/m^2 as tolerated. Dose for next cycle may be increased to 1,500 mg/m^2. **Note:** May increase dose provided the absolute granulocyte count (AGC) and platelet nadirs exceed $1,500 \times 10^6$/L and $100,00 \times 10^6$/L, respectively.

Dose Reduction Guidelines

AGC (10^6/L)		Platelets (10^6/L)	% Full Dose
1,000	and	100,000	100
500–999	or	50,000–99,000	75
<500	or	<50,000	Hold

SIDE EFFECTS

FREQUENT: Nausea and vomiting (69%), generalized pain (48%), fever (41%), mild to moderate pruritic rash (30%), mild to moderate dyspnea, constipation (23%), peripheral edema (20%). ***OCCASIONAL*** (10–19%): Diarrhea, petachiae, alopecia, usually minimal, stomatitis (burning/erythema of oral mucosa, sore throat, difficulty swallowing), infection, somnolence, paresthesia, petechiae. ***RARE:*** Sweating, rhinitis, insomnia, malaise.

ADVERSE REACTIONS/TOXIC EFFECTS

Severe bone marrow suppression evidenced by anemia, thrombocytopenia, leukopenia occurs commonly.

NURSING IMPLICATIONS

BASELINE ASSESSMENT:

CBC, renal and hepatic function lab tests should be performed prior to initiation of therapy and periodically thereafter. Drug should be suspended or dose modified if bone marrow suppression is detected.

INTERVENTION/EVALUATION:

Assess all lab results before each dose is given. Monitor for dyspnea, fever, pruritic rash, dehydration due to vomiting. Assess oral mucosa for mucosal erythema, ulceration at inner margin of lips, sore throat, difficulty swallowing (stomatitis). Assess skin for rash. Monitor for and report diarrhea. Provide antiemetics as needed.

PATIENT/FAMILY TEACHING:

Avoid crowds and exposure to infection. Maintain fastidious oral hygiene. Promptly report fever, sore throat, signs of local infection, easy bruising, rash. Contact physician if nausea/vomiting continues at home.

gemfibrozil

gem-**fie**-bro-zill
(Lopid)

▶CLASSIFICATION

PHARMACOTHERAPEUTIC: Fibric acid derivative. ***CLINICAL:*** Antihyperlipoproteinemic (see p. 50C)

ACTION/*THERAPEUTIC EFFECT*

Inhibits lipolysis of fat in adipose tissue; decreases liver uptake of free fatty acids (reduces hepatic triglyceride production). Inhibits synthesis of VLDL carrier apolipoprotein B. *Lowers serum cholesterol and triglycerides (decreases VLDL, LDL, increases HDL).*

PHARMACOKINETICS

Well absorbed from GI tract. Metabolized in liver. Primarily excreted in urine. Not removed by hemodialysis. Half-life: 1.5 hrs.

USES

Treatment of hyperlipidemia, decreases risk of coronary heart disease in pts with type IIB hyperlipidemia. Treatment of severe primary hyperlipidemia (types IV, V).

PRECAUTIONS

CONTRAINDICATIONS: Hepatic dysfunction (including primary biliary cirrhosis), severe renal dysfunction, preexisting gallbladder disease. **CAUTIONS:** Hypothyroidism, diabetes mellitus, estrogen or anticoagulant therapy.
▷**LIFESPAN CONSIDERATIONS:**
Pregnancy/Lactation: Unknown if drug crosses placenta or is distributed in breast milk. Decision to discontinue nursing or drug should be based on potential for serious adverse effects. **Pregnancy Category C. Children:** Not recommended in those <2 yrs of age (cholesterol necessary for normal development). **Elderly:** Age-related renal impairment may require dosage adjustment.

INTERACTIONS

DRUG: May increase effect of **warfarin.** May cause rhabdomyolysis, leading to acute renal failure with **lovastatin. HERBAL:** None known. **FOOD:** None known. **LAB VALUES:** May increase SGOT (AST), SGPT (ALT), alkaline phosphatase, bilirubin, creatinine kinase, LDH. May decrease hemoglobin, hematocrit, potassium, leukocyte counts.

AVAILABILITY (Rx)

TABLETS: 600 mg.

ADMINISTRATION/HANDLING

PO:
• Give 30 min before morning and evening meals.

INDICATIONS/ROUTES/DOSAGE

Hyperlipidemia:
PO: Adults, elderly: 900 mg to 1.5 g/day in 2 divided doses.

SIDE EFFECTS

FREQUENT (20%): Dyspepsia. **OCCASIONAL** (2–10%): Abdominal pain, diarrhea, nausea, vomiting, fatigue. **RARE** (<2%): Constipation, acute appendicitis, vertigo, headache, rash, altered taste.

ADVERSE REACTIONS/TOXIC EFFECTS

Cholelithiasis, cholecystitis, acute appendicitis, pancreatitis, malignancy occur rarely.

NURSING IMPLICATIONS

BASELINE ASSESSMENT:

Assess baseline lab results: serum glucose, triglyceride, cholesterol levels, liver function tests, CBC.

INTERVENTION/EVALUATION:

Determine pattern of bowel activity. Monitor LDL, VLDL, serum triglyceride, and cholesterol lab results for therapeutic response. Assess for rash, pruritus. Check

G

for headache and dizziness, blurred vision. Monitor liver function and hematology tests. Assess for pain, esp. right upper quadrant/epigastric pain suggestive of adverse gallbladder effects. Monitor serum glucose for those receiving insulin or oral antihyperglycemics.

PATIENT/FAMILY TEACHING:

Follow special diet (important part of treatment). Periodic lab tests are essential part of therapy. Notify physician in event of abdominal/epigastric pain.

gemtuzumab ozogamicin

gem-**too**-zoo-mab
(Mylotarg)

▶CLASSIFICATION

PHARMACOTHERAPEUTIC:
Monoclonal antibody. **CLINI-CAL:** Antineoplastic (see p. 71C)

ACTION/*THERAPEUTIC EFFECT*

Composed of an antibody cojoined with a cytotoxic antitumor antibody. The antibody portion binds to an antigen expressed on surface of leukemic blast in >80% of pts with AML, resulting in formation of a complex. This releases the antibiotic inside the lysosomes of the myeloid cells *binding to DNA resulting in DNA double-strand breaks and cell death. Produces inhibition of colony formation in cultures of adult leukemic bone marrow cells.*

PHARMACOKINETICS

After first infusion elimination half-life is 45 hrs; after second dose, elimination half-life increased to 60 hrs.

USES

Treatment of pts with CD33 positive acute myeloid leukemia (AML) in first relapse who are >60 yrs of age and not considered candidates for cytotoxic chemotherapy.

PRECAUTIONS

CONTRAINDICATIONS: None significant. ***CAUTIONS:*** Liver impairment.
▷***LIFESPAN CONSIDERATIONS:***
Pregnancy/Lactation: May cause fetal harm. Not known if excreted in breast milk. **Pregnancy Category D. Children:** Safety and efficacy not established. **Elderly:** No age-related precautions noted.

INTERACTIONS

DRUG: None significant. ***HERBAL:*** None known. ***FOOD:*** None known. ***LAB VALUES:*** May decrease WBCs, hemoglobin, hematocrit, platelet count, potassium, magnesium. May increase bilirubin, SGOT (AST), SGPT (ALT), transaminase.

AVAILABILITY (Rx)

POWDER FOR INJECTION: 5 mg.

ADMINISTRATION/HANDLING

IV 🏥

Storage:

• Protect from direct and indirect sunlight and unshielded fluorescent light during preparation and administration. • Refrigerate, do not freeze. • Following reconstitution in vial, stable for 8 hrs if refrigerated and protected from light. • Once diluted with 100 ml 0.9% NaCl, use immediately.

Reconstitution:

• Prepare in a biologic safety hood with fluorescent light off. •

Allow vials to come to room temperature. • Reconstitute each vial with 5 ml Sterile water for Injection using sterile syringes to provide concentration of 1 mg/ml. • Gently swirl; inspect for particulate matter/discoloration. • Withdraw desired volume from each vial and inject into 100 ml 0.9% NaCl and place into a UV protectant bag.

Rate of administration:

• Do not give IV push or bolus. • Infuse over 2 hrs. • Use separate line equipped with a low protein binding 1.2 micron filter. • May give through peripheral or central line.

IV INCOMPATIBILITY ⊘

Do not mix with any other medications.

INDICATIONS/ROUTES/DOSAGE
AML:

IV INFUSION: Adults ≥60 yrs: 9 mg/m^2; repeat in 14 days for total of 2 doses.

Note: Diphenhydramine 50 mg and acetaminophen 650–1,000 mg given 1 hr before administering; follow by acetaminophen 650–1,000 mg q4h for 2 doses, then q4h as needed. Full recovery from hematologic toxicities is not a requirement for giving second dose.

SIDE EFFECTS

Note: Most pts experience a postinfusion symptom complex of fever (85%), chills (73%), nausea (70%), vomiting (63%) that resolves within 2–4 hrs with supportive therapy. **FREQUENT** (31–44%): Asthenia (loss of strength, energy), diarrhea, abdominal pain, headache, stomatitis (burning/erythema of oral mucosa, ulceration, sore throat, difficulty swallowing), dyspnea, epistaxis. **OCCASIONAL** (15–25%): Constipation, neutropenic fever, nonspecific rash, herpes simplex, hypertension, hypotension, petechiae, peripheral edema, dizziness, insomnia, back pain. **RARE** (10–14%): Pharyngitis, ecchymosis, dyspepsia, tachycardia, hematuria, rhinitis.

ADVERSE REACTIONS/TOXIC EFFECTS

Severe myelosuppression occurs in 98% of all pts characterized as neutropenia, anemia, thrombocytopenia. Sepsis occurs in 25% of pts. Hepatotoxicity may occur.

NURSING IMPLICATIONS

BASELINE ASSESSMENT:

Obtain baseline CBC. Hepatic function studies, blood serum chemistry for comparison to expected myelosuppression. Use strict aseptic technique to protect pt from infection.

INTERVENTION/EVALUATION:

Monitor CBC, blood chemistries, WBC, hepatic function studies. Monitor for myelosuppression (fever, sore throat, signs of local infection, easy bruising or unusual bleeding from any site), symptoms of anemia (excessive tiredness, weakness). Assess for impending stomatitis. Monitor B/P for hyper/hypotension.

PATIENT/FAMILY TEACHING:

Do not have immunizations without physician's approval (drug lowers body's resistance). Avoid contact with those who have recently received live virus vaccine. Promptly report fever, sore throat, signs of local infection, easy bruising or unusual bleeding from any site.

gentamicin sulfate

jen-tah-**my**-sin
(Alcomicin♣, Cidomycin♣, Garamycin, Genoptic, Gentacidin, Jenamicin)

▶CLASSIFICATION

PHARMACOTHERAPEUTIC: Aminoglycoside. **CLINICAL:** Antibiotic (see p. 17C)

ACTION/*THERAPEUTIC EFFECT*

Bactericidal. Irreversibly binds to protein of bacterial ribosomes, *interfering in protein synthesis of susceptible microorganisms.*

PHARMACOKINETICS

Rapid, complete absorption after IM administration. Protein binding: <10%. Widely distributed (does not cross blood-brain barrier, low concentrations in CSF). Excreted unchanged in urine. Removed by hemodialysis. Half-life: 2–4 hrs (half-life increased with impaired renal function, neonates; decreased in cystic fibrosis, burn or febrile pts).

USES/*UNLABELED*

Parenteral: Treatment of skin/skin structure, bone, joint, respiratory tract, intra-abdominal, complicated urinary tract, and acute pelvic infections; postop, burns, septicemia, meningitis. **Ophthalmic:** Ointment/solution for superficial eye infections. **Topical:** Cream/ointment for superficial skin infections. Ophthalmic or topical applications may be combined with systemic administration for serious, extensive infections. **Topical:** *Prophylaxis of minor bacterial skin infections, treatment of dermal ulcer.*

PRECAUTIONS

CONTRAINDICATIONS: Hypersensitivity to gentamicin, other aminoglycosides (cross sensitivity). Sulfite sensitivity may result in anaphylaxis, esp. in asthmatics. **CAUTIONS:** Elderly, neonates because of renal insufficiency or immaturity; neuromuscular disorders (potential for respiratory depression), prior hearing loss, vertigo, renal impairment. Cumulative effects may occur with concurrent systemic administration and topical application to large areas.

▷**LIFESPAN CONSIDERATIONS:** **Pregnancy/Lactation:** Readily crosses placenta, not known if distributed in breast milk. **Children:** Caution in neonates: Immature renal function, increasing half-life and toxicity. **Elderly:** Age-related renal impairment may require dosage adjustment.

INTERACTIONS

DRUG: Other **aminoglycosides, nephrotoxic, ototoxic-producing medications** may increase toxicity. May increase effects of **neuromuscular blocking agents.** **HERBAL:** None known. **FOOD:** None known. **LAB VALUES:** May increase BUN, SGPT (ALT), SGOT (AST), bilirubin, creatinine, LDH concentrations; may decrease serum calcium, magnesium, potassium, sodium concentrations. Therapeutic blood serum level: Peak 6–10 mcg/ml; trough: 0.5–2 mcg/ml. Toxic blood serum level: Peak: >10 mcg/ml; trough: >2 mcg/ml.

AVAILABILITY (Rx)

INJECTION: 10 mg/ml, 40 mg/ml,

2 mg/ml (Intrathecal). **OPHTHAL-MIC SOLUTION:** 3 mg/ml. **OPHTHALMIC OINTMENT:** 3 mg/g. **CREAM:** 0.5%. **OINTMENT:** 0.1%.

ADMINISTRATION/HANDLING

IM:

• To minimize discomfort, give deep IM slowly. • Less painful if injected into gluteus maximus rather than lateral aspect of thigh.

IV 🔳

Storage:

• Store vials at room temperature. • Solution appears clear or slightly yellow. • Intermittent IV infusion (piggyback) is stable for 24 hrs at room temperature. • Discard if precipitate forms.

Reconstitution:

• Dilute with 50–200 ml D_5W or 0.9% NaCl. Amount of diluent for infants, children depends on individual needs.

Rate of administration:

• Infuse over 30–60 min for adults, older children, and over 60–120 min for infants, young children.

Intrathecal:

• Use only 2 mg/ml intrathecal preparation without preservative. • Mix with 10% estimated CSF volume or NaCl. • Use intrathecal forms immediately after preparation. Discard unused portion. • Give over 3–5 min.

Ophthalmic:

• Place finger on lower eyelid and pull out until a pocket is formed between eye and lower lid • Hold dropper above pocket and place correct number of drops ($1/4$–$1/2$ inch ointment) into pocket. Close eye gently. • **Solution:** Apply digital pressure to lacrimal sac for 1–2 min (minimizes drainage into nose and throat, reducing risk of systemic effects). • **Ointment:** Close eye for 1–2 min, rolling eyeball (increases contact area of drug to eye). • Remove excess solution or ointment around eye with tissue.

IV INCOMPATIBILITIES ⊘

Allopurinol (Aloprim), amphotericin B complex (Abelcet, Ambisome, Amphotec), furosemide (Lasix), heparin, hetastarch (Hespan), idarubicin (Idamycin), indomethacin (Indocin), propofol (Diprivan).

IV COMPATIBILITIES

Amiodarone (Cordarone), diltiazem (Cardizem), insulin, lorazepam (Ativan), magnesium, midazolam (Versed), multivitamins.

INDICATIONS/ROUTES/DOSAGE

Note: Space parenteral doses evenly around the clock. Dosage based on ideal body weight. Peak, trough level determined periodically to maintain desired serum concentrations (minimizes risk of toxicity). **Recommended peak level:** 4–10 mcg/ml; **trough level:** 1–2 mcg/ml.

Usual dosage:

IM/IV: Adults, elderly: 3–6 mg/kg/day in divided doses q8h or 4–6.6 mg/kg once daily. **Children 5–12 yrs:** 2–2.5 mg/kg/dose q8h. **Children <5 yrs:** 2.5 mg/kg/dose q8h. **Neonates:** 2.5–3.5 mg/kg/dose q8–12h.

Hemodialysis:

IM/IV: Adults, elderly: 0.5–0.7 mg/kg/dose postdialysis. **Children:** 1.25–1.75 mg/kg/dose postdialysis.

Intrathecal:

Adults: 4–8 mg/day. **Children 3 mos–12 yrs:** 1–2 mg/day. **Neonates:** 1 mg/day.

Usual ophthalmic dosage:

OINTMENT:* Adults, elderly:** Thin strip to conjunctiva 2–3 times/day. ***SOLUTION: 1–2 drops q2–4h up to 2 drops qh.

Usual topical dosage:

Adults, elderly: Apply 3–4 times/day.

SIDE EFFECTS

OCCASIONAL: Pain, induration at IM injection site; phlebitis, thrombophlebitis with IV administration; hypersensitivity reactions: rash, fever, urticaria, pruritus. ***Ophthalmic:*** Burning, tearing, itching, blurred vision. ***Topical:*** Redness, itching. ***RARE:*** Alopecia, hypertension, weakness.

ADVERSE REACTIONS/TOXIC EFFECTS

Nephrotoxicity (evidenced by increased BUN and serum creatinine, decreased creatinine clearance) may be reversible if drug stopped at first sign of symptoms; irreversible ototoxicity (tinnitus, dizziness, ringing/roaring in ears, reduced hearing) and neurotoxicity (headache, dizziness, lethargy, tremors, visual disturbances) occur occasionally. Risk is greater with higher dosages, prolonged therapy, or if solution is applied directly to mucosa. Superinfections, particularly with fungi, may result from bacterial imbalance via any route of administration. Ophthalmic application may cause paresthesia of conjunctiva, mydriasis.

> ### NURSING IMPLICATIONS

BASELINE ASSESSMENT:

Dehydration must be treated before parenteral therapy is begun. Establish baseline hearing acuity. Question for history of allergies, esp. to aminoglycosides and sulfite (and parabens for topical/ophthalmic routes).

INTERVENTION/EVALUATION:

Monitor I&O (maintain hydration), urinalysis (casts, RBCs, WBCs, decrease in specific gravity). Be alert to ototoxic and neurotoxic symptoms (see Adverse Reactions/Toxic Effects). Check IM injection site for induration. Evaluate IV site for phlebitis (heat, pain, red streaking over vein). Assess for rash (**ophthalmic:** Assess for redness, burning, itching, tearing; **topical:** Assess for redness, itching). Be alert for superinfection, particularly genital/anal pruritus, changes in oral mucosa, diarrhea. When treating those with neuromuscular disorders, assess respiratory response carefully. Therapeutic blood serum level: Peak 6–10 mcg/ml; trough: 0.5–2 mcg/ml. Toxic blood serum level: Peak: >10 mcg/ml; trough: >2 mcg/ml.

PATIENT/FAMILY TEACHING:

Discomfort may occur with IM injection. Blurred vision or tearing may occur briefly after each ophthalmic dose. Notify physician in event of any hearing, visual, balance, urinary problems, even after therapy is completed. ***Ophthalmic:*** Contact physician if tearing, redness, or irritation continues. ***Topical:*** Cleanse area gently before applying; notify physician if redness, itching occurs.

---

ginger

Also known as black ginger, race ginger, zingiber

▶CLASSIFICATION
HERBAL

ACTION/*EFFECT*
Possesses antipyretic, analgesic, antitussive, sedative properties. Increases GI motility; may act on serotonin receptors, primarily $5HT_3$, *reducing nausea and vomiting.*

USES
Prevention of nausea and vomiting caused by motion sickness or early pregnancy, dyspepsia; treatment of rheumatoid arthritis.

PRECAUTIONS
CONTRAINDICATIONS: None significant. *CAUTIONS:* Pregnancy, pts with bleeding conditions, diabetes (may cause hypoglycemia).
▷*LIFESPAN CONSIDERATIONS:*
Pregnancy/Lactation: Use during pregnancy is controversial. Avoid use (large amounts act as an abortifacient). **Children:** Safety and efficacy not established. **Elderly:** No age-related precautions noted.

INTERACTIONS
DRUG: Large amounts may increase risk of bleeding with **anticoagulants, antiplatelets. HERBAL: Feverfew, garlic, ginkgo, ginseng** may increase risk of bleeding. *FOOD:* None significant. *LAB VALUES:* None significant.

AVAILABILITY
CAPSULES: 470 mg, 550 mg. *ROOT:* 470 mg, 550 mg. *EXTRACT. POWDER. TABLETS. TEA. TINCTURE.*

INDICATIONS/ROUTES/DOSAGE
Morning sickness:
PO: **Adults:** 250 mg 4 times/day. **Maximum:** 4 g/day.

Motion sickness:
PO: **Adults:** 1 g (dried powder root) 30 min prior to travel.

Nausea:
PO: **Adults:** 550–1,100 mg 3 times/day.

SIDE EFFECTS
Abdominal discomfort, heartburn, diarrhea, hypersensitivity reaction, nausea.

ADVERSE REACTIONS/TOXIC EFFECTS
CNS depression, arrhythmias.

G

NURSING IMPLICATIONS

BASELINE ASSESSMENT
Assess for use of anticoagulants, antiplatelets (may increase risk of bleeding).

INTERVENTION/EVALUATION
Monitor for hypersensitivity reaction.

PATIENT/FAMILY TEACHING
Avoid use during pregnancy/breast-feeding.

ginkgo biloba

Also known as fossil tree, maidenhair tree, tanakan

▶CLASSIFICATION
HERBAL

ACTION/*EFFECT*
Possesses antioxidant and free radical scavenging properties, *protecting tissues from oxidative damage and preventing progression of tissue degeneration in pts with dementia.* Inhibits platelet-

activating factor bonding at numerous cells, *decreasing platelet aggregation, smooth muscle contraction; may also increase cardiac contractility and coronary blood flow.* Decreases blood viscosity, *improving circulation by relaxing vascular smooth muscle.* Increases cerebral and peripheral blood flow and reduces vascular permeability. May influence neurotransmitter system (e.g., cholinergic).

USES

Dementia syndromes, including Alzheimer's. Improves circulation in the brain and peripherally. Improves conditions associated with cerebral vascular insufficiency (e.g., memory loss, difficulty concentrating, vertigo, tinnitus). Improves cognitive behavior/sleep patterns in pts with depression. Acts as an antioxidant.

PRECAUTIONS

CONTRAINDICATIONS: Pregnancy/lactation. ***CAUTIONS:*** Pts with bleeding disorders, diabetes, epileptic pts or those prone to seizures. Avoid use in couples having difficulty conceiving.

▷***LIFESPAN CONSIDERATIONS:*** **Pregnancy/Lactation:** Contraindicated. **Children:** Safety and efficacy not established. Avoid use. **Elderly:** No age-related precautions noted.

INTERACTIONS

DRUG: May increase effect of **MAOIs.** May increase bleeding with **anti-coagulants, antiplatelets (e.g., warfarin, aspirin, heparin, clopidogrel).** ***HERBAL:*** **Feverfew, ginger, garlic, ginseng** may increase risk of bleeding. ***FOOD:*** None significant. ***LAB VALUES:*** May alter blood glucose levels.

AVAILABILITY (OTC)

CAPSULES: 40 mg, 60 mg. ***TABLETS:*** 40 mg, 60 mg. ***FLUID EXTRACT. TINCTURE.***

INDICATIONS/ROUTES/DOSAGE
Dementia:
PO: Adults, elderly: 120–240 mg/day ***(extract)*** in 2–3 doses.

Vertigo, tinnitus:
PO: Adults, elderly: 120–160 mg/day.

SIDE EFFECTS

Headache, dizziness, palpitations, constipation, allergic skin reactions. Large doses may cause nausea, vomiting, diarrhea, weakness, lack of muscle tone.

ADVERSE REACTIONS/TOXIC EFFECTS

None significant.

NURSING IMPLICATIONS

BASELINE ASSESSMENT:
Assess for use of anticoagulants/antiplatelets, MAOIs. Determine if pt has any bleeding disorders, diabetes, history of seizures.

INTERVENTION/EVALUATION:
Monitor for hypersensitivity reaction, blood glucose levels.

PATIENT/FAMILY TEACHING:
Avoid use with anticoagulants/antiplatelets. May take up to 6 mos before it becomes effective. Do not use during pregnancy/breast-feeding. Avoid use in children.

✐ - see color pill atlas   <u>underscored</u> - top 100 prescribed drug

ginseng

Also known as Asian ginseng, Chinese ginseng, red ginseng

▶CLASSIFICATION
HERBAL

ACTION/EFFECT

Affects the hypothalamic-pituitary-adrenal axis, *reducing stress.* Appears to stimulate natural killer cell action, *affecting the immune function.* Increases antioxidant activity, interferes with platelet aggregation, has analgesic, anti-inflammatory effects.

USES

Increases resistance to stress, boosts energy, enhances brain activity, increases physical endurance, aids in blood sugar control, improves cognitive function, concentration, memory, work efficiency.

PRECAUTIONS

CONTRAINDICATIONS: Pts with bleeding tendencies or thrombosis. Avoid use during pregnancy/lactation. **CAUTIONS:** Pts with cardiac disorders, diabetes, hormone-sensitive cancers (e.g., breast, uterine, ovarian), endometriosis, uterine fibroids.
▷**LIFESPAN CONSIDERATIONS:**
Pregnancy/Lactation: Insufficient information. Do not use. **Children:** Safety and efficacy not established. **Elderly:** No age-related precautions noted.

INTERACTIONS

DRUG: May increase bleeding with **anticoagulants, antiplatelets (e.g., aspirin, clopidogrel,** enoxaparin, heparin, warfarin).** May increase effect of **oral antidiabetic agents, insulin.** May decrease effect of **furosemide.** May interfere with immunosuppressant drugs (e.g., **cyclosporine, prednisone),** *HERBAL:* **Chamomile, feverfew, garlic, ginger, ginkgo** may increase risk of bleeding. *FOOD:* **Coffee, tea** may increase effect. *LAB VALUES:* May prolong APTT, decrease glucose.

AVAILABILITY (OTC)

CAPSULES: 100 mg, 250 mg, 410 mg, 500 mg. **TABLETS:** 250 mg, 1,000 mg. **DRIED ROOT. EXTRACT. POWDER. TEA (usually 1,500 mg/bag). TINCTURE.**

INDICATIONS/ROUTES/DOSAGE
Usual dosage:

PO: **Adults, elderly:** *(tablets/capsules):* 200–600 mg/day. *(Powder root):* 0.6–3 g 1–3 times/day. *(Tea—1,500mg):* 1–3 times/day.

SIDE EFFECTS

FREQUENT: Insomnia. **OCCASIONAL:** Vaginal bleeding, amenorrhea, palpitations, hypertension, diarrhea, headache, allergic reactions.

ADVERSE REACTIONS/TOXIC EFFECTS

None significant.

NURSING IMPLICATIONS

BASELINE ASSESSMENT:

Determine if pt is pregnant/breast-feeding. Assess if pt is diabetic, taking oral hypoglycemic agents, insulin; taking anticoagulants, immunosuppressant agents. Determine baseline blood glucose.

INTERVENTION/EVALUATION:
Monitor coagulation studies, glucose levels. Assess for hypersensitivity reaction, rash.

PATIENT/FAMILY TEACHING:
Avoid use in pregancy/breastfeeding, children. Avoid continuous use for >3 mos.

glatiramer

glah-**tie**-rah-mir
(Copaxone)
Do not confuse with Compazine.

▶CLASSIFICATION

PHARMACOTHERAPEUTIC:
Immunosuppressive. **CLINICAL:**
Neurologic agent

ACTION/*THERAPEUTIC EFFECT*
Exact mechanism unknown. May act by modifying immune processes thought to be responsible for pathogenesis of multiple sclerosis. *Slows progression of multiple sclerosis.*

PHARMACOKINETICS
Substantial fraction of glatirimer is hydrolyzed locally. Some fraction of injected material enters lymphatic circulation, reaching regional lymph nodes; some may enter systemic circulation intact.

USES
Treatment of relapsing, remitting multiple sclerosis.

PRECAUTIONS
CONTRAINDICATIONS: Hypersensitivity to glatiramer or mannitol. **CAUTIONS:** Immediate postinjection reaction (flushing, chest pain, palpitations, anxiety, dyspnea, urticaria).

▷**LIFESPAN CONSIDERATIONS:**
Pregnancy/Lactation: Unknown if distributed in breast milk. **Pregnancy Category B. Children:** Safety and efficacy not established. **Elderly:** Information not available.

INTERACTIONS
DRUG: None significant. **HERBAL:** None known. **FOOD:** None known. **LAB VALUES:** None significant.

AVAILABILITY (Rx)
INJECTION: 20 mg/ml.

ADMINISTRATION/HANDLING
SubQ:
• Refrigerate (diluent may be stored at room temperature). • Reconstitute with diluent provided by manufacturer (Sterile Water for Injection). • Gently swirl and let stand at room temperature until solid material is completely dissolved. • Use immediately following reconstitution.

INDICATIONS/ROUTES/DOSAGE
Multiple sclerosis:
SubQ: **Adults, elderly:** 20 mg once daily.

SIDE EFFECTS
COMMON (40–73%): Pain, erythema, inflammation, pruritus at injection site, asthenia (loss of strength, energy). **FREQUENT** (18–27%): Arthralgia, vasodilation, anxiety, hypertonia, nausea, transient chest pain, dyspnea, flu syndrome, rash, pruritus. **OCCASIONAL** (10–17%): Palpitations, back pain, sweating, rhinitis, diarrhea, urinary urgency. **RARE** (6–8%): Anorexia, fever, neck pain,

peripheral edema, ear pain, facial edema, vertigo, vomiting.

ADVERSE REACTIONS/TOXIC EFFECTS

Infection occurs commonly. Lymphadenopathy occurs occasionally.

NURSING IMPLICATIONS

INTERVENTION/EVALUATION:

Assess injection site for reaction. Monitor for fever, chills (evidence of infection) and treat accordingly.

PATIENT/FAMILY TEACHING:

Report difficulty in breathing or swallowing, rash, or itching, swelling of lower extremities, weakness. Avoid pregnancy.

glimepiride

glim-**eh**-purr-eyd
(Amaryl)

▶CLASSIFICATION

PHARMACOTHERAPEUTIC:
Second-generation sulfonylurea.
CLINICAL: Hypoglycemic (see p. 39C)

ACTION/THERAPEUTIC EFFECT

Promotes release of insulin from beta cells of pancreas, increases insulin sensitivity at peripheral sites, *lowering blood glucose concentration.*

PHARMACOKINETICS

	Onset	Peak	Duration
PO	—	2–3 hrs	24 hrs

Completely absorbed from GI tract. Protein binding: >99%. Me-tabolized in liver. Excreted in urine and eliminated in feces. Half-life: 5–9.2 hrs.

USES

Adjunct to diet/exercise in management of noninsulin-dependent diabetes mellitus (type 2, NIDDM). Use in combination with insulin or metformin in pts not controlled by diet/exercise in conjunction with oral hypoglycemic agent.

PRECAUTIONS

CONTRAINDICATIONS: Sole therapy for type I diabetes mellitus, diabetic complications (ketosis, acidosis, diabetic coma), stress situations (severe infection, trauma, surgery), severe renal or hepatic impairment. **CAUTIONS:** Severe diarrhea, intestinal obstruction, prolonged vomiting, liver disease, hyperthyroidism (not controlled), impaired renal function, adrenal insufficiency, debilitation, malnutrition, pituitary insufficiency.

▷**LIFESPAN CONSIDERATIONS:**
Pregnancy/Lactation: Not recommended for use during pregnancy. Unknown if distributed in breast milk. **Pregnancy Category C. Children:** Safety and efficacy not established. **Elderly:** Hypoglycemia may be difficult to recognize. Age-related renal impairment may increase sensitivity to glucose lowering effect.

INTERACTIONS

DRUG: May increase effect of **oral anticoagulants. Fluconazole, cimetidine, ranitidine, ciprofloxacin, MAO inhibitors, quinidine, salicylates** (large doses) may increase effect. **Beta-blockers** may increase hypoglycemic effect, mask signs of hypoglycemia. **Corticosteroids, thiazide diuretics, lithium** may decrease effect. ***HERBAL:*** None known. ***FOOD:*** None known. ***LAB VALUES:*** May increase alkaline phosphatase, SGOT (AST), LDH, creatinine, BUN.

AVAILABILITY (Rx)
TABLETS: 1 mg, 2 mg, 4 mg.

ADMINISTRATION/HANDLING
PO:
• Give with breakfast or first main meal.

INDICATIONS/ROUTES/DOSAGE
Diabetes mellitus:
PO: Adults: Initially, 1–2 mg once daily, with breakfast or first main meal. **Maintenance:** 1–4 mg once daily. After dose of 2 mg is reached, dosage should be increased in increments of up to 2 mg q1–2wks, based on blood glucose response. **Maximum:** 8 mg/day.

Combination therapy with insulin:
PO: Adults: 8 mg once daily with breakfast or first main meal with low-dose insulin.

Renal function impairment:
PO: Adults: 1 mg once/day.

SIDE EFFECTS
FREQUENT: Altered taste sensation, dizziness, drowsiness, weight gain, constipation, diarrhea, heartburn, nausea, vomiting, stomach fullness, headache. ***OCCASIONAL:*** Increased sensitivity of skin to sunlight, peeling of skin, itching, rash.

ADVERSE REACTIONS/TOXIC EFFECTS
Hypoglycemia may occur due to overdosage, insufficient food intake esp. with increased glucose demands. GI hemorrhage, cholestatic hepatic jaundice, leukopenia, thrombocytopenia, pancytopenia, agranulocytosis, aplastic or hemolytic anemia occurs rarely.

NURSING IMPLICATIONS

BASELINE ASSESSMENT:
Check blood glucose level. Discuss lifestyle to determine extent of learning, emotional needs. Assure follow-up instruction if pt/family do not thoroughly understand diabetes management or glucose-testing technique.

INTERVENTION/EVALUATION:
Monitor blood glucose and food intake. Assess for hypoglycemia (cool wet skin, tremors, dizziness, anxiety, headache, tachycardia, numbness in mouth, hunger, diplopia) or hyperglycemia (polyuria, polyphagia, polydipsia, nausea, vomiting, dim vision, fatigue, deep rapid breathing). Be alert to conditions that alter glucose requirements: fever, increased activity or stress, surgical procedure.

PATIENT/FAMILY TEACHING:
Prescribed diet is principal part of treatment; do not skip or delay meals. Carry candy, sugar packets, or other sugar supplements for immediate response to hypoglycemia. Wear medical alert identification. Check with physician when glucose demands are altered (e.g., fever, infection, trauma, stress, heavy physical activity).

glipizide

glip-ih-zide
(Glucotrol, <u>Glucotrol XL</u>)
Do not confuse with glimepiride, glyburide.

▶CLASSIFICATION

PHARMACOTHERAPEUTIC:
Second-generation sulfonylurea.
CLINICAL: Hypoglycemic (see
p. 39C)

ACTION/THERAPEUTIC EFFECT

Promotes release of insulin from
beta cells of pancreas, increases
insulin sensitivity at peripheral
sites, *lowering blood glucose concentration.*

PHARMACOKINETICS

Onset	Peak	Duration
PO		
10–30 min	0.5–2 hrs	24 hrs

Well absorbed from GI tract. Protein binding: 99%. Metabolized in
liver. Excreted in urine. Half-life:
2–4 hrs.

USES

Adjunct to diet/exercise in management of stable, mild to moderately severe noninsulin-dependent
diabetes mellitus (type 2, NIDDM).
May be used to supplement insulin in those with type I diabetes
mellitus.

PRECAUTIONS

CONTRAINDICATIONS: Sole
therapy for type I diabetes mellitus, diabetic complications (ketosis, acidosis, diabetic coma),
stress situations (severe infection,
trauma, surgery), severe renal or
hepatic impairment. **CAUTIONS:**
Severe diarrhea, intestinal obstruction, prolonged vomiting,
liver disease, hyperthyroidism
(not controlled), impaired renal
function, adrenal insufficiency, debilitation, malnourishment, pituitary insufficiency.

▷**LIFESPAN CONSIDERATIONS:**
Pregnancy/Lactation: Insulin is
drug of choice during pregnancy;
glipizide given within 1 mo of delivery may produce neonatal hypoglycemia. Drug crosses placenta; distributed in breast milk.
**Pregnancy Category C. Chil-
dren:** Safety and efficacy not established. **Elderly:** Hypoglycemia
may be difficult to recognize. Age-
related renal impairment may increase sensitivity to glucose lowering effect.

INTERACTIONS

DRUG: May increase effect of **oral
anticoagulants. Fluconazole,
cimetidine, ranitidine, ciprofloxacin, MAO inhibitors, quinidine, salicylates** (large doses)
may increase effect. **Beta-blockers** may increase hypoglycemic
effect, mask signs of hypoglycemia. **Corticosteroids, thiazide diuretics, lithium** may decrease effect. **HERBAL:** None
known. **FOOD:** None known. **LAB
VALUES:** May increase alkaline
phosphatase, SGOT (AST), LDH,
creatinine, BUN.

AVAILABILITY (Rx)

TABLETS: 5 mg, 10 mg. **TABLETS
(extended-release):** 2.5 mg, 5 mg,
10 mg.

ADMINISTRATION/HANDLING

PO:

• May give with food (response
better if taken 15–30 min before
meals). • Do not crush extended-
release tablets.

INDICATIONS/ROUTES/DOSAGE

Diabetes mellitus:

PO: Adults: Initially, 5 mg/day (2.5
mg in geriatric or those with liver
disease). Adjust dosage in 2.5–5

mg increments at intervals of several days. **Maximum single dose:** 15 mg. **Maximum dose/day:** 40 mg. **Maintenance:** 10 mg/day.

Usual elderly dosage:

PO: Initially, 2.5–5 mg/day. May increase by 2.5–5 mg/day q1–2wks.

SIDE EFFECTS

FREQUENT: Altered taste sensation, dizziness, drowsiness, weight gain, constipation, diarrhea, heartburn, nausea, vomiting, stomach fullness, headache. *OCCASIONAL:* Increased sensitivity of skin to sunlight, peeling of skin, itching, rash.

ADVERSE REACTIONS/TOXIC EFFECTS

Hypoglycemia may occur because of overdosage, insufficient food intake esp. with increased glucose demands. GI hemorrhage, cholestatic hepatic jaundice, leukopenia, thrombocytopenia, pancytopenia, agranulocytosis, aplastic or hemolytic anemia occurs rarely.

NURSING IMPLICATIONS

BASELINE ASSESSMENT:

Check blood glucose level. Discuss lifestyle to determine extent of learning, emotional needs. Assure follow-up instruction if pt/family do not thoroughly understand diabetes management or glucose-testing technique.

INTERVENTION/EVALUATION:

Monitor blood glucose and food intake. Assess for hypoglycemia (cool wet skin, tremors, dizziness, anxiety, headache, tachycardia, numbness in mouth, hunger, diplopia) or hyperglycemia (polyuria, polyphagia, polydipsia, nausea, vomiting,

dim vision, fatigue, deep rapid breathing). Be alert to conditions that alter glucose requirements: fever, increased activity or stress, surgical procedure.

PATIENT/FAMILY TEACHING:

Prescribed diet is principal part of treatment; do not skip or delay meals. Carry candy, sugar packets, or other sugar supplements for immediate response to hypoglycemia. Wear medical alert identification. Check with physician when glucose demands are altered (e.g., fever, infection, trauma, stress, heavy physical activity).

glucagon hydrochloride *

glue-ka-gon
(Glucagon Emergency Kit)
Do not confuse with Glaucon.

▶CLASSIFICATION

PHARMACOTHERAPEUTIC: Glucose elevating agent. *CLINICAL:* Antihypoglycemic, antispasmodic, antidote

ACTION/*THERAPEUTIC EFFECT*

Promotes hepatic glycogenolysis, gluconeogenesis. Stimulates enzyme to increase production of cAMP, *resulting in increased plasma glucose concentration, relaxant effect on smooth muscle, and inotropic myocardial effect.*

USES/*UNLABELED*

Treatment of severe hypoglycemia in diabetic pts. Not for use in chronic hypoglycemia or hypoglycemia due to starvation, adrenal insufficiency, since liver glycogen unavailable. Diagnostic aid in radiographic examination of

GI tract. *Treatment of toxicity associated with beta-blockers, calcium channel blockers; esophageal obstruction due to foreign bodies.*

PRECAUTIONS

CONTRAINDICATIONS: Pheochromocytoma, hypersensitivity to glucagon (protein). **CAUTIONS:** History of insulinoma or pheochromocytoma.

INTERACTIONS

DRUG: May increase **anticoagulant** effect. **HERBAL:** None known. **FOOD:** None known. **LAB VALUES:** May decrease potassium.

AVAILABILITY (Rx)

POWDER FOR INJECTION: 1 mg, 10 mg.

ADMINISTRATION/HANDLING

Note: Place pt on side to avoid potential aspiration (glucagon, as well as hypoglycemia, may produce nausea and vomiting).

SubQ/IM/IV:

• Store vial at room temperature. • After reconstitution, is stable for 48 hrs if refrigerated. If reconstituted with Sterile Water for Injection, use immediately. Do not use glucagon solution unless clear. • Reconstitute powder with manufacturer's diluent when preparing 2 mg doses or less. For doses exceeding 2 mg, dilute with Sterile Water for Injection. • To provide 1 mg glucagon/ml, use 1 ml diluent. For 1 mg vial of glucagon, use 10 ml diluent for 10 mg vial. • Pt will usually awaken in 5–20 min. Although 1–2 additional doses may be administered, the concern for effects of continuing cerebral hypoglycemia requires consideration of parenteral glucose. • When pt awakens, give supplemental carbohydrate to restore liver glycogen and prevent secondary hypoglycemia. If pt fails to respond to glucagon, IV glucose is necessary.

IV INCOMPATIBILITY ⊘

Do not mix with any other medications.

INDICATIONS/ROUTES/DOSAGE

Note: Administer IV dextrose if pt fails to respond to glucagon.

Hypoglycemia:

SubQ/IM/IV: Adults, elderly: 0.5–1 mg (0.5–1 unit). May repeat 1–2 additional doses if response is delayed. **Children <20 kg:** 0.5 mg.

Diagnostic aid:

IM/IV: Adults, elderly: 0.25–2 mg (0.25–2 units).

SIDE EFFECTS

OCCASIONAL: Nausea, vomiting. **RARE:** Allergic reaction (urticaria, respiratory distress, hypotension).

ADVERSE REACTIONS/TOXIC EFFECTS

Overdose may produce continuing nausea, vomiting, hypokalemia (severe weakness, decreased appetite, irregular heartbeat, muscle cramps).

NURSING IMPLICATIONS

BASELINE ASSESSMENT:

Obtain immediate assessment, including history, clinical signs, and symptoms. If hypoglycemic coma is established, give glucagon promptly as described above.

INTERVENTION/EVALUATION:

Monitor response time carefully. Have IV dextrose readily available in event pt does not awaken within 5–20 min. Assess for possible allergic reaction (urticaria, respiratory difficulty, hypotension). When pt is conscious, give carbohydrate.

PATIENT/FAMILY TEACHING:

Recognize significance of identifying symptoms of hypoglycemia: pale cool skin, anxiety, difficulty concentrating, headache, hunger, nausea, nervousness, shakiness, sweating, unusual tiredness, weakness, unconsciousness. Instruct pt, family, or friend to give sugar form first (orange juice, honey, hard candy, sugar cubes, or table sugar dissolved in water or juice) if symptoms of hypoglycemia develop, followed by cheese and crackers or half a sandwich or glass of milk.

glucosamine/ chondroitin

▶CLASSIFICATION
HERBAL

ACTION/EFFECT

Glucosamine: Necessary for synthesis of mucopolysaccharides, which comprise the body's tendons, ligaments, cartilage, synovial fluid. May decrease glucose-induced insulin secretion, *relieving symptoms of osteoarthritis.* *Chondroitin:* Endogenously found in cartilage tissue, substrate for forming joint matrix structure. May have some anticoagulant properties, *relieving symptoms of osteoarthritis.*

USES

Treatment of osteoarthritis.

PRECAUTIONS

CONTRAINDICATIONS: None significant. *CAUTIONS: Glucosamine:* Diabetes (may increase insulin resistance). *Chondroitin:* None significant.

▷*LIFESPAN CONSIDERATIONS:* **Pregnancy/Lactation:** Avoid use. **Children:** Safety and efficacy not established. **Elderly:** No age-related precautions noted.

INTERACTIONS

DRUG: (Glucosamine): None significant. *(Chondroitin):* Monitor anticoagulant therapy. *HERBAL:* None significant. *FOOD:* None significant. *LAB VALUES: (Glucosamine):* May increase glucose. *(Chondroitin):* May increase anti-factor Xa level.

AVAILABILITY (OTC)

Glucosamine: CAPSULES: 500 mg. *TABLETS:* 500 mg.

Chondroitin: CAPSULES: 250 mg. **Note:** There are many combination products available.

INDICATIONS/ROUTES/DOSAGE
Osteoarthritis:

PO: **Adults, elderly:** *(Glucosamine):* 500 mg 3 times/day or 1–2 g/day. *(Chondroitin):* 200–400 mg 2–3 times/day.

SIDE EFFECTS

(Glucosamine): Mild GI symptoms (e.g., gas, bloating, cramps). *(Chondroitin):* Well tolerated. May cause nausea, diarrhea, constipation, edema, alopecia, allergic reactions.

ADVERSE REACTIONS/TOXIC EFFECTS

None significant.

NURSING IMPLICATIONS

BASELINE ASSESSMENT:

Assess if pt is taking anticoagulants/antiplatelets, antidiabetic drugs. Determine if pt is pregnant/breast-feeding.

EVALUATION/INTERVENTION:

Monitor effectiveness of therapy in relieving osteoarthritis symptoms, blood glucose levels.

PATIENT/FAMILY TEACHING:

Avoid use in pregnancy/breast-feeding, children. May take several mos of therapy to be effective. Glucosamine may alter glucose levels.

glyburide

glye-byoo-ride
(Diabeta, Euglucon✤, Micronase)
Do not confuse with Micro-K, Micronor, Zebeta.

FIXED-COMBINATION(S)

With metformin, an antidiabetic **(Glucovance)**

▶CLASSIFICATION

PHARMACOTHERAPEUTIC: Second-generation sulfonylurea. **CLINICAL:** Hypoglycemic (see p. 39C)

ACTION/THERAPEUTIC EFFECT

Promotes release of insulin from beta cells of pancreas, increases insulin sensitivity at peripheral sites, *lowering blood glucose concentration*.

PHARMACOKINETICS

Onset	Peak	Duration
PO		
0.25–1 hr	1–2 hrs	24 hrs

Well absorbed from GI tract. Protein binding: 99%. Metabolized in liver to weakly active metabolite. Primarily excreted in urine. Not removed by hemodialysis. Half-life: 10 hrs.

USES

Adjunct to diet/exercise in management of stable, mild to moderately severe noninsulin-dependent diabetes mellitus (type 2, NIDDM). May be used to supplement insulin in those with type 1 diabetes mellitus.

PRECAUTIONS

CONTRAINDICATIONS: Sole therapy for type I diabetes mellitus, diabetic complications (ketosis, acidosis, diabetic coma), stress situations (severe infection, trauma, surgery), severe renal or hepatic impairment. ***CAUTIONS:*** Severe diarrhea, intestinal obstruction, prolonged vomiting, liver disease, hyperthyroidism (not controlled), impaired renal function, adrenal insufficiency, debilitation, malnourishment, pituitary insufficiency.

▷*LIFESPAN CONSIDERATIONS:* **Pregnancy/Lactation:** Crosses placenta, distributed in breast milk. May produce neonatal hypoglycemia if given within 2 wks of delivery. **Pregnancy Category C. Children:** Safety and efficacy not established. **Elderly:** Hypoglycemia may be difficult to recognize. Age-related renal impairment may increase sensitivity to glucose lowering effect.

INTERACTIONS

DRUG: May increase effect of **oral anticoagulants. Fluconazole, cimetidine, ranitidine, ciprofloxacin, MAO inhibitors, quinidine, salicylates** (large doses) may increase effect. **Beta blockers** may increase hypoglycemic effect, mask signs of hypoglycemia. **Corticosteroids, thiazide diuretics, lithium** may decrease effect. ***HERBAL:*** None known. ***FOOD:*** None known. ***LAB VALUES:*** May increase alkaline phosphatase, SGOT (AST), LDH, creatinine, BUN.

AVAILABILITY (Rx)

TABLETS: 1.25 mg, 2.5 mg, 5 mg.

ADMINISTRATION/HANDLING
PO:

• May give with food (response better if taken 15–30 min before meals).

INDICATIONS/ROUTES/DOSAGE
Diabetes mellitus:

PO: Adults: Initially, 2.5 mg up to 20 mg/day. **Range:** 1.25–20 mg/day as a single or in divided doses. **Maintenance:** 7.5 mg/day.

Usual elderly dosage:

PO: Initially, 1.25–2.5 mg/day. May increase by 1.25–2.5 mg/day q1–3wks.

SIDE EFFECTS

FREQUENT: Altered taste sensation, dizziness, drowsiness, weight gain, constipation, diarrhea, heartburn, nausea, vomiting, stomach fullness, headache. ***OCCASIONAL:*** Increased sensitivity of skin to sunlight, peeling of skin, itching, rash.

ADVERSE REACTIONS/TOXIC EFFECTS

Overdosage, insufficient food intake may produce hypoglycemia, esp. with increased glucose demands. Cholestatic jaundice, leukopenia, thrombocytopenia, pancytopenia, agranulocytosis, aplastic or hemolytic anemia occurs rarely.

NURSING IMPLICATIONS

BASELINE ASSESSMENT:

Check blood glucose level. Discuss lifestyle to determine extent of learning, emotional needs. Assure follow-up instruction if pt/family do not thoroughly understand diabetes management or glucose-testing technique.

INTERVENTION/EVALUATION:

Monitor blood glucose and food intake. Assess for hypoglycemia (cool wet skin, tremors, dizziness, anxiety, headache, tachycardia, numbness in mouth, hunger, diplopia) or hyperglycemia (polyuria, polyphagia, polydipsia, nausea, vomiting, dim vision, fatigue, deep rapid breathing). Be alert to conditions that alter glucose requirements: fever, increased activity or stress, surgical procedure.

PATIENT/FAMILY TEACHING:

Prescribed diet is principal part of treatment; do not skip or delay meals. Carry candy, sugar packets, or other sugar supplements for immediate response to hypoglycemia. Wear medical alert identification. Check with physician when glucose demands are altered (e.g., fever, infection, trauma, stress, heavy physical activity).

---

glycopyrrolate

gly-ko-**pie**-roll-ate
(Robinul✦)

►CLASSIFICATION

PHARMACOTHERAPEUTIC:
Quaternary anticholinergic.
CLINICAL: Antimuscarinic, antiarrhythmic, cholinergic adjunct

ACTION/*THERAPEUTIC EFFECT*

Inhibits action of acetylcholine on structures innervated by postganglionic sites: smooth, cardiac muscle; SA, AV nodes; exocrine glands. Larger doses may decrease motility, secretory activity of GI system, tone of ureter, urinary bladder. *Reduces salivation and excessive secretions of respiratory tract; reduces gastric secretions, acidity.*

USES

Inhibits salivation and excessive secretions of the respiratory tract. Reverses the muscarinic effects of cholinergic agents (e.g., neostigmine).

PRECAUTIONS

CONTRAINDICATIONS: Narrow-angle glaucoma, severe ulcerative colitis, toxic megacolon, obstructive disease of GI tract, paralytic ileus, intestinal atony, bladder neck obstruction due to prostatic hypertrophy, myasthenia gravis in pts not treated with neostigmine, tachycardia secondary to cardiac insufficiency or thyrotoxicosis, cardiospasm, unstable cardiovascular status in acute hemorrhage. **EXTREME CAUTION:** Autonomic neuropathy, known or suspected GI infections, diarrhea, mild to moderate ulcerative colitis. **CAUTIONS:** Hyperthyroidism, hepatic or renal disease, hypertension, tachyarrhythmias, CHF, coronary artery disease, gastric ulcer, esophageal reflux or hiatal hernia associated with reflux esophagitis, infants, elderly, pts with COPD.

INTERACTIONS

DRUG: Antacids, antidiarrheals may decrease absorption. **Anticholinergics** may increase effects. May decrease absorption of **ketoconazole.** May increase severity of GI lesions with **potassium chloride** (wax matrix). **HERBAL:** None known. **FOOD:** None known. **LAB VALUES:** May decrease uric acid.

AVAILABILITY (Rx)

INJECTION: 0.2 mg/ml.

INDICATIONS/ROUTES/DOSAGE
Preop:

IM: Adults, elderly: 4.4 mcg/kg 30–60 min before procedure. **Children >2 yrs:** 4.4 mcg/kg. **Children <2 yrs:** 4.4–8.8 mcg/kg.

Block effects of anticholinesterase agents:

IV: Adults, elderly: 0.2 mg for each 1 mg neostigmine or 5 mg pyridostigmine.

SIDE EFFECTS

FREQUENT: Dry mouth (sometimes severe), decreased sweating, constipation. **OCCASIONAL:** Blurred vision, bloated feeling, urinary hesitancy, drowsiness (with high dosage), headache, intolerance to light, loss of taste, nervousness, flushing, insomnia, impotence, mental confusion/

excitement (particularly in elderly, children). Parenteral form may produce temporary lightheadedness, local irritation. ***RARE:*** Dizziness, faintness.

ADVERSE REACTIONS/TOXIC EFFECTS

Overdosage may produce temporary paralysis of ciliary muscle, pupillary dilation, tachycardia, palpitation, hot/dry/flushed skin, absence of bowel sounds, hyperthermia, increased respiratory rate, EKG abnormalities, nausea, vomiting, rash over face/upper trunk, CNS stimulation, psychosis (agitation, restlessness, rambling speech, visual hallucination, paranoid behavior, delusions), followed by depression.

NURSING IMPLICATIONS

BASELINE ASSESSMENT:

Before giving medication, instruct pt to void (reduces risk of urinary retention).

INTERVENTION/EVALUATION:

Monitor daily bowel activity and stool consistency. Palpate bladder for urinary retention. Monitor changes in B/P, temperature. Assess skin turgor, mucous membranes to evaluate hydration status (encourage adequate fluid intake), bowel sounds for peristalsis. Be alert for fever (increased risk of hyperthermia).

PATIENT/FAMILY TEACHING:

Take 30 min before meals (food decreases absorption of medication). Use care not to become overheated during exercise in hot weather (may result in heat stroke). Avoid hot baths, saunas. Avoid tasks that require alertness, motor skills until response

to drug is established. Do not take antacids or medicine for diarrhea within 1 hr of taking this medication (decreased effectiveness).

gold sodium thiomalate

gold sodium thigh-oh-**mal**-ate (Aurolate, Myochrysine ♦)

▶**CLASSIFICATION**

PHARMACOTHERAPEUTIC: Gold compound. ***CLINICAL:*** Antirheumatic, anti-inflammatory

ACTION/*THERAPEUTIC EFFECT*

Inhibits phagocytosis, lysomal enzyme activity, decreasing concentration of rheumatoid factor, immunoglobulins. *Decreases synovial inflammation, retards cartilage and bone destruction (suppresses or prevents, but does not cure, arthritis, synovitis).*

USES/*UNLABELED*

Management of rheumatoid arthritis in pts with insufficient therapeutic response to nonsteroidal anti-inflammatory agents. *Treatment of psoriatic arthritis.*

PRECAUTIONS

CONTRAINDICATIONS: History of gold-induced pathoses (necrotizing enterocolitis, exfoliative dermatitis, pulmonary fibrosis, blood dyscrasias), hepatic dysfunction or history of hepatitis, uncontrolled diabetes or CHF, urticaria, eczema, colitis, hemorrhagic conditions, systemic lupus erythematosus, recent radiation therapy. ***CAUTIONS:*** Renal/hepatic disease, inflammatory bowel disease.

INTERACTIONS

DRUG: **Bone marrow depressants, hepatotoxic, nephrotoxic medications** may increase toxicity. **Penicillamine** may increase risk of adverse hematologic or renal effects. ***HERBAL:*** None known. ***FOOD:*** None known. ***LAB VALUES:*** May decrease hemoglobin, hematocrit, platelets, WBCs. May alter liver function tests. May increase urine protein.

AVAILABILITY (Rx)

INJECTION: 10 mg/ml, 25 mg/ml, 50 mg/ml.

INDICATIONS/ROUTES/DOSAGE

Rheumatoid arthritis:

Note: Give as weekly injections.

IM: **Adults, elderly:** Initially, 10 mg, then 25 mg for second dose. Follow with 25–50 mg/wk until improvement noted or total of 1 g administered. **Maintenance:** 25–50 mg q2wks for 2–20 wks; if stable, may increase to q3–4wk intervals. **Children:** Initially, 10 mg, then 1 mg/kg/wk. **Maximum single dose:** 50 mg.

SIDE EFFECTS

FREQUENT: Pruritic dermatitis, stomatitis (erythema, redness, shallow ulcers of oral mucous membranes, sore throat, difficulty swallowing), diarrhea/loose stools, abdominal pain, nausea. ***OCCASIONAL:*** Vomiting, anorexia, flatulence, dyspepsia, conjunctivitis, photosensitivity. ***RARE:*** Constipation, urticaria, rash.

ADVERSE REACTIONS/TOXIC EFFECTS

Signs of gold toxicity: decreased hemoglobin, leukopenia (WBC below 4,000 mm^3), reduced granulocyte counts (below 150,000/mm^3), proteinuria, hematuria, blood dyscrasias (anemia, leukopenia, thrombocytopenia, eosinophilia), glomerulonephritis, nephrotic syndrome, cholestatic jaundice.

NURSING IMPLICATIONS

BASELINE ASSESSMENT:

Rule out pregnancy before beginning treatment; CBC, urinalysis, renal and liver function tests should be performed before therapy begins.

INTERVENTION/EVALUATION:

Monitor daily bowel activity and stool consistency. Assess urine tests for proteinuria or hematuria. Monitor CBC, renal and hepatic function studies. Assess skin daily for rash, purpura, or ecchymoses. Assess oral mucous membranes, borders of tongue, palate, pharynx for ulceration, complaint of metallic taste sensation (signs of stomatitis). Evaluate for therapeutic response: relief of pain, stiffness, swelling, increase in joint mobility, reduced joint tenderness, improved grip strength.

PATIENT/FAMILY TEACHING:

Therapeutic response may take 6 mos or longer. Avoid exposure to sunlight (gray to blue pigment may appear). Maintain diligent oral hygiene.

gonadorelin

go-nad-oh-**rell**-in
(Factrel, Lutrepulse, Relisom✿)
Do not confuse with
gonadotropin, guanadrel, Sectral.

►CLASSIFICATION

PHARMACOTHERAPEUTIC:
Gonadotropin-releasing hormone. **CLINICAL:** Diagnostic agent

ACTION/*THERAPEUTIC EFFECT*

Stimulates synthesis, release of luteinizing hormone (LH), follicle-stimulating hormone (FSH) from anterior pituitary. Stimulates release of gonadotropin-releasing hormone from hypothalamus.

USES/*UNLABELED*

As a single dose, evaluates the functional capacity and response of gonadotropes of anterior pituitary in suspected gonadotropic deficiency (does not differentiate between hypothalamus or pituitary disorders). Multiple injection testing is used to evaluate residual gonadotropic function of pituitary after removal of a pituitary tumor by surgery and/or irradiation. Induction of ovulation in women with primary hypothalamic amenorrhea. **Acetate:** *Treatment of delayed puberty, infertility.*

PRECAUTIONS

CONTRAINDICATIONS: *Gonadorelin acetate:* Women with any condition exacerbated by pregnancy, ovarian cysts, or causes of anovulation other than hypothalamic in origin. **CAUTIONS:** None significant.

INTERACTIONS

DRUG: None significant. **HERBAL:** None known. **FOOD:** None known. **LAB VALUES:** None significant.

AVAILABILITY (Rx)

POWDER FOR INJECTION: 100 mcg, 500 mcg.

INDICATIONS/ROUTES/DOSAGE

Note: Test should be conducted in the absence of other drugs that affect pituitary secretion of gonadotropins.

GONADORELIN ACETATE:

Primary hypothalamic amenorrhea:

IV PUMP: Adults: 5 mcg q90min (range 1–20 mcg); treatment interval 21 days. Refer to manufacturer's manual for proper dilutions/settings on pump. Response usually occurs 2–3 wks after initiation. Continue additional 2 wks after ovulation occurs (maintains corpus luteum).

GONADORELIN HYDROCHLORIDE:

Diagnostic agent:

IV/*SubQ*: Adults: 100 mcg. In females, perform test in early follicular phase of menstrual cycle.

SIDE EFFECTS

OCCASIONAL: Gonadorelin acetate: Multiple pregnancy, inflammation, infection, mild phlebitis, hematoma at catheter site. **Gonadorelin hydrochloride:** Swelling, pain, or itching at injection site with SubQ administration. Local or generalized skin rash with chronic SubQ administration. **RARE: Gonaorelin acetate:** Ovarian hyperstimulation. **Gonadorelin hydrochloride:** Headache, nausea, lightheadedness, abdominal discomfort, hypersensitivity reactions (bronchospasm, tachycardia, flushing, urticaria), induration at injection site.

ADVERSE REACTIONS/TOXIC EFFECTS

Anaphylactic reaction occurs rarely.

NURSING IMPLICATIONS

BASELINE ASSESSMENT:

Before test is started, ensure that pt understands procedure. *Gonadorelin acetate:* Pt instructions included with kit from manufacturer. *Gonadorelin hydrochloride:* Venous blood sample (for LH) to be drawn immediately before administration.

INTERVENTION/EVALUATION:

Gonadorelin acetate: With baseline pelvic ultrasound, perform follow-up studies. *Gonadorelin hydrochloride:* Change cannula and IV site at 48 hr intervals. Assure protocol for test is maintained: usually venous blood samples (for LH) drawn after administration at intervals of 15, 30, 45, 60, and 120 min.

goserelin acetate

gos-**er**-ah-lin
(Zoladex)

▶CLASSIFICATION

PHARMACOTHERAPEUTIC: Gonadotropin-releasing hormone analog. *CLINICAL:* Antineoplastic (see pp. 71C, 87C)

ACTION/*THERAPEUTIC EFFECT*

Synthetic luteinizing hormone-releasing hormone analogue. Stimulates release of luteinizing hormone (LH), follicle-stimulating hormone (FSH) from anterior pituitary *(increases testosterone concentrations). After initial increase, decreases release of LH, FSH, testosterone.*

USES

Treatment of advanced carcinoma of prostate as alternative when orchiectomy or estrogen therapy is either not indicated or unacceptable to pt. In combination with flutamide prior to and during radiation therapy for early stages of prostate cancer. Management of endometriosis. Treatment of advanced breast cancer in premenopausal and perimenopausal women. Endometrial thinning before ablation for dysfunctional uterine bleeding.

PRECAUTIONS

CONTRAINDICATIONS: Pregnancy. *CAUTIONS:* None significant.

INTERACTIONS

DRUG: None significant. *HERBAL:* None known. *FOOD:* None known. *LAB VALUES:* May increase serum acid phosphatase, testosterone concentrations.

AVAILABILITY (Rx)

IMPLANT: 3.6 mg, 10.8 mg.

INDICATIONS/ROUTES/DOSAGE

Prostatic carcinoma:

SubQ IMPLANT: **Adults >18 yrs, elderly:** 3.6 mg q28days or 10.8 mg q12wks into upper abdominal wall.

Breast carcinoma, endometriosis:

SubQ/IMPLANT: **Adults:** 3.6 mg q28days into upper abdominal wall.

Endometrial thinning:

SubQ: **Adults:** 3.6 mg once or 4 wks apart in 2 doses.

SIDE EFFECTS

FREQUENT: Headache (60%), hot flashes (55%), depression (54%), sweating (45%), sexual dysfunction (21%), decreased erection (18%), lower urinary tract symptoms (13%). **OCCASIONAL** (5–10%): Nausea, pain, lethargy, dizziness, insomnia, anorexia, nausea, rash, upper respiratory infection, hair growth, abdominal pain. **RARE:** Pruritus.

ADVERSE REACTIONS/TOXIC EFFECTS

Arrhythmias, CHF, hypertension occur rarely. Ureteral obstruction, spinal cord compression observed (immediate orchiectomy may be necessary).

NURSING IMPLICATIONS

INTERVENTION/EVALUATION:

Monitor pt closely for worsening signs and symptoms of prostatic cancer, esp. during first mo of therapy.

PATIENT/FAMILY TEACHING:

Use contraceptive measures during therapy. Inform physician if regular menstruation persists, become pregnant. Breakthrough menstrual bleeding may occur if dose is missed. Use nonhormonal methods of contraception.

granisetron

gran-**is**-eh-tron
(Kytril)

▶CLASSIFICATION

PHARMACOTHERAPEUTIC: Serotonin receptor antagonist. **CLINICAL:** Antiemetic

ACTION/THERAPEUTIC EFFECT

Selectively blocks serotonin stimulation at receptor sites on abdominal vagal afferent nerve and chemoreceptor trigger zone, *preventing nausea, vomiting.*

PHARMACOKINETICS

Rapidly, widely distributed to tissues. Protein binding: 65%. Metabolized in liver to active metabolite. Excreted in urine, eliminated in feces. Half-life: 10–12 hrs (half-life increased in elderly).

USES/UNLABELED

Prevents nausea, vomiting associated with emetogenic cancer therapy (includes high-dose cisplatin). *Prophylaxis of nausea/vomiting associated with cancer radiotherapy.* **PO:** Prevention of nausea/vomiting associated with radiation therapy.

PRECAUTIONS

CONTRAINDICATIONS: None significant. **CAUTIONS:** Safety in children <2 yrs not established.
▷**LIFESPAN CONSIDERATIONS:** **Pregnancy/Lactation:** Unknown if drug is distributed in breast milk. **Pregnancy Category B. Children:** Safety and efficacy not established in pts <2 yrs of age. **Elderly:** No age-related precautions noted.

INTERACTIONS

DRUG: Hepatic enzyme inducers may decrease effect. **HERBAL:** None known. **FOOD:** None known. **LAB VALUES:** May increase SGOT (AST), SGPT (ALT).

AVAILABILITY (Rx)

TABLETS: 1 mg, 2 mg. **INJECTION:** 1 mg/ml. **ORAL SOLUTION.**

ADMINISTRATION/HANDLING

IV 💉

Storage:

• Appears as a clear, colorless solution. • Store at room temperature. • After dilution, is stable for at least 24 hrs at room temperature. • Inspect for particulates, discoloration.

Reconstitution:

• May be given undiluted or dilute with 20–50 ml 0.9% NaCl or D_5W. Do not mix with other medications.

Rate of administration:

• May give undiluted as IV push over 30 sec. • For IV piggyback, infuse over 5–20 min. depending on volume of diluent used.

IV INCOMPATIBILITY $\oslash$

Amphotericin B (Fungizone).

IV COMPATIBILITIES

Allopurinol (Aloprim), bumetanide (Bumex), calcium gluconate, carboplatin (Paraplatin), cisplatin (Platinol), cyclophosphamide (Cytoxan), cytarabine (ARA-C), dacarbazine (DTIC), dexamethasone (Decadron), diphenylhydramine (Benadryl), docetaxel (Taxotere), doxorubicin (Adriamycin), etoposide (Vepesid), gemcitabine (Gemzar), magnesium, mitoxantrone (Novantrone), paclitaxel (Taxol), potassium.

INDICATIONS/ROUTES/DOSAGE

Antiemetic:

IV: Adults, elderly, children >2 yrs: 10 mcg/kg beginning within 30 min before initiating chemotherapy.

PO: Adults, elderly: 1 mg up to 1 hr before chemotherapy and 12 hrs after first dose or 2 mg once 1 hr prior to chemotherapy. Give only on days that chemotherapy is administered.

Postop nausea/vomiting:

PO: Adults, elderly, children ≥4 yrs: 20–40 mcg/kg as a single postop dose.

SIDE EFFECTS

FREQUENT (14–21%): Headache, constipation, asthenia (loss of strength), **OCCASIONAL** (6–8%): Diarrhea, abdominal pain. **RARE** (<2%): Altered taste, hypersensitivity reaction.

ADVERSE REACTIONS/TOXIC EFFECTS

None significant.

G

NURSING IMPLICATIONS

BASELINE ASSESSMENT:

Assure granisetron is given within 30 min of start of chemotherapy.

INTERVENTION/EVALUATION:

Monitor for therapeutic effect. Assess for headache. Monitor frequency and consistency of stools.

PATIENT/FAMILY TEACHING:

Granisetron is effective shortly after administration; prevents nausea, vomiting. Explain that transitory taste disorder may occur.

griseofulvin ✱

griz-ee-oh-**full**-vin
(Fulvicin ♣, Grisactin, Grisovin-FP ♣, GrisPEG)

▶CLASSIFICATION

CLINICAL: Antifungal

ACTION/THERAPEUTIC EFFECT

Inhibits fungal cell mitosis by disrupting mitotic spindle structure. Fungistatic.

USES

Treatment of tineas (ringworm): *t. capitis, t. corporis, t. cruris, t. pedis, t. unguium.*

PRECAUTIONS

CONTRAINDICATIONS: Porphyria, hepatocellular failure. ***CAUTIONS:*** Exposure to sun or ultraviolet light (photosensitivity), hypersensitivity to penicillins.

INTERACTIONS

DRUG: May decrease effects of warfarin, oral contraceptives. ***HERBAL:*** None known. ***FOOD:*** None known. ***LAB VALUES:*** None significant.

AVAILABILITY (Rx)

TABLETS (microsize): 250 mg, 500 mg. ***CAPSULES:*** 250 mg. ***ORAL SUSPENSION:*** 125 mg/5 ml. ***TABLETS (ultramicrosize):*** 125 mg, 165 mg, 250 mg, 330 mg.

INDICATIONS/ROUTES/DOSAGE

Usual dosage:

Note: Duration depends on the site of infection.

Adults (microsize): 500–1,000 mg as single or divded doses. **Children:** 10–12 mg/kg/day.

Adults (ultramicrosize): 330–750 mg/day as single or divded doses. **Children >2 yrs:** 5–10 mg/kg/day.

SIDE EFFECTS

OCCASIONAL: Hypersensitivity reaction (rash, pruritus, urticaria), headache, nausea, diarrhea, excessive thirst, flatulence, oral thrush, dizziness, insomnia. ***RARE:*** Paresthesia of hands/feet, proteinuria.

ADVERSE REACTIONS/TOXIC EFFECTS

Granulocytopenia should cause discontinuation of drug.

BASELINE ASSESSMENT:

Question for history of allergies, esp. to griseofulvin, penicillins.

INTERVENTION/EVALUATION:

Assess skin for rash and response to therapy. Determine pattern of bowel activity and stool consistency. Question presence of headache: onset, location, type of discomfort. Assess mental status for dizziness.

PATIENT/FAMILY TEACHING:

Prolonged therapy (wks or mos) is usually necessary. Do not miss a dose; continue therapy as long as ordered. Avoid alcohol (may produce tachycardia, flushing). Maintain good hygiene (prevents superinfection). Separate personal items in direct contact with affected areas. Keep areas dry; wear light clothing for ventilation. Take with foods high in fat such as milk, ice cream (reduces GI upset and assists absorption).

guaifenesin (glyceryl guaiacolate)

guay-**fen**-ah-sin
(Balminil❄, Benylin E❄, Glycotuss, Humibid, Robitussin)

FIXED-COMBINATION(S)

With phenylephrine and phenylpropanolamine, sympathomimetics **(Entex)**

▶ CLASSIFICATION

CLINICAL: Expectorant

ACTION/*THERAPEUTIC EFFECT*

Enhances fluid output of respiratory tract by decreasing adhesiveness and surface tension, *promoting removal of viscous mucus.*

PHARMACOKINETICS

Well absorbed from GI tract. Metabolized in liver. Excreted in urine.

USES

Symptomatic relief of cough in presence of mucus in respiratory tract. Not for use with persistent cough due to smoking, asthma, emphysema or cough accompanied by excessive secretions.

PRECAUTIONS

CONTRAINDICATIONS: None significant. ***CAUTIONS:*** None significant.

▷***LIFESPAN CONSIDERATIONS:***
Pregnancy/Lactation: Not known if drug crosses placenta or is distributed in breast milk. **Pregnancy Category C. Children/Elderly:** No age-related precautions noted. Caution advised in pts <2 yrs with persistent cough.

INTERACTIONS

DRUG: None significant. ***HERBAL:*** None known. ***FOOD:*** None known. ***LAB VALUES:*** None significant.

AVAILABILITY (OTC)

TABLETS: 100 mg, 200 mg. ***TABLETS (sustained-release):*** 600 mg. ***CAPSULES:*** 200 mg. ***CAPSULES (sustained-release):*** 300 mg. ***SYRUP:*** 100 mg/5 ml. ***LIQUID:*** 200 mg/5 ml.

ADMINISTRATION/HANDLING

PO:

• Store syrup, liquid, capsules at room temperature. • Give without regard to meals. • Do not crush or break sustained-release capsule. May sprinkle contents on soft food, then swallow without crushing/chewing.

INDICATIONS/ROUTES/DOSAGE

Note: Give extended-release capsules at 12-hr intervals.

Expectorant:

PO: Adults, elderly, children >12 yrs: 200–400 mg q4h. **Maximum:** 2.4 g/day. **Children 6–12 yrs:** 100–200 mg q4h. **Maximum:** 1.2 g/day. **Children 2–6 yrs:** 50–100 mg q4h. **Maximum:** 600 mg/day. **Children <2 yrs:** 12 mg/kg/day in 6 divded doses.

SIDE EFFECTS

RARE: Dizziness, headache, rash, diarrhea, nausea, vomiting, stomach pain.

ADVERSE REACTIONS/TOXIC EFFECTS

Excessive dosage may produce nausea, vomiting.

NURSING IMPLICATIONS

BASELINE ASSESSMENT:

Assess type, severity, frequency of cough and productions. Increase fluid intake and environmental humidity to lower viscosity of lung secretions.

INTERVENTION/EVALUATION:

Initiate deep breathing and coughing exercises, particularly in pts with impaired pulmonary function. Assess for clinical improvement and record onset of relief of cough.

PATIENT/FAMILY TEACHING:

Avoid tasks that require alertness, motor skills until response to drug is established. Do not take for chronic cough. Inform physician if cough persists or if fever, rash, headache, or sore throat is present with cough. Maintain adequate hydration.

guanabenz

(Wytensin)

See Classification section under: Antihypertensives (p. 51C)

guanadrel

(Hylorel)

See Classification section under: Antihypertensives

guanfacine

(Tenex)

See Classification section under: Antihypertensives (p. 51C)

halcinonide

(Halog)

See Classification section under: Corticosteroids: topical

halobetasol

(Ultravate)

See Classification section under: Corticosteroids: topical (p. 81C)

haloperidol

hal-oh-**pear**-ih-dawl
(Apo-Haloperidol✤, Haldol, Novoperidol✤, Peridol✤)
Do not confuse with Halcion, Halog, Stadol.

▶CLASSIFICATION

CLINICAL: Antipsychotic, antiemetic, antidyskinetic (see p. 55C)

ACTION/THERAPEUTIC EFFECT

Competitively blocks postsynaptic dopamine receptors, interrupts impulse movement, and increases turnover of brain dopamine, *producing tranquilizing effect.* Strong extrapyramidal, antiemetic effects, weak anticholinergic, sedative effects.

PHARMACOKINETICS

Readily absorbed from GI tract. Protein binding: 92%. Extensively metabolized in liver. Primarily excreted in urine. Not removed by hemodialysis. Half-life: *PO:* 12–37 hrs; *IM:* 17–25 hrs, *IV:* 10–19 hrs.

USES/*UNLABELED*

Management of psychotic disorders, control of tics, vocal utterances in Tourette's syndrome. Used in management of severe behavioral problems in children, short-term treatment of hyperactivity in children. *Treatment of infantile autism, Huntington's chorea, nausea/vomiting associated with cancer chemotherapy.*

PRECAUTIONS

CONTRAINDICATIONS: Coma, alcohol ingestion, Parkinson's disease, thyrotoxicosis. **CAUTIONS:** Impaired respiratory/hepatic/cardiovascular function, alcohol withdrawal, history of seizures, urinary retention, glaucoma, prostatic hypertrophy, elderly.
▷*LIFESPAN CONSIDERATIONS:*
Pregnancy/Lactation: Crosses placenta; distributed in breast milk. **Pregnancy Category C.**

Children: More susceptible to dystonias; not recommended in those <3 yrs of age. **Elderly:** More susceptible to orthostatic hypotension, anticholinergic effects and sedation, increased risk for extrapyramidal effects. Decreased dosage recommended.

INTERACTIONS

DRUG:* Alcohol, CNS depressants** may increase CNS depression. **Epinephrine** may block alpha-adrenergic effects. **Extrapyramidal symptom (EPS)-producing medications** may increase EPS. **Lithium** may increase neurologic toxicity. ***HERBAL: None known. ***FOOD:*** None known. ***LAB VALUES:*** None significant. Therapeutic blood serum level: 0.2–1 mcg/ml; toxic blood serum level: >1 mcg/ml.

AVAILABILITY (Rx)

TABLETS: 0.5 mg, 1 mg, 2 mg, 5 mg, 10 mg, 20 mg. ***ORAL CONCENTRATE:*** 2 mg/ml. ***INJECTION:*** 5 mg/ml. ***INJECTION (Decanoate):*** 50 mg/ml, 100 mg/ml.

ADMINISTRATION/HANDLING

PO:

• Give without regard to meals. • Scored tablets may be crushed.

IM:

Parenteral administration: Pt must remain recumbent for 30–60 min in head-low position with legs raised to minimize hypotensive effect.

• Prepare Decanoate IM injection using 21 gauge needle. • Do not exceed maximum volume of 3 ml per IM injection site. • Inject slow, deep IM into upper outer quadrant of gluteus maximus.

IV

Note: Only haloperidol lactate is given IV.

Storage:

• Discard if precipitate forms, discoloration occurs. • Store at room temperature. • Protect from light, do not freeze.

Reconstitution:

• May give undiluted. • Flush with at least 2 ml 0.9% NaCl before and after administration. • May add to 30–50 ml most solutions (D_5W preferred)

Rate of administration:

• Give IV push at rate of 5 mg/min. • Infuse IV piggyback over 30 min. • For IV infusion, up to 25 mg/hr has been used (titrated to pt response).

IV INCOMPATIBILITIES ⊘

Allopurinol (Aloprim), amphotericin B complex (Abelcet, AmbiSome, Amphotec), cefepime (Maxipime), fluconazole (Diflucan), foscarnet (Foscavir), heparin, nitroprusside (Nipride), piperacillin-tazobactam (Zosyn).

IV COMPATIBILITIES

Dobutamine (Dobutrex), dopamine (Intropin), lorazepam (Ativan), midazolam (Versed), propofol (Diprivan).

INDICATIONS/ROUTES/DOSAGE

Usual adult dosage:

PO: 0.5–5 mg 2–3 times/day. **Maximum:** 100 mg/day.

IM (lactate): 2–5 mg q4–8h as needed.

IM (decanoate): 10–15 times stabilized oral dose given at 3–4 wk intervals.

Usual dosage for children:

PO: (3–12 yrs, 15–40 kg): Initially, 0.25–0.5 mg/day in divided doses. May increase by 0.25–0.5 mg q5–7days. **Maximum:** 0.15 mg/kg/day.

IM (lactate): (6–12 yrs): 1–3 mg/dose q4–8h. **Maximum:** 0.15 mg/kg/day.

SIDE EFFECTS

FREQUENT: Blurred vision, constipation, orthostatic hypotension, dry mouth, swelling or soreness of female breasts, peripheral edema. ***OCCASIONAL:*** Allergic reaction, difficulty urinating, decreased thirst, dizziness, decreased sexual ability, drowsiness, nausea, vomiting, photosensitivity, lethargy.

ADVERSE REACTIONS/TOXIC EFFECTS

Extrapyramidal symptoms appear to be dose related and may be noted in first few days of therapy. Marked drowsiness and lethargy, excessive salivation, fixed stare may be mild to severe in intensity. Less frequently seen are severe akathisia (motor restlessness) and acute dystonias: torticollis (neck muscle spasm), opisthotonos (rigidity of back muscles), and oculogyric crisis (rolling back of eyes). Tardive dyskinesia (protrusion of tongue, puffing of cheeks, chewing/puckering of the mouth) may occur during long-term administration or following drug discontinuance, and may be irreversible. Risk is greater in female geriatric pts. Abrupt withdrawal following long-term therapy may provoke transient dyskinesia signs.

NURSING IMPLICATIONS

BASELINE ASSESSMENT:

Assess behavior, appearance, emotional status, response to environment, speech pattern, thought content.

INTERVENTION/EVALUATION:

Supervise suicidal risk pt closely during early therapy (as depression lessens, energy level improves, causing increased suicide potential). Monitor for rigidity, tremor, masklike facial expression, fine tongue movement. Assess for therapeutic response (interest in surroundings, improvement in self-care, increased ability to concentrate, relaxed facial expression). Therapeutic blood serum level: 0.2–1 mcg/ml; toxic blood serum level: >1 mcg/ml.

PATIENT/FAMILY TEACHING:

Full therapeutic effect may take up to 6 wks. Do not abruptly withdraw from long-term drug therapy. Sugarless gum, sips of tepid water may relieve dry mouth. Drowsiness generally subsides during continued therapy. Avoid tasks that require alertness, motor skills until response to drug is established. Avoid alcohol. Report muscle stiffness. Avoid exposure to sunlight, overheating, and dehydration (increased risk of heat stroke).

haloprogin

(Halotex)

See Classification section under: Antifungals: topical

heparin sodium

hep-ah-rin
(Hepalean✤, Liquaemin)
Do not confuse with Hespan.

▶CLASSIFICATION

PHARMACOTHERAPEUTIC:
Blood modifier. ***CLINICAL:*** Anticoagulant (see p. 29C)

ACTION/*THERAPEUTIC EFFECT*

Interferes with blood coagulation by blocking conversion of prothrombin to thrombin and fibrinogen to fibrin. *Prevents further extension of existing thrombi or new clot formation.* No effect on existing clots.

PHARMACOKINETICS

Well absorbed after SubQ administration. Protein binding: Very high. Metabolized in liver, removed from circulation by uptake by reticuloendothelial system. Primarily excreted in urine. Not removed by hemodialysis. Half-life: 1–6 hrs.

USES

Prophylaxis, treatment of venous thrombosis, pulmonary embolism, peripheral arterial embolism, atrial fibrillation with embolism. Prevention of thromboembolus in cardiac and vascular surgery, dialysis procedures, blood transfusions, and blood sampling for laboratory purposes. Adjunct in treatment of coronary occlusion with acute MI. Maintains patency of indwelling intravascular devices. Diagnoses and treatment of acute/chronic consumptive coagulation pathology (e.g., DIC). Prevents cerebral thrombosis in progressive strokes.

PRECAUTIONS

CONTRAINDICATIONS: Bleeding abnormalities, vitamin K insufficiency, chronic alcoholism, severe hepatic/renal disease, salicylate therapy, severe hypertension, pregnancy, ergot alkaloids, lidocaine; peripheral artery disease, coronary insufficiency, angina, sepsis, thrombocytopenia, brain/spinal cord surgery, spinal anesthesia, eye surgery, oral anticoagulants. ***CAUTIONS:*** Severe hypertension, peripheral vascular disease, indwelling catheters, those >60 yrs, factors increasing risk of hemorrhage, diabetes, mild hepatic/renal disease.

▷***LIFESPAN CONSIDERATIONS:***
Pregnancy/Lactation: Use with caution, particularly during last trimester, immediate postpartum period (increased risk of maternal hemorrhage). Does not cross placenta; not distributed in breast milk. **Pregnancy Category B. Children:** No age-related precautions noted. Benzyl alcohol preservative may cause gasping syndrome in infants. **Elderly:** More susceptible to hemorrhage. Age-related decreased renal function may increase risk of bleeding.

INTERACTIONS

DRUG: **Anticoagulants, platelet aggregation inhibitors, thrombolytics** may increase risk of bleeding. **Antithyroid medications, cefoperazone, cefotetan, valproic acid** may cause hypoprothrombinemia. **Probenecid** may increase effect. ***HERBAL:*** **Feverfew, ginkgo biloba** may have additive effect. ***FOOD:*** None known. ***LAB VALUES:*** May increase free fatty acids, SGOT (AST), SGPT (ALT). May decrease triglycerides, cholesterol.

AVAILABILITY (Rx)

INJECTION: 10 units/ml, 100 units/ml, 1,000 units/ml, 2,500 units/ml, 5,000 units/ml, 7,500 units/ml, 10,000 units/ml, 20,000 units/ml, 40,000 units/ml, 25,000 units/500 ml infusion.

ADMINISTRATION/HANDLING

Note: Do *not* give by IM injection (pain, hematoma, ulceration, erythema).

SubQ:

Note: Used in low-dose therapy.

• After withdrawal of heparin from vial, change needle before injection (prevents leakage along needle track). • Inject above iliac crest or in abdominal fat layer. Do not inject within 2 inches of umbilicus, or any scar tissue. • Withdraw needle rapidly, apply prolonged pressure at injection site. Do not massage. • Rotate injection sites.

IV 💊

Note: Used in full-dose therapy. Intermittent IV produces higher incidence of bleeding abnormalities. Continuous IV preferred.

Storage:

• Store at room temperature.

Reconstitution:

• Dilute IV infusion in isotonic sterile saline, D_5W, or lactated Ringer's. • Invert container at least 6 times (ensures mixing, prevents pooling of medication).

Rate of administration:

• Use constant-rate IV infusion pump or microdrip.

IV INCOMPATIBILITIES ⊘

Amiodarone (Cordarone), amphotericin B complex (Abelcet, Ambisome, Amphotec), ciprofloxacin (Cipro), dacarbazine (DTIC), diazepam (Valium), dobutamine (Dobutrex), doxorubicin (Adriamycin), droperidol (Inapsine), filgrastim (Neupogen), gentamicin (Garamycin), haloperidol (Haldol), idarubicin (Idamycin), labetalol (Trandate), nicardipine (Cardene), phenytoin (Dilantin), quinidine, tobramycin (Nebcin), vancomycin (Vancocin).

IV COMPATIBILITIES

Ampicillin/sulbactam (Unasyn), aztreonam (Azactam), calcium gluconate, cafazolin (Ancef), ceftazidime (Fortaz), ceftriaxone (Rocephin), digoxin, dopamine (Intropin), enalpril (Vasotec), famotidine (Pepcid), furosemide (Lasix), insulin, labetalol (Normodyne, Trandate), lidocaine, magnesium, methylprednisolone (Solu-Medtrol), metoclopramide (Reglan), midazolam (Versed), piperacillin/tazobactam (Zosyn), potassium, propofol (Diprivan).

INDICATIONS/ROUTES/DOSAGE

Line flushing:

IV: **Adults, elderly, children:** 100 units q6–8h. **Infants (<10 kg):** 10 units q6–8h.

Usual Adult Dosage:

Prophylaxis

SubQ: 5,000 units q8–12h.

Treatment:

INTERMITTENT IV: Initially, 10,000 units, then 50–70 units/kg (5,000–10,000 units) q4–6h

IV INFUSION: Loading dose: 80 units/kg, then 18 units/kg/hr with adjustments according to APTT. **Range:** 10–30 units/kg/hr.

Usual dosage for children:

INTERMITTENT IV: **>1 yr:** Initially, 50–100 units/kg, then 50–100 units q4h.

IV INFUSION: Loading dose: 75 units/kg, then 20 units/kg/hr with adjustments according to APTT.

IV INFUSION: <1 yr: Loading dose: 75 units/kg, then 28 units/kg/hr.

SIDE EFFECTS

OCCASIONAL: Itching, burning, particularly on soles of feet (due to vasospastic reaction). **RARE:** Pain, cyanosis of extremity 6–10 days after initial therapy, lasts 4–6 hrs; hypersensitivity reaction (chills, fever, pruritus, urticaria, asthma, rhinitis, lacrimation, headache).

ADVERSE REACTIONS/TOXIC EFFECTS

Bleeding complications ranging from local ecchymoses to major hemorrhage occur more frequently in high-dose therapy, intermittent IV infusion, and in women >60 yrs. **Antidote:** Protamine sulfate 1–1.5 mg for every 100 units heparin SubQ if overdosage occurred before 30 min, 0.5–0.75 mg for every 100 units heparin SubQ if overdosage occurred within 30–60 min, 0.25–0.375 mg for every 100 units heparin SubQ if 2 hrs have elapsed since overdosage, 25–50 mg if heparin given by IV infusion.

NURSING IMPLICATIONS

BASELINE ASSESSMENT:

Cross-check dose with coworker. Determine activated partial thromboplastin time (APTT) before administration and 24 hrs after initiation of therapy, then 24–48 hrs for first week of therapy or until mainte-nance dose is established. Follow with APTT determinations 1–2 times weekly for 3–4 wks. In long-term therapy, monitor 1–2 times/mo.

INTERVENTION/EVALUATION:

Monitor APTT (therapeutic dosage at 1.5–2.5 times normal) diligently. Assess hematocrit, platelet count, urine/stool culture for occult blood, SGOT (AST), SGPT (ALT), regardless of route of administration. Assess for decrease in B/P, increase in pulse rate, complaint of abdominal or back pain, severe headache (may be evidence of hemorrhage). Question for increase in amount of discharge during menses. Check peripheral pulses; skin for bruises, petechiae. Check for excessive bleeding from minor cuts, scratches. Assess gums for erythema, gingival bleeding. Assess urine output for hematuria. Avoid IM injections of other medications due to potential for hematomas. When converting to coumadin therapy, monitor PT results (will be 10–20% higher while heparin is given concurrently).

PATIENT/FAMILY TEACHING:

Use electric razor, soft toothbrush to prevent bleeding. Report any sign of red or dark urine, black or red stool, coffee-ground vomitus, red-speckled mucus from cough. Do not use any OTC medication without physician approval (may interfere with platelet aggregation). Wear/carry identification that notes anticoagulant therapy. Inform dentist, other physicians of heparin therapy.

H

---

hepatitis A vaccine

(Havrix, Vaqta)

USES

Active immunization of persons >2 yrs against disease caused by hepatitis A virus.

DOSAGE

IM: Adults (>18 yrs): Havrix: 1,440 ELU, Vaqta: 50 U. **Children (2–18 yrs):** Havrix: 720 ELU, Vaqta: 25 U. Booster shot varies from 6 to 18 mos (provides persistent antibody concentration).

SIDE EFFECTS

OCCASIONAL (1–10%): Injection site soreness, pain, tenderness, induration, redness, swelling, fatigue, fever, malaise, nausea, anorexia, headache.

hepatitis B immune globulin (Human)

(Nabi-HB)

▶CLASSIFICATION

CLINICAL: Immunization agent

ACTION/*THERAPEUTIC EFFECT*

Immune globulin of inactivated hepatitis B virus, *providing passive immunization against hepatitis B virus.*

USES

Treatment of acute exposure to blood containing hepatitis B surface antigen (HbsAg), prenatal exposure of infants born to HbsAg-positive mothers, sexual exposure to HbsAg-positive partners, house-

hold exposure to those with acute hepatitis B virus infection.

AVAILABILITY (Rx)

INJECTION: 5 ml vial.

INDICATIONS/ROUTES/DOSAGE

Acute exposure:

IM: 0.06 ml/kg, ideally within 24 hrs.

Infants born to HbsAg-positive mothers:

IM: 0.5 ml, ideally within 12 hrs of birth.

Sexual exposure:

IM: 0.06 ml/kg within 14 days of last sexual contact or if sexual contact is to continue.

Household exposure:

IM: 0.5 ml.

SIDE EFFECTS

FREQUENT: Headache (26%), local pain (12%). **OCCASIONAL** (5%): Malaise, nausea, myalgia.

hetastarch

het-ah-starch
(Hespan, Hextend)
Do not confuse with Heparin.

▶CLASSIFICATION

CLINICAL: Plasma volume expander

ACTION/*THERAPEUTIC EFFECT*

Exerts osmotic pull on tissue fluids; *reducing hemoconcentration and blood viscosity, increasing circulating blood volume.*

PHARMACOKINETICS

Smaller molecules (<50,000 molecular weight) rapidly excreted by kidneys; larger molecules (>50,000 molecular weight) slowly degraded to smaller sized molecules, then excreted. Half-life: 17 days.

USES

Fluid replacement and plasma volume expansion in treatment of shock due to hemorrhage, burns, surgery, sepsis, trauma, leukapheresis.

PRECAUTIONS

CONTRAINDICATIONS: Severe bleeding disorders, severe CHF, oliguria, anuria. ***CAUTIONS:*** Thrombocytopenia, elderly or very young, pulmonary edema, CHF, impaired renal function, hepatic disease, those on sodium restriction.

▷***LIFESPAN CONSIDERATIONS:***
Pregnancy/Lactation: Do not use in pregnancy unless benefits outweigh risk to fetus. **Pregnancy Category C. Children:** Safety and efficacy not established. **Elderly:** No age-related precautions noted.

INTERACTIONS

DRUG: None significant. ***HERBAL:*** None known. ***FOOD:*** None known. ***LAB VALUES:*** May prolong prothrombin time (PT), partial thromboplastin time (PTT), bleeding, and clotting times; decrease hematocrit.

AVAILABILITY (Rx)

INJECTION: 6 g/100 ml 0.9% NaCl (500 ml infusion container).

ADMINISTRATION/HANDLING
IV 🖫

Storage:
• Store solutions at room temperature. • Solution should appear clear, pale yellow to amber. Do not use if discolored (deep turbid brown) or if precipitate forms.

Rate of administration:
• Administer only by IV infusion. • Do not add drugs or mix with other IV fluids. • In acute hemorrhagic shock, administer at rate approaching 1.2 g/kg (20 ml/kg) per hr. Use slower rates for burns, septic shock. • Monitor central venous pressure (CVP) when given by rapid infusion. If there is a precipitous rise in CVP, immediately discontinue drug (overexpansion of blood volume).

IV INCOMPATIBILITIES ⊘

Amikacin (Amikin), ampicillin (Polycillin), cefazolin (Ancef, Kefzol), cefotaxime (Claforan), cefoxitin (Mefoxin), gentamicin (Garamycin), ranitidine (Zantac), tobramycin (Nebcin).

IV COMPATIBILITIES

Cimetidine (Tagamet), diltiazem (Cardizem), enalapril (Vasotec).

INDICATIONS/ROUTES/DOSAGE
Plasma volume expansion:

IV: Adults, elderly: 500–1,000 ml/day up to 1,500 ml/day (20 mg/kg) at a rate up to 20 ml/kg/hr in hemorrhagic shock (slower rates for burns or septic shock). **Children:** 10 ml/kg/dose. **Maximum total daily dose:** Not to exceed 20 ml/kg.

Leukapheresis:

IV: Adults, elderly: 250–700 ml infused at constant rate, usually 1:8 to venous whole blood.

SIDE EFFECTS

RARE: Allergic reaction resulting in vomiting, mild temperature elevation, chills, itching; submaxillary and parotid gland enlargement, peripheral edema of lower extremities, mild flulike symptoms: headache, muscle aches.

H

✤ - Canadian trade name   ✳ - see also www.wbsaunders.com/SIMON/SaundersNDH

ADVERSE REACTIONS/TOXIC EFFECTS

Fluid overload (headache, weakness, blurred vision, behavioral changes, incoordination, isolated muscle twitching) and pulmonary edema (rapid breathing, rales, wheezing, coughing, increased B/P, distended neck veins) may occur. Anaphylactoid reaction may be observed as periorbital edema, urticaria, wheezing.

NURSING IMPLICATIONS

INTERVENTION/EVALUATION:

Monitor for fluid overload (peripheral and/or pulmonary edema, impending CHF symptoms). Assess lung sounds for wheezing, rales. During leukapheresis, monitor CBC, leukocyte and platelet counts, differential, hemoglobin, hematocrit, PT, PTT, I&O. Monitor central venous B/P (detects overexpansion of blood volume). Monitor urine output closely (increase in output generally occurs in oliguric pts after administration). Assess for periorbital edema, itching, wheezing, urticaria (allergic reaction). Monitor for oliguria, anuria, any change in output ratio. Monitor for bleeding from surgical or trauma sites.

hyaluronate sodium

hi-al-**your**-on-ate
(Hyalgan, Synvisc)

▶CLASSIFICATION
CLINICAL: Anti-arthritic

ACTION/*THERAPEUTIC EFFECT*

Naturally occurring; maintains viscosity of synovial fluid, supports lubricating/shock-absorbing properties of auricular cartilage.

USES

Treatment of pain associated with osteoarthritis of the knee.

AVAILABILITY (Rx)
SOLUTION: 20 mg/2 ml, 16 mg/2 ml.

INDICATIONS/ROUTES/DOSAGE
Osteoarthritis:

INTRA-ARTICULAR: **Adults:** *Hyalgan:* 5 injections/treatment cycle. *Synvisc:* 3 injections/treatment cycle.

SIDE EFFECTS
OCCASIONAL: *Hyalgan* (7–23%): Injection site pain, skin reaction (ecchymosis, rash), pruritus, headache. *Synvisc* (1–3%): Knee pain/swelling, rash, pruritus, calf cramps, muscle pain.

hydralazine hydrochloride

hy-**dral**-ah-zeen
(Apresoline, Novohylazin✦)

FIXED-COMBINATION(S)

With hydrochlorothiazide, a diuretic **(Apresodex, Apresoline-Esidrex, Apresazide, Hydralazine PLUS, Hydrazide);** with reserpine, an antihypertensive **(Serpasil-Apresoline);** with hydrochlorothiazide and reserpine **(Cherapas, Ser-Ap-Es, Serathide)**

Do not confuse with hydroxyzine.

► CLASSIFICATION

PHARMACOTHERAPEUTIC:
Vasodilator. ***CLINICAL:*** Antihypertensive (see p. 52C)

ACTION/*THERAPEUTIC EFFECT*

Directly relaxes vascular smooth muscle (greater effect on arterioles), *reducing B/P.* Produces decreased peripheral vascular resistance, increased heart rate, cardiac output. Decreases afterload (increases CO, decreases systemic resistance).

PHARMACOKINETICS

Onset	Peak	Duration
PO		
10–20 min	0.5–2 hrs	2–4 hrs

Well absorbed from GI tract. Widely distributed. Protein binding: 85–90%. Metabolized in liver to active metabolite. Primarily excreted in urine. Not removed by hemodialysis. Half-life: 3–7 hrs (half-life increased with impaired renal function).

USES/*UNLABELED*

Management of moderate/severe hypertension. *Treatment of congestive heart failure.*

PRECAUTIONS

CONTRAINDICATIONS: Coronary artery disease, rheumatic heart disease, lupus erythematosus. ***CAUTIONS:*** Impaired renal function, cerebrovascular disease.
▷***LIFESPAN CONSIDERATIONS:***
Pregnancy/Lactation: Drug crosses placenta; unknown if drug is distributed in breast milk. Thrombocytopenia, leukopenia, petechial bleeding, hematomas have occurred in newborns (resolved within 1–3 wks). **Pregnancy Cate-**

gory C. **Children:** No age-related precautions noted. **Elderly:** More sensitive to hypotensive effects. Age-related renal impairment may require dosage adjustment.

INTERACTIONS

DRUG: **Diuretics, other hypotensives** may increase hypotensive effect. ***HERBAL:*** None known. ***FOOD:*** None known. ***LAB VALUES:*** May produce positive direct Coomb's' test.

AVAILABILITY (Rx)

TABLETS: 10 mg, 25 mg, 50 mg, 100 mg. ***INJECTION:*** 20 mg/ml.

ADMINISTRATION/HANDLING

PO:
• Best given with food or regularly spaced meals. • Tablets may be crushed.

IV ▥

Storage:
• Store at room temperature.

Rate of administration:
• May give undiluted. • Give single dose over 1 min.

IV INCOMPATIBILITIES ⊘

Aminophylline, ampicillin (Polycillin), furosemide (Lasix).

IV COMPATIBILITIES

Heparin, potassium, vitamins.

INDICATIONS/ROUTES/DOSAGE

Hypertension:
PO: **Adults:** Initially, 10 mg 4 times/day. May increase by 10–25 mg/dose q2–5days. **Maximum:** 300 mg/day. **Children:** Initially, 0.75–1 mg/kg/day in 2–4 divided doses, not to exceed 25 mg/dose. May increase over 3–4 wks. **Maximum:** 7.5 mg/kg/day (5 mg/kg/day in infants).

H

IM/IV: Adults, elderly: Initially, 10–20 mg/dose q4–6h. May increase to 40 mg/dose. **Children:** Initially, 0.1–0.2 mg/kg/dose (maximum 20 mg) q4–6h as needed up to 1.7–3.5 mg/kg/day in divided doses q4–6h.

Dosage in renal impairment:

Creatinine Clearance	Dosage Interval
10–50 ml/min	q8h
<10 ml/min	q8–24h

SIDE EFFECTS

FREQUENT: Headache, palpitations, tachycardia (generally disappears in 7–10 days). ***OCCASIONAL:*** GI disturbance (nausea, vomiting, diarrhea), paresthesia, fluid retention, peripheral edema, dizziness, flushed face, nasal congestion.

ADVERSE REACTIONS/TOXIC EFFECTS

High dosage may produce lupus erythematosis–like reaction (fever, facial rash, muscle and joint aches, splenomegaly). Severe orthostatic hypotension, skin flushing, severe headache, myocardial ischemia, cardiac arrhythmias may develop. Profound shock may occur in cases of severe overdosage.

NURSING IMPLICATIONS

BASELINE ASSESSMENT:

Obtain B/P, pulse immediately before each dose administration, in addition to regular monitoring (be alert to fluctuations). Keep tissues readily available at pt's bedside for lacrimation, nasal congestion.

INTERVENTION/EVALUATION:

Monitor for headache, palpitations, tachycardia. Assess for peripheral edema of hands, feet (usually, first area of low extremity swelling is behind medial malleolus in ambulatory, sacral area in bedridden). Monitor pattern of daily bowel activity and stool consistency.

PATIENT/FAMILY TEACHING:

To reduce hypotensive effect, rise slowly from lying to sitting position and permit legs to dangle from bed momentarily before standing. Unsalted crackers, dry toast may relieve nausea. If taking high-dose therapy, report muscle and joint aches, fever (lupus-like reaction).

hydrochlorothiazide

high-drow-chlor-oh-**thigh**-ah-zide (Apo-Hydro ♣, Esidrix, HydroDIURIL, Microzide, Oretic)

FIXED-COMBINATION(S)

With methyldopa, an antihypertensive **(Aldoril)**; with propranolol, a beta-blocker **(Inderide)**; with hydralazine, a vasodilator **(Apresazide)**; with captopril, an ACE inhibitor **(Capozide)**; with enalapril, an ACE inhibitor **(Vaseretic)**; with irbesartan, an angiotensin II inhibitor **(Avalide)**; with losartan, an angiotensin II inhibitor **(Hyzaar)**; with metoprolol, a beta-blocker **(Lopressor HCT)**; with moexipril, an ACE inhibitor **(Uniretic)**; with quinapril, an ACE inhibitor **(Accuretic)**; with telmisartan, an angiotensin II inhibitor **(Micardis HCT)**; with candesartan, an angiotensin II inhibitor **(Atacand HCT)**; with timolol, a beta-blocker **(Timolide)**; with labetolol, an alpha-beta blocker

(Normozide); with potassium-sparing diuretics (amiloride) **[Moduretic];** (spironolactone) **[Aldactazide]** (triamterene) **[Dyazide, Maxzide];** with valsartan, an angiotensin II inhibitor **(Diovan HCT)**

▶CLASSIFICATION

PHARMACOTHERAPEUTIC: Sulfonamide derivative. **CLINICAL:** Thiazide diuretic, antihypertensive (see p. 83C)

ACTION/*THERAPEUTIC EFFECT*

Diuretic: Blocks reabsorption of water, electrolytes (sodium, potassium) at cortical diluting segment of distal tubule, *promoting renal excretion.* **Antihypertensive:** Reduces plasma, extracellular fluid volume, decreases peripheral vascular resistance (PVR) by direct effect on blood vessels, *reducing B/P.*

PHARMACOKINETICS

Onset	Peak	Duration
PO [diuretic]		
2 hrs	4–6 hrs	6–12 hrs

Variably absorbed from GI tract. Primarily excreted unchanged in urine. Not removed by hemodialysis. Half-life: 5.6–14.8 hrs.

USES/*UNLABELED*

Adjunctive therapy in edema associated with CHF, hepatic cirrhosis, corticoid or estrogen therapy, renal impairment. In treatment of hypertension, may be used alone or with other antihypertensive agents. *Treatment of diabetes insipidus; prevents calcium-containing renal stones.*

PRECAUTIONS

CONTRAINDICATIONS: History of hypersensitivity to sulfonamides or thiazide diuretics, renal decompensation, anuria. **CAUTIONS:** Severe renal disease, impaired hepatic function, diabetes mellitus, elderly/debilitated, thyroid disorders.

▷*LIFESPAN CONSIDERATIONS:*
Pregnancy/Lactation: Crosses placenta; small amount distributed in breast milk; nursing not advised. **Pregnancy Category D. Children:** No age-related precautions noted except jaundiced infants may be at risk for hyperbilirubinemia. **Elderly:** May be more sensitive to hypotensive and electrolyte effects. Age-related renal impairment may require caution.

INTERACTIONS

DRUG: Cholestyramine, colestipol may decrease absorption, effects. May increase **digoxin** toxicity (due to hypokalemia). May increase **lithium** toxicity. **HERBAL:** None known. **FOOD:** None known. **LAB VALUES:** May increase bilirubin, serum calcium, LDL, cholesterol, triglycerides, creatinine, glucose, uric acid. May decrease urinary calcium, magnesium, potassium, sodium.

AVAILABILITY [Rx]

CAPSULES: 12.5 mg, **TABLETS:** 25 mg, 50 mg, 100 mg. **ORAL SOLUTION:** 50 mg/5 ml.

ADMINISTRATION/HANDLING
PO:

• May give with food or milk if GI upset occurs, preferably with breakfast (may prevent nocturia).

INDICATIONS/ROUTES/DOSAGE
Edema:
PO: Adults: 12.5–100 mg/day.

H

Maximum: 200 mg/day. **Children (6 mos–12 yrs):** 2 mg/kg/day. **Maximum:** 200 mg/day. **Children (<6 mos):** 2–4 mg/kg/day. **Maximum:** 37.5 mg/day.

Usual dosage for children:

PO: 37.5–100 mg/day. **Children <2 yrs:** 12.5–37.5 mg/day.

SIDE EFFECTS

EXPECTED: Increase in urine frequency/volume. ***FREQUENT:*** Potassium depletion. ***OCCASIONAL:*** Postural hypotension, headache, GI disturbances, photosensitivity reaction.

ADVERSE REACTIONS/TOXIC EFFECTS

Vigorous diuresis may lead to profound water loss and electrolyte depletion, resulting in hypokalemia, hyponatremia, dehydration. Acute hypotensive episodes may occur. Hyperglycemia may be noted during prolonged therapy. GI upset, pancreatitis, dizziness, paresthesias, headache, blood dyscrasias, pulmonary edema, allergic pneumonitis, dermatologic reactions occur rarely. Overdosage can lead to lethargy, coma without changes in electrolytes or hydration.

NURSING IMPLICATIONS

BASELINE ASSESSMENT:

Check vital signs, esp. B/P for hypotension prior to administration. Assess baseline electrolytes; particularly check for low potassium. Evaluate edema, skin turgor, mucous membranes for hydration status. Assess muscle strength, mental status. Note skin temperature, moisture. Obtain baseline weight. Initiate I&O.

INTERVENTION/EVALUATION:

Continue to monitor B/P, vital signs, electrolytes, I&O, weight. Note extent of diuresis. Watch for changes from initial assessment (hypokalemia may result in weakness, tremor, muscle cramps, nausea, vomiting, change in mental status, tachycardia; hyponatremia may result in confusion, thirst, cold/clammy skin). Be esp. alert for potassium depletion in pts taking digoxin (cardiac arrhythmias). Potassium supplements are frequently ordered. Check for constipation (may occur with exercise diuresis).

PATIENT/FAMILY TEACHING:

Expect increased frequency and volume of urination. To reduce hypotensive effect, rise slowly from lying to sitting position and permit legs to dangle momentarily before standing. Eat foods high in potassium such as whole grains (cereals), legumes, meat, bananas, apricots, orange juice, potatoes (white, sweet), raisins. Protect skin from sun/ultraviolet rays (photosensitivity may occur).

hydrocodone bitartrate

high-drough-**koe**-doan
(Hycodan✿, Robidone✿)

FIXED-COMBINATION(S)

With acetaminophen (**Anexsia, Lortab, Vicodin, Vicodin HP, Zydone);** with aspirin (**Lortab ASA);** with chlorpheniramine, an antihistamine (**Tussionex);** with ibuprofen, a NSAID (**Vicoprofen);** with phenypropanolamine, a sympathomimetic (**Hycomine)**

▶CLASSIFICATION

PHARMACOTHERAPEUTIC:
Opioid agonist **(Schedule III).**
CLINICAL: Narcotic analgesic,
antitussive (see p. 116C)

ACTION/*THERAPEUTIC EFFECT*

Binds at opiate receptor sites in
CNS. *Reduces intensity of pain
stimuli incoming from sensory
nerve endings, altering pain perception and emotional response to
pain; suppresses cough reflex.*

PHARMACOKINETICS

Onset	Peak	Duration
PO (analgesic)		
10–20 min	30–60min	4–6 hrs
PO (antitussive)		
—	—	4–6 hrs

Well absorbed from GI tract. Metabolized in liver. Primarily excreted in urine. Half-life: 3.8 hrs
(increased in elderly).

USES

Relief of moderate to moderately
severe pain, nonproductive cough.

PRECAUTIONS

CONTRAINDICATIONS: None
significant. ***EXTREME CAUTION:***
CNS depression, anoxia, hypercapnia, respiratory depression, seizures, acute alcoholism, shock, untreated myxedema, respiratory
dysfunction. ***CAUTIONS:*** Increased
intracranial pressure, impaired hepatic function, acute abdominal
conditions, hypothyroidism, prostatic hypertrophy, Addison's disease,
urethral stricture, COPD.
▷*LIFESPAN CONSIDERATIONS:*
Pregnancy/Lactation: Readily
crosses placenta; distributed in breast
milk. May prolong labor if administered in latent phase of first stage of

labor, or before cervical dilation of
4–5 cm has occurred. Respiratory depression may occur in neonate if
mother received opiates during
labor. Regular use of opiates during
pregnancy may produce withdrawal
symptoms (irritability, excessive crying, tremors, hyperactive reflexes,
fever, vomiting, diarrhea, yawning,
sneezing, seizures) in the neonate.
Pregnancy Category C (Category D
if used for prolonged periods or high
doses at term). **Children:** Those <2
yrs of age may be more susceptible
to respiratory depression. **Elderly:**
May be more susceptible to respiration depression, may cause paradoxical excitement. Age-related renal impairment, prostatic hypertrophy or
obstruction may increase risk of urinary retention; dosage adjustment
recommended.

INTERACTIONS

***DRUG:* Alcohol, CNS depres-
sants** may increase CNS or respiratory depression, hypotension.
MAO inhibitors may produce severe, fatal reaction (reduce dose
to ¼ usual dose). ***HERBAL:*** None
known. ***FOOD:*** None known. ***LAB
VALUES:*** May increase amylase, lipase plasma concentrations.

ADMINISTRATION/HANDLING

PO:

• Give without regard to meals. •
Tablets may be crushed.

INDICATIONS/ROUTES/DOSAGE

Analgesia:

***PO:* Adults, children >12 yrs:**
5–10 mg q4–6h. **Elderly:** 2.5–5
mg q4–6h.

Antitussive:

***PO:* Adults:** 5–10 mg q4–6h as
needed. **Maximum:** 15 mg/dose.
Children: 0.6 mg/kg/day in 3–4
divided doses at intervals of no

less than 4 hrs. **Maximum single dose in children 2–12 yrs:** 5 mg. **Maximum single dose in children <2 yrs:** 1.25 mg.

Extended-release:

PO: **Adults:** 10 mg q12h. **Children 6–12 yrs:** 5 mg q12h.

SIDE EFFECTS

Note: Effects are dependent on dosage amount but occur infrequently with oral antitussives. Ambulatory pts and those not in severe pain may experience dizziness, nausea, vomiting, hypotension more frequently than those who are in supine position or having severe pain.

FREQUENT: Sedation, decreased B/P, increased sweating, flushed face, dizziness, drowsiness, hypotension. *OCCASIONAL:* Decreased urination, blurred vision, constipation, dry mouth, headache, nausea, vomiting, difficult/painful urination, euphoria, dysphoria.

ADVERSE REACTIONS/TOXIC EFFECTS

Overdosage results in respiratory depression, skeletal muscle flaccidity, cold clammy skin, cyanosis, extreme somnolence progressing to convulsions, stupor, coma. Tolerance to analgesic effect, physical dependence may occur with repeated use. Prolonged duration of action, cumulative effect may occur in those with impaired hepatic, renal function.

NURSING IMPLICATIONS

BASELINE ASSESSMENT:

Obtain vital signs before giving medication. If respirations are 12/min or lower (20/min or lower in children), withhold medication, contact physician. *Analgesic:* Assess onset, type, location, and duration of pain. Effect of medication is reduced if full pain recurs before next dose. *Antitussive:* Assess type, severity, frequency of cough, and productions.

INTERVENTION/EVALUATION:

Palpate bladder for urinary retention. Monitor pattern of daily bowel activity and stool consistency. Initiate deep breathing and coughing exercises, particularly in those with impaired pulmonary function. Assess for clinical improvement and record onset of relief of pain or cough.

PATIENT/FAMILY TEACHING:

Change positions slowly to avoid orthostatic hypotension. Avoid tasks that require alertness, motor skills until response to drug is established. Tolerance/dependence may occur with prolonged use of high doses. Avoid alcohol. Report nausea, vomiting, constipation, shortness of breath, difficulty breathing. May take with food.

hydrocortisone ✳

high-droe-**core**-tah-sewn
(Cortef♣, Cort-Dome, Cortenema, Hydrocortone, Hytone, Locoid, Pandel)

hydrocortisone acetate

(Cortaid, Cortamed♣, Corticaine, Proctocort)

hydrocortisone sodium phosphate

(Hydrocortone Phosphate)

hydrocortisone sodium succinate

(A-HydroCort, Solu-Cortef)

hydrocortisone valerate

(WestCort)

FIXED-COMBINATION(S)

With neomycin, an antibiotic **(NeoCort-Dome);** with bacitracin, neomycin, polymyxin B, anti-infectives **(Cortisporin);** hydrocortisone acetate with neomycin, an antibiotic **(Neo-Cortef);** with ciprofloxacin, an antibiotic **(Cipro HC Otic)**

▶CLASSIFICATION

PHARMACOTHERAPEUTIC: Adrenal corticosteroid. **CLINICAL:** Glucocorticoid (see pp. 79C, 82C)

ACTION/*THERAPEUTIC EFFECT*

Inhibits accumulation of inflammatory cells at inflammation sites, phagocytosis, lysosomal enzyme release and synthesis and/or release of mediators of inflammation. *Prevents/suppresses cell-mediated immune reactions. Decreases/prevents tissue response to inflammatory process.*

PHARMACOKINETICS

Well absorbed after IM administration. Widely distributed. Metabolized in liver. Half-life: *plasma:* 1.5–2 hrs; *biologic:* 8–12 hrs.

USES

Management of adrenocortical insufficiency; relief of inflammation of corticosteroid-responsive dermatoses; adjunctive treatment of ulcerative colitis.

PRECAUTIONS

CONTRAINDICATIONS: Hypersensitivity to any corticosteroid or sulfite, systemic fungal infection, peptic ulcer (except life-threatening situations). Avoid live virus vaccine such as smallpox. **Topical:** Marked circulation impairment. Do not instill ocular solution when topical corticosteroids are being used on eyelids or surrounding skin. **CAUTIONS:** Thromboembolic disorders, history of tuberculosis (may reactivate disease), hypothyroidism, cirrhosis, nonspecific ulcerative colitis, CHF, hypertension, psychosis, renal insufficiency, seizure disorders. Prolonged therapy should be discontinued slowly. **Topical:** Do not apply to extensive areas.

▷*LIFESPAN CONSIDERATIONS:* **Pregnancy/Lactation:** Crosses placenta, distributed in breast milk. May produce cleft palate if used chronically during first trimester. Nursing contraindicated. **Pregnancy Category D. Children:** Prolonged treatment or high doses may decrease short-term growth rate, cortisol secretion. **Elderly:** May be more susceptible to developing hypertension or osteoporosis.

INTERACTIONS

DRUG: Amphotericin may increase hypokalemia. May decrease effect of **oral hypoglycemics, insulin, diuretics, potassium supplements.** May increase **digoxin** toxicity (due to hypokalemia). **Hepatic enzyme inducers** may decrease effect. **Live virus vaccines** may potentiate virus replication, increase vaccine side effects, decrease pt's antibody response to vaccine. **HERBAL:** None known. **FOOD:** None known. **LAB VALUES:**

May decrease calcium, potassium, thyroxine. May increase cholesterol, lipids, glucose, sodium, amylase.

AVAILABILITY (Rx)

Hydrocortisone: **GEL:** 0.5%, 1% (OTC). **LOTION:** 0.25%, 0.5%, 1%, 2%, 2.5%. **CREAM:** 0.5%, 1% (OTC), 2.5%. **OINTMENT:** 0.5%, 1% (OTC), 2.5%. **TOPICAL SOLUTION:** 1%. **Cypionate:** **ORAL SUSPENSION:** 10 mg/5 ml.

Sodium phosphate: **INJECTION:** 50 mg/ml

Sodium succinate: **INJECTION:** 100 mg, 250 mg, 500 mg, 1,000 mg.

Acetate: **INJECTION:** 25 mg/ml, 50 mg/ml. **SUPPOSITORY:** 10 mg, 25 mg, 30 mg. **CREAM:** 0.5%, 1%. **OINTMENT:** 0.5%, 1%.

Valerate: **CREAM:** 0.2%.

ADMINISTRATION/HANDLING
IV 💉

Storage:

• Store at room temperature. • *Hydrocortisone sodium succinate:* After reconstitution, use solution within 72 hrs. Use immediately if further diluted with D_5W, 0.9% NaCl, or other compatible diluent. • Once reconstituted, solution is stable for 72 hrs at room temperature.

Reconstitution:

• May further dilute with D_5W or 0.9% NaCl.

Rate of administration:

• Give IV push over 1 min.

Topical:

• Gently cleanse area prior to application. • Use occlusive dressings only as ordered. • Apply sparingly and rub into area thoroughly.

Rectal:

• Shake homogeneous suspension well. • Instruct pt to lie on left side with left leg extended, right leg flexed. • Gently insert applicator tip into rectum, pointed slightly toward navel (umbilicus) and slowly instill medication.

IV INCOMPATIBILITIES ⊘

Ciprofloxacin (Cipro), diazepam (Valium), idarubicin (Idamycin), medazolam (Versed), phenytoin (Dilantin).

IV COMPATIBILITIES

Aminophylline, amphotericin, calcium gluconate, diltiazem (Cardizem), dopamine (Intropin), heparin, insulin, lidocaine, lorazepam (Ativan), magnesium, propofol (Diprivan).

INDICATIONS/ROUTES/DOSAGE
Acute adrenal insufficiency:

IV: **Adults, elderly:** 100 mg IV bolus, then 300 mg/day in divided doses q8h. **Children:** 1–2 mg/kg IV bolus, then 150–250 mg/day in divided doses q6–8h. **Infants:** 1–2 mg/kg/dose IV bolus, then 25–150 mg/day in divided doses q6–8h.

Anti-inflammatory/ immunosuppression:

IM/IV: **Adults, elderly:** 15–240 mg q12h. **Children:** 1–5 mg/kg/day in divided doses q12h.

Physiologic replacement:

IM: **Children:** 0.25–0.35 mg/kg/day as a single daily dose.

PO: **Children:** 0.5–0.75 mg/kg/day in divided doses q8h.

Status asthmaticus:

IV: **Adults, elderly:** 100–500 mg q6h. **Children:** 2 mg/kg/dose q6h.

Shock:

IV: **Adults, elderly, children >12 yrs:** 100–500 mg q6h. **Children**

<12 yrs: 50 mg/kg. May repeat in 4 hrs, then q24h as needed.

Usual rectal dosage:

***RECTAL:* Adults, elderly:** 100 mg at bedtime for 21 nights or until clinical and proctologic remission occurs (may require 2–3 mos therapy).

***CORTIFOAM:* Adults, elderly:** 1 applicator 1–2 times/day for 2–3 wks, then every second day thereafter.

Usual topical dosage:

Adults, elderly: Apply sparingly 2–4 times/day.

SIDE EFFECTS

FREQUENT: Insomnia, heartburn, nervousness, abdominal distention, increased sweating, acne, mood swings, increased appetite, facial flushing, delayed wound healing, increased susceptibility to infection, diarrhea/constipation. ***OCCASIONAL:*** Headache, edema, change in skin color, frequent urination. ***Topical:*** Itching, redness, irritation. ***RARE:*** Tachycardia, allergic reaction (rash, hives), psychic changes, hallucinations, depression. ***Topical:*** Allergic contact dermatitis, purpura. Systemic absorption more likely with occlusive dressings or extensive application in young children.

ADVERSE REACTIONS/TOXIC EFFECTS

Long-term therapy: Hypocalcemia, hypokalemia, muscle wasting (esp. arms, legs), osteoporosis, spontaneous fractures, amenorrhea, cataracts, glaucoma, peptic ulcer, CHF. ***Abrupt withdrawal following long-term therapy:*** Anorexia, nausea, fever, headache, sudden severe joint pain, rebound inflammation, fatigue, weakness, lethargy, dizziness, orthostatic hypotension.

NURSING IMPLICATIONS

BASELINE ASSESSMENT:

Obtain baseline values for weight, B/P, glucose, cholesterol, electrolytes. Check results of initial tests, e.g., TB skin test, x-rays, EKG.

INTERVENTION/EVALUATION:

Assess for edema. Be alert to infection (reduced immune response): sore throat, fever, or vague symptoms. Evaluate bowel activity. Monitor electrolytes. Watch for hypocalcemia (muscle twitching, cramps) or hypokalemia (weaknes, numbness/tingling esp. lower extremities, nausea and vomiting, irritability, EKG changes). Assess emotional status, ability to sleep.

PATIENT/FAMILY TEACHING:

Notify physician of fever, sore throat, muscle aches, sudden weight gain/swelling. Do not take aspirin or any other medication without consulting physician. Inform dentist, physicians of cortisone therapy now or within past 12 mos. Caution against overuse of joints injected for symptomatic relief. ***Topical:*** Apply after shower or bath for best absorption. Do not cover unless physician orders; do not use tight diapers, plastic pants, or coverings. Avoid contact with eyes.

H

hydromorphone hydrochloride

high-dro-**more**-phone
(Dilaudid, Dilaudid HP, Hydromorph Contin♣)

FIXED-COMBINATION(S)

With guaifenesin, an expectorant **(Dilaudid Cough Syrup)**

▶CLASSIFICATION

PHARMACOTHERAPEUTIC:
Opioid agonist **(Schedule II).**
CLINICAL: Narcotic analgesic, antitussive (see p. 116C).

ACTION/THERAPEUTIC EFFECT

Binds at opiate receptor sites in CNS. *Reduces intensity of pain stimuli incoming from sensory nerve endings, altering pain perception and emotional response to pain; suppresses cough reflex.*

PHARMACOKINETICS

Onset	Peak	Duration
PO		
30 min	90–120 min	4 hrs
SubQ		
15 min	30–90 min	4 hrs
IM		
15 min	30–60 min	4–5 hrs
IV		
10–15 min	15–30 min	2–3 hrs
Rectal		
15–30 min	—	—

Well absorbed from GI tract, after IM administration. Widely distributed. Metabolized in liver. Excreted in urine. Half-life: 1–3 hrs.

USES

Relief of moderate to severe pain, persistent nonproductive cough.

PRECAUTIONS

CONTRAINDICATIONS: None significant. **EXTREME CAUTION:** CNS depression, anoxia, hypercapnia, respiratory depression, seizures, acute alcoholism, shock, untreated myxedema, respiratory dysfunction. **CAUTIONS:** Increased intracranial pressure, impaired hepatic function, acute abdominal conditions, hypothyroidism, prostatic hypertrophy, Addison's disease, urethral stricture, COPD.

▷**LIFESPAN CONSIDERATIONS:**
Pregnancy/Lactation: Readily crosses placenta; unknown if distributed in breast milk. May prolong labor if administered in latent phase of first stage of labor or before cervical dilation of 4–5 cm has occurred. Respiratory depression may occur in neonate if mother receives opiates during labor. Regular use of opiates during pregnancy may produce withdrawal symptoms in the neonate (irritability, excessive crying, tremors, hyperactive reflexes, fever, vomiting, diarrhea, yawning, sneezing, seizures). **Pregnancy Category B** (Category D if used for prolonged periods or in high doses at term). **Children:** Those <2 yrs of age may be more susceptible to respiratory depression. **Elderly:** May be more susceptible to respiration depression, may cause paradoxical excitement. Age-related renal impairment, prostatic hypertrophy or obstruction may increase risk of urinary retention; dosage adjustment recommended.

INTERACTIONS

DRUG: Alcohol, CNS depressants may increase CNS or respiratory depression, hypotension. **MAO inhibitors** may produce severe, fatal reaction (reduce dose to 1/4 usual dose). **HERBAL:** None known. **FOOD:** None known. **LAB VALUES:** May increase amylase, lipase plasma concentrations.

AVAILABILITY (Rx)

TABLETS: 1 mg, 2 mg, 3 mg, 4 mg, 8 mg. **LIQUID:** 5 mg/5 ml. **IN-**

JECTION: 1 mg/ml, 2 mg/ml, 3 mg/ml, 4 mg/ml, 10 mg/ml. ***POWDER FOR INJECTION:*** 250 mg. ***SUPPOSITORY:*** 3 mg.

ADMINISTRATION/HANDLING

PO:

• Give without regard to meals. • Tablets may be crushed.

SubQ/IM:

• Use short 30 gauge needle for SubQ injection. • Administer slowly, rotating injection sites. • Pts with circulatory impairment experience higher risk of overdosage because of delayed absorption of repeated administration.

IV 🐾

Note: High concentration injection (10 mg/ml) should be used only in those tolerant to opiate agonists, currently receiving high doses of another opiate agonist for severe, chronic pain due to cancer.

Storage:

• Store at room temperature; protect from light. • Slight yellow discoloration of parenteral form does not indicate loss of potency.

Reconstitution:

• May give undiluted. • May further dilute with 5 ml Sterile Water for Injection or 0.9% NaCl.

Rate of administration:

• Administer IV push very slowly (over 2–5 min). • Rapid IV increases risk of severe adverse reactions (chest wall rigidity, apnea, peripheral circulatory collapse, anaphylactoid effects, cardiac arrest).

Rectal:

• Refrigerate suppositories. • Moisten suppository with cold water before inserting well up into rectum.

IV INCOMPATIBILITIES ⊘

Amphotericin B complex (Abelcet, Ambisome, Amphotec), cefazolin (Ancef, Kefzol), diazepam (Valium), phenobarbital, phenytoin (Dilantin).

IV COMPATIBILITIES

Dobutamine (Dobutrex), dopamine (Intropin), heparin, lorazepam (Ativan), magnesium, midazolam (Versed), milrinone (Primacor), propofol (Diprivan).

INDICATIONS/ROUTES/DOSAGE   H

Analgesia:

PO/SubQ/IM/IV: **Adults, elderly, children >12 yrs:** 1–4 mg/dose q4–6h.

IV: **Children <12 yrs:** 0.015 mg/kg/dose q4–6h.

PO: **Children <12 yrs:** 0.03–0.08 mg/kg/dose q4–6h. **Maximum:** 5 mg.

RECTAL: **Adults, elderly:** 3 mg q6–8h.

Antitussive:

PO: **Adults, children >12 yrs, elderly:** 1 mg q3–4h. **Children 6–12 yrs:** 0.5 mg q3–4h.

Usual PCA dosage:

Adults, elderly: Loading dose: 0.5–1 mg. ***BOLUS:*** 0.1–0.5 mg. Lockout interval: 5–10 min. Continuous infusion: 0.2–0.5 mg/hr.

Usual epidural dosage:

Adults, elderly: 0.15–0.3 mg bolus, then 0.15–0.3 mg/hr. Lockout interval: 15–30 min.

SIDE EFFECTS

Note: Effects are dependent on dosage amount, route of administration but occur infrequently with oral antitussives. Ambulatory pts and those not in severe pain may experience dizziness, nausea,

---

vomiting, hypotension more frequently than those in supine position or having severe pain. **FREQUENT:** Drowsiness, dizziness, hypotension, decreased appetite. **OCCASIONAL:** Confusion, diaphoresis, facial flushing, urinary retention, constipation, dry mouth, nausea, vomiting, headache, pain at injection site. **RARE:** Allergic reaction, depression.

ADVERSE REACTIONS/TOXIC EFFECTS

Overdosage results in respiratory depression, skeletal muscle flaccidity, cold clammy skin, cyanosis, extreme somnolence progressing to convulsions, stupor, coma. Tolerance to analgesic effect, physical dependence may occur with repeated use. Prolonged duration of action, cumulative effect may occur in those with impaired hepatic, renal function.

NURSING IMPLICATIONS

BASELINE ASSESSMENT:

Obtain vital signs before giving medication. If respirations are 12/min or lower (20/min or lower in children), withhold medication, contact physician. **Analgesic:** Assess onset, type, location, and duration of pain. Effect of medication is reduced if full pain recurs before next dose. **Antitussive:** Assess type, severity, frequency of cough and productions.

INTERVENTION/EVALUATION:

Monitor B/P, pulse, respirations. Assess cough, lung sounds. Increase fluid intake and environmental humidity to improve viscosity of lung secretions. To prevent pain cycles, instruct pt to request pain medication as soon

as discomfort begins. Check for constipation (esp. in long-term use) and increase fiber, fluids, and exercise as appropriate. Initiate deep breathing and coughing exercises, particularly in those with impaired pulmonary function. Assess for clinical improvement and record onset of relief of pain or cough.

PATIENT/FAMILY TEACHING:

Discomfort may occur with injection. Change positions slowly to avoid orthostatic hypotension. Avoid tasks that require alertness, motor skills until response to drug is established. Tolerance/dependence may occur with prolonged use of high doses. Report difficulty breathing.

hydroxychloroquine sulfate

hi-drocks-ee-**klor**-oh-kwin
(Plaquenil❦, Plaquenil Sulfate)

▶CLASSIFICATION

CLINICAL: Antimalarial, antirheumatic

ACTION/THERAPEUTIC EFFECT

Concentrates in parasite acid vesicles, interfering with parasite protein synthesis, increasing pH *(inhibits parasite growth)*. Antirheumatic action unknown, but may involve suppressing formation of antigens responsible for hypersensitivity reactions.

USES/UNLABELED

Treatment of falciparum malaria (terminates acute attacks and cures nonresistant strains), suppression of acute attacks and prolongation of interval between treatment/relapse in vivax, ovale, malariae malaria. Treatment of discoid or systematic lupus erythematosus, acute and chronic rheumatoid arthritis. *Treatment of juvenile arthritis, sarcoid-associated hypercalcemia.*

PRECAUTIONS

CONTRAINDICATIONS: Retinal or visual field changes, long-term therapy for children, psoriasis, porphyria. After weighing risk/benefit ratio, physician may still elect to use drug, esp. with plasmodial forms. **CAUTIONS:** Alcoholism, hepatic disease, G-6-PD deficiency. Children are esp. susceptible to hydroxychloroquine fatalities.

INTERACTIONS

DRUG: May increase concentration of **penicillamine,** increase risk of hematologic/renal or severe skin reaction. **HERBAL:** None known. **FOOD:** None known. **LAB VALUES:** None significant.

AVAILABILITY (Rx)

TABLETS: 200 mg (155 mg base).

INDICATIONS/ROUTES/DOSAGE

Note: 200 mg hydroxychloroquine = 155 mg base.

Suppression of malaria:

PO: Adults: 310 mg base weekly on same day each week. **Children:** 5 mg base/kg/wk. Begin 2 wks prior to exposure; continue 6–8 wks after leaving endemic area or if therapy is not begun prior to exposure.

PO: Adults: 620 mg base. **Children:** 10 mg base/kg given in 2 divided doses 6 hrs apart.

Treatment of malaria (acute attack): Dose (mg base):

Dose	Times	Adults	Children
Initial	Day 1	620 mg	10 mg/kg
Second	6 hrs later	310 mg	5 mg/kg
Third	Day 2	310 mg	5 mg/kg
Fourth	Day 3	310 mg	5 mg/kg

Rheumatoid arthritis:

PO: Adults: Initially, 400–600 mg (310–465 mg base) daily for 5–10 days; gradually increase dose to optimum response level. **Maintenance (usually within 4–12 wks):** Decrease dose by 50%, continue at level of 200–400 mg/day. Maximum effect may not be seen for several mos.

Lupus erythematosus:

PO: Adults: Initially, 400 mg 1–2 times/day for several wks or mos. **Maintenance:** 200–400 mg/day.

SIDE EFFECTS

FREQUENT: Mild transient headache, anorexia, nausea, vomiting. **OCCASIONAL:** Visual disturbances; nervousness; fatigue; pruritus (esp. of palms, soles, scalp); irritability, personality changes, diarrhea. **RARE:** Stomatitis dermatitis, reduced hearing.

ADVERSE REACTIONS/TOXIC EFFECTS

Ocular toxicity (esp. retinopathy, which may progress even after drug is discontinued). **Prolonged therapy:** Peripheral neuritis, neuromyopathy, hypotension, EKG changes, agranulocytosis, aplastic anemia, thrombocytopenia, convulsions, psychosis. **Overdosage:** Headache, vomiting, visual disturbance, drowsiness, convulsions, hypokalemia followed by cardiovascular collapse, death.

H

NURSING IMPLICATIONS

BASELINE ASSESSMENT:

Evaluate CBC, hepatic function results.

INTERVENTION/EVALUATION:

Monitor and report any visual disturbances promptly. Evaluate for GI distress: Give dose with food (for malaria). Monitor hepatic function tests. Assess skin and buccal mucosa; inquire about pruritus. Report reduced hearing immediately.

PATIENT/FAMILY TEACHING:

Continue drug for full length of treatment. In long-term therapy therapeutic response may not be evident for up to 6 mos. Immediately notify physician of *any* new symptom of visual difficulties, muscular weakness, decreased hearing, tinnitus.

hydroxyurea ✳

high-**drocks**-ee-your-e-ah
(Droxia, Hydrea, Mylocel)

▶CLASSIFICATION

PHARMACOTHERAPEUTIC:
Synthetic urea analog. ***CLINICAL:*** Antineoplastic (see p. 71C)

ACTION/*THERAPEUTIC EFFECT*

Cell cycle-specific for S phase. Inhibits DNA synthesis without interfering with RNA synthesis or protein, *interfering with the normal repair process of cells damaged by irradiation.*

USES/*UNLABELED*

Treatment of melanoma, resistant chronic myelocytic leukemia, recurrent, metastatic, or inoperable ovarian carcinoma. Also used in combination with radiation therapy for local control of primary squamous cell carcinoma of head and neck, excluding lip. Treatment of sickle-cell anemia. *Treatment of cervical carcinoma, polycythemia vera. Long-term suppression of HIV.*

PRECAUTIONS

CONTRAINDICATIONS: WBC less than 2,500/mm^3 or platelet count <100,000/mm^3. ***CAUTIONS:*** Previous irradiation therapy, other cytotoxic drugs, impaired renal, hepatic function.

INTERACTIONS

DRUG: May decrease effect of **antigout medications. Bone marrow depressants** may increase bone marrow depression. **Live virus vaccines** may potentiate virus replication, increase vaccine side effects, decrease pt's antibody response to vaccine. ***HERBAL:*** None known. ***FOOD:*** None known. ***LAB VALUES:*** May increase BUN, creatinine, uric acid.

AVAILABILITY (Rx)

CAPSULES: 200 mg, 300 mg, 400 mg, 500 mg. ***TABLETS:*** 1,000 mg.

INDICATIONS/ROUTES/DOSAGE

Note: Dosage individualized based on clinical response, tolerance to adverse effects. When used in combination therapy, consult specific protocols for optimum dosage, sequence of drug administration. Dosage based on actual or ideal body weight, whichever is less. Therapy interrupted when platelets fall below 100,000/mm^3 or leukocytes fall below 2,500/mm^3. Resume when counts rise toward normal.

Solid tumors:

PO: Adults, elderly: 80 mg/kg q3days or 20–30 mg/kd/day as a single dose daily.

Therapy with irradiation:

PO: Adults, elderly: 80 mg/kg q3days beginning at least 7 days before starting irradiation.

Resistant chronic myelocytic leukemia (CML):

PO: Adults, elderly: 20–30 mg/kg once daily. **Children:** Initially, 10–20 mg/kg once daily.

HIV infection:

PO: Adults, elderly: 500 mg 2 times/day (with didanosine).

Sickle cell anemia:

PO: Adults, elderly, children: Initially, 15 mg/kg once daily. May increase by 5 mg/kg/day. **Maximum:** 35 mg/kg/wk.

SIDE EFFECTS

FREQUENT: Nausea, vomiting, anorexia, constipation/diarrhea. ***OCCASIONAL:*** Mild reversible rash, facial flushing, pruritus, fever, chills, malaise. ***RARE:*** Alopecia, headache, drowsiness, dizziness, disorientation.

ADVERSE REACTIONS/TOXIC EFFECTS

Bone marrow depression manifested as hematologic toxicity (leukopenia, and to lesser extent, thrombocytopenia, anemia).

NURSING IMPLICATIONS

BASELINE ASSESSMENT:

Obtain bone marrow studies, liver, kidney function tests before therapy begins, periodically thereafter. Obtain hemoglobin, WBC, platelet count weekly during therapy. Those with marked renal impairment may develop visual, auditory hallucinations, marked hematologic toxicity.

INTERVENTION/EVALUATION:

Assess pattern of daily bowel activity and stool consistency. Monitor for hematologic toxicity (fever, sore throat, signs of local infection, easy bruising, or unusual bleeding from any site), symptoms of anemia (excessive tiredness, weakness). Assess skin for rash, erythema.

PATIENT/FAMILY TEACHING:

Promptly report fever, sore throat, signs of local infection, easy bruising, or unusual bleeding from any site.

hydroxyzine hydrochloride

high-**drox**-ih-zeen
(Apo-Hydroxyzine✤, Atarax, Novohydroxyzin✤, Vistaril)

hydroxyzine pamoate

(Vistaril)
Do not confuse with hydralazine.

▶CLASSIFICATION

PHARMACOTHERAPEUTIC:
Piperazine derivative. ***CLINICAL:*** Antihistamine, antianxiety, antispasmotic, antiemetic, antipruritic (see p. 48C)

ACTION/THERAPEUTIC EFFECT

Suppresses activity at subcortical levels of CNS, *producing anticholinergic, antihistaminic, analgesic effects, skeletal muscle relaxation.* Diminishes vestibular stimulation and depresses labyrinthine function, *controlling nausea, vomiting.*

PHARMACOKINETICS

	Onset	Peak	Duration
PO	15–30 min	—	—

Well absorbed from GI tract, parenteral administration. Metabolized in liver. Primarily excreted in urine. Not removed by hemodialysis. Half-life: 20–25 hrs (half-life increased in elderly).

USES

Relief of anxiety, tension; pruritus caused by allergic conditions, preop and postop sedation, control of muscle spasm, nausea, and vomiting.

PRECAUTIONS

CONTRAINDICATIONS: None significant. **CAUTIONS:** None significant.

▷**LIFESPAN CONSIDERATIONS:** **Pregnancy/Lactation:** Unknown if drug crosses placenta or is distributed in breast milk. **Pregnancy Category C. Children:** Not recommended in newborns/premature infants (increased risk of anticholinergic effects). Paradoxical excitement may occur. **Elderly:** Increased risk of dizziness, sedation, confusion; hypotension, hyperexcitability may occur.

INTERACTIONS

DRUG: **Alcohol, CNS depressants** may increase CNS depressant effects. **MAO inhibitors** may increase anticholinergic, CNS depressant effects. **HERBAL:** None known. **FOOD:** None known. **LAB VALUES:** May cause false positives with 17-hydroxy corticosteroid determinations.

AVAILABILITY (Rx)

TABLETS: 10 mg, 25 mg, 50 mg, 100 mg. **CAPSULES:** 25 mg, 50 mg, 100 mg. **SYRUP:** 10 mg/5 ml. **ORAL SUSPENSION:** 25 mg/5 ml. **INJECTION:** 25 mg/ml, 50 mg/ml.

ADMINISTRATION/HANDLING
PO:

• Shake oral suspension well. • Scored tablets may be crushed; do not crush or break capsule.

IM:

Note: Significant tissue damage, thrombosis, gangrene may occur if injection is given SubQ, intra-arterial, or by IV. • IM may be given undiluted. • Use Z-track technique of injection to prevent SubQ infiltration. • Inject deep IM into gluteus maximus or midlateral thigh in adults, midlateral thigh in children.

INDICATIONS/ROUTES/DOSAGE
Antiemetic

IM: **Adults, elderly:** 25–100 mg/dose q4–6h.

Anxiety:

PO: **Adults, elderly:** 25–100 mg 4 times/day. **Maximum:** 600 mg/day.

Pruritus:

PO: **Adults, elderly:** 25 mg 3–4 times/day..

Usual children's dosage:

PO: 2 mg/kg/day in divided doses q6–8h.

IM: 0.5–1 mg/kg/dose q4–6h.

SIDE EFFECTS

Side effects are generally mild and transient. **FREQUENT:** Drowsiness, dry mouth, marked discomfort with IM injection. **OCCASIONAL:** Dizziness, ataxia (muscular incoordination), weakness, slurred speech, headache, agitation, increased anxiety. ***RARE:*** Paradoxical CNS hyperactivity/nervousness in children, excitement/restlessness in elderly/debilitated pts (generally noted during first 2 wks of therapy, particularly noted in presence of uncontrolled pain).

ADVERSE REACTIONS/TOXIC EFFECTS

Hypersensitivity reaction (wheezing, dyspnea, tightness of chest).

NURSING IMPLICATIONS

BASELINE ASSESSMENT:

Anxiety: Offer emotional support to anxious pt. Assess motor responses (agitation, trembling, tension) and autonomic responses (cold, clammy hands, sweating). ***Antiemetic:*** Assess for dehydration (poor skin turgor, dry mucous membranes, longitudinal furrows in tongue).

INTERVENTION/EVALUATION:

For those on long-term therapy, liver/renal function tests, blood counts should be performed periodically. Monitor lung sounds for signs of hypersensitivity reaction. Monitor serum electrolytes in those with severe vomiting. Assess for paradoxical reaction, particularly during early therapy. Assist with ambulation if drowsiness, lightheadedness occurs.

PATIENT/FAMILY TEACHING:

Marked discomfort may occur with IM injection. Sugarless gum, sips of tepid water may relieve dry mouth. Drowsiness usually diminishes with continued therapy. Avoid tasks that require alertness, motor skills until response to drug is established.

hyoscyamine

high-oh-**sigh**-ah-meen
(Anaspaz, Buscopan✢,
Cystospaz, Levsin, Levsinex,
Neoquess, Nulev)
Do not confuse with Anaprox.

FIXED-COMBINATION(S)

With phenobarbital, a sedative-hypnotic **(Levsinex with PB, Anaspaz PB)**

▶**CLASSIFICATION**

PHARMACOTHERAPEUTIC:
Anticholinergic. ***CLINICAL:*** Antimuscarinic, antispasmodic

ACTION/*THERAPEUTIC EFFECT*

Inhibits action of acetylcholine at postganglionic (muscarinic) receptor sites, *decreasing secretions (bronchial, salivary, sweat glands, gastric juices). Reduces motility of GI and urinary tract.*

USES

Treatment of GI tract disorders caused by spasm. Adjunct in treatment of peptic ulcer disease, GI hypermotility, infant colic, hypermotility of lower urinary tract.

PRECAUTIONS

CONTRAINDICATIONS: Narrow-angle glaucoma, severe ulcerative colitis, toxic megacolon, obstructive disease of GI tract, paralytic ileus, intestinal atony, bladder neck obstruction due to prostatic hypertrophy, myasthenia gravis in those not treated with neostigmine, tachycardia secondary to cardiac insufficiency or thyrotoxicosis, cardiospasm, unstable cardiovascular status in acute hemorrhage. ***EXTREME CAUTION:*** Autonomic neuropathy, known or suspected GI infections, diarrhea, mild to moderate ulcerative colitis, bronchial asthma. **CAUTIONS:** Hyperthyroidism, hepatic or renal disease, hypertension, tachyarrhythmias, CHF, coronary artery disease, gastric ulcer, esophageal reflux or hiatal hernia associated with reflux esophagitis, infants, elderly, COPD.

INTERACTIONS

DRUG: Antacids, antidiarrheals may decrease absorption. **Anticholinergics** may increase effects. May decrease absorption of **ketoconazole.** May increase severity of GI lesions with **potassium chloride (wax matrix).** **HERBAL:** None known. **FOOD:** None known. **LAB VALUES:** None significant.

AVAILABILITY (Rx)

TABLETS: 0.125 mg, 0.15 mg. **CAPSULES (timed-release):** 0.375 mg. **ORAL SOLUTION:** 0.125 mg/ml. **ELIXIR:** 0.125 mg/5 ml. **INJECTION:** 0.5 mg/ml. **OPHTHALMIC SOLUTION:** 0.25%.

ADMINISTRATION/HANDLING
PO:

• Give without regard to meals. • Tablets may be crushed, chewed. • Extended-release capsule should be swallowed whole.

Parenteral:

• May give undiluted.

INDICATIONS/ROUTES/DOSAGE
GI tract disorders:

IM/SubQ: Adults, elderly, children >12 yrs: 0.25–0.5 mg q4h for 1–4 doses.

PO/SUBLINGUAL: Adults, elderly, children >12 yrs: 0.125–0.25 mg q4h. **Maximum:** 1.5 or 0.375–0.75 mg q12h **(timed-relase capsule).**

Children 2–12 yrs: 0.0625–0.125 mg q4h as needed. **Maximum:** 0.75 mg/day. **Children <2 yrs:** Drops dose q4h (using drop formulation).

Hypermotility of lower urinary tract:

PO/SUBLINGUAL: Adults, elderly: 0.15–0.3 mg 4 times/day or 0.375 mg q12h **(timed-relase capsule).**

Duodenography:

IV: Adults, elderly: 0.25–0.5 mg 10 min prior to procedure.

Preop:

IM: Adults, elderly: 0.5 mg (0.005 mg/kg) 30–60 min prior to induction of anesthesia or administration of preop medications.

SIDE EFFECTS

FREQUENT: Dry mouth (sometimes severe), decreased sweating, constipation. **OCCASIONAL:** Blurred vision, bloated feeling, urinary hesitancy, drowsiness (with high dosage), headache, intolerance to light, loss of taste, nervousness, flushing, insomnia, impotence, mental confusion/excitement (particularly in elderly, children). Parenteral form may produce temporary lightheadedness, local irritation. **RARE:** Dizziness, faintness.

ADVERSE REACTIONS/TOXIC EFFECTS

Overdosage may produce temporary paralysis of ciliary muscle, pupillary dilation, tachycardia, palpitation, hot/dry/flushed skin, absence of bowel sounds, hyperthermia, increased respiratory rate, EKG abnormalities, nausea, vomiting, rash over face/upper trunk, CNS stimulation, psychosis (agitation, restlessness, rambling speech, visual hallucination, paranoid behavior, delusions), followed by depression.

NURSING IMPLICATIONS

BASELINE ASSESSMENT:

Before giving medication, instruct pt to void (reduces risk of urinary retention).

INTERVENTION/EVALUATION:

Monitor daily bowel activity and stool consistency. Palpate bladder for urinary retention. Monitor changes in B/P, temperature. Assess skin turgor, mucous membranes to evaluate hydration status (encourage adequate fluid intake), bowel sounds for peristalsis. Be alert for fever (increased risk of hyperthermia).

PATIENT/FAMILY TEACHING:

Do not become overheated during exercise in hot weather (may result in heat stroke). Avoid hot baths, saunas. Avoid tasks that require alertness, motor skills until response to drug is established. Sugarless gum, sips of tepid water may relieve dry mouth. Do not take antacids or medicine for diarrhea within 1 hr of taking this medication (decreased effectiveness).

ibuprofen

eye-byew-**pro**-fen
(Advil, Motrin, Novoprofen✦, Nuprin, Rufen, Trendar)

FIXED-COMBINATION(S)

With hydrocodone, an opioid analgesic **(Vicoprofen)**

▶**CLASSIFICATION**

PHARMACOTHERAPEUTIC:
Nonsteroidal anti-inflammatory.
CLINICAL: Antirheumatic, analgesic, antipyretic, antidysmenorrheal, vascular headache suppressant (see p. 106C)

ACTION/*THERAPEUTIC EFFECT*

Produces analgesic and anti-inflammatory effect by inhibiting prostaglandin synthesis, *reducing inflammatory response and intensity of pain stimulus reaching sensory nerve endings.* Antipyresis produced by effect on hypothalamus, producing vasodilation, *thereby decreasing elevated body temperature.*

PHARMACOKINETICS

Onset	Peak	Duration
PO (analgesic)		
0.5 hrs	—	4–6 hrs
PO (antirheumatic)		
2 days	1–2 wks	—

Rapidly absorbed from GI tract. Protein binding: >90%. Metabolized in liver. Primarily excreted in urine. Not removed by hemodialysis. Half-life: 2–4 hrs.

USES/*UNLABELED*

Symptomatic treatment of acute/chronic rheumatoid arthritis and osteoarthritis; reduces fever. Relief of mild to moderate pain, primary dysmenorrhea. Temporary relief of minor aches/pain associated with common cold, headache, toothache, muscular aches, backaches, menstrual cramps. *Treatment of psoriatic arthritis, vascular headaches.*

PRECAUTIONS

CONTRAINDICATIONS: Active

peptic ulcer, GI ulceration, chronic inflammation of GI tract, GI bleeding disorders, history of hypersensitivity to aspirin or NSAIDs. **CAUTIONS:** Impaired renal/hepatic function, history of GI tract disease, predisposition to fluid retention.

▷**LIFESPAN CONSIDERATIONS:**
Pregnancy/Lactation: Unknown if drug crosses placenta or is distributed in breast milk. Avoid use during third trimester (may adversely affect fetal cardiovascular system: premature closure of ductus arteriosus). **Pregnancy Category B** (Category D if used in third trimester or near delivery). **Children:** Safety and efficacy not established in those <6 mos of age. **Elderly:** GI bleeding or ulceration more likely to cause serious adverse effects. Age-related renal impairment may increase risk of liver or renal toxicity; reduced dosage recommended.

INTERACTIONS
DRUG: May increase effects of **oral anticoagulants, heparin, thrombolytics.** May decrease effect of **antihypertensives, diuretics. Salicylates, aspirin** may increase risk of GI side effects, bleeding. **Bone marrow depressants** may increase risk of hematologic reactions. May increase concentration, toxicity of **lithium.** May increase **methotrexate** toxicity. **Probenecid** may increase concentration. **HERBAL: Feverfew** effect may be decreased. **Ginkgo biloba** may increase risk of bleeding. **FOOD:** None known. **LAB VALUES:** May prolong bleeding time. May alter blood glucose. May increase BUN, creatinine, potassium, liver function tests. May decrease hemoglobin, hematocrit.

AVAILABILITY (Rx)
TABLETS: 100 mg, 200 mg **(OTC),** 400 mg, 600 mg, 800 mg. **TABLETS (chewable):** 50 mg, 100 mg. **ORAL SUSPENSION:** 100 mg/5 ml **(OTC), ORAL DROPS:** 40 mg/ml.

ADMINISTRATION/HANDLING
PO:
• Do not crush or break enteric-coated form. • Give with food, milk, or antacids if GI distress occurs.

INDICATIONS/ROUTES/DOSAGE
Acute/chronic rheumatoid arthritis, osteoarthritis:
PO: Adults, elderly: 300–800 mg 3–4 times/day. **Maximum:** 3.2 g.

Mild to moderate pain, primary dysmenorrhea:
PO: Adults, elderly: 400 mg q4–6h.

Fever, minor aches/pain:
PO: Adults, elderly: 200–400 mg q4–6h. **Maximum:** 1.2 g/day. **Children:** 5–10 mg/kg/dose q6–8h. **Maximum:** 40 mg/kg/day. **OTC:** 7.5 mg/kg/dose q6–8h. **Maximum:** 30 mg/kg/day.

Juvenile arthritis:
PO: Children: 30–70 mg/kg/day in 3–4 divided doses.

SIDE EFFECTS
OCCASIONAL (3–9%): Nausea (with or without vomiting), dyspepsia (heartburn, indigestion, epigastric pain), dizziness, rash. **RARE** (<3%): Diarrhea/constipation, flatulence, abdominal cramping/pain, itching.

ADVERSE REACTIONS/TOXIC EFFECTS
Acute overdosage may result in metabolic acidosis. Peptic ulcer,

GI bleeding, gastritis, severe hepatic reaction (cholestasis, jaundice) occur rarely. Nephrotoxicity (dysuria, hematuria, proteinuria, nephrotic syndrome) and severe hypersensitivity reaction (particularly those with systemic lupus erythematosus, other collagen diseases) occur rarely.

NURSING IMPLICATIONS

BASELINE ASSESSMENT:

Assess onset, type, location, and duration of pain or inflammation. Inspect appearance of affected joints for immobility, deformities, and skin condition.

INTERVENTION/EVALUATION:

Monitor for evidence of nausea, dyspepsia. Monitor pattern of daily bowel activity and stool consistency. Assess skin for evidence of rash. Evaluate for therapeutic response: relief of pain, stiffness, swelling, increase in joint mobility, reduced joint tenderness, improved grip strength.

PATIENT/FAMILY TEACHING:

Avoid aspirin, alcohol during therapy (increases risk of GI bleeding). If GI upset occurs, take with food, milk, or antacids. Do not crush or chew enteric-coated tablet.

ibutilide fumarate

eye-**byewt**-ih-lied
(Corvert)

▶CLASSIFICATION

CLINICAL: Antiarrhythmic (see p. 14C)

ACTION/*THERAPEUTIC EFFECT*

Prolongs both atrial and ventricular action potential duration and increases atrial and ventricular refractory period. Activates slow, inward current (sodium), produces mild slowing of sinus rate and AV conduction, dose-related prolongation of QT interval. Converts arrhythmias to sinus rhythm.

PHARMACOKINETICS

After IV administration, highly distributed, rapidly cleared. Protein binding: 40%. Primarily excreted in urine as metabolite. Half-life: 2–12 hrs (avg: 6 hrs).

USES/*UNLABELED*

Rapid conversion of atrial fibrillation or flutter of recent onset to sinus rhythm (arrhythmias of longer duration less likely to respond to therapy).

PRECAUTIONS

CONTRAINDICATIONS: None significant. **CAUTIONS:** Abnormal liver function, heart block.

▷**LIFESPAN CONSIDERATIONS:**
Pregnancy/Lactation: Teratogenic, embryocidal in animals. Discourage breast feeding during therapy. **Pregnancy Category C. Children:** Safety and efficacy not established. **Elderly:** No age-related precautions noted.

INTERACTIONS

DRUG: Do not give concurrently with **class Ia (disopyramide, quinidine, procainamide, moricizine)** or **class III (amiodarone, sotalol, bretylium) antiarrhythmics** or within 4 hrs postinfusion of ibutilide. **Phenothiazines, tricyclic and tetracyclic antidepressants, H₁ receptor antagonists** may prolong QT interval. **HERBAL:** None

known. **FOOD:** None known. **LAB VALUES:** None significant.

AVAILABILITY (Rx)

INJECTION: 0.1 mg/ml solution.

ADMINISTRATION/HANDLING

IV 💊

Storage:

• Compatible with D₅W, 0.9% NaCl. Compatible with polyvinyl chloride plastic and polyolefin bag admixtures. • Admixtures with diluent are stable at room temperature for 24 hrs, 48 hrs if refrigerated.

Reconstitution:

• Give undiluted or may dilute in 50 ml diluent.

Rate of administration: • Give infusion over 10 min. • Monitor pt with continuous EKG reading for at least 4 hrs following infusion or until QT interval has returned to baseline.

IV INCOMPATIBILITY ⊘

No information available for Y-site administration.

INDICATIONS/ROUTES/DOSAGE

Atrial arrhythmias:

IV INFUSION: Adults, elderly ≥60 kg (132 lbs): One vial (1 mg) given over 10 min. If arrhythmia does not stop within 10 min after end of initial infusion, a second 10 min infusion may be given 10 min after completion of first infusion. **Adults, elderly <60 kg (132 lbs):** 0.1 ml/kg (0.01 mg/kg) given over 10 min. If arrhythmia does not stop within 10 min after end of initial infusion, a second 10 min infusion may be given 10 min after completion of first infusion.

SIDE EFFECTS

Generally well tolerated. **OCCASIONAL:** Ventricular extrasystoles (5.1%), ventricular tachycardia (4.9%), headache (3.6%), hypotension, postural hypotension (2%). **RARE:** Bundle-branch block, AV block, bradycardia, hypertension.

ADVERSE REACTIONS/TOXIC EFFECTS

Sustained polymorphic ventricular tachycardia, occasionally with QT prolongation (torsades de pointes) occurs rarely. Overdosage results in CNS toxicity (CNS depression, rapid gasping breathing, seizures). May exaggerate expected prolongation of repolarization. May worsen existing arrhythmias or produce new arrhythmias.

NURSING IMPLICATIONS

BASELINE ASSESSMENT:

Those with atrial fibrillation of >2–3 days duration must be treated with anticoagulants generally for at least 2 wks prior to ibutilide therapy. Cardiac monitoring equipment, intracardiac pacing facility, cardioverter/defibrillator, medications for treatment of sustained ventricular tachycardia (VT), including polymorphic VT, must be available during and after administration. Anticipate proarrhythmic events.

INTERVENTION/EVALUATION:

Observe pt with continuous EKG monitoring for at least 4 hrs following infusion or until QT interval has returned to baseline. If any arrhythmic activity is noted, continue EKG monitoring. Monitor for symptoms of electrolyte abnormalities, esp. magnesium and potassium, and overdrive cardiac pacing, electrical cardioversion, or defibrillation.

idarubicin hydrochloride

eye-dah-**roo**-bi-sin
(Idamycin, Idamycin PFS)
Do not confuse with
Adriamycin, doxorubicin.

▶CLASSIFICATION

PHARMACOTHERAPEUTIC:
Anthracycline antibiotic. **CLINICAL:** Antineoplastic (see p. 71C)

ACTION/*THERAPEUTIC EFFECT*

Inhibits nucleic acid synthesis by interacting with the enzyme topoisomerase II (an enzyme promoting DNA strand supercoiling), *producing death of rapidly dividing cells.*

PHARMACOKINETICS

Widely distributed. Protein binding: 97%. Rapidly metabolized in liver to active metabolite. Primarily eliminated via biliary excretion. Not removed by hemodialysis. Half-life: 4–46 hrs; metabolite: 8–92 hrs.

USES

Treatment of acute myeloid leukemia (AML) in adults.

PRECAUTIONS

CONTRAINDICATIONS: None significant. **EXTREME CAUTION:** Preexisting myelosuppression, cardiac disease, impaired hepatic/renal function.
▷**LIFESPAN CONSIDERATIONS:**
Pregnancy/Lactation: If possible, avoid use during pregnancy (may be embryotoxic). Unknown if drug is distributed in breast milk (advise to discontinue nursing before drug initiation). **Pregnancy Category D. Children:** Safety and efficacy not established. **Elderly:** Cardiotoxicity may be more fre-

quent, Caution in those with inadequate bone marrow reserves. Age-related renal impairment may require dosage adjustment.

INTERACTIONS

DRUG: May decrease effect of **antigout medications. Bone marrow depressants** may increase bone marrow depression. **Live virus vaccines** may potentiate virus replication, increase vaccine side effects, decrease pt's antibody response to vaccine. **HERBAL:** None known. **FOOD:** None known. **LAB VALUES:** May increase uric acid, SGOT (AST), SGPT (ALT), alkaline phosphatase, bilirubin. May cause EKG changes.

AVAILABILITY (Rx)

INJECTION: 5 mg, 10 mg, 20 mg.

ADMINISTRATION/HANDLING

Note: Give by free-flowing IV infusion (*never* SubQ or IM). Gloves, gowns, eye goggles recommended during preparation and administration of medication. If powder or solution comes in contact with skin, wash thoroughly. Avoid small veins, swollen or edematous extremities, and areas overlying joints, tendons.

IV

Storage:

• Reconstituted solution is stable for 72 hrs (3 days) at room temperature or 168 hrs (7 days) if refrigerated. • Discard unused solution.

Note: Idamycin PFS does not require reconstitution and is stored refrigerated.

Reconstitution:

• Reconstitute each 10 mg vial with 10 ml 0.9% NaCl (5 ml/5 mg vial) to provide a concentration of 1 mg/ml.

Rate of administration:

• Administer into tubing of freely running IV infusion of D_5W or 0.9% NaCl, preferably via butterfly needle, *slowly* (>10–15 min). • Extravasation produces immediate pain, severe local tissue damage. Terminate infusion immediately. Apply cold compresses for $1/2$ hr immediately, then $1/2$ hr 4 times/day for 3 days. Keep extremity elevated.

IV INCOMPATIBILITIES ⊘

Acyclovir (Zovirax), allopurinol (Aloprim), ampicillin-sulbactam (Unasyn), cefazolin (Ancef, Kefzol), cefepime (Maxipime), ceftazidime (Fortaz), clindamycin (Cleocin), dexamethasone (Decadron), furosemide (Lasix), hydrocortisone (Solu-Cortef), lorazepam (Ativan), meperidine, methotrexate, piperacillin/tazobactam (Zosyn), sodium bicarbonate, teniposide (Vumon), vancomycin (Vancocin), vincristine (Oncovin).

IV COMPATIBILITIES

Diphenhydramine (Benadryl), granisetron (Kytril), magnesium, potassium.

INDICATIONS/ROUTES/DOSAGE

Note: Dosage individualized based on clinical response, tolerance to adverse effects. When used in combination therapy, consult specific protocols for optimum dosage, sequence of drug administration.

Usual dose:

IV: Adults: 12 mg/m^2/day for 3 days (combined with Ara-C). **Children (solid tumor):** 5 mg/m^2 once daily for 3 days. *(Leukemia):* 10–12 mg/m^2 once daily for 3 days.

Dosage in hepatic/renal impairment:

	Dose Reduction
Serum creatinine ≥2	25%
Bilirubin >2.5	50%
Bilirubin >5	Do not give

SIDE EFFECTS

FREQUENT: Nausea, vomiting (82%), complete alopecia (scalp, axillary, pubic hair) (77%), abdominal cramping, diarrhea (73%), mucositis (50%). **OCCASIONAL:** Hyperpigmentation of nailbeds, phalangeal and dermal creases (46%), fever (36%), headache (20%). **RARE:** Conjunctivitis, neuropathy.

ADVERSE REACTIONS/TOXIC EFFECTS

Bone marrow depression manifested as hematologic toxicity (principally leukopenia and, to lesser extent, anemia, thrombocytopenia) generally occurs within 10–15 days, returns to normal levels by third week. Cardiotoxicity noted as either acute, transient abnormal EKG findings and/or cardiomyopathy manifested as CHF may occur.

NURSING IMPLICATIONS

BASELINE ASSESSMENT:

Determine baseline renal and hepatic function, CBC results. Obtain EKG before therapy. Antiemetic before and during therapy may prevent, relieve nausea, vomiting. Inform pt of high potential for alopecia.

INTERVENTION/EVALUATION:

Monitor for hematologic toxicity (fever, sore throat, signs of local infection, easy bruising, or unusual bleeding from any site), symptoms of anemia (excessive tiredness, weakness). Avoid IM injections, rectal temperatures, and other trauma that may precipitate bleeding. Check infusion site frequently for extravasation (causes severe local necrosis). Assess for potentially fatal CHF dyspnea, rales, edema, and life-threatening arrhythmias.

PATIENT/FAMILY TEACHING:

Total body alopecia is frequent but reversible. Assist with ways to cope with hair loss. New hair growth resumes 2–3 mos after last therapy dose and may have different color, texture. Maintain fastidious oral hygiene. Avoid crowds, those with infections. Teach pt and family the early signs of bleeding and infection.

ifosfamide

eye-**fos**-fah-mid
(Ifex)

▶CLASSIFICATION

PHARMACOTHERAPEUTIC:
Alkylating agent. **CLINICAL:**
Antineoplastic (see p. 71C)

ACTION/*THERAPEUTIC EFFECT*

Converted to active metabolite, binds with intracellular structures. Action primarily due to cross-linking strands of DNA, RNA, *inhibiting protein synthesis.*

PHARMACOKINETICS

Metabolized in liver to active metabolite. Crosses blood-brain barrier (limited). Primarily excreted in urine. Removed by hemodialysis. Half-life: 15 hrs.

USES/*UNLABELED*

Third-line chemotherapy of germ cell testicular carcinoma (used in combination with agents that protect against hemorrhagic cystitis). *Treatment of soft tissue sarcoma, Ewing's sarcoma, non-Hodgkin's lymphomas, lung, pancreatic carcinoma.*

PRECAUTIONS

CONTRAINDICATIONS: Severely depressed bone marrow function. ***CAUTIONS:*** Impaired renal, liver function, compromised bone marrow function.
▷***LIFESPAN CONSIDERATIONS:***
Pregnancy/Lactation: If possible, avoid use during pregnancy, esp. first trimester. May cause fetal damage. Drug is distributed in breast milk. Breast feeding not recommended. **Pregnancy Category D. Children:** Not intended for this pt population. **Elderly:** Age-related renal impairment may require dosage adjustment.

INTERACTIONS

DRUG: **Bone marrow depressants** may increase bone marrow depression. **Live virus vaccines** may potentiate virus replication, increase vaccine side effects, decrease pt's antibody response to vaccine. ***HERBAL:*** None known. ***FOOD:*** None known. ***LAB VALUES:*** May increase BUN, creatinine, uric acid, SGOT (AST), SGPT (ALT), LDH, bilirubin.

AVAILABILITY (Rx)

POWDER FOR INJECTION: 1 g, 3 g.

ADMINISTRATION/HANDLING

Note: May be carcinogenic, mutagenic, or teratogenic. Handle with extreme care during preparation/administration.

IV 🔳

Storage:
• Store vial at room temperature. • After reconstitution with Bacteriostatic Water for Injection, solution is stable for 1 wk at room temperature, 3 wks if refrigerated (further diluted solution is stable for 6 wks if refrigerated). • Solution prepared with other diluents should be used within 6 hrs.

Reconstitution:
• Reconstitute 1 g vial with 20 ml Sterile Water for Injection or Bacteriostatic Water for Injection to provide a concentration of 50 mg/ml. Shake to dissolve. • Further dilute with D_5W or 0.9% NaCl to provide concentration of 0.6–20 mg/ml.

Rate of administration:
• Infuse over a minimum of 30 min. • Give with at least 2,000 ml PO or IV fluid (prevents bladder toxicity). • Give with a protectant against hemorrhagic cystitis (e.g., mesna).

IV INCOMPATIBILITIES ⊘

Cefepime (Maxipime), methotrexate.

IV COMPATIBILITIES

Granisetron (Kytril), ondansetron (Zofran).

INDICATIONS/ROUTES/DOSAGE

Note: Dosage individualized based on clinical response, tolerance to adverse effects. When used in combination therapy, consult specific protocols for optimum dosage, sequence of drug administration.

Germ cell testicular carcinoma:

IV: **Adults:** 700–2,000 mg/m^2/day for 5 consecutive days. Repeat q3wks or after recovery from hematologic toxicity. Administer with mesna.

Usual pediatric dosage:

IV: 1,200–1,800 mg/m^2/day for 5 days q21–28days.

SIDE EFFECTS

FREQUENT: Alopecia (83%), nausea, vomiting (58%). **OCCASIONAL** (5–15%): Confusion, somnolence, hallucinations, infection. **RARE** (<5%): Dizziness, seizures, disorientation, fever, malaise, stomatitis (mucosal irritation, glossitis, gingivitis).

ADVERSE REACTIONS/TOXIC EFFECTS

Hemorrhagic cystitis with hematuria, dysuria occurs frequently if a pretective agent (mesna) is not used. Myelosuppression characterized as leukopenia, and, to a lesser extent, thrombocytopenia, occurs frequently. Pulmonary toxicity, hepatotoxicity, nephrotoxicity, cardiotoxicity, CNS toxicity (confusion, hallucinations, somnolence, coma) may require discontinuation of therapy.

NURSING IMPLICATIONS

BASELINE ASSESSMENT:
Obtain urinalysis before each dose. If hematuria occurs (>10 RBCs per field), therapy should be withheld until resolution occurs. Obtain WBC, platelet count, hemoglobin before each dose.

INTERVENTION/EVALUATION:
Monitor hematologic studies,

urinalysis diligently. Assess for fever, sore throat, signs of local infection, easy bruising, unusual bleeding from any site, symptoms of anemia (excessive tiredness, weakness).

PATIENT/FAMILY TEACHING:

Maintain copious daily fluid intake (protects against cystitis). Do not have immunizations without physician's approval (drug lowers body's resistance). Avoid contact with those who have recently received live virus vaccine. Avoid crowds, those with infections. Report unusual bleeding/bruising, fever, chills, sore throat, joint pain, sores in mouth or on lips, yellowing skin/eyes.

imatinib mesylate

ih-**mah**-tin-ib
(Gleevec)

▶CLASSIFICATION

PHARMACOTHERAPEUTIC: Protein-tyrosine kinase inhibitor. **CLINICAL:** Antineoplastic (see p. 71C)

ACTION/*THERAPEUTIC EFFECT*

Inhibits the Bcr-Abl tyrosine kinase, a translocation-created enzyme, created by the Philadelphia chromosome abnormality noted in chronic myeloid leukemia (CML), *inhibiting proliferation and inhibiting tumor growth during the three stages of CML: CML in myeloid blast crisis, CML in accelerated phase, or CML in chronic phase.*

PHARMACOKINETICS

Well absorbed following oral administration. Binds to plasma proteins, particularly albumin. Metabolized in the liver. Eliminated mainly in the feces as metabolites. Half-life: 18 hrs.

USES

Treatment of pts with chronic myeloid leukemia (CML) in blast crisis, accelerated phase, or chronic phase after failure of intereferon-alpha therapy.

PRECAUTIONS

CONTRAINDICATIONS: Known hypersensitivity to imatinib. **CAUTIONS:** Hepatic, renal impairment.

▷**LIFESPAN CONSIDERATIONS: Pregnancy/Lactation:** Has potential for severe teratogenic effects. Avoid breast-feeding. **Pregnancy Category D. Children:** Safety and efficacy not established. **Elderly:** Increased frequency of fluid retention noted.

INTERACTIONS

DRUG: Ketoconazole, itraconazole, erythromycin, clarithromycin increase imatinib plasma concentration. **Dexamethasone, phenytoin, carbamazepine, rifampicin, phenobarbital** decrease imatinib plasma concentration. Increases **simvastatin, triazolobenzodiazepines, dihydropyridine, calcium channel blockers** concentration. May alter **cyclosporine, pimozide** therapeutic effect Reduces **warfarin** effect. **HERBAL: St. John's wort** decreases imatinib concentration. **FOOD:** None known. **LAB VALUES:** May decrease WBC, platelets, potassium. May increase transaminase, bilirubin.

AVAILABILITY (Rx)

CAPSULES: 100 mg.

ADMINISTRATION/HANDLING
PO:

• Give with a meal and a large glass of water.

INDICATIONS/ROUTES/DOSAGE
Chronic myeloid leukemia (CML):
PO: Adults, elderly: 400 mg/day for pts in chronic phase CML; 600 mg/day for pts in accelerated phase or blast crisis. May increase dose 400–600 mg/day in those in chronic phase or 600–800 mg (given as 400 mg twice/day) in pts in accelerated phase or blast crisis in absence of severe drug reaction or severe neutropenia or thrombocytopenia in the following circumstances: Progression of the disease, failure to achieve satisfactory hematologic response after ≥ 3 mo treatment, or loss of previously achieved hematologic response.

SIDE EFFECTS
FREQUENT (24–68%): Nausea, diarrhea, vomiting, headache, fluid retention (periorbital, lower extremities), rash, musculoskeletal pain, muscle cramps, arthralgia. **OCCASIONAL** (10–23%): Abdominal pain, cough, myalgia, fatigue, pyrexia, anorexia, dyspepsia (heartburn, gastric upset), constipation, night sweats, pruritus. **RARE** (<10%): Nasopharyngitis, petechiae, weakness, epistaxis.

ADVERSE REACTIONS/TOXIC EFFECTS
Severe fluid retention (pleural effusion, pericardial effusion, pulmonary edema, ascites), hepatotoxicity occurs rarely. Neutropenia, thrombocytopenia are expected responses to the drug. Respiratory toxicity is manifested as dyspnea, pneumonia.

NURSING IMPLICATIONS

BASELINE ASSESSMENT:
Obtain CBC weekly for first mo, biweekly for second mo, and periodically thereafter. Monitor liver function tests (transaminase, bilirubin, alkaline phosphatase) before treatment begins and monthly thereafter.

INTERVENTION/EVALUATION:
Assess eye area, lower extremities for early evidence of fluid retention. Weigh and monitor for unexpected rapid weight gain. Offer antiemetics to control nausea, vomiting. Monitor stool frequency and consistency. Monitor CBC for evidence of neutropenia, thrombocytopenia; assess liver function tests for hepatotoxicity. Duration of neutropenia and thrombocytopenia ranges from 2 to 4 wks.

PATIENT/FAMILY TEACHING:
Avoid crowds, those with known infection. Avoid contact with anyone who recently received live virus vaccine; do not receive vaccinations. Take with food and a full glass of water.

imiglucerase

im-ih-**gloo**-sir-ace
(Cerezyme)
Do not confuse with Cerebyx.

▶CLASSIFICATION
CLINICAL: Enzyme

ACTION/THERAPEUTIC EFFECT
Analogue of enzyme beta-glucocerebrosidase, which catalyzes hydrolysis of glycolipid gluco-

cerebroside to glucose and ceramide, *minimizing conditions (e.g., anemia, bone disease) associated with Gaucher's disease.*

USES

Enzyme. Secondary hematologic sequelae include severe anemia, thrombocytopenia, progressive hepatosplenomegaly, skeletal complications.

AVAILABILITY (Rx)

POWDER FOR INJECTION: 200 units, 400 units.

ADMINISTRATION/HANDLING

IV 🖼

Storage:
• Refrigerate. • Once reconstituted, stable for 24 hrs if refrigerated.

Reconstitution:
• Reconstitute with 5.1 ml sterile water to provide concentration of 40 units/ml. • Further dilute with 100–200 ml 0.9% NaCl.

Rate of administration:
• Infuse over 1–2 hrs.

IV INCOMPATIBILITY

Do not mix with any other medication.

INDICATIONS/ROUTES/DOSAGE

Gaucher's disease:

IV INFUSION (over 1–2 hrs): **Adults, elderly, children:** Initially, 2.5 units/kg 3 times/wk up to 60 units/kg/wk. **Maintenance:** Progressive reduction in dosage while monitoring pt response.

SIDE EFFECTS

FREQUENT (3%): Headache. ***OCCASIONAL*** (1–<3%): Nausea, abdominal discomfort, dizziness, pruritus, rash, small decrease in B/P or urinary frequency.

imipenem/cilastatin sodium

im-ih-**peh**-nem/sill-as-**tah**-tin (Primaxin)

▶CLASSIFICATION

PHARMACOTHERAPEUTIC: Fixed-combination cabapenem. ***CLINICAL:*** Antibiotic

ACTION/*THERAPEUTIC EFFECT*

Imipenem: Bactericidal. Binds to bacterial membranes, *inhibiting bacterial cell wall synthesis.* **Cilastatin:** Prevents renal metabolism of imipenem.

PHARMACOKINETICS

Readily absorbed after IM administration. Widely distributed. Protein binding: 13–21%. Metabolized in kidney. Primarily excreted in urine. Removed by hemodialysis. Half-life: 1 hr (half-life increased with impaired renal function).

USES

Treatment of respiratory tract, skin/skin structure, gynecologic, bone/joint, intra-abdominal, complicated/uncomplicated urinary tract infections, endocarditis, polymicrobic infections, septicemia; serious nosocomial infections.

PRECAUTIONS

CONTRAINDICATIONS: Hypersensitivity to beta-lactams. ***IM:*** Hypersensitivity to any local anesthetics of amide type; severe shock or heart block (due to use of lidocaine diluent). ***CAUTIONS:*** Hypersensitivity to penicillins, cephalosporins, other allergens; renal dysfunction, CNS disorders, particularly with history of seizures.

▷**LIFESPAN CONSIDERATIONS:**
Pregnancy/Lactation: Crosses placenta; distributed in cord blood, amniotic fluid, breast milk. **Pregnancy Category C. Children:** No precautions in those <12 yrs of age. **Elderly:** Age-related renal function impairment may require dosage adjustment.

INTERACTIONS

DRUG: None significant. **HERBAL:** None known. **FOOD:** None known. **LAB VALUES:** May increase SGOT (AST), SGPT (ALT), alkaline phosphatase, LDH, bilirubin, BUN, creatinine. May decrease hemoglobin, hematocrit.

AVAILABILITY (Rx)

INJECTION FOR IM: 500 mg, 750 mg. **INJECTION FOR IV:** 250 mg, 500 mg.

ADMINISTRATION/HANDLING

IM:

• Prepare with 1% lidocaine without epinephrine; 500 mg vial with 2 ml, 750 mg vial with 3 ml lidocaine HCl. • Administer suspension within 1 hr of preparation. • Do not mix with any other medications. • Inject deep in large muscle; aspirate to decrease risk of injection into a blood vessel.

IV 🔳

Storage:

• Solution appears colorless to yellow; discard if solution turns brown. • IV infusion (piggyback) is stable for 4 hrs at room temperature, 24 hrs if refrigerated. • Discard if precipitate forms.

Reconstitution:

• Dilute each 250 mg or 500 mg vial with 100 ml D_5W; $D_{10}W$, 0.9% NaCl.

Rate of administration:

• Give by intermittent IV infusion (piggyback). Do not give IV push.
• Infuse over 20–30 min (1 g dose >40–60 min). • Observe pt during first 30 min of infusion to observe for possible hypersensitivity reaction.

IV INCOMPATIBILITIES ⊘

Allopurinol (Aloprim), amphotericin B complex (Abelcet, Ambisome, Amphotec), fluconazole (Diflucan).

IV COMPATIBILITIES

Diltiazem (Cardizem), insulin, propofol (Diprivan).

INDICATIONS/ROUTES/DOSAGE

Serious infections:

IV: Adults, elderly: 2–4 g/day in divided doses q6h.

Mild to moderate infections:

IV: Adults, elderly: 1–2 g/day in divided doses q6–8h..

Usual pediatric dosage:

IV: ≥3 mos–12 yrs: 60–100 mg/kg/day in divided doses q6h. **Maximum:** 4 g/day. **1–3 mos:** 100 mg/kg/day in divided doses q6h. **<1 mo:** 20–25 mg/kg/dose q8–24h.

Dosage in renal impairment:

Dose and/or frequency is modified based on creatinine clearance and/or severity of infection.

Creatinine Clearance	Dosage
31–70 ml/min	500 mg q8h
21–30 ml/min	500 mg q12h
0–20 ml/min	250 mg q12h

SIDE EFFECTS

OCCASIONAL (2–3%): Diarrhea, nausea, vomiting. **RARE** (1–2%): Rash.

ADVERSE REACTIONS/TOXIC EFFECTS

Antibiotic-associated colitis, other superinfections may occur. Anaphylactic reactions in those receiving beta-lactams have occurred.

NURSING IMPLICATIONS

BASELINE ASSESSMENT:

Question pt for history of allergies, particularly to beta-lactams, penicillins, cephalosporins. Inquire about history of seizures.

INTERVENTION/EVALUATION:

Evaluate for phlebitis (heat, pain, red streaking over vein), pain at IV injection site. Assess for GI discomfort, nausea, vomiting. Determine pattern of bowel activity and stool consistency. Assess skin for rash. Be alert to tremors and possible seizures.

PATIENT/FAMILY TEACHING:

Do not take any other medication unless approved by physician. Notify physician in event of tremors, seizures, rash, diarrhea, or other new symptom.

imipramine

ih-**mih**-prah-meen
(Api-Imipramine ✦, Janimine, Tofranil, Tofranil-PM)
Do not confuse with desipramine.

▶**CLASSIFICATION**

PHARMACOTHERAPEUTIC: Tricyclic. **CLINICAL:** Antidepressant, antinuritic, antipanic, antineuralgic, antinarcolepsy adjunct, anticataplectic, antibulimic (see p. 35C)

ACTION/*THERAPEUTIC EFFECT*

Blocks reuptake of neurotransmitters (norepinephrine, serotonin) at presynaptic membranes, increasing concentration at postsynaptic receptor sites, *resulting in antidepressant effect*. Anticholinergic effect *controls nocturnal enuresis*.

USES/*UNLABELED*

Treatment of various forms of depression, often in conjunction with psychotherapy. Treatment of nocturnal enuresis in children >6 yrs. *Treatment of panic disorder, neurogenic pain, attention deficit hyperactivity disorder (ADHD), cataplexy associated with narcolepsy.*

PRECAUTIONS

CONTRAINDICATIONS: Acute recovery period following MI, within 14 days of MAO inhibitor ingestion. ***CAUTIONS:*** Prostatic hypertrophy, history of urinary retention or obstruction, glaucoma, diabetes mellitus, history of seizures, hyperthyroidism, cardiac/hepatic/renal disease, schizophrenia, increased intraocular pressure, hiatal hernia.

INTERACTIONS

DRUG: **Alcohol, CNS depressants** may increase CNS, respiratory depression, hypotensive effects. **Antithyroid agents** may increase risk of agranulocytosis. **Phenothiazines** may increase sedative, anticholinergic effects. **Cimetidine** may increase concentration, toxicity. May decrease effects of **clonidine, guanadrel.** May increase cardiac effects with **sympathomimetics.** May increase risk of hypertensive crisis, hyperpyretic, convulsions with **MAO inhibitors.** **Phenytoin** may decrease concentrations. ***HERBAL:*** **Ginkgo biloba**

may decrease seizure threshold. **St. John's wort** may have additive effect. **FOOD:** None known. **LAB VALUES:** May alter EKG readings, glucose. Therapeutic blood serum level: 225–300 ng/ml; toxic blood serum level: >500 ng/ml.

AVAILABILITY (Rx)

TABLETS: 10 mg, 25 mg, 50 mg. **INJECTION:** 25 mg/ml. **CAPSULES:** 75 mg, 100 mg, 125 mg, 150 mg.

ADMINISTRATION/HANDLING
PO:

• Give with food or milk if GI distress occurs. • Do not crush or break film-coated tablets.

IM:

• Parenteral form takes on yellow or reddish hue when exposed to light. Slight discoloration does not affect potency but marked discoloration is associated with potency loss. • Give by IM only if PO administration is not feasible. • Crystals may form with injectable form. Redissolve by immersing ampule in hot water for 1 min. • Give deep IM slowly.

INDICATIONS/ROUTES/DOSAGE
Depression:

PO: Adults: Initially, 75–100 mg daily. Dosage may be gradually increased to 300 mg daily for hospitalized pts, 200 mg for outpts, then reduce dosage to effective maintenance level (50–150 mg daily). **Elderly:** Initially, 10–25 mg/day at bedtime. May increase by 10–25 mg q3–7days. **Range:** 50–150 mg. **Children:** 1.5 mg/kg/day. May increase 1 mg/kg q3–4days. **Maximum:** 5 mg/kg/day.

IM: Adults: Do not exceed 100 mg/day, administered in divided doses.

Childhood enuresis:

PO: Children >6 yrs: Initially, 10–25 mg at bedtime. May increase by 25 mg/day. **Maximum (6–12 yrs):** 50 mg. **(>12 yrs):** 75 mg.

SIDE EFFECTS

FREQUENT: Drowsiness, fatigue, dry mouth, blurred vision, constipation, delayed micturition, postural hypotension, excessive sweating, disturbed concentration, increased appetite, urinary retention. **OCCASIONAL:** GI disturbances (nausea, metallic taste sensation). **RARE:** Paradoxical reaction (agitation, restlessness, nightmares, insomnia), extrapyramidal symptoms (particularly fine hand tremor).

ADVERSE REACTIONS/TOXIC EFFECTS

High dosage may produce cardiovascular effects (severe postural hypotension, dizziness, tachycardia, palpitations, arrhythmias) and seizures. May also result in altered temperature regulation (hyperpyrexia or hypothermia). Abrupt withdrawal from prolonged therapy may produce headache, malaise, nausea, vomiting, vivid dreams.

NURSING IMPLICATIONS

BASELINE ASSESSMENT:

For those on long-term therapy, liver/renal function tests, blood counts should be performed periodically.

INTERVENTION/EVALUATION:

Supervise suicidal risk pt closely during early therapy (as depression lessens, energy level improves, causing increased suicide potential). Assess appearance, behavior, speech pattern, level of interest, mood. Monitor pattern of daily bowel activity and stool consistency. Monitor B/P, pulse for hypotension, arrhythmias. Assess for urinary retention by bladder palpation. Therapeutic blood serum level: 225–300 ng/ml; toxic blood serum level: >500 ng/ml.

PATIENT/FAMILY TEACHING:

Change positions slowly to avoid hypotensive effect. Tolerance to postural hypotension, sedative, and anticholinergic effects usually develops during early therapy. Therapeutic effect may be noted within 2–5 days, maximum effect within 2–3 wks. Dry mouth may be relieved by sugarless gum, sips of tepid water. Do not abruptly discontinue medication. Avoid tasks that require alertness, motor skills until response to drug is established.

immune globulin IV (IGIV)

(Gamimune N, Gammagard, Gammar-IV, Iveegam, Polygam, Sandoglobulin, Venoglobulin-I)
Do not confuse with
Sandimmune, Sandostatin.

▶CLASSIFICATION
CLINICAL: Immune serum

ACTION/*THERAPEUTIC EFFECT*

Increases antibody titer and antigen-antibody reaction, *providing passive immunity against infection. Induces rapid increase in platelet counts. Produces anti-inflammatory effect.*

PHARMACOKINETICS

Evenly distributed between in-travascular and extravascular space. Half-life: 21–23 days.

USES/*UNLABELED*

Treatment of pts with primary immunodeficiency syndromes, idiopathic thrombocytopenia purpura (ITP), Kawasaki disease, prevention of recurrent bacterial infections in pts with hypogammaglobulinemia associated with B-cell chronic lymphocytic leukemia (CLL). Treatment adjuct in bone marrow transplantation. *Prevents acute infections in immunosuppressed pts, controls/prevents infections in infants/children immunosuppressed in association with AIDs or ARC. Prophylaxis/treatment of infections in high-risk, preterm, low birth weight neonates, treatment of chronic inflammatory demyelinating polyneuropathies. Treatment of multiple sclerosis.*

PRECAUTIONS

CONTRAINDICATIONS: History of allergic response to gamma globulin or anti-immunoglobulin A (IgA) antibodies, allergic response to thimerosal, those with isolated immunoglobulin A (IgA) deficiency. IM also contraindicated in those who have severe thrombocytopenia and any coagulation disorder. ***CAUTIONS:*** Prior systemic allergic reactions following administration of human immunoglobulin preparations. Pre-existing renal dysfunction, diabetes; those >65 are at increased risk of acute renal failure.

▷*LIFESPAN CONSIDERATIONS:*
Pregnancy/Lactation: Unknown if drug crosses placenta or is distributed in breast milk. **Pregnancy Category C. Children/Elderly:** No age-related precautions noted.

INTERACTIONS

DRUG: Live virus vaccines may potentiate virus replication, increase vaccine side effects, decrease pt's antibody response to vaccine. **HERBAL:** None known. **FOOD:** None known. **LAB VALUES:** None significant.

AVAILABILITY (Rx)

INJECTION: 5%, 10%. **POWDER FOR INJECTION:** 50 mg/ml, 1 g, 3 g, 6 g, 12 g.

ADMINISTRATION/HANDLING
IV 💊

Storage:

• Refer to individual IV preparations for storage requirements, stability after reconstitution.

Reconstitution:

• Reconstitute only with diluent provided by manufacturer. • Discard partially used or turbid preparations.

Rate of administration:

• Give by infusion only. • After reconstituted, administer via separate tubing. • Avoid mixing with other medication/IV infusion fluids. • Rate of infusion varies with product used. • Monitor vital signs and B/P diligently during and immediately following IV administration (precipitous fall in B/P may produce picture of anaphylactic reaction). Stop infusion immediately. Epinephrine should be readily available.

IV INCOMPATIBILITY ⊘

Do not mix with any other medications.

INDICATIONS/ROUTES/DOSAGE
Primary immunodeficiency syndrome:

IV INFUSION: Adults, elderly, children: 200–400 mg/kg q1mo.

ITP:

IV INFUSION: Adults, elderly, children: 400 mg/kg/day for 2–5 days.

Kawasaki disease:

IV INFUSION: Adults, elderly, children: 2 g/kg as a single dose.

CLL:

IV INFUSION: Adults, elderly, children: 400 mg/kg q3–4wks.

SIDE EFFECTS

FREQUENT: Tachycardia, backache, headache, joint or muscle pain. **OCCASIONAL:** Fatigue, wheezing, rash or pain at injection site, leg cramps, hives, bluish color of lips/nailbeds, lightheadedness.

ADVERSE REACTIONS/TOXIC EFFECTS

Anaphylactic reactions occur rarely but increased incidence when given large IM doses or in those receiving repeated injections of immune globulin. Epinephrine should be readily available. Overdose may produce chest tightness, chills, diaphoresis, dizziness, flushed face, nausea, vomiting, fever, hypotension.

NURSING IMPLICATIONS

BASELINE ASSESSMENT:

Inquire about history of exposure to disease for both pt and family as appropriate. Have epinephrine readily available. Well hydrate pt prior to use.

INTERVENTION/EVALUATION:

Control rate of IV infusion carefully; too rapid infusion increases risk of precipitous fall in B/P and signs of anaphylaxis (facial flushing, chest tightness, chills, fever, nausea, vomiting, diaphoresis). Assess pt closely during infusion, esp. first hour; monitor vital signs continuously. Stop infusion temporarily if above signs noted. For treatment of ITP, monitor platelets.

PATIENT/FAMILY TEACHING:
Explain rationale for therapy. Rapid response, lasts 1–3 mos. Local pain or muscle tenderness may occur at IM injection site.

indapamide

in-**dap**-ah-myd
(Lozide✤, Lozol)
Do not confuse with iodamide, iopamidol.

▶**CLASSIFICATION**

PHARMACOTHERAPEUTIC: Thiazide. **CLINICAL:** Diuretic, antihypertensive (see p. 83C)

ACTION/THERAPEUTIC EFFECT
Diuretic: Blocks reabsorption of water, electrolytes (sodium, potassium) at cortical diluting segment of distal tubule, *promoting renal excretion.* **Antihypertensive:** Reduces plasma, extracellular fluid volume, decreases peripheral vascular resistance (PVR) by direct effect on blood vessels, *reducing B/P.*

PHARMACOKINETICS

Onset	Peak	Duration
PO		
1–2 hrs	<2 hrs	Up to 36 hrs (diuretic)

Completely absorbed from GI tract. Protein binding: 71–79%. Metabolized in liver. Primarily excreted in urine. Not removed by hemodialysis. Half-life: 14–18 hrs.

USES
Treatment of hypertension and edema associated with CHF. May be used alone or with antihypertensive agents.

PRECAUTIONS
CONTRAINDICATIONS: None significant. **CAUTIONS:** History of hypersensitivity to sulfonamides or thiazide diuretics, renal decompensation, anuria. Severe renal disease, impaired hepatic function, diabetes mellitus, elderly/debilitated, thyroid disorders.

▷**LIFESPAN CONSIDERATIONS:**
Pregnancy/Lactation: Crosses placenta; small amount distributed in breast milk; nursing not advised. **Pregnancy Category D. Children:** Safety and efficacy not established. **Elderly:** More sensitive to hypotensive, electrolyte effects. Age-related impaired renal function may require caution.

INTERACTIONS
DRUG: May increase risk of **digoxin** toxicity (due to hypokalemia). May decrease clearance, increase toxicity of **lithium. HERBAL:** None known. **FOOD:** None known. **LAB VALUES:** May increase plasma renin activity. May decrease calcium, protein-bound iodine, potassium, sodium.

AVAILABILITY (Rx)
TABLETS: 1.25 mg, 2.5 mg.

ADMINISTRATION/HANDLING
PO:
• Give with food or milk if GI upset occurs, preferably with breakfast (may prevent nocturia).
• Do not crush or break tablets.

INDICATIONS/ROUTES/DOSAGE
Edema:

PO: Adults: Initially, 2.5 mg/day, may increase to 5 mg/day in 1 wk.

Hypertension:

PO: Adults: Initially, 1.25 mg, may increase to 2.5 mg/day in 4 wks or 5 mg/day after additional 4 wks.

Usual elderly dosage:

PO: Initially 1.25 mg/day or every other day. May increase up to 5 mg/day.

SIDE EFFECTS

FREQUENT (>5%): Fatigue, numbness of extremities, tension, irritability, agitation, headache, dizziness, lightheadedness, insomnia, muscle cramping. ***OCCASIONAL*** (<5%): Tingling of extremities, frequent urination, polyuria, hives, rhinorrhea, flushing, weight loss, orthostatic hypotension, depression, blurred vision, nausea, vomiting, diarrhea/constipation, dry mouth, impotence, rash, pruritus.

ADVERSE REACTIONS/TOXIC EFFECTS

Vigorous diuresis may lead to profound water loss and electrolyte depletion, resulting in hypokalemia, hyponatremia, dehydration. Acute hypotensive episodes may occur. Hyperglycemia may be noted during prolonged therapy. GI upset, pancreatitis, dizziness, paresthesias, headache, blood dyscrasias, pulmonary edema, allergic pneumonitis, dermatologic reactions occur rarely. Overdosage can lead to lethargy, coma without changes in electrolytes or hydration.

NURSING IMPLICATIONS

BASELINE ASSESSMENT:

Check vital signs, esp. B/P for hypotension prior to administration. Assess baseline electrolytes, particularly check for low potassium. Assess edema, skin turgor, mucous membranes for hydration status. Assess muscle strength, mental status. Note skin temperature, moisture. Obtain baseline weight. Initiate I&O.

INTERVENTION/EVALUATION:

Continue to monitor B/P, vital signs, electrolytes, I&O, weight. Note extent of diuresis. Watch for electrolyte disturbances (hypokalemia may result in weakness, tremor, muscle cramps, nausea, vomiting, change in mental status, tachycardia; hyponatremia may result in confusion, thirst, cold/clammy skin).

PATIENT/FAMILY TEACHING:

Expect increased frequency and volume of urination. To reduce hypotensive effect, rise slowly from lying to sitting position and permit legs to dangle momentarily before standing. Eat foods high in potassium such as whole grains (cereals), legumes, meat, bananas, apricots, orange juice, potatoes (white, sweet), raisins.

indinavir

in-**din**-oh-vir
(Crixivan)
Do not confuse with Denavir.

►CLASSIFICATION

PHARMACOTHERAPEUTIC: Protease inhibitor. ***CLINICAL:*** Antiviral (see pp. 58C, 96C)

ACTION/*THERAPEUTIC EFFECT*

Suppresses human immunodeficiency virus (HIV) protease, an

enzyme necessary for splitting viral polyprotein precursors into mature and infectious virus particles. *Resultant effect interrupts HIV replication, forms immature noninfectious viral particles.*

PHARMACOKINETICS

Rapidly absorbed following PO administration. Protein binding: 60%. Metabolized in liver. Primarily excreted in urine. Unknown if removed by hemodialysis. Half-life: 1.8 hrs (half-life increased with impaired liver function).

USES/*UNLABELED*

Treatment of human immunodeficiency virus (HIV) when antiretroviral therapy is warranted. *Prophylaxis following occupational exposure to HIV.*

PRECAUTIONS

CONTRAINDICATIONS: Hypersensitivity to indinavir; nephrolithiasis. ***CAUTIONS:*** Renal, hepatic function impairment.
▷***LIFESPAN CONSIDERATIONS:*** **Pregnancy/Lactation:** Unknown if excreted in breast milk. HIV-infected women not to breast-feed. **Pregnancy Category C. Children:** Safety and efficacy not established. **Elderly:** Information not available.

INTERACTIONS

DRUG: Avoid concurrent administration of indinavir with **triazolam, midazolam** (potential for arrhythmias, prolonged sedation). ***HERBAL:*** **St. John's wort** may decrease concentration, effect. ***FOOD:*** Avoid meals high in fat, calories and protein. ***LAB VALUES:*** May increase bilirubin (occurs in 10% of pts), SGOT (AST), SGPT (ALT).

AVAILABILITY [Rx]

CAPSULES: 200 mg, 333 mg, 400 mg.

ADMINISTRATION/HANDLING

PO:

• Store at room temperature. • Protect from moisture (capsules sensitive to moisture; keep in original bottle). • Best given without food but with water only (optimal absorption) 1 hr before or 2 hrs after a meal but may give with water, skim milk, juice, coffee or tea, or with light meal (e.g., dry toast with jelly, juice and coffee with skim milk and sugar; or cornflakes, skim milk and sugar). • Do not give with meal high in fat, calories, and protein. • If indinavir and didanosine are given concurrently, give at least 1 hr apart on an empty stomach.

INDICATIONS/ROUTES/DOSAGE

HIV infection:

PO: **Adults:** 800 mg (two 400 mg capsules) q8h.

Dosage with hepatic insufficiency:

PO: **Adults:** 600 mg q8h.

SIDE EFFECTS

FREQUENT: Nausea (12%), abdominal pain (9%), headache (6%), diarrhea (5%). ***OCCASIONAL:*** Vomiting, asthenia, fatigue (4%), insomnia, accumulation of fat in waist, abdomen, or back of neck. ***RARE:*** Abnormal taste sensation, heartburn, symptomatic urinary tract disease, transient kidney dysfunction.

ADVERSE REACTIONS/TOXIC EFFECTS

Nephrolithiasis (flank pain with or without hematuria) occurs in 4% of pts.

NURSING IMPLICATIONS

BASELINE ASSESSMENT:

Offer emotional support. Establish baseline lab values. Emphasize need for close monitoring of renal function (urinalysis, serum creatinine) during therapy.

INTERVENTION/EVALUATION:

Encourage adequate hydration. Pt should drink 48 oz (1.5 L) of liquid for each 24 hrs during therapy. Monitor for evidence of nephrolithiasis (flank pain, hematuria) and contact physician if symptoms occur (therapy should be interrupted for 1–3 days). Monitor stool frequency and consistency (watery, loose, soft). Assess for abdominal discomfort, headache.

PATIENT/FAMILY TEACHING:

Advise that indinavir is not cure for HIV, and condition may progress in spite of treatment. If dose is missed, take next dose at regularly scheduled time (do *not* double the dose). Best taken without food but water only (optimal absorption) 1 hr before or 2 hrs after a meal but may take with water, skim milk, juice, coffee or tea, or with light meal.

indomethacin

in-doe-**meth**-ah-sin
(Apo-Indomethacin✤,
Indocid✤, Indocin, Indocin-SR,
Indotec✤, Novomethacin✤)

indomethacin sodium trihydrate

(Indocin IV)

▶CLASSIFICATION

PHARMACOTHERAPEUTIC:
Nonsteroidal anti-inflammatory.
CLINICAL: Anti-inflammatory,
analgesic (see p. 106C)

ACTION/*THERAPEUTIC EFFECT*

Produces analgesic and anti-inflammatory effect by inhibiting prostaglandin synthesis, *reducing inflammatory response and intensity of pain stimulus reaching sensory nerve endings.* **Patent ductus:** Inhibits prostaglandin synthesis, increases sensitivity of premature ductus to dilating effects of prostaglandins, *causing closure of patent ductus arteriosus.*

USES/*UNLABELED*

Treatment of active stages of rheumatoid arthritis, osteoarthritis, ankylosing spondylitis, acute gouty arthritis, acute painful shoulder. Relief of acute bursitis and/or tendinitis of shoulder. For closure of hemodynamically significant patent ductus arteriosus of premature infants weighing 500–1,750 g. *Treatment of psoriatic arthritis, rheumatic complications associated with Paget's disease of bone, fever due to malignancy, vascular headache, pericarditis.*

PRECAUTIONS

CONTRAINDICATIONS: History of allergic reaction to aspirin or other NSAIDs, history of recurrent or active GI lesions. *Suppository:* History of proctitis or recent rectal bleeding. ***CAUTIONS:*** Impaired renal/hepatic function, elderly, volume depletion, CHF, sepsis, epilepsy, parkinsonism, psychiatric disturbances, coagulation defects.

INTERACTIONS

DRUG: May increase effects of **oral**

anticoagulants, heparin, thrombolytics. May decrease effect of **antihypertensives, diuretics.** Do not give concurrently with **triamterene** (may potentiate acute renal failure). **Salicylates, aspirin** may increase risk of GI side effects, bleeding. **Bone marrow depressants** may increase risk of hematologic reactions. May increase concentration, toxicity of **lithium.** May increase **methotrexate** toxicity. **Probenecid** may increase concentration. May increase concentration of **aminoglycosides** in neonates. *HERBAL:* **Feverfew** effect may be decreased. **Ginkgo biloba** may increase risk of bleeding. *FOOD:* None known. *LAB VALUES:* May prolong bleeding time. May alter blood glucose. May increase BUN, creatinine, potassium, liver function tests. May decrease sodium, platelet count.

AVAILABILITY (Rx)

CAPSULES: 25 mg, 50 mg. *CAPSULES (sustained-release):* 75 mg. *ORAL SUSPENSION:* 25 mg/5 ml. *SUPPOSITORY:* 50 mg. *POWDER FOR INJECTION:* 1 mg.

ADMINISTRATION/HANDLING

PO:

• Give after meals or with food or antacids. • Do not crush sustained-release capsules.

Rectal:

• If suppository is too soft, chill for 30 min in refrigerator or run cold water over foil wrapper. • Moisten suppository with cold water before inserting well up into rectum.

Note: IV injection preferred for patent ductus arteriosus in neonate (may give dose PO via NG tube or rectally).

IV 🔲

Storage:

• IV solutions made without preservatives should be used immediately. • Use IV immediately after reconstitution. IV solution appears clear; discard if cloudy or if precipitate forms. • Discard unused portion.

Reconstitution:

• To 1 mg vial, add 1–2 ml preservative-free Sterile Water for Injection or 0.9% NaCl to provide concentration of 1 mg or 0.5 mg/ml, respectively. • Do not further dilute.

Rate of administration:

• Administer over 5–10 sec. • Restrict fluid intake.

IV INCOMPATIBILITIES ⊘

Amino acid injection, calcium gluconate, cimetidine (Tagamet), dobutamine (Dobutrex), dopamine (Intropin), gentamicin (Garamycin), tobramycin (Nebcin).

IV COMPATIBILITIES

Insulin, potassium.

INDICATIONS/ROUTES/DOSAGE

Moderate to severe rheumatoid arthritis, osteoarthritis, ankylosing spondylitis:

PO: **Adults, elderly:** Initially, 25 mg 2–3 times/day. Increase by 25–50 mg/wk up to 150–200 mg/day. **Children:** 1–2 mg/kg/day. **Maximum:** 150–200 mg/day. *EXTENDED-RELEASE:* **Adults, elderly:** Initially, 75 mg/day up to 75 mg two times/day.

Acute gouty arthritis:

PO: **Adults, elderly:** Initially, 100 mg, then 50 mg three times/day.

Acute painful shoulder:

PO: **Adults, elderly:** 75–150 mg/day in 3–4 divided doses.

Usual rectal dosage:

Adults, elderly: 50 mg four times/

day. **Children:** Initially, 1.5–2.5 mg/kg/day, up to 4 mg/kg/day. Do not exceed 150–200 mg/day.

Patent ductus arteriosus:

Note: May give up to 3 doses at 12–24 hr intervals.

IV: Neonates: Initially, 0.2 mg/kg. **>7 days old:** 0.25 mg/kg for 2nd and 3rd doses. **Age 2–7 days:** 0.2 mg/kg for 2nd and 3rd doses. **<48 hrs old:** 0.1 mg/kg for 2nd and 3rd doses.

SIDE EFFECTS

FREQUENT (3–11%): Headache, nausea, vomiting, dyspepsia (heartburn, indigestion, epigastric pain), dizziness. **OCCASIONAL** (<3%): Depression, ringing in ears, increased sweating, drowsiness, constipation, diarrhea. **Patent ductus arteriosus:** Bleeding disturbances. **RARE:** Increased B/P, confusion, hives, itching, rash, blurred vision.

ADVERSE REACTIONS/TOXIC EFFECTS

Ulceration of esophagus, stomach, duodenum, or small intestine, paralytic ileus may occur. In those with impaired renal function, hyperkalemia along with worsening of impairment may occur. May aggravate depression or psychiatric disturbances, epilepsy, parkinsonism. Nephrotoxicity (dysuria, hematuria, proteinuria, nephrotic syndrome) occurs rarely. **Patent ductus arteriosus:** Acidosis, apnea, bradycardia, alkalosis occur rarely.

NURSING IMPLICATIONS

BASELINE ASSESSMENT:

May mask signs of infection. Assess onset, type, location, and duration of pain, fever, or inflammation. Inspect appearance of affected joints for immobility, deformities, and skin condition.

INTERVENTION/EVALUATION:

Monitor for evidence of nausea, dyspepsia. Assist with ambulation if dizziness occurs. Evaluate for therapeutic response: relief of pain, stiffness, swelling, increase in joint mobility, reduced joint tenderness, improved grip strength.

PATIENT/FAMILY TEACHING:

Avoid aspirin, alcohol during therapy (increases risk of GI bleeding). If GI upset occurs, take with food, milk. Avoid tasks that require alertness, motor skills until response to drug is established. Swallow capsule whole; do not crush or chew.

infliximab

in-**flicks**-ih-mab
(Remicade)

▶CLASSIFICATION

PHARMACOTHERAPEUTIC: Monoclonal antibody. **CLINICAL:** Gastrointestinal anti-inflammatory

ACTION/THERAPEUTIC EFFECT

Binds to soluble and transmembrane cytokines, inhibiting receptor binding and functional activity, *reducing infiltration of inflammatory cells, decreasing inflamed areas of the intestine.*

PHARMACOKINETICS

Absorbed into GI tissue; primarily distributed in the vascular compartment. Half-life: 9.5 days.

USES

Treatment of moderate-to-severe Crohn's disease, treatment of those with fistulizing Crohn's disease for the reduction in number of draining enterocutaneous fistula(s). Treatment of rheumatoid arthritis (with methotrexate).

PRECAUTIONS

CONTRAINDICATIONS: Hypersensitivity to murine. ***CAUTIONS:*** Elderly, those on immunosuppressive therapy, CHF. Increases risk of tuberculosis.

▷***LIFESPAN CONSIDERATIONS:*** **Pregnancy/Lactation:** Unknown if distributed in breast milk. **Pregnancy Category C. Children:** Safety and efficacy not established. **Elderly:** Use cautiously due to a higher rate of infection.

INTERACTIONS

DRUG: None significant. ***HERBAL:*** None known. ***FOOD:*** None known. ***LAB VALUES:*** None significant.

AVAILABILITY (Rx)

POWDER FOR INJECTION: 100 mg.

ADMINISTRATION/HANDLING

IV 🔟

Storage:

• Store at room temperature.

Reconstitution:

• Reconstitute each vial with 10 ml Sterile Water for Injection, using 21 gauge or smaller needle. Direct the stream of sterile water to the glass wall of the vial. • Swirl the vial gently to dissolve the contents. Do not shake. • Allow the solution to stand for 5 min. • Because infliximab is a protein, the solution may develop a few translucent particles; do not use if particles are opaque or foreign particles are present. • Solution should appear colorless to light yellow and opalescent; do not use if discolored. • Withdraw a volume of 0.9% NaCl from a 250 ml bag to equal the volume of reconstituted solution to be injected into the 250 ml bag (approximately 10 ml). Total dose to be infused should equal 250 ml. • Slowly add the reconstituted infliximab solution to the 250 ml infusion bag. Gently mix. Infusion concentration should range between 0.4 and 4 mg/ml. • Begin infusion within 3 hrs after reconstitution.

Rate of administration:

• Administer IV infusion >2 hrs, using set with a low-protein-binding filter.

IV INCOMPATIBILITY 🚫

Do not infuse infliximab concurrently in the same IV line with other agents.

INDICATIONS/ROUTES/DOSAGE

Moderate-to-severe Crohn's disease:

IV INFUSION: Adults, elderly: 5 mg/kg as a single IV infusion.

Fistulizing Crohn's disease:

IV INFUSION: Adults, elderly: Initially, 5 mg/kg followed with additional 5 mg/kg doses at 2 and 6 wks after the first infusion.

Rheumatoid arthritis:

IV INFUSION: Adults, elderly: 3 mg/kg; follow with additional doses at 2 and 6 wks after the first infusion: Then q8wks thereafter.

SIDE EFFECTS

FREQUENT (10–22%): Headache, nausea, fatigue, fever. ***OCCASIONAL*** (5–9%): Fever/chills during infusion, pharyngitis, vomiting, pain, dizziness, bronchitis, rash, rhinitis, coughing, pruritus, sinusitis, myalgia, back pain. ***RARE*** (1–4%): Hypo/

hypertension, paresthesia, anxiety, depression, insomnia, diarrhea, urinary tract infection.

ADVERSE REACTIONS/TOXIC EFFECTS

Potential for hypersensitivity reaction, lupuslike syndrome.

NURSING IMPLICATIONS

BASELINE ASSESSMENT:

Determine pattern of bowel activity. Check baseline hydration status: skin turgor, mucous membranes for dryness, urinary status.

INTERVENTION/EVALUATION:

Monitor stool frequency and consistency (watery, loose, soft, semisolid, solid). Assess bowel sounds for peristaltic activity. Encourage adequate fluid intake.

insulin

in-sull-in

Rapid acting:
INSULIN LISPRO:
(Humalog)

INSULIN ASPART:
(Novolog)

REGULAR INSULIN:
(Regular Iletin II, Humulin R, Novolin R, Velosulin BR)

Intermediate acting:
NPH:
(Pork NPH Iletin II, Humulin N, Novolin N)

LENTE:
(Lente Helin II, Humulin L, Novolin L)

NPH/regular mixture (70%/30%):
HUMULIN 70/30, NOVOLIN 70/30
NPH/regular mixture (50%/50%):
HUMULIN 50/50

NPH/Lispro mixture (75%/25%):
HUMALOG MIX 75/25

Long acting:
ULTRALENTE:
(Humulin U Ultralente)

INSULIN GLARGINE:
(Lantus)

▶CLASSIFICATION

PHARMACOTHERAPEUTIC:
Exogenous insulin. ***CLINICAL:***
Antidiabetic (see p. 38C)

ACTION/*THERAPEUTIC EFFECT*

Facilitates passage of glucose, K, Mg across cellular membranes of skeletal and cardiac muscle, adipose tissue; controls storage and metabolism of carbohydrates, protein, fats. Promotes conversion of glucose to glycogen in liver.

PHARMACOKINETICS

	Onset (hrs)	Peak (hrs)	Duration (hrs)
Lispro	1/4	1/2–1½	4–5
Insulin aspart	1/6	1–3	3–5
Regular	1/2–1	2–4	5–7
NPH	1–2	6–14	24+
Lente	1–3	6–14	24+
Ultralente	6	18–24	36+
Insulin glargine	—	—	24

USES

Treatment of insulin-dependent type I diabetes mellitus; noninsulin-dependent type II diabetes mellitus when diet/weight control therapy has failed to maintain satisfactory blood glucose levels or in event of pregnancy, surgery, trauma, infection, fever, severe renal, hepatic, or endocrine dysfunction. Regular insulin used in emergency treatment of ketoacidosis, to promote passage of glucose across cell membrane in hyperalimentation, to facilitate intracellular shift of K+ in hyperkalemia.

PRECAUTIONS

CONTRAINDICATIONS: Hypersensitivity or insulin resistance may require change of type or species source of insulin.

▷*LIFESPAN CONSIDERATIONS:* **Pregnancy/Lactation:** Insulin is drug of choice for diabetes in pregnancy; close medical supervision is needed. Following delivery, insulin needs may drop for 24–72 hrs, then rise to prepregnancy levels. Not secreted in breast milk; lactation may decrease insulin requirements. **Pregnancy Category B. Children:** No age-related precautions noted. **Elderly:** Decreased vision, shakiness may lead to inaccurate dosage.

INTERACTIONS

DRUG: **Glucocorticoids, thiazide diuretics** may increase blood glucose. **Alcohol** may increase insulin effect. **Beta-adrenergic blockers** may increase risk of hypo/hyperglycemia, mask signs of hypoglycemia, prolong period of hypoglycemia. ***HERBAL:*** None known. ***FOOD:*** None known. ***LAB VALUES:*** May decrease potassium, magnesium, phosphate concentrations.

AVAILABILITY (OTC)

REGULAR, NPH, 70/30, 50/50, LENTE, ULTRALENTE: all 100 units/ml.

ADMINISTRATION/HANDLING

SubQ:

• Store currently used insulin at room temperature (avoid extreme temperatures, direct sunlight). Store extra vials in refrigerator. • Discard unused vials if not used for several wks. No insulin should have precipitate or discoloration. • Give SubQ only. (Regular insulin is the *only* insulin that may be given IV, IM for ketoacidosis or other specific situations.) • Do not give cold insulin; warm to room temperature. • Rotate vial gently between hands; do not shake. Regular insulin should be clear; no insulin should have precipitate or discoloration. • Usually administered approximately 30 min before a meal (Insulin lispro is given up to 15 min before meals). Check blood glucose concentration before administration; dosage highly individualized. • When insulin is mixed, regular insulin is always drawn up first. Mixtures must be administered at once (binding can occur within 5 min). Humalog may be mixed with Humulin N, Humulin L. • SubQ injections may be given in thigh, abdomen, upper arm, buttocks, or upper back if there is adequate adipose tissue. • Rotation of injection sites is essential; maintain careful record. • For home situations, prefilled syringes are stable for 1 wk under refrigeration (this includes mixtures once they have stabilized, e.g., 15 min for NPH/Regular, 24 hrs for Lente/Regular). Prefilled syringes should be stored in vertical or oblique position to avoid plugging; plunger should be pulled back slightly and the syringe rocked to remix the solution before injection.

IV (Regular):

• Use only if solution is clear. • May give undiluted.

IV INCOMPATIBILITIES ⊘

Digoxin (Lanoxin), diltiazem (Cardizem), dopamine (Intropin), nafcillin (Nafcil).

IV COMPATIBILITIES

Amiodarone (Cordarone), ampicillin/sulbactam (Unasyn), cefazolin (Ancef), dobutamine (Dobutrex), famotidine (Pepcid), heparin, magnesium, midazolam (Versed), milrinone (Primacor), potassium, propofol (Diprivan), vancomycin (Vancocin).

INDICATIONS/ROUTES/DOSAGE

Dosage for insulin is individualized/monitored.

Usual dosage guidelines:

Note: Adjust dosage to achieve premeal and bedtime glucose level of 80–140 mg/dl (children <5 yrs: 100–200 mg/dl).

SubQ: **Adults, elderly, children:** 0.5–1 unit/kg/day. **Adolescents (during growth spurt):** 0.8–1.2 units/kg/day.

SIDE EFFECTS

OCCASIONAL: Local redness, swelling, itching (due to improper injection technique or allergy to cleansing solution or insulin). ***INFREQUENT:*** Somogyi effect (rebound hyperglycemia) with chronically excessive insulin doses. Systemic allergic reaction (rash, angioedema, anaphylaxis), lipodystrophy (depression at injection site due to breakdown of adipose tissue), lipohypertrophy (accumulation of SubQ tissue at injection site due to lack of adequate site rotation). ***RARE:*** Insulin resistance.

ADVERSE REACTIONS/TOXIC EFFECTS

Severe hypoglycemia (due to hyperinsulinism) may occur in overdose of insulin, decrease or delay of food intake, excessive exercise, or those with brittle diabetes. Diabetic ketoacidosis may result from stress, illness, omission of insulin dose, or long-term poor insulin control.

NURSING IMPLICATIONS

BASELINE ASSESSMENT:

Check blood glucose level. Discuss lifestyle to determine extent of learning, emotional needs.

INTERVENTION/EVALUATION:

Assess for hypoglycemia (refer to pharmacokinetics table for peak times/duration): cool wet skin, tremors, dizziness, headache, anxiety, tachycardia, numbness in mouth, hunger, diplopia. Check sleeping pt for restlessness or diaphoresis. Check for hyperglycemia: polyuria (excessive urine output), polyphagia (excessive food intake), polydipsia (excessive thirst), nausea and vomiting, dim vision, fatigue, deep rapid breathing. Be alert to conditions altering glucose requirements: fever, increased activity or stress, surgical procedure.

PATIENT/FAMILY TEACHING:

Prescribed diet is essential part of treatment; do not skip or delay meals. Carry candy, sugar packets, other sugar supplements for immediate response to hypoglycemia. Wear/carry medical alert identification. Check with physician when insulin demands are altered, e.g., fever, infection, trauma, stress, heavy physical activity. Do not take other medication without consulting physician. Weight control, exercise, hygiene (including foot care), and not smoking are integral part of therapy. Protect skin, limit sun exposure. Inform dentist, physician, or surgeon of medication before any treatment is given.

interferon alfa-2a

inn-ter-**fear**-on
(Roferon-A)
Do not confuse with interferon alfa-2b.

▶CLASSIFICATION

PHARMACOTHERAPEUTIC: Biologic response modifier. **CLINICAL:** Antineoplastic (see p. 71C).

ACTION/*THERAPEUTIC EFFECT*

Inhibits viral replication in virus-infected cells, *suppressing cell proliferation, increasing phagocytic action of macrophages; augments specific lymphocytic cell toxicity.*

PHARMACOKINETICS

Well absorbed after IM, SubQ administration. Undergoes proteolytic degradation during reabsorption in kidney. Half-life: *IM* 6–8 hrs; *IV* 3.7–8.5 hrs.

USES/*UNLABELED*

Treatment of hairy cell leukemia, AIDS-related Kaposi's sarcoma, chronic myelogenous leukemia (CML), chronic hepatitis C. *Treatment of active, chronic hepatitis; bladder, renal carcinoma, non-Hodgkin's lymphoma, malignant melanoma, multiple myeloma, mycosis fungoides.*

PRECAUTIONS

CONTRAINDICATIONS: None

significant. **CAUTIONS:** Renal, hepatic impairment, seizure disorders, compromised CNS function, cardiac disease, history of cardiac abnormalities, myelosuppression.

▷*LIFESPAN CONSIDERATIONS:*
Pregnancy/Lactation: If possible, avoid use during pregnancy. Breast feeding not recommended. **Pregnancy Category C. Children:** Safety and efficacy not established. **Elderly:** Neurotoxicity, cardiotoxicity may occur more frequently. Age-related renal impairment may require caution.

INTERACTIONS

DRUG: Bone marrow depressants may have additive effect. **HERBAL:** None known. **FOOD:** None known. **LAB VALUES:** May increase SGOT (AST), SGPT (ALT), alkaline phosphatase, LDH. May decrease hemoglobin, hematocrit, leukocyte, platelet counts.

AVAILABILITY (Rx)

INJECTION: 3 million units/ml, 6 million units/ml, 9 million units/ml, 36 million units/ml. **POWDER FOR INJECTION:** 6 million units/ml (18 million units vial).

ADMINISTRATION/HANDLING
SubQ/IM:

Note: SubQ preferred for thrombocytopenic pts, those at risk for bleeding.

• Refrigerate. • Do not shake vial. • Reconstituted solution is stable for 30 days if refrigerated. Solution appears colorless. Do not use if precipitate or discoloration occurs. • Reconstitute 18 million unit vial with 3 ml diluent (provided by manufacturer) to provide concentration of 6 million units/ml (3 million units/0.5 ml).

INDICATIONS/ROUTES/DOSAGE

Note: Dosage individualized based on clinical response, tolerance to adverse effects. When used in combination therapy, consult specific protocols for optimum dosage, sequence of drug administration. If severe adverse reactions occur, modify dose or temporarily discontinue medication.

Hairy cell leukemia:

SUBQ/IM: **Adults:** Initially, 3 million units/day for 16–24 wks. **Maintenance:** 3 million units 3 times/wk. Do not use 36 million unit vial.

CML:

SUBQ/IM: **Adults:** 9 million units daily.

AIDS-related Kaposi's sarcoma:

SUBQ/IM: **Adults:** Initially, 36 million units/day for 10–12 wks (may give 3 million units on day 1; 9 million units on day 2; 18 million units on day 3; then begin 36 million units/day for remainder of 10–12 wks). **Maintenance:** 36 million units/day 3 times/wk.

Chronic hepatitis C:

SUBQ/IM: **Adults:** Initially, 6 million units once daily for 3 wks, then 3 million units 3 times/wk for 6 mos.

SIDE EFFECTS

FREQUENT (>20%): Flulike symptoms (fever, fatigue, headache, aches, pains, anorexia, chills), nausea, vomiting, coughing, dyspnea, hypotension, edema, chest pain, dizziness, diarrhea, weight loss, taste change, abdominal discomfort, confusion, paresthesia, depression, visual and sleep disturbances, sweating, lethargy. *OCCASIONAL* (5–20%): Partial alopecia, rash, dry throat/skin, pruritus, flatulence, constipation, hypertension, palpitations, sinusitis. *RARE* (<5%): Hot flashes, hypermotility, Raynaud's syndrome, bronchospasm, earache, ecchymosis.

ADVERSE REACTIONS/TOXIC EFFECTS

Arrhythmias, stroke, transient ischemic attacks, CHF, pulmonary edema, myocardial infarction occur rarely.

NURSING IMPLICATIONS

BASELINE ASSESSMENT:
CBC and platelet counts, blood chemistries, urinalysis, renal and liver function tests should be performed prior to initial therapy and routinely thereafter.

INTERVENTION/EVALUATION:
Offer emotional support. Monitor all levels of clinical function (numerous side effects). Encourage ample fluid intake, particularly during early therapy.

PATIENT/FAMILY TEACHING:
Clinical response may take 1–3 mos. Flulike symptoms tend to diminish with continued therapy. Contact physician if nausea/vomiting continues at home. Do not change brands without consulting physician. Avoid alcohol. Use caution driving, performing tasks requiring mental alertness.

interferon alfa-2b

inn-ter-**fear**-on
(Intron-A)
Do not confuse with interferon alfa-2a.

FIXED-COMBINATION(S)

With ribavirin, an antiviral **(Rebetron)**

▶CLASSIFICATION

PHARMACOTHERAPEUTIC:
Biologic response modifier.
CLINICAL: Antineoplastic (see p. 71C)

ACTION/*THERAPEUTIC EFFECT*

Inhibits viral replication in virus-infected cells, suppresses cell proliferation, *increases phagocytic action of macrophages, augments specific cytotoxicity of lymphocytes.*

PHARMACOKINETICS

Well absorbed after IM, SubQ administration. Undergoes proteolytic degradation during reabsorption in kidney. Half-life: 2–3 hrs.

USES/*UNLABELED*

Treatment of hairy cell leukemia, condylomata acuminata (genital, venereal warts), AIDS-related Kaposi's sarcoma, chronic hepatitis non-A, non-B/C, chronic hepatitis B (including children ≥1 yr), non-Hodgkin's lymphoma. *Treatment of bladder, cervical, renal carcinoma, chronic myelocytic leukemia, laryngeal papillomatosis, multiple myeloma, mycosis fungoides.*

PRECAUTIONS

CONTRAINDICATIONS: None significant. **CAUTIONS:** Renal, hepatic impairment, seizure disorders, compromised CNS function, cardiac diseases, history of cardiac abnormalities, myelosuppression.

▷*LIFESPAN CONSIDERATIONS:*
Pregnancy/Lactation: If possible, avoid use during pregnancy. Breast feeding not recommended. **Pregnancy Category C. Children:** Safety and efficacy not es-

tablished. **Elderly:** Neurotoxicity, cardiotoxicity may occur more frequently. Age-related renal impairment may require caution.

INTERACTIONS

DRUG: Bone marrow depressants may have additive effect. **HERBAL:** None known. **FOOD:** None known. **LAB VALUES:** May increase SGOT (AST), SGPT (ALT), alkaline phosphatase, LDH, prothrombin time, partial thromboplastin time. May decrease hemoglobin, hematocrit, leukocyte, platelet counts.

AVAILABILITY (Rx)

INJECTION (solution): 5 million units/ml. **POWDER FOR INJECTION:** 3 million units, 5 million units, 10 million units, 18 million units, 25 million units, 50 million units.

ADMINISTRATION/HANDLING

SubQ/IM:

• Do not give IM if platelets <50,000/m^3; give SubQ. • For hairy cell leukemia, reconstitute each 3 million IU vial with 1 ml Bacteriostatic Water for Injection to provide concentration of 3 million IU/ml (1 ml to 5 million IU vial; 2 ml to 10 million IU vial; 5 ml to 25 million IU vial provides concentration of 5 million IU/ml). • For condylomata acuminata, reconstitute each 10 million IU vial with 1 ml Bacteriostatic Water for Injection to provide concentration of 10 million IU/ml. • For AIDS-related Kaposi's sarcoma, reconstitute 50 million IU vial with 1 ml Bacteriostatic Water for Injection to provide concentration of 50 million IU/ml. • Agitate vial gently, withdraw with sterile syringe.

IV ▥

Storage:

• Refrigerate unopened vials (stable for 7 days at room temperature).

Reconstitution:

• Prepare immediately before use.
• Reconstitute with diluent provided by manufacturer. • Withdraw desired dose and further dilute with 100 ml 0.9% NaCl to provide final concentration at least 10 million IU/100 ml.

Rate of administration:

• Administer over 20 min.

IV INCOMPATIBILITY ⊘

No information available. Do not mix with other medications via Y-site administration.

INDICATIONS/ROUTES/DOSAGE

Note: Dosage individualized based on clinical response, tolerance to adverse effects. When used in combination therapy, consult specific protocols for optimum dosage, sequence of drug administration.

Hairy cell leukemia:

IM/SubQ: **Adults:** 2 million IU/m² 3 times/wk. If severe adverse reactions occur, modify dose or temporarily discontinue.

Condylomata acuminata:

INTRALESIONAL: **Adults:** 1 million IU/lesion 3 times/wk for 3 wks. Use only 10 million IU vial, reconstitute with no more than 1 ml diluent. Use TB syringe with 25 or 26 gauge needle. Give in evening with acetaminophen (alleviates side effects).

AIDS-related Kaposi's sarcoma:

IM/SubQ: **Adults:** 30 million IU/m² 3 times/wk. Use only 50 million IU vials. If severe adverse reactions occur, modify dose or temporarily discontinue.

Chronic hepatitis non-A, non-B/C:

IM/SubQ: **Adults:** 3 million IU 3 times/wk for up to 6 mos (for up to 18–24 mos for chronic hepatitis C).

Chronic hepatitis B:

IM/SubQ: **Adults:** 30–35 million IU/wk (5 million IU/day or 10 million IU 3 times/wk).

Malignant melanoma:

IV: **Adults:** Initially, 20 million units 5 times/wk for 4 wks. **Maintenance:** 10 million units IM/SubQ for 48 wks.

SIDE EFFECTS

Note: Dose-related effects. *FREQUENT:* Flulike symptoms (fever, fatigue, headache, aches, pains, anorexia, chills), rash (hairy cell leukemia, Kaposi's sarcoma only). *Kaposi's sarcoma:* All previously mentioned side effects plus depression, dyspepsia, dry mouth/thirst, alopecia, rigors. *OCCASIONAL:* Dizziness, pruritus, dry skin, dermatitis, alteration in taste. *RARE:* Confusion, leg cramps, back pain, gingivitis, flushing, tremor, nervousness, eye pain.

ADVERSE REACTIONS/TOXIC EFFECTS

Hypersensitivity reaction occurs rarely. Severe adverse reactions of flulike symptoms appear dose related.

NURSING IMPLICATIONS

BASELINE ASSESSMENT:

CBC, platelet counts, blood chemistries, urinalysis, renal and liver function tests should be performed prior to initial therapy and routinely thereafter.

INTERVENTION/EVALUATION:

Offer emotional support. Monitor all levels of clinical function (numerous side effects). Encourage ample fluid intake, particularly during early therapy.

PATIENT/FAMILY TEACHING:

Clinical response occurs in 1–3 mos. Flulike symptoms tend to diminish with continued therapy. Some symptoms may be alleviated or minimized by bedtime doses. Do not have immunizations without physician's approval (drug lowers body's resistance). Avoid contact with those who have recently received live virus vaccine.

interferon alfacon-1

inn-ter-**fear**-on
(Infergen)

▶CLASSIFICATION

PHARMACOTHERAPEUTIC:
Biologic response modifier.
CLINICAL: Antiviral

ACTION/*THERAPEUTIC EFFECT*

Stimulates immune system, *inhibiting hepatitis C virus.*

USES

Treatment of chronic hepatitis C viral (HCV) infections in pts with compensated liver disease who have anti-HCV serum antibodies and/or presence of HCV RNA.

AVAILABILITY (Rx)

INJECTION: 15 mcg vials, 9 mcg vials

INDICATIONS/ROUTES/DOSAGE

Hepatits C:

SubQ: **Adults:** 9 mcg 3 times/wk for 24 wks. May increase to 15 mcg in pts tolerating 9 mcg dose and not responding adequately. **Note:** At least 48 hrs should elapse between doses.

SIDE EFFECTS

FREQUENT (>50%): Headache, fatigue, fever, depression.

interferon alfa-n3

inn-ter-**fear**-on
(Alferon N)

▶CLASSIFICATION

PHARMACOTHERAPEUTIC:
Biologic response modifier.
CLINICAL: Antineoplastic

ACTION/*THERAPEUTIC EFFECT*

Inhibits viral replication in virus-infected cells, *suppresses cell proliferation, increases phagocytic action of macrophages, augments specific cytotoxicity of lymphocytes.*

USES/*UNLABELED*

Treatment of refractory or recurring condylomata acuminata (genital, venereal warts). Treatment of active chronic hepatitis, *bladder carcinoma, chronic myelocytic leukemia, laryngeal papillomatosis, non-Hodgkin's lymphoma, malignant melanoma, multiple myeloma, mycosis fungoides.*

PRECAUTIONS

CONTRAINDICATIONS: Previous history of anaphylactic reaction to mouse immunoglobulin (IgG), egg protein, or neomycin. ***CAUTIONS:*** Unstable angina, uncontrolled CHF, severe pulmonary disease, diabetes mellitus with ketoacidosis, thrombophlebitis, pulmonary embolism, hemophilia, severe myelosuppression, seizure disorders.

INTERACTIONS

DRUG: **Bone marrow depressants** may have additive effect. ***HERBAL:*** None known. ***FOOD:*** None known. ***LAB VALUES:*** May increase SGOT (AST), SGPT (ALT), alkaline phosphatase, LDH. May decrease hemoglobin, hematocrit, leukocyte, platelet counts.

AVAILABILITY (Rx)

INJECTION: 5 million units.

ADMINISTRATION/HANDLING

Intralesional:

• Refrigerate vial. Do not freeze or shake. • Inject into base of each wart with 30 gauge needle.

INDICATIONS/ROUTES/DOSAGE

Condylomata acuminata:

INTRALESIONAL: **Adults >18 yrs:** 0.05 ml (250,000 IU) per wart 2 times/wk up to 8 wks. **Maximum dose/treatment session:** 0.5 ml (2.5 million IU). Do not repeat for 3 mos after initial 8 wks unless warts enlarge or new warts appear.

SIDE EFFECTS

FREQUENT: Flulike symptoms (fever, fatigue, headache, aches, pains, anorexia, chills). ***OCCASIONAL:*** Dizziness, pruritus, dry skin, dermatitis, alteration in taste.

RARE: Confusion, leg cramps, back pain, gingivitis, flushing, tremor, nervousness, eye pain.

ADVERSE REACTIONS/TOXIC EFFECTS

Hypersensitivity reaction occurs rarely. Severe adverse reactions of flulike symptoms appear dose related.

NURSING IMPLICATIONS

INTERVENTION/EVALUATION:

Monitor all levels of clinical function (numerous side effects). Encourage ample fluid intake, particularly during early therapy.

PATIENT/FAMILY TEACHING:

Flulike symptoms tend to diminish with continued therapy. Some symptoms may be alleviated or minimized by bedtime doses.

interferon beta-1a

inn-ter-**fear**-on
(Avonex, Refib ♣)
Do not confuse with Avelox, interferon beta-1b.

▶CLASSIFICATION

PHARMACOTHERAPEUTIC: Biologic response modifier. ***CLINICAL:*** Multiple sclerosis agent

ACTION/*THERAPEUTIC EFFECT*

Interacts with specific cell receptors found on surface of human cells. *Possesses antiviral and immunoregulatory activities.*

PHARMACOKINETICS

Following IM administration, peak serum levels attained in 3–15 hrs. Biological markers increase within

12 hrs and remain elevated for 4 days. Half-life: 10 hrs (IM).

USES/*UNLABELED*

Treatment of relapsing multiple sclerosis to slow progression of physical disability, decrease frequency of clinical exacerbations. *Treatment of AIDS, AIDS-related Kaposi's sarcoma, renal cell carcinoma, malignant melanoma, acute non-A, non-B hepatitis.*

PRECAUTIONS

CONTRAINDICATIONS: Hypersensitivity to interferon, albumin. ***CAUTIONS:*** Chronic progressive multiple sclerosis, children <18 yrs.

▷*LIFESPAN CONSIDERATIONS:* **Pregnancy/Lactation:** Interferon beta-1a has abortifacient potential. Unknown distributed in breast milk. **Pregnancy Category C. Children:** Safety and efficacy not established. **Elderly:** No information available.

INTERACTIONS

DRUG: None significant. ***HERBAL:*** None known. ***FOOD:*** None known. ***LAB VALUES:*** May increase SGOT (AST), SGPT (ALT), bilirubin, alkaline phosphatase, BUN, calcium, glucose. May decrease hemoglobin, platelets, WBCs, neutrophils.

AVAILABILITY (Rx)

POWDER FOR INJECTION: 33 mcg (6.6 million units).

ADMINISTRATION/HANDLING
IM:

• Refrigerate vials. • Following reconstitution, use within 6 hrs if refrigerated. Discard if discolored, contains a precipitate. • Reconstitute 33 mcg (6.6 million IU) vial with 1.1 ml diluent (supplied by manufacturer). • Gently swirl to dissolve medication; do not shake. • Discard if discolored, contains particulate matter. • Discard unused portion (contains no preservative).

INDICATIONS/ROUTES/DOSAGE
Relapsing-remitting multiple sclerosis:
IM: **Adults:** 30 mcg once weekly.

SIDE EFFECTS

FREQUENT: Headache (67%), flu-like symptoms (61%), myalgia (34%), upper respiratory infection (31%), pain (24%), asthenia, chills (21%), sinusitis (18%), infection (11%). ***OCCASIONAL:*** Abdominal pain, arthralgia (9%), chest pain, dyspnea (6%), malaise, syncope (4%). ***RARE:*** Injection site reaction, hypersensitivity reaction (3%).

ADVERSE REACTIONS/TOXIC EFFECTS

Anemia occurs in 8% of pts.

NURSING IMPLICATIONS

BASELINE ASSESSMENT:

Obtain hemoglobin, CBC, platelet count, blood chemistries including liver function tests. Assess home situation for support of therapy.

INTERVENTION/EVALUATION:

Assess for headache, flulike symptoms, muscle ache (see Side Effects). Periodically monitor lab results and reevaluate injection technique. Assess for depression and suicidal ideation.

PATIENT/FAMILY TEACHING:

Do not change schedule or dosage without consultation with physician. Instruct on correct reconstitution of product and administration, including aseptic technique. Provide puncture-resistant container for used needles, syringes, and explain proper disposal. Explain that injection site reactions may occur. These do not require discontinuation of therapy, but note type and extent carefully. Depression or suicidal ideation must be reported immediately.

interferon beta-1b

inn-ter-**fear**-on
(Betaseron)
Do not confuse with interferon beta-1a.

▶CLASSIFICATION

PHARMACOTHERAPEUTIC: Biological response modifier. ***CLINICAL:*** Multiple sclerosis, cancer, AIDs agent

ACTION/*THERAPEUTIC EFFECT*

Interacts with specific cell receptors found on surface of human cells. *Possesses antiviral and immunoregulatory activities.*

PHARMACOKINETICS

Half-life: 8 min–4.3 hrs.

USES/*UNLABELED*

Reduces frequency of clinical exacerbations with pts with relapsing-remitting multiple sclerosis (recurrent attacks of neurologic dysfunction). *Treatment of AIDS, AIDS-related Kaposi's sarcoma, renal cell carcinoma, malignant melanoma, acute non-A, non-B hepatitis.*

PRECAUTIONS

CONTRAINDICATIONS: Hypersensitivity to interferon, albumin. ***CAUTIONS:*** Chronic progressive multiple sclerosis, children <18 yrs of age.

▷***LIFESPAN CONSIDERATIONS:***
Pregnancy/Lactation: Unknown whether distributed in breast milk. **Pregnancy Category C. Children:** Safety and efficacy not established. **Elderly:** No information available.

INTERACTIONS

DRUG: None significant. ***HERBAL:*** None known. ***FOOD:*** None known. ***LAB VALUES:*** May increase SGOT (AST), SGPT (ALT), bilirubin, alkaline phosphatase, BUN, calcium, glucose. May decrease hemoglobin, platelets, WBCs, neutrophils.

AVAILABILITY (Rx)

POWDER FOR INJECTION: 0.3 mg (9.6 million units).

ADMINISTRATION/HANDLING
SubQ:

• Refrigerate vials. • After reconstitution is stable for 3 hrs if refrigerated. • Use within 3 hrs of reconstitution. • Discard if discolored, contains a precipitate. • Reconstitute 0.3 mg (9.6 million IU) vial with 1.2 ml diluent (supplied by manufacturer) to provide concentration of 0.25 mg/ml (8 million U/ml). • Gently swirl to dissolve medication; do not shake. • Discard if discolored, contains particulate matter. • Withdraw 1 ml solution and inject SubQ into arms, abdomen, hips, or thighs using 27 gauge needle. • Discard unused portion (contains no preservative).

INDICATIONS/ROUTES/DOSAGE

Relapsing-remitting multiple sclerosis:

SubQ: **Adults:** 0.25 mg (8 million IU) every other day.

SIDE EFFECTS

FREQUENT: Injection site reaction (85%), headache (84%), flulike symptoms (76%), fever (59%), pain (52%), asthenia (49%), myalgia (44%), sinusitis (36%), diarrhea, dizziness (35%), mental symptoms (29%), constipation (24%), diaphoresis (23%), vomiting (21%). **OCCASIONAL:** Malaise (15%), somnolence (6%), alopecia (4%).

ADVERSE REACTIONS/TOXIC EFFECTS

Seizures occur rarely.

NURSING IMPLICATIONS

BASELINE ASSESSMENT:

Obtain hemoglobin, CBC, platelet count, blood chemistries including liver function tests. Assess home situation for support of therapy.

INTERVENTION/EVALUATION:

Periodically monitor lab results and reevaluate injection technique. Assess for nausea (high incidence). Monitor sleep pattern. Monitor stool frequency and consistency (watery, loose, soft). Assist with ambulation if dizziness occurs. Question for evidence of heartburn, epigastric discomfort. Monitor food intake. Assess for depression and suicidal ideation.

PATIENT/FAMILY TEACHING:

Inform physician of flulike symptoms (occur commonly but decreases over time). Wear sunscreens, protective clothing if exposed to ultraviolet light or sunlight until tolerance known.

interferon gamma-1b

inn-ter-**fear**-on
(Actimmune)

▶CLASSIFICATION

PHARMACOTHERAPEUTIC:
Biologic response modifier.
CLINICAL: Immunlogivc agent

ACTION/THERAPEUTIC EFFECT

Induces activation of macrophages in blood monocytes to phagocytes (necessary in cellular immune response to intracellular and extracellular pathogens). *Enhances phagocytic function, antimicrobial activity of monocytes.*

PHARMACOKINETICS

Slowly absorbed following SubQ administration.

USES

Reduces frequency, severity of serious infections due to chronic granulomatous disease. Treatment of severe, malignant osteopetrosis.

PRECAUTIONS

CONTRAINDICATIONS: Hypersensitivity to *Escherichia coli* products. **CAUTIONS:** Seizure disorders, compromised CNS function, preexisting cardiac disease (including ischemia, CHF, arrhythmia), myelosuppression.

▷**LIFESPAN CONSIDERATIONS:**
Pregnancy/Lactation: Unknown if drug crosses placenta or is distributed in breast milk. **Pregnancy Category C. Children:** Safety and efficacy not established in those <1 yr of age. Flulike symptoms may occur more frequently. **Elderly:** No information available.

INTERACTIONS

DRUG:* Bone marrow depressants** may increase bone marrow depression. ***HERBAL: None known. ***FOOD:*** None known. ***LAB VALUES:*** None significant.

AVAILABILITY (Rx)

INJECTION: 100 mcg (3 million units).

ADMINISTRATION/HANDLING

Note: Avoid excessive agitation of vial; do not shake.

SubQ:

• Refrigerate vials. Do not freeze. • Do not keep at room temperature >12 hrs; discard if left out longer. • Vials are single dose; discard unused portion. • Clear, colorless solution. Do not use if discolored, precipitate formed. • When given 3 times/week, give in left deltoid, right deltoid, and anterior thigh.

INDICATIONS/ROUTES/DOSAGE

Chronic granulomatous disease, osteopetrosis:

SubQ: **Adults, children >1 yr:** 50 mcg/m^2 (1.5 million units/m^2) in pts with body surface area (BSA) >0.5 m^2; 1.5 mcg/kg/dose in pts with BSA ≤0.5 m^2. Give 3 times/wk.

SIDE EFFECTS

FREQUENT: Fever (52%), headache (33%), rash (17%), chills, fatigue, diarrhea (14%). ***OCCASIONAL*** (10–13%): Vomiting, nausea, ***RARE*** (3–6%): Weight loss, myalgia, anorexia.

ADVERSE REACTIONS/TOXIC EFFECTS

May exacerbate preexisting CNS, cardiac abnormalities demonstrated as decreased mental status, gait disturbance, dizziness.

NURSING IMPLICATIONS

BASELINE ASSESSMENT:

CBC, platelet, blood chemistries, urinalysis, renal and liver function tests should be performed prior to initial therapy and at 3 mo intervals during course of treatment.

INTERVENTION/EVALUATION:

Monitor for flulike symptoms (fever, chills, fatigue, muscle aches). Assess skin for evidence of rash.

PATIENT/FAMILY TEACHING:

Flulike symptoms (fever, chills, fatigue, muscle aches) are generally mild and tend to disappear as treatment continues. Symptoms may be minimized by bedtime administration. Avoid tasks that require alertness, motor skills until response to drug is established. If home use prescribed, instruct in proper technique of administration, care in proper disposal of needles, syringes. Vial should remain refrigerated.

interleukin-2 (aldesleukin)

in-tur-**lew**-kin
(IL-2, Proleukin)
Do not confuse with interferon 2.

▶CLASSIFICATION

PHARMACOTHERAPEUTIC: Biological response modifier. ***CLINICAL:*** Antineoplastic (see p. 67C)

ACTION/*THERAPEUTIC EFFECT*

A highly purified protein (lymphokine) is modified, *providing enhancement of lymphocyte mitogenesis, enhancement of lymphocyte cytotoxicity, induction of natural killer cells and interferon gamma production. Activates cellular immunity, inhibits tumor growth.*

PHARMACOKINETICS

Distributed to extravascular, extracellular space. Metabolized in kidney (to amino acids in cells lining the proximal convoluted tubule). Excreted in urine. Half-life: 30–120 min.

USES/*UNLABELED*

Treatment of metastatic renal cell carcinoma, metastatic melanoma. *Kaposi's sarcoma, colorectal cancer, non-Hodgkins lymphoma.*

PRECAUTIONS

CONTRAINDICATIONS: Abnormal thallium stress test or pulmonary function tests, organ allografts, retreatment in those who experience the following toxicities: sustained ventricular tachycardia, cardiac rhythm disturbances uncontrolled or unresponsive, recurrent chest pain with EKG changes, angina, MI; intubation >72 hrs, pericardial tamponade, renal dysfunction requiring dialysis >72 hrs, coma or toxic psychosis >48 hrs, repetitive or difficult-to-control seizures, bowel ischemia/perforation, GI bleeding requiring surgery. *EXTREME CAUTION:* Those with normal thallium stress tests and pulmonary function tests who have history of prior cardiac or pulmonary disease. *CAUTIONS:* Those with fixed requirements for large volumes of fluid

(e.g., those with hypercalcemia), history of seizures.

▷*LIFESPAN CONSIDERATIONS:*
Pregnancy/Lactation: Avoid use in those of either sex not practicing effective contraception. **Pregnancy Category C. Children:** Safety and efficacy not established. **Elderly:** Age-related decreased renal function may require caution. Do not tolerate toxicity.

INTERACTIONS

DRUG: **Antihypertensives** may increase hypotensive effect. **Glucocorticoids** may decrease effects. **Cardiotoxic, hepatotoxic, nephrotoxic, myelotoxic** producing medications may increase toxicity. *HERBAL:* None known. *FOOD:* None known. *LAB VALUES:* May increase bilirubin, BUN, serum creatinine, transaminase, alkaline phosphatase. May decrease magnesium, calcium, phosphorus, potassium, sodium.

AVAILABILITY (Rx)

POWDER FOR INJECTION: 22 million units (1.3 mg).

ADMINISTRATION/HANDLING

Note: Hold administration in those who develop moderate to severe lethargy or somnolence (continued administration may result in coma).

IV 🦠

Storage:
• Refrigerate vial before and after reconstitution. • Reconstituted solution stable for 48 hrs. • Discard solution that does not appear clear, colorless to slightly yellow. Discard unused portion.

Reconstitution:
• Reconstitute 22 million unit vial

with 1.2 ml Sterile Water for Injection to provide concentration of 18 million units/ml. Do not use Bacteriostatic Water for Injection or 0.9% NaCl. • During reconstitution, direct the Sterile Water for Injection at the side of vial. Swirl contents gently to avoid foaming. Do not shake.

Rate of administration:

• Further dilute dose in 50 ml D_5W and infuse over 15 min. Do not use an in-line filter. • Solution should be warmed to room temperature before pt infusion. • Monitor diligently for drop in mean arterial B/P (sign of capillary leak syndrome [CLS]). Continued treatment may result in significant hypotension (<90 mm Hg or a 20 mm Hg drop from baseline systolic pressure), edema, pleural effusion, mental status changes.

IV INCOMPATIBILITIES ⊘

Bacteriostatic Water for Injection or NaCl should not be used to reconstitute because of increased aggregation. Ganciclovir (Cytovene), lorazepam (Ativan), pentamidine (Pentam), prochlorperazine (Compazine), promethazine (Phenergan).

IV COMPATIBILITIES

Calcium gluconate, dopamine (Intropin), heparin, lorazepam (Ativan), magnesium, potassium.

INDICATIONS/ROUTES/DOSAGE

Note: Restrict therapy to those with normal cardiac and pulmonary functions as defined by thallium stress testing, pulmonary function testing. Dosage individualized based on clinical response, tolerance to adverse effects.

Metastatic melanoma, metastatic renal cell carcinoma:

IV: **Adults >18:** 600,000 IU/kg q8h for 14 doses; rest 9 days, repeat 14 doses. Total: 28 doses. May repeat treatment no sooner than 7 wks from date of hospital discharge.

SIDE EFFECTS

Note: Side effects generally self-limiting and reversible within 2–3 days after discontinuation of therapy. ***FREQUENT*** (48–89%): Fever, chills, nausea, vomiting, hypotension, diarrhea, oliguria/anuria, mental status changes, irritability, confusion, depression), sinus tachycardia, pain (abdomen, chest, back), fatigue, dyspnea, pruritus. ***OCCASIONAL*** (17–47%): Edema, erythema, rash, stomatitis, anorexia, weight gain, infection (urinary tract, injection site, catheter tip), dizziness. ***RARE*** (4–15%): Dry skin, sensory disorders (vision, speech, taste), dermatitis, headache, arthralgia, myalgia, weight loss, hematuria, conjunctivitis, proteinuria.

ADVERSE REACTIONS/TOXIC EFFECTS

Anemia, thrombocytopenia, leukopenia occur commonly. GI bleeding, pulmonary edema occur occasionally. Capillary leak syndrome results in hypotension (<90 mm Hg or a 20 mm Hg drop from baseline systolic pressure) and extravasation of plasma proteins and fluid into extravascular space and loss of vascular tone. May result in cardiac arrhythmias, angina, MI, respiratory insufficiency. Fatal malignant hyperthermia, cardiac arrest or stroke, pulmonary emboli as well as bowel perforation/gangrene, severe depression leading to suicide have occurred in <1% of pts.

NURSING IMPLICATIONS

BASELINE ASSESSMENT:

Those with bacterial infection and those with indwelling central lines should be treated with antibiotic therapy before treatment begins. All pts should be neurologically stable with a negative CT scan before treatment begins. CBC, blood chemistries including electrolytes, renal and hepatic function tests, chest x-ray should be performed before therapy begins and daily thereafter.

INTERVENTION/EVALUATION:

Determine serum amylase concentration frequently during therapy. Discontinue medication at first sign of hypotension and hold for moderate to severe lethargy (physician must decide whether therapy should continue). Assess mental status changes (irritability, confusion, depression), weight gain or loss. Maintain strict I&O. Assess for extravascular fluid accumulation: rales in lungs, edema in dependent areas.

PATIENT/FAMILY TEACHING:

Nausea may decrease during therapy. At home, increase fluid intake (protects against renal impairment). Do not have immunizations without physician's approval (drug lowers body resistance); avoid contact with those who have recently taken live virus vaccine.

ipecac syrup

ip-eh-**kak**
(PMS Ipecac Syrup♣)

►CLASSIFICATION

PHARMACOTHERAPEUTIC:
Antidote. ***CLINICAL:*** Antidote

ACTION/*THERAPEUTIC EFFECT*

Acts centrally by stimulating medullary chemoreceptor trigger zone and locally by irritating gastric mucosa, *producing emesis.*

USES

Induces vomiting in early treatment of unabsorbed oral poisons, drug overdosage.

PRECAUTIONS

CONTRAINDICATIONS: Ingestion of petroleum distillates (paint thinner, gasoline, kerosene), alkali (lye), acids, strychnine. ***CAUTIONS:*** Impaired cardiac function, pathologic blood vessel disease.

INTERACTIONS

DRUG: Antiemetics may decrease effect. Avoid carbonated beverages (causes stomach distention), milk or milk products (decreases effectiveness). ***HERBAL:*** None known. ***FOOD:*** None known. ***LAB VALUES:*** None significant.

AVAILABILITY (OTC)
SYRUP: 70 mg/ml.

INDICATIONS/ROUTES/DOSAGE

Note: If vomiting has not occurred within 20 min after first dose, repeat with 15 ml. If vomiting has not occurred within 30 min after last dose, initiate gastric lavage, activated charcoal.

Emetic:

PO: Adults, elderly, children >12 yrs: 15–30 ml; give with 3–4 glasses water immediately following administration. **Children 1–12 yrs:** 15 ml; follow with 1–2 glasses water. **Children 6 mos–1 yr:** 5–10 ml; follow with 1 glass water. If vomiting has not occurred within 30 min, repeat initial dosage.

SIDE EFFECTS

EXPECTED RESPONSE: Nausea, vomiting. After vomiting, diarrhea and CNS symptoms (drowsiness, mild CNS depression) commonly occur.

ADVERSE REACTIONS/TOXIC EFFECTS

Cardiotoxicity may occur if ipecac syrup is not vomited (noted as hypotension, tachycardia, precordial chest pain, pulmonary congestion, dyspnea, ventricular tachycardia and fibrillation, cardiac arrest). Overdose may produce diarrhea, fast/irregular heartbeat, nausea continuing >30 min, stomach pain, respiratory difficulty, unusually tired, aching/stiff muscles.

NURSING IMPLICATIONS

BASELINE ASSESSMENT:

Do not administer to semiconscious, unconscious, or convulsing pt. Gastric lavage, activated charcoal is necessary if vomiting does not occur within 30 min of second dosage to avoid drug toxicity (bloody stools, vomitus, abdominal pain, hypotension, dyspnea, shock, cardiac disturbances, seizures, coma). Main-

tain pt in upright position to enhance emetic effect.

INTERVENTION/EVALUATION:

Closely monitor vital signs, EKG during and after drug is administered. Watch for changes from initial assessment. Check for reversal of poisoning or overdosage symptoms. Monitor daily bowel activity and stool consistency (watery, loose, soft, semisolid, solid) and record time of evacuation. Assess for dehydration in excessive vomiting: poor skin turgor, dry mucous membranes, longitudinal furrows in tongue.

ipratropium bromide

ih-prah-**trow**-pea-um
(<u>Atrovent</u>)

FIXED-COMBINATION(S)

With albuterol, a bronchodilator **(Combivent, DuoNeb)** **Do not confuse with** Alupent.

▶**CLASSIFICATION**

PHARMACOTHERAPEUTIC: Antiocholinergic. ***CLINICAL:*** Bronchodilator

ACTION/*THERAPEUTIC EFFECT*

Inhibits vagal mediated response by reversing action of acetylcholine, *producing smooth muscle relaxation, bronchodilating response*. Produces significant increase in forced vital lung capacity.

PHARMACOKINETICS

Onset	Peak	Duration
Inhalation		
<15 min	1–2 hrs	3–4 hrs

Minimal systemic absorption. Metabolized in liver (systemic absorption). Primarily eliminated in feces. Half-life: 1.5–4 hrs.

USES

Maintenance treatment of bronchospasm due to chronic obstructive airway disease, including bronchitis, emphysema. Adjunct to bronchodilators for maintenance treatment of bronchial asthma. Not to be used for immediate bronchospasm relief. *Nasal spray:* Rhinorrhea (0.03% associated with perineal rhinitis, 0.06% associated with common cold).

PRECAUTIONS

CONTRAINDICATIONS: History of hypersensitivity to atropine. *CAUTIONS:* Narrow-angle glaucoma, prostatic hypertrophy, bladder neck obstruction.
▷*LIFESPAN CONSIDERATIONS:* **Pregnancy/Lactation:** Unknown if distributed in breast milk. **Pregnancy Category B. Children/Elderly:** No age-related precautions noted.

INTERACTIONS

DRUG: Avoid mixing with **cromolyn inhalation** solution (forms precipitate). *HERBAL:* None known. *FOOD:* None known. *LAB VALUES:* None significant.

AVAILABILITY (Rx)

ORAL INHALATION: 18 mcg/actuation. *AEROSOL SOLUTION FOR INHALATION:* 0.02% (500 mcg vial). *NASAL SPRAY:* 0.03%, 0.06%.

ADMINISTRATION/HANDLING

Inhalation:

• Shake container well, exhale completely through mouth; place mouthpiece into mouth and close lips, holding inhaler upright. • Inhale deeply through mouth while fully depressing the top of canister. Hold breath as long as possible before exhaling slowly. • Wait 2 min before inhaling second dose (allows for deeper bronchial penetration). • Rinse mouth with water immediately after inhalation (prevents mouth/throat dryness).

INDICATIONS/ROUTES/DOSAGE

Bronchospasm:

INHALATION: **Adults, elderly:** 2 inhalations 4 times/day. Wait 1–10 min before administering second inhalation. **Maximum:** 12 inhalations/24 hrs. **Children 3–12 yrs:** 1–2 inhalations 3 times/day. **Maximum:** 6 inhalations/24 hrs.

NEBULIZATION: **Adults, elderly:** 500 mcg 3–4 times/day. **Children:** 125–250 mcg 3 times/day. **Neonates:** 25 mcg/kg/dose 3 times/day.

Rhinorrhea:

INTRANASAL: **Adults, children >6 yrs:** *0.03%:* 2 sprays 2–3 times/day. **Adults, children >12 yrs:** *0.06%:* 2 sprays 3–4 times/day.

SIDE EFFECTS

FREQUENT: Inhalation (3–6%): Cough, dry mouth, headache, nausea. *Nasal:* Dry nose/mouth, headache, nasal irritation. *OCCASIONAL: Inhalation* (2%): Dizziness, transient increased bronchospasm. *RARE* (<1%): Hypotension, insomnia, metallic/unpleasant taste, palpitations, urinary retention. *Nasal:* Diarrhea/constipation, dry throat, stomach pain, stuffy nose.

ADVERSE REACTIONS/TOXIC EFFECTS

Worsening of narrow-angle glaucoma, acute eye pain, hypotension occur rarely.

BASELINE ASSESSMENT:

Offer emotional support (high incidence of anxiety due to difficulty in breathing and sympathomimetic response to drug).

INTERVENTION/EVALUATION:

Monitor rate, depth, rhythm, type of respiration; quality and rate of pulse. Assess lung sounds for rhonchi, wheezing, rales. Monitor arterial blood gases. Observe lips, fingernails for blue or dusky color in light-skinned pts; gray in dark-skinned pts. Observe for clavicular retractions, hand tremor. Evaluate for clinical improvement (quieter, slower respirations, relaxed facial expression, cessation of clavicular retractions).

PATIENT/FAMILY TEACHING:

Increase fluid intake (decreases lung secretion viscosity). Do not take more than 2 inhalations at any one time (excessive use may produce paradoxical bronchoconstriction or a decreased bronchodilating effect). Rinsing mouth with water immediately after inhalation may prevent mouth/throat dryness. Avoid excessive use of caffeine derivatives (chocolate, coffee, tea, cola, cocoa).

irbesartan

ir-beh-**sar**-tan
(Avapro)

FIXED-COMBINATION(S)

With hydrochlorothiazide, a diuretic **(Avalide)**

▶**CLASSIFICATION**

PHARMACOTHERAPEUTIC:
Angiotensin II receptor antagonist.
CLINICAL: Antihypertensive
(see p. 7C)

ACTION/_THERAPEUTIC EFFECT_

Potent vasodilator. An angiotensin II receptor (type AT1) antagonist; blocks vasoconstrictor and aldosterone-secreting effects of angiotensin II, inhibiting the binding of angiotensin II to the AT1 receptors, _producing vasodilation, decreased peripheral resistance, decrease in B/P._

PHARMACOKINETICS

Rapidly and completely absorbed following PO administration. Protein binding: 90%. Undergoes hepatic metabolism to inactive metabolite. Recovered primarily in feces and, to a lesser extent, in urine. Not removed by hemodialysis. Half-life: 11–15 hrs.

USES/_UNLABELED_

Treatment of hypertension alone or in combination with other antihypertensives. _Treatment of heart failure._

PRECAUTIONS

CONTRAINDICATIONS: None significant. **_CAUTIONS:_** Renal/hepatic function impairment, renal arterial stenosis.

▷**_LIFESPAN CONSIDERATIONS:_**
Pregnancy/Lactation: Category C (first trimester), **Category D** (second and third trimester). Unknown if distributed in breast

milk. May cause fetal/neonatal morbidity/mortality. **Children:** Safety and efficacy not established. **Elderly:** No age-related precautions noted.

INTERACTIONS

DRUG: **Hydrochlorothiazide** produces further reduction in B/P. ***HERBAL:*** None known. ***FOOD:*** None known. ***LAB VALUES:*** Minor increase in BUN, serum creatinine. May decrease hemoglobin.

AVAILABILITY (Rx)

TABLETS: 75 mg, 150 mg, 300 mg.

ADMINISTRATION/HANDLING
PO:

• Give without regard to meals.

INDICATIONS/ROUTES/DOSAGE

Note: May be given concurrently with other antihypertensives. If B/P is not controlled by irbesartan alone, a diuretic may be added.

Hypertension:

PO: Adults, elderly, mildly impaired renal or hepatic function: 150 mg once daily in pts who are not volume depleted. May be titrated to 300 mg once daily.

SIDE EFFECTS

OCCASIONAL (3–9%): Upper respiratory infection, fatigue, diarrhea, cough. ***RARE*** (1–2%): Heartburn, dizziness, headache, nausea, rash.

ADVERSE REACTIONS/TOXIC EFFECTS

Overdosage may manifest as hypotension and tachycardia; bradycardia occurs less often. Institute supportive measures.

NURSING IMPLICATIONS

BASELINE ASSESSMENT:

Obtain B/P and apical pulse immediately before each dose, in addition to regular monitoring (be alert to fluctuations). If excessive reduction in B/P occurs, place pt in supine position, feet slightly elevated. Question possibility of pregnancy (see Pregnancy Category). Assess medication history (esp. diuretic).

INTERVENTION/EVALUATION:

Maintain hydration (offer fluids frequently). Assess for evidence of upper respiratory infection. Assist with ambulation if dizziness occurs. Monitor all blood serum levels. Assess B/P for hypertension/hypotension.

PATIENT/FAMILY TEACHING:

Inform female pt regarding consequences of second-and third-trimester exposure to irbesartan. Avoid tasks that require alertness, motor skills (possible dizziness effect). Report any sign of infection (sore throat, fever). Need for lifelong control. Caution against exercising during hot weather (risk of dehydration, hypotension).

irinotecan

eye-rin-**oh**-teh-can
(Camptosar)

►CLASSIFICATION

PHARMACOTHERAPEUTIC: DNA topoisomerase inhibitor. ***CLINICAL:*** Antineoplastic (see p. 71C)

ACTION/*THERAPEUTIC EFFECT*

Interacts with topoisomerase I, an enzyme, which relieves torsional strain in DNA by inducing reversible single-strand breaks. Binds to topoisomerase-DNA complex preventing relegation of these single-strand breaks. *Produces cytotoxic effect due to double-strand DNA damage produced during DNA synthesis.*

PHARMACOKINETICS

Following IV administration, metabolized to active metabolite in liver. Protein binding (metabolite): 95%. Excreted in urine and eliminated via biliary route. Half-life: 6 hrs (metabolite: 10 hrs).

USES

Treatment of metastatic carcinoma of colon/rectum in pts whose disease has recurred or progressed following 5-fluorouracil-based therapy.

PRECAUTIONS

CONTRAINDICATIONS: None significant. **CAUTIONS:** Pt previously receiving pelvic/abdominal irradiation (increased risk of myelosuppression, elderly >65 yrs).
▷*LIFESPAN CONSIDERATIONS:* **Pregnancy/Lactation:** May cause fetal harm. Unknown if distributed in breast milk; discontinue nursing. **Pregnancy Category D. Children:** Safety and efficacy not established. **Elderly:** Risk of diarrhea significantly increased.

INTERACTIONS

DRUG: Other myelosuppressants may increase risk of myelosuppression. May increase akathisia with **prochlorperazone. Laxatives** may increase severity of diarrhea. **Diuretics** may increase risk of dehydration (due to vomiting/diarrhea with irinotecan therapy). **Live virus vaccines** may potentiate virus replication, increase vaccine side effects, decrease antibody response to vaccine. **HERBAL:** None known. **FOOD:** None known. **LAB VALUES:** May increase SGOT (AST), alkaline phosphatase.

AVAILABILITY (Rx)

INJECTION: 20 mg/ml vial.

ADMINISTRATION/HANDLING

IV 📷

Storage:
• Store vials at room temperature, protect from light. • Solution diluted in D_5W is stable for 48 hrs if refrigerated. • Use within 24 hrs if refrigerated or 6 hrs if kept at room temperature. • Do not refrigerate solution if diluted with 0.9% NaCl.

Reconstitution:
• Dilute in D_5W(preferred) or 0.9% NaCl to concentration of 0.12 to 1.1 mg/ml.

Rate of administration:
• Administer all doses as IV infusion over 90 min. • Assess for extravasation (flush site with sterile water, apply ice if extravasation occurs).

IV INCOMPATIBILITY ⊘

Gemcitabine (Gemzar).

INDICATIONS/ROUTES/DOSAGE

Carcinoma of colon/rectum:

IV INFUSION: Adults, elderly: Initially, 125 mg/m² once weekly for 4 wks. Rest 2 wks. Additional courses may be repeated q6wks. Subsequent doses adjusted in

25–50 mg/m^2 increments as high as 150 mg/m^2, as low as 50 mg/m^2.

Note: Do not begin a new course until granulocyte count recovered to >1,500/mm^3, platelet count recovered to >100,000/mm^3, and treatment-related diarrhea fully resolved.

SIDE EFFECTS

COMMON: Nausea (64%), alopecia (49%), vomiting (45%), diarrhea (32%). ***FREQUENT:*** Constipation, fatigue (29%), fever (28%), asthenia (loss of strength, energy) (25%), skeletal pain (23%) abdominal pain, dyspnea (22%). ***OCCASIONAL:*** Anorexia (19%), headache, stomatitis (18%), rash (16%).

ADVERSE REACTIONS/TOXIC EFFECTS

Expect myelosuppression characterized as neutropenia in 97% of pts, neutrophil count <500/mm^3 in 78%. Thrombocytopenia, anemia sepsis occur frequently.

NURSING IMPLICATIONS

BASELINE ASSESSMENT:

Offer emotional support to pt and family. Assess hydration status, electrolytes, CBC before each dose. Premedicate with antiemetics on day of treatment, starting at least 30 min prior to administration.

INTERVENTION/EVALUATION:

Assess for early signs of diarrhea (preceded by complaints of diaphoresis and abdominal cramping). Monitor hydration status, I+O, electrolytes, CBC, hemoglobin, platelets. Monitor infusion site for signs of inflammation. Inform pt of possibility of alopecia. Assess skin for evidence of rash.

PATIENT/FAMILY TEACHING:

Inform pt of possible late diarrhea causing dehydration, electrolyte depletion. Provide antiemetic/antidiarrheal regimen for subsequent use. Do not have immunizations without physician's approval (drug lowers body's resistance). Avoid contact with those who have recently received live virus vaccine. Avoid crowds, those with infections.

iron dextran

iron **dex**-tran
(Dexiron✤, Infed, Infufer✤)

▶CLASSIFICATION

PHARMACOTHERAPEUTIC: Trace element. ***CLINICAL:*** Hematinic iron preparation

ACTION/THERAPEUTIC EFFECT

Essential component of formation of hemoglobin, *replenishes hemoglobin and depleted iron stores.* Necessary for effective erythropoiesis and O$_2$ transport capacity of blood. Serves as cofactor of several essential enzymes.

PHARMACOKINETICS

Readily absorbed after IM administration. Major portion of absorption occurs within 72 hrs; remainder within 3–4 wks. Iron is bound to protein to form hemosiderin, ferritin, or transferrin. No physiologic system of elimination. Small amounts lost daily in shedding of skin, hair, and nails, and in feces, urine, and perspiration. Half-life: 5–20 hrs.

USES

Treatment of established iron deficiency anemia. Use only when PO administration is not feasible or when rapid replenishment of iron is warranted.

PRECAUTIONS

CONTRAINDICATIONS: All anemias except iron deficiency anemia (eliminates pernicious, aplastic, normocytic, refractory). **EXTREME CAUTION:** Serious liver impairment. **CAUTIONS:** History of allergies, bronchial asthma, rheumatoid arthritis.

▷**LIFESPAN CONSIDERATIONS:** **Pregnancy/Lactation:** May cross placenta in some form (unknown); trace distributed in breast milk. **Pregnancy Category C. Children/ Elderly:** No age-related precautions noted.

INTERACTIONS

DRUG: None significant. **HERBAL:** None significant. **FOOD:** None significant. **LAB VALUES:** None significant.

AVAILABILITY (Rx)

INJECTION: 50 mg/ml.

ADMINISTRATION/HANDLING

Note: Test dose is generally given before the full dosage; stay with pt for several mins after injection due to potential for anaphylactic reaction.

IM:

• Draw up medication with one needle, use new needle for injection (minimizes skin staining). • Administer deep IM in upper outer quadrant of buttock only. • Use Z-tract technique (displacement of SubQ tissue lateral to injection site before inserting needle) to minimize skin staining.

IV

Storage:

• Store at room temperature.

Reconstitution:

• May give undiluted or dilute in 0.9% NaCl for infusion.

Rate of administration:

• Do not exceed IV administration rate of 50 mg/min (1 ml/min). A too rapid IV rate may produce flushing, chest pain, shock, hypotension, tachycardia. • Pt must remain recumbent 30–45 min following IV administration (avoid postural hypotension).

IV INCOMPATIBILITY ⊘

No information available via Y-site administration.

INDICATIONS/ROUTES/DOSAGE

Note: Discontinue oral iron form before administering iron dextran. Dosage expressed in terms of milligrams of elemental iron. Dosage individualized based on degree of anemia, pt weight, presence of any bleeding. Use periodic hematologic determinations as guide to therapy.

Iron deficiency anemia (no blood loss):

IM/IV: Adults, elderly: Mg iron = $0.66 \times$ weight (kg) $\times$ (100 − hemoglobin <g/dl>/14.8).

Replacement secondary to blood loss:

IM/IV: Adults, elderly: Replacement iron (mg) = blood loss (ml) $\times$ hematocrit.

SIDE EFFECTS

FREQUENT: Allergic reaction (rash, itching), backache, muscle pain, chills, dizziness, headache, fever, nausea, vomiting, flushed skin, pain or redness at injection site, brown discoloration of skin, metallic taste.

ADVERSE REACTIONS/TOXIC EFFECTS

Anaphylaxis has occurred during the first few mins after injection, causing death on rare occasions. Leukocytosis, lymphadenopathy occur rarely.

NURSING IMPLICATIONS

BASELINE ASSESSMENT:

Do not give concurrently with oral iron form (excessive iron may produce excessive iron storage [hemosiderosis]). Be alert to those with rheumatoid arthritis or iron deficiency anemia (acute exacerbation of joint pain and swelling may occur). Inguinal lymphadenopathy may occur with IM injection. Assess for adequate muscle mass before injecting medication.

INTERVENTION/EVALUATION:

Monitor IM site for abscess formation, necrosis, atrophy, swelling, brownish color to skin. Question pt regarding soreness, pain, inflammation at or near IM injection site. Check IV site for phlebitis. Monitor serum ferritin levels.

PATIENT/FAMILY TEACHING:

Pain and brown staining may occur at injection site. Oral iron should not be taken when receiving iron injections. Stools frequently become black with iron therapy; this is harmless unless accompanied by red streaking, sticky consistency of stool, abdominal pain or cramping, which should be reported to physician. Oral hygiene, hard candy, or gum may reduce metallic taste. Notify physician immediately if fever, back pain, headache occur.

iron sucrose

iron **sue**-crose
(Venofer)

▶CLASSIFICATION

PHARMACOTHERAPEUTIC:
Trace element. ***CLINICAL:***
Hematinic iron preparation

ACTION/*THERAPEUTIC EFFECT*

Replenishes body iron stores in pts on chronic hemodialysis who have iron deficiency anemia and are receiving erythropoietin.

USES/*UNLABELED*

Treatment of iron deficiency anemia in pts undergoing chronic hemodialysis who are receiving supplemental erythropoietin therapy. *Treatment of dystrophic epidermolysis bullosa.*

PRECAUTIONS

CONTRAINDICATIONS: All anemias except iron deficiency anemia (eliminates pernicious, aplastic, normocytic, refractory anemia), evidence of iron overload. ***CAUTIONS:*** History of allergies, bronchial asthma; hepatic, renal, or cardiac dysfunction.

INTERACTIONS

DRUG: None significant. ***HERBAL:*** None significant. ***FOOD:*** None significant. ***LAB VALUES:*** Increases **Hgb, Hct, serum ferritin, serum transferrin saturation.**

AVAILABILITY (Rx)

INJECTION: 20 mg/ml (100 mg elemental iron) in 5 ml single dose vial.

ADMINISTRATION/HANDLING

Note: Administer directly into dialysis line during hemodialysis.

IV

Storage:

• Store at room temperature.

Reconstitution:

• May give undiluted as slow IV injection or IV infusion. For IV infusion, dilute each vial in maximum of 100 ml 0.9% NaCl immediately prior to infusion.

Rate of administration:

• For IV injection, administer into the dialysis line at a rate of 1 ml (20 mg iron) undiluted solution per min (5 min per vial). Do not exceed 1 vial per injection. • For IV infusion, administer into dialysis line (reduces risk of hypotensive episodes) at a rate of 100 mg iron over at least 15 min.

IV INCOMPATIBILITIES ⊘

Do not mix with other medication or add to parenteral nutrition solution for IV infusion.

INDICATIONS/ROUTES/DOSAGE

Note: Dosage expressed in terms of milligrams of elemental iron.

Iron deficiency anemia:

IV: Adults, elderly: 5 ml iron sucrose (100 mg elemental iron) delivered by IV during dialysis; administer 1–3 times/wk to total dose of 1,000 mg in 10 doses. Give no more than 3 times/wk.

SIDE EFFECTS

FREQUENT (23–36%): Hypotension, leg cramps, diarrhea.

ADVERSE REACTIONS/TOXIC EFFECTS

A too rapid IV administration may produce severe hypotension, headache, vomiting, nausea, dizziness, paresthesia, abdominal and muscle pain, edema, cardiovascular collapse. Hypersensitivity reaction occurs rarely.

NURSING IMPLICATIONS

INTERVENTION/EVALUATION:

Initially, monitor Hgb, Hct, serum ferritin, serum transferrin levels monthly then every 2–3 mos thereafter. Reliable serum iron values can be obtained 48 hrs after administration.

isoetharine hydrochloride

eye-sew-**eth**-ah-reen
(Bronkosol, Dey-Dose)

isoetharine mesylate

(Bronkometer)
Do not confuse with Bronkodyl.

▶**CLASSIFICATION**

PHARMACOTHERAPEUTIC:
Sympathomimetic (adrenergic agonist). ***CLINICAL:*** Bronchodilator (see p. 63C).

ACTION/*THERAPEUTIC EFFECT*

Stimulates beta$_2$-adrenergic receptors in lungs, resulting in relaxation of bronchial smooth muscle, *relieving bronchospasm; reduces airway resistance.*

USES

Relief of acute bronchial asthma,

bronchospasm associated with chronic bronchitis, emphysema.

PRECAUTIONS

CONTRAINDICATIONS: History of hypersensitivity to symphomimetics. ***CAUTIONS:*** Hypertension, cardiovascular disease, hyperthyroidism, diabetes mellitus.

INTERACTIONS

DRUG: May decrease effects of **beta-blockers.** Digoxin may increase risk of arrhythmias. ***HERBAL:*** None known. ***FOOD:*** None known. ***LAB VALUES:*** May decrease serum potassium levels.

AVAILABILITY (Rx)

SOLUTION FOR NEBULIZATION: 0.125%, 0.251%, 0.5%, 1%. ***INHALATION:*** 1%.

INDICATIONS/ROUTES/DOSAGE

Bronchospasm:

INHALATION: Adults, elderly: 1–2 inhalations q4h as needed.

NEBULIZATION: Adults, elderly: 0.5–1 ml of a 0.5% solution. **Children:** 0.01 ml/kg of 1% solution. **Maximum:** 0.5 ml.

SIDE EFFECTS

OCCASIONAL: Tremor, nausea, nervousness, palpitations, tachycardia, peripheral vasodilation, dryness of mouth, throat, dizziness, vomiting, headache, increased B/P, insomnia.

ADVERSE REACTIONS/TOXIC EFFECTS

Excessive sympathomimetic stimulation may cause palpitations, extrasystoles, tachycardia, chest pain, slight increase in B/P followed by a substantial decrease, chills, sweating, and blanching of skin. Too frequent or excessive use may lead to loss of bronchodilating effectiveness and/or severe, paradoxical bronchoconstriction.

NURSING IMPLICATIONS

BASELINE ASSESSMENT:

Offer emotional support (high incidence of anxiety due to difficulty in breathing and sympathomimetic response to drug).

INTERVENTION/EVALUATION:

Assess lung sounds for rhonchi, wheezing, rales. Monitor arterial blood gases. Observe lips, fingernails for blue or dusky color in light-skinned pts; gray in dark-skinned pts. Observe for clavicular retractions, hand tremor. Evaluate for clinical improvement (quieter, slower respirations, relaxed facial expression, cessation of clavicular retractions).

PATIENT/FAMILY TEACHING:

Increase fluid intake (decreases lung secretion viscosity). Rinsing mouth with water immediately after inhalation may prevent mouth/throat dryness. Avoid excessive use of caffeine derivatives (chocolate, coffee, tea, cola, cocoa).

isoflurophate

(Floropryl)

See Classification section under: Antiglaucoma

isoniazid

eye-sew-**nye**-ah-zid
(INH, Isotamine✤, Laniazid,
Nydrazid, PMS Isoniazid✤)

FIXED-COMBINATION(S)

With rifampin, an antitubercular
(Rifamate); with pyrazinamide
and rifampin, antituberculars
(Rifater)

▶CLASSIFICATION

PHARMACOTHERAPEUTIC:
Isonicotinic acid derivative.
CLINICAL: Antitubercular

ACTION/THERAPEUTIC EFFECT

Inhibits mycolic acid synthesis
that *causes disruption of bacterial
cell wall and loss of acid-fast properties in susceptible mycobacteria.*
Active only during cell division.
Bactericidal.

PHARMACOKINETICS

Readily absorbed from GI tract.
Protein binding: 10–15%. Widely
distributed (including CSF). Metabolized in liver. Primarily excreted in urine. Removed by hemodialysis. Half-life: 0.5–5 hrs.

USES

Drug of choice in tuberculosis
prophylaxis. Used in combination
with one or more other antitubercular agents for treatment of all
forms of active tuberculosis.

PRECAUTIONS

CONTRAINDICATIONS: Acute
liver disease, history of hypersensitivity reactions or hepatic injury
with previous isoniazid therapy.
CAUTIONS: Chronic liver disease
or alcoholism, severe renal impairment. May be cross sensitive

with nicotinic acid or other chemically related medications.
▷**LIFESPAN CONSIDERATIONS:**
Pregnancy/Lactation: Prophylaxis usually postponed until after
delivery. Crosses placenta; distributed in breast milk. **Pregnancy Category C. Children:** No
age-related precautions noted. **Elderly:** More susceptible to develop hepatitis.

INTERACTIONS

DRUG: Alcohol may increase hepatotoxicity, metabolism. May increase toxicity of **carbamazepine,
phenytoin.** May decrease **ketoconazole** concentrations. **Disulfiram** may increase CNS effects.
Hepatotoxic medications may increase hepatotoxicity. **HERBAL:**
None known. **FOOD:** None known.
LAB VALUES: May increase SGOT
(AST), SGPT (ALT), bilirubin.

AVAILABILITY (Rx)

TABLETS: 50 mg, 100 mg, 300
mg. **SYRUP:** 50 mg/5 ml. **INJEC-
TION:** 100 mg/ml.

ADMINISTRATION/HANDLING

PO:

• Give 1 hr before or 2 hrs after
meals (may give with food to decrease GI upset, but will delay absorption). • Administer at least 1
hr before antacids, esp. those containing aluminum.

INDICATIONS/ROUTES/DOSAGE

Tuberculosis (treatment):

PO/IM: Adults, elderly: 5 mg/kg/
day (maximum 300 mg/day) as
single dose. **Children:** 10–15 mg/
kg/day (maximum 300 mg/day) as
single dose.

Tuberculosis (prevention):

PO/IM: Adults, elderly: 300

mg/day as single dose. **Children:** 10 mg/kg/day (maximum 300 mg/day) as single dose.

SIDE EFFECTS

FREQUENT: Nausea, vomiting, diarrhea, abdominal pain. **RARE:** Pain at injection site, hypersensitivity reaction.

ADVERSE REACTIONS/TOXIC EFFECTS

Neurotoxicity (clumsiness or unsteadiness, numbness, tingling, burning or pain in hands/feet), optic neuritis, hepatotoxicity occur rarely.

NURSING IMPLICATIONS

BASELINE ASSESSMENT:

Question for history of hypersensitivity reactions or hepatic injury from isoniazid, sensitivity to nicotinic acid or chemically related medications. Assure collection of specimens for culture, sensitivity. Evaluate initial hepatic function results.

INTERVENTION/EVALUATION:

Monitor hepatic function test results and assess for hepatitis: anorexia, nausea, vomiting, weakness, fatigue, dark urine, jaundice (hold INH and inform physician promptly). Assess for tingling, numbness, or burning of extremities (those esp. at risk for neuropathy may be given pyridoxine prophylactically: malnourished, elderly, diabetics, those with chronic liver disease, including alcoholics). Be alert for fever, skin eruptions (hypersensitivity reaction).

PATIENT/FAMILY TEACHING:

Do not skip doses; continue taking isoniazid for full length of therapy (6–24 mos). Take preferably 1 hr before or 2 hrs after meals (with food if GI upset). Avoid alcohol during treatment. Do not take any other medications without consulting physician, including antacids; must take isoniazid at least 1 hr before antacid. Avoid tuna, sauerkraut, aged cheeses, smoked fish (provide list of tyramine-containing foods) that may cause reaction such as red/itching skin, pounding heartbeat, lightheadedness, hot or clammy feeling, headache; contact physician. Notify physician of any new symptom, immediately for vision difficulties, nausea/vomiting, dark urine, yellowing of skin/eyes, fatigue, numbness or tingling of hands or feet.

isoproterenol hydrochloride

eye-sew-pro-**tear**-en-all
(Isuprel)
Do not confuse with Isordil.

►CLASSIFICATION

PHARMACOTHERAPEUTIC: Sympathomimetic (adrenergic agonist). **CLINICAL:** Cardiac stimulant

ACTION/THERAPEUTIC EFFECT

Stimulates beta$_1$-adrenergic receptors, *increasing myocardial contractility, stroke volume, cardiac output.*

USES

Treatment of carotid sinus hypersensitivity, Adams-Stokes syndrome, ventricular arrhythmias due to AV nodal block, diagnosis of coronary artery disease; adjunct in treatment of shock.

PRECAUTIONS

CONTRAINDICATIONS: Tachycardia due to digitalis toxicity, preexisting arrhythmias, angina, precordial distress. **CAUTIONS:** Hypersensitivity to sulfite, elderly/debilitated, hypertension, cardiovascular disease, impaired renal function, hyperthyroidism, diabetes mellitus, prostatic hypertrophy, glaucoma. Safety and efficacy in children not established.

INTERACTIONS

DRUG: Tricyclic antidepressants may increase cardiovascular effects. May decrease effects of **beta-blockers. Digoxin** may increase risk of arrhythmias. **HERBAL:** Ma huang (ephedra) increases CNS stimulation. **FOOD:** None known. **LAB VALUES:** May decrease serum potassium levels.

AVAILABILITY (Rx)

INJECTION: 1:5,000 (0.2 mg/ml).

ADMINISTRATION/HANDLING
IV 💉

Storage:
• Do not use if solution is pink to brown, contains a precipitate, or appears cloudy.

Reconstitution:
• For IV push, dilute 0.2 mg (1 ml) of 1:5,000 solution to a volume of 10 ml 0.9% NaCl or D$_5$W. • For IV infusion, dilute 0.2–2 mg (1–10 ml) of 1:5,000 solution in 500 ml D$_5$W to provide a solution of 0.4–4 mcg/ml.

Rate of administration:
• Administer IV push at rate of 1 ml/min, regulated by EKG monitoring. • Rate of IV infusion determined by pt's heart rate, central venous pressure, systemic B/P, and urine flow measurements. • Use microdrip (60 drops/ml) or infusion pump to administer drug. • If EKG changes occur, heart rate exceeds 110 beats/min, or premature beats occur, consider reducing rate of infusion or temporarily stopping infusion.

IV INCOMPATIBILITY ⊘

No information available via Y-site administration.

IV COMPATIBILITIES

Amiodarone (Cordarone), heparin, potassium, propofol (Diprivan).

INDICATIONS/ROUTES/DOSAGE
Usual parenteral dosage:

IV INFUSION: Adults, elderly: 2–20 mcg/min. **Children:** 0.05–2 mcg/kg/min.

SIDE EFFECTS

FREQUENT (10–20%): Palpitations, tachycardia, restlessness, nervousness, tremor, insomnia, anxiety. **OCCASIONAL** (<10%): Increased sweating, headache, nausea, flushed skin, dizziness, coughing.

ADVERSE REACTIONS/TOXIC EFFECTS

Excessive sympathomimetic stimulation may cause palpitations, extrasystoles, tachycardia, chest pain, slight increase in B/P followed by a substantial decrease, chills, sweating, and blanching of skin. Ventricular arrhythmias may occur if heart rate is above 130 beats/min. Parotid gland swelling may occur with prolonged use.

Onset	Peak	Duration
Extended-release		
Up to 4 hrs	—	6–8 hrs
Tablets, capsules		
20–40 min	45–120 min	4–6 hrs
Mononitrate		
30–60 min	—	—

Poorly absorbed from GI tract; well absorbed after SubQ administration. Protein binding: <4%. Metabolized in liver (undergoes first-pass effect). Primarily excreted in urine. Not removed by hemodialysis. Half-life: **PO:** 4 hrs, **SubQ:** 1 hr. **Mononitrate:** Not subjected to first-pass metabolism in liver. Removed by hemodialysis.

USES

Treatment and prevention of angina pectoris. Chronic prophylaxis of angina. **Mononitrate:** Prevention of angina pectoris due to coronary artery disease.

PRECAUTIONS

CONTRAINDICATIONS: Hypersensitivity to nitrates, severe anemia, closed-angle glaucoma, postural hypotension, head trauma, increased intracranial pressure. ***Extended-release:*** GI hypermotility/malabsorption, severe anemia. ***CAUTIONS:*** Acute MI, hepatic/renal disease, glaucoma (contraindicated in closed-angle glaucoma), blood volume depletion from diuretic therapy, systolic B/P below 90 mm Hg.
▷***LIFESPAN CONSIDERATIONS:*** **Pregnancy/Lactation:** Unknown if drug crosses placenta or is distributed in breast milk. **Pregnancy Category C. Children:** Safety and efficacy not established. **Elderly:** May be more sensitive to hypotensive effects. Age-related decreased renal function may require cautious use.

BASELINE ASSESSMENT:
Be alert to anginal pain or precordial distress, pulse rate exceeding 110 beats/min.

INTERVENTION/EVALUATION:
Monitor EKG, blood Pco_2 or bicarbonate and blood pH, central venous pressure, pulse, systemic B/P, urine output.

isosorbide dinitrate

eye-sew-**sore**-bide
(Apo-ISDN♣, Cedocard♣, Dilatrate, Isordil, Sorbitrate)

isosorbide mononitrate

(Imdur, ISMO, Isuprel, Monoket) **Do not confuse with** Inderal, Isuprel, K-Dur, Plendil.

▶CLASSIFICATION

PHARMACOTHERAPEUTIC: Nitrate. ***CLINICAL:*** Antianginal (see p. 104C)

ACTION/*THERAPEUTIC EFFECT*

Decreases myocardial O_2 demand, increases myocardial O_2 supply, reducing wall tension by venous dilation (preload) and arterial dilation (afterload). *Dilates coronary arteries; improves collateral blood flow to ischemic areas within myocardium.*

PHARMACOKINETICS

Onset	Peak	Duration
Chewable		
5–20 min	15–60 min	1–4 hrs
Sublingual		
5–20 min	15–60 min	1–4 hrs

INTERACTIONS
DRUG:* Alcohol, antihypertensives, vasodilators** may increase risk of orthostatic hypotension. ***HERBAL: None known. ***FOOD:*** None known. ***LAB VALUES:*** May increase urine catecholamines, urine VMA (vanilmandelic acid).

AVAILABILITY (Rx)
DINITRATE: TABLETS: 5 mg, 10 mg, 20 mg, 30 mg, 40 mg. ***TABLETS (sublingual):*** 2.5 mg, 5 mg, 10 mg. ***TABLETS (chewable):*** 5 mg, 10 mg. ***TABLETS (sustained-release):*** 40 mg. ***CAPSULES (sustained-release):*** 40 mg.

MONONITRATE: TABLETS: 10 mg, 20 mg. ***TABLETS (extended-release):*** 60 mg.

ADMINISTRATION/HANDLING
PO:
• Best if taken on an empty stomach. • Oral tablets may be crushed. • Do not crush or break sublingual or extended-release form. • Do not crush chewable form before administering.

SubQ:
• Do not crush/chew sublingual tablets. • Dissolve tablets under tongue; do not swallow.

INDICATIONS/ROUTES/DOSAGE
Note: Patch: Allow 10–12 hr drug-free interval.

Acute angina, prophylactic management in situations likely to provoke attack:
SUBLINGUAL/CHEWABLE:
Adults, elderly: Initially, 2.5–5 mg. Repeat at 5–10 min intervals. No more than 3 doses in 15–30 min period.

Acute prophylactic management of angina:
SUBLINGUAL/CHEWABLE:
Adults, elderly: 5–10 mg q2–3h.

Long-term prophylaxis of angina:
***PO:* Adults, elderly:** Initially, 5–20 mg 3–4 times/day. **Maintenance:** 10–40 mg q6h. Consider 2–3 times/day, last dose no later than 7 PM to minimize intolerance.

***MONONITRATE:* Adults, elderly:** 20 mg 2 times/day, 7 hrs apart. First dose upon awakening in morning.

***EXTENDED-RELEASE:* Adults, elderly:** Initially, 40 mg. **Maintenance:** 40–80 mg 2–3 times/day. Consider 1–2 times/day, last dose at 2 PM to minimize intolerance.

IMDUR: 60–120 mg/day as single dose.

SIDE EFFECTS
FREQUENT: Headache (may be severe) occurs mostly in early therapy, diminishes rapidly in intensity, usually disappears during continued treatment; transient flushing of face and neck, dizziness (esp. if pt is standing immobile or is in a warm environment), weakness, postural hypotension, nausea, vomiting, restlessness. ***SUBLINGUAL:*** Burning, tingling sensation at oral point of dissolution. ***OCCASIONAL:*** GI upset, blurred vision, dry mouth.

ADVERSE REACTIONS/TOXIC EFFECTS
Drug should be discontinued if blurred vision, dry mouth occurs. Severe postural hypotension manifested by fainting, pulselessness, cold/clammy skin, profuse sweating. Tolerance may occur with repeated, prolonged therapy (minor

tolerance with intermittent use of sublingual tablets). Tolerance may not occur with extended-release form. High dose tends to produce severe headache.

NURSING IMPLICATIONS

BASELINE ASSESSMENT:
Record onset, type (sharp, dull, squeezing), radiation, location, intensity, and duration of anginal pain, and precipitating factors (exertion, emotional stress). If headache occurs during management therapy, administer medication with meals.

INTERVENTION/EVALUATION:
Assist with ambulation if light-headedness, dizziness occurs. Assess for facial/neck flushing. Monitor B/P for hypotension.

PATIENT/FAMILY TEACHING:
Rise slowly from lying to sitting position and dangle legs momentarily before standing. Take oral form on empty stomach (however, if headache occurs during management therapy, take medication with meals). Dissolve sublingual tablet under tongue; do not swallow. Take at first signal of angina. If not relieved within 5 min, dissolve second tablet under tongue. Repeat if no relief in another 5 min. If pain continues, contact physician. Expel from mouth any remaining sublingual tablet after pain is completely relieved. Do not change from one brand of drug to another. Avoid alcohol (intensifies hypotensive effect). If alcohol is ingested soon after taking nitroglycerin, possible acute hypotensive episode (marked drop in B/P, vertigo, pallor) may occur.

isotretinoin

eye-sew-**tret**-ih-noyn
(Accutane, Isotrex✤)
Do not confuse with Accupril, Accurbron..

▶CLASSIFICATION
PHARMACOTHERAPEUTIC:
Keratinization stabilizer. ***CLINICAL:*** Antiacne, antirosacea agent

ACTION/*THERAPEUTIC EFFECT*
Reduces sebaceous gland size, inhibiting its activity. *Produces antikeratinizing, anti-inflammatory effects.*

USES/*UNLABELED*
Treatment of severe, recalcitrant cystic acne that is unresponsive to conventional acne therapies. *Treatment of g-negative folliculitis, severe rosacea, correcting severe keratinization disorders.*

PRECAUTIONS
CONTRAINDICATIONS: Hypersensitivity to isotretinoin or parabens (component of capsules). ***CAUTIONS:*** Renal, hepatic dysfunction.
▷***LIFESPAN CONSIDERATIONS:***
Pregnancy/Lactation: Contraindicated in females who are or may become pregnant while undergoing treatment. Extremely high risk of major deformities in infant if pregnancy occurs while taking any amount of isotretinoin, even for short periods. Pt must be capable of understanding and carrying out instructions and of complying with mandatory contraception. Excretion in milk unknown; due to potential for serious adverse effects, not recommended

I

during nursing. **Pregnancy Category X.**

INTERACTIONS

DRUG: Etretinate, tretinoin, vitamin A may increase toxic effects. Tetracycline may increase potential of pseudotumor cerebri. **HERBAL:** None known. **FOOD:** None known. **LAB VALUES:** May increase triglycerides, cholesterol, SGPT (ALT), SGOT (AST), alkaline phosphatase, LDH, sedimentation rate, fasting blood glucose, uric acid; may decrease HDL.

AVAILABILITY (Rx)

CAPSULES: 10 mg, 20 mg, 40 mg.

INDICATIONS/ROUTES/DOSAGE
Recalcitrant cystic acne:

PO: Adults: Initially, 0.5–2 mg/kg/day divided in 2 doses for 15–20 wks. May repeat after at least 2 mos of therapy.

SIDE EFFECTS

FREQUENT: Cheilitis (inflammation of lips) (90%); skin/mucous membrane dryness (80%); skin fragility, pruritus, epistaxis, dry nose/mouth; conjunctivitis (40%); hypertriglyceridemia (25%); nausea, vomiting, abdominal pain (20%). **OCCASIONAL:** Musculoskeletal symptoms (16%) including bone or joint pain, arthralgia, generalized muscle aches; photosensitivity (5–10%). **RARE:** Decreased night vision, depression.

ADVERSE REACTIONS/TOXIC EFFECTS

Inflammatory bowel disease and pseudotumor cerebri (benign intracranial hypertension) have been associated with isotretinoin therapy.

NURSING IMPLICATIONS

BASELINE ASSESSMENT:
Assess baselines for blood lipids and glucose.

INTERVENTION/EVALUATION:
Assess acne for decreased cysts. Evaluate skin and mucous membranes for excessive dryness. Monitor blood glucose, lipids.

PATIENT/FAMILY TEACHING:
A transient exacerbation of acne may occur during initial period. May have decreased tolerance to contact lenses during and after therapy. Do not take vitamin supplements with vitamin A due to additive effects. Notify physician immediately of onset of abdominal pain, severe diarrhea, rectal bleeding (possible inflammatory bowel disease), or headache, nausea and vomiting, visual disturbances (possible pseudotumor cerebri). Decreased night vision may occur suddenly; take caution with night driving. Avoid prolonged exposure to sunlight; use sunscreens, protective clothing. Do not donate blood during or for 1 mo after treatment. **Women:** Explain the serious risk to fetus if pregnancy occurs (both oral and written warnings are given, with pt acknowledging in writing that she understands the warnings and consents to treatment). Must have a negative serum pregnancy test within 2 wks prior to starting therapy; therapy will begin on the second or third day of the next normal menstrual period. Effective contraception (using 2 reliable forms of contraception simultaneously) must be used for at least 1 mo before, during, and for at least 1 mo after therapy.

isradipine

iss-**rah**-dih-peen
(DynaCirc, DynaCirc CR)
Do not confuse with Dynabec,
Dynacin.

▶CLASSIFICATION

PHARMACOTHERAPEUTIC:
Calcium channel blocker. **CLIN-ICAL:** Antihypertensive (see p.
66C)

ACTION/*THERAPEUTIC EFFECT*

Inhibits calcium movement across
cardiac, vascular smooth muscle.
Potent peripheral vasodilator (does
not depress SA, AV nodes). *In-creases myocardial contractility,
heart rate, cardiac output; decreases
peripheral vascular resistance.*

PHARMACOKINETICS

	Onset	Peak	Duration
PO	2–3 hrs	—	—

Well absorbed from GI tract. Protein
binding: 95%. Metabolized in liver
(undergoes first-pass effect). Primar-ily excreted in urine. Not removed
by hemodialysis. Half-life: 8 hrs.

USES/*UNLABELED*

Management of hypertension.
May be used alone or with thi-azide-type diuretics. *Treatment of
chronic angina pectoris, Raynaud's
phenomena.*

PRECAUTIONS

CONTRAINDICATIONS: Sick-sinus
syndrome/second-or third-degree
AV block (except in presence of
pacemaker). **CAUTIONS:** Impaired
renal/hepatic function, CHF.
▷**LIFESPAN CONSIDERATIONS:**
Pregnancy/Lactation: Unknown if

drug crosses placenta or is dis-tributed in breast milk. **Pregnancy
Category C. Children:** Safety and
efficacy not established. **Elderly:**
Age-related renal impairment may
require cautious use.

INTERACTIONS

DRUG: **Beta-blockers** may have
additive effect. **HERBAL:** None
known. **FOOD:** **Grapefruit/grape-fruit juice** may increase absorp-tion. **LAB VALUES:** None significant.

AVAILABILITY (Rx)

CAPSULES: 2.5 mg, 5 mg. **EX-TENDED-RELEASE CAPSULES:** 5
mg, 10 mg.

ADMINISTRATION/HANDLING

PO:
• Do not crush or break capsule.

INDICATIONS/ROUTES/DOSAGE

Hypertension:
PO: Adults, elderly: Initially, 2.5 mg
2 times/day. May increase by 5 mg
q2–4wks. **Maximum:** 20 mg/day.

SIDE EFFECTS

FREQUENT (4–7%): Peripheral
edema, palpitations (higher fre-quency in females). **OCCA-SIONAL** (3%): Facial flushing,
cough. **RARE** (1–2%): Angina,
tachycardia, rash, pruritus.

ADVERSE REACTIONS/TOXIC EFFECTS

CHF occurs rarely. Overdosage
produces nausea, drowsiness,
confusion, slurred speech.

NURSING IMPLICATIONS

BASELINE ASSESSMENT:

Assess baseline renal/liver func-tion tests. Assess B/P, apical
pulse immediately before drug

is administered (if pulse is 60/min or below, or systolic B/P is below 90 mm Hg, withhold medication, contact physician).

INTERVENTION/EVALUATION:

Assess for peripheral edema behind medial malleolus (sacral area in bedridden pts). Monitor pulse rate for bradycardia. Assess skin for flushing.

PATIENT/FAMILY TEACHING:

Do not abruptly discontinue medication. Compliance with therapy regimen is essential to control hypertension. To avoid hypotensive effect, rise slowly from lying to sitting position, wait momentarily before standing. Contact physician/nurse if irregular heartbeat, shortness of breath, pronounced dizziness, or nausea occurs. Avoid use of grapefruit/grapefruit juice.

itraconazole

eye-tra-**con**-ah-zoll
(Sporanox)
Do not confuse with Suprax.

▶CLASSIFICATION
CLINICAL: Antifungal

ACTION/*THERAPEUTIC EFFECT*

Inhibits synthesis of ergosterol (vital component of fungal cell formation), damaging fungal cell membrane. *Fungistatic.*

PHARMACOKINETICS

Moderately absorbed from GI tract (increased with food). Protein binding: 99%. Widely distributed (primarily in liver, kidney, fatty tissue). Metabolized in liver to active metabolite. Primarily excreted in urine. Not removed by hemodialysis. Half-life: 21 hrs; metabolite: 12 hrs.

USES/*UNLABELED*

Treatment of blastomycosis (pulmonary, extrapulmonary), histoplasmosis, aspergillosis, onychomycosis, dermatophyte skin infections, tinea pedis in pts unable to take topical therapy. *Solution:* Oral, esophageal candidiasis. *Suppresses histoplasmosis; treatment of fungal pneumonia/septicemia, disseminated sporotrichosis, ringworm of hand.*

PRECAUTIONS

CONTRAINDICATIONS: Coadministration of terfenadine. Hypersensitivity to itraconazole, fluconazole, ketoconazole, miconazole. ***CAUTIONS:*** Hepatitis, HIV-infected pts, pts with achlorhydria, hypochlorhydria (decreases absorption), impaired liver function.

▷*LIFESPAN CONSIDERATIONS:*
Pregnancy/Lactation: Distributed in breast milk. **Pregnancy Category C. Children:** Safety and efficacy not established. **Elderly:** Age-related renal impairment may require dosage adjustment.

INTERACTIONS

DRUG: May increase **buspirone, cyclosporine, digoxin, lovastatin, simvastatin** concentrations. May increase effect of **oral anticoagulants. Phenytoin, rifampin** may decrease concentrations. **Antacids, H$_2$ antagonists, didanosine** may decrease absorption. ***HERBAL:*** None known. ***FOOD:*** **Grapefruit juice** may alter absorption. ***LAB VALUES:*** May increase SGOT (AST), SGPT (ALT), alkaline phosphatase, LDH, bilirubin. May decrease potassium.

AVAILABILITY (Rx)

CAPSULES: 100 mg. ***ORAL SOLUTION:*** 10 mg/ml. ***INJECTION:*** 10 mg/ml, 25 ml amp.

ADMINISTRATION/HANDLING
PO:

• Give capsules with food (increases absorption). • Give solution on an empty stomach.

IV 💡
Storage:

• Store at room temperature. Do not freeze.

Reconstitution:

• Use only components provided by manufacturer. • Do not dilute with any other diluent. • Add full contents of amp (250 mg/10 ml) to infusion bag provided (50 ml 0.9% NaCl). • Mix gently.

Rate of administration:

• Infuse over 60 min using extension line and infusion set provided. • Following administration, flush infusion set with 15–20 ml 0.9% NaCl over 30 sec to 15 min. • Discard entire infusion line.

IV INCOMPATIBILITIES ⊘

Note: Dilution compatibility other than 0.9% NaCl unknown. Do not mix with D_5W or lactated Ringer's. Do not give any medication in same bag of itraconazole or through same IV line. Not for IV bolus administration. Do not mix with any other medication.

INDICATIONS/ROUTES/DOSAGE

Note: Doses >200 mg is given in 2 divided doses.

Blastomycosis, histoplasmosis:

PO: Adults, elderly: Initially, 200 mg/day with food. May increase in 100 mg increments. **Maximum:** 400 mg/day.

Aspergillosis:

PO: Adults, elderly: 200–400 mg/day.

Onychomycosis:

PO: Adults, elderly: 200 mg/day for 12 consecutive wks or 200 mg twice daily for 1 wk; 3 wk rest period; repeat.

Life-threatening infection:

PO: Adults, elderly: Initially, 200 mg 3 times/day for 3 days as loading dose. **Maintenance:** 200–400 mg/day in 2 divided doses.

Oral candidiasis:

PO: Adults: 200 mg daily for 1–2 wks.

Esophageal candidiasis:

PO: Adults: 100–200 mg daily for 3 wks.

Usual IV dosage:

IV: Adults: 200 mg 2 times/day for 4 doses; then 200 mg/day. Infuse over 1 hr.

SIDE EFFECTS

FREQUENT (9–11%): Nausea, rash. ***OCCASIONAL*** (3–5%): Vomiting, headache, diarrhea, hypertension, headache, peripheral edema, fatigue, fever. ***RARE*** (≤2%): Abdominal pain, dizziness, anorexia, pruritus.

ADVERSE REACTIONS/TOXIC EFFECTS

Hepatitis (anorexia, abdominal pain, unusual tiredness/weakness, jaundice, dark urine) occurs rarely.

NURSING IMPLICATIONS

BASELINE ASSESSMENT:
Determine baseline temperature, liver function tests. Assess allergies.

INTERVENTION/EVALUATION:

Assess for signs and symptoms of liver dysfunction and monitor hepatic enzyme test results in pts with preexisting liver dysfunction.

PATIENT/FAMILY TEACHING:

Take capsules with food, solution on empty stomach. Therapy will continue for at least 3 mos and until lab tests and clinical presentation indicate infection is controlled. Report the following at once: unusual fatigue, yellow skin, dark urine, pale stool, anorexia/nausea/vomiting.

kanamycin sulfate

can-ah-**my**-sin
(Kantrex)

▶CLASSIFICATION

PHARMACOTHERAPEUTIC:
Aminoglycoside. *CLINICAL:*
Antibiotic

ACTION/THERAPEUTIC EFFECT

Irreversibly binds to protein on bacterial ribosome, *interfering in protein synthesis of susceptible microorganisms.*

USES

Treatment of wound and surgical site irrigation.

AVAILABILITY (Rx)

INJECTION: 1 g/3 ml.

INDICATIONS/ROUTES/DOSAGE

Irrigation:

Adults: 0.25% solution to irrigate

pleural space, ventricular or abscess cavities, wounds, or surgical sites.

SIDE EFFECTS

OCCASIONAL: Phlebitis; hypersensitivity reactions: rash, fever, urticaria, pruritus. *RARE:* Headache.

kaolin/pectin

kay-oh-lyn
(Kaopectate, Kapectolin)
Do not confuse with Kayexelate.

FIXED-COMBINATION(S)

With atropine, hyoscyamine, scopolamine, belladonna alkaloids, opium **(Donnagel PG, Kapectolin PG);** with opium **(Parepectolin)**

▶CLASSIFICATION

PHARMACOTHERAPEUTIC:
Magnesium/aluminum silicate.
CLINICAL: Antidiarrheal (see p. 41C)

ACTION/THERAPEUTIC EFFECT

Adsorbent, protectant *(adsorbs bacteria, toxins, reduces water loss).*

PHARMACOKINETICS

Not absorbed orally. Up to 90% of pectin decomposed in GI tract.

USES

Symptomatic treatment of mild to moderate acute diarrhea.

PRECAUTIONS

CONTRAINDICATIONS: None significant. *CAUTIONS:* None significant.

▷*LIFESPAN CONSIDERATIONS:*
Pregnancy/Lactation: Unknown if drug crosses placenta or is dis-

tributed in breast milk. **Pregnancy Category C. Children:** Not recommended in those <3 yrs of age. **Elderly:** More sensitive to fluid and electrolyte loss; use caution.

INTERACTIONS

DRUG: May decrease absorption of **digoxin. HERBAL:** None known. ***FOOD:*** None known. ***LAB VALUES:*** None significant.

AVAILABILITY (OTC)
ORAL SUSPENSION.

ADMINISTRATION/HANDLING
PO:
• Shake suspension well before administration.

INDICATIONS/ROUTES/DOSAGE
Antidiarrheal:

***PO:* Adults, elderly:** 60–120 ml after each loose bowel movement (LBM). **Children >12 yrs:** 60 ml after each LBM. **6–12 yrs:** 30–60 ml after each LBM. **3–6 yrs:** 15–30 ml after each LBM.

SIDE EFFECTS
RARE: Constipation.

ADVERSE REACTIONS/TOXIC EFFECTS
None significant.

NURSING IMPLICATIONS

INTERVENTION/EVALUATION:
Encourage adequate fluid intake. Assess bowel sounds for peristalsis. Assess stools for frequency and consistency (watery, loose, soft, semisolid, solid).

PATIENT/FAMILY TEACHING:
Do not use >2 days or with high fever.

---

kava kava

Also known as ava, kew, sakau, tonga, yagona
Note: May be removed from market.

►CLASSIFICATION
HERBAL

ACTION/*EFFECT*

Exact mechanism of action unknown, but possesses CNS effects, including *anxiolytic, sedative and analgesic.*

USES

Treatment of anxiety disorders, stress, and restlessness. Also used for sedation and sleep enhancement.

PRECAUTIONS

CONTRAINDICATIONS: Pregnancy, lactation (may cause loss of uterine tone). ***CAUTIONS:*** Depression, history of recurrent hepatitis.
▷*LIFESPAN CONSIDERATIONS:*
Pregnancy/Lactation: Contraindicated. **Children:** Safety and efficacy not established. **Elderly:** No age-related precautions noted.

INTERACTIONS

DRUG:* Alcohol, benzodiazepine** may increase risk of drowsiness. **HERBAL: Chamomile, goldenseal, melatonin, St. John's wort, ginseng, valerian** may increase risk of excessive drowsiness. ***FOOD: None significant. ***LAB VALUES:*** May increase liver function tests.

AVAILABILITY (OTC)

CAPSULES: 140 mg, 150 mg, 250 mg, 300 mg, 425 mg, 500 mg. ***LIQUID. EXTRACT. TINCTURE.***

INDICATIONS/ROUTES/DOSAGE

Anxiety:

PO: Adults, elderly: 100 mg 3 times/day or 1 cup of the tea 3 times/day.

SIDE EFFECTS

Gastrointestinal upset, headache, dizziness, vision changes (blurred vision, red eyes), allergic skin reactions, dermopathy (dry, flaky skin, yellowing of the eyes, skin, hair, nails), nausea, vomiting, weight loss, shortness of breath.

ADVERSE REACTIONS/TOXIC EFFECTS

None significant.

NURSING IMPLICATIONS

BASELINE ASSESSMENT

Assess if pregnant/breast-feeding (contraindicated). Determine baseline liver function tests. Assess for use of other CNS depressants.

INTERVENTION/EVALUATION

Monitor liver function tests. Assess for allergic skin reactions.

PATIENT/FAMILY TEACHING

Avoid use if pregnant, planning to become pregnant, or breast-feeding, children <12 yrs. Avoid driving, operating machinery. Avoid using for longer than 3 mos (may be habit forming).

ketamine hydrochloride

key-tah-meen
(Ketalar)

▶CLASSIFICATION

CLINICAL: Rapid-acting general anesthetic (see p. 2C)

ACTION/*THERAPEUTIC EFFECT*

Selectively blocks afferent impulses, interacts with CNS transmitter systems *producing an anesthetic state characterized by profound analgesia, normal pharyngeal-laryngeal reflexes.*

PHARMACOKINETICS

	Onset	Peak	Duration
IM	3–4 min	—	12–25 min
IV	15–30 sec	—	5–10 min

Rapidly distributed. Metabolized in liver. Primarily excreted in urine. Half-life: distribution: 10–15 min, elimination: 2–3 hrs.

USES

Sole anesthetic for short diagnostic and surgical procedures that do not require skeletal muscle relaxation. Induction of anesthesia prior to administering other general anesthetics. Used to supplement low-potency agents.

PRECAUTIONS

CONTRAINDICATIONS: Those in whom a significant increase in B/P would be hazardous, psychiatric disorders (schizophrenia, acute psychoses), known intolerance to drug. **CAUTIONS:** Hypertension, cardiac decompensation, chronic alcoholism, acute alcohol intoxication, debilitated, impaired respiratory, circulatory, renal, hepatic, endocrine function.

▷*LIFESPAN CONSIDERATIONS:* **Pregnancy/Lactation:** Not recommended; safety not established. **Pregnancy Category C.**

Children/Elderly: No age-related precautions noted.

INTERACTIONS

DRUG: Antihypertensives, CNS depressants may increase risk of hypotension or respiratory depression. **HERBAL:** None known. **FOOD:** None known. **LAB VALUES:** May increase intraocular pressure.

AVAILABILITY (Rx)

INJECTION: 10 mg/ml, 50 mg/ml, 100 mg/ml.

ADMINISTRATION/HANDLING

IM:

• Use 10 mg/ml vial.

IV 🔟

Reconstitution:

• For induction anesthesia using IV push, dilute 100 mg/ml with equal volume Sterile Water for Injection, D_5W, or 0.9% NaCl. • For maintenance IV infusion, dilute 50 mg/ml vial (10 ml) or 100 mg/ml vial (5 ml) to 250–500 ml D_5W or 0.9% NaCl to provide a concentration of 1–2 mg/ml.

Rate of administration:

• Administer IV push slowly over 60 sec (too rapid IV may produce severe hypotension, respiratory depression). • Administer IV infusion at rate of 0.5 mg/kg/min.

IV INCOMPATIBILITY ⊘

No information available via Y-site administration.

IV COMPATIBILITY

Propofol (Diprivan).

INDICATIONS/ROUTES/DOSAGE

Usual dosage:

IM: Adults, elderly: 3–8 mg/kg. **Children:** 3–7 mg/kg.

IV: Adults, elderly: 1–4.5 mg/kg. **Children:** 0.5–2 mg/kg.

SIDE EFFECTS

FREQUENT: Increase in B/P, pulse. Emergence reaction occurs frequently (12%), resulting in dreamlike state, vivid imagery, hallucination, delirium, occasionally with confusion, excitement, irrational behavior. Lasts from few hrs to 24 hrs after administration. **OCCASIONAL:** Pain at injection site. **RARE:** Rash.

ADVERSE REACTIONS/TOXIC EFFECTS

Continuous or repeated intermittent infusion may result in extreme somnolence, respiratory/circulatory depression. A too-rapid IV may produce marked severe hypotension, respiratory depression, irregular muscular movements.

K

NURSING IMPLICATIONS

BASELINE ASSESSMENT:

Resuscitative equipment, endotracheal tube, suction, O_2 must be available. Obtain vital signs before induction.

INTERVENTION/EVALUATION:

Monitor vital signs q3–5min during and after administration until recovery is achieved. Assess for emergence reaction (hypnotic/barbiturate may be needed). Keep verbal, tactile, visual stimulation at minimum during recovery.

PATIENT/FAMILY TEACHING:

Do not drive or operate machinery for 24 hrs after anesthesia.

ketoconazole

keet-oh-**con**-ah-zol
(Apo-Ketoconazole ✤, Nizoral,
Nizoral AD)
Do not confuse with Nasarel.

▶CLASSIFICATION

PHARMACOTHERAPEUTIC:
Imidizole derivative. **CLINICAL:**
Antifungal (see p. 42C)

ACTION/*THERAPEUTIC EFFECT*

Inhibits synthesis of ergosterol
(vital component of fungal cell formation), damaging fungal cell
membrane. *Fungistatic.*

USES/*UNLABELED*

Treatment of histoplasmosis, blastomycosis, candidiasis, chronic mucocutaneous candidiasis, coccidioidomycosis, paracoccidioidomycosis,
chromomycosis, seborrheic dermatitis, tineas (ringworm): corporis, capitis,
manus, cruris, pedis, unguium (onychomycosis), oral thrush, candiduria.
Shampoo: Reduces scaling due to
dandruff. Treatment of tinea versicolor.
Topical: Treatment of tineas, pityriasis
versicolor, cutaneous candidiasis, seborrheic dermatitis, dandruff. *Systemic:*
*Treatment of fungal pneumonia, sep-
ticemia, prostate cancer.*

PRECAUTIONS

CONTRAINDICATIONS: None
significant. **CAUTIONS:** Hepatic
impairment.

INTERACTIONS

**DRUG: Alcohol, hepatotoxic med-
ications** may increase hepatotoxicity. **Antacids, anticholinergics, H₂
antagonists, omeprazole** may decrease absorption (allow 2 hr interval). May increase concentration,
toxicity of **cyclosporine, lovas-**
tatin, simvastatin. Isoniazid, rifampin** may decrease concentration. **HERBAL: Echinacea** may
have additive hepatotoxic effects.
FOOD: None known. **LAB VALUES:**
May increase SGOT (AST), SGPT
(ALT), alkaline phosphatase, b: iliru-
bin. May decrease corticosteroid,
testosterone concentrations.

AVAILABILITY (Rx)

TABLETS: 200 mg. **CREAM:** 2%.
SHAMPOO: 2%, 1% (OTC).

ADMINISTRATION/HANDLING

PO:
• Give with food to minimize GI irritation. • Tablets may be crushed.
• Ketoconazole requires acidity;
give antacids, anticholinergics, H₂
blockers *at least* 2 hrs after dosing.

Shampoo:
• Apply to wet hair, massage for 1
min, rinse thoroughly, reapply for
3 min, rinse.

Topical:
• Apply and rub gently into af-
fected/surrounding area.

INDICATIONS/ROUTES/DOSAGE

Usual oral dosage:

Adults, elderly: 200–400 mg/day.
Children: 3.3–6.6 mg/kg/day.
Maximum: 800 mg/day in 2 di-
vided doses.

Usual topical dosage:

Adults, elderly: Apply 1–2 times/
day for 2–4 wks.

Dandruff:

SHAMPOO: Adults, elderly: 2
times/wk for 4 wks, allowing at
least 3 days between shampooing. Intermittent use to maintain
control.

SIDE EFFECTS

OCCASIONAL (3–10%): Nausea,

vomiting. ***RARE*** (<2%): Abdominal pain, diarrhea, headache, dizziness, photophobia, pruritus. Topical application may cause itching, burning, irritation.

ADVERSE REACTIONS/TOXIC EFFECTS

Hematologic toxicity occurs occasionally (thrombocytopenia, hemolytic anemia, leukopenia). Hepatotoxicity may occur within first week to several mos of therapy. Anaphylaxis occurs rarely.

NURSING IMPLICATIONS

BASELINE ASSESSMENT:

Confirm that a culture or histologic test was done for accurate diagnosis; therapy may begin before results known.

INTERVENTION/EVALUATION:

Monitor hepatic function tests; be alert for hepatotoxicity: dark urine, pale stools, fatigue, anorexia/nausea/vomiting (unrelieved by giving medication with food). Monitor CBC for evidence of hematologic toxicity. Determine pattern of bowel activity, stool consistency. Assess for dizziness and provide assistance as needed. Evaluate skin for rash, urticaria, itching. ***Topical:*** Check for local burning, itching, irritation.

PATIENT/FAMILY TEACHING:

Prolonged therapy (wks or mos) is usually necessary. Do not miss a dose; continue therapy as long as directed. Avoid alcohol (due to potential liver problem). Do not drive car, machinery if dizziness occurs. Take any antacids/antiulcer medications at least 2 hrs after ketoconazole. Notify physician of dark urine, pale stool, yellow skin/eyes, increased irritation in topical use, or onset of other new symptom. ***Topical:*** Rub well into affected areas. Avoid contact with eyes. Keep skin clean, dry; wear light clothing for ventilation. Separate personal items in direct contact with affected area. ***Shampoo:*** Initially use twice weekly for 4 wks with at least 3 days between shampooing; frequency then determined by response.

ketoprofen

key-toe-**pro**-fen
(Actron, Apo-Keto ♣, Orafen ♣, Orudis, Orudis KT, Oruvail, Rhodis ♣)

▶CLASSIFICATION

PHARMACOTHERAPEUTIC: Nonsteroidal anti-inflammatory. ***CLINICAL:*** Antirheumatic, analgesic, antidysmenorrheal, vascular headache suppressant (see p. 106C)

ACTION/*THERAPEUTIC EFFECT*

Produces analgesic and anti-inflammatory effect by inhibiting prostaglandin synthesis, *reducing inflammatory response and intensity of pain stimulus reaching sensory nerve endings.*

PHARMACOKINETICS

Rapid, complete absorption from GI tract. Protein binding: 99%. Primarily metabolized in liver, excreted in urine. Not removed by hemodialysis. Half-life: 1.5–4 hrs.

USES/*UNLABELED*

Symptomatic treatment of acute and chronic rheumatoid arthritis

K

and osteoarthritis. Relief of mild to moderate pain, primary dysmenorrhea. *Treatment of ankylosing spondylitis, psoriatic arthritis, acute gouty arthritis, vascular headache.*

PRECAUTIONS

CONTRAINDICATIONS: Active peptic ulcer, GI ulceration, chronic inflammation of GI tract, GI bleeding disorders, history of hypersensitivity to aspirin or NSAIDs. **CAUTIONS:** Impaired renal/hepatic function, history of GI tract disease, predisposition to fluid retention.

▷**LIFESPAN CONSIDERATIONS:**
Pregnancy/Lactation: Unknown if drug is distributed in breast milk. Avoid use during third trimester (may adversely affect fetal cardiovascular system: premature closure of ductus arteriosus). **Pregnancy Category B** (Category D if used in third trimester or near delivery). **Children:** Safety and efficacy not established. **Elderly:** GI bleeding or ulceration more likely to cause serious adverse effects. Age-related renal impairment may increase risk of liver or renal toxicity; decreased dosage recommended.

INTERACTIONS

DRUG: May increase effects of **oral anticoagulants, heparin, thrombolytics.** May decrease effect of **antihypertensives, diuretics. Salicylates, aspirin** may increase risk of GI side effects, bleeding. **Bone marrow depressants** may increase risk of hematologic reactions. May increase concentration, toxicity of **lithium.** May increase methotrexate toxicity. **Probenecid** may increase concentration. **HERBAL: Feverfew** effects may be decreased. **Ginkgo**

biloba may increase risk of bleeding. **FOOD:** None known. **LAB VALUES:** May prolong bleeding time. May increase alkaline phosphatase, LDH, liver function tests. May decrease sodium, hemoglobin, hematocrit.

AVAILABILITY (Rx)

TABLETS: (OTC): 12.5 mg. **CAPSULES:** 25 mg, 50 mg, 75 mg. **CAPSULES (extended-release):** 100 mg, 150 mg, 200 mg.

ADMINISTRATION/HANDLING

PO:
• May give with food, milk, or full glass (8 oz) water (minimizes potential GI distress). • Do not break, chew extended-release capsules.

INDICATIONS/ROUTES/DOSAGE

Note: Do not exceed 300 mg/day. Oruvail not recommended as initial therapy in pts who are small, >75 yrs of age, or renally impaired.

Acute and chronic rheumatoid arthritis, osteoarthritis:

PO: Adults: Initially, 75 mg three times/day or 50 mg four times/day. **Elderly:** Initially, 25–50 mg 3–4 times/day. **Maintenance:** 150–300 mg/day in 3–4 divided doses. *Extended-release:* 100–200 mg/day as single dose.

Mild to moderate pain, dysmenorrhea:

PO: Adults: 25–50 mg q6–8h.

SIDE EFFECTS

FREQUENT (11%): Dyspepsia (heartburn, indigestion, epigastric pain). **OCCASIONAL** (>3%): Nausea, diarrhea/constipation, flatulence, abdominal cramping, headache. **RARE** (<2%): Anorexia, vomiting, visual disturbances, fluid retention.

ADVERSE REACTIONS/TOXIC EFFECTS

Peptic ulcer, GI bleeding, gastritis, severe hepatic reaction (cholestasis, jaundice) occur rarely. Nephrotoxicity (dysuria, hematuria, proteinuria, nephrotic syndrome) and severe hypersensitivity reaction (bronchospasm, angiofacial edema) occur rarely.

NURSING IMPLICATIONS

BASELINE ASSESSMENT:

Assess onset, type, location, and duration of pain or inflammation. Inspect appearance of affected joints for immobility, deformities, skin condition.

INTERVENTION/EVALUATION:

Monitor for evidence of nausea, dyspepsia. Monitor pattern of daily bowel activity and stool consistency. Evaluate for therapeutic response: relief of pain, stiffness, swelling, increase in joint mobility, reduced joint tenderness, improved grip strength.

PATIENT/FAMILY TEACHING:

Avoid aspirin, alcohol during therapy (increases risk of GI bleeding). If GI upset occurs, take with food, milk. Swallow capsule whole; do not crush or chew.

ketorolac tromethamine

key-**tore**-oh-lack
(Acular, Acular PF, Toradol)
Do not confuse with Acthar.

▶CLASSIFICATION

PHARMACOTHERAPEUTIC:
Nonsteroidal anti-inflammatory.
CLINICAL: Analgesic, intraocular anti-inflammatory (see p. 107C)

ACTION/THERAPEUTIC EFFECT

Produces analgesic effect by inhibiting prostaglandin synthesis, *reducing intensity of pain stimulus reaching sensory nerve endings.* Reduces prostaglandin levels in aqueous humor, *reducing intraocular inflammation.*

PHARMACOKINETICS

	Onset	Peak	Duration
IM	10 min	1–2 hrs	4–6 hrs
IV	10 min	1–2 hrs	4–6 hrs

Readily absorbed from GI tract, after IM administration. Protein binding: >99%. Partially metabolized primarily in kidneys. Primarily excreted in urine. Not removed by hemodialysis. Half-life: 3.8–6.3 hrs (half-life increased with impaired renal function, in elderly).

USES/UNLABELED

Short-term relief of mild to moderate pain. **Ophthalmic:** Relief of ocular itching due to seasonal allergic conjunctivitis. Treatment postop for inflammation following cataract extraction, pain following incisional refractive surgery. **Ophthalmic:** *Prophylaxis/treatment of ocular inflammation.*

PRECAUTIONS

CONTRAINDICATIONS: Active peptic ulcer, GI ulceration, chronic inflammation of GI tract, GI bleeding disorders, history of hypersensitivity to aspirin or NSAIDs. **CAUTIONS:** Impaired renal/hepatic function, history of GI tract disease, predisposition to fluid retention.

▷**LIFESPAN CONSIDERATIONS:**
Pregnancy/Lactation: Unknown if drug is excreted in breast milk. Avoid use during third trimester (may adversely affect fetal cardiovascular system: premature closure of ductus arteriosus). **Pregnancy Category C** (Category D if used in third trimester). **Children:** Safety and efficacy not established, but doses of 0.5 mg/kg have been used. **Elderly:** GI bleeding or ulceration more likely to cause serious adverse effects. Age-related renal impairment may increase risk of liver or renal toxicity; decreased dosage recommended.

INTERACTIONS

DRUG: May increase effects of **oral anticoagulants, heparin, thrombolytics.** May decrease effect of **antihypertensives, diuretics. Salicylates, aspirin** may increase risk of GI side effects, bleeding. **Bone marrow depressants** may increase risk of hematologic reactions. May increase concentration, toxicity of **lithium.** May increase methotrexate toxicity. **Probenecid** may increase concentration. **HERBAL: Feverfew** effects may be decreased. **Ginkgo biloba** may increase risk of bleeding. **FOOD:** None known. **LAB VALUES:** May prolong bleeding time. May increase liver function tests.

AVAILABILITY (Rx)

TABLETS: 10 mg. **INJECTION:** 15 mg/ml, 30 mg/ml. **OPHTHALMIC SOLUTION:** 0.5%.

ADMINISTRATION/HANDLING

PO:
• Give with food, milk, or antacids if GI distress occurs.

IM:
• Give deep IM slowly into large muscle mass.

IV 🅦
• Give undiluted as IV push. • Give over at least 15 sec.

Ophthalmic:
• Place finger on lower eyelid and pull out until pocket is formed between eye and lower lid. Hold dropper above pocket and place prescribed number of drops in pocket. • Close eye gently. Apply digital pressure to lacrimal sac for 1–2 min (minimized drainage into nose and throat, reducing risk of systemic effects). • Remove excess solution with tissue.

IV INCOMPATIBILITY ⊘

No information available via Y-site administration.

INDICATIONS/ROUTES/DOSAGE

Note: Combined duration of IM/IV and PO not to exceed 5 days. May give as single dose, regular, or as needed schedule.

Analgesic (multiple dosing):

PO: Adults, elderly: 10 mg q4–6h. **Maximum:** 40 mg/24 hrs.

IV/IM: Adults <65 yrs: 30 mg q6h. **Maximum:** 120 mg/24 hrs. **>65 yrs, renally impaired, <50 kg:** 15 mg q6h. **Maximum:** 60 mg/24 hrs. **Children (2–16 yrs):** 0.5 mg/kg q6h.

Analgesic (single dose):

IM: Adults <65 yrs: 60 mg; **>65 yrs, renally impaired, <50 kg:** 30 mg. **Children (2–16 yrs):** 0.4–1 mg/kg.

IV: Adults <65 yrs: 30 mg; **>65 yrs, renally impaired, <50 kg:** 15 mg. **Children:** 0.4–1 mg/kg.

Usual ophthalmic dosage:
Adults, elderly: 1 drop 4 times/day.

SIDE EFFECTS

Note: Age increases possibility of side effects.

FREQUENT (12–17%): Headache, nausea, abdominal cramping/pain, dyspepsia (heartburn, indigestion, epigastric pain). **OCCASIONAL** (3–9%): Diarrhea. **Ophthalmic:** Transient stinging and burning. **RARE** (1–3%): Constipation, vomiting, flatulence, stomatitis. **Ophthalmic:** Ocular irritation, allergic reactions, superficial ocular infection, keratitis.

ADVERSE REACTIONS/TOXIC EFFECTS

GI bleeding, peptic ulcer occur infrequently. Nephrotoxicity (glomerular nephritis, interstitial nephritis, and nephrotic syndrome) may occur in those with preexisting impaired renal function. Acute hypersensitivity reaction (fever, chills, joint pain) occurs rarely.

NURSING IMPLICATIONS

BASELINE ASSESSMENT:

Assess onset, type, location, and duration of pain.

INTERVENTION/EVALUATION:

Monitor stool frequency, consistency. Evaluate for therapeutic response: relief of pain, stiffness, swelling, increase in joint mobility, reduced joint tenderness, improved grip strength. Be alert to signs of bleeding (may also occur with ophthalmic route due to systemic absorption).

PATIENT/FAMILY TEACHING:

Avoid aspirin, alcohol during therapy with oral or ophthalmic ketorolac (increases tendency to bleed). If GI upset occurs, take with food, milk. Avoid tasks that require alertness, motor skills until response to drug is established. **Ophthalmic:** Transient stinging and burning may occur upon instillation. Do not administer while wearing soft contact lenses.

ketotifen fumarate

key-**tow**-tih-fen
(Zaditor)

K

▶CLASSIFICATION

PHARMACOTHERAPEUTIC:
Ophthalmic decongestant agent.
CLINICAL: Antiallergic

ACTION/*THERAPEUTIC EFFECT*

Selective histamine H_1-antagonist and mast cell stabilizer, suppresses release of mediators from cells involved in hypersensitivity reactions, decreases chemotaxis and activation of eosinophils. *Reduces symptoms of allergic conjunctivitis.*

USES

Temporary relief of itching of the eye due to allergic conjunctivitis.

AVAILABILITY (Rx)

OPHTHALMIC SOLUTION: 0.025%.

INDICATIONS/ROUTES/DOSAGE

Allergic conjunctivitis:

OPHTHALMIC: Adults, elderly, children >3 yrs: 1 drop in affected eye q8–12hrs.

SIDE EFFECTS

FREQUENT (10–25%): Conjunctival infection, headache, rhinitis. **OCCASIONAL** (1–5%): Allergic reaction, burning, stinging, eyelid disorder, flulike syndrome, keratitis, mydriasis, ocular discharge/pain, pharyngitis, photophobia, rash.

labetolol hydrochloride

lah-**bet**-ah-lol
(Normodyne, Trandate)

FIXED-COMBINATION(S)

With hydrochlorothiazide, a diuretic **(Normozide)**
Do not confuse with Trental.

▶CLASSIFICATION

PHARMACOTHERAPEUTIC:
Alpha, beta-adrenergic blocker.
CLINICAL: Antihypertensive

ACTION/*THERAPEUTIC EFFECT*

Selectively blocks beta$_1$-adrenergic receptors, *slowing sinus heart rate, decreasing cardiac output, decreasing B/P* (exact mechanism unknown but may block peripheral adrenergic receptors, decrease sympathetic outflow from CNS or decrease renin release from kidney). Large dose blocks beta$_2$-adrenergic receptors, *increasing airway resistance.* Alpha blockage *causes vasodilation, decreased peripheral vascular resistance.*

PHARMACOKINETICS

	Onset	Peak	Duration
PO	0.5–2 hrs	2–4 hrs	8–12 hrs
IV	2–5 min	5–15 min	2–4 hrs

Completely absorbed from GI tract. Protein binding: 50%. Undergoes first-pass metabolism. Metabolized in liver. Primarily excreted in urine. Not removed by hemodialysis. Half-life: PO: 6–8 hrs; IV: 5.5 hrs.

USES/*UNLABELED*

Management of mild, moderate, severe hypertension. May be used alone or in combination with other antihypertensives. *Treatment of chronic angina pectoris; produces controlled hypotension during surgery.*

PRECAUTIONS

CONTRAINDICATIONS: Bronchial asthma, uncontrolled CHF, second-or third-degree heart block, severe bradycardia, cardiogenic shock. **CAUTIONS:** Drug-controlled CHF, nonallergic bronchospastic disease (chronic bronchitis, emphysema), impaired hepatic, cardiac function, pheochromocytoma, diabetes mellitus.

▷**LIFESPAN CONSIDERATIONS:**
Pregnancy/Lactation: Drug crosses placenta; small amount distributed in breast milk. **Pregnancy Category C** (Category D if used in second or third trimester). **Children:** Safety and efficacy not established. **Elderly:** Age-related peripheral vascular disease may increase susceptibility to decreased peripheral circulation.

INTERACTIONS

DRUG: Diuretics, other hypotensives may increase hypotensive effect; **sympathomimetics, xanthines** may mutually inhibit effects; may mask symptoms of hypoglycemia, prolong hypoglycemic effect of **insulin, oral hypoglycemics. MAO inhibitors** may produce hypertension.

HERBAL: None known. **FOOD:** None known. **LAB VALUES:** May increase ANA titer, SGOT (AST), SGPT (ALT), alkaline phosphatase, LDH, bilirubin, BUN, creatinine, potassium uric acid, lipoproteins, triglycerides.

AVAILABILITY (Rx)

TABLETS: 100 mg, 200 mg, 300 mg. **INJECTION:** 5 mg/ml.

ADMINISTRATION/HANDLING
PO:

• Give without regard to food. • Tablets may be crushed.

IV 🖾

Note: Pt must be in supine position for IV administration and for 3 hrs after receiving medication (substantial drop in B/P upon standing should be expected).

Storage:

• Store at room temperature. • After dilution, IV solution is stable for 24 hrs. • Solution appears clear, colorless to light yellow. • Discard if precipitate forms or discoloration occurs.

Reconstitution:

• For IV infusion, dilute 200 mg in 160 ml D_5W, 0.9% NaCl, lactated Ringer's or any combination thereof to provide concentration of 1 mg/ml.

Rate of administration:

• For IV push, give over 2 min at 10 min intervals. • For IV infusion, administer at rate of 2 mg/min (2 ml/min) initially. Rate is adjusted according to B/P. • Monitor B/P immediately before, and q5–10min during IV administration (maximum effect occurs within 5 min).

IV INCOMPATIBILITIES ⊘

Amphotericin B complex (Abel-cet, Ambisome, Amphotec), ceftriaxone (Rocephin), furosemide (Lasix), heparin, nafcillin (Nafcil), thiopental.

IV COMPATIBILITIES

Amiodarone (Cordarone), calcium gluconate, dobutamine (Dobutrex), dopamine (Intropin), lidocaine, lorazepam (Ativan), magnesium, midazolam (Versed), milrinone (Primacor), nitroglycerin, norepinephrine (Levophed), potassium chloride, propofol (Diprivan).

INDICATIONS/ROUTES/DOSAGE
Hypertension:

PO: Adults: Initially, 100 mg 2 times/day adjusted in increments of 100 mg 2 times/day q2–3days. **Maintenance:** 200–400 mg 2 times/day. **Maximum:** 2.4 g/day.

Usual elderly dosage:

PO: Initially, 100 mg 1–2 times/day. May increase as needed.

Severe hypertension, hypertensive emergency:

IV: Adults: Initially, 20 mg. Additional doses of 20–80 mg may be given at 10 min intervals, up to total dose of 300 mg.

IV INFUSION: Adults: Initially, 2 mg/min up to total dose of 300 mg.

PO: Adults: (after IV therapy): Initially, 200 mg; then, 200–400 mg in 6–12 hrs. Increase dose at 1 day intervals to desired level.

SIDE EFFECTS

FREQUENT: Drowsiness, trouble sleeping, unusually tired or weak, decreased sexual ability, transient scalp tingling. **OCCASIONAL:** Dizziness, difficulty breathing, swelling of hands/feet, depression, anxiety, constipation, diarrhea, nasal congestion, nausea, vomit-

L

ing, stomach discom-fort. **RARE:** Altered taste, dry eyes, increased urination, numbness or tingling in fingers, toes, or scalp.

ADVERSE REACTIONS/TOXIC EFFECTS

May precipitate or aggravate CHF (due to decreased myocardial stimulation). Abrupt withdrawal may precipitate ischemic heart disease, producing sweating, palpitations, headache, tremor. Beta-blockers may mask signs, symptoms of acute hypoglycemia (tachycardia, B/P changes) in diabetic pts.

NURSING IMPLICATIONS

BASELINE ASSESSMENT:

Assess baseline renal/liver function tests. Assess B/P, apical pulse immediately before drug is administered (if pulse is 60/min or below, or systolic B/P is below 90 mm Hg, withhold medication, contact physician).

INTERVENTION/EVALUATION:

Monitor B/P for hypotension. Assess pulse for strength/weakness, irregular rate, bradycardia. Monitor EKG for cardiac arrhythmias. Monitor stool frequency and consistency. Assist with ambulation if dizziness occurs. Assess for evidence of CHF: dyspnea (particularly on exertion or lying down), night cough, peripheral edema, distended neck veins. Monitor I&O (increase in weight, decrease in urine output may indicate CHF).

PATIENT/FAMILY TEACHING:

Do not discontinue drug except upon advice of physician (abrupt discontinuation may precipitate heart failure). Compliance with therapy regimen is essential to control hypertension, arrhythmias. Avoid tasks that require alertness, motor skills until response to drug is established. Report shortness of breath, excessive fatigue, weight gain, prolonged dizziness or headache. Do not use nasal decongestants, OTC cold preparations (stimulants) without physician approval.

lactulose

lack-tyoo-lows
(Acilac❧, Chronulac, Duphalac❧, Evalose, Heptalac, Kristalose, Laxilose❧)
Do not confuse with lactose.

▶**CLASSIFICATION**

PHARMACOTHERAPEUTIC: Lactose derivative. *CLINICAL:* Hyperosmotic laxative, ammonia detoxicant (see p. 101C)

ACTION/*THERAPEUTIC EFFECT*

Retains ammonia in colon (decreases blood ammonia concentration), producing osmotic effect. *Promotes increased peristalsis, bowel evacuation (expelling ammonia from colon).*

PHARMACOKINETICS

Onset	Peak	Duration
PO		
24–48 hrs	—	—
Rectal		
30–60 min	—	—

Poorly absorbed from GI tract. Acts in colon. Primarily excreted in feces.

USES

Prevention/treatment of portal systemic encephalopathy (including hepatic precoma, coma); treatment of constipation.

PRECAUTIONS

CONTRAINDICATIONS: Those on galactose-free diet, abdominal pain, nausea, vomiting, appendicitis. ***CAUTIONS:*** Diabetes mellitus.
▷***LIFESPAN CONSIDERATIONS:***
Pregnancy/Lactation: Unknown if drug crosses placenta or is distributed in breast milk. **Pregnancy Category B. Children:** Avoid use in children <6 yrs of age (usually unable to describe symptoms). **Elderly:** No age-related precautions noted.

INTERACTIONS

DRUG: May decrease transit time of concurrently administered **oral medication,** decreasing absorption. ***HERBAL:*** None known. ***FOOD:*** None known. ***LAB VALUES:*** May decrease potassium concentration.

AVAILABILITY (Rx)

SYRUP: 10 g/15 ml.

ADMINISTRATION/HANDLING

PO:

• Store solution at room temperature. • Solution appears pale yellow to yellow, sweet, viscous liquid. Cloudiness, darkened solution does not indicate potency loss. • Drink water, juice, or milk with each dose (aids stool softening, increases palatability).

Rectal:

• Lubricate anus with petroleum jelly before enema insertion. • Insert carefully (prevents damage to rectal wall) with nozzle toward navel. • Squeeze container until entire dose expelled. • Retain until definite lower abdominal cramping felt.

INDICATIONS/ROUTES/DOSAGE

Constipation:

PO: Adults, elderly: 15–30 ml/day up to 60 ml/day. **Children:** 7.5 ml/day after breakfast.

Portal-systemic encephalopathy:

PO: Adults, elderly: Initially, 30–45 ml every hr. Then, 30–45 ml 3–4 times/day. Adjust dose q1–2days to produce 2–3 soft stools/day. **Children:** 40–90 ml/day in divided doses. **Infants:** 2.5–10 ml/day in divided doses.

Usual rectal dosage (as retention enema):

Adults, elderly: 300 ml with 700 ml water or saline; retain 30–60 min; repeat q4–6hrs. (If evacuation occurs too promptly, repeat immediately.)

SIDE EFFECTS

OCCASIONAL: Cramping, flatulence, increased thirst, abdominal discomfort. ***RARE:*** Nausea, vomiting.

ADVERSE REACTIONS/TOXIC EFFECTS

Diarrhea indicates overdosage. Long-term use may result in laxative dependence, chronic constipation, loss of normal bowel function.

NURSING IMPLICATIONS

INTERVENTION/EVALUATION:

Encourage adequate fluid intake. Assess bowel sounds for peristalsis. Monitor daily bowel activity and stool consistency (watery, loose, soft, semisolid, solid) and record time of evacuation. Assess for abdominal disturbances. Monitor serum electrolytes in those exposed to prolonged, frequent, or excessive use of medication.

PATIENT/FAMILY TEACHING:

Evacuation occurs in 24–48 hrs of initial dose. Institute measures to promote defecation: Increase fluid intake, exercise, high-fiber diet.

lamivudine

lah-**mih**-view-deen
(Epivir, 3TC✦)
Do not confuse with lamotrigine.

FIXED-COMBINATIONS

With zidovudine, an antiviral **(Combivir),** with abacavir, and zidovudine, antivirals **(Trizivir)**

►CLASSIFICATION

PHARMACOTHERAPEUTIC: Nucleoside reverse transcriptase inhibitor. **CLINICAL:** Antiviral (see pp. 58C, 94C)

ACTION/*THERAPEUTIC EFFECT*

Inhibits HIV reverse transcriptase via viral DNA chain termination. Also inhibits RNA-and DNA-dependent DNA polymerase, an enzyme necessary for viral HIV replication, *slowing HIV replication, reducing progression of HIV infection.*

PHARMACOKINETICS

Rapidly, completely absorbed from GI tract. Protein binding: <36%. Widely distributed (crosses blood-brain barrier). Primarily excreted unchanged in urine. Not removed by hemo/peritoneal dialysis. Half-life: 11–15 hrs (intracellular); serum (adults) 2–11 hrs, (children) 1.7–2

hrs. Half-life increased with impaired renal function.

USES/*UNLABELED*

Used in combination with zidovudine for treatment of HIV infection when therapy is necessary based on clinical or immunologic evidence of disease. Treatment for chronic hepatitis B. *Prophylaxis in health-care workers at risk of acquiring HIV after occupational exposure to virus.*

PRECAUTIONS

CONTRAINDICATIONS: None significant. **CAUTIONS:** Peripheral neuropathy or history of peripheral neuropathy, history of pancreatitis in children, impaired renal function.

▷**LIFESPAN CONSIDERATIONS:**
Pregnancy/Lactation: Drug crosses placenta; unknown if distributed in breast milk. Breast feeding not recommended (possibility of HIV transmission). **Pregnancy Category C. Children:** Safety and efficacy not established in those <3 mos of age. **Elderly:** Age-related renal impairment may require dosage adjustment.

INTERACTIONS

DRUG: Trimethoprim-sulfamethoxazole increases lamivudine concentration. **HERBAL: St. John's wort** may decrease concentration, effect. **FOOD:** None known. **LAB VALUES:** May increase neutrophil count, SGOT (AST), SGPT (ALT), amylase serum level, hemoglobin.

AVAILABILITY (Rx)

TABLETS: 100 mg, 150 mg. **ORAL SOLUTION:** 5 mg/ml, 10 mg/ml.

ADMINISTRATION/HANDLING

PO:

* Give without regard to meals.

INDICATIONS/ROUTES/DOSAGE

Note: Complete prescribing information for zidovudine should be consulted before concurrent therapy with lamivudine and zidovudine is begun.

HIV infection:

PO: Adults, children 12–16 yrs, >50 kg (>100 lbs): 150 mg twice daily in combination with zidovudine. **Adults <50 kg:** 2 mg/kg twice daily in combination with zidovudine. **Children 3 mos–12 yrs:** 4 mg/kg twice daily (up to 150 mg) in combination with zidovudine.

Chronic hepatitis B:

PO: Adults, children ≥17 yrs: 100 mg daily. **Children <17 yrs:** 3 mg/kg/day. **Maximum:** 100 mg/day.

Dosage in renal impairment:

Dose and/or frequency is modified based on creatinine clearance.

Creatinine Clearance	Dosage
50	150 mg twice daily
30–49	150 mg once daily
15–29	150 mg first dose, then 100 mg once daily
5–14	150 mg first dose, then 50 mg once daily
<5	50 mg first dose, then 25 mg once daily

SIDE EFFECTS

FREQUENT: Headache (35%), nausea (33%), malaise/fatigue (27%), nasal disturbances (20%), diarrhea, cough (18%), musculoskeletal pain, neuropathy (12%), insomnia (11%), anorexia, dizziness, fever/chills (10%). *OCCASIONAL:* Depression, (9%), myalgia (8%), abdominal cramps (6%), dyspepsia, arthralgia (5%).

ADVERSE REACTIONS/TOXIC EFFECTS

Pancreatitis occurs in 13% of pediatric pts. Anemia, neutropenia, thrombocytopenia occur rarely.

NURSING IMPLICATIONS

BASELINE ASSESSMENT:

Establish baseline lab values, esp. renal function. Advise parents to closely monitor pediatric pts for symptoms of pancreatitis (severe, steady abdominal pain often radiating to the back, clammy skin, reduced B/P; nausea and vomiting may accompany abdominal pain).

INTERVENTION/EVALUATION:

Monitor amylase, lipase, BUN, serum creatinine. Assess for headache, nausea, cough. Determine pattern of bowel activity and stool consistency. Modify diet, or administer laxative as needed. Assess for dizziness, sleep pattern. If pancreatitis in children occurs, movement aggravates abdominal pain; sitting up or flexion at the waist relieves the pain.

PATIENT/FAMILY TEACHING:

Continue therapy for full length of treatment. Doses should be evenly spaced. Inform pt lamivudine is not a cure and pt may continue to experience illnesses, including opportunistic infections. Do not drive, use machinery, or engage in other activities that require mental acuity if experiencing dizziness.

L

lamotrigine

lam-**oh**-trih-geen
(Lamictal)
Do not confuse with
lamivudine.

▶CLASSIFICATION

CLINICAL: Anticonvulsant (see
p. 33C)

ACTION/*THERAPEUTIC EFFECT*

Exact mechanism unknown. May
be due to inhibition of voltage-
sensitive sodium channels, stabilizing neuronal membranes and
regulating presynaptic transmitter
release of excitatory amino acids,
producing anticonvulsant activity.

PHARMACOKINETICS

Rapidly, completely absorbed
following PO administration (not affected by food). Protein binding:
55%. Binds to melanin-containing
tissue (e.g., eye, pigmented skin).
Metabolized in liver. Primarily excreted unchanged in urine. Not removed by hemodialysis. Half-life:
7.5–12.5 hrs (half-life increased in
those receiving other anticonvulsants).

USES

Adjunctive therapy in adults with
partial seizures, adults and children in treatment of generalized
seizures of Lennox-Gastaut syndrome. Conversion to monotherapy in adults treated with another
enzyme-inducing antiepileptic
drug (EIAED).

PRECAUTIONS

CONTRAINDICATIONS: None
significant. **CAUTIONS:** Renal/he-
patic function impairment, cardiac
function impairment.

▷*LIFESPAN CONSIDERATIONS:*
Pregnancy/Lactation: Reduced
fetal weight, delayed ossification
noted in animals. Distributed in breast
milk. Breast feeding not recommended. **Pregnancy Category C.**
Children: No age-related precautions noted in those >2 yrs of age. **El-**
derly: Age-related renal impairment
may require dosage adjustment;
lower doses recommended.

INTERACTIONS

DRUG: May increase **carbamaze-**
pine, valproic acid serum levels.
Phenobarbital, primidone, phe-
nytoin, carbamazepine, valproic
acid decreases lamotrigine concentration. **HERBAL:** None known.
FOOD: None known. **LAB VALUES:**
None significant.

AVAILABILITY (Rx)

TABLETS: 25 mg, 100 mg, 150
mg, 200 mg. **CHEWABLE TAB-**
LETS: 2 mg, 5 mg, 25 mg.

ADMINISTRATION/HANDLING
PO:

• Give without regard to food.

INDICATIONS/ROUTES/DOSAGE

Note: If pt currently on valproic
acid, reduce lamotrigine dosage to
less than half the normal dosage.

Seizure control in pts receiving
enzyme-inducing antiepileptic
drugs (AEDs), but not valproate:
PO: Adults, elderly, children >12
yrs: Recommended as add-on
therapy: 50 mg once/day for 2
wks, followed by 100 mg/day in 2
divided doses for 2 wks. **Mainte-**
nance: Dose may be increased
by 100 mg/day every week, up to
300–500 mg/day in 2 divided
doses. **Children (2–12 yrs):** 0.6
mg/kg/day in 2 divided doses for
2 wks; then 1.2 mg/kg/day in 2 di-

vided doses for wks 3 and 4. **Maintenance:** 5–15 mg/kg/day. **Maximum:** 400 mg/day.

Seizure control in pts receiving combination therapy of valproic acid and enzyme-inducing antiepileptic drugs (AEDs):

PO: **Adults, elderly, children >12 yrs:** 25 mg every other day for 2 wks, followed by 25 mg once/day for 2 wks. **Maintenance:** Dose may be increased by 25–50 mg/day q1–2wks, up to 150 mg/day in 2 divided doses. **Children (2–12 yrs):** 0.15 mg/kg/day in 2 divided doses for 2 wks; then 0.3 mg/kg/day in 2 divided doses for wks 3 and 4. **Maintenance:** 1–5 mg/kg/day in 2 divided doses. **Maximum:** 200 mg/day.

Conversion to monotherapy:

PO: **Adults, children >12 yrs:** Add lamotrigine 50 mg/day for 2 wks; then 100 mg/day during wks 3 and 4; then increase by 100 mg/day q1–2wks until maintenance dosage achieved (300–500 mg/day in 2 divided doses/day). Gradually discontinue other EIAED over 4 wks once maintenance dose achieved.

Renal function impairment:

Note: Same dosage as combination therapy (see above).

Discontinuation therapy:

Note: A reduction in dosage over at least 2 wks (approx. 50% per week) is recommended.

SIDE EFFECTS

FREQUENT: Dizziness (38%), double vision (28%), headache (29%), ataxia [muscular incoordination] (22%), nausea (19%), blurred vision (16%), somnolence, rhinitis (14%). ***OCCASIONAL*** (5–10%): Rash, pharyngitis, vomiting, cough, flu syndrome, diarrhea, dysmenorrhea, fever, insomnia, dyspepsia. ***RARE:*** Constipation, tremor, anxiety, pruritus, vaginitis.

ADVERSE REACTIONS/TOXIC EFFECTS

Abrupt withdrawal may increase seizure frequency.

NURSING IMPLICATIONS

BASELINE ASSESSMENT:

Review history of seizure disorder (type, onset, intensity, frequency, duration, LOC), drug history (esp. other anticonvulsants), other medical conditions (e.g., renal function impairment). Provide safety precautions, quiet, dark environment.

INTERVENTION/EVALUATION:

Report to physician promptly if evidence of rash occurs (drug discontinuation may be necessary). Assist with ambulation if dizziness, ataxia occurs. Assess for clinical improvement (decrease in intensity/frequency of seizures). Assess for visual abnormalities, headache.

PATIENT/FAMILY TEACHING:

Take medication only as prescribed; do not abruptly withdraw medication after long-term therapy. Avoid tasks that require alertness, motor skills until response to drug is established. Avoid alcohol. Carry identification card/bracelet to note anticonvulsant therapy. Strict maintenance of drug therapy is essential for seizure control. If noncompliance is an issue in causing acute seizures, discuss reasons for noncompliance and address it. Report first sign of rash to physician.

L

lansoprazole

lan-sew-**prah**-zoll
(Prevacid)
Do not confuse with Pravachol,
Prevpac.

▶CLASSIFICATION

CLINICAL: Gastric acid pump
inhibitor (see p. 122C)

ACTION/THERAPEUTIC EFFECT

Converted to active metabolites that
irreversibly bind to and inhibit
H+/K+ ATPase (an enzyme on surface of gastric parietal cells). Inhibits hydrogen ion transport into
gastric lumen, *increasing gastric pH,
reducing gastric acid production.*

PHARMACOKINETICS

	Onset	Peak	Duration
15 mg	2–3 hrs	—	24 hrs
30 mg	1–2 hrs	—	>24 hrs

Once leaving stomach, rapid and
complete absorption (food may decrease absorption). Protein binding: 97%. Distributed primarily to
gastric parietal cells, converted to
two active metabolites. Extensively
metabolized in liver. Eliminated
from body in bile and urine. Not removed by hemodialysis. Half-life:
1.5 hrs (half-life increased in elderly, those with liver impairment).

USES

Short-term treatment (up to 4 wks)
for healing and symptomatic relief
of active duodenal ulcer, short-
term treatment (up to 8 wks) for
healing and symptomatic relief of
erosive esophagitis. Long-term
treatment of pathologic hypersecretory conditions including
Zollinger-Ellison syndrome. Short-
term treatment (up to 8 wks) of active gastric ulcer. *H. pylori*–associated duodenal ulcer, maintenance
treatment for healed duodenal
ulcer. Treatment for gastroesophageal reflux disease (GERD),
NSAID-associated gastric ulcer.

PRECAUTIONS

CONTRAINDICATIONS: None
significant. **CAUTIONS:** Impaired
hepatic function.
▷**LIFESPAN CONSIDERATIONS:**
Pregnancy/Lactation: Unknown
if distributed in breast milk. **Pregnancy Category B. Children:**
Safety and efficacy not established. **Elderly:** No age-related
precautions noted but doses >30
mg not recommended.

INTERACTIONS

DRUG: May interfere with **ketoconazole, ampicillin, iron salts,
digoxin** absorption. **Sucralfate**
may delay lansoprazole absorption
(give lansoprazole 30 min before
sucralfate). **HERBAL:** None known.
FOOD: None known. **LAB VALUES:**
May increase SGOT (AST), SGPT
(ALT), serum creatinine, alkaline
phosphatase, bilirubin, triglycerides, uric acid, LDH, cholesterol.
May produce abnormal WBC, RBC
and platelet counts, albumin/globu-
lin ratio, electrolyte balance. May
increase hematocrit, hemoglobin.

AVAILABILITY (Rx)

CAPSULES (extended-release): 15
mg, 30 mg. **ORAL SUSPENSION.**

ADMINISTRATION/HANDLING
PO:

• Give while fasting or before
meals (food diminishes absorption). • Do not chew or crush delayed-release capsules. • If pt has
difficulty swallowing capsules,
open capsules and sprinkle gran-

ules on 1 tablespoon of apple-sauce and swallow immediately.

INDICATIONS/ROUTES/DOSAGE
Duodenal ulcer:
PO: Adults, elderly: 15–30 mg/day, before eating, preferably in AM, for up to 4 wks.

Erosive esophagitis:
PO: Adults, elderly: 30 mg/day, before eating, for up to 8 wks. If healing does not occur within 8 wks (5–10%), may give for additional 8 wks.

Gastric ulcer:
PO: Adults: 30 mg/day for up to 8 wks.

Healed duodenal ulcer, GERD:
PO: Adults: 15 mg/day.

H. pylori:
PO: Adults: 30 mg 2 times/day for 10 days (with amoxicillin, clarithromycin).

Pathologic hypersecretory conditions (including Zollinger-Ellison syndrome):
PO: Adults, elderly: 60 mg/day. Individualize dosage according to pt needs and for as long as clinically indicated. May increase to >120 mg/day in divided doses.

Usual dosage for children:
3 mos–14 yrs, <10 kg: 7.5 mg; **10–20 kg:** 15 mg; **>20 kg:** 30 mg.

SIDE EFFECTS
OCCASIONAL (2–3%): Diarrhea, abdominal pain, rash, pruritus, altered appetite. ***RARE*** (1%): Nausea, headache.

ADVERSE REACTIONS/TOXIC EFFECTS
Bilirubinemia, eosinophilia, hyperlipemia occur rarely.

NURSING IMPLICATIONS

BASELINE ASSESSMENT:
Obtain baseline lab values. Assess drug history, esp. use of sucralfate.

INTERVENTION/EVALUATION:
Monitor ongoing laboratory results. Assess for therapeutic response, i.e., relief of GI symptoms. Question if diarrhea, abdominal pain, nausea occur.

PATIENT/FAMILY TEACHING:
Do not chew or crush delayed-release capsules. For those who have difficulty swallowing capsules, open capsules and sprinkle granules on 1 tablespoon of applesauce and swallow immediately.

---

latanoprost

See Classification section under: Antiglaucoma agents (p. 45C)

---

leflunomide

lee-**flew**-no-mide
(Arava)

▶CLASSIFICATION

PHARMACOTHERAPEUTIC: Immunomodulatory agent. ***CLINICAL:*** Anti-inflammatory

ACTION/*THERAPEUTIC EFFECT*

Extends the immune response exhibited in rheumatoid synovium, hinders proliferation of lymphocytes, possesses anti-inflammatory action. *Reduces signs and symptoms of rheumatoid arthritis and retards structural damage.*

PHARMACOKINETICS

Well absorbed following PO administration. Protein binding: >99%. Metabolized to active metabolite in GI wall and liver. Mechanisms of excretion include both renal and biliary systems. Not removed by hemodialysis. Half-life: 16 days.

USES

Treatment of active rheumatoid arthritis.

PRECAUTIONS

CONTRAINDICATIONS: Pregnancy or planning to become pregnant (Pregnancy Category X). ***CAUTIONS:*** Impaired hepatic/renal function, positive hepatitis B or C serology, those with immunodeficiency or bone marrow dysplasias, nursing mothers.
▷***LIFESPAN CONSIDERATIONS:*** **Pregnancy/Lactation:** Can cause fetal harm. Unknown if excreted in breast milk. Avoid use in nursing mothers. **Pregnancy Category X. Children:** Safety and efficacy not established in those <18 yrs of age. **Elderly:** No age-related precautions noted.

INTERACTIONS

DRUG: **Rifampin** increases concentration of leflunomide. ***HERBAL:*** None known. ***FOOD:*** None known. ***LAB VALUES:*** May increase liver enzymes (esp. ALT, AST).

AVAILABILITY (Rx)

TABLETS: 10 mg, 20 mg.

ADMINISTRATION/HANDLING
PO:

• Give without regard to food.

INDICATIONS/ROUTES/DOSAGE
Rheumatoid arthritis:

PO: Adults, elderly: Initially 100 mg daily for 3 days, then 10–20 mg daily.

SIDE EFFECTS

FREQUENT (10–20%): Diarrhea, respiratory tract infection, hair loss, rash, nausea.

ADVERSE REACTIONS/TOXIC EFFECTS

Transient thrombocytopenia and leukopenia occur rarely.

NURSING IMPLICATIONS

BASELINE ASSESSMENT:

Question for possibility of pregnancy (Pregnancy Category X). Assess limitations in activities of daily living due to rheumatoid arthritis.

INTERVENTION/EVALUATION:

Monitor tolerance to medication. Assess symptomatic relief of rheumatoid arthritis.

PATIENT/FAMILY TEACHING:

May take without regard to food. Improvement may take >8 wks.

lepirudin

leh-**pier**-ruh-din
(Refludan)

►CLASSIFICATION

PHARMACOTHERAPEUTIC: Thrombin inhibitor. ***CLINICAL:*** Anticoagulant

ACTION/*THERAPEUTIC EFFECT*
Inhibits thrombogenic action of

thrombin, *producing an increase in activated partial thromboplastin time (APTT)*. Action independent of antithrombin II and not inhibited by platelet factor 4.

PHARMACOKINETICS

Distributed primarily in extracellular fluid. Primarily eliminated by kidneys. Half-life 1.3 hrs (half-life increased with impaired renal function). Removed by hemodialysis.

USES

Anticoagulant in those with heparin-induced thrombocytopenia and associated thromboembolic disease to prevent further thromboembolic complications.

PRECAUTIONS

CONTRAINDICATIONS: None significant. **CAUTIONS:** Conditions associated with increased risk of bleeding (e.g., bacterial endocarditis, recent major bleeding, CVA, stroke, intracerebral surgery, hemorrhagic diathesis, severe hypertension, severe renal/liver function impairment, recent major surgery).

▷**LIFESPAN CONSIDERATIONS:** **Pregnancy/Lactation:** Unknown if distributed in breast milk or crosses placenta. **Pregnancy Category B. Children:** Safety and efficacy not established. **Elderly:** Age-related renal function impairment may require dosage adjustment.

INTERACTIONS

DRUG: Warfarin, platelet aggregation inhibitors, thrombolytics may increase risk of bleeding complications. **HERBAL: Ginkgo biloba** may increase risk of bleeding. **FOOD:** None known.

LAB VALUES: Increases APTT, thrombin time.

AVAILABILITY (Rx)

POWDER FOR INJECTION: 50 mg.

ADMINISTRATION/HANDLING

IV 🏧

Storage:
• Store unreconstituted vials at room temperature. • Reconstituted solution to be used immediately • IV infusion stable for up to 24 hrs at room temperature.

Reconstitution:
• Add 1 ml Sterile Water for Injection or 0.9% NaCl to 50 mg vial. • Shake gently. • Produces a clear, colorless solution (do not use if cloudy). • For IV push, further dilute by transferring to syringe and adding sufficient Sterile Water for Injection, 0.9% NaCl or D_5W to produce concentration of 5 mg/ml. • For IV infusion, add contents of 2 vials (100 mg) to 250 ml or 500 ml 0.9% NaCl or D_5W, providing a concentration of 0.4 or 0.2 mg/ml, respectively.

Rate of administration:
• Give IV push given over 15–20 sec. • Adjust IV infusion based on APTT or pt's body weight.

IV INCOMPATIBILITY ⊘

Do not mix with any other medication.

INDICATIONS/ROUTES/DOSAGE

Note: Give initial dose as soon as possible after surgery but not more than 24 hrs after surgery.

Anticoagulant:
Note: Dose adjusted according to APTT ratio with target range of 1.5–2.5 normal.

IV/IV INFUSION: **Adults, elderly:** 0.2–0.4 mg/kg, IV slowly over 15–20 sec, followed by IV infusion of 0.15 mg/kg/hr for 2–10 days or longer. **Note:** For pts >110 kg, maximum initial dose is 44 mg, with maximum rate of 16.5 mg/hr.

Dosage in renal impairment:

Initial dose decreased to 0.2 mg/kg with infusion rate adjusted based on creatinine clearance (Ccr)

Ccr (ml/min)	% of Standard Infusion Rate	Infusion Rate (mg/kg/hr)
45–60	50	0.075
30–44	30	0.045
15–29	15	0.0225

SIDE EFFECTS

FREQUENT (5–14%): Bleeding (from puncture sites/wound), hematuria, fever, GI and rectal bleeding. *OCCASIONAL* (1–3%): Epistaxis, allergic reaction (rash, pruritis, vaginal bleeding).

ADVERSE REACTIONS/TOXIC EFFECTS

Overdosage is characterized by excessively high APTT values. Intracranial bleeding occurs rarely. Abnormal liver function occurs in 6% of pts.

NURSING IMPLICATIONS

BASELINE ASSESSMENT:

Assess CBC, including platelet count. Determine initial B/P. Assess renal/liver function.

INTERVENTION/EVALUATION:

Monitor APTT diligently. Assess hematocrit, platelet count, urine/stool culture for occult blood, SGOT (AST), SGPT (ALT), renal function studies. Assess for decrease in B/P, increase in pulse rate, complaint of abdominal or back pain, severe headache (may be evidence of hemorrhage). Question for increase in amount of discharge during menses. Check peripheral pulses; skin for bruises, petechiae. Check for excessive bleeding from minor cuts, scratches. Assess gums for erythema, gingival bleeding. Assess urine output for hematuria.

PATIENT/FAMILY TEACHING:

Report bleeding, bruising, dizziness or lightheadedness, rash, itching, fever, swelling, breathing difficulty.

letrozole

leh-troe-zoll
(Femara)

▶CLASSIFICATION

PHARMACOTHERAPEUTIC: Aromatase inhibitor, hormone. *CLINICAL:* Antineoplastic (see p. 72C)

ACTION/*THERAPEUTIC EFFECT*

Decreases circulating estrogen by inhibiting aromatase, an enzyme that catalyzes the final step in estrogen production. Since growth of many breast cancers are stimulated by estrogens, *drug suppresses estrogen biosynthesis in hormonally responsive breast cancers.*

PHARMACOKINETICS

Rapidly and completely absorbed. Metbolized in liver. Primarily eliminated via the kidneys. Unknown if removed by hemodialysis. Half-life: approx. 2 days.

USES

Treatment of advanced breast cancer in postmenopausal women whose disease progressed after antiestrogen therapy. First-line treatment of advanced breast cancer.

PRECAUTIONS

CONTRAINDICATIONS: None significant. **CAUTIONS:** Renal or liver impairment.

▷**LIFESPAN CONSIDERATIONS:**
Pregnancy/Lactation: Unknown if distributed in breast milk. **Pregnancy Category D. Children:** Safety and efficacy not established. **Elderly:** No age-related precautions noted.

INTERACTIONS

DRUG: None significant. **HERBAL:** None known. **FOOD:** None known. **LAB VALUES:** May increase serum calcium cholesterol, ALT (SGPT), AST (SGOT), GGT.

AVAILABILITY (Rx)

TABLETS: 2.5 mg.

ADMINISTRATION/HANDLING
PO:

• Give without regard to food.

INDICATIONS/ROUTES/DOSAGE
Breast cancer:

PO: Adults, elderly: 2.5 mg daily. Continue until tumor progression is evident.

SIDE EFFECTS

FREQUENT (9–21%): Musculoskeletal pain (back, arm, leg), nausea, headache. **OCCASIONAL** (5–8%): Constipation, arthralgia, fatigue, vomiting, hot flashes, diarrhea, abdominal pain, cough, rash, anorexia, hypertension, peripheral edema. **RARE** (1–4%): Asthenia (loss of strength, energy), somnolence, dyspepsia (heartburn, indigestion, epigastric pain), weight increase, pruritus.

ADVERSE REACTIONS/TOXIC EFFECTS

None significant.

NURSING IMPLICATIONS

INTERVENTION/EVALUATION:

Monitor for and assist with ambulation if asthenia/dizziness occurs. Assess for headache. Offer antiemetic for nausea/vomiting. Monitor for evidence of musculoskeletal pain; offer analgesics for pain relief.

PATIENT/FAMILY TEACHING:

Notify physician if nausea, asthenia, hot flashes become unmanageable.

L

leucovorin calcium (folinic acid, citrovorum factor)

lou-**koe**-vor-in
(Lederle✤, Leucovorin✤, Wellcovorin)
Do not confuse with Wellbutrin, Wellferon.

▶CLASSIFICATION

PHARMACOTHERAPEUTIC: Folic acid antagonist. **CLINICAL:** Antidote

ACTION/THERAPEUTIC EFFECT

Competes with methotrexate for same transport processes into cells (limits methotrexate action on normal cells). *Allows purine, DNA, RNA, protein synthesis.*

PHARMACOKINETICS

Readily absorbed from GI tract. Widely distributed. Primarily concentrated in liver. Metabolized in liver, intestinal mucosa to active metabolite. Primarily excreted in urine. Half-life: 6.2 hrs.

USES/*UNLABELED*

Prophylzxis and treatment of methotrexate, pyrimethamine, trimethoprim toxicity. Treatment of folate-deficient megaloblastic anemia of infancy, sprue, pregnancy, colorectal carcinoma. *Treatment adjunct for head/neck carcinoma, Ewing's sarcoma, non-Hodgkin's lymphoma, gestational trophoblastic neoplasms.*

PRECAUTIONS

CONTRAINDICATIONS: Pernicious anemia, other megaloblastic anemias secondary to vitamin B_{12} deficiency. ***CAUTIONS:*** History of allergies, sprue, bronchial asthma. ***With 5-fluorouracil:*** Those with GI toxicities (more common/severe).

▷*LIFESPAN CONSIDERATIONS:* **Pregnancy/Lactation:** Unknown if drug crosses placenta or is distributed in breast milk. **Pregnancy Category C. Children:** May increase risk of seizures by counteracting anticonvulsant effects of barbiturate, hydantoins. **Elderly:** Age-related renal impairment may require dosage adjustment when used in rescue from effects of high-dose methotrexate therapy.

INTERACTIONS

DRUG: May decrease effect of **anticonvulsants.** May increase effect, toxicity of **5-fluorouracil.** ***HERBAL:*** None known. ***FOOD:*** None known. ***LAB VALUES:*** None significant.

AVAILABILITY (Rx)

TABLETS: 5 mg, 10 mg, 15 mg, 25 mg. ***INJECTION:*** 10 mg/ml. ***POWDER FOR INJECTION:*** 50 mg, 100 mg, 200 mg, 350 mg, 500 mg.

ADMINISTRATION/HANDLING
PO:

• Scored tablets may be crushed.

IV 🔳
Storage:

• Store vials for parenteral use at room temperature. • Injection appears as clear, yellowish solution. • Use immediately if reconstituted with Sterile Water for Injection; is stable for 7 days if reconstituted with Bacteriostatic Water for Injection.

Reconstitution:

• Reconstitute each 50 mg vial with 5 ml Sterile Water for Injection or Bacteriostatic Water for Injection containing benzyl alcohol to provide concentration of 10 mg/ml. • Due to benzyl alcohol in 1 mg ampule and in Bacteriostatic Water for Injection, reconstitute doses >10 mg/m^2 with Sterile Water for Injection. • Further dilute with D_5W or 0.9% NaCl.

Rate of administration:

• Do not exceed 160 mg/min if given by IV infusion (because of calcium content).

IV INCOMPATIBILITIES ⃠

Amphotericin B complex (Abelcet, Ambisome, Amphotec), droperidol (Inapsine), foscarnet (Foscavir).

IV COMPATIBILITIES

Etoposide (VP-16, Vepesid), fluorouracil, methotrexate.

INDICATIONS/ROUTES/DOSAGE

Antidote, prevention/treatment of hematopoietic effects of folic acid antagonists:

Note: For rescue therapy in cancer chemotherapy, refer to specific protocol being used for optimal dosage and sequence of leucovorin administration.

Conventional rescue dosage:

10 mg/m^2 parenterally one time then q6h orally until serum methotrexate <10^{-8}M. If 24 hr serum creatinine increased by 50% or more over baseline or methotrexate >5 × 10^{-6}M or 48 hr level >9 × 10^{-7}M, increase to 100 mg/m^2 IV q3h until methotrexate level <10^{-8}M.

Megaloblastic anemia:

IM: Adults: Up to 1 mg/day.

Advanced colorectal cancer:

IV: Adults: 200 mg/m^2 over minimum of 3 min (follow with 5-fluorouracil 370 mg/m^2 by IV injection) or 20 mg/m^2 (follow with 5-fluorouracil 425 mg/m^2). Repeat daily for 5 days; repeat cycle at 4 wk intervals for 2 cycles; then, at 4–5 wk intervals.

Note: Do not start next cycle until pt recovered from prior treatment course (until WBC are 4,000/mm^3 and platelets are 130,000/mm^3).

Pyrimethamine/ trimethoprim toxicity:

(Prevention): **IV/PO: Adults, elderly:** 0.4–5 mg with each dose of folic acid antagonist.

(Treatment): **PO: Adults, elderly, children:** 2–15 mg/day.

SIDE EFFECTS

FREQUENT: With 5-fluorouracil: Diarrhea, stomatitis, nausea, vomiting, lethargy/malaise/fatigue, alopecia, anorexia. **OCCASIONAL:** Urticaria, dermatitis.

ADVERSE REACTIONS/TOXIC EFFECTS

Excessive dosage may negate chemotherapeutic effect of folic acid antagonists. Anaphylaxis occurs rarely. Diarrhea may cause rapid clinical deterioration and death.

NURSING IMPLICATIONS

BASELINE ASSESSMENT:

Give as soon as possible, preferably within 1 hr, for treatment of accidental overdosage of folic acid antagonists.

INTERVENTION/EVALUATION:

Monitor for vomiting—may need to change from oral to parenteral therapy. Observe elderly and debilitated closely because of risk of severe toxicities. Assess CBC, differential, platelet count (also electrolytes and liver function tests for combination with 5-fluorouracil).

PATIENT/FAMILY TEACHING:

Explain purpose of medication in treatment of cancer. Report allergic reaction, vomiting.

leuprolide acetate

leu-pro-lied
(Lupron, Lupron Depot Ped)
Do not confuse with Lopurin, Nuprin.

▶CLASSIFICATION

PHARMACOTHERAPEUTIC: Gonadotropin-releasing hormone analog. **CLINICAL:** Antineoplastic (see p. 72C, 87C)

ACTION/*THERAPEUTIC EFFECT*

Initial or intermittent administration stimulates release of luteinizing hormone (LH) and follicle-stimulating hormone (FSH) from anterior pituitary, increasing (within 1 wk) testosterone level in males, estradiol in premenopausal women. Continuous daily administration suppresses secretion of gonadotropin-releasing hormone, *producing fall (within 2–4 wks) in testosterone levels to castrate level in males, estrogen level in premenopausal women to postmenopausal levels. In central precocious puberty, gonadotropins reduced to prepubertal levels.*

PHARMACOKINETICS

Rapidly, well absorbed after SubQ administration. Slow absorption after IM administration. Protein binding: 7–15%. Half-life: 3–4 hrs.

USES

Treatment of advanced prostatic carcinoma, endometriosis, central precocious puberty, uterine fibroid tumors, anemia caused by uterine leiomyomata.

PRECAUTIONS

CONTRAINDICATIONS: None significant. ***EXTREME CAUTION:*** Pts with life-threatening disease when rapid symptomatic relief is necessary. ***CAUTIONS:*** Hypersensitivity to benzyl alcohol. Risk of osteoporosis in men treated for prostate cancer.

▷***LIFESPAN CONSIDERATIONS:*** **Pregnancy/Lactation:** *Depot:* Contraindicated in pregnancy. May cause spontaneous abortion. **Pregnancy Category X. Children/Elderly:** No age-related precautions noted.

INTERACTIONS

DRUG: None significant. ***HERBAL:*** None known. ***FOOD:*** None known. ***LAB VALUES:*** May increase serum acid phosphatase. Initially increases testosterone, then decreases testosterone concentration.

AVAILABILITY (Rx)

INJECTION: 5 mg/ml. ***LYPHOLIZED MICROSPHERES FOR INJECTION:*** 3.75 mg, 7.5 mg, 11.25 mg, 15 mg, 22.5 mg, 30 mg.

ADMINISTRATION/HANDLING

Note: May be carcinogenic, mutagenic, or teratogenic. Handle with extreme care during preparation/administration.

SubQ:

• Injection appears clear, colorless. • Refrigerate. • Store opened vial at room temperature. • Discard if precipitate forms or solution appears discolored. • *Depot vials:* Store at room temperature. Reconstitute only with diluent provided; use immediately. Do not use needles <22 gauge. • Use syringes provided by manufacturer (0.5 ml low-dose insulin syringe may be used as alternative).

INDICATIONS/ROUTES/DOSAGE

Prostatic carcinoma:

SᴜʙQ: **Adults, elderly:** 1 mg daily.

IM: Adults, elderly: *Depot:* 7.5 mg q28–33days or 22.5 mg q3mos or 30 mg q4mos.

Endometriosis, uterine leiomyomata:

IM: Adults: *Depot:* 3.75 mg monthly or 11.25 mg as single injection.

Central precocious puberty:

SᴜʙQ: **Children:** Initially, 35–50 mcg/kg/day; if down regulation not achieved, titrate upward by 10 mcg/kg/day.

IM: Children: Initially, 0.15–0.3 mg/kg/4 wks (minimum: 7.5 mg); if down regulation not achieved, titrate upward in 3.75 mg increments q4wks.

SIDE EFFECTS

FREQUENT: Hot flashes (ranging from mild flushing to sweating). **Females:** Amenorrhea, spotting. **OCCASIONAL:** Arrhythmias, palpitations, blurred vision, dizziness, edema, headache, burning/itching, swelling at injection site, nausea, insomnia, increased weight. **Females:** Deepening voice, increased hair growth, decreased libido, increased breast tenderness, vaginitis, altered mood. **Males:** Constipation, decreased testicle size, gynecomastia, impotence, decreased appetite, angina. **RARE: Males:** Thrombophlebitis.

ADVERSE REACTIONS/TOXIC EFFECTS

Occasionally, a worsening of signs/ symptoms of prostatic carcinoma occurs 1–2 wks after initial dosing (subsides during continued therapy). Increased bone pain and less frequently dysuria or hematuria, weakness or paresthesia of lower extremities may be noted. Myocardial infarction, pulmonary embolism occur rarely.

NURSING IMPLICATIONS

BASELINE ASSESSMENT:

Question for possibility of pregnancy before initiating therapy (Pregnancy Category X). Obtain serum testosterone, prostatic acid phosphatase (PAP) levels periodically during therapy.

Serum testosterone and PAP levels should increase during first week of therapy. Testosterone level then should decrease to baseline level or less within 2 wks, PAP level within 4 wks.

INTERVENTION/EVALUATION:

Monitor for arrhythmias, palpitations. Assess for peripheral edema behind medial malleolus (sacral area in bedridden pts). Assess sleep pattern. Monitor for visual difficulties. Assist with ambulation if dizziness occurs. Offer antiemetics if nausea occurs.

PATIENT/FAMILY TEACHING:

Hot flashes tend to decrease during continued therapy. A temporary exacerbation of signs/ symptoms of disease may occur during first few wks of therapy. Use contraceptive measures during therapy. Inform physician if regular menstruation persists, become pregnant.

levalbuterol

lee-val-**bwet**-err-all
(Xopenex)
Do not confuse with Xanax.

▶CLASSIFICATION

PHARMACOTHERAPEUTIC: Sympathomimetic. **CLINICAL:** Bronchodilator (see p. 63C)

ACTION/THERAPEUTIC EFFECT

Stimulates beta$_2$-adrenergic receptors in the lungs resulting in relaxation of bronchial smooth muscle. *Relieves bronchospasm, reduces airway resistance.*

PHARMACOKINETICS

Onset	Peak	Duration
Inhalation		
10–17 min	1.5 hrs	5–6 hrs

USES

Treatment and prevention of brochospasm due to reversible obstructive airway disease.

PRECAUTIONS

CONTRAINDICATIONS: History hypersensitivity to sympathomimetics. **CAUTIONS:** Cardiovascular disorders (e.g., cardiac arrhythmias), seizures, hypertension, diabetes mellitus.

▷**LIFESPAN CONSIDERATIONS:**
Pregnancy/Lactation: Crosses placenta; unknown if distributed in breast milk. **Pregnancy Category C. Children:** Safety and efficacy not established in those <12 yrs of age. **Elderly:** Lower initial doses recommended.

INTERACTIONS

DRUG: Beta-adrenergic blocking agents (beta-blockers) antagonize effects. May increase risk of arrhythmias with **digoxin. MAO inhibitors, tricyclic antidepressants** may potentiate cardiovascular effects. **HERBAL: Ma Huang (Ephedra)** may increase CNS stimulation. **FOOD:** None known. **LAB VALUES:** May increase potassium.

AVAILABILITY (Rx)

SOLUTION FOR NEBULIZATION:
0.63 mg in 3 ml vials; 1.25 mg in 3 ml vials.

ADMINISTRATION/HANDLING
Nebulization:

• No diluent necessary. • Protect from light/excessive heat. Store at room temperature. • Once foil is opened, use within 2 wks. • Discard if solution is not colorless. • Do not mix with other medications. • Give over 5–15 min.

INDICATIONS/ROUTES/DOSAGE
Bronchospasm:

NEBULIZATION: Adults, children >12 yrs: 0.63–1.25 mg q6–8hrs (three times/day). **Maximum:** 1.25 mg three times/day.

Elderly: 0.63 mg q6–8 hrs (three times/day).

SIDE EFFECTS

FREQUENT: Tremor, nervousness, headache, throat dryness/irritation. **OCCASIONAL:** Dry, irritated mouth or throat, coughing, bronchial irritation. **RARE:** Drowsiness, diarrhea, dry mouth, flushing, sweating, anorexia.

ADVERSE REACTIONS/TOXIC EFFECTS

Excessive sympathomimetic stimulation may produce palpitations, extrasystoles, tachycardia, chest pain, slight increase in B/P followed by substantial decrease, chills, sweating, blanching of skin. Too frequent or excessive use may lead to loss of bronchodilating effectiveness and/or severe, paradoxical bronchoconstriction.

NURSING IMPLICATIONS

BASELINE ASSESSMENT:

Offer emotional support (high incidence of anxiety due to difficulty in breathing and sympathomimetic response to drug).

INTERVENTION/EVALUATION:

Monitor rate, depth, rhythm, type of respiration; quality and rate of pulse, EKG, serum potassium,

ABG determinations. Assess lung sounds for wheezing (bronchoconstriction) and rales.

PATIENT/FAMILY TEACHING:
Increase fluid intake (decreases lung secretion viscosity). Rinsing mouth with water immediately after inhalation may prevent mouth/throat dryness. Avoid excessive use of caffeine derivatives (chocolate, coffee, tea, cola, cocoa).

levetiracetam

leave-ty-rah-**see**-tam
(Keppra)

►CLASSIFICATION
CLINICAL: Anticonvulsant

ACTION/THERAPEUTIC EFFECT
Inhibits burst firing without affecting normal neuronal excitability, *preventing seizure activity.*

USES
Adjunctive therapy in treatment of partial onset seizures in adults with epilepsy.

PRECAUTIONS
CONTRAINDICATIONS: Hypersensitivity reaction. ***CAUTIONS:*** Renal function impairment.

INTERACTIONS
DRUG: None significant. ***HERBAL:*** None significant. ***FOOD:*** None significant. ***LAB VALUES:*** May increase Hgb/Hct, RBC, WBC.

AVAILABILITY (Rx)
TABLETS: 250 mg, 500 mg, 750 mg.

INDICATIONS/ROUTES/DOSAGE
Partial onset seizures:
PO: Adults, elderly: Initially, 500 mg q12hrs. May increase by 1,000 mg/day q2wks. **Maximum:** 3,000 mg/day.

Dosage in renal impairment:

Creatinine Clearance (ml/min)	Dosage
80	500–1500 mg q12hrs
50–80	500–1000 mg q12hrs
30–50	250–750 mg q12hrs
<30	250–500 mg q12hrs
ESRD using dialysis	500–1000 mg q12hrs (following dialysis, a 250–500 mg supplemental dose is recommended).

SIDE EFFECTS
FREQUENT (10–15%): Somnolence, asthenia (loss of strength, energy), headache, infection. ***OCCASIONAL*** (3–9%): Dizziness, pharyngitis, pain, depression, nervousness, vertigo, rhinitis, anorexia. ***RARE*** (<3%): Amnesia, anxiety, emotional lability, cough, sinusitis, anorexia, diplopia.

ADVERSE REACTIONS/TOXIC EFFECTS
None significant.

NURSING IMPLICATIONS

BASELINE ASSESSMENT:
Assess for hypersensitivity to levetiractem, renal function.

INTERVENTION/EVALUATION:
Monitor renal function

PATIENT/FAMILY TEACHING:
Use caution driving or performing tasks requiring alertness (may

cause dizziness/somnolence). Do not discontinue abruptly.

levobunolol hydrochloride

(Betagan Liquifilm)

See Classification section under: Antiglaucoma agents (p. 46C)

levobupivacaine

(Chirocaine)

See Classification section under: Local anesthetics (p. 5C)

levofloxacin

leave-oh-**flocks**-ah-sin (Levaquin, Quixin)

►CLASSIFICATION

PHARMACOTHERAPEUTIC: Fluoroquinolone. **CLINICAL:** Antibiotic (see p. 22C)

ACTION/*THERAPEUTIC EFFECT*

Inhibits the DNA enzyme, gyrase, in susceptible microorganisms, interfering with bacterial DNA replication and repair, *producing bactericidal activity.*

PHARMACOKINETICS

Well absorbed following both PO and IV administration. Protein binding: 24–38%. Penetrates rapidly and extensively into leuko-cytes, epithelial cells, and macrophages. Lung concentrations are 2–5 times higher than those of plasma. Eliminated unchanged in the urine. Partially removed by hemodialysis. Half-life: 8 hrs.

USES

Treatment of acute bacterial exacerbation of chronic bronchitis, community-acquired pneumonia, acute maxillary sinusitis, complicated urinary tract infections, acute pyelonephritis, uncomplicated mild to moderate skin and skin-structure infections. *Ophthalmic:* Treatment superficial infections to conjunctiva or cornea.

PRECAUTIONS

CONTRAINDICATIONS: History of hypersensitivity to fluoroquinolone, antibiotics, cinoxacin, nalidixic acid. **CAUTIONS:** Impaired renal/hepatic function, diabetes mellitus.

▷*LIFESPAN CONSIDERATIONS:* **Pregnancy/Lactation:** Excreted in breast milk. Avoid use in pregnancy. **Pregnancy Category C. Children:** Safety and efficacy not established in those <18 yrs of age. **Elderly:** Age-related renal impairment may require dosage adjustment.

INTERACTIONS

DRUG: Antacids, sucralfate, iron preparations decrease levofloxacin absorption. **NSAIDs** may increase risk of CNS stimulation/seizures. **HERBAL:** None known. **FOOD:** None known. **LAB VALUES:** May alter blood glucose concentrations.

AVAILABILITY (Rx)

TABLETS: 250 mg, 500 mg, 750 mg. **INJECTION:** 500 mg/20 ml vials. **PREMIX:** 250 mg/50 ml, 500 mg/100 ml, 750 mg/100 ml. ***OPH-THALMIC SOLUTION:*** 0.5%.

ADMINISTRATION/HANDLING
PO:
• Do not administer antacids (aluminum, magnesium), sucralfate, iron and multivitamin preparations with zinc within 2 hrs of levofloxacin administration (significantly reduces levofloxacin absorption). • Encourage use of cranberry juice, citrus fruits (acidifies urine). • Give without regard to food.

IV 🎇
Storage:
• Available in single-dose 20 ml (500 mg) vials and premixed with D_5W; ready to infuse.

Reconstitution:
• For infusion using single-dose vial, withdraw desired amount (10 ml for 250 mg, 20 ml for 500 mg). Dilute each 10 ml (250 mg) with minimum 40 ml 0.9% NaCl, D_5W, D_5W/0.9% NaCl, D_5W/lactated Ringer's, plasma-lyte 56/D_5W, D_5W/0.45% NaCl, 0.15% KCl, or sodium lactate.

Rate of administration:
• Administer slowly, over not less than 60 min.

Ophthalmic:
• Place finger on lower eyelid and pull out until a pocket is formed between eye and lower lid. Hold dropper above pocket and place correct number of drops into pocket. • Close eye gently. Apply digital pressure to lacrimal sac for 1–2 min (minimizes drainage into nose and throat, reducing risk of systemic effects).

IV INCOMPATIBILITY ⊘
No information available via Y-site administration.

IV COMPATIBILITIES
Dobutamine (Dobutrex), dopamine (Intron), lidocaine, lorazepam (Ativan).

INDICATIONS/ROUTES/DOSAGE
Bronchitis:
PO/IV: **Adults, elderly:** 500 mg q24h for 7 days.

Pneumonia:
PO/IV: **Adults, elderly:** 500 mg q24h for 7–14 days.

Acute maxillary sinusitis:
PO/IV: **Adults, elderly:** 500 mg q24h for 10–14 days.

Skin, skin-structure:
PO/IV: **Adults, elderly:** 500 mg q24h for 7–10 days.

Urinary tract infection, acute pyelonephritis:
PO/IV: **Adults, elderly:** 250 mg q24h for 10 days.

Dosage in renal impairment:
Bronchitis, pneumonia, sinusitis, skin, skin-structure infections:

Creatinine Clearance	Dosage
50–80 ml/min	No change
20–49 ml/min	500 mg initially, then 250 mg q24h
10–19 ml/min	500 mg initially, dialysis then 250 mg q48h

Urinary tract infection, pyelonephritis:

Creatinine Clearance	Dosage
20 ml/min	No change
10–19 ml/min	250 mg initially, then 250 mg q48h

Bacterial conjunctivitis:
OPHTHALMIC: **Adults, elderly, children <1 yr:** 1–2 drops q2h for

2 days (up to 8 times/day), then 1–2 drops q4h for 5 days.

SIDE EFFECTS

OCCASIONAL (1–3%): Diarrhea, nausea, stomach pain, dizziness, drowsiness, headache, lightheadedness. ***Ophthalmic:*** Local burning/discomfort, margin crusting, crystals/scales, foreign body sensation, itching, bad taste. ***RARE*** (<1%): Flatulence, taste perversion, pain, inflammation or swelling in calves, hands, or shoulder. ***Ophthalmic:*** Corneal staining, keratitis, allergic reaction, lid edema, tearing, reduced vision.

ADVERSE REACTIONS/TOXIC EFFECTS

Pseudomembranous colitis (severe abdominal pain/cramps, severe watery diarrhea, fever) may occur. Superinfection (genital-anal pruritus, ulceration or changes in oral mucosa, moderate to severe diarrhea) may occur. Hypersensitivity reactions, including photosensitivity (rash, pruritus, blistering, swelling, sensation of skin burning), have occurred in those receiving fluoroquinolone therapy.

NURSING IMPLICATIONS

BASELINE ASSESSMENT:
Question for hypersensitivity to levofloxacin or other fluoroquinolones.

INTERVENTION/EVALUATION:
Report hypersensitivity reaction: skin rash, urticaria, pruritus, photosensitivity promptly. Be alert for superinfection (e.g., genital-anal pruritus, ulceration or changes in oral mucosa, moderate to severe diarrhea, new or increased fever). Provide symptomatic relief for nausea. Evalu-

ate food tolerance, change in taste sensation.

PATIENT/FAMILY TEACHING:
Continue medication for full length of treatment. Check with physician if no improvement within a few days. Discontinue at first sign of skin rash or other allergic reaction. ***Ophthalmic:*** Do not touch eyelids or surrounding areas with dropper tip of bottle.

levorphanol tartrate

leh-**vor**-phan-ole
(Levo-Dromoran)

▶CLASSIFICATION

PHARMACOTHERAPEUTIC:
Opioid agonist **(Schedule II).**
CLINICAL: Narcotic analgesic (see p. 116C)

ACTION/*THERAPEUTIC EFFECT*

Binds at opiate receptor sites in CNS. *Reduces intensity of pain stimuli incoming from sensory nerve endings, altering pain perception and emotional response to pain.*

USES

Relief of moderate to severe pain. Used preoperatively to produce sedation, and as adjunct with nitrous oxide/O_2 anesthesia.

PRECAUTIONS

CONTRAINDICATIONS: None significant. ***EXTREME CAUTION:*** CNS depression, anoxia, hypercapnia, respiratory depression, seizures, acute alcoholism, shock, untreated myxedema, respiratory dysfunction. ***CAUTIONS:*** Increased intracranial pressure, impaired hepatic function, acute abdominal conditions, hypothyroidism, prostatic hypertrophy, Addison's disease, urethral stricture, COPD.

INTERACTIONS

DRUG: Alcohol, CNS depressants may increase CNS or respiratory depression, hypotension. **MAO inhibitors** may produce severe, fatal reaction (reduce dose to usual $1/4$ dose). **HERBAL:** None known. **FOOD:** None known. **LAB VALUES:** May increase amylase, lipase plasma concentrations.

AVAILABILITY (Rx)

TABLETS: 2 mg. **INJECTION:** 2 mg/ml.

INDICATIONS/ROUTES/DOSAGE

Note: Reduce initial dosage in those with hypothyroidism, Addison's disease, renal insufficiency, elderly/debilitated, those on concurrent CNS depressants.

PO/SubQ: Adults, elderly: 2 mg. May be increased to 3 mg, if needed.

IV: Adults: Optimum dosage not established.

SIDE EFFECTS

Note: Effects are dependent on dosage amount, route of administration. Ambulatory pts and those not in severe pain may experience dizziness, nausea, vomiting, hypotension more frequently than those in supine position or having severe pain.

FREQUENT: Dizziness, drowsiness, hypotension, nausea, vomiting. **OCCASIONAL:** Shortness of breath, confusion, decreased urination, stomach cramps, altered vision, constipation, dry mouth,

headache, difficult or painful urination. **RARE:** Allergic reaction (rash, itching), histamine reaction (decreased B/P, increased sweating, flushed face, wheezing).

ADVERSE REACTIONS/TOXIC EFFECTS

Overdosage results in respiratory depression, skeletal muscle flaccidity, cold clammy skin, cyanosis, extreme somnolence progressing to convulsions, stupor, coma. Tolerance to analgesic effect, physical dependence may occur with repeated use. Paralytic ileus may occur with prolonged use.

NURSING IMPLICATIONS

BASELINE ASSESSMENT:

Pt should be in a recumbent position before drug is administered by parenteral route. Assess onset, type, location, and duration of pain. Obtain vital signs before giving medication. If respirations are 12/min or lower (20/min or lower in children), withhold medication, contact physician.

INTERVENTION/EVALUATION:

Monitor vital signs after parenteral administration for decreased B/P, a change in rate or quality of pulse, decreased respirations. Assess for adequate voiding, possible constipation. Assess therapeutic response and contact physician if pain relief is inadequate.

PATIENT/FAMILY TEACHING:

Promptly report recurrence of pain (effect of medication is reduced if full pain recurs before next dose). Tolerance/dependence may occur with prolonged use of high doses.

L

levothyroxine 🖊

lee-voe-thye-**rox**-een
(Eltroxin, Levotec✚, Levothroid,
Levoxyl, Synthroid, Unithroid)
Do not confuse with
liothyronine.

FIXED-COMBINATION(S)
With liothyronine, T₃ **(Thyrolar)**

► CLASSIFICATION

PHARMACOTHERAPEUTIC:
Synthetic isomer of thyroxine.
CLINICAL: Thyroid hormone
(T₄) (see p. 126C)

ACTION/THERAPEUTIC EFFECT

Involved in normal metabolism,
growth and development (esp.
CNS of infants). Possesses catabolic and anabolic effects. *Increases basal metabolic rate, enhances gluconeogenesis, stimulates
protein synthesis.*

PHARMACOKINETICS

Variable, incomplete absorption
from GI tract. Protein binding:
>99%. Widely distributed. Deiodi-
nated in peripheral tissues, minimal metabolism in liver. Eliminated by biliary excretion.
Half-life: 6–7 days.

USES

Replacement in decreased or absent thyroid function (partial or
complete absence of gland, primary atrophy, functional deficiency, effects of surgery, radiation
or antithyroid agents, pituitary or
hypothalamic hypothyroidism);
management of simple (nontoxic)
goiter and chronic lymphocytic
thyroiditis; treatment of thyrotoxicosis (with antithyroid drugs) to
prevent goitrogenesis and hypothyroidism. Management of thyroid cancer. Diagnostic in thyroid
suppression tests.

PRECAUTIONS

CONTRAINDICATIONS: Thyrotoxicosis and myocardial infarction
uncomplicated by hypothy-
roidism, hypersensitivity to any
component (with tablets: tartrazine, allergy to aspirin, lactose
intolerance), treatment of obesity.
CAUTIONS: Elderly, angina pectoris, hypertension or other cardiovascular disease.

▷ **LIFESPAN CONSIDERATIONS:**
Pregnancy/Lactation: Drug
does not cross placenta; minimal
excretion in breast milk. **Pregnancy Category A. Children:** No
age-related precautions noted.
Caution in neonates in interpret-
ing thyroid function tersts. **Elderly:** May be more sensitive to
thyroid effects; individualized
dosage recommended.

INTERACTIONS

DRUG: May alter effect of **oral anticoagulants. Cholestyramine,
colestipol** may decrease absorption. **Sympathomimetics** may increase effects, coronary insufficiency. **HERBAL:** None known.
FOOD: None known. **LAB VALUES:**
None significant.

AVAILABILITY (Rx)

TABLETS: 0.025 mg, 0.05 mg,
0.075 mg, 0.088 mg, 0.1 mg, 0.112
mg, 0.125 mg, 0.137 mg, 0.15 mg,
0.175 mg, 0.2 mg, 0.3 mg. **INJEC-
TION:** 200 mcg, 500 mcg.

ADMINISTRATION/HANDLING

Note: Do not interchange brands
because there have been problems with bioequivalence between manufacturers.

🖊 - see color pill atlas

PO:

• Give at same time each day to maintain hormone levels. • Administer before breakfast to prevent insomnia. • Tablets may be crushed.

IV 💉

Storage:

• Store vials at room temperature.

Reconstitution:

• Reconstitute 200 mcg or 500 mcg vial with 5 ml 0.9% NaCl to provide a concentration of 40 or 100 mcg/ml, respectively; shake until clear.

Rate of administration:

• Use immediately and discard unused portions. • Give each 100 mcg or less over 1 min.

IV INCOMPATIBILITIES ⊘

Do not use or mix with other IV solutions.

INDICATIONS/ROUTES/DOSAGE

Note: Begin therapy with small doses; gradually increase.

Hypothyroidism:

PO: **Adults, elderly:** Initially, 0.05 mg/day. Increase by 0.025 mg q2–3wks. **Maintenance:** 0.1–0.2 mg/day.

Myxedema coma or stupor (medical emergency):

IV: **Adults, elderly:** Initially, 0.4 mg. Follow with daily supplements of 0.1–0.2 mg. **Maintenance:** 0.05–0.1 mg/day.

Thyroid suppression therapy:

PO: **Adults, elderly:** 2–6 mcg/kg/day for 7–10 days.

TSH suppression in thyroid cancer, nodules, euthyroid goiters:

PO: **Adults, elderly:** Use larger doses than that used for replacement therapy.

Congenital hypothyroidism:

PO: **Children >12 yrs:** >0.15 mg/day; **Children 6–12 yrs:** 0.1–0.15 mg/day; **Children 1–5 yrs:** 0.075–0.1 mg/day; **Children 6–12 mos:** 0.05–0.075 mg/day; **Infants 0–6 mos:** 0.025–0.05 mg/day.

Usual parenteral dosage:

IV: **Adults, elderly, children:** Initial dosage approximately one-half the previously established oral dosage.

SIDE EFFECTS

OCCASIONAL: Children may have reversible hair loss upon initiation. ***RARE:*** Dry skin, GI intolerance, skin rash, hives, pseudotumor cerebri (severe headache in children).

ADVERSE REACTIONS/TOXIC EFFECTS

Excessive dosage produces signs/symptoms of hyperthyroidism: weight loss, palpitations, increased appetite, tremors, nervousness, tachycardia, increased B/P, headache, insomnia, menstrual irregularities. Cardiac arrhythmias occur rarely.

NURSING IMPLICATIONS

BASELINE ASSESSMENT:

Question for hypersensitivity to tartrazine, aspirin, lactose. Obtain baseline weight, vital signs. Signs and symptoms of diabetes mellitus, diabetes insipidus, adrenal insufficiency, hypopituitarism may become intensified. Treat with adrenocortical steroids prior to thyroid therapy in coexisting hypothyroidism and hypoadrenalism.

INTERVENTION/EVALUATION:

Monitor pulse for rate, rhythm (report pulse of 100 or marked increase). Assess for tremors, nervousness. Check appetite and sleep pattern.

PATIENT/FAMILY TEACHING:

Do not discontinue; replacement for hypothyroidism is lifelong. Follow-up office visits and thyroid function tests are essential. Take medication at the same time each day, preferably in the morning. Monitor pulse, report marked increase, pulse of 100 or above, change of rhythm. Do not change brands. Notify physician promptly of chest pain, weight loss, nervousness or tremors, insomnia. Children may have reversible hair loss or increased aggressiveness during the first few mos of therapy. Full therapeutic effect may take 1–3 wks.

lidocaine hydrochloride

lie-doe-cane
(LidoPen, Xylocaine, Xylocard✦, Zilactin-L✦)

FIXED-COMBINATION(S)

With epinephrine, a sympathomimetic **(Lidocaine with Epinephrine, Xylocaine with Epinephrine)**

▶**CLASSIFICATION**

PHARMACOTHERAPEUTIC: Amide anesthetic. *CLINICAL:* Antiarrhythmic, anesthetic (see pp. 5C, 12C)

ACTION/*THERAPEUTIC EFFECT*

Anesthetic: Inhibits conduction of nerve impulses, *causing tempo-rary loss of feeling and sensation.* *Antiarrhythmic:* Decreases depolarization, automaticity, excitability of ventricle during diastole by direct action, *reversing ventricular arrhythmias.*

PHARMACOKINETICS

Onset	Peak	Duration
IV		
30–90 sec	—	10–20 min
Local anesthetic		
2.5 min	—	30–60 min

Completely absorbed after IM administration. Protein binding: 60–80%. Widely distributed. Metabolized in liver. Primarily excreted in urine. Minimally removed by hemodialysis. Half-life: 1–2 hrs.

USES

Antiarrhythmic: Rapid control of acute ventricular arrhythmias following myocardial infarction, cardiac catheterization, cardiac surgery, digitalis-induced ventricular arrhythmias. *Local anesthetic:* Infiltration or nerve block for dental or surgical procedures, childbirth. *Topical anesthetic:* Local skin disorders (minor burns, insect bites, prickly heat, skin manifestations of chickenpox, abrasions). Mucous membranes (local anesthesia of oral, nasal, and laryngeal mucous membranes, respiratory or urinary tracts; relieves discomfort of pruritus ani, hemorrhoids, pruritus vulvae). *Dermal patch:* Treatment of shingles-related skin pain.

PRECAUTIONS

CONTRAINDICATIONS: Hypersensitivity to amide-type local anesthetics, Adams-Stokes syndrome, supraventricular arrhythmias, Wolff-Parkinson-White syndrome. Spinal anesthesia contraindicated in septicemia. ***CAUTIONS:*** Dosage should be reduced for elderly, debilitated, acutely ill; safety in children not established. Severe renal/hepatic disease, hypovolemia, CHF, shock, heart block, marked hypoxia, severe respiratory depression, bradycardia, incomplete heart block. Anesthetic solutions containing epinephrine should be used with caution in peripheral or hypertensive vascular disease, and during or following potent general anesthesia. Sulfite sensitivity or asthma for some local and topical anesthetic preparations. Tartrazine or aspirin sensitivity with some topical preparations.

▷***LIFESPAN CONSIDERATIONS:***
Pregnancy/Lactation: Crosses placenta; distributed in breast milk. **Pregnancy Category C. Children:** No age-related precautions noted. **Elderly:** More sensitive to adverse effects. Dose and rate of infusion should be reduced. Age-related renal impairment may require dosage adjustment.

INTERACTIONS

DRUG: May increase cardiac effects with **other antiarrhythmics. Anticonvulsants** may increase cardiac depressant effects. **Beta-adrenergic blockers** may increase risk of toxicity. ***HERBAL:*** None known. ***FOOD:*** None known. ***LAB VALUES:*** IM lidocaine may increase CPK level (used in diagnostic test for presence of acute MI). Therapeutic blood serum level: 1.5–6 mcg/ml; toxic blood serum level: >6 mcg/ml.

AVAILABILITY (Rx)

INJECTION: IM: 300 mg/3 ml. ***DIRECT IV:*** 10 mg/ml, 20 mg/ml. ***IV***
ADMIXTURE: 40 mg/ml, 100 mg/ml, 200 mg/ml. ***IV INFUSION:*** 2 mg/ml, 4 mg/ml, 8 mg/ml. ***INJECTION (anesthesia):*** 0.5%, 1%, 1.5%, 2%, 4%.

TOPICAL: LIQUID: 2.5%, 5%. ***OINTMENT:*** 2.5%, 5%. ***CREAM:*** 0.5%. ***GEL:*** 0.5%, 2.5%. ***SPRAY:*** 0.5%. ***SOLUTION:*** 2%, 4%. ***JELLY:*** 2%. ***DERMAL PATCH:*** 5%.

ADMINISTRATION/HANDLING

Note: Resuscitative equipment and drugs (including O_2) must always be readily available when administering lidocaine by any route.

IM:

• Use 10% (100 mg/ml); clearly identify lidocaine that is *for IM use.*
• Give in deltoid muscle (blood level is significantly higher than if injection is given in gluteus muscle or lateral thigh).

IV 🔟

Note: Use only lidocaine without preservative, clearly marked *for IV use.*

Storage:

• Store at room temperature.

Reconstitution:

• For IV infusion, prepare solution by adding 1 g to 1 L D_5W to provide concentration of 1 mg/ml (0.1%). • Commercially available preparations of 0.2%, 0.4%, and 0.8% may be used for IV infusion. Maximum concentration: 4 g/250 ml.

Rate of administration:

• For IV push, use 1% (10 mg/ml) or 2% (20 mg/ml). • Administer IV push at rate of 25–50 mg/min. • Administer for IV infusion at rate of 1–4 mg/min (1–4 ml); use volume control IV set.

Topical:

• Not for ophthalmic use. • For skin disorders, apply directly to affected area or put on gauze or bandage, which is then applied to the skin. • For mucous membrane use, apply to desired area using manufacturer's insert. • Administer the lowest dose possible that still provides anesthesia.

IV INCOMPATIBILITIES $\oslash$

Amphotericin B complex (Abelcet, Ambisome, Amphotec), thiopental.

IV COMPATIBILITIES

Amiodarone (Cordarone), calcium gluconate, diltiazem (Cardizem), dobutamine (Dobutrex), dopamine (Intropin), enalapril (Vasotec), haloperidol (Haldol), labetalol (Normodyne, Trandate), potassium, propofol (Diprivan).

INDICATIONS/ROUTES/DOSAGE

Ventricular arrhythmias:

***IM:* Adults, elderly:** 300 mg (or 4.3 mg/kg). May repeat in 60–90 min.

***IV:* Adults, elderly:** Initially, 50–100 mg (1 mg/kg) IV bolus at rate of 25–50 mg/min. May repeat in 5 min. Give no more than 200–300 mg in 1 hr. **Maintenance:** 20–50 mcg/kg/min (1–4 mg/min) as IV infusion. **Children, infants:** Initially, 0.5–1 mg/kg IV bolus; may repeat but total dose not to exceed 3–5 mg/kg. **Maintenance:** 10–50 mcg/kg/min as IV infusion.

Usual local anesthetic dosage:

Dose varies with procedure, degree of anesthesia, vascularity, duration. **Maximum dose:** 4.5 mg/kg. Do not repeat within 2 hrs.

Usual topical dosage:

TOPICAL:* Adults, elderly:** Apply to affected areas as needed. ***DERMAL PATCH: Apply to intact skin over most painful area (up to 3 patches once for up to 12 hrs in a 24 hr period).

SIDE EFFECTS

CNS effects generally dose related and of short duration. ***OCCASIONAL: IM:*** Pain at injection site. ***Topical:*** Burning, stinging, tenderness. ***RARE:*** Generally with high dose: Drowsiness, dizziness, disorientation, lightheadedness, tremors, apprehension, euphoria, sensation of heat/cold/numbness, blurred/double vision, ringing/roaring in ears (tinnitus), nausea.

ADVERSE REACTIONS/TOXIC EFFECTS

Although serious adverse reactions to lidocaine are uncommon, high dosage by any route may produce cardiovascular depression: bradycardia, somnolence, hypotension, arrhythmias, heart block, cardiovascular collapse, cardiac arrest. Potential for malignant hyperthermia. CNS toxicity may occur, esp. with regional anesthesia use, progressing rapidly from mild side effects to tremors, convulsions, vomiting, respiratory depression. Methemoglobinemia (evidenced by cyanosis) has occurred following topical application of lidocaine for teething discomfort and laryngeal anesthetic spray. Overuse of oral lidocaine has caused seizures in children. Allergic reactions are rare.

NURSING IMPLICATIONS

BASELINE ASSESSMENT:

Question for hypersensitivity to lidocaine, amide anesthetics.

Obtain baseline B/P, pulse, respirations, EKG, and electrolytes.

INTERVENTION/EVALUATION:

Monitor EKG, vital signs closely during and after drug is administered for cardiac performance. If EKG shows arrhythmias, prolongation of PR interval or QRS complex, inform physician immediately. Assess pulse for irregularity, strength/weakness, bradycardia. Assess B/P for evidence of hypotension. Monitor for therapeutic serum level (1.5–6 mcg/ml). For lidocaine given by all routes, monitor vital signs and pt's state of consciousness. Drowsiness should be considered a warning sign of high blood levels of lidocaine. Therapeutic blood serum level: 1.5–6 mcg/ml; toxic blood serum level: >6 mcg/ml.

PATIENT/FAMILY TEACHING:

Local anesthesia: Assure that pt understands loss of feeling, sensation and need for protection until anesthetic wears off (e.g., no ambulation, including special positions for some regional anesthesia; not chewing gum, eating, or drinking following administration to oral area, etc.). **Topical anesthesia:** Do not eat, drink, or chew gum for 1 hr following application (swallowing reflex may be impaired increasing risk of aspiration; numbness of tongue or buccal mucosa may lead to biting trauma).

linezolid

lyn-eh-**zoe**-lid
(Zyvox)
Do not confuse with Vioxx.

▶**CLASSIFICATION**

PHARMACOTHERAPEUTIC: Oxalodinone. ***CLINICAL:*** Antibiotic

ACTION/*THERAPEUTIC EFFECT*

Binds to a site on bacterial 23S ribosomal RNA, preventing formation of complex that is an essential component of bacterial translation process. *Bacteriostatic against Enterococci and Staphylococci, bactericidal against streptococci.*

PHARMACOKINETICS

Rapidly, extensively absorbed following PO administration. Protein binding: Low. Metabolized in liver by oxidation. Excreted in urine. Half-life: 4–5.4 hrs.

USES

Treatment of vancomycin-resistant *Enterococcus faecium* (VRE) infections, nosocomial pneumonia, uncomplicated/complicated skin/skin structure infections, community-acquired pneumonia (CAP).

PRECAUTIONS

CONTRAINDICATIONS: None significant. ***CAUTIONS:*** Renal function impairment.
▷***LIFESPAN CONSIDERATIONS:***
Pregnancy/Lactation: Unknown if distributed in breast milk. **Children:** Safety and efficacy not established. **Elderly:** No age-related precautions noted.

INTERACTIONS

DRUG: Decreases effect of **MAOIs. Adrenergic agents (sympathomimetics)** increase effect. ***HERBAL:*** None known. ***FOOD:*** None known. ***LAB VALUES:*** May decrease platelets, hemoglobin, WBC, ALT (SGPT).

AVAILABILITY (Rx)

TABLETS: 400 mg, 600 mg. **POWDER FOR RECONSTITUTION (oral):** 100 mg/5 ml. **INJECTION:** 2 mg/ml in 100 ml, 200 ml, 300 ml bags.

ADMINISTRATION/HANDLING

PO:

• Give without regard to meals. • Use suspension within 21 days after reconstitution.

IV 💹

Storage:

• Store at room temperature • Protect from light. • Yellow color does not affect potency.

Rate of administration:

• Infuse over 30–120 min.

IV INCOMPATIBILITIES ⊘

Do not mix with other medications. If same line is used, flush with compatible fluid (D_5W, 0.9% NaCl, lactated Ringer's). Amphotericin B complex (Abelcet, Ambisome, Amphotec), chlorpromazine (Thorazine), diazepam (Valium), erythromycin (Erythrocin), pentamidine (Pentam IV), phenytoin (Dilantin), sulfamethoxazole-trimethoprim (Bactrim).

INDICATIONS/ROUTES/DOSAGE

VRE:

PO/IV: Adults: 600 mg q12hrs for 14–28 days.

Nosocomial pneumonia, CAP, complicated skin infections:

PO/IV: Adults: 600 mg q12hrs for 10–14 days.

Uncomplicated skin infections:

PO/IV: Adults: 400 mg q12hrs for 10–14 days.

SIDE EFFECTS

OCCASIONAL (2–5%): Diarrhea, nausea, headache. **RARE** (<2%): Taste alteration, vaginal candidiasis (itching, discharge), fungal infection, dizziness, tongue discoloration.

ADVERSE REACTIONS/TOXIC EFFECTS

Thrombocytopenia occurs rarely. Myelosuppression. Antibiotic-associated colitis (severe abdominal pain and tenderness, fever, watery and severe diarrhea) may result from altered bacterial balance.

NURSING IMPLICATIONS

INTERVENTION/EVALUATION:

Monitor bowel activity and stool consistency carefully; mild GI effects may be tolerable, but increasing severity may indicate onset of antibiotic-associated colitis. Be alert for superinfection: severe genital/anal pruritus, abdominal pain, severe mouth soreness, moderate to severe diarrhea. Monitor CBC weekly.

PATIENT/FAMILY TEACHING:

Continue therapy for full length of treatment. Doses should be evenly spaced. May cause GI upset (may take with food or milk).

liothyronine ✳

lye-oh-**thigh**-roe-neen
(Cytomel)
Do not confuse with levothyroxine.

FIXED-COMBINATION(S)

With levothyroxine, T_4 **(Thyrolar)**

▶CLASSIFICATION

PHARMACOTHERAPEUTIC: Synthetic form thyroid hormone T_3. **CLINICAL:** Thyroid hormone (see p. 126C)

ACTION/*THERAPEUTIC EFFECT*

Involved in normal metabolism, growth and development (esp. CNS of infants). Possesses catabolic and anabolic effects. *Increases basal metabolic rate, enhances gluconeogenesis, stimulates protein synthesis.*

USES

PO: Replacement in decreased or absent thyroid function (partial or complete absence of gland, primary atrophy, functional deficiency, effects of surgery, radiation or antithyroid agents, pituitary or hypothalamic hypothyroidism). Management of simple (nontoxic) goiter; diagnostically in T_3 suppression test (differentiates hyperthyroidism from euthyroidism). *IV:* Myxedema coma, precoma.

PRECAUTIONS

CONTRAINDICATIONS: Thyrotoxicosis and MI uncomplicated by hypothyroidism, treatment of obesity. ***CAUTIONS:*** Elderly, angina pectoris, hypertension, or other cardiovascular disease.

INTERACTIONS

DRUG: May alter effect of **oral anticoagulants. Cholestyramine, colestipol** may decrease absorption. **Sympathomimetics** may increase effects, coronary insufficiency. ***HERBAL:*** None known. ***FOOD:*** None known. ***LAB VALUES:*** None significant.

AVAILABILITY (Rx)

TABLETS: 5 mcg, 25 mcg, 50 mcg. ***INJECTION:*** 10 mcg/ml.

INDICATIONS/ROUTES/DOSAGE
Hypothyroidism:

PO: **Adults:** Initially, 25 mcg/day. Increase by 12.5–25 mcg q1–

2wks. **Elderly:** Initially, 5 mcg/day. May increase by 5 mcg/day q1–2wks. **Maintenance:** 25–75 mcg/day. **Children:** 5 mcg/day. May increase by 5 mcg q1–2wks. **Maintenance:** 15–20 mcg/day.

Myxedema:

PO: **Adults, elderly:** Initially, 5 mcg/day. Increase by 5–10 mcg q1–2wks (after 25 mcg/day reached, may increase by 12.5 mcg increments). **Maintenance:** 50–100 mcg/day.

Nontoxic goiter:

PO: **Adults, elderly:** Initially, 5 mcg/day. Increase by 5–10 mcg/day q1–2wks. When 25 mcg/day obtained, may increase by 12.5–25 mcg/day q1–2wks. **Maintenance:** 75 mcg/day. **Children:** 5 mcg/day. May increase by 5 mcg q1–2wks. **Maintenance:** 15–20 mcg/day.

Congenital hypothyroidism:

PO: **Children:** Initially, 5 mcg/day. Increase by 5 mcg/day q3–4days. **Maintenance: (Infants):** 20 mcg/day. **(1 yr):** 50 mcg/day. **(>3 yrs):** Full adult dosage.

T_3 suppression test:

PO: **Adults, elderly:** 75–100 mcg/day for 7 days, then repeat I^{131} thyroid uptake test.

Myxedema coma, precoma:

Note: Initial and subsequent dosage based on pt's clinical status, response. Administer IV dose at least 4 hrs but no longer than 12 hrs apart.

IV: **Adults, elderly:** Initially, 25–50 mcg (10–20 mcg in pts with cardiovascular disease). Total dose at least 65 mcg/day.

SIDE EFFECTS

OCCASIONAL: Children may have reversible hair loss upon initiation. ***RARE:*** Dry skin, GI intolerance, skin rash, hives, pseudotumor cerebri (severe headache in children).

ADVERSE REACTIONS/TOXIC EFFECTS

Excessive dosage produces signs/symptoms of hyperthyroidism: weight loss, palpitations, increased appetite, tremors, nervousness, tachycardia, increased B/P, headache, insomnia, menstrual irregularities. Cardiac arrhythmias occur rarely.

NURSING IMPLICATIONS

BASELINE ASSESSMENT:

Question for hypersensitivity to tartrazine, aspirin. Obtain baseline weight, vital signs. Signs and symptoms of diabetes mellitus, diabetes insipidus, adrenal insufficiency, hypopituitarism may become intensified. Treat with adrenocortical steroids prior to thyroid therapy in coexisting hypothyroidism and hypoadrenalism.

INTERVENTION/EVALUATION:

Monitor pulse for rate, rhythm (report pulse >100 or marked increase). Assess for tremors, nervousness. Assess appetite and sleep pattern.

PATIENT/FAMILY TEACHING:

Do not discontinue; replacement for hypothyroidism is lifelong. Follow-up office visits and thyroid function tests are essential. Take medication at the same time each day, preferably in morning. Teach pt or family to take pulse correctly, report marked increase, pulse of 100 or above, change of rhythm. Notify physician promptly of chest pain, weight loss, nervousness or tremors, insomnia. Children may have reversible hair loss or increased aggressiveness during first few mos of therapy.

---

lisinopril

lih-**sin**-oh-prill
(<u>Prinivil</u>, <u>Zestril</u>)
Do not confuse with Desyrel, fosinopril, Lioresal, Plendil, Prilosec, Proventil, Restoril, Zostrix.

FIXED-COMBINATION(S)

With hydrochlorothiazide, a diuretic **(Prinzide, <u>Zestoretic</u>)**

▶CLASSIFICATION

PHARMACOTHERAPEUTIC:
Angiotensin-converting enzyme (ACE) inhibitor. ***CLINICAL:*** Antihypertensive (see p. 6C)

ACTION/*THERAPEUTIC EFFECT*

Suppresses renin-angiotensin-aldosterone system (prevents conversion of angiotensin I to angiotensin II, a potent vasoconstrictor; may also inhibit angiotensin II at local vascular and renal sites). Decreases plasma angiotensin II, increases plasma renin activity, decreases aldosterone secretion. *Reduces peripheral arterial resistance, B/P (afterload), pulmonary capillary wedge pressure (preload), pulmonary vascular resistance.* In those with heart failure, *also decreases heart size, increases cardiac output, exercise tolerance time.*

PHARMACOKINETICS

	Onset	Peak	Duration
PO	1 hr	6 hrs	24 hrs

Incompletely absorbed from GI tract. Protein binding: 25%. Primarily excreted unchanged in urine.

Removed by hemodialysis. Half-life: 12 hrs (half-life prolonged with impaired renal function).

USES/*UNLABELED*

Treatment of hypertension. Used alone or in combination with other antihypertensives. Adjunctive therapy in management of heart failure. Improves survival in pts who had myocardial infarction. *Treatment of hypertension/renal crises with scleroderma.*

PRECAUTIONS

CONTRAINDICATIONS: MI, coronary insufficiency, angina, evidence of coronary artery disease, hypersensitivity to phentolamine, history of angioedema with previous treatment with ACEIs. ***CAUTIONS:*** Renal impairment, those with sodium depletion or on diuretic therapy, dialysis, hypovolemia, coronary or cerebrovascular insufficiency.

▷*LIFESPAN CONSIDERATIONS:*
Pregnancy/Lactation: Crosses placenta; unknown if distributed in breast milk. **Pregnancy Category D.** Has caused fetal/neonatal mortality, morbidity. **Children:** Safety and efficacy not established. **Elderly:** May be more sensitive to hypotensive effects.

INTERACTIONS

DRUG: **Alcohol, diuretics, hypotensive agents** may increase effects. NSAIDs may decrease effect. **Potassium-sparing diuretics, potassium supplements** may cause hyperkalemia. May increase **lithium** concentration, toxicity. ***HERBAL:*** None known. ***FOOD:*** None known. ***LAB VALUES:*** May increase potassium, SGOT (AST), SGPT (ALT), alkaline phosphatase, bilirubin, BUN, creatinine. May decrease sodium. May cause positive ANA titer.

AVAILABILITY (Rx)

TABLETS: 2.5 mg, 5 mg, 10 mg, 20 mg, 40 mg.

ADMINISTRATION/HANDLING
PO:
• Give without regard to food. • Tablets may be crushed.

INDICATIONS/ROUTES/DOSAGE
Hypertension (used alone):
PO: Adults: Initially, 10 mg/day. **Maintenance:** 20–40 mg/day as single dose.

Hypertension (combination therapy):
Note: Discontinue diuretic 2–3 days prior to initiating lisinopril therapy.
PO: Adults: Initially, 5 mg/day titrated to pt's needs.

Heart failure:
PO: Adults: Initially, 5 mg/day (2.5 mg/day in pts with hyponatremia). **Range:** 5–20 mg/day.

Myocardial infarction:
PO: Adults, elderly: Initially, 5 mg, then 5 mg after 24 hrs, 10 mg after 48 hrs, then 10 mg/day for 6 wks. (Pts with low systolic B/P: 2.5 mg/day for 3 days, then 2.5–5 mg/day.)

Usual elderly dosage:
PO: Initially, 2.5–5 mg/day. May increase by 2.5–5 mg/day at 1–2 wk intervals. **Maximum:** 40 mg/day.

Dosage in renal impairment:
Titrate to pt's needs after giving the following initial dose:

Creatinine Clearance	% Normal Dose
>30 ml/min	100
10–30 ml/min	50
<10 ml/min	25

SIDE EFFECTS

FREQUENT (5–12%): Headache, dizziness, postural hypotension. ***OCCASIONAL*** (2–4%): Chest discomfort, fatigue, rash, abdominal pain, nausea, diarrhea, upper respiratory infection. ***RARE*** (≤1%): Palpitations, tachycardia, peripheral edema, insomnia, paresthesia, confusion, constipation, dry mouth, muscle cramps.

ADVERSE REACTIONS/TOXIC EFFECTS

Excessive hypotension ("first-dose syncope") may occur in those with CHF, severely salt/volume depleted. Angioedema (swelling of face/lips), hyperkalemia occurs rarely. Agranulocytosis, neutropenia may be noted in those with impaired renal function or collagen vascular disease (systemic lupus erythematosus, scleroderma). Nephrotic syndrome may be noted in those with history of renal disease.

NURSING IMPLICATIONS

BASELINE ASSESSMENT:

Obtain B/P and apical pulse immediately before each dose, in addition to regular monitoring (be alert to fluctuations). If excessive reduction in B/P occurs, place pt in supine position, feet slightly elevated. In those with renal impairment, autoimmune disease, or taking drugs that affect leukocytes or immune response, CBC and differential count should be performed before therapy begins and q2wks for 3 mos, then periodically thereafter.

INTERVENTION/EVALUATION:

Assess for edema; check lungs for rales. Monitor I&O; weigh daily. Assess stools for frequency and consistency; prevent constipation. Assist with ambulation if dizziness occurs. Therapeutic blood serum level: 0.6–1.2 mEq/L; toxic blood serum level: >1.5 mEq/L.

PATIENT/FAMILY TEACHING:

To reduce hypotensive effect, rise slowly from lying to sitting position and permit legs to dangle from bed momentarily before standing. Full therapeutic effect may take 2–4 wks. Report any sign of infection (sore throat, fever), swelling of hands or feet or face, chest pain, difficulty breathing or swallowing. Skipping doses or voluntarily discontinuing drug may produce severe, rebound hypertension. Do not take cold preparations, nasal decongestants. Restrict sodium and alcohol as ordered.

lithium carbonate

lith-ee-um
(Carbolith✦, Duralith✦, Eskalith, Lithane, Lithobid)

lithium citrate

(Cibalith-S)
Do not confuse with Levbid, Lithostat, Lithotabs.

▶CLASSIFICATION

PHARMACOTHERAPEUTIC: Psychotherapeutic. ***CLINICAL:*** Antimanic, antidepressant, vascular headache prophylactic

ACTION/*THERAPEUTIC EFFECT*

Affects storage, release, reuptake of neurotransmitters. Antimanic effect may be result of increase in norepinephrine reuptake and increase in serotonin receptor sensitivity, *producing antimanic, antidepressant effects.*

PHARMACOKINETICS

Rapid, complete absorption from GI tract. Primarily excreted unchanged in urine. Removed by hemodialysis. Half-life: 18–24 hrs (half-life increased in elderly).

USES/UNLABELED

Prophylaxis, treatment of acute mania, manic phase of bipolar disorder (manic-depressive illness). *Treatment of mental depression, prophylaxis of vascular headache, treatment of neutropenia.*

PRECAUTIONS

CONTRAINDICATIONS: Severe cardiovascular disease, severe renal disease, severe dehydration/sodium depletion, debilitated pts. ***CAUTIONS:*** Cardiovascular disease, thyroid disease, elderly.
▷***LIFESPAN CONSIDERATIONS:*** **Pregnancy/Lactation:** Freely crosses placenta; distributed in breast milk. **Pregnancy Category D. Children:** May increase bone formation or density (alter parathyroid hormone concentrations). **Elderly:** More susceptible to develop lithium-induced goiter/clinical hypothyroidism, CNS toxicity. Increased thirst, urination more frequent; lower dosage recommended.

INTERACTIONS

DRUG: May increase effects of **antithyroid medication, iodinated glycerol, potassium iodide. NSAIDs** may increase concentration, toxicity. May decrease absorption of **phenothiazines. Phenothiazines** may increase intracellular concentration, increase renal excretion, extrapyramidal symptoms (EPS), delirium, mask early signs of lithium toxicity. **Diuretics** may increase concentration, toxicity. **Haloperidol** may increase EPS, neurologic toxicity. **Molindone** may increase risk of neurotoxic symptoms. ***HERBAL:*** None known. ***FOOD:*** None known. ***LAB VALUES:*** May increase blood glucose, calcium, immunoreactive parathyroid hormone. Therapeutic blood serum level: 0.6–1.2 mEq/L; toxic blood serum level: >1.5 mEq/L.

AVAILABILITY (Rx)

CAPSULES: 150 mg, 300 mg, 600 mg. ***TABLETS:*** 300 mg. ***TABLETS (slow-release):*** 300 mg, 450 mg. ***SYRUP:*** 300 mg/5 ml.

ADMINISTRATION/HANDLING

PO:

• Preferable to administer with meals or milk. • Do not crush, chew, or break extended-release or film-coated tablets.

INDICATIONS/ROUTES/DOSAGE

Note: During acute phase, therapeutic serum lithium concentration of 1–1.4 mEq/L is required. Desired level during long-term control: 0.5–1.3 mEq/L. Monitor serum concentrations, clinical response to determine proper dosage.

Usual dosage:

PO: Adults: 300 mg 3–4 times/day. **Maximum:** 2.4 g/day or 450–900 mg slow-release form 2 times/day. **Elderly:** 300 mg 2 times/day. May increase by 300 mg/day q1wk. **Maintenance:** 900–1,200 mg/day. **Children >12 yrs:** 600–1,800 mg/day in 3–4 divided doses (2 doses/day for slow-release). **Children <12 yrs:** 15–60 mg/kg/day in 3–4 divided doses.

SIDE EFFECTS

Note: Effects are dose related and seldom occur at serum lithium levels <1.5 mEq/L.

OCCASIONAL: Fine hand tremor, polydipsia (excessive thirst), polyuria (increased urination), mild nausea. *RARE:* Weight gain, fast/slow heartbeat, acne, rash, muscle twitching, blue hue in fingers/toes, coldness in arms/legs, pseudotumor cerebri (eye pain, headache, vision problems, noises in ears).

ADVERSE REACTIONS/TOXIC EFFECTS

Serum lithium concentration of 1.5–2.0 mEq/L may produce vomiting, diarrhea, drowsiness, incoordination, coarse hand tremor, muscle twitching, EKG T-wave depression, mental confusion. Serum lithium concentration of 2.0–2.5 mEq/L may result in ataxia, giddiness, tinnitus, blurred vision, clonic movements, severe hypotension. Acute toxicity characterized by seizures, oliguria, circulatory failure, coma, death.

NURSING IMPLICATIONS

BASELINE ASSESSMENT:

Serum lithium levels should be tested q3–4days during initial phase of therapy, q1–2mos thereafter, and weekly if there is no improvement of disorder or adverse effects occur.

INTERVENTION/EVALUATION:

Lithium serum testing should be performed as close as possible to 12th hr after last dose. Besides serum lithium concentration levels, clinical assessment of therapeutic effect or tolerance to drug effect is necessary for correct dosing-level management. Assess behavior, appearance, emotional status, response to environment, speech pattern, thought content. Monitor serum lithium concentrations, differential count, urinalysis, creatinine clearance. Assess for increased urine output, persistent thirst. Report polyuria, prolonged vomiting, diarrhea, fever to physician (may need to temporarily reduce or discontinue dosage). Monitor for signs of lithium toxicity. Assess for therapeutic response (interest in surroundings, improvement in self-care, increased ability to concentrate, relaxed facial expression). Therapeutic blood serum level: 0.6–1.2 mEq/L; toxic blood serum level: >1.5 mEq/L.

PATIENT/FAMILY TEACHING:

Do not engage in activities requiring alert response until effects of drug are known. Thirst, frequent urination may occur. A fluid intake of 2–3 quarts liquid per day and maintenance of a normal salt intake are necessary during initial phase of treatment to avoid dehydration. GI disturbances generally disappear during continued therapy. Thyroid function tests should be performed q6–12mos in elderly pts (increased incidence of goiter, hypothyroidism). Therapeutic improvement noted in 1–3 wks.

lomefloxacin hydrochloride

low-meh-**flocks**-ah-sin
(Maxaquin)

▶CLASSIFICATION

PHARMACOTHERAPEUTIC: Quinolone. *CLINICAL:* Anti-infective (see p. 22C)

ACTION/*THERAPEUTIC EFFECT*

Inhibits the enzyme DNA-gyrase in susceptible microorganisms, *interfering with bacterial DNA replication and repair. Bactericidal.*

PHARMACOKINETICS

Well absorbed from GI tract. Protein binding: 10%. Widely distributed. Metabolized in liver. Primarily excreted in urine. Not removed by hemodialysis. Half-life: 4–6 hrs (half-life increased with impaired renal function, elderly).

USES

Treatment of infections of urinary tract, lower respiratory tract, postop prophylaxis in pts undergoing transurethral procedures.

PRECAUTIONS

CONTRAINDICATIONS: Hypersensitivity to quinolones. *CAUTIONS:* Renal impairment, CNS disorders, seizures, those taking theophylline or caffeine.

▷*LIFESPAN CONSIDERATIONS:* **Pregnancy/Lactation:** Unknown if distributed in breast milk. If possible, do not use during pregnancy/lactation (risk of arthropathy to fetus/infant). **Pregnancy Category C. Children:** Safety and efficacy not established. **Elderly:** Age-related renal impairment may require dosage adjustment.

INTERACTIONS

DRUG: **Antacids, iron prep, sucralfate** may decrease absorption. Decreases clearance, may increase concentration, toxicity of **theophylline.** May increase effects of **oral anticoagulants.** *HERBAL:* None known. *FOOD:* None known. *LAB VALUES:* May increase SGOT (AST), SGPT (ALT), alkaline phosphatase, LDH, serum bilirubin, BUN, serum creatinine concentration.

AVAILABILITY (Rx)

TABLETS: 400 mg.

ADMINISTRATION/HANDLING

PO:
• May be given without regard to meals (preferred dosing time: 2 hrs after meals). • Do not administer antacids (aluminum, magnesium) within 2 hrs of lomefloxacin. • Encourage cranberry juice, citrus fruits (to acidify urine).

INDICATIONS/ROUTES/DOSAGE

Urinary tract infections:
PO: Adults, elderly: 400 mg/day for 10–14 days.

Uncomplicated UTI:
PO: Adults (females): 400 mg/day for 3 days.

Lower respiratory tract infections:
PO: Adults, elderly: 400 mg/day for 10 days.

Postop prophylaxis:
PO: Adults, elderly: 400 mg 2–6 hrs prior to surgery.

Dosage in renal impairment:
The dose and/or frequency is modified in pts based on severity of renal impairment.

Creatinine Clearance	Dosage
>40 ml/min	No change
10–40 ml/min	400 mg initially, then 200 mg/day for 10–14 days

SIDE EFFECTS

OCCASIONAL (2–3%): Nausea, headache, photosensitivity, dizziness ***RARE*** (1%): Diarrhea.

ADVERSE REACTIONS/TOXIC EFFECTS

Antibiotic-associated colitis (severe abdominal pain and tenderness, fever, watery and severe diarrhea), fungal overgrowth may result from altered bacterial balance.

NURSING IMPLICATIONS

BASELINE ASSESSMENT:

Question for history of hypersensitivity to lomefloxacin, quinolones.

INTERVENTION/EVALUATION:

Check for dizziness, headache. Be alert for superinfection, e.g., genital pruritus, vaginitis, fever, oral candidiasis.

PATIENT/FAMILY TEACHING:

Do not skip dose; take full course of therapy. Do not take antacids (reduces/destroys effectiveness). Avoid sunlight/ultraviolet exposure; wear sunscreen, protective clothing if photosensitivity develops.

---

lomustine

low-**meuw**-steen
(CeeNU)

▶CLASSIFICATION

PHARMACOTHERAPEUTIC:
Alkylating agent (nitrosurea).
CLINICAL: Antineoplastic (see p. 72C)

ACTION/*THERAPEUTIC EFFECT*

Inhibits DNA, RNA synthesis by cross-linking with DNA, RNA strands, preventing cellular division, *interfering with DNA/RNA function.* Cell cycle-phase nonspecific.

USES/*UNLABELED*

Treatment of primary and metastatic brain tumors, disseminated Hodgkin's disease. *Treatment of gastrointestinal, lung, renal, breast carcinoma, multiple myeloma, malignant melanoma.*

PRECAUTIONS

CONTRAINDICATIONS: None significant. ***CAUTIONS:*** Depressed platelet, leukocyte, erythrocyte counts.

INTERACTIONS

DRUG:* Bone marrow depressants** may increase bone marrow depression. **Live virus vaccines** may potentiate virus replication, increase vaccine side effects, decrease pt's antibody response to vaccine. ***HERBAL: None known. ***FOOD:*** None known. ***LAB VALUES:*** May increase liver function tests.

AVAILABILITY (Rx)

CAPSULES: 10 mg, 40 mg, 100 mg.

INDICATIONS/ROUTES/DOSAGE

Note: Dosage is individualized based on clinical response and tolerance to adverse effects. When used in combination therapy, consult specific protocols for optimum dosage, sequence of drug administration.

Usual dosage:

PO: Adults, elderly: 100–130 mg/m^2 as single dose. Repeat dose at intervals of at least 6 wks but not until circulating blood elements have returned to acceptable levels. Adjust dose based on hematologic response to previous dose. **Children:** 75–150 mg/m² as single dose.

SIDE EFFECTS

FREQUENT: Nausea, vomiting occur 45 min–6 hrs after dosing, lasts 12–24 hrs. Anorexia often follows for 2–3 days. **OCCASIONAL:** Neurotoxicity (confusion, slurred speech), stomatitis, darkening of skin, diarrhea, skin rash, itching, hair loss.

ADVERSE REACTIONS/TOXIC EFFECTS

Bone marrow depression manifested as hematologic toxicity (principally leukopenia, mild anemia, thrombocytopenia). Leukopenia occurs at about 6 wks, thrombocytopenia at about 4 wks, and persists for 1–2 wks. Refractory anemia, thrombocytopenia occur commonly if therapy continued longer than 1 yr. Hepatotoxicity occurs infrequently. Large cumulative doses may result in renal damage.

NURSING IMPLICATIONS

BASELINE ASSESSMENT:

Manufacturer recommends weekly blood counts; experts recommend first blood count obtained 2–3 wks after initial therapy, subsequent blood counts indicated by prior toxicity. Antiemetics can reduce duration, frequency of nausea, vomiting.

INTERVENTION/EVALUATION:

Monitor hematologic status, liver function tests. Monitor for stomatitis (burning/erythema of oral mucosa at inner margin of lips, sore throat, difficulty swallowing). Monitor for hematologic toxicity (fever, sore throat, signs of local infection, easy bruising, unusual bleeding from any site), symptoms of anemia (excessively tired, weak).

PATIENT/FAMILY TEACHING:

Nausea, vomiting abates generally in <1 day. Fasting prior to therapy can reduce frequency/duration of GI effects. Maintain fastidious oral hygiene. Do not have immunizations without physician's approval (drug lowers body's resistance). Avoid crowds and those with known illness. Promptly report fever, sore throat, signs of local infection, easy bruising or unusual bleeding from any site, swelling of legs and feet, yellow skin.

L

loperamide hydrochloride

low-**pear**-ah-myd
(Apo-Loperamide✤, Imodium, Imodium A-D, Loperacap✤, Novo-Loperamide✤)
Do not confuse with Ionamin.

FIXED-COMBINATION(S)

With simethicone, an antiflatulent **(Imodium Advanced)**

▶ CLASSIFICATION

CLINICAL: Antidiarrheal (see p. 41C)

ACTION/THERAPEUTIC EFFECT

Direct effect on intestinal wall muscles; *slows intestinal motility, prolongs transit time of intestinal contents (reduces fecal volume, diminishes loss of fluid/electrolytes, increases viscosity, bulk).*

PHARMACOKINETICS

Poorly absorbed from GI tract. Protein binding: 97%. Metabolized in liver. Eliminated in feces, excreted in urine. Not removed by hemodialysis. Half-life: 9.1–14.4 hrs.

USES

Controls, provides symptomatic relief of acute nonspecific diarrhea; chronic diarrhea associated with inflammatory bowel disease; traveler's diarrhea. Reduces volume of discharge from ileostomy.

PRECAUTIONS

CONTRAINDICATIONS: Those who must avoid constipation, diarrhea associated with pseudomembranous enterocolitis due to broad-spectrum antibiotics or with organisms that invade intestinal mucosa (*Escherichia coli,* shigella, salmonella), acute ulcerative colitis (may produce toxic megacolon). **CAUTIONS:** Those with fluid/electrolyte depletion, hepatic impairment.

▷**LIFESPAN CONSIDERATIONS:**
Pregnancy/Lactation: Unknown if drug crosses placenta or is distributed in breast milk. **Pregnancy Category B. Children:** Not recommended in those <6 yrs of age (infants <3 mos more susceptible to CNS effects). **Elderly:** May mask dehydration and electrolyte depletion.

INTERACTIONS

DRUG: Opioid (narcotic) analgesics may increase risk of constipation. **HERBAL:** None known. **FOOD:** None known. **LAB VALUES:** None significant.

AVAILABILITY (OTC)

TABLETS: 2 mg. **CAPSULES (Rx):** 2 mg. **LIQUID:** 1 mg/5 ml.

INDICATIONS/ROUTES/DOSAGE
Acute diarrhea (capsules):

PO: Adults, elderly: Initially, 4 mg, then 2 mg after each unformed stool. **Maximum:** 16 mg/day. **Children, 8–12 yrs, >30 kg:** Initially, 2 mg 3 times/day for 24 hrs; **5–8 yrs, 20–30 kg:** Initially, 2 mg 2 times/day for 24 hrs; **2–5 yrs, 13–20 kg:** Initially, 1 mg 3 times/day for 24 hrs. **Maintenance:** 1 mg/10 kg only after loose stool.

Chronic diarrhea:

PO: Adults, elderly: Initially, 4 mg, then 2 mg after each unformed stool until diarrhea is controlled.

Traveler's diarrhea:

PO: Adults, elderly: Initially, 4 mg, then 2 mg after each loose bowel movement (LBM). **Maximum:** 8 mg/day for 2 days. **Children 9–11 yrs:** Initially 2 mg, then 1 mg after each LBM. **Maximum:** 6 mg/day for 2 days. **Children 6–8 yrs:** Initially, 1 mg, then 1 mg after each LBM. **Maximum:** 4 mg/day for 2 days.

SIDE EFFECTS

RARE: Dry mouth, drowsiness, abdominal discomfort, allergic reaction (rash, itching).

ADVERSE REACTIONS/TOXIC EFFECTS

Toxicity results in constipation, GI irritation including nausea, vomiting, CNS depression. Treatment: Activated charcoal.

NURSING IMPLICATIONS

BASELINE ASSESSMENT:

Do not administer in presence of bloody diarrhea or temperature >101°F.

INTERVENTION/EVALUATION:

Encourage adequate fluid intake. Assess bowel sounds for peristalsis. Monitor stool frequency and consistency (watery, loose, soft, semisolid, solid). Withhold drug and notify physician promptly in event of abdominal pain, distention, or fever.

PATIENT/FAMILY TEACHING:

Do not exceed prescribed dose. Avoid tasks that require alertness, motor skills until response to drug is established. Notify physician if diarrhea does not stop within 3 days, if abdominal distention or pain occurs, or if fever develops.

lopinavir/ritonavir

low-**pin**-ah-veer/rih-**ton**-ah-veer
(Kaletra)

►CLASSIFICATION

PHARMACOTHERAPEUTIC:
Protease inhibitor combination.
CLINICAL: Antiretroviral (see pp. 58C, 96C)

ACTION/THERAPEUTIC EFFECT

Lopinavir prevents cleavage of a polyprotein, *resulting in production of immature, noninfectious viral particles*. Ritonavir inhibits metabolism of lopinivir, providing increased lopinavir plasma levels.

PHARMACOKINETICS

Readily absorbed following PO administration (increased when taken with food). Protein binding: 98–99%. Metabolized in liver. Primarily eliminated in feces. Not removed by hemodialysis. Half-life: 5–6 hrs.

USES

In combination with other antiretroviral agents for the treatment of HIV infection.

PRECAUTIONS

CONTRAINDICATIONS: Hypersensitivity to lopinavir or ritonavir. Concomitant use of flecainide, pimozide, propafenone (increased risk of serous cardiac arrhythmias), midazolam, triazolam (increases sedation or respiratory depression), ergot derivatives (peripheral vasospasm, ischemia of extremities). ***CAUTIONS:*** Impaired liver function, hepatitis B or C. High-dose itraconazole, ketoconazole not recommended. May cause disulfiram reaction with oral solution (contains alcohol) with disulfiram, metronidazole.

▷***LIFESPAN CONSIDERATIONS:***
Pregnancy/Lactation: Unknown if excreted in breast milk. Not recommended that HIV-infected mothers breast-feed. **Pregnancy Category C. Children:** Safety and efficacy not established in those <6 mos of age. **Elderly:** Age-related renal or liver impairment, cardiac function impairment requires caution.

INTERACTIONS

DRUG: **Carbamazepine, corticosteroids, efavirenz, nevirapine, phenobarbital, phenytoin, rifampin** may decrease concentration, effect. May increase concentration, effect of **clarithromycin, felodipine, immunosuppresants, nicardipine, nifedipine, rifabuton.** May decrease concentration, effect of **atovaquone, methadone, oral contraceptives.** May increase concentration, risk of myopathy with **atorvastatin, cerivastatin. HERBAL:** St. **John's wort** may decrease concentrations, effect. ***FOOD:*** None known. ***LAB VALUES:*** May increase glucose, uric acid, AST (SGOT), ALT (SGPT), GGT, total cholesterol, triglycerides.

AVAILABILITY (Rx)

CAPSULES: 133.3 mg lopinavir/ 33.3 mg ritonavir. **ORAL SOLUTION:** 80 mg lopinavir/20 mg ritonavir per ml.

ADMINISTRATION/HANDLING
PO:

• Refrigerate until dispensed. • Avoid exposure to excessive heat. • If stored at room temperature, use within 2 mos. • Give with food.

INDICATIONS/ROUTES/DOSAGE
HIV:

PO: Adults: 400/100 mg of lopinavir/ritonavir (3 capsules or 5 ml) twice daily. Increase to 533/133 mg (4 capsules or 6.5 ml) when taken with efavirenz or nevirapine. **Children 7 to <15 kg without efavirenz or nevirapine:** 12 mg/kg 2 times/day. **15–40 kg:** 10 mg/kg 2 times/day. **Children 7–<15 kg with efavirenz or nevirapine:** 13 mg/kg 2 times/day. **15–50 kg:** 11 mg/kg 2 times/day.

SIDE EFFECTS

FREQUENT (14%): Diarrhea (mild to moderate severity). **OCCASIONAL** (2–6%): Nausea, asthenia (loss of strength, energy), abdominal pain, headache, vomiting. **RARE** (<2%): Insomnia, rash.

ADVERSE REACTIONS/TOXIC EFFECTS

Anemia, leukopenia, lymphadenopathy, deep vein thrombosis, Cushing's syndrome, pancreatitis, hemorrhagic colitis occur rarely.

NURSING IMPLICATIONS

BASELINE ASSESSMENT:

Obtain baseline values for CBC, renal and hepatic function tests, weight.

INTERVENTION/EVALUATION:

Monitor consistency and frequency of stools. Assess for opportunistic infections: onset of fever, oral mucosa changes, cough, or other respiratory symptoms. Check weight at least twice a week. Assess for nausea, vomiting.

PATIENT/FAMILY TEACHING:

Explain correct administration of medication. Eat small, frequent meals to offset nausea, vomiting. Medication is not a cure for HIV infection, nor does it reduce risk of transmission to others.

loracarbef

laur-ah-**car**-bef
(Lorabid)
Do not confuse with Lortab.

▶CLASSIFICATION

PHARMACOTHERAPEUTIC: Cephalosporin. **CLINICAL:** Antibiotic (see p. 20C)

ACTION/THERAPEUTIC EFFECT

Bactericidal. Binds to bacterial membranes, *inhibiting bacterial cell wall synthesis.*

USES

Treatment of bronchitis, otitis media, pharyngitis, pneumonia, sinusitis, skin and soft tissue infections, urinary tract infections (uncomplicated cystitis, pyelonephritis).

PRECAUTIONS

CONTRAINDICATIONS: History of hypersensitivity to cephalosporins, anaphylactic reaction to penicillins. ***CAUTIONS:*** Renal impairment.

INTERACTIONS

DRUG:* Probenecid** increases serum concentrations, half-life of loracarbef. ***HERBAL: None known. ***FOOD:*** None known. ***LAB VALUES:*** May increase SGOT (AST), SGPT (ALT), alkaline phosphatase, BUN, creatinine. May decrease leukocytes, platelets.

AVAILABILITY (Rx)

CAPSULES: 200 mg. ***POWDER FOR ORAL SUSPENSION:*** 100 mg/5 ml.

ADMINISTRATION/HANDLING

PO:

• Give 1 hr before or 2 hrs after meal. • After reconstitution, powder for suspension may be kept at room temperature for 14 days. Discard unused portion after 14 days. • Shake oral suspension well before using.

INDICATIONS/ROUTES/DOSAGE

Bronchitis:

***PO:* Adults, elderly, children >12 yrs:** 200–400 mg q12h for 7 days.

Pharyngitis:

***PO:* Adults, elderly, children >12 yrs:** 200 mg q12h for 10 days. **Children 6 mos–12 yrs:** 7.5 mg/kg q12h for 10 days.

Pneumonia:

***PO:* Adults, elderly, children >12 yrs:** 400 mg q12h for 14 days.

Sinusitis:

***PO:* Adults, elderly, children >12 yrs:** 400 mg q12h for 10 days. **Children: 6 mos–12 yrs:** 15 mg/kg q12h for 10 days.

Skin, soft tissue infections:

***PO:* Adults, elderly, children >12 yrs:** 200 mg q12h for 7 days. **Children 6 mos–12 yrs:** 7.5 mg/kg q12h for 7 days.

Urinary tract infections:

***PO:* Adults, elderly, children 6 mos–12 yrs:** 200–400 mg q12h for 7–14 days.

Otitis media:

***PO:* Children 6 mos–12 yrs:** 15 mg/kg q12h for 10 days.

SIDE EFFECTS

FREQUENT: Abdominal pain, anorexia, nausea, vomiting, diarrhea. ***OCCASIONAL:*** Skin rash, itching. ***RARE:*** Dizziness, headache, vaginitis.

ADVERSE REACTIONS/TOXIC EFFECTS

Antibiotic-associated colitis, other superinfections may result from altered bacterial balance. Hypersensitivity reactions (ranging from rash, urticaria, fever to anaphylaxis) occur in less than 5%, generally those with history of allergies, esp. penicillin.

NURSING IMPLICATIONS

BASELINE ASSESSMENT:

Question history of allergies, particularly cephalosporins, penicillins.

INTERVENTION/EVALUATION:

Assess for nausea, vomiting. Check stool frequency and consistency. Assess skin for rash (diaper area in children). Monitor I&O, urinalysis, renal function reports for nephrotoxicity. Be alert for superinfection: genital/anal pruritus, moniliasis, abdominal pain, sore mouth or tongue, moderate to severe diarrhea.

loratadine 🔍

low-**rah**-tah-deen
(<u>Claritin</u>, Claritin Reditabs)

FIXED-COMBINATION(S)

With pseudoephedrine, a sympathomimetic **(Claritin-D)**

▶**CLASSIFICATION**

PHARMACOTHERAPEUTIC: H_1 antagonist. **CLINICAL:** Antihistamine (see p. 48C)

ACTION/THERAPEUTIC EFFECT

Long acting with selective peripheral histamine H_1 receptor antagonist action. Competes with histamine for receptor site *to prevent allergic responses mediated by histamine (urticaria, pruritus)*. Has no significant anticholinergic effects.

PHARMACOKINETICS

Onset	Peak	Duration
PO		
1–3 hrs	8–12 hrs	24 hrs

Rapidly, almost completely absorbed from GI tract. Protein binding: 97% (metabolite: 73–77%). Distributed mainly in liver, lungs, GI tract, bile. Metabolized in liver to active metabolite (undergoes extensive first-pass metabolism). Excreted in urine, eliminated in feces. Not removed by hemodialysis. Half-life: 3–20 hrs; metabolite: 28 hrs (half-life increased in elderly, liver disease).

USES/*UNLABELED*

Relief of nasal and non-nasal symptoms of seasonal allergic rhinitis (hay fever). Treatment of idiopathic chronic urticaria (hives). *Adjunct treatment of bronchial asthma.*

PRECAUTIONS

CONTRAINDICATIONS: Hypersensitivity to loratadine or any ingredient. **CAUTIONS:** Liver impairment. Safety in children <6 yrs not known.

▷**LIFESPAN CONSIDERATIONS:**
Pregnancy/Lactation: Excreted in breast milk. **Pregnancy Category B. Children/Elderly:** More sensitive to anticholinergic effects (e.g., dry mouth, nose, throat).

INTERACTIONS

DRUG: Ketoconazole, erythromycin may increase concentrations. **HERBAL:** None known. **FOOD:** None known. **LAB VALUES:** May suppress wheal and flare reactions to antigen skin testing, unless antihistamines are discontinued 4 days before testing.

AVAILABILITY (Rx)

TABLETS: 10 mg. **SYRUP:** 10 mg/10 ml.

ADMINISTRATION/HANDLING
PO:

• Preferably give on an empty stomach (food delays absorption).

INDICATIONS/ROUTES/DOSAGE
Allergic rhinitis, hives:

PO: Adults, elderly, children >6 yrs: 10 mg once daily. **Children 2–5 yrs:** 5 mg once daily. **Hepatic function impairment:** 10 mg every other day.

SIDE EFFECTS

FREQUENT (8–12%): Headache, fatigue, drowsiness. **OCCASION-AL** (3%): Dry mouth, nose, throat.

ADVERSE REACTIONS/TOXIC EFFECTS

None significant.

NURSING IMPLICATIONS

BASELINE ASSESSMENT:

Assess lung sounds, skin for urticaria, other allergy symptoms.

INTERVENTION/EVALUATION:

For upper respiratory allergies, increase fluids to maintain thin secretions and offset thirst, loss of fluids from increased sweating. Monitor symptoms for therapeutic response.

PATIENT/FAMILY TEACHING:

Take loratadine on an empty stomach. Does not cause drowsiness; however, if blurred vision or eye pain occurs, do not drive or perform activities requiring visual acuity. Avoid alcohol during antihistamine therapy.

lorazepam

low-**raz**-ah-pam
(Alzapam, Apo-Lorazepam✷,
Ativan, Novolorazepam✷)
Do not confuse with Alprazolam.

▶CLASSIFICATION

PHARMACOTHERAPEUTIC:
Benzodiazepine **(Schedule IV).
Clinical:** Antianxiety, sedative-hypnotic, antiemetic, skeletal muscle relaxant, amnesiac, anticonvulsant, antitremor (see p. 11C)

ACTION/*THERAPEUTIC EFFECT*

Enhances inhibitory neurotransmitter gamma-aminobutyric acid (GABA) neurotransmission at CNS, affecting memory, motor, sensory, and cognitive functions, *producing anxiolytic, muscle relaxation, anticonvulsant, sedative, antiemetic effect.*

PHARMACOKINETICS

	Onset	Peak	Duration
IM	15–30 min	—	12–24 hrs
IV	1–5 min	—	12–24 hrs

Well absorbed after PO, IM administration. Protein binding: 85%. Widely distributed. Metabolized in liver. Primarily excreted in urine. Not removed by hemodialysis. Half-life: 10–20 hrs.

USES/*UNLABELED*

Management of anxiety disorders associated with depressive symptoms. Parenteral form used preoperatively to provide sedation, relieve anxiety, and produce anterograde amnesia. Treatment of status epilepticus. *Treatment of alcohol withdrawal, adjunct to endoscopic procedures (diminishes pt recall), panic disorders, skeletal muscle spasms, cancer chemotherapy–induced nausea/vomiting, tension headache, tremors.*

PRECAUTIONS

CONTRAINDICATIONS: Acute narrow-angle glaucoma, acute alcohol intoxication. **CAUTIONS:** Impaired kidney/liver function.
▷*LIFESPAN CONSIDERATIONS:*
Pregnancy/Lactation: May cross placenta; may be distributed in breast milk. May increase risk of fetal abnormalities if administered

L

during first trimester of pregnancy. Chronic ingestion during pregnancy may produce fetal toxicity, withdrawal symptoms, CNS depression in neonates. **Pregnancy Category D. Children:** Safety and efficacy not established in those <12 yrs. **Elderly:** Use small initial doses with gradual increases to avoid ataxia or excessive sedation.

INTERACTIONS

DRUG: Alcohol, CNS depressants may increase CNS depressant effect. **HERBAL: Kava kava, valerian** may increase CNS depression. **FOOD:** None known. **LAB VALUES:** None significant. Therapeutic blood serum level: 50–240 ng/ml; toxic blood serum level: N/A.

AVAILABILITY (Rx)

TABLETS: 0.5 mg, 1 mg, 2 mg. **INJECTION:** 2 mg/ml, 4 mg/ml.

ADMINISTRATION/HANDLING
PO:

• Give with food. • Tablets may be crushed.

IM:

• Give deep IM into large muscle mass.

IV 💉

Storage:

• Refrigerate parenteral form. • Do not use if precipitate forms or solution appears discolored. • Avoid freezing.

Reconstitution:

• Dilute with equal volume of Sterile Water for Injection, 0.9% NaCl, or D_5W. • To dilute prefilled syringe, remove air from half-filled syringe, aspirate equal volume of diluent, pull plunger back slightly to allow for mixing, and gently invert syringe several times (do not shake vigorously).

Rate of administration:

• Give by IV push into tubing of free-flowing IV infusion (0.9% NaCl, D_5W) at rate of infusion not to exceed 2 mg/min.

IV INCOMPATIBILITIES ⊘

Aldesleukin (Proleukin), aztreonam (Azactam), idarubicin (Idamycin), ondansetron (Zofran), sufentanil (Sufenta).

IV COMPATIBILITIES

Bumetanide (Bumex), cefepime (Maxipime), diltiazem (Cardizem), dobutamine (Dobutrex), dopamine (Intropin), heparin, labetalol (Normodyne, Trandate), milrinone (Primacor), norepinephrine (Levophed), piperacill/tazobactam (Zosyn), potassium, propofol (Diprivan).

INDICATIONS/ROUTES/DOSAGE
Anxiety:

PO: Adults: 1–10 mg/day in 2–3 divided doses. **Average:** 2–6 mg/day. **Elderly:** Initially, 0.5–1 mg/day. May increase gradually.

IV: Adults, elderly: Titrate to desired effect.

PO/IV: Children: 0.05 mg/kg/dose q4–8h. **Range:** 0.02–0.1 mg/kg. **Maximum:** 2 mg/dose.

Insomnia due to anxiety:

PO: Adults: 2–4 mg at bedtime. **Elderly:** 0.5–1 mg at bedtime.

Preop:

IM: Adults, elderly: 0.05 mg/kg given 2 hrs before procedure. Do not exceed 4 mg.

IV: Adults, elderly: 0.044 mg/kg (up to 2 mg total) 15–20 min before surgery.

Status epilepticus:

***IV:* Adults, elderly:** 4 mg/dose over 2–5 min. May repeat in 10–15 min (8 mg maximum in 12-hr period). **Children:** 0.1 mg/kg over 2–5 min. **Maximum:** 4 mg. May repeat second dose of 0.05 mg/kg in 15–20 min. **Neonate:** 0.05 mg/kg. May repeat in 10–15 min.

SIDE EFFECTS

FREQUENT: Drowsiness, ataxia (incoordination), confusion. Morning drowsiness may occur initially. ***OCCASIONAL:*** Blurred vision, slurred speech, hypotension, headache. ***RARE:*** Paradoxical CNS restlessness, excitement in elderly/debilitated.

ADVERSE REACTIONS/TOXIC EFFECTS

Abrupt or too rapid withdrawal may result in pronounced restlessness, irritability, insomnia, hand tremors, abdominal/muscle cramps, sweating, vomiting, seizures. Overdosage results in somnolence, confusion, diminished reflexes, coma.

NURSING IMPLICATIONS

BASELINE ASSESSMENT:

Offer emotional support to anxious pt. Pt must remain recumbent for up to 8 hrs (individualized) after parenteral administration to reduce hypotensive effect. Assess motor responses (agitation, trembling, tension) and autonomic responses (cold, clammy hands, sweating).

INTERVENTION/EVALUATION:

For those on long-term therapy, liver/renal function tests, blood counts should be performed periodically. Assess for paradoxical reaction, particularly during early therapy. Evaluate for therapeutic response: a calm facial expression, decreased restlessness and/or insomnia. Therapeutic blood serum level: 50–240 ng/ml; toxic blood serum level: N/A.

PATIENT/FAMILY TEACHING:

Drowsiness usually disappears during continued therapy. Avoid tasks that require alertness, motor skills until response to drug is established. Smoking reduces drug effectiveness. Do not abruptly withdraw medication after long-term therapy. Do not use alcohol or CNS depressants. Contraception recommended for long-term therapy. Notify physician at once if pregnancy is suspected.

losartan

loh-**sar**-tan
(Cozaar)
Do not confuse with Zocor.

FIXED-COMBINATION(S)

With hydrochlorothiazide, a thiazide diuretic **(Hyzaar)**

▶CLASSIFICATION

PHARMACOTHERAPEUTIC: Angiotensin II receptor antagonist. ***CLINICAL:*** Antihypertensive (see pg. 7C)

ACTION/*THERAPEUTIC EFFECT*

Potent vasodilator. An angiotensin II receptor (type AT_1) antagonist, blocks vasoconstrictor and aldosterone-secreting effects of angiotensin II, inhibiting the binding of angiotensin II to the AT_1 receptors, *causing vasodilation, de-*

---

creased peripheral resistance, decrease in B/P.

PHARMACOKINETICS

	Onset	Peak	Duration
PO	—	6 hrs	24 hrs

Well absorbed following PO administration. Proteing binding: >98%. Undergoes first-pass metabolism in liver to active metabolites. Excreted in urine and via biliary system. Not removed by hemodialysis. Half-life: 2 hrs.

USES

Treatment of hypertension. Used alone or in combination with other antihypertensives.

PRECAUTIONS

CONTRAINDICATIONS: None significant. **CAUTIONS:** Renal/hepatic function impairment, renal arterial stenosis.

▷**LIFESPAN CONSIDERATIONS:** **Pregnancy/Lactation:** Has caused fetal/neonatal morbidity, mortality. Potential for adverse effects on nursing infant. Do not breastfeed. **Pregnancy Category C:** First trimester. **Pregnancy Category D:** Second and third trimesters (fetal/neonatal morbidity/mortality). **Children:** Safety and efficacy not established. **Elderly:** No age-related precautions noted.

INTERACTIONS

DRUG: **Cimetidine** may increase effects. **Phenobarbital, rifampin** may decrease effects. May inhibit effects of **ketoconazole, troleandomycin.** May increase concentration, toxicity of **lithium. HERBAL:** None known. **FOOD:** **Grapefruit juice** may alter absorption. **LAB VALUES:** May increase BUN, serum creatinine, SGOT (AST), SGPT (ALT), alkaline phosphatase, bilirubin. May decrease hemoglobin, hematocrit.

AVAILABILITY (Rx)

TABLETS: 25 mg, 50 mg.

ADMINISTRATION/HANDLING
PO:
• May give without regard to food.
• Do not crush or break tablets.

INDICATIONS/ROUTES/DOSAGE

Hypertension:

PO: Adults, elderly: Initially, 50 mg once daily. **Maximum:** May be given once or twice daily with total daily doses ranging from 25 to 100 mg.

Hepatic function impairment:

PO: Initially, 25 mg daily.

SIDE EFFECTS

FREQUENT (8%): Upper respiratory infection. **OCCASIONAL** (2–4%): Dizziness, diarrhea, cough. **RARE** (≤1%): Insomnia, dyspepsia, heartburn, back/leg pain, muscle cramps/ache, nasal congestion, sinusitis.

ADVERSE REACTIONS/TOXIC EFFECTS

Overdosage may manifest as hypotension and tachycardia; bradycardia occurs less often. Institute supportive measurement.

NURSING IMPLICATIONS

BASELINE ASSESSMENT:

Obtain B/P and apical pulse immediately before each dose, in addition to regular monitoring (be alert to fluctuations). If excessive reduction in B/P occurs, place pt in supine position, feet slightly elevated. Question possibility of pregnancy (see Pregnancy/Lactation). Assess medication history (esp. diuretic).

INTERVENTION/EVALUATION:

Maintain hydration (offer fluids frequently). Assess for evidence of upper respiratory infection, cough. Assist with ambulation if dizziness occurs. Monitor stool frequency and consistency (watery, loose, soft).

PATIENT/FAMILY TEACHING:

Inform female pt regarding consequences of second-and third-trimester exposure to losartan. Report pregnancy to physician as soon as possible. Avoid tasks that require alertness, motor skills (possible dizziness effect). Report any sign of infection (sore throat, fever), chest pain. Do not take cold preparations, nasal decongestants. Do not stop taking medication. Need for lifelong control.

lovastatin

low-vah-**stah**-tin
(Mevacor)
Do not confuse with Levstatin, Livostin, Mivacron.

▶**CLASSIFICATION**

PHARMACOTHERAPEUTIC:
HMG-CoA reductase inhibitor.
CLINICAL: Antihyperlipidemic
(see p. 50C)

ACTION/*THERAPEUTIC EFFECT*

Inhibits HMG-CoA reductase, the enzyme that catalyzes the early step in cholesterol synthesis. *Decreases LDL cholesterol, VLDL cholesterol, plasma triglycerides; increases HDL cholesterol.*

PHARMACOKINETICS

Incompletely absorbed from GI tract (increased on empty stomach). Protein binding: >95%. Hydrolyzed in liver to active metabolite. Primarily eliminated in feces. Not removed by hemodialysis. Half-life: 3 hrs.

USES

Treatment of hypercholesterolemia and coronary atherosclerosis. Reduces risk of myocardial infarction, unstable angina, need for revascularization procedures in those without symptomatic cardiovascular disease, with average to moderately elevated total cholesterol and LDL cholesterol levels and below average HDL cholesterol levels.

PRECAUTIONS

CONTRAINDICATIONS: Active liver disease, unexplained elevated liver function tests. ***CAUTIONS:*** Anticoagulant therapy, history of liver disease, substantial alcohol consumption. Withholding/discontinuing lovastatin may be necessary when pt is at risk for renal failure (secondary to rhabdomyolysis); major surgery, severe acute infection, trauma, hypotension, severe metabolic, endocrine or electrolyte disorders, or uncontrolled seizures.

▷***LIFESPAN CONSIDERATIONS:***
Pregnancy/Lactation: Contraindicated in pregnancy (suppression of cholesterol biosynthesis may cause fetal toxicity) and lactation. Unknown if drug is distributed in breast milk. **Pregnancy Category X. Children:** Safety and efficacy not established. **Elderly:** No age-related precautions noted.

INTERACTIONS

DRUG: Increased risk of rhabdomyolysis, acute renal failure with **cyclosporine, erythromycin, gemfibrozil, niacin, other immunosuppressants. Erythromycin, itraconazole, ketoconazole** may increase concentration causing severe muscle pain, inflammation, weakness. **HERBAL:** None known. **FOOD:** Large amounts of **grapefruit juice** may increase risk of side effects (e.g., muscle pain, weakness). **LAB VALUES:** May increase creatinine kinase, serum transaminase concentrations.

AVAILABILITY (Rx)

TABLETS: 10 mg, 20 mg, 40 mg.

ADMINISTRATION/HANDLING
PO:
• Give with meals.

INDICATIONS/ROUTES/DOSAGE
Hyperlipoproteinemia:

PO: Adults, elderly: Initially: 20–40 mg/day with evening meal. Increase at 4 wk intervals up to maximum of 80 mg/day. **Maintenance:** 20–80 mg/day in single or divided doses.

SIDE EFFECTS

Generally well tolerated. Side effects usually mild and transient. **FREQUENT** (5–9%): Headache, flatulence, diarrhea, abdominal pain or cramps, rash/pruritus. **OCCASIONAL** (3–4%): Nausea, vomiting, constipation, dyspepsia. **RARE** (1–2%): Dizziness, heartburn, myalgia, blurred vision, eye irritation.

ADVERSE REACTIONS/TOXIC EFFECTS

Potential for cataracts.

NURSING IMPLICATIONS

BASELINE ASSESSMENT:

Question for possibility of pregnancy before initiating therapy (Pregnancy Category X). Assess baseline lab results: cholesterol, triglycerides, liver function tests.

INTERVENTION/EVALUATION:

Determine pattern of bowel activity. Check for headache, dizziness, blurred vision. Assess for rash, pruritus. Monitor cholesterol and triglyceride lab results for therapeutic response. Be alert for malaise, muscle cramping or weakness. Monitor temperature at least twice a day.

PATIENT/FAMILY TEACHING:

Take with meals. Follow special diet (important part of treatment). Periodic lab tests are essential part of therapy. Report promptly any muscle pain or weakness, esp. if accompanied by fever or malaise. Avoid drinking large amounts of grapefruit juice.

---

loxapine hydrochloride

lox-ah-peen
(Apo-Loxapine✦, Loxapac✦, Loxitane)

loxapine succinate
(Loxitane)

►CLASSIFICATION

PHARMACOTHERAPEUTIC: Dibenzodiazepine derivative. **CLINICAL:** Antipsychotic (see p. 55C)

✎ - see color pill atlas   <u>underscored</u> - top 100 prescribed drug

ACTION/*THERAPEUTIC EFFECT*

Blocks dopamine at postsynaptic receptor sites in brain. *Suppresses locomotor activity, produces tranquilization.* Strong anticholinergic effects.

USES/*UNLABELED*

Symptomatic management of psychotic disorders. *Management anxiety associated with mental depression.*

PRECAUTIONS

CONTRAINDICATIONS: Severe CNS depression, comatose states. ***EXTREME CAUTION:*** History of seizures. ***CAUTIONS:*** Cardiovascular disorders, glaucoma, history of urinary retention, prostatic hypertrophy.

INTERACTIONS

DRUG: Alcohol, CNS depressants may increase CNS depression. Antacids, antidiarrheals may decrease absorption. Extrapyramidal symptom (EPS)-producing medications may increase risk of EPS. ***HERBAL:*** None known. ***FOOD:*** None known. ***LAB VALUES:*** None significant.

AVAILABILITY (Rx)

CAPSULES: 5 mg, 10 mg, 25 mg, 50 mg. ***ORAL SOLUTION:*** 25 mg/ml.

INDICATIONS/ROUTES/DOSAGE

Psychotic disorders:

PO: **Adults:** Initially, 10 mg 2 times/day. **Maintenance range:** 15–25 mg 2–4 times/day. **Elderly:** Initially, 3–5 mg 2 times/day.

SIDE EFFECTS

FREQUENT: Blurred vision, confusion, drowsiness, dry mouth, dizziness, lightheadedness. ***OCCASIONAL:*** Allergic reaction (rash, itching), decreased urination, constipation, decreased sexual ability, enlarged breasts, headache, photosensitivity, nausea, vomiting, insomnia, weight gain.

ADVERSE REACTIONS/TOXIC EFFECTS

Extrapyramidal symptoms frequently noted are akathisia (motor restlessness, anxiety). Less frequently noted are akinesia (rigidity, tremor, salivation, mask-like facial expression, reduced voluntary movements). Infrequently noted dystonias: torticollis (neck muscle spasm), opisthotonos (rigidity of back muscles), and oculogyric crisis (rolling back of eyes). Tardive dyskinesia (protrusion of tongue, puffing of cheeks, chewing/puckering of mouth) occurs rarely but may be irreversible. Risk is greater in female elderly pts. Grand mal seizures may occur in epileptic pts (risk higher with IM administration).

NURSING IMPLICATIONS

BASELINE ASSESSMENT:

Assess behavior, appearance, emotional status, response to environment, speech pattern, thought content.

INTERVENTION/EVALUATION:

Supervise suicidal risk pt closely during early therapy (as depression lessens, energy level improves, and suicide potential increases). Assess stool consistency and frequency. Monitor for rigidity, tremor, masklike facial expression (esp. in those receiving IM injection). Assess for therapeutic response (interest in surroundings, improvement in self-care, increased ability to concentrate, relaxed facial expression).

PATIENT/FAMILY TEACHING:
Full therapeutic effect may take up to 6 wks. Report visual disturbances. Sugarless gum, sips of tepid water may relieve dry mouth. Drowsiness generally subsides during continued therapy. Avoid tasks that require alertness, motor skills until response to drug is established. Avoid alcohol, CNS depressants, OTC medications. Describe signs and symptoms of extrapyramidal involvement and tardive dyskinesia for pt to report immediately.

mafenide acetate

ma-fe-nide
(Sulfamylon)

▶CLASSIFICATION

PHARMACOTHERAPEUTIC: Topical anti-infective. **CLINICAL:** Burn preparation

ACTION/THERAPEUTIC EFFECT

Decreases number of bacteria in avascular tissue of second- and third-degree burns. *Bacteriostatic. Promotes spontaneous healing of deep partial-thickness burns.*

USES

Adjunctive therapy for second- and third-degree burns to prevent infection, septicemia; protection against conversion from partial-to full-thickness wounds (infection causes extended tissue destruction). **Solution:** Adjunct agent to control bacterial infection when used under moist dressing over meshed autografts on excised burn wounds.

PRECAUTIONS

CONTRAINDICATIONS: Hypersensitivity to mafenide or sulfite. **CAUTIONS:** Impaired renal function that increases risk of metabolic acidosis. Cross-sensitivity to sulfonamides not certain.

INTERACTIONS

DRUG: None significant. **HERBAL:** None known. **FOOD:** None known. **LAB VALUES:** None significant.

AVAILABILITY (Rx)

CREAM. TOPICAL POWDER.

INDICATIONS/ROUTES/DOSAGE

Usual topical dosage:

Adults, elderly: Apply 1–2 times/day.

SIDE EFFECTS

Difficult to distinguish side effects and effects of severe burn. **FREQUENT:** Pain, burning upon application. **OCCASIONAL:** Allergic reaction (usually 10–14 days after initiation of mafenide): Itching, rash, facial edema, swelling; unexplained syndrome of marked hyperventilation with respiratory alkalosis. **RARE:** Delay in eschar separation, excoriation of new skin.

ADVERSE REACTIONS/TOXIC EFFECTS

Hemolytic anemia, porphyria, bone marrow depression, superinfections (esp. with fungi), metabolic acidosis occurs rarely.

NURSING IMPLICATIONS

BASELINE ASSESSMENT:

Evaluate arterial blood gases (ABGs) for acid-base balance, renal function tests and CBC for baseline.

INTERVENTION/EVALUATION:

Be alert to fluid balance and renal function: Monitor I&O, renal function tests, urinary pH, and promptly report changes. Watch for signs/symptoms of metabolic acidosis: Kussmaul's respirations, nausea, vomiting, diarrhea, headache, tremors, weakness and cardiac arrhythmias (due to associated hyperkalemia), sensorium changes, decreased PCO_2, blood pH, and HCO_3. Assess burns, surrounding skin areas for allergic reaction or superinfection: rash, excoriation, swelling, itching, increased pain, purulent exudate.

PATIENT/FAMILY TEACHING:

Application may cause temporary pain or burning; burn areas must be completely covered by cream. Therapy must not be interrupted (attempts will be made to reduce adverse reaction before considering discontinuance of drug). Bathe burn area daily.

magnesium

magnesium chloride

(Citro-Mag♣, Phillips' Magnesia Tablets♣, Slow-Mag)

magnesium citrate

(Citrate of Magnesia, Citroma, Citro-Nesia)

magnesium hydroxide

(MOM)

magnesium oxide

(Mag-Ox 400, Maox)

magnesium protein complex

(Mg-PLUS)

magnesium sulfate

(Epsom salt, magnesium sulfate injection)
Do not confuse with manganese sulfate.

FIXED-COMBINATION(S)

With aluminum, an antacid **(Aludrox, Delcid, Gaviscon, Maalox)**; with aluminum and simethicone, an antiflatulent **(Di-Gel, Gelusil, Maalox Plus, Mylanta, Silain-Gel)**; with aluminum and calcium, an antacid **(Camalox)**; with mineral oil, a lubricant laxative **(Haley's MO)**; with magnesium oxide and aluminum oxide, antacids **(Riopan)**

▶**CLASSIFICATION**

CLINICAL: Antacid, anticonvulsant, electrolyte, laxative (see pp. 9C, 100C)

ACTION/*THERAPEUTIC EFFECT*

Antacid: Acts in stomach to neutralize *gastric acid, increase pH*. **Laxative:** Osmotic effect primarily in small intestine. Draws water into intestinal lumen, produces *distention, promotes peristalsis, bowel evacuation*. **Systemic (dietary supplement, replacement):** Found primarily in intracellular fluids. Essential *for enzyme activity, nerve conduction, and muscle contraction*. **Anticonvulsant:** Blocks neuromuscular transmission, amount of acetylcholine released at motor end plate, *producing seizure control*.

M

PHARMACOKINETICS

Antacid, laxative: Minimal absorption through intestine. Absorbed dose primarily excreted in urine. *Systemic:* Widely distributed. Primarily excreted in urine.

USES

Treatment/prevention of hypomagnesemia. Treatment of hypertension, torsade de pointes, encephalopathy, seizures associated with acute nephritis, constipation, hyperacidity.

PRECAUTIONS

CONTRAINDICATIONS: Antacids: Severe renal impairment, appendicitis or symptoms of appendicitis, ileostomy, intestinal obstruction. *Laxative:* Appendicitis, undiagnosed rectal bleeding, CHF, intestinal obstruction, hypersensitivity, colostomy, ileostomy. *Systemic:* Heart block, myocardial damage, renal failure. *CAUTIONS:* Safety in children <6 yrs not known. *Antacids:* Undiagnosed gastrointestinal or rectal bleeding, ulcerative colitis, colostomy, diverticulitis, chronic diarrhea. *Laxative:* Diabetes mellitus or pts on low-salt diet (some products contain sugar, sodium). *Systemic:* Severe renal impairment.

▷*LIFESPAN CONSIDERATIONS:*
Pregnancy/Lactation: *Antacid:* Unknown if distributed in breast milk. **Pregnancy Category C.** *Parenteral:* Readily crosses placenta; distributed in breast milk for 24 hrs after magnesium therapy is discontinued. Continuous IV infusion increases risk of magnesium toxicity in neonate. IV administration should not be used 2 hrs preceding delivery. **Pregnancy Category B** (anticonvulsant/laxative). **Children:** No age-related precautions noted. **Elderly:** Increased risk of developing magnesium deficiency (e.g., poor diet, decreased absorption, medications).

INTERACTIONS

DRUG: Antacids: May decrease absorption of **ketoconazole, tetracyclines.** May decrease effect of **methenamine.** *Antacids, laxatives:* May decrease effects of **oral anticoagulants, digoxin, phenothiazines.** May form nonabsorbable complex with **tetracyclines.** *Systemic:* **Calcium** may neutralize effects. CNS depression-producing medications may increase CNS depression. May cause changes in cardiac conduction/heart block with **digoxin.** *HERBAL:* None known. *FOOD:* None known. *LAB VALUES: Antacid:* May increase gastrin, pH. *Laxative:* May decrease potassium. *Systemic:* None significant.

AVAILABILITY (OTC)

TABLETS: 400 mg, 500 mg. *TABLETS (chewable):* 311 mg. *TABLETS (sustained-release):* 535 mg. *CAPSULES:* 140 mg. *LIQUID:* 54 mg/5 ml, 400 mg/5 ml, 800 mg/5 ml. *MOM:* 30 ml, 60 ml. *INJECTION (Rx):* 10%, 12.5%, 20%, 50%.

ADMINISTRATION/HANDLING

PO [Antacid]:

• Shake suspension well before use. • Chewable tablets should be chewed thoroughly before swallowing and follow with full glass of water.

PO [Laxative]:

• Drink full glass of liquid (8 oz) with each dose (prevents dehydration). • Flavor may be improved by following with fruit juice or citrus carbonated beverage. •

𝓵 - see color pill atlas · <u>underscored</u> - top 100 prescribed drug

Refrigerate citrate of magnesia (retains potency, palatability).

IM:

• For adults, elderly, use 250 mg/ml (25%) or 500 mg/ml (50%) magnesium sulfate concentration.
• For infants, children, do not exceed 200 mg/ml (20%).

IV 📋

Storage:

• Store at room temperature.

Reconstitution:

• Must dilute (do not exceed 20 mg/ml concentration).

Rate of administration:

• For IV infusion, do not exceed magnesium sulfate concentration 200 mg/ml (20%). • Do not exceed IV infusion rate of 150 mg/min.

IV INCOMPATIBILITIES ⃠

Amphotericin B complex (Abelcet, Ambisome, Amphotec), cefepime (Maxipime).

IV COMPATIBILITIES

Amikacin (Amikin), cefazolin (Ancef), dobutamine (Dobutrex), enalapril (Vasotec), gentamicin (Garamycin), heparin, insulin, labetalol (Normodyne, Trandate), milrinone (Primacor), piperacillin/tazobactam (Zosyn), potassium, propofol (Diprivan), tobramycin (Nebcin), vancomycin (Vancocin).

INDICATIONS/ROUTES/DOSAGE

Hypomagnesemia (magnesium sulfate):

***IM/IV:* Adults, elderly:** 1 g q6h for 4 doses. **Children:** 25–50 mg/kg/dose q4–6h for 3–4 doses.

***PO:* Adults, elderly:** 3 g q6h for 4 doses. **Children:** 10–20 mg/kg (elemental magnesium)/dose 4 times/day.

Hypertension, seizures (magnesium sulfate):

***IM/IV:* Adults, elderly:** 1 g q6h for 4 doses as needed. **Children:** 20–100 mg/kg/dose q4–6h as needed.

Torsade de pointes (magnesium sulfate):

***IV:* Children, neonates:** 25–50 mg/kg/dose. **Maximum:** 2 g

LAXATIVE:

Magnesium citrate:

***PO:* Adults, elderly, children >12 yrs:** 150–300 ml. **Children 6–12 yrs:** 100–150 ml. **Children <6 yrs:** 2–4 ml/kg.

Magnesium hydroxide:

***PO:* Adults, elderly, children >12 yrs:** 30–60 ml/day. **Children 6–11 yrs:** 15–30 ml/day. **Children 2–5 yrs:** 5–15 ml/day. **Children <2 yrs:** 0.5 ml/kg/dose.

ANTACID:

Magnesium hydroxide

Note: Up to 4 times/day.

***PO:* Adults, elderly:** *(Tablet):* 622–1,244 mg/dose. *(Liquid concentrate):* 2.5–7.5 ml/dose. *(Liquid):* 5–15 ml/dose. **Children:** *(Liquid):* 2.5–5 ml/dose.

SIDE EFFECTS

FREQUENT: Antacid: Chalky taste, diarrhea, laxative effect. ***OCCASIONAL: Antacid:*** Nausea, vomiting, stomach cramps. ***Antacid, laxative:*** Prolonged use or large dose with renal impairment may cause increased magnesium (dizziness, irregular heartbeat, mental changes, tiredness, weakness). ***Laxative:*** Cramping, diarrhea, increased thirst, gas. ***Systemic:*** Reduced respiratory rate, decreased reflexes, flushing, hypotension, decreased heart rate.

M

ADVERSE REACTIONS/TOXIC EFFECTS

Antacid, laxative: None significant. **Systemic:** May produce prolonged PQ interval, widening of QRS intervals. May cause loss of deep tendon reflexes, heart block, respiratory paralysis, and cardiac arrest. **Antidote:** 10–20 ml 10% calcium gluconate (5–10 mEq of calcium).

NURSING IMPLICATIONS

BASELINE ASSESSMENT:

Assess if pt is sensitive to magnesium. **Antacid:** Assess GI pain (duration, location, time of occurrence, relief with food or caused by food or alcohol, constant or sporadic, worsened when lying down or bending over). **Laxative:** Assess color, amount, consistency of stool. Assess bowel habits (usual pattern), bowel sound for peristalsis. Assess pt for any abdominal pain, weight loss, nausea, vomiting, history of recent abdominal surgery. **Systemic:** Assess renal function, magnesium level.

INTERVENTION/EVALUATION:

Antacid: Assess for relief of gastric distress. Monitor renal function (esp. if dosing is long term or frequent). **Laxative:** Monitor stools for diarrhea or constipation. Maintain adequate fluid intake. **Systemic:** Monitor renal function, magnesium levels, EKG for cardiac function. Test patellar reflex or knee jerk reflexes before giving repeat parenteral doses (used as indication of CNS depression; suppressed reflex may be sign of impending respiratory arrest). Patellar reflex must be present, respiratory rate >16/min before each parenteral dose. Provide seizure precautions.

PATIENT/FAMILY TEACHING:

Antacid: Give at least 2 hrs apart from other medication. Do not take >2 wks unless directed by physician. For peptic ulcer take 1 and 3 hrs after meals and at bedtime for 4–6 wks. Chew tablets thoroughly followed with glass of water; shake suspensions well. Repeat dosing/large doses may have laxative effect. **Laxative:** Drink full glass (8 oz) liquid to aid stool softening. Use only for short term. Do not use if abdominal pain, vomiting, nausea are present. **Systemic:** Inform physician of any signs of hypermagnesemia (confusion, irregular heartbeat, cramping, unusual tiredness or weakness, lightheadedness, or dizziness).

mannitol

man-ih-toll
(Osmitrol)

▶CLASSIFICATION

CLINICAL: Osmotic diuretic, antiglaucoma, antihemolytic

ACTION/*THERAPEUTIC EFFECT*

Elevates osmotic pressure of glomerular filtrate, increases flow of water into interstitial fluid and plasma, inhibiting renal tubular reabsorption of sodium, chloride, *producing diuresis.* Enhances flow of water from eye into plasma, *reducing intraocular pressure (IOP).*

PHARMACOKINETICS

Remains in extracellular fluid. Primarily excreted in urine. Removed by hemodialysis. Half-life: 100 min. Onset diuresis occurs in 1–3 hrs, decreases intraocular pressure in 0.5–1 hr, duration 4–6 hrs. Decreases cerebral spinal fluid pressure in 15 min, duration 3–8 hrs.

USES

Prevention, treatment of oliguric phase of acute renal failure (before evidence of permanent renal failure). Reduces increased intracranial pressure due to cerebral edema, edema of injured spinal cord, intraocular pressure due to acute glaucoma. Promotes urinary excretion of toxic substances (aspirin, bromides, imipramine, barbiturates).

PRECAUTIONS

CONTRAINDICATIONS: Increasing oliguria or anuria, CHF, pulmonary edema, organic CNS disease, severe dehydration, fluid overload, active intracranial bleeding (except during craniotomy), severe electrolyte depletion. **CAUTIONS:** Impaired renal, hepatic function.

▷**LIFESPAN CONSIDERATIONS:**
Pregnancy/Lactation: Unknown if drug crosses placenta or is distributed in breast milk. **Pregnancy Category C. Children:** Safety and efficacy not established in those <12 yrs of age. **Elderly:** Age-related renal impairment may require caution.

INTERACTIONS

DRUG: May increase **digoxin** toxicity (due to hypokalemia). **HERBAL:** None known. **FOOD:** None known. **LAB VALUES:** May de-

crease phosphate, potassium, sodium.

AVAILABILITY (Rx)

INJECTION: 5%, 10%, 15%, 20%, 25%.

ADMINISTRATION/HANDLING

Note: Assess IV site for patency before each dose. Extravasation noted with pain, thrombosis.

IV 💯

Storage:

• Store at room temperature. • If crystals are noted in solution, warm bottle in hot water and shake vigorously at intervals. Cool to body temperature before administration. Do not use if crystals remain after warming procedure.

Rate of administration:

• Administer by IV infusion over 30–90 min. • Rate of administration should be titrated to promote urinary output of 30–50 ml/hr. • Use filter for infusion of 20% or more concentration. • Do not add KCl or NaCl to mannitol 20% or greater. Do not add to whole blood for transfusion.

IV INCOMPATIBILITIES ⊘

Cefepime (Amxipime), doxorubicin liposome (Doxil), filgrastim (Neupogen).

IV COMPATIBILITIES

Cisplatin (Platinol), ondansetron (Zofran), propofol (Diprivan).

INDICATIONS/ROUTES/DOSAGE

Usual IV dosage:

Note: Test dose of 12.5 g for adults (200 mg/kg for children) over 3–5 min to produce a urine flow of at least 30–50 ml/hr over 2–3 hrs (1 ml/kg/hr for children).

Adults, elderly, children: Initially,

0.5–1 g/kg, then 0.25–0.5 g/kg q4–6h.

SIDE EFFECTS

FREQUENT: Dry mouth, thirst. **OCCASIONAL:** Blurred vision, increased urination, headache, arm pain, backache, nausea, vomiting, urticaria (hives), dizziness, hypotension, hypertension, tachycardia, fever, anginalike chest pain.

ADVERSE REACTIONS/TOXIC EFFECTS

Fluid and electrolyte imbalance may occur because of rapid administration of large doses or inadequate urinary output resulting in overexpansion of extracellular fluid. Circulatory overload may produce pulmonary edema, CHF. Excessive diuresis may produce hypokalemia, hyponatremia. Fluid loss in excess of electrolyte excretion may produce hypernatremia, hyperkalemia.

NURSING IMPLICATIONS

BASELINE ASSESSMENT:

Check B/P, pulse before giving medication. Assess skin turgor, mucous membranes, mental status, muscle strength. Obtain baseline weight. Initiate I&O.

INTERVENTION/EVALUATION:

Monitor urinary output to ascertain therapeutic response. Monitor electrolyte, BUN, renal, hepatic reports. Assess vital signs, skin turgor, mucous membranes. Weigh daily. Signs of hyponatremia include confusion, drowsiness, thirst or dry mouth, cold/clammy skin. Signs of hypokalemia include changes in muscle strength, tremors, muscle cramps, changes in mental status, cardiac arrhyth-

mias. Signs of hyperkalemia include colic, diarrhea, muscle twitching followed by weakness or paralysis, arrhythmias.

PATIENT/FAMILY TEACHING:

Expect increased frequency and volume of urination.

maprotiline hydrochloride

mah-**pro**-tih-leen
(Ludiomil)

▶CLASSIFICATION

PHARMACOTHERAPEUTIC: Tetracyclic. **CLINICAL:** Antidepressant

ACTION/*THERAPEUTIC EFFECT*

Blocks reuptake of norepinephrine by CNS presynaptic neuronal membranes, increasing availability at postsynaptic neuronal receptor sites. Resulting enhancement of synaptic activity *produces antidepressant effect.* Moderate anticholinergic activity.

USES/*UNLABELED*

Relief of depressive-affective (mood) disorders, including depressive neurosis, major depression. Also used for depression phase of bipolar disorder (manic-depressive illness). *Treatment of neurogenic pain.*

PRECAUTIONS

CONTRAINDICATIONS: Acute recovery period following MI, within 14 days of MAO inhibitor ingestion, known or suspected seizure disorders. **CAUTIONS:** Prostatic hypertrophy, history of urinary retention or obstruction, glaucoma, diabetes mellitus, history of seizures, hyperthyroidism, cardiac/hepatic/renal disease, schizophrenia, increased intraocular pressure, hiatal hernia.

INTERACTIONS

DRUG:* Alcohol, CNS depressants** may increase effect. **MAO inhibitors** may increase risk of hypertensive crisis, severe convulsions. **Sympathomimetics** may increase cardiovascular effects (arrhythmias, tachycardia, severe hypertension). ***HERBAL: None known. ***FOOD:*** None known. ***LAB VALUES:*** None significant.

AVAILABILITY (Rx)

TABLETS: 25 mg, 50 mg, 75 mg.

INDICATIONS/ROUTES/DOSAGE

Mild to moderate depression:

***PO:* Adults:** 75 mg/day to start, in 1–4 divided doses. **Elderly:** 50–75 mg/day. In 2 wks, increase dosage gradually in 25 mg increments until therapeutic response is achieved. Reduce to lowest effective maintenance level.

Severe depression:

***PO:* Adults:** 100–150 mg/day in 1–4 divided doses. May increase gradually to maximum 225 mg/day.

Usual elderly dosage:

PO: Initially, 25 mg at bedtime. May increase by 25 mg q3–7days. **Maintenance:** 50–75 mg/day.

SIDE EFFECTS

FREQUENT: Drowsiness, fatigue, dry mouth, blurred vision, constipation, delayed micturition, postural hypotension, excessive sweating, disturbed concentration, increased appetite, urinary reten-

tion. ***OCCASIONAL:*** GI disturbances (nausea, GI distress, metallic taste sensation), photosensitivity. ***RARE:*** Paradoxical reaction (agitation, restlessness, nightmares, insomnia), extrapyramidal symptoms (particularly fine hand tremor).

ADVERSE REACTIONS/TOXIC EFFECTS

Higher incidence of seizures than with tricyclic antidepressants (esp. in those with no previous history of seizures). High dosage may produce cardiovascular effects (severe postural hypotension, dizziness, tachycardia, palpitations, arrhythmias) and seizures. May also result in altered temperature regulation (hyperpyrexia or hypothermia). Abrupt withdrawal from prolonged therapy may produce headache, malaise, nausea, vomiting, vivid dreams.

M

NURSING IMPLICATIONS

BASELINE ASSESSMENT:

For those on long-term therapy, liver/renal function tests, blood counts should be performed periodically.

INTERVENTION/EVALUATION:

Supervise suicidal risk pt closely during early therapy (as depression lessens, energy level improves, increasing suicide potential). Assess appearance, behavior, speech pattern, level of interest, mood. Monitor B/P, pulse for hypotension, arrhythmias. Assess for urinary retention.

PATIENT/FAMILY TEACHING:

Tolerance to postural hypotension, sedative and anticholinergic effects usually develops during early therapy. Therapeutic effect may be noted within 3–7 days, maximum effect within 2–3 wks. Wear protective clothing, use sunscreen to protect skin from ultraviolet light or sunlight. Dry mouth may be relieved by sugarless gum, sips of tepid water. Report visual disturbances. Do not abruptly discontinue medication. Avoid tasks that require alertness, motor skills until response to drug is established.

mechlorethamine hydrochloride

(Mustargen)

See Classification section under: Antineoplastics (p. 72C)

meclizine

mek-lih-zeen
(Antivert, Bonamine✦, Bonine)

▶CLASSIFICATION

PHARMACOTHERAPEUTIC:
Anticholinergic. ***CLINICAL:*** Antiemetic, antivertigo

ACTION/*THERAPEUTIC EFFECT*

Reduces labyrinth excitability, diminishes vestibular stimulation of labyrinth, affecting chemoreceptor trigger zone (CTZ), *reducing nausea, vomiting, vertigo.* Anticholinergic activity.

PHARMACOKINETICS

Onset	Peak	Duration
PO		
30–60 min	—	12–24 hrs

Well absorbed from GI tract. Widely distributed. Metabolized in liver. Primarily excreted in urine. Half-life: 6 hrs.

USES

Prevention and treatment of nausea, vomiting, vertigo due to motion sickness. Treatment of vertigo associated with diseases affecting vestibular system.

PRECAUTIONS

CONTRAINDICATIONS: None significant. ***CAUTIONS:*** Narrow-angle glaucoma, prostatic hypertrophy, pyloroduodenal or bladder obstruction, asthma, COPD, increased intraocular pressure, cardiovascular disease, hyperthyroidism, hypertension, seizure disorders.
▷*LIFESPAN CONSIDERATIONS:*
Pregnancy/Lactation: Unknown whether drug crosses placenta or is distributed in breast milk (may produce irritability in nursing infants). **Pregnancy Category B. Children/Elderly:** May be more sensitive to anticholinergic effects (e.g., dry mouth).

INTERACTIONS

DRUG:* Alcohol, CNS depression–producing medications** may increase CNS depressant effect. ***HERBAL: None known. ***FOOD:*** None known. ***LAB VALUES:*** May suppress wheal, flare reactions to antigen skin testing, unless meclizine discontinued 4 days before testing.

AVAILABILITY (Rx)

TABLETS: 12.5 mg, 25 mg, 50 mg.
TABLETS (chewable): 25 mg.
CAPSULES: 25 mg.

ADMINISTRATION/HANDLING

PO:

• Give without regard to meals. • Scored tablets may be crushed. • Do not crush or break capsule form.

INDICATIONS/ROUTES/DOSAGE

Motion sickness:

PO: Adults, elderly, children >12 yrs: 25–50 mg 1 hr before exposure to motion. Repeat q24h as needed.

Vertigo:

PO: Adults, elderly, children >12 yrs: 25–100 mg/day in divided doses as needed.

SIDE EFFECTS

Note: Elderly (>60 yrs) tend to develop sedation, dizziness, hypotension, mental confusion, disorientation, agitation, psychoticlike symptoms.

FREQUENT: Drowsiness. ***OCCASIONAL:*** Blurred vision, dry mouth, nose, or throat.

ADVERSE REACTIONS/TOXIC EFFECTS

Children may experience dominant paradoxical reaction (restlessness, insomnia, euphoria, nervousness, tremors). Overdosage in children may result in hallucinations, convulsions, death. Hypersensitivity reaction (eczema, pruritus, rash, cardiac disturbances, photosensitivity) may occur. Overdosage may vary from CNS depression (sedation, apnea, cardiovascular collapse, death) to severe paradoxical reaction (hallucinations, tremor, seizures).

NURSING IMPLICATIONS

INTERVENTION/EVALUATION:

Monitor B/P, esp. in elderly (increased risk of hypotension). Monitor children closely for paradoxical reaction. Monitor serum electrolytes in those with severe vomiting. Assess skin turgor, mucous membranes to evaluate hydration status.

PATIENT/FAMILY TEACHING:

Tolerance to sedative effect may occur. Avoid tasks that require alertness, motor skills until response to drug is established. Dry mouth, drowsiness, dizziness may be an expected response of drug. Avoid alcoholic beverages during therapy. Sugarless gum, sips of tepid water may relieve dry mouth. Coffee or tea may help reduce drowsiness.

---

meclofenamate sodium

(Meclodium, Meclomen)

See Classification section under: Nonsteroidal Anti-Inflammatory Drugs (NSAIDs)

M

---

medroxyprogesterone acetate

meh-drocks-ee-pro-**jes**-ter-own
(Amen, Curretab, Depo-Provera, Novo-Medrone✣, Provera)
Do not confuse with Ambien, hydroxyprogesterone, methylprednisolone, methytestosterone.

FIXED-COMBINATION(S)

With conjugated estrogens **(Lunelle, Premphase, Prempro)**

▶CLASSIFICATION

PHARMACOTHERAPEUTIC: Hormone. ***CLINICAL:*** Progestin, antineoplastic

---

ACTION/*THERAPEUTIC EFFECT*

Transforms endometrium from proliferative to secretory (in an estrogen-primed endometrium); inhibits secretion of pituitary gonadotropins, *preventing follicular maturation and ovulation.* Stimulates growth of mammary alveolar tissue; relaxes uterine smooth muscle. *Restores hormonal imbalance.*

PHARMACOKINETICS

Slow absorption after IM administration. Protein binding: 90%. Metabolized in liver. Primarily excreted in urine.

USES/*UNLABELED*

PO: Prevention of endometrial hyperplasia (concurrently given with estrogen to women with intact uterus), treatment of secondary amenorrhea, abnormal uterine bleeding. **IM:** Adjunctive therapy, palliative treatment of inoperable, recurrent, metastatic endometrial carcinoma, renal carcinoma; prevention of pregnancy. *Treatment of endometriosis, hormonal replacement therapy in estrogen-treated menopausal women.*

PRECAUTIONS

CONTRAINDICATIONS: History of or active thrombotic disorders (cerebral apoplexy, thrombophlebitis, thromboembolic disorders), hypersensitivity to progestins, severe liver dysfunction, estrogen-dependent neoplasia, undiagnosed abnormal genital bleeding, missed abortion, use as pregnancy test, undiagnosed vaginal bleeding, carcinoma of breast, known or suspected pregnancy. **CAUTIONS:** Those with conditions aggravated by fluid retention (asthma, seizures, migraine, cardiac or renal dysfunction), diabetes, history of mental depression.

▷*LIFESPAN CONSIDERATIONS:*

Pregnancy/Lactation: Avoid use during pregnancy, esp. first 4 mos (congenital heart, limb reduction defects may occur). Distributed in breast milk. **Pregnancy Category D. Children:** Safety and efficacy not established. **Elderly:** No age-related precautions noted.

INTERACTIONS

DRUG: May interfere with effects of **bromocriptine. HERBAL:** None known. **FOOD:** None known. **LAB VALUES:** May increase alkaline phosphatase, LDL. May decrease HDL cholesterol.

AVAILABILITY (Rx)

TABLETS: 2.5 mg, 5 mg, 10 mg. **INJECTION:** 150 mg/ml, 400 mg/ml.

ADMINISTRATION/HANDLING

PO:

• Give without regard to meals.

IM:

• Shake vial immediately before administering (ensures complete suspension). • Rarely, a residual lump, change in skin color, or sterile abscess occurs at injection site.

INDICATIONS/ROUTES/DOSAGE

Endometrial hyperplasia:

PO: Adults: 2–10 mg/day for 14 days.

Secondary amenorrhea:

PO: Adults: 5–10 mg/day for 5–10 days (begin at any time during menstrual cycle) or 2.5 mg/day.

Abnormal uterine bleeding:

PO: Adults: 5–10 mg/day for 5–10 days (begin on calculated day 16 or day 21 of menstrual cycle).

Endometrial, renal carcinoma:
IM: **Adults, elderly:** Initially, 400–1,000 mg, repeat at 1 wk intervals. If improvement occurs, disease stabilized, begin maintenance with as little as 400 mg/mo.

Pregnancy prevention:
IM: **Adults:** 150 mg q3 mos.

SIDE EFFECTS

FREQUENT: Transient menstrual abnormalities (spotting, change in menstrual flow or cervical secretions, amenorrhea) at initiation of therapy. *OCCASIONAL:* Edema, weight change, breast tenderness, nervousness, insomnia, fatigue, dizziness. *RARE:* Alopecia, mental depression, dermatologic changes, headache, fever, nausea.

ADVERSE REACTIONS/TOXIC EFFECTS

Thrombophlebitis, pulmonary or cerebral embolism, retinal thrombosis occurs rarely.

NURSING IMPLICATIONS

BASELINE ASSESSMENT:

Question for hypersensitivity to progestins, possibility of pregnancy before initiating therapy (Pregnancy Category X). Obtain baseline weight, blood glucose, B/P.

INTERVENTION/EVALUATION:

Check weight daily; report weekly gain of 5 lbs or more. Check B/P periodically. Assess skin for rash, hives. Report immediately the development of chest pain, sudden shortness of breath, sudden decrease in vision, migraine headache, pain (esp. with swelling, warmth, and redness) in calves, numbness of an arm or leg (thrombotic disorders).

PATIENT/FAMILY TEACHING:

Notify physician of abnormal vaginal bleeding or other symptoms. Stop taking medication and contact physician at once if pregnancy is suspected.

megestrol acetate

meh-**geh**-stroll
(Megace)

▶CLASSIFICATION

PHARMACOTHERAPEUTIC: Hormone. *CLINICAL:* Antineoplastic (see p. 72C)

M

ACTION/*THERAPEUTIC EFFECT*

Suppresses release of luteinizing hormone from anterior pituitary by inhibiting pituitary function, *regressing tumor size. Increases appetite* (mechanism unknown).

PHARMACOKINETICS

Well absorbed from GI tract. Metabolized in liver; excreted in urine.

USES/*UNLABELED*

Palliative management of recurrent, inoperable, or metastatic endometrial or breast carcinoma. Treatment of anorexia, cachexia, or unexplained significant weight loss in pts with AIDS. *Treatment of hormonally dependent/advanced prostate carcinoma.*

PRECAUTIONS

CONTRAINDICATIONS: None significant. *CAUTIONS:* History of thrombophlebitis.

▷**LIFESPAN CONSIDERATIONS:**
Pregnancy/Lactation: If possible, avoid use during pregnancy, esp. first 4 mos. Breast feeding not recommended. **Pregnancy Category X. Children:** Safety and efficacy not established. **Elderly:** No age-related precautions noted.

INTERACTIONS
DRUG: None significant. **HERBAL:** None known. **FOOD:** None known. **LAB VALUES:** May increase serum glucose levels.

AVAILABILITY (Rx)
TABLETS: 20 mg, 40 mg. **SUSPENSION:** 40 mg/ml.

INDICATIONS/ROUTES/DOSAGE
Palliative treatment of advanced breast cancer:
PO: Adults, elderly: 160 mg/day in 4 equally divided doses.

Palliative treatment of advanced endometrial carcinoma:
PO: Adults, elderly: 40–320 mg/day in divided doses. **Maximum:** 800 mg/day.

Anorexia, cachexia, weight loss:
PO: Adults, elderly: 800 mg (20 ml)/day.

SIDE EFFECTS
FREQUENT: Weight gain secondary to increased appetite. **OCCASIONAL:** Nausea, breakthrough bleeding, backache, headache, breast tenderness, carpal tunnel syndrome. **RARE:** Feeling of coldness.

ADVERSE REACTIONS/TOXIC EFFECTS
Thrombophlebitis, pulmonary embolism occurs rarely.

NURSING IMPLICATIONS

BASELINE ASSESSMENT:
Question for possibility of pregnancy before initiating therapy (Pregnancy Category X). Provide support to pt, family, recognizing this drug is palliative, not curative.

PATIENT/FAMILY TEACHING:
Importance of contraception. Notify physician if headache, nausea, breast tenderness, or other symptom persists.

melatonin

Also known as pineal hormone.

▶**CLASSIFICATION**
HERBAL

ACTION/EFFECT
Hormone synthesized endogenously by the pineal gland. Interacts with melatonin receptors in the brain *to regulate the body's circadian rhythm, sleep patterns.* Acts as an antioxidant, *protecting cells from oxidative damage by free radicals.*

USES
Treatment for insomnia, jet lag. Also used as an antioxidant.

PRECAUTIONS
CONTRAINDICATIONS: Pregnancy/breast-feeding. **CAUTIONS:** Depression (may worsen dysphoria), seizures (may increase incidence), cardiovascular or hepatic disease.

▷**LIFESPAN CONSIDERATIONS:**
Pregnancy/Lactation: Contrain-

dicated. **Children:** Safety and efficacy not established. **Elderly:** No age-related precautions noted.

INTERACTIONS:

DRUG: May be additive with **alcohol, benzodiazepines.** May interfere with **immunosuppressants.** May enhance effects of **isoniazid.** **HERBAL:** Chamomile, ginseng, goldenseal, kava kava, valerian may increase sedative effects. **FOOD:** None significant. **LAB VALUES:** May increase human growth hormone levels. May decrease LH levels.

AVAILABILITY (OTC)

LOZENGES: 3 mg. **POWDER. TABLETS:** 0.5 mg, 3 mg.

INDICATIONS/ROUTES/DOSAGE

Insomnia:

PO: Adults, elderly: 0.5–5 mg at bedtime.

Jet lag:

PO: Adults, elderly: 5 mg/day beginning 3 days before flight and 3 days after flight.

SIDE EFFECTS

Headache, transient depression, fatigue, drowsiness, dizziness, abdominal cramps/irritability, decreased alertness, hypersensitivity reaction, tachycardia, nausea, vomiting, anorexia, changes in sleep patterns, confusion.

ADVERSE REACTIONS/TOXIC EFFECTS

None significant.

NURSING IMPLICATIONS

BASELINE ASSESSMENT

Assess if pregnant/breast-feeding (avoid use). Determine if pt has history of seizures or depression. Assess sleep patterns if used for insomnia. Determine medication usage (esp. CNS depressants).

INTERVENTION/EVALUATION

Monitor effectiveness in improving insomnia. Assess for hypersensitivity reactions, CNS effects.

PATIENT/FAMILY TEACHING

Do not use if pregnant, planning to become pregnant, or breast-feeding. Avoid driving or operating machinery.

meloxicam

meh-**locks**-ih-cam
(Mobic)

▶CLASSIFICATION

PHARMACOTHERAPEUTIC: Nonsteroidal anti-inflammatory. **CLINICAL:** Anti-inflammatory, analgesic (see p. 107C)

ACTION/THERAPEUTIC EFFECT

Produces analgesic and anti-inflammatory effect by inhibiting prostaglandin synthesis, *reducing inflammatory response and intensity of pain stimulus reaching sensory nerve endings.*

PHARMACOKINETICS

Onset	Peak	Duration
PO analgesic		
30 min	4–5 hrs	—

Well absorbed following PO administration. Protein binding: 99%. Metabolized in liver. Eliminated via the kidney/feces. Not removed by hemodialysis. Half-life: 15–20 hours.

USES

Relief of signs and symptoms of osteoarthritis.

PRECAUTIONS

CONTRAINDICATIONS: Aspirin-induced nasal polyps associated with bronchospasm. ***CAUTIONS:*** Bleeding conditions (e.g., hemophilia, Crohn's disease, diverticulitis, peptic ulcer, ulcerative colitis), renal impairment.
▷***LIFESPAN CONSIDERATIONS:***
Pregnancy/Lactation: Excreted in breast milk. **Pregnancy Category C. Children:** Safety and efficacy not established. **Elderly:** Age-related renal impairment may require dosage adjustment. More susceptible to GI toxicity; lower dosage recommended.

INTERACTIONS

DRUG: None significant. ***HERBAL:*** **Ginkgo biloba** may increase risk of bleeding. ***FOOD:*** None known. ***LAB VALUES:*** May increase serum creatinine, SGOT, SGPT.

AVAILABILITY (Rx)

TABLETS: 7.5 mg.

ADMINISTRATION/HANDLING

PO:

* Give without regard to meals.

INDICATIONS/ROUTES/DOSAGE

Osteoarthritis:

PO: Adults: Initially, 7.5 mg/day. **Maximum:** 15 mg/day.

SIDE EFFECTS

FREQUENT (7–9%): Dyspepsia (heartburn, indigestion, epigastric pain), headache, diarrhea, nausea. ***OCCASIONAL:*** (3–4%): Dizziness, insomnia, rash, pruritus, flatulence, constipation, vomiting.

RARE (<2%): Somnolence/drowsiness, urticaria, photosensitivity.

ADVERSE REACTIONS/TOXIC EFFECTS

In those treated chronically, peptic ulcer, GI bleeding, gastritis, severe hepatic reaction (jaundice), nephrotoxicity (hematuria, dysuria, proteinuria), severe hypersensitivity reaction (bronchospasm, angiofacial edema) occur rarely.

NURSING IMPLICATIONS

BASELINE ASSESSMENT:

Assess onset, type, location, duration of pain or inflammation. Inspect appearance of affected joints for immobility, deformities, skin condition.

INTERVENTION/EVALUATION:

Evaluate for therapeutic response: relief of pain, stiffness, swelling, increase in joint mobility, reduced joint tenderness, improved grip strength.

PATIENT/FAMILY TEACHING:

Avoid aspirin, alcohol during therapy (increases risk of GI bleeding). Report GI distress, diarrhea, nausea.

melphalan

mel-fah-lan
(Alkeran)
Do not confuse with Leukeran, Mephyton, Myleran.

▶CLASSIFICATION

PHARMACOTHERAPEUTIC: Alkylating agent. ***CLINICAL:*** Antineoplastic (see p. 72C)

ACTION/*THERAPEUTIC EFFECT*

Primarily cross-links strands of DNA, RNA, *inhibiting protein synthesis, producing cell death.* Cell cycle-phase nonspecific.

USES/*UNLABELED*

Treatment of multiple myeloma, nonresectable epithelial carcinoma of ovary. *Treatment of breast, testicular carcinoma, neuroblastoma, rhabdomyosarcoma.*

PRECAUTIONS

CONTRAINDICATIONS: Resistance to previous therapy with drug. ***CAUTIONS:*** Bone marrow depression, chickenpox (present or recent), herpes zoster, infection, decreased renal function, history of gout.

INTERACTIONS

DRUG: May decrease effect of **antigout** medications. **Bone marrow depressants** may increase bone marrow depression. **Live virus vaccines** may potentiate virus replication, increase vaccine side effects, decrease pt's antibody response to vaccine. ***HERBAL:*** None known. ***FOOD:*** None known. ***LAB VALUES:*** May increase uric acid.

AVAILABILITY (Rx)

TABLETS: 2 mg. ***POWDER FOR INJECTION:*** 50 mg.

ADMINISTRATION/HANDLING:

IV 🔟

Storage:

• Store at room temperature; protect from light. • Once reconstituted, stable for 90 min at room temperature (do not refrigerate).

Reconstitution:

• Reconstitute 50 mg vial with diluent supplied by manufacturer to yield a 5 mg/ml solution. • Further dilute with 0.9% NaCl to final concentration, not to exceed 2 mg/ml (central line) or 0.45 mg/ml (peripheral line).

Rate of administration:

• Infuse over 15–30 min at a rate not to exceed 10 mg/min.

IV INCOMPATIBILITY ⊘

Do not mix with any other medications.

INDICATIONS/ROUTES/DOSAGE

Note: May be carcinogenic, mutagenic, or teratogenic. Handle with extreme care during administration. Dosage individualized based on clinical response, tolerance to adverse effects. When used in combination therapy, consult specific protocols for optimum dosage, sequence of drug administration. Leukocyte count usually maintained between 3,000–4,000/mm^3.

Ovarian carcinoma:

PO: Adults, elderly: 0.2 mg/kg/day for 5 successive days. Repeat at 4–6 wk intervals.

Multiple myeloma:

PO: Adults: 6 mg once daily, initially adjusted as indicated or 0.15 mg/kg/day for 7 days or 0.25 mg/kg/day for 4 days. Repeat at 4–6 wk intervals.

IV: Adults: 16 mg/m^2/dose q2wks for 4 doses; then repeat monthly as per protocol.

Note: Decrease dose by 50% in pts with BUN >30 or serum creatinine >1.

SIDE EFFECTS

FREQUENT: Nausea, vomiting (may be severe with large dose). ***OCCASIONAL:*** Diarrhea, stomatitis (burning/erythema of oral mucosa, sore throat, difficulty swallowing, oral ulceration), rash, pruritus, alopecia.

ADVERSE REACTIONS/TOXIC EFFECTS

Bone marrow depression manifested as hematologic toxicity (principally leukopenia, thrombocytopenia, and, to lesser extent, anemia, pancytopenia, agranulocytosis). Leukopenia may occur as early as 5 days. WBC, platelet counts return to normal levels during fifth wk, but leukopenia or thrombocytopenia may last >6 wks after discontinuing drug. Hyperuricemia noted by hematuria, crystalluria, flank pain.

NURSING IMPLICATIONS

BASELINE ASSESSMENT:

Obtain blood counts weekly. Dosage may be decreased or discontinued if WBC falls below 3,000/mm^3 or platelet count falls below 100,000/mm^3. Antiemetics may be effective in preventing, treating nausea, vomiting.

INTERVENTION/EVALUATION:

Monitor for stomatitis. Monitor for hematologic toxicity (fever, sore throat, signs of local infection, easy bruising, unusual bleeding from any site), symptoms of anemia (excessive tiredness, weakness), signs of hyperuricemia (hematuria, flank pain). Avoid IM injections, rectal temperatures, other traumas that may induce bleeding.

PATIENT/FAMILY TEACHING:

Increase fluid intake (may protect against hyperuricemia). Maintain fastidious oral hygiene. Alopecia is reversible, but new hair growth may have different color or texture. Avoid crowds and those with infections.

menotropins

(Humegon, Pergonal, Repronex)

See Classification section under: Fertility agents (p. 87C)

meperidine hydrochloride

meh-**pear**-ih-deen
(Demerol)

▶CLASSIFICATION

PHARMACOTHERAPEUTIC:
Narcotic agonist. ***CLINICAL:***
Opiate analgesic **(Schedule II)** (see p. 116C)

ACTION/*THERAPEUTIC EFFECT*

Binds with opioid receptors within CNS, *altering processes affecting pain perception, emotional response to pain.*

PHARMACOKINETICS

Onset	Peak	Duration
PO		
15 min	60 min	2–4 hrs
SubQ		
10–15 min	30–50 min	2–4 hrs
IM		
10–15 min	30–50 min	2–4 hrs
IV		
1 min	5–7 min	2–4 hrs

Variably absorbed from GI tract, well absorbed after IM administration. Protein binding: 60–80%. Widely distributed. Metabolized in liver to active metabolite. Primarily excreted in urine. Not removed by hemodialysis. Half-life: 2.4–4 hrs (half-life increased in elderly).

USES

Relief of moderate to severe pain, preop sedation, obstetrical support, anesthesia adjunct.

PRECAUTIONS

CONTRAINDICATIONS: Those receiving MAO inhibitors in past 14 days, diarrhea due to poisoning, delivery of premature infant. **EXTREME CAUTION:** Impaired renal, hepatic function, elderly/debilitated, supraventricular tachycardia, cor pulmonale, history of seizures, acute abdominal conditions, increased intracranial pressure, respiratory abnormalities.
▷**LIFESPAN CONSIDERATIONS:** **Pregnancy/Lactation:** Crosses placenta; distributed in breast milk. Respiratory depression may occur in neonate if mother received opiates during labor. Regular use of opiates during pregnancy may produce withdrawal symptoms in neonate (irritability, excessive crying, tremors, hyperactive reflexes, fever, vomiting, diarrhea, yawning, sneezing, seizures). **Pregnancy Category B** (Category D if used for prolonged periods or in high doses at term). **Children:** Paradoxical excitement may occur. Those <2 yrs of age more susceptible to respiratory depressant effects. **Elderly:** More susceptible to respiratory depressant effects. Age-related renal impairment may increase risk of urinary retention.

INTERACTIONS

DRUG: **Alcohol, CNS depressants** may increase CNS or respiratory depression, hypotension. **MAO inhibitors** may produce severe, fatal reaction (reduce dose to $1/4$ usual dose). **HERBAL:** **Valerian** may increase CNS depression. **FOOD:** None known. **LAB VALUES:** May increase amylase, lipase. Therapeutic blood serum level: 100–550 ng/ml; toxic blood serum level: >1,000 ng/ml.

AVAILABILITY (Rx)

TABLETS: 50 mg, 100 mg. **SYRUP:** 50 mg/5 ml. **INJECTION:** 10 mg/ml, 25 mg/ml, 50 mg/ml, 75 mg/ml, 100 mg/ml.

ADMINISTRATION/HANDLING

PO:
• Give without regard to meals. • Dilute syrup in glass of water (prevents anesthetic effect on mucous membranes).

SubQ/IM:
Note: IM preferred over SubQ route (SubQ produces pain, local irritation, induration).

• Administer slowly. • Those with circulatory impairment experience higher risk of overdosage due to delayed absorption of repeated administration.

IV
Note: Give by slow IV push or IV infusion.

Storage:
• Store at room temperature.

Reconstitution:
• May give undiluted or may dilute in D_5W, lactated Ringer's, dextrose-saline combination (2.5%, 5%, or 10% dextrose in water—0.45% or 0.9% NaCl), Ringer's, lactated Ringer's, or molar sodium lactate diluent for IV injection or infusion.

M

Rate of administration:

• IV dosage must always be administered very slowly, over 2–3 min. • Rapid IV increases risk of severe adverse reactions (chest wall rigidity, apnea, peripheral circulatory collapse, anaphylactoid effects, cardiac arrest).

IV INCOMPATIBILITIES ⊘

Allopurinol (Aloprim), amphotericin B complex (Abelcet, Ambisome, Amphotec), cefepime (Maxipime), cefoperazone (Cefobid), doxorubicin liposome (Doxil), furosemide (Lasix), idarubicin (Idamycin), nafcillin (Nafcil).

IV COMPATIBILITIES

Bumetanide (Bumex), diltiazem (Cardizem), dobutamine (Dobutrex), dopamine (Intropin), heparin, insulin, lidocaine, magnesium, oxytocin (Pitocin), potassium.

INDICATIONS/ROUTES/DOSAGE

Pain:

PO/IM/SuBQ: **Adults, elderly:** 50–150 mg q3–4h. **Children:** 1.1–1.5 mg/kg q3–4h. Do not exceed single pediatric dose 100 mg.

Usual PCA dosage for adults:

LOADING DOSE: 50–100 mg. *INTERMITTENT BOLUS:* 5–30 mg. *LOCKOUT INTERVAL:* 10–20 min. *CONTINUOUS INFUSION:* 5–40 mg/hr. *4 HR LIMIT:* 200–300 mg.

Dosage in renal impairment:

Creatinine Clearance	% Normal Dose
10–50 ml/min	75
<10 ml/min	50

SIDE EFFECTS

Note: Effects are dependent on dosage amount, route of administration. Ambulatory pts and those not in severe pain may experience dizziness, nausea, vomiting more frequently than those in supine position or having severe pain.

FREQUENT: Sedation, decreased B/P, diaphoresis, flushed face, dizziness, nausea, vomiting, constipation. **OCCASIONAL:** Confusion, irregular heartbeat, tremors, decreased urination, abdominal pain, dry mouth, headache, irritation at injection site, euphoria, dysphoria. **RARE:** Allergic reaction (rash, itching), insomnia.

ADVERSE REACTIONS/TOXIC EFFECTS

Overdosage results in respiratory depression, skeletal muscle flaccidity, cold clammy skin, cyanosis, extreme somnolence progressing to convulsions, stupor, coma. Antidote: 0.4 mg naloxone (Narcan). Tolerance to analgesic effect, physical dependence may occur with repeated use.

NURSING IMPLICATIONS

BASELINE ASSESSMENT:

Pt should be in recumbent position before drug is administered by parenteral route. Assess onset, type, location, duration of pain. Obtain vital signs before giving medication. If respirations are 12/min or lower (20/min or lower in children), withhold medication, contact physician. Effect of medication is reduced if full pain recurs before next dose.

INTERVENTION/EVALUATION:

Monitor vital signs 15–30 min after SubQ/IM dose, 5–10 min after IV dose (monitor for decreased B/P, change in rate/quality of pulse). Monitor stools; avoid constipation. Check for adequate voiding. Initiate deep breathing and coughing exercises, particularly in those with impaired pulmonary function. Therapeutic blood serum level: 100–550 ng/ml; toxic blood serum level: >1,000 ng/ml.

PATIENT/FAMILY TEACHING:

Medication should be taken before pain fully returns, within ordered intervals. Discomfort may occur with injection. Change positions slowly to avoid orthostatic hypotension. Increase fluids, bulk to prevent constipation. Tolerance/dependence may occur with prolonged use of high doses. Avoid alcohol and other CNS depressants.

mepivacaine hydrochloride

(Carbocaine, Polocaine)
FIXED-COMBINATION(S)

With levonordefrin, a vasoconstrictor **(Isocaine)**

See Classification section under: Anesthetics: local (p. 5C)

mercaptopurine

(Purinethol)

See Classification section under: Antineoplastics (p. 72C)

meropenem

murr-**oh**-pen-em
(Merrem IV)

▶CLASSIFICATION

PHARMACOTHERAPEUTIC: Cabapenem. **CLINICAL:** Antibiotic

ACTION/*THERAPEUTIC EFFECT*

Penetrates most g-positive and g-negative cell walls, *inhibiting bacterial cell wall synthesis. Bactericidal.*

PHARMACOKINETICS

Following IV administration, widely distributed into tissues/fluid including cerebrospinal fluid. Protein binding: 2%. Primarily excreted unchanged in urine. Removed by hemodialysis. Half-life: 1 hr.

USES/*UNLABELED*

Treatment of intra-abdominal infections, bacterial meningitis (pediatric pts ≥3 mos only). Cystic fibrosis. *Lowers respiratory infections, febrile neutropenia, obstetric/gynecologic infections, sepsis.*

PRECAUTIONS

CONTRAINDICATIONS: None significant. **CAUTIONS:** Hypersensitivity to penicillins, cephalosporins, other allergens; renal function impairment, CNS disorders, particularly with history of seizures.

▷*LIFESPAN CONSIDERATIONS:*
Pregnancy/Lactation: Unknown if distributed in breast milk. **Pregnancy Category B. Children:** Safety and efficacy not established in those <3 mos of age. **Elderly:** Age-related renal impairment may require dosage - adjustment.

INTERACTIONS

DRUG: Probenecid inhibits renal excretion of meropenem (do not use concurrently). **HERBAL:** None known. **FOOD:** None known. **LAB VALUES:** May increase SGOT (AST), SGPT (ALT), alkaline phosphatase, LDH, bilirubin, BUN, crea-

M

tinine. May decrease hemoglobin, hematocrit, potassium.

AVAILABILITY (Rx)

POWDER FOR INJECTION: 500 mg, 1 g.

ADMINISTRATION/HANDLING

IV 🏺

Storage:

• Store vials at room temperature. • After reconstitution with 0.9% NaCl, stable for 2 hrs at room temperature, 18 hrs if refrigerated (with D_5W, stable for 1 hr at room temperature, 8 hrs if refrigerated).

Reconstitution:

• Reconstitute each 500 mg with 10 ml Sterile Water for Injection to provide a concentration of 50 mg/ml. • Shake to dissolve until clear. • May further dilute with 100 ml 0.9% NaCl or D_5W.

Rate of administration:

• May give by IV push or IV intermittent infusion (piggyback). • If administering as IV intermittent infusion (piggyback), give over 15–30 min; if administered by IV push (5–20 ml), give over 3–5 min.

IV INCOMPATIBILITIES ⊘

Acyclovir (Zovirax), amphotericin B (Fungizone), diazepam (Valium), doxycycline (Vibramycin), metronidazole (Flagyl), ondansetron (Zofran).

IV COMPATIBILITIES

Dobutamine (Dobutrex), dopamine (Intropin), heparin, magnesium.

INDICATIONS/ROUTES/DOSAGE

Note: Space doses evenly around the clock.

Usual parenteral dosage:

***IV:* Adults, elderly:** 1 g q8h.

Intra-abdominal (pediatric):

***IV:* Children ≥3 mos:** 20 mg/kg q8h. **Children >50 kg:** 1 g q8h. **Maximum:** 2 g q8h.

Meningitis (pediatric):

***IV:* Children ≥3 mos:** 40 mg/kg q8h. **Children >50 kg:** 2 g q8h. **Maximum:** 2 g q8h.

Dosage in renal impairment:

Reduce dosage in pts with creatinine clearance <50 ml/min.

Creatinine Clearance	Dosage	Interval
26–50 ml/ min	Recommended dose (1,000 mg)	q12h
10–25 ml/ min	½ recommended dose	q12h
<10 ml/ min	½ recommended dose	q24h

SIDE EFFECTS

FREQUENT (3–5%): Diarrhea, nausea, vomiting, headache, inflammation at injection site. ***OCCASIONAL*** (2%): Oral moniliasis, rash, pruritus. ***RARE*** (<2%): Constipation, glossitis.

ADVERSE REACTIONS/TOXIC EFFECTS

Antibiotic-associated colitis, other superinfections may occur. Anaphylactic reactions in those receiving beta lactams have occurred. Seizures may occur in those with CNS disorders (brain lesions, history of seizures) or with bacterial meningitis or impaired renal function.

NURSING IMPLICATIONS

BASELINE ASSESSMENT:

Inquire about history of seizures.

INTERVENTION/EVALUATION:

Monitor daily bowel activity and stool consistency (watery, loose, soft). Monitor for nausea, vomiting. Evaluate hydration status. Evaluate for inflammation at IV injection site. Assess skin for rash. Monitor I&O, renal function tests. Check mental status; be alert to tremors and possible seizures. Assess temperature, B/P twice daily, more often if necessary. Monitor electrolytes, esp. potassium.

PATIENT/FAMILY TEACHING:

Notify physician in event of tremors, seizures, rash, diarrhea, or other new symptom.

mesalamine (5-aminosalicylic acid, 5-ASA)

mess-**al**-ah-meen
(Asacol, Canasa, Fiv-ASA, Mesasal♣, Pentasa, Quintasa♣, Rowasa, Salofalk♣)
Do not confuse with Os-cal.

▶**CLASSIFICATION**

PHARMACOTHERAPEUTIC:
Salicylic acid derivative. ***CLINICAL:*** Anti-inflammatory agent

ACTION/THERAPEUTIC EFFECT

Produces local inhibitory effect on arachidonic acid metabolite production (increased in pts with chronic inflammatory bowel disease). *Blocks prostaglandin production, diminishes inflammation in colon.*

PHARMACOKINETICS

Poorly absorbed from colon. Moderately absorbed from GI tract. Metabolized in liver to active metabolite. Unabsorbed portion eliminated in feces; absorbed portion excreted in urine. Unknown if removed by hemodialysis. Half-life: 0.5–1.5 hrs; metabolite: 5–10 hrs.

USES

Treatment of active mild to moderate distal ulcerative colitis, proctosigmoiditis, or proctitis. ***Asacol:*** Maintenance of remission of ulcerative colitis.

PRECAUTIONS

CONTRAINDICATIONS: None significant. ***CAUTIONS:*** Preexisting renal disease, sulfasalazine sensitivity.

▷***LIFESPAN CONSIDERATIONS:***
Pregnancy/Lactation: Unknown whether drug crosses placenta or is distributed in breast milk. **Pregnancy Category B. Children:** Safety and efficacy not established. **Elderly:** Age-related renal impairment may require cautious use.

INTERACTIONS

DRUG: None significant. ***HERBAL:*** None known. ***FOOD:*** None known. ***LAB VALUES:*** May increase SGOT (AST), SGPT (ALT), alkaline phosphatase, BUN, serum creatinine.

AVAILABILITY (Rx)

TABLETS (delayed-release): 400 mg. ***CAPSULES (controlled-release):*** 250 mg. ***SUPPOSITORY:*** 500 mg. ***RECTAL SUSPENSION:*** 4 g/60 ml.

ADMINISTRATION/HANDLING

Note: Store rectal suspension, suppository, oral forms at room temperature.

PO:

• Have pt swallow whole; do not break outer coating of tablet. • Give without regard to food.

M

Rectal:

• Shake bottle well. • Instruct pt to lie on left side with lower leg extended, upper leg flexed forward. • Knee-chest position may also be used. • Insert applicator tip into rectum, pointing toward umbilicus. • Squeeze bottle steadily until contents are emptied.

INDICATIONS/ROUTES/DOSAGE

Ulcerative colitis, proctosigmoiditis, proctitis:

PO: **Adults, elderly:** *(Asacol):* 800 mg 3 times/day for 6 wks. **Children:** 50 mg/kg/day q8–12h. *(Pentasa):* 1 g 4 times/day for 8 wks. **Children:** 50 mg/kg/day q6–12h.

RECTAL: (retention enema): **Adults, elderly:** 60 ml (4 g) at bedtime; retain overnight, about 8 hrs, for 3–6 wks.

(Suppository): **Adults, elderly:** 1 suppository (500 mg) 2 times/day, retain 1–3 hrs for 3–6 wks.

Maintenance of remission, ulcerative colitis:

PO: **Adults, elderly:** 1.6 g/day in divided doses.

SIDE EFFECTS

Note: Generally well tolerated, with only mild and transient effects. *FREQUENT* (>6%): *PO:* Abdominal cramps/pain, diarrhea, dizziness, headache, nausea, vomiting, rhinitis, unusual tiredness. *Rectal:* Abdominal/stomach cramps, flatulence, headache, nausea. *OCCASIONAL* (2–6%): *PO:* Hair loss, decreased appetite, back/joint pain, flatulence, acne. *Rectal:* Hair loss. *RARE* (<2%): *Rectal:* Anal irritation.

ADVERSE REACTIONS/TOXIC EFFECTS

Sulfite sensitivity in susceptible pts noted as cramping, headache, diarrhea, fever, rash, hives, itching, wheezing. Discontinue drug immediately. Hepatitis, pancreatitis, pericarditis occur rarely with oral dosage.

NURSING IMPLICATIONS

INTERVENTION/EVALUATION:

Encourage adequate fluid intake. Assess bowel sounds for peristalsis. Monitor daily bowel activity and stool consistency (watery, loose, soft, semisolid, solid) and record time of evacuation. Assess for abdominal disturbances. Assess skin for rash, hives. Discontinue medication if rash, fever, cramping, or diarrhea occurs.

PATIENT/FAMILY TEACHING:

Avoid tasks that require alertness, motor skills until response to drug is established.

mesna

mess-nah
(Mesnex, Uromitexan ♣)

►**CLASSIFICATION**

PHARMACOTHERAPEUTIC: Cytoprotective agent. *CLINICAL:* Antineoplastic adjunct, antidote

ACTION/*THERAPEUTIC EFFECT*

Reduced to free thiol compound, mesna, which reacts with urotoxic ifosfamide metabolites (detoxification). *Inhibits ifosfamide-induced hemorrhagic cystitis.*

PHARMACOKINETICS

Rapidly metabolized after IV administration to mesna disulfide, which is reduced to mesna in kidney. Excreted in urine. Half-life: 0.36 hrs.

USES
To decrease incidence of ifosfamide-induced hemorrhagic cystitis.

PRECAUTIONS
CONTRAINDICATIONS: None significant. ***CAUTIONS:*** None significant.

▷***LIFESPAN CONSIDERATIONS:***
Pregnancy/Lactation: Unknown whether drug crosses placenta or is distributed in breast milk. **Pregnancy Category B. Children:** Safety and efficacy not established. **Elderly:** Information not available.

INTERACTIONS
DRUG: None significant. ***HERBAL:*** None known. ***FOOD:*** None known. ***LAB VALUES:*** May produce false-positive test for urinary ketones.

AVAILABILITY (Rx)
INJECTION: 100 mg/ml.

ADMINISTRATION/HANDLING
IV 🔟
Storage:
• Store parenteral form at room temperature. • After dilution, is stable for 24 hrs at room temperature (recommended use within 6 hrs). Discard unused medication.

Reconstitution:
• Dilute each 100 mg with D_5W or 0.9% NaCl to provide concentration of 20 mg/ml.

Rate of administration:
• Give at rate of ifosfamide if given together.

IV INCOMPATIBILITIES ⊘
Amphotericin B complex (Abelcet, Ambisome, Amphotec).

IV COMPATIBILITIES
Allopurinol (Aloprim), etoposide (VP-16, Vepesid), granisetron (Kytril), ondansetron (Zofran)

INDICATIONS/ROUTES/DOSAGE
Hemorrhagic cystitis (ifosfamide):
IV: Adults, elderly: 20% of ifosfamide dose at time of ifosfamide administration and 4 and 8 hrs after each dose of ifosfamide. Total dose: 60% of ifosfamide dosage.

Hemorrhagic cystitis (cyclophosphamide):
IV: Adults, elderly: 20% of cyclophosphamide dose at time of cyclophosphamide administration and q3h for 3–4 doses.

PO: 40% of antineoplastic agent dose in 3 doses at 4 hr intervals.

SIDE EFFECTS
FREQUENT (>17%): Bad taste in mouth, soft stools. ***Large doses:*** Diarrhea, limb pain, headache, fatigue, nausea, hypotension, allergic reaction.

ADVERSE REACTIONS/TOXIC EFFECTS
Hematuria occurs rarely.

NURSING IMPLICATIONS

BASELINE ASSESSMENT:
Each dose must be administered with ifosfamide.

INTERVENTION/EVALUATION:
Assess morning urine specimen for hematuria. If such occurs, dosage reduction or discontinuation may be necessary. Monitor

M

---

daily bowel activity and stool consistency (watery, loose, soft, semisolid, solid) and record time of evacuation. Monitor B/P for hypotension.

PATIENT/FAMILY TEACHING:

Inform physician/nurse if headache, limb pain, or nausea occurs.

mesoridazine besylate

mess-oh-**rid**-ah-zeen (Serentil)
Do not confuse with Serevent.

▶CLASSIFICATION

PHARMACOTHERAPEUTIC: Phenothiazine. **CLINICAL:** Antipsychotic (see p. 55C)

ACTION/THERAPEUTIC EFFECT

Blocks dopamine at postsynaptic receptor sites in brain. *Suppresses behavioral response in psychosis.* Strong anticholinergic, sedative effects.

USES

Symptomatic management of psychotic disorders, treatment of hyperactivity, uncooperativeness associated with mental deficiency, chronic brain syndrome; as adjunctive treatment of alcohol dependence, management of anxiety /tension associated with neurosis.

PRECAUTIONS

CONTRAINDICATIONS: Severe CNS depression, comatose states, severe cardiovascular disease, bone marrow depression, subcortical brain damage. **CAUTIONS:** Impaired respiratory/hepatic/ renal/cardiac function, alcohol withdrawal, history of seizures, urinary retention, glaucoma, prostatic hypertrophy.

INTERACTIONS

DRUG: **Alcohol, CNS depressants** may increase CNS, respiratory depression, hypotensive effects. **Tricyclic antidepressants, MAO inhibitors** may increase sedative, anticholinergic effects. **Antithyroid** agents may increase risk of agranulocytosis. Extrapyramidal symptoms (EPS) may increase **with EPS-producing medications. Hypotensives** may increase hypotension. May decrease **levodopa** effects. **Lithium** may decrease absorption, produce adverse neurologic effects. **HERBAL:** None known. **FOOD:** None known. **LAB VALUES:** May produce false-positive pregnancy test, PKU. EKG changes may occur, including Q and T wave disturbances.

AVAILABILITY (Rx)

TABLETS: 10 mg, 25 mg, 50 mg, 100 mg. **INJECTION:** 25 mg/ml.

INDICATIONS/ROUTES/DOSAGE
Usual adult dosage:

PO: 30–150 mg/day in 2–3 divided doses.

IM: 25–100 mg/day.

SIDE EFFECTS

FREQUENT: Orthostatic hypotension, dizziness, and fainting occur frequently after first injection, occasionally after subsequent injections, and rarely with oral dosage. **OCCASIONAL:** Drowsiness during early therapy, dry mouth, blurred vision, lethargy, constipation or diarrhea, nasal congestion, peripheral edema, urinary reten-

---

tion. **RARE:** Ocular changes, skin pigmentation (those on high doses for prolonged periods).

ADVERSE REACTIONS/TOXIC EFFECTS

Abrupt withdrawal following long-term therapy may precipitate nausea, vomiting, gastritis, dizziness, tremors. Blood dyscrasias, particularly agranulocytosis, mild leukopenia (sore mouth/gums/throat) may occur. May lower seizure threshold.

NURSING IMPLICATIONS

BASELINE ASSESSMENT:

Avoid skin contact with solution (contact dermatitis). Assess behavior, appearance, emotional status, response to environment, speech pattern, thought content.

INTERVENTION/EVALUATION:

Assess for orthostatic hypotension. Monitor stool frequency and consistency (watery, loose, soft, semisolid, solid). Supervise suicidal risk pt closely during early therapy (as depression lessens, energy level improves, increasing suicide potential). Assess for therapeutic response (interest in surroundings, improvement in self-care, increased ability to concentrate, relaxed facial expression).

PATIENT/FAMILY TEACHING:

Full therapeutic effect may take up to 6 wks. Urine may become pink, reddish brown. Do not abruptly withdraw from long-term drug therapy. Report visual disturbances. Drowsiness generally subsides during continued therapy. Do not use alcohol or other CNS depressants.

metaproterenol sulfate

met-ah-pro-**tair**-in-all
(Alupent, Metaprel)
Do not confuse with Atrovent, metipranolol, metoprolol.

▶CLASSIFICATION

PHARMACOTHERAPEUTIC: Sympathomimetic (adrenergic agonist). ***CLINICAL:*** Bronchodilator (see p. 63C)

ACTION/*THERAPEUTIC EFFECT*

Stimulates beta$_2$-adrenergic receptors resulting in relaxation of bronchial smooth muscle, *relieving bronchospasm; reduces airway resistance.*

USES

Relief of reversible bronchospasm due to bronchial asthma, bronchitis, emphysema.

PRECAUTIONS

CONTRAINDICATIONS: Preexisting arrhythmias. ***CAUTIONS:*** Impaired cardiac function, diabetes mellitus, hypertension, hyperthyroidism.

INTERACTIONS

DRUG: **Tricyclic antidepressants** may increase cardiovascular effects. **MAO inhibitors** may increase risk of hypertensive crises. May decrease effects of **beta-blockers. Digoxin, other sympathomimetics** may increase risk of arrhythmias. ***HERBAL:*** **Ma Huang (Ephedra)** may increase CNS effects. ***FOOD:*** None known. ***LAB VALUES:*** May decrease serum potassium levels.

INDICATIONS/ROUTES/DOSAGE

Bronchospasm:
METERED-DOSE INHALATION:

M

Adults, elderly, children >12 yrs: 2–3 inhalations as single dose. Wait 2 min before administering second dose. Do not repeat for 3–4 hrs. **Maximum:** 12 inhalations/day.

PO: Adults, children >9 yrs or >60 lbs: 20 mg 3–4 times/day. **Children 6–9 yrs or <60 lbs:** 10 mg 3–4 times/day. **Children 2–6 yrs:** 1.3–2.6 mg/kg/day in divided doses q6–8h. **Children <2 yrs:** 0.4 mg/kg/dose 3–4 times/day.

NEBULIZATION: Adults, elderly: 0.2–0.3 ml (10–15 mg) of 5% solution q4–6h. **Children:** 0.01–0.02 ml/kg (0.5–1 mg/kg) of 5% solution q4–6h. **Maximum dose:** 0.3 ml (15 mg).

Usual elderly dosage:

PO: Initially, 10 mg 3–4 times/day. May increase up to 20 mg 3–4 times/day.

SIDE EFFECTS

FREQUENT (>10%): Shakiness, nervousness, nausea, dry mouth. **OCCASIONAL** (1–9%): Dizziness, vertigo, weakness, headache, GI distress, vomiting, cough, dry throat. **RARE** (<1%): Drowsiness, diarrhea, unusual taste.

ADVERSE REACTIONS/TOXIC EFFECTS

Excessive sympathomimetic stimulation may cause palpitations, extrasystoles, tachycardia, chest pain, slight increase in B/P followed by a substantial decrease, chills, sweating, and blanching of skin. Too frequent or excessive use may lead to loss of bronchodilating effectiveness and/or severe, paradoxical bronchoconstriction.

NURSING IMPLICATIONS

BASELINE ASSESSMENT:
Offer emotional support (high incidence of anxiety because of difficulty in breathing and sympathomimetic response to drug).

INTERVENTION/EVALUATION:
Monitor rate, depth, rhythm, type of respiration; quality and rate of pulse. Assess lung sounds for rhonchi, wheezing, rales. Monitor arterial blood gases. Observe lips, fingernails for blue or dusky color in light-skinned pts; gray in dark-skinned pts. Evaluate for clinical improvement (quieter, slower respirations, relaxed facial expression, cessation of clavicular retractions).

PATIENT/FAMILY TEACHING:
Increase fluid intake (decreases lung secretion viscosity). Do not take more than 2 inhalations at any one time (excessive use may produce paradoxical bronchoconstriction or a decreased bronchodilating effect). Avoid excessive use of caffeine derivatives (chocolate, coffee, tea, cola, cocoa).

metaraminol bitartrate

(Aramine)

See Classification section under: Sympathomimetics

metformin hydrochloride   🅿

met-**for**-min
(Glucophage, Novo-Metformin ♣)

FIXED-COMBINATION(S)

With glyburide, an antidiabetic **(Glucovance)**

▶CLASSIFICATION

PHARMACOTHERAPEUTIC:
Antihyperglycemic. *CLINICAL:*
Antidiabetic (see p. 40C)

ACTION/*THERAPEUTIC EFFECT*

Lowers both basal and postprandial plasma glucose by decreasing hepatic glucose production, intestinal absorption of glucose and improves insulin sensitivity. *Provides improvement in glycemic control, stabilizes or decreases body weight, improves lipid profile.*

PHARMACOKINETICS

Slowly, incompletely absorbed following PO administration (food delays/decreases extent of absorption). Protein binding: Negligible. Primarily distributed to intestinal mucosa, salivary glands. Primarily excreted unchanged in urine. Removed by hemodialysis. Half-life: 8.9–19 hrs.

USES/*UNLABELED*

Adjunct to diet in management of noninsulin-dependent diabetes mellitus (type II, NIDDM) whose hyperglycemia cannot be managed by diet alone. May be used concurrently with a sulfonylurea antidiabetic agent or insulin when diet and metformin or a sulfonylurea alone do not result in adequate glycemic control. *Treatment of metabolic complications of AIDS, weight reduction.*

PRECAUTIONS

CONTRAINDICATIONS: History of lactic acidosis, conditions associated with hypoxemia (e.g., CHF), hyper-sensitivity to metformin, renal disease or dysfunction (serum creatinine >1.5 mg/dl [males], >1.4 mg/dl [females]) or abnormal creatinine clearance (Ccr), acute or chronic metabolic acidosis, including diabetic ketoacidosis, with or without coma. Temporarily withhold metformin therapy in pts undergoing radiologic studies involving parenteral iodinated contrast material (alters renal function). *CAUTIONS:* Conditions delaying food absorption (e.g., diarrhea, gastroparesis, vomiting), causing hyperglycemia (e.g., high fever) or hypoglycemia (e.g., malnutrition), uncontrolled hypo/hyperthyroidism, cardiovascular pts, concurrent drugs that affect renal function, hepatic impairment, elderly, malnourished, or debilitated, pts with decreased renal function, CHF, excessive alcohol intake, chronic respiratory difficulty.

▷*LIFESPAN CONSIDERATIONS:*
Pregnancy/Lactation: Insulin is drug of choice during pregnancy. Distributed in breast milk in animals. **Pregnancy Category B. Children:** Safety and efficacy not established. **Elderly:** Age-related renal impairment or peripheral vascular disease may require dosage adjustment or discontinuation.

INTERACTIONS

DRUG: **Alcohol, amiloride, digoxin, morphine, procainamide, quinidine, quinine, ranitidine, triamterene, trimethoprim, vancomycin, cimetidine, furosemide, nifedipine** increases metformin concentration. **Furosemide, hypoglycemia-causing medication** may decrease dosage of metformin needed. **Iodinated contrast studies** may produce acute renal failure (increases risk of lactic acidosis). *HERBAL:* None

M

known. **FOOD:** None known. **LAB VALUES:** None significant.

AVAILABILITY (Rx)

TABLETS: 500 mg, 850 mg. **TABLETS (extended-release):** 500 mg.

ADMINISTRATION/HANDLING
PO:

• When transferring pts from oral hypoglycemic agents other than chlorpropamide, no transition period necessary. When transferring from chlorpropamide, exercise care during first 2 wks (prolonged retention of chlorpropamide) as overlapping drug effects, possible hypoglycemia may occur. • If no adequate response to maximum dose of metformin within 4 wks, gradually add oral sulfonylurea antidiabetic agent while continuing metformin at maximum dose.
• Do not crush film-coated tablets.
• Give with meals.

INDICATIONS/ROUTES/DOSAGE
Diabetes mellitus (500 mg tablet):

PO: Adults, elderly: Initially, 500 mg twice daily (with morning and evening meals). May increase dosage in 500 mg increments every week, in divided doses. Can be given twice daily up to 2,000 mg/day (e.g., 1,000 mg twice daily with morning and evening meals). If 2,500 mg/day dose is required, give 3 times/day with meals. **Maximum dose/day:** 2,500 mg/day. **Children 10–16 yrs:** Initially, 500 mg 2 times/day. May increase by 500 mg/day at weekly intervals. **Maximum:** 2,000 mg/day.

Diabetes mellitus (850 mg tablet):

PO: Adults, elderly: Initially, 850 mg/day, with morning meal. May increase dosage in 850 mg incre-

ments every *other* week, in divided doses. **Maintenance:** 850 mg twice daily (with morning and evening meals). **Maximum dose/day:** 2,550 mg (850 mg 3 times/day).

Diabetes mellitus (extended-release tablets):

PO: Adults, elderly: Initially, 500 mg once daily. May increase by 500 mg/day at weekly intervals. **Maximum:** 2,000 mg/day once daily.

SIDE EFFECTS

OCCASIONAL (>3%): GI disturbances are transient and resolve spontaneously during therapy (diarrhea, nausea, vomiting, abdominal bloating, flatulence, anorexia). **RARE** (1–3%): Unpleasant or metallic taste (resolves spontaneously during therapy).

ADVERSE REACTIONS/TOXIC EFFECTS

Lactic acidosis occurs rarely (0.03 cases/1,000 pts) but is a serious, often fatal (50%) complication. Characterized by increase in blood lactate levels (>5 mmol/L), decrease in blood pH, electrolyte disturbances. Symptoms include unexplained hyperventilation, myalgia, malaise, somnolence. May advance to cardiovascular collapse (shock), acute CHF, acute MI, prerenal azotemia.

NURSING IMPLICATIONS

BASELINE ASSESSMENT:

Inform pt of potential risks and advantages of therapy (see Adverse Reactions/Toxic Effects) and of alternative modes of therapy. Before initiation of therapy and annually thereafter, assess hemoglobin, hematocrit, RBC, and serum creatinine.

INTERVENTION/EVALUATION:

Monitor folic acid, renal function tests for evidence of early lactic acidosis. If pt is on concurrent oral sulfonylureas, assess for hypoglycemia (cool wet skin, tremors, dizziness, anxiety, headache, tachycardia, numbness in mouth, hunger, diplopia). Be alert to conditions that alter glucose requirements: fever, increased activity or stress, surgical procedure.

PATIENT/FAMILY TEACHING:

Discontinue metformin and contact physician immediately if evidence of lactic acidosis appears (unexplained hyperventilation, muscle aches, extreme tiredness, unusual sleepiness). Prescribed diet is principal part of treatment; do not skip or delay meals. Diabetes mellitus requires lifelong control.

methadone hydrochloride

meth-ah-doan
(Dolophine)

▶CLASSIFICATION

PHARMACOTHERAPEUTIC:
Narcotic agonist. **CLINICAL:**
Opioid analgesic **(Schedule II)**
(see p. 116C)

ACTION/THERAPEUTIC EFFECT

Binds with opioid receptors within CNS, *altering processes affecting analgesia, emotional response to acute withdrawal syndrome.*

PHARMACOKINETICS

Onset	Peak	Duration
PO		
30–60 min	0.5–1 hr	4–6 hrs
SubQ		
10–15 min	—	4–6 hrs
IM		
10–15 min	—	4–6 hrs

Well absorbed after IM injection. Protein binding: 80–85%. Metabolized in liver. Primarily excreted in urine. Not removed by hemodialysis. Half-life: 15–25 hrs.

USES

Relief of severe pain, detoxification, and temporary maintenance treatment of narcotic abstinence syndrome.

PRECAUTIONS

CONTRAINDICATIONS: Hypersensitivity to narcotics, diarrhea due to poisoning, delivery of premature infant, during labor. **EXTREME CAUTION:** Impaired renal, hepatic function, elderly/debilitated, supraventricular tachycardia, cor pulmonale, history of seizures, acute abdominal conditions, increased intracranial pressure, respiratory abnormalities.

▷**LIFESPAN CONSIDERATIONS:**
Pregnancy/Lactation: Crosses placenta; distributed in breast milk. Respiratory depression may occur in neonate if mother received opiates during labor. Regular use of opiates during pregnancy may produce withdrawal symptoms in neonate (irritability, excessive crying, tremors, hyperactive reflexes, fever, vomiting, diarrhea, yawning, sneezing, seizures). Pregnancy **Category B** (Category D if used for prolonged periods or in high doses at term). **Children:** Paradoxical excitement may occur. Those

M

<2 yrs more susceptible to respiratory depressant effects. **Elderly:** More susceptible to respiratory depressant effects. Age-related renal impairment may increase risk of urinary retention.

INTERACTIONS

DRUG:* Alcohol, CNS depressants** may increase CNS or respiratory depression, hypotension. **MAO inhibitors** may produce severe, fatal reaction (reduce dose to $1/4$ usual dose). ***HERBAL:* Valerian** may increase CNS depression. ***FOOD: None known. ***LAB VALUES:*** May increase amylase, lipase.

AVAILABILITY (Rx)

TABLETS: 5 mg, 10 mg. ***TABLETS (dispersable):*** 40 mg. ***ORAL SOLUTION:*** 5 mg/5 ml, 10 mg/5 ml. ***ORAL CONCENTRATE:*** 10 mg/ml. ***INJECTION:*** 10 mg/ml.

ADMINISTRATION/HANDLING
PO:

• Give without regard to meals. • Dilute syrup in glass of H_2O (prevents anesthetic effect on mucous membranes).

SubQ/IM:

Note: IM preferred over SubQ route (SubQ produces pain, local irritation, induration).

• Do not use if solution appears cloudy or contains a precipitate. • Administer slowly. • Those with circulating impairment experience higher risk of overdosage due to delayed absorption of repeated administration.

INDICATIONS/ROUTES/DOSAGE
Analgesia:

***PO/IM/IV/SubQ:* Adults, elderly:** 2.5–10 mg q3–8h as needed up to 5–20 mg q6–8h. **Children:** Initially, 0.1 mg/kg/dose q4h for 2–3 doses, then q6–12h. **Maximum:** 10 mg/dose.

Detoxification:

***PO:* Adults, elderly:** 15–40 mg/day.

Maintenance of opiate dependence:

***PO:* Adults, elderly:** 20–120 mg/day.

SIDE EFFECTS

FREQUENT: Sedation, decreased B/P, increased sweating, flushed face, constipation, dizziness, nausea, vomiting. ***OCCASIONAL:*** Confusion, decreased urination, pounding heartbeat, stomach cramps, visual changes, dry mouth, headache, decreased appetite, nervousness, inability to sleep. ***RARE:*** Allergic reaction (rash, itching).

ADVERSE REACTIONS/TOXIC EFFECTS

Overdosage results in respiratory depression, skeletal muscle flaccidity, cold clammy skin, cyanosis, extreme somnolence progressing to convulsions, stupor, coma. ***Antidote:*** 0.4 mg naloxone (Narcan). Tolerance to analgesic effect, physical dependence may occur with repeated use.

NURSING IMPLICATIONS

BASELINE ASSESSMENT:

Pt should be in recumbent position before drug is administered by parenteral route. Obtain vital signs before giving medication. If respirations are 12/min or lower (20/min or lower in children), withhold medication, contact physician.

INTERVENTION/EVALUATION:
Monitor vital signs 15–30 min

after SubQ/IM dose, 5–10 min after IV dose. Oral medication is one-half as potent as parenteral. Assess for adequate voiding. Assess for clinical improvement and record onset of relief of pain. Provide support to pt in detoxification program; monitor for withdrawal symptoms.

PATIENT/FAMILY TEACHING:
Discomfort may occur with injection. Avoid tasks that require alertness, motor skills until response to drug is established.

methimazole

meth-**im**-ah-zole
(Tapazole)

▶CLASSIFICATION
PHARMACOTHERAPEUTIC: Thiomidazole derivative. **CLINICAL:** Antithyroid

ACTION/*THERAPEUTIC EFFECT*
Inhibits synthesis of thyroid hormone by interfering with incorporation of iodine into tyrosyl residues, *effective in treatment of hyperthyroidism.*

USES
Treatment of hyperthyroidism; adjunct to relieve hyperthyroidism in preparation for surgical treatment or radioactive iodine therapy.

PRECAUTIONS
CONTRAINDICATIONS: None significant. **CAUTIONS:** Pts >40 yrs or in combination with other agranulocytosis-inducing drugs, impaired liver function.

INTERACTIONS
DRUG: Amiodarone, iodinated glycerol, iodine, potassium iodide may decrease response. May decrease effect of **oral anticoagulants.** May increase concentration of **digoxin** (as pt becomes euthyroid). May decrease thyroid uptake of I^{131}. **HERBAL:** None known. **FOOD:** None known. **LAB VALUES:** May increase SGOT (AST), SGPT (ALT), alkaline phosphatase, LDH, bilirubin, prothrombin time. May decrease prothrombin level, WBC count.

AVAILABILITY (Rx)
TABLETS: 5 mg, 10 mg.

INDICATIONS/ROUTES/DOSAGE
Hyperthyroidism:
PO: Adults, elderly: Initially, 15–60 mg/day in 3 divided doses. **Maintenance:** 5–15 mg/day. **Children:** Initially, 0.4 mg/kg/day in 3 divided doses. **Maintenance:** One-half the initial dose.

SIDE EFFECTS
FREQUENT (3–5%): Fever, rash, pruritus. **OCCASIONAL** (1–3%): Dizziness, loss of taste, nausea, vomiting, stomach pain, peripheral neuropathy (numbness in fingers, toes, face). **RARE** (<1%): Swollen lymph nodes/salivary glands.

ADVERSE REACTIONS/TOXIC EFFECTS
Agranulocytosis (which may occur as long as 4 mos after therapy); pancytopenia and hepatitis have occurred.

NURSING IMPLICATIONS

BASELINE ASSESSMENT:
Obtain baseline weight, pulse.

INTERVENTION/EVALUATION:
Monitor pulse and weight daily. Assess skin for rash, pruritus, swollen lymph glands. Monitor hematology results for bone

M

marrow suppression; check for signs of infection or bleeding.

PATIENT/FAMILY TEACHING:

Do not exceed ordered dose. Space evenly around the clock. Take resting pulse daily to monitor therapeutic results. Seafood and iodine products may be restricted. Report illness, unusual bleeding, or bruising immediately.

methocarbamol

(Robaxin)

FIXED-COMBINATION(S)

With aspirin, a salicylate **(Robaxisal)**

See Classification section under: Skeletal muscle relaxants

methohexital sodium

(Brevital)

See Classification section under: Anesthetics: general (p. 2C)

methotrexate sodium

meth-oh-**trex**-ate
(Folex, Mexate, Rheumatrex)

▶CLASSIFICATION

PHARMACOTHERAPEUTIC: Antimetabolite. **CLINICAL:** Antineoplastic, antiarthritic, antipsoriatic (see p. 72C)

ACTION/*THERAPEUTIC EFFECT*

Inhibits DNA, RNA, protein synthesis by competing with enzyme necessary to reduce folic acid to tetrahydrofolic acid, a component essential to DNA, RNA, protein synthesis. Cell cycle-specific for S phase of cell division. Mild immunosuppressant activity.

PHARMACOKINETICS

Variably absorbed from GI tract. Protein binding: 50–60%. Widely distributed. Metabolized in liver, intracellularly. Primarily excreted in urine. Removed by hemodialysis; not removed by peritoneal dialysis. Half-life: 3–10 hrs (high doses: 8–15 hrs).

USES/*UNLABELED*

Treatment of trophoblastic neoplasms (gestational choriocarcinoma, chorioadenoma destruens, hydatidiform mole), acute leukemias, breast cancer, epidermoid cancers of head and neck, lung cancer, advanced stages of lymphosarcoma, mycosis fungoides, meningeal leukemia, severe psoriasis, rheumatoid arthritis. *Treatment of cervical, ovarian, bladder, renal, prostatic, testicular carcinoma, acute myelocytic leukemia, psoriatic arthritis, systemic dermatomyositis.*

PRECAUTIONS

CONTRAINDICATIONS: Impaired renal function. **Psoriasis:** Poor nutritional status, severe renal/hepatic disease, preexisting blood dyscrasias. **EXTREME CAUTION:** Infection, peptic ulcer, ulcerative colitis, very young, elderly, debilitated, preexisting liver damage, impaired hepatic function, preexisting bone marrow depression. **CAUTIONS:** Impaired renal, hepatic function, peptic ulcer, ulcerative colitis.

▷*LIFESPAN CONSIDERATIONS:*
Pregnancy/Lactation: Avoid

pregnancy during methotrexate therapy and minimum 3 mos after therapy in males or at least one ovulatory cycle after therapy in females. May cause fetal death, congenital anomalies. Drug is distributed in breast milk. Breast feeding not recommended. **Pregnancy Category D.** *Psoriasis or rheumatoid arthritis pts:* **Pregnancy Category X. Children/Elderly:** Decreased renal/liver function requires caution; may require dosage adjustment.

INTERACTIONS

DRUG: **Parenteral acyclovir** may increase neurotoxicity. **Alcohol, hepatotoxic medications** may increase hepatotoxicity. **NSAIDs** may increase toxicity. **Asparaginase** may decrease effects of methotrexate. **Bone marrow depressants** may increase bone marrow depression. **Probenecid, salicylates** may increase concentration, toxicity. **Live virus vaccines** may potentiate virus replication, increase vaccine side effects, decrease pt's antibody response to vaccine. ***HERBAL:*** None known. ***FOOD:*** None known. ***LAB VALUES:*** May increase uric acid, SGOT (AST).

AVAILABILITY (Rx)

TABLETS: 2.5 mg, 5 mg, 7.5 mg, 10 mg, 15 mg. ***POWDER FOR INJECTION:*** 20 mg, 50 mg, 100 mg, 1 g. ***INJECTION:*** 2.5 mg/ml, 25 mg/ml. ***INJECTION (preservative-free):*** 25 mg/ml.

ADMINISTRATION/HANDLING

Note: May be carcinogenic, mutagenic, or teratogenic. Handle with extreme care during preparation/administration. Wear gloves when preparing solution. If powder or solution comes in contact with skin, wash immediately, thoroughly with soap, water. May give IM, IV, intra-arterially, intrathecally.

IV

Storage:
• Store vials at room temperature.

Reconstitution:
• Reconstitute each 5 mg with 2 ml Sterile Water for Injection or 0.9% NaCl to provide a concentration of 2.5 mg/ml. Maximum concentration 25 mg/ml. • May further dilute with D_5W or 0.9% NaCl. • For intrathecal use, dilute with preservative-free 0.9% NaCl to provide a 1 mg/ml concentration.

Rate of administration:
• Give IV push at rate of 10 mg/min. • Give IV infusion over 30 min to 4 hrs.

IV INCOMPATIBILITIES

Chlorpromazine (Thorazine), droperidol (Inapsine), gemcitabine (Gemzar), idarubicin (Idamycin), midazolam (Versed), nalbuphine (Nubain).

IV COMPATIBILITIES

Cyclophosphamide (Cytoxan), doxorubicin (Adria), etoposide (VP-16, Vepesid), fluorouracil, granisetron (Kytril), ondansetron (Zofran).

INDICATIONS/ROUTES/DOSAGE

Note: Refer to individual protocols.

Trophoblastic neoplasms:
PO/IM: Adults, elderly: 15–30 mg/day for 5 days; repeat in 7 days for 3–5 courses.

Head/neck cancer:
PO/IM/IV: Adults, elderly: 25–50 mg/m² once weekly.

Rheumatoid arthritis:

PO: Adults, elderly: 7.5 mg once weekly or 2.5 mg q12h for 3 doses/wk. **Maximum:** 20 mg/wk.

Psoriasis:

PO: Adults, elderly: 2.5–5 mg/dose q12h for 3 doses/wk given once weekly.

PO/IM: 10–25 mg once weekly.

Choriocarcinoma, chorioadenoma destruens, hydatidiform mole:

IM/PO: Adults, elderly: 15–30 mg/day for 5 days; repeat 3–5 times with 1–2 wks between courses.

ALL:

IM/IV/PO: Adults, elderly: Induction: 3.3 mg/m^2/day (in combination).

IM/PO: Maintenance: 30 mg/m^2/wk in divided doses.

IV: 2.5 mg/kg q14days.

Burkitt's lymphoma:

PO: Adults: 10–25 mg/day for 4–8 days; repeat with 7–10 day rest between courses.

Lymphosarcoma:

PO: Adults, elderly: 0.625–2.5 mg/kg/day.

Mycosis fungoides:

PO: Adults, elderly: 2.5–10 mg/day.

IM: 50 mg/wk or 25 mg 2 times/wk.

Juvenile rheumatoid arthritis:

PO/IM/SubQ: Children: 5–15 mg/m^2/wk as a single dose or in 3 divided doses given 12 hrs apart.

Usual antineoplastic dosage for children:

Note: Refer to individual protocols.

PO/IM: 7.5–30 mg/m^2/wk or q2wks.

IV: 10–33,000 mg/m^2 bolus or continuous infusion over 6–42 hrs.

SIDE EFFECTS

FREQUENT (3–10%): Nausea, vomiting, stomatitis. In psoriatic pts, burning, erythema at psoriatic site. ***OCCASIONAL*** (1–3%): Diarrhea, rash, dermatitis, pruritis, alopecia, dizziness, anorexia, malaise, headache, drowsiness, blurred vision.

ADVERSE REACTIONS/TOXIC EFFECTS

High potential for various, severe toxicity. GI toxicity may produce oral ulcers of mouth, gingivitis, glossitis, pharyngitis, stomatitis, enteritis, hematemesis. Hepatotoxicity occurs more frequently with frequent, small doses than with large, intermittent doses. Pulmonary toxicity characterized as interstitial pneumonitis. Hematologic toxicity resulting from marked bone marrow depression may be manifested as leukopenia, thrombocytopenia, anemia, hemorrhage (may develop rapidly). Skin toxicity produces rash, pruritus, urticaria, pigmentation, photosensitivity, petechiae, ecchymosis, pustules. Severe nephropathy produces azotemia, hematuria, renal failure.

NURSING IMPLICATIONS

BASELINE ASSESSMENT:

Question for possibility of pregnancy before initiating therapy (Pregnancy Category X) in those with psoriasis or rheumatoid arthritis. Obtain all functional tests before therapy and repeat throughout therapy. Antiemetics may prevent nausea, vomiting.

INTERVENTION/EVALUATION:

Monitor hepatic and renal function tests, hemoglobin, hematocrit, WBC, differential, platelet count, urinalysis, chest radiographs, serum uric acid level. Monitor for hematologic toxicity (fever, sore throat, signs of local infection, easy bruising, unusual bleeding from any site), symptoms of anemia (excessive tiredness, weakness). Assess skin for evidence of dermatologic toxicity. Keep pt well hydrated, urine alkaline. Avoid IM injections, rectal temperatures, traumas that induce bleeding. Apply 5 full min of pressure to IV sites.

PATIENT/FAMILY TEACHING:

Maintain fastidious oral hygiene. Do not have immunizations without physician's approval (drug lowers body's resistance). Avoid crowds, those with infection. Avoid alcohol, salicylates. Avoid sunlamp and sunlight exposure. Use contraceptive measures during therapy and for 3 mos (males) or one ovulatory cycle (females) after therapy. Promptly report fever, sore throat, signs of local infection, easy bruising, unusual bleeding from any site. Alopecia is reversible, but new hair growth may have different color or texture. Contact physician if nausea/vomiting continues at home.

methylcellulose

meth-ill-**cell**-you-los
(Citrucel, Cologel)
Do not confuse with Citracal, Citrucel.

▶ CLASSIFICATION

CLINICAL: Bulk-forming laxative (see p. 100C)

ACTION/*THERAPEUTIC EFFECT*

Dissolves and expands in water, *providing increased bulk, moisture content in stool, increasing peristalsis, bowel motility.*

PHARMACOKINETICS

	Onset	Peak	Duration
PO	12–24 hrs	—	—

Full effect may not be evident for 2–3 days. Acts in small/large intestine.

USES

Prophylaxis in those who should not strain during defecation. Facilitates defecation in those with diminished colonic motor response.

PRECAUTIONS

CONTRAINDICATIONS: Abdominal pain, nausea, vomiting, symptoms of appendicitis, partial bowel obstruction, dysphagia. **CAUTIONS:** None significant.

▷ *LIFESPAN CONSIDERATIONS:* **Pregnancy/Lactation:** Safe for use in pregnancy. **Pregnancy Category C. Children:** Safety and efficacy not established in those <6 yrs of age. Not recommended in this age group. **Elderly:** No age-related precautions noted.

INTERACTIONS

DRUG: May interfere with effects of potassium-sparing diuretics, potassium supplements. May decrease effect of oral anticoagulants, digoxin, salicylates by decreasing absorption. **HERBAL:** None known. **FOOD:** None known. **LAB VALUES:** May increase glucose. May decrease potassium.

AVAILABILITY (OTC)
POWDER.

M

ADMINISTRATION/HANDLING

PO:

• Instruct pt to drink 6–8 glasses of water/day (aids stool softening).
• Not to be swallowed in dry form; mix with at least 1 full glass (8 oz) liquid.

INDICATIONS/ROUTES/DOSAGE

Laxative:

PO: Adults, elderly: 1 tbsp (15 ml) in 8 oz water 1–3 times/day. **Children 6–12 yrs:** 1 tsp (5 ml) in 4 oz water 3–4 times/day.

SIDE EFFECTS

RARE: Some degree of abdominal discomfort, nausea, mild cramps, griping, faintness.

ADVERSE REACTIONS/TOXIC EFFECTS

Esophageal or bowel obstruction may occur if administered with insufficient liquid (less than 250 ml or 1 full glass).

NURSING IMPLICATIONS

INTERVENTION/EVALUATION:

Encourage adequate fluid intake. Assess bowel sounds for peristalsis. Monitor daily bowel activity and stool consistency (watery, loose, soft, semisolid, solid) and record time of evacuation. Monitor serum electrolytes in those exposed to prolonged, frequent, or excessive use of medication.

PATIENT/FAMILY TEACHING:

Institute measures to promote defecation: increase fluid intake, exercise, high-fiber diet.

---

methyldopa ✳

meth-ill-**doe**-pah
(Aldomet, Apo-Methyldopa♣, Novomedopa♣)
Do not confuse with Anzemet.

FIXED-COMBINATION(S)

With hydrochlorothiazide, a diuretic **(Aldoril);** with chlorothiazide, a diuretic **(Aldoclor)**

▶CLASSIFICATION

PHARMACOTHERAPEUTIC: Alpha-adrenergic agonist. ***CLINICAL:*** Antihypertensive (see p. 52C)

ACTION/*THERAPEUTIC EFFECT*

Stimulates central inhibitory alpha-adrenergic receptors (lowers arterial pressure, reduces plasma renin activity). *Reduces standing and supine B/P.*

USES

Management of moderate to severe hypertension.

PRECAUTIONS

CONTRAINDICATIONS: Acute hepatitis, active cirrhosis. ***CAUTIONS:*** Impaired hepatic function.

INTERACTIONS

DRUG: **Tricyclic antidepressants, NSAIDs** may decrease effect. **Hypotensive-producing medications** may increase effect. May increase risk of toxicity of **lithium.** May cause hyperexcitability with **MAO inhibitors. Sympathomimetics** may decrease effects. ***HERBAL:*** None known. ***FOOD:*** None known. ***LAB VALUES:*** May increase SGOT (AST), SGPT (ALT), alkaline phosphatase, bilirubin, BUN, creatinine,

---

potassium, sodium, prolactin, uric acid. May produce false-positive Coomb's test, prolong prothrombin time.

AVAILABILITY (Rx)

TABLETS: 125 mg, 250 mg, 500 mg. **ORAL SUSPENSION:** 250 mg/5 ml. **INJECTION:** 250 mg/5 ml.

INDICATIONS/ROUTES/DOSAGE

Hypertension:

PO: Adults: Initially, 250 mg 2–3 times/day for 2 days. Adjust dosage at intervals of 2 days (minimum). **Elderly:** Initially, 125 mg 1–2 times/day. May increase by 125 mg q2–3days. **Maintenance:** 500 mg to 2 g/day in 2–4 divided doses. **Children:** Initially, 10 mg/kg/day in 2–4 divided doses. Adjust dose at intervals of 2 days (minimum). **Maximum:** 65 mg/kg/day or 3 g/day, whichever is less.

IV: Adults: 250–500 mg q6h up to 1 g q6h. **Children:** 20–40 mg/kg/day in divided doses q6h. **Maximum:** 65 mg/kg/day or 3 g/day, whichever is less.

SIDE EFFECTS

FREQUENT: Peripheral edema, drowsiness, headache, dry mouth. **OCCASIONAL:** Mental changes (e.g., anxiety, depression), decreased sexual ability or interest, diarrhea, swelling of breasts, nausea, vomiting, lightheadedness, numbness in hands/feet, rhinitis.

ADVERSE REACTIONS/TOXIC EFFECTS

Hepatotoxicity (abnormal liver function tests, jaundice, hepatitis), hemolytic anemia, unexplained fever and flulike symptoms: Discontinue medication, contact physician.

NURSING IMPLICATIONS

BASELINE ASSESSMENT:

Obtain baseline B/P, pulse, weight.

INTERVENTION/EVALUATION:

Monitor B/P, pulse closely q30min until stabilized. Monitor weight daily during initial therapy. Monitor liver function tests. Assess for peripheral edema of hands, feet (usually, first area of low extremity swelling is behind medial malleolus in ambulatory, sacral area in bedridden).

PATIENT/FAMILY TEACHING:

Urine may darken in color. Avoid sudden or prolonged standing, exercise, hot environment or hot shower, alcohol ingestion. Full therapeutic effect of oral administration may take 2–3 days. Drowsiness usually disappears during continued therapy.

M

methylergonovine

meth-ill-er-go-**noe**-veen
(Methergine)

▶CLASSIFICATION

PHARMACOTHERAPEUTIC: Ergot alkaloid. **CLINICAL:** Uterine stimulant

ACTION/THERAPEUTIC EFFECT

Stimulates alpha-adrenergic, serotonin receptors, producing arterial vasoconstriction. Causes vasospasm of coronary arteries. Directly stimulates uterine muscle *(increases strength, frequency of contractions, decreases uterine bleeding)*.

PHARMACOKINETICS

	Onset	Peak	Duration
PO	5–10 min	—	—
IM	2–5 min	—	—
IV	Immediate	—	3 hrs

Rapidly absorbed from GI tract, after IM administration. Distributed rapidly to plasma, extracellular fluid, tissues. Metabolized in liver (undergoes first-pass effect). Primarily excreted in urine.

USES/*UNLABELED*

Prevents and treats postpartum, postabortion hemorrhage due to atony or involution (not for induction or augmentation of labor). *Treatment of incomplete abortion.*

PRECAUTIONS

CONTRAINDICATIONS: Hypertension, pregnancy, toxemia, untreated hypocalcemia. ***CAUTIONS:*** Renal or hepatic impairment, coronary artery disease, occlusive peripheral vascular disease, sepsis.
▷*LIFESPAN CONSIDERATIONS:*
Pregnancy/Lactation: Contraindicated during pregnancy. Small amounts in breast milk. **Pregnancy Category C. Children/Elderly:** No information available.

INTERACTIONS

DRUG: **Vasoconstrictors, vasopressors** may increase effect. ***HERBAL:*** None known. ***FOOD:*** None known. ***LAB VALUES:*** May decrease prolactin concentration.

AVAILABILITY (Rx)

TABLETS: 0.2 mg. ***INJECTION:*** 0.2 mg/ml.

ADMINISTRATION/HANDLING

Note: May give PO, IM, or IV.

Storage:
• Refrigerate ampules. • Initial dose may be given parenterally, followed by oral regimen. • IV use in life-threatening emergencies only.

Reconstitution:
•Dilute to volume of 5 ml with 0.9% NaCl .
Rate of administration:
• Give over at least 1 min, carefully monitoring B/P.

IV INCOMPATIBILITY ⊘

No information available for Y-site administration.

IV COMPATIBILITIES

Heparin, potassium.

INDICATIONS/ROUTES/DOSAGE

Usual oral dosage:

PO: **Adults:** 0.2–0.4 mg 2–4 times/day (q6–12h) until danger of uterine atony and hemorrhage has passed.

Usual parenteral dosage:

IM/IV: **Adults:** Initially, 0.2 mg. May repeat no more often than q2–4h for no more than 5 doses total.

SIDE EFFECTS

FREQUENT: Nausea, uterine cramping, vomiting. ***OCCASIONAL:*** Abdominal/stomach pain, diarrhea, dizziness, sweating, ringing in ears, bradycardia, chest pain. ***RARE:*** Allergic reaction (rash, itching), dyspnea, sudden/severe hypertension.

ADVERSE REACTIONS/TOXIC EFFECTS

Severe hypertensive episodes may result in cerebrovascular accident, serious arrhythmias, seizures; hypertensive effects more frequent with pt susceptibility, rapid IV administration, concurrent regional anesthesia or vasoconstrictors. Peripheral ischemia may lead to gangrene.

NURSING IMPLICATIONS

BASELINE ASSESSMENT:

Determine calcium, B/P, and pulse baselines. Assess bleeding prior to administration.

INTERVENTION/EVALUATION:

Monitor uterine tone, bleeding, B/P, and pulse q15min until stable (about 1–2 hrs). Assess extremities for color, warmth, movement, pain. Report chest pain promptly. Provide support with ambulation if dizziness occurs.

PATIENT/FAMILY TEACHING:

Avoid smoking because of added vasoconstriction. Report increased cramping, bleeding, or foul-smelling lochia. Pale, cold hands or feet should be reported (possibility of decreased circulation).

methylphenidate hydrochloride 🖉

meh-thyl-**fen**-ih-date
(Concerta, Metadate, Methylin, Ritalin, Ritalin LA, Ritalin SR)
Do not confuse with Rifadin.

▶CLASSIFICATION

PHARMACOTHERAPEUTIC:
Piperidine derivative B **(Schedule II).** ***CLINICAL:*** CNS stimulant

ACTION/*THERAPEUTIC EFFECT*

Blocks reuptake mechanisms of dopaminergic neurons. *Decreases motor restlessness, enhances ability to pay attention. Increases motor activity, mental alertness; diminishes sense of fatigue, enhances spirit, produces mild euphoria.*

PHARMACOKINETICS

	Onset	Peak	Duration
PO (tablets)	—	—	3–6 hrs
PO (extended-release)	—	—	8 hrs

Slowly, incompletely absorbed from GI tract. Protein binding: 15%. Metabolized in liver. Excreted in urine, eliminated in feces via biliary system. Unknown if removed by hemodialysis. Half-life: 2–4 hrs.

USES/*UNLABELED*

Adjunct to treatment of attention deficit hyperactivity disorder (ADHD) with moderate to severe distractability, short attention spans, hyperactivity, emotional impulsivity in children >6 yrs. Management of narcolepsy in adults. *Treatment of secondary mental depression.*

PRECAUTIONS

CONTRAINDICATIONS: History of marked anxiety, tension, agitation; glaucoma, those with motor tics, family history of Tourette's disorder.

▷*LIFESPAN CONSIDERATIONS:*
Pregnancy/Lactation: Unknown if drug crosses placenta or is distributed in breast milk. **Pregnancy Category C. Children:** May be more susceptible to develop anorexia, insomnia, stomach pain, decreased weight. Chronic use may inhibit growth. **Elderly:** No age-related precautions noted.

M

INTERACTIONS

DRUG: CNS stimulants may have additive effect. **MAO inhibitors** may increase effects. **HERBAL: Ma Huang (Ephedra)** may increase CNS stimulation. **FOOD:** None known. **LAB VALUES:** None significant.

AVAILABILITY (Rx)

TABLETS: *(Methylin, Ritalin):* 5 mg, 10 mg, 20 mg. **CAPSULES (extended-release):** *(Metadate CD):* 20 mg. **TABLETS (extended-release):** *(Metadate ER, Methylin ER):* *10 mg,* 20 mg. *(Concerta):* 18 mg, 36 mg, 54 mg.

ADMINISTRATION/HANDLING

PO:

• Do not give drug in afternoon or evening (drug causes insomnia). • Do not crush or break sustained-release capsules. • Tablets may be crushed. • Give dose 30–45 min before meals.

INDICATIONS/ROUTES/DOSAGE

ADHD:

PO: Children >6 yrs: Initially, 2.5–5 mg before breakfast and lunch. May increase by 5–10 mg/day at weekly intervals. **Maximum:** 60 mg/day.

Note: Sustained-release forms *(Methylin, Metadate SR, Ritalin SR)* may be given once the daily dose is titrated; the regular tablets and the titrated 8 hr dosage correspond to sustained-release size.

Concerta: Initially, 18 mg once daily; may increase by 18 mg/day at weekly intervals. **Maximum:** 54 mg/day.

Narcolepsy:

PO: Adults, elderly: 10 mg 2–3 times/day. **Range:** 10–60 mg/day.

SIDE EFFECTS

FREQUENT: Nervousness, insomnia, anorexia. **OCCASIONAL:** Dizziness, drowsiness, headache, nausea, stomach pain, fever, rash, joint pain. **RARE:** Blurred vision, Tourette's syndrome (uncontrolled vocal outbursts, repeated body movements).

ADVERSE REACTIONS/TOXIC EFFECTS

Prolonged administration to children with attention deficit disorder may produce a temporary suppression of normal weight gain pattern. Overdose may produce tachycardia, palpitations, cardiac irregularities, chest pain, psychotic episode, seizures, coma. Hypersensitivity reactions, blood dyscrasias occur rarely.

NURSING IMPLICATIONS

INTERVENTION/EVALUATION:

CBC, differential, and platelet count should be performed routinely during therapy. If paradoxical return of attention deficit occurs, dosage should be reduced or discontinued.

PATIENT/FAMILY TEACHING:

Avoid tasks that require alertness, motor skills until response to drug is established. Dry mouth may be relieved by sugarless gum, sips of tepid water. Report any increase in seizures. Take last dose early in evening to avoid insomnia. Report nervousness, palpitations, fever, vomiting, skin rash.

methylprednisolone

meth-ill-pred-**niss**-oh-lone
(Medrol)

methylprednisolone sodium succinate

(Solu-Medrol, A-Methapred)

methylprednisolone acetate

(Depo-Medrol, Duralone)
Do not confuse with Mebaril, medroxyprogesterone.

FIXED-COMBINATIONS

Methylprednisolone acetate with Neomycin, an anti-infective **(Neo-Medrol)**

▶CLASSIFICATION

PHARMACOTHERAPEUTIC: Adrenal corticosteroid. *CLINI-CAL:* Glucocorticoid (see p. 79C)

ACTION/*THERAPEUTIC EFFECT*

Inhibits accumulation of inflammatory cells at inflammation sites, phagocytosis, lysosomal enzyme release and synthesis and/or release of mediators of inflammation. *Prevents/suppresses cell-mediated immune reactions. Decreases/prevents tissue response to inflammatory process.*

PHARMACOKINETICS

Well absorbed from GI tract, after IM administration. Widely distributed. Metabolized in liver. Excreted in urine. Removed by hemodialysis. Half-life: >3.5 hrs.

USES

Substitution therapy of deficiency states: acute/chronic adrenal insufficiency, congenital adrenal hyperplasia, adrenal insufficiency secondary to pituitary insufficiency. *Nonendocrine disorders:* arthritis, rheumatic carditis, allergic, collagen, intestinal tract, liver, ocular, renal, and skin diseases, bronchial asthma, cerebral edema, malignancies.

PRECAUTIONS

CONTRAINDICATIONS: Hypersensitivity to any corticosteroid, systemic fungal infection, peptic ulcers (except life-threatening situations). Avoid immunizations, smallpox vaccination. *CAUTIONS:* History of tuberculosis (may reactivate disease), hypothyroidism, cirrhosis, nonspecific ulcerative colitis, CHF, hypertension, psychosis, renal insufficiency. Prolonged therapy should be discontinued slowly.

▷*LIFESPAN CONSIDERATIONS:* **Pregnancy/Lactation:** Crosses placenta, distributed in breast milk. May cause cleft palate (chronic use first trimester). Nursing contraindicated. **Pregnancy Category C. Children:** Prolonged treatment or high doses may decrease short-term growth rate, cortisol secretion. **Elderly:** No age-related precaution noted.

INTERACTIONS

DRUG: **Amphotericin** may increase hypokalemia. May decrease effect of **oral hypoglycemics, insulin, diuretics, potassium supplements.** May increase **digoxin** toxicity (due to hypokalemia). **Hepatic enzyme inducers** may decrease effect. **Live virus vaccines** may potentiate virus replication, increase vaccine side effects, decrease pt's antibody response to vaccine. *HERBAL:* None known. *FOOD:* None known. *LAB VALUES:* May decrease calcium, potassium, thyroxine. May increase cholesterol, lipids, glucose, sodium, amylase.

AVAILABILITY (Rx)

TABLETS: 2 mg, 4 mg, 8 mg, 16

M

mg, 24 mg, 32 mg. *SUCCINATE: POWDER FOR INJECTION:* 40 mg, 125 mg, 500 mg, 1 g, 2 g. *ACETATE: INJECTION:* 20 mg/ml, 40 mg/ml, 80 mg/ml.

ADMINISTRATION/HANDLING

PO:
* Give with food or milk. * Give single doses before 9 AM; give multiple doses at evenly spaced intervals.

IM:
* Methylprednisolone acetate should not be further diluted. * Methylprednisolone sodium succinate should be reconstituted with Bacteriostatic Water for Injection. * Give deep IM in gluteus maximus.

IV ▩

Storage:
* Store vials at room temperature.

Reconstitution:
* Follow directions with Mix-o-vial.
* For infusion, add to D$_5$W, 0.9% NaCl, or D$_5$With 0.9% NaCl.

Rate of administration:
* Give IV push over 2–3 min. * Give IV piggyback over 10–20 min. * Do *not* give methylprednisolone acetate IV.

IV INCOMPATIBILITIES ⊘

Ciprofloxacin (Cipro), diltiazem (Cardizem), docetaxel (Taxotere), etoposide (Vepesed), filgrastim (Neupogen), gemcitabine (Gemzar), paclitaxel (Taxol), potassium chloride, propofol (Diprivan), venorelbine (Navelbine).

IV COMPATIBILITIES

Dopamine (Intropin), heparin, midazolam (Versed), theophylline.

INDICATIONS/ROUTES/DOSAGE

Note: Individualize dose based on disease, pt, and response.

ORAL METHYLPREDNISOLONE:

PO: **Adults, elderly:** Initially, 4–48 mg/day.

METHYLPREDNISOLONE SODIUM SUCCINATE:

IV: **Adults, elderly: (High dose):** 30 mg/kg over at least 30 min. Repeat q4–6h for 48–72 hrs.

IV: **Adults, elderly:** 40–250 mg q4–6h

METHYLPREDNISOLONE ACETATE:

IM: **Adults, elderly:** 10–80 mg/day.

INTRA-ARTICULAR, INTRALESIONAL: 4–40 mg, up to 80 mg q1–5wks.

SIDE EFFECTS

FREQUENT: Insomnia, heartburn, nervousness, abdominal distention, increased sweating, acne, mood swings, increased appetite, facial flushing, GI distress, delayed wound healing, increased susceptibility to infection, diarrhea/constipation. *OCCASIONAL:* Headache, edema, tachycardia, change in skin color, frequent urination, depression. *RARE:* Psychosis, increased blood coagulability, hallucinations.

ADVERSE REACTIONS/TOXIC EFFECTS

Long-term therapy: Muscle wasting (esp. arms, legs), osteoporosis, spontaneous fractures, amenorrhea, cataracts, glaucoma, peptic ulcer, CHF. *Abrupt withdrawal following long-term therapy:* Anorexia, nausea, fever, headache, severe joint pain, rebound inflammation, fatigue, weakness, lethargy, dizziness, orthostatic hypotension.

NURSING IMPLICATIONS

BASELINE ASSESSMENT:

Question for hypersensitivity to any of the corticosteroids, components. Obtain baselines for height, weight, B/P, glucose, electrolytes. Check results of initial tests, e.g., TB skin test, x-rays, EKG.

INTERVENTION/EVALUATION:

Monitor I&O, weight; assess for edema. Evaluate bowel activity; report hyperacidity promptly. Check vital signs at least 2 times/day. Be alert to infection: sore throat, fever, or vague symptoms. Monitor electrolytes. Watch for hypocalcemia (muscle twitching, cramps, positive Trousseau's or Chvostek's signs) or hypokalemia (weakness and muscle cramps, numbness/tingling [esp. lower extremities], nausea and vomiting, irritability, EKG changes). Assess emotional status, ability to sleep. Check lab results for blood coagulability and clinical evidence of thromboembolism.

PATIENT/FAMILY TEACHING:

Take oral dose with food or milk. Do not change dose/schedule or stop taking drug; must taper off gradually under medical supervision. Notify physician of fever, sore throat, muscle aches, sudden weight gain/swelling. Maintain careful personal hygiene, avoid exposure to disease or trauma. Severe stress (serious infection, surgery or trauma) may require increased dosage. Follow-up visits, lab tests are necessary; children must be assessed for growth retardation. Inform dentist or other physicians of methylprednisolone therapy now or within past 12 mos.

methysergide maleate

meth-ih-**sir**-guide
(Sansert)

▶CLASSIFICATION

PHARMACOTHERAPEUTIC:
Ergotamine derivative. ***CLINICAL:*** Antimigraine

ACTION/*THERAPEUTIC EFFECT*

Directly stimulates smooth muscle leading to vasoconstriction, *preventing or aborting vascular headaches.*

USES

Treatment of vascular headaches (e.g., migraine, cluster headaches).

PRECAUTIONS

CONTRAINDICATIONS: Pregnancy, peripheral vascular disease (thromboangiitis obliterans, leutic arteritis, severe arteriosclerosis, Raynaud's disease), phlebitis or cellulitis of lower limbs, pulmonary disease, collagen diseases, fibrotic disease, impaired renal or hepatic function, severe pruritus, valvular heart disease, coronary artery disease, severe hypertension, debilitated, malnutrition. ***CAUTIONS:*** None significant.

INTERACTIONS

DRUG: Ergot alkaloids, systemic vasoconstrictors (e.g., norepinephrine) may increase vasoconstrictor effect. ***HERBAL:*** None known. ***FOOD:*** None known. ***LAB VALUES:*** May increase BUN.

M

AVAILABILITY (Rx)

TABLETS: 2 mg.

INDICATIONS/ROUTES/DOSAGE

Vascular headache:

PO: Adults: 4–8 mg/day in divided doses. Do not give continuously >6 mos without 3–4 wk drug-free interval between courses of therapy. Discontinue gradually over 2–3 wks (avoids rebound headache).

SIDE EFFECTS

FREQUENT: Dizziness, diarrhea. ***OCCASIONAL:*** Changes in vision, peripheral edema, flushed face, rash, constipation, insomnia.

ADVERSE REACTIONS/TOXIC EFFECTS

Prolonged administration or excessive dosage may produce ergotamine poisoning: nausea, vomiting, weakness of legs, pain in limb muscles, numbness and tingling of fingers/toes, precordial pain, tachycardia or bradycardia, hyper/hypotension. Feet and hands will become cold, pale, numb. Muscle pain occurs when walking and, later, even at rest. Gangrene may occur. Occasionally, confusion, depression, drowsiness, convulsions may appear.

NURSING IMPLICATIONS

BASELINE ASSESSMENT:

Question pt regarding onset, location, and duration of migraine, and possible precipitating symptoms.

INTERVENTION/EVALUATION:

Monitor closely for evidence of ergotamine overdosage as result of prolonged administration or excessive dosage (see Adverse Reactions/Toxic Effects).

PATIENT/FAMILY TEACHING:

Initiate therapy at first sign of migraine attack. Inform physician if need to progressively increase dose in order to relieve vascular headaches or if irregular heartbeat, nausea, vomiting, numbness or tingling of fingers or toes or if pain or weakness of extremities is noted.

metipranolol

(OptiPranolol)

See Classification section under: Antiglaucoma agents (p. 46C)

metoclopramide

meh-tah-**klo**-prah-myd
(Apo-Metoclop✶, Maxeran✶, Reglan)
Do not confuse with Renagel.

▶CLASSIFICATION

PHARMACOTHERAPEUTIC: Dopamine receptor antagonist. ***CLINICAL:*** GI emptying adjunct, peristaltic stimulant, antiemetic

ACTION/*THERAPEUTIC EFFECT*

Stimulates motility of upper GI tract, *accelerates intestinal transit and gastric emptying.* Decreases reflux into esophagus. Raises threshold activity of chemoreceptor trigger zone, *producing antiemetic activity.*

PHARMACOKINETICS

Well absorbed from GI tract. Metabolized in liver. Protein binding: 30%. Primarily excreted in urine. Not removed by hemodialysis. Half-life: 4–6 hrs.

USES/*UNLABELED*

To facilitate small bowel intubation, stimulate gastric emptying, intestinal transit. Relieves symptoms of acute, recurrent gastroparesis (nausea, vomiting, persistent fullness after meals). Prevents nausea, vomiting associated with cancer chemotherapy. Treatment of heartburn, delayed gastric emptying secondary to reflux esophagitis. *Treatment of slow gastric emptying, vascular headaches, persistent hiccups, drug-related postop nausea/ vomiting. Prophylaxis of aspiration pneumonia.*

PRECAUTIONS

CONTRAINDICATIONS: Pheochromocytoma, history of seizure disorders, concurrent use of medications likely to produce extrapyramidal reactions, GI obstruction or perforation, GI hemorrhage. ***CAUTIONS:*** Impaired renal function, CHF, cirrhosis.

▷*LIFESPAN CONSIDERATIONS:*
Pregnancy/Lactation: Crosses placenta; distributed in breast milk. **Pregnancy Category B. Children:** More susceptible to having dystonia reactions. **Elderly:** More likely to have parkinsonism and tardive dyskinesias after long-term therapy.

INTERACTIONS

DRUG:* Alcohol** may increase CNS depressant effect. **CNS depressants** may increase sedative effect. ***HERBAL: None known. ***FOOD:*** None known. ***LAB VALUES:*** May increase aldosterone, prolactin concentrations.

AVAILABILITY (Rx)

TABLETS: 5 mg, 10 mg. ***SYRUP:*** 5 mg/5 ml. ***INJECTION:*** 5 mg/ml.

ADMINISTRATION/HANDLING

PO:

• Give 30 min before meals and at bedtime. • Tablets may be crushed.

IV 🔟

Storage:

• Store vials at room temperature. • After dilution, IV infusion (piggyback) is stable for 48 hrs.

Reconstitution:

• Dilute doses >10 mg in 50 ml D_5W, 0.9% NaCl, or lactated Ringer's.

Rate of administration:

• Infuse >15 min. • May give slow IV push at rate of 10 mg over 1–2 min. • A too-rapid IV injection may produce intense feeling of anxiety or restlessness, followed by drowsiness.

IV INCOMPATIBILITIES ⊘

Allopurinol (Aloprim), cefepime (Maxipime), doxorubicin liposome (Doxil), furosemide (Lasix), propofol (Diprivan).

IV COMPATIBILITIES

Diltiazem (Cardizem), heparin, lidocaine, magnesium, midazolam (Versed).

INDICATIONS/ROUTES/DOSAGE

Note: May give PO, IM, direct IV, IV infusion.

Diabetic gastroparesis:

***PO/IV:* Adults:** 10 mg before meals and at bedtime for 2–8 wks.

***PO:* Elderly:** Initially, 5 mg before meals and at bedtime. May increase to 10 mg.

IV: Elderly: 5 mg over 1–2 min. May increase to 10 mg.

Symptomatic gastroesophageal reflux:

PO: Adults: 10–15 mg up to 4 times/day; single doses up to 20 mg, as needed. **Elderly:** Initially, 5 mg 4 times/day. May increase to 10 mg. **Children:** 0.4–0.8 mg/kg/day in 4 divided doses.

Prevention of cancer chemotherapy–induced nausea and vomiting:

IV: Adults, elderly, children: 1–2 mg/kg 30 min prior to chemotherapy; repeat q2h for 2 doses, then q3h, as needed.

To facilitate small bowel intubation (single dose):

IV: Adults, elderly: 10 mg. **Children 6–14 yrs:** 2.5–5 mg. **Children <6 yrs:** 0.1 mg/kg.

Postop nausea/vomiting:

IV: Adults, elderly, children >14 yrs: 10 mg; repeat q6–8h as needed. **Children <14 yrs:** 0.1–0.2 mg/kg/dose; repeat q6–8 h as needed.

SIDE EFFECTS

Note: Doses of 2 mg/kg or higher or length of therapy may result in a greater incidence of side effects. **FREQUENT** (10%): Drowsiness, restlessness, fatigue, lassitude. **OCCASIONAL** (3%): Dizziness, anxiety, headache, insomnia, breast tenderness, altered menstruation, constipation, rash, dry mouth, galactorrhea, gynecomastia. **RARE** (<3%): Hypotension, hypertension, tachycardia.

ADVERSE REACTIONS/TOXIC EFFECTS

Extrapyramidal reactions occur most frequently in children and young adults (age 18–30) receiving high doses (2 mg/kg) during cancer chemotherapy, and is usually limited to akathisia (motor restlessness), involuntary limb movement, and facial grimacing.

NURSING IMPLICATIONS

BASELINE ASSESSMENT:

Antiemetic: Assess for dehydration (poor skin turgor, dry mucous membranes, longitudinal furrows in tongue).

INTERVENTION/EVALUATION:

Monitor for anxiety, restlessness, extrapyramidal symptoms during IV administration. Monitor pattern of daily bowel activity and stool consistency. Assess for periorbital edema. Assess skin for rash, hives. Evaluate for therapeutic response from gastroparesis (nausea, vomiting, persistent fullness after meals).

PATIENT/FAMILY TEACHING:

Avoid tasks that require alertness, motor skills until drug response is established. Report involuntary eye, facial, or limb movement (extrapyramidal reaction). Avoid alcohol.

metolazone

me-**toh**-lah-zone
(Diulo, Mykrox, Zaroxolyn)
Do not confuse with
methazolamide, metoprolol, Zarontin.

▶CLASSIFICATION

PHARMACOTHERAPEUTIC: Thiazide-like. **CLINICAL:** Diuretic, antihypertensive (see p. 84C)

ACTION/*THERAPEUTIC EFFECT*

Diuretic: Blocks reabsorption of sodium, potassium, chloride at distal convoluted tubule, promoting delivery of sodium to potassium side, increasing potassium excretion (Na-K) exchange, *producing renal excretion.* ***Antihypertensive:*** Reduces plasma, extracellular fluid volume. *Decreases peripheral vascular resistance, reduced B/P by direct effect on blood vessels.*

PHARMACOKINETICS

Onset	Peak	Duration
PO (diuretic)		
1 hr	2 hrs	12–24 hrs

Incompletely absorbed from GI tract. Protein binding: 95%. Primarily excreted unchanged in urine. Not removed by hemodialysis. Half-life: 14 hrs.

USES

Diulo, Zaroxolyn: Treatment of mild to moderate essential hypertension, edema of renal disease, edema due to CHF. ***Mykrox:*** Treatment of mild to moderate hypertension.

PRECAUTIONS

CONTRAINDICATIONS: History of hypersensitivity to sulfonamides or thiazide diuretics, renal decompensation, anuria, hepatic coma or precoma. ***CAUTIONS:*** Severe renal disease, impaired hepatic function, diabetes mellitus, elderly/debilitated, thyroid disorders.

▷*LIFESPAN CONSIDERATIONS:* **Pregnancy/Lactation:** Crosses placenta; small amount distributed in breast milk—nursing not advised. **Pregnancy Category D. Children:** No age-related precautions noted. **Elderly:** May be more sensitive to hypotensive/electrolyte effects. Age-related renal impairment may require caution.

INTERACTIONS

DRUG: **Cholestyramine, colestipol** may decrease absorption, effects. May increase **digoxin** toxicity (due to hypokalemia). May increase **lithium** toxicity. ***HERBAL:*** None known. ***FOOD:*** None known. ***LAB VALUES:*** May increase bilirubin, serum calcium, LDL, cholesterol, triglycerides, creatinine, glucose, uric acid. May decrease urinary calcium, magnesium, potassium, sodium.

AVAILABILITY (Rx)

TABLETS: 2.5 mg, 5 mg, 10 mg. ***TABLETS (Mykrox):*** 0.5 mg.

ADMINISTRATION/HANDLING

PO:

• May give with food or milk if GI upset occurs, preferably with breakfast (may prevent nocturia).

INDICATIONS/ROUTES/DOSAGE

DIULO, ZAROXOLYN:

Edema:

PO: Adults: 5–10 mg once daily in morning. Reduce dose to lowest maintenance level when dry weight is achieved (nonedematous state).

Edema due to renal disease:

PO: Adults: 5–20 mg once daily in morning. Reduce dose to lowest maintenance level when dry weight is achieved (nonedematous state).

Hypertension:

PO: Adults: 2.5–5 mg once daily in morning.

M

Usual elderly dosage (Diulo, Zaroxolyn):

PO: Initially, 2.5 mg/day or every other day.

MYKROX:

Hypertension:

PO: Adults: 0.5 mg once daily in morning. Dose may be increased to 1 mg once daily if B/P response is insufficient.

Usual dosage for children:

PO: 0.2–0.4 mg/kg/day in divided doses q12–24h.

SIDE EFFECTS

EXPECTED: Increase in urine frequency/volume. **FREQUENT** (9–10%): Dizziness, lightheadedness, headache. **OCCASIONAL** (4–6%): Muscle cramps/spasm, fatigue, lethargy. **RARE** (<2%): Weakness, palpitations, depression, nausea, vomiting, abdominal bloating, constipation, diarrhea, urticaria.

ADVERSE REACTIONS/TOXIC EFFECTS

Vigorous diuresis may lead to profound water loss and electrolyte depletion, resulting in hypokalemia, hyponatremia, dehydration. Acute hypotensive episodes may occur. Hyperglycemia may be noted during prolonged therapy. GI upset, pancreatitis, dizziness, paresthesias, headache, blood dyscrasias, pulmonary edema, allergic pneumonitis, dermatologic reactions occur rarely. Overdosage can lead to lethargy, coma without changes in electrolytes or hydration.

NURSING IMPLICATIONS

BASELINE ASSESSMENT:

Check vital signs, esp. B/P for hypotension prior to administration. Assess baseline electrolytes; particularly check for low potassium. Assess edema, skin turgor, mucous membranes for hydration status. Assess muscle strength, mental status. Note skin temperature, moisture. Obtain baseline weight. Initiate I&O.

INTERVENTION/EVALUATION:

Continue to monitor B/P, vital signs, electrolytes, I&O, weight. Note extent of diuresis. Watch for electrolyte disturbances (hypokalemia may result in weakness, tremor, muscle cramps, nausea, vomiting, change in mental status, tachycardia; hyponatremia may result in confusion, thirst, cold/clammy skin).

PATIENT/FAMILY TEACHING:

Expect increased frequency and volume of urination. To reduce hypotensive effect, rise slowly from lying to sitting position and permit legs to dangle momentarily before standing. Eat foods high in potassium such as whole grains (cereals), legumes, meat, bananas, apricots, orange juice, potatoes (white, sweet), raisins.

metoprolol tartrate

meh-**toe**-pro-lol
(Apo-Metoprolol♦, Betaloc♦, Lopressor, Novometoprol♦, Toprol XL)
Do not confuse with
metaproterenol, metolazone.

FIXED-COMBINATION(S)

With hydrochlorothiazide, a diuretic **(Lopressor HCT)**

▶CLASSIFICATION

PHARMACOTHERAPEUTIC:
Beta₁-adrenergic blocker. **CLINICAL:** Antianginal, antihypertensive, MI adjunct (see p. 61C)

ACTION/*THERAPEUTIC EFFECT*

Selectively blocks beta₁-adrenergic receptors, *slowing sinus heart rate, decreasing cardiac output, decreasing B/P* (exact mechanism unknown but may block peripheral adrenergic receptors, decrease sympathetic outflow from CNS, or decrease renin release from kidney). Large dose may block beta₂-adrenergic receptors, *increasing airway resistance. Decreases myocardial ischemia* severity by decreasing O_2 requirements.

PHARMACOKINETICS

	Onset	Peak	Duration
PO	10–15 min	—	6 hrs
IV	—	20 min	5–8 hrs

Well absorbed from GI tract. Protein binding: 12%. Widely distributed. Metabolized in liver (undergoes significant first-pass metabolism). Primarily excreted in urine. Removed by hemodialysis. Half-life: 3–7 hrs.

USES/*UNLABELED*

Management of mild to moderate hypertension. Used alone or in combination with diuretics, esp. thiazide type. Management of chronic stable angina pectoris. Reduces cardiovascular mortality in those with definite or suspected acute MI. **Extended-release:** Management of hypertension, long-term treatment of angina pectoris. Treatment of heart failure. *Treatment/prophylaxis of cardiac arrhythmias, hypertrophic cardiomyopathy, pheochromocytoma, vascular headache, tremors, anxiety, thyrotoxicosis, mitral valve prolapse syndrome.* Increases survival rate in diabetics with heart disease.

PRECAUTIONS

CONTRAINDICATIONS: Overt cardiac failure, cardiogenic shock, heart block greater than first degree, sinus bradycardia. ***Myocardial infarction:*** Heart rate <45 beats/min, systolic B/P <100 mm Hg. ***CAUTIONS:*** Bronchospastic disease, impaired renal function, peripheral vascular disease, hyperthyroidism, diabetes, inadequate cardiac function.

▷*LIFESPAN CONSIDERATIONS:*
Pregnancy/Lactation: Crosses placenta; distributed in breast milk. Avoid use during first trimester. May produce bradycardia, apnea, hypoglycemia, hypothermia during delivery, small birth weight infants. **Pregnancy Category C** (Category D if used in second or third trimester). **Children:** Safety and efficacy not established. **Elderly:** Age-related peripheral vascular disease may increase susceptibility to decreased peripheral circulation.

INTERACTIONS

DRUG:* Diuretics, other hypotensives** may increase hypotensive effect**; sympathomimetics, xanthines** may mutually inhibit effects; may mask symptoms of hypoglycemia, prolong hypoglycemic effect of **insulin, oral hypoglycemics; NSAIDs** may decrease antihypertensive effect; **cimetidine** may increase concentration. ***HERBAL: None known. ***FOOD:*** None known. **LAB VALUES:** May increase ANA titer, SGOT (AST), SGPT (ALT), alkaline phosphatase, LDH, bilirubin, BUN, creatinine, potassium, uric acid, lipoproteins, triglycerides.

AVAILABILITY (Rx)

TABLETS: 50 mg, 100 mg. ***TAB-***

M

LETS (extended-release): 25 mg, 50 mg, 100 mg, 200 mg. **INJECTION:** 1 mg/ml.

ADMINISTRATION/HANDLING
PO:
• Tablets may be crushed; do not crush or break extended-release tablets. • Give at same time each day. • May be given with or immediately after meals (enhances absorption).

IV 🏵
Storage:
• Store at room temperature.

Rate of administration:
• May give undiluted. • Administer IV injection over 1 min. • Monitor EKG during administration.

IV INCOMPATIBILITIES ⊘
Amphotericin B complex (Abelcet, Ambisome, Amphotec).

IV COMPATIBILITY
Alteplase (Activase).

INDICATIONS/ROUTES/DOSAGE
Hypertension, angina pectoris:
PO: Adults: Initially, 100 mg/day as single or divided dose. Increase at weekly (or longer) intervals. **Maintenance:** 100–450 mg/day.

Usual elderly dosage:
PO: Initially, 25 mg/day. **Range:** 25–300 mg/day.

Usual dosage for extended-release tablets:
PO: Adults: Hypertension: 50–100 mg/day as single dose. May increase at least at weekly intervals until optimum B/P attained. **Angina:** Initially, 100 mg/day as single dose. May increase at least at weekly intervals until optimum clinical response achieved. **Heart failure:** Initially, 25 mg/day. May double dose q2wks. **Maximum:** 200 mg/day.

Myocardial infarction (early treatment):
IV: Adults: 5 mg q2min for 3 doses, followed by 50 mg orally q6h for 48 hrs. Begin oral dose 15 min after last IV dose. Alternatively, in those who do not tolerate full IV dose, give 25–50 mg orally q6h, 15 min after last IV dose.

Myocardial infarction (late treatment, maintenance):
PO: Adults: 100 mg 2 times/day for at least 3 mos.

SIDE EFFECTS
Generally well tolerated, with transient and mild side effects. **FREQUENT:** Decreased sexual ability, drowsiness, insomnia, unusual tiredness/weakness. **OCCASIONAL:** Anxiety, nervousness, diarrhea, constipation, nausea, vomiting, nasal congestion, stomach discomfort, dizziness, difficulty breathing, cold hands/feet. **RARE:** Altered taste, dry eyes, nightmares, numbness in fingers/feet, allergic reaction (rash, pruritus).

ADVERSE REACTIONS/TOXIC EFFECTS
Excessive dosage may produce profound bradycardia, hypotension, bronchospasm. Abrupt withdrawal may result in sweating, palpitations, headache, tremulousness, exacerbation of angina, MI, ventricular arrhythmias. May precipitate CHF, MI in those with cardiac disease, thyroid storm in those with thyrotoxicosis, peripheral ischemia in those with existing peripheral vascular disease. Hypoglycemia may occur in previously controlled diabetics.

BASELINE ASSESSMENT:

Assess baseline renal/liver function tests. Assess B/P, apical pulse immediately before drug is administered (if pulse is 60/min or below, or systolic B/P is below 90 mm Hg, withhold medication, contact physician). *Antianginal:* Record onset, type (sharp, dull, squeezing), radiation, location, intensity, and duration of anginal pain, and precipitating factors (exertion, emotional stress).

INTERVENTION/EVALUATION:

Measure B/P near end of dosing interval (determines if B/P is controlled throughout day). Monitor B/P for hypotension, respiration for shortness of breath. Assess pulse for strength/weakness, irregular rate, bradycardia. Assess for evidence of CHF: dyspnea (particularly on exertion or lying down), night cough, peripheral edema, distended neck veins. Monitor I&O (increase in weight, decrease in urine output may indicate CHF). Therapeutic response to hypertension noted in 1–2 wks.

PATIENT/FAMILY TEACHING:

Do not abruptly discontinue medication. Compliance with therapy regimen is essential to control hypertension, arrhythmias. If a dose is missed, take next scheduled dose (do not double dose). To avoid hypotensive effect, rise slowly from lying to sitting position, wait momentarily before standing. Report excessive fatigue, dizziness. Do not use nasal decongestants, OTC cold preparations (stimulants) without physician ap-proval. Outpts should monitor B/P, pulse before taking medication. Restrict salt, alcohol intake.

metronidazole hydrochloride

meh-trow-**nye**-dah-zoll
(Apo-Metronidazole✽, Flagyl, MetroCream, MetroGel, MetroLotion, NidaGel✽, Noritate, Novonidazol✽, Protostat, Satric)

FIXED-COMBINATION(S)

With bismuth subsalicylate and tetracycline, an anti-infective **(Helidac, Noritate)**

▶CLASSIFICATION

PHARMACOTHERAPEUTIC: Nitroimidazole derivative. *CLINICAL:* Antibacterial, antiprotozoal

ACTION/*THERAPEUTIC EFFECT*

Taken up by cells in susceptible microorganisms. Disrupts DNA, inhibits nucleic acid synthesis *producing bactericidal, amebicidal, trichomonacidal effects*. Produces anti-inflammatory, immunosuppressive effects when applied topically.

PHARMACOKINETICS

Well absorbed from GI tract, minimal absorption after topical application. Protein binding: <20%. Widely distributed, crosses blood-brain barrier. Metabolized in liver to active metabolite. Primarily excreted in urine; partially eliminated in feces. Removed by hemodialysis. Half-life: 8 hrs (half-life increased in alcoholic liver disease, neonates).

USES/*UNLABELED*

Treatment of anaerobic infections (skin/skin structure, CNS, lower respiratory tract, bone and joints, intra-abdominal, gynecologic, endocarditis, septicemia). Treatment of trichomoniasis, amebiasis, perioperatively for contaminated/potentially contaminated intra-abdominal surgery, antibiotic–associated pseudomembranous colitis (AAPC). Treatment of *H. pylori-associated gastritis/duodenal ulcer. Topical application in treatment of acne rosacea. Also used in treatment of grade III, IV decubitus ulcers with anaerobic infection. Treatment of bacterial vaginosis.* Treatment of inflammatory bowel disease.

PRECAUTIONS

CONTRAINDICATIONS: Hypersensitivity to metronidazole or other nitroimidazole derivatives (also parabens with topical application). ***CAUTIONS:*** Blood dyscrasias, severe hepatic dysfunction, CNS disease, predisposition to edema, concurrent corticosteroid therapy. Safety and efficacy of topical administration in those <21 yrs of age not established.

▷***LIFESPAN CONSIDERATIONS:*** **Pregnancy/Lactation:** Readily crosses placenta; distributed in breast milk. Contraindicated during first trimester in those with trichomoniasis. Topical use during pregnancy or lactation discouraged. **Pregnancy Category B. Children:** No age-related precautions noted. **Elderly:** Age-related liver impairment may require dosage adjustment.

INTERACTIONS

DRUG:* Alcohol** may cause disulfiram-type reaction. May increase effect of **oral anticoagulants.** May increase toxicity with **disulfiram.** ***HERBAL: None known. ***FOOD:*** None known. ***LAB VALUES:*** May increase SGOT (AST), SGPT (ALT), LDH.

AVAILABILITY (Rx)

TABLETS: 250 mg, 500 mg. ***TABLETS (extended-release):*** 750 mg. ***CAPSULES:*** 375 mg. ***POWDER FOR INJECTION:*** 500 mg. ***INJECTION (infusion):*** 500 mg/100 ml. ***LOTION:*** 0.75% ***VAGINAL GEL:*** 0.75%. ***TOPICAL GEL:*** 0.75%. ***TOPICAL CREAM:*** 1%.

ADMINISTRATION/HANDLING

PO:

• Give without regard to meals. Give with food to decrease GI irritation.

IV 🎨

Storage:

• Store at room temperature (ready to use infusion bags).

Rate of administration:

• Infuse >30–60 min. Do not give bolus. • Avoid prolonged use of indwelling catheters.

IV INCOMPATIBILITIES ⊘

Amphotericin B complex (Abelcet, Ambisome, Amphotec), filgrastim (Neupogen).

IV COMPATIBILITIES

Diltiazem (Cardizem), dopamine (Intropin), heparin, lorazepam (Ativan), magnesium, midazolam (Versed).

INDICATIONS/ROUTES/DOSAGE

Amebiasis:

***PO:* Adults, elderly:** 500–750 mg q8h. **Children:** 35–50 mg/kd/day in divided doses q8h.

Parasitic infections:

***PO:* Adults, elderly:** 250 mg q8h or 2 g as a single dose. **Children:** 15–30 mg/kg/day in divided doses q8h.

Anaerobic infections:

***PO/IV:* Adults, elderly, children:** 30 mg/kd/day in divided doses q6h. **Maximum:** 4 g/day.

AAPC:

***PO:* Adults, elderly:** 250–500 mg 3–4 times/day for 10–14 days. **Children:** 30 mg/kg/day in divided doses q6h for 7–10 days.

H. pylori:

***PO:* Adults, elderly:** 250–500 mg 3 times/day (in combination). **Children:** 15–20 mg/kg/day in 2 divided doses.

Bacterial vaginosis:

***INTRAVAGINAL:* Adults:** One applicatorful 2 times/day or once daily at bedtime for 5 days.

***PO:* Adults:** 750 mg at bedtime for 7 days.

Rosacea:

TOPICAL:* Adults:** Thin application 2 times/day to affected area. ***CREAM: Once daily. ***LOTION:*** Apply twice daily.

SIDE EFFECTS

FREQUENT: Anorexia, nausea, dry mouth, metallic taste. ***Vaginal:*** Symptomatic cervicitis/vaginitis, abdominal cramps, uterine pain. ***OCCASIONAL:*** Diarrhea or constipation, vomiting, dizziness, erythematous rash, urticaria, reddish brown or dark urine. ***Topical:*** Transient redness, mild dryness, burning, irritation, stinging (also tearing when applied too close to eyes). ***Vaginal:*** Vaginal, perineal, vulvar itching, vulvar swelling.

RARE: Mild, transient leukopenia, thrombophlebitis with IV therapy.

ADVERSE REACTIONS/TOXIC EFFECTS

Oral therapy may result in furry tongue, glossitis, cystitis, dysuria, pancreatitis, flattening of T waves with EKG readings. Peripheral neuropathy (numbness, tingling, paresthesia) is usually reversible if treatment is stopped immediately upon appearance of neurologic symptoms. Seizures occur occasionally.

NURSING IMPLICATIONS

BASELINE ASSESSMENT:

Question for history of hypersensitivity to metronidazole or other nitroimidazole derivatives (and parabens with topical). Obtain specimens for diagnostic tests before giving first dose (therapy may begin before results are known).

INTERVENTION/EVALUATION:

Determine pattern of bowel activity. Monitor I&O and assess for urinary problems. Be alert to neurologic symptoms: dizziness, numbness, tingling or paresthesia of extremities. Assess for rash, urticaria. Watch for onset of superinfection: ulceration or change of oral mucosa, furry tongue, vaginal discharge, genital/anal pruritus.

PATIENT/FAMILY TEACHING:

Urine may be red-brown or dark. Avoid alcohol and alcohol-containing preparations, e.g., cough syrups, elixirs. If dizziness occurs, do not drive or use machines that require alertness. If taking metronidazole for trichomoniasis, refrain from sexual intercourse until physician advises. For amebiasis, frequent stool specimen checks will be necessary. *Topical:* Avoid contact with eyes. May apply cosmetics after application. Metronidazole acts on redness, papules, and pustules but has no effect on rhinophyma (hypertrophy of nose), telangiectasia, or ocular problems (conjunctivitis, keratitis, blepharitis). Other recommendations for rosacea include avoidance of hot or spicy foods, alcohol, extremes of hot or cold temperatures, excessive sunlight.

mexiletine hydrochloride

(Mexitil)

See Classification section under: Anti-arrhythmic (p. 12C)

miconazole nitrate

mih-**kon**-nah-zoll
(Micatin, Micozole✿, Monistat✿, Monistat 3, 7, Monistat-Derm)
Do not confuse with Micronase, Micronor.

▶CLASSIFICATION

PHARMACOTHERAPEUTIC: Imidazole derivative. *CLINICAL:* Antifungal (see p. 42C)

ACTION/*THERAPEUTIC EFFECT*

Inhibits synthesis of ergosterol (vital component of fungal cell formation), damaging fungal cell membrane. *Fungistatic; may be fungicidal, depending on concentration.*

PHARMACOKINETICS

Topical: No systemic absorption following application to intact skin.

Intravaginal: Small amount absorbed systemically.

USES

Vaginal: Vulvovaginal candidiasis. *Topical:* Cutaneous candidiasis, tinea cruris, t. corporis, t. pedis, t. versicolor.

PRECAUTIONS

CONTRAINDICATIONS: Children <1 yr; topically, children <2 yrs. *CAUTIONS:* Hepatic insufficiency.
▷*LIFESPAN CONSIDERATIONS:* **Pregnancy/Lactation:** Unknown if drug crosses placenta or is distributed in breast milk. **Pregnancy Category C. Children/Elderly:** No age-related precautions noted.

INTERACTIONS

DRUG: May increase effects of **oral anticoagulants, oral hypoglycemics. Isoniazid, rifampin** may decrease concentrations. *HERBAL:* None known. *FOOD:* None known. *LAB VALUES:* None significant.

AVAILABILITY (Rx)

VAGINAL SUPPOSITORY: 100 mg, 200 mg. *TOPICAL CREAM:* 2%. *VAGINAL CREAM:* 2%. *TOPICAL POWDER:* 2%. *TOPICAL SPRAY:* 2%.

INDICATIONS/ROUTES/DOSAGE

Vulvovaginal candidiasis:

INTRAVAGINAL: **Adults, elderly:** One 200 mg suppository at bedtime for 3 days; one 100 mg suppository or one applicatorful at bedtime for 7 days.

Topical fungal infections, cutaneous candidiasis:

TOPICAL: **Adults, elderly:** Apply liberally 2 times/day, morning and evening.

SIDE EFFECTS

Topical: Itching, burning, stinging, erythema, urticaria. **Vaginal** *(2%)*: Vulvovaginal burning, itching, irritation, headache, skin rash.

ADVERSE REACTIONS/TOXIC EFFECTS

None significant.

NURSING IMPLICATIONS

BASELINE ASSESSMENT:

Topical: Avoid occlusive dressing. Apply only a small amount to cover area completely. **Spray:** Shake well before using.

INTERVENTION/EVALUATION:

Topical/vaginal: Assess for burning, itching, irritation.

PATIENT/FAMILY TEACHING:

Vaginal preparation: Base interacts with certain latex products such as contraceptive diaphragm. Ask physician about douching, sexual intercourse. **Topical:** Rub well into affected areas. Avoid getting in eyes. Keep areas clean, dry; wear light clothing for ventilation. Separate personal items in contact with affected areas.

midazolam hydrochloride

my-**day**-zoe-lam
(Versed)
Do not confuse with VePesid.

▶CLASSIFICATION

PHARMACOTHERAPEUTIC: Benzodiazepine **(Schedule IV).** **CLINICAL:** Sedative (see p. 3C)

ACTION/*THERAPEUTIC EFFECT*

Enhances action of gamma-aminobutyric acid (GABA) neurotransmission at CNS, *producing sedative, anxiolytic effect due to CNS depressant action.* Inhibits spinal afferent pathways, *producing skeletal muscle relaxation.* Directly depresses motor nerve, muscle function effects.

PHARMACOKINETICS

	Onset	Peak	Duration
IM	5–15 min	45 min	1–6 hrs
IV	1–5 min	5–7 min	20–30 min

Well absorbed after IM administration. Protein binding: 97%. Metabolized in liver to active metabolite. Primarily excreted in urine. Not removed by hemodialysis. Half-life: 1–5 hrs.

USES

Sedation, anxiolytic, amnesia prior to procedure or induction of anesthesia, conscious sedation prior to diagnostic/radiographic procedure, continuous IV sedation of intubated and mechanically ventilated pts, status epilepticus.

PRECAUTIONS

CONTRAINDICATIONS: Shock, comatose pts, acute alcohol intoxication, acute narrow-angle glaucoma. **CAUTIONS:** Acute illness, severe fluid/electrolyte imbalance, impaired renal function, CHF, treated open-angle glaucoma.

▷*LIFESPAN CONSIDERATIONS:* **Pregnancy/Lactation:** Crosses placenta; unknown if drug is distributed in breast milk. **Pregnancy Category D. Children:** Neonates more likely to have respiratory depression. **Elderly:** Age-related renal impairment may require dosage adjustment.

M

INTERACTIONS

DRUG: Alcohol, CNS depressants may increase CNS, respiratory depression, hypotensive effects. **Hypotension-producing medications** may increase hypotensive effects. **HERBAL: Kava kava, valerian** may increase CNS depression. **FOOD: Grapefruit juice** increases oral absorption. **LAB VALUES:** None significant.

AVAILABILITY (Rx)

INJECTION: 1 mg/ml, 2 mg/ml, 5 mg/ml. **SYRUP:** 2 mg/ml.

ADMINISTRATION/HANDLING

IM:

• Give deep IM into large muscle mass.

IV

Storage:

• Store vials at room temperature.

Rate of administration:

• May give undiluted or as infusion. • O_2, resuscitative equipment must be readily available before IV is administered. • Administer by slow IV injection, in incremental dosages: Give each incremental dose over 2 or more mins at intervals of at least 2 min. • Reduce IV rate in those >60 yrs, and/or debilitated, those with chronic disease states, and/or impaired pulmonary function. • A too-rapid IV rate, excessive doses, or a single large dose increases risk of respiratory depression/arrest.

IV INCOMPATIBILITIES ⊘

Albumin, ampicillin/sulbactam (Unasyn), amphotericin B complex (Abelcet, Ambisome, Amphotec), ampicillin (Polycillin), bumetanide (Bumex), dexamethasone (Decadron), fosphenytoin (Cerebyx), furosemide (Lasix), hydrocortisone (Solu Cortef), methotrexate, nafcillin (Nafcil), sodium bicarbonate, sodium pentothal (Thiopental), sulfamethoxazole-trimethoprim (Bactrim).

IV COMPATIBILITIES

Amiodarone (Cordarone), calcium gluconate, diltiazem (Cardizem), dopamine (Intropin), fentanyl, heparin, insulin, milrinone (Primacor), nitroglycerin, norepinephrine (Levophed), potassium.

INDICATIONS/ROUTES/DOSAGE

Note: Dose must be individualized based on age, underlying disease, medications, desired effect.

Preop sedation:

IM: Adults, elderly: 0.07–0.08 mg/kg 30–60 min prior to surgery. **Children:** 0.1–0.15 mg/kg 30–60 min prior to surgery. **Maximum total dose:** 10 mg.

IV: Children 6–12 yrs: 0.025–0.05 mg/kg. **Children 6 mos–5 yrs:** 0.05–0.1 mg/kg.

PO: Children: 0.25–0.5 mg/kg. **Maximum:** 20 mg.

Conscious sedation for procedures:

IV: Adults, elderly: 1–2.5 mg over 2 min. Titrate as needed. **Total dose:** 2.5–5 mg.

Consious sedation during mechanical ventilation:

IV: Adults, elderly: 0.01–0.5 mg/kg; may repeat at 10–15 min intervals until adequately sedated, then continuous infusion: intially, 0.02–0.1 mg/kg/hr (1–7 mg/hr). **Children >32 wks:** Initially, 1 mcg/kg/min as continuous infusion. **Children <32 wks:** Initially, 0.5 mcg/kg/min as continuous infusion.

Status epilepticus:

IV: Children >2 mos: Loading dose of 0.15 mg/kg followed by continuous infusion of 1 mcg/kg/min. Titrate. **Range:** 1–18 mcg/kg/min.

SIDE EFFECTS

FREQUENT (4–10%): Decreased respiratory rate, tenderness at IM/IV injection site, pain during injection, desaturation, hiccups. *OCCASIONAL* (2–3%): Pain at IM injection site, hypotension, paradoxical reaction. *RARE* (<2%): Nausea, vomiting, headache, coughing, hypotensive episodes.

ADVERSE REACTIONS/TOXIC EFFECTS

Too much or too little dosage, improper administration, or cerebral hypoxia may result in agitation, involuntary movements, hyperactivity, combativeness. Underventilation/apnea may produce hypoxia, cardiac arrest. A too-rapid IV rate, excessive doses, or a single large dose increases risk of respiratory depression/arrest.

NURSING IMPLICATIONS

BASELINE ASSESSMENT:

Resuscitative equipment, endotracheal tube, suction, O_2 must be available. Obtain vital signs before administration.

INTERVENTION/EVALUATION:

Monitor respiratory rate continuously during parenteral administration for underventilation, apnea. Monitor vital signs q3–5min during recovery period.

midodrine

my-doe-dreen
(ProAmatine)
Do not confuse with protamine.

▶CLASSIFICATION

PHARMACOTHERAPEUTIC: Vasopressor. *CLINICAL:* Orthostatic hypotension adjunct

ACTION/*THERAPEUTIC EFFECT*

Forms active metabolite desglymidodrine, which is an alpha$_1$ agonist, activating alpha receptors of arteriolar and venous vasculature. *Increases vascular tone, B/P.*

PRECAUTIONS

CONTRAINDICATIONS: Severe cardiac disease, persistent hypertension, pheochromocytoma, thyrotoxicosis, acute renal function impairment, urinary retention. *CAUTIONS:* Renal, liver impairment, history of visual problems.

INTERACTIONS

DRUG: **Digoxin** may have additive bradycardiac effects. **Sodium-retaining steroids** (e.g., **fludrocortisone**) may increase sodium retention. **Vasoconstrictors** may be additive. *HERBAL:* None significant. *FOOD:* None significant. *LAB VALUES:* None significant.

USES

Treatment of symptomatic orthostatic hypotension.

AVAILABILITY (Rx)

TABLETS: 2.5 mg, 5 mg.

INDICATIONS/ROUTES/DOSAGE

Orthostatic hypotension:

PO: Adults, elderly: 10 mg 3 times/day. Give during day when pt is up-

M

right (upon arising, midday, late afternoon not later than 6 PM).

SIDE EFFECTS

FREQUENT (7–20%): Paresthesia, piloerection, pruritus, dysuria, supine hypertension. **OCCASIONAL** (1–7%): Pain, rash, chills, headache, facial flushing, confusion, dry mouth, anxiety.

ADVERSE REACTIONS/TOXIC EFFECTS

None significant.

NURSING IMPLICATIONS

BASELINE ASSESSMENT:

Assess sensitivity to midodrine, taking of other medications (esp. digoxin sodium-retaining vasoconstrictors. Assess medical problems, including acute renal function impairment, severe hypertension, cardiac disease.

INTERVENTION/EVALUATION:

Monitor blood pressure, renal and liver function.

PATIENT/FAMILY TEACHING:

Do not take last dose of the day after evening meal or <3 hrs prior to bedtime. Do not give if pt will be supine. Avoid use of other medication, esp. nonprescription sympathomimetics.

mifepristone

my-fih-**priss**-tone
(Mifeprex)
Do not confuse with Mirapex.

▶CLASSIFICATION
CLINICAL: Abortifacient

ACTION/THERAPEUTIC EFFECT

Has antiprogestational activity resulting from competitive interaction with progesterone; inhibits the activity of endogenous or exogenous progesterone. Also has antiglucocorticoid and weak antiandrogenic activity. *Terminating pregnancy.*

USES/UNLABELED

Termination of intrauterine pregnancy. *Postcoital contraception/contragestation; intrauterine fetal death/nonviable early pregnancy, unresectable meningioma, endometriosis, Cushing's syndrome.*

PRECAUTIONS

CONTRAINDICATIONS: Confirmed/suspected ectopic pregnancy, IUD in place, chronic adrenal failure, concurrent long-term steroid or anticoagulant therapy, hemorrhagic disorders, inherited porphyries. **CAUTIONS:** Treatment of women >35 yrs or smoke >10 cigarettes/day. Cardiovascular disease, hypertension, liver/renal impairment, diabetes, severe anemia.

INTERACTIONS

DRUG: Ketoconazole, itraconazole, erythromycin may inhibit metabolism. **Rifampin, phenytoin, phenobarbital, carbamazepine** may increase metabolism. **HERBAL: St. John's wort** may increase metabolism. **FOOD: Grapefruit** may inhibit metabolism. **LAB VALUES:** May decrease Hgb/Hct and RBC count.

AVAILABILITY (Rx)
TABLETS: 200 mg.

INDICATIONS/ROUTES/DOSAGE
Note: Treatment with mifepristone and misoprostil requires three office visits.

Termination of pregnancy:

PO: Adults: *Day 1:* 600 mg as single dose. *Day 3:* 400 mcg misoprostil. *Day 14:* Post-treatment examination.

SIDE EFFECTS

FREQUENT (>10%): Headache, dizziness, abdominal pain, nausea, vomiting, diarrhea, fatigue. **OCCASIONAL** (3–10%): Uterine hemorrhage, back pain, insomnia, vaginitis, dyspepsia, back pain, fever, viral infections, rigors (chills/shaking). **RARE:** (1–2%): Anxiety, syncope, anemia, asthenia, leg pain, sinusitis, leukorrhea.

ADVERSE REACTIONS/TOXIC EFFECTS

None significant.

> #### NURSING IMPLICATIONS
>
> **BASELINE ASSESSMENT:**
>
> Assess for use of ketoconazole, itraconazole, erythromycin, rifampin, anticonvulsants.
>
> **INTERVENTION/EVALUATION:**
> Monitor Hgb/Hct.
>
> **PATIENT/FAMILY TEACHING:**
>
> Advise pts of treatment procedure and effects, need for follow-up visit. Vaginal bleeding/uterine cramping may occur. Advise pt what to do in an emergency.

---

miglitol

mig-lih-toll
(Glyset)

▶CLASSIFICATION

PHARMACOTHERAPEUTIC:
Alpha-glucosidase inhibitor. **CLIN-ICAL:** Antidiabetic (see p. 39C)

ACTION/*THERAPEUTIC EFFECT*

An oral alpha-glucosidase inhibitor that delays the digestion of ingested carbohydrates into simple sugars such as glucose. *Produces smaller rise in blood glucose concentration following meals.*

USES

Treatment of type II noninsulin-dependent diabetes mellitus.

PRECAUTIONS

CONTRAINDICATIONS: Diabetic ketoacidosis, inflammatory bowel disease, colonic ulceration, partial intestinal obstruction, hypersensitivity to miglitol. **CAUTIONS:** Renal function impairment.

INTERACTIONS

DRUG: May decrease concentration/effect of **digoxin, propranolol, ranitidine. HERBAL:** None significant. **FOOD:** None significant. **LAB VALUES:** None significant.

AVAILABILITY [Rx]

TABLETS: 25 mg, 50 mg.

INDICATIONS/ROUTES/DOSAGE

Antidiabetic:

PO: Adults, elderly: Initially, 25 mg 3 times/day (with first bite of each main meal). **Maintenance:** 50 mg 3 times/day. **Maximum:** 100 mg 3 times/day.

SIDE EFFECTS

FREQUENT (10–40%): Flatulence, soft stools, diarrhea, abdominal pain. **OCCASIONAL** (5%): Rash.

> #### NURSING IMPLICATIONS
>
> **BASELINE ASSESSMENT:**
>
> Check blood glucose levels. Determine use of medications, esp. digoxin, propranolol, ranitidine.

M

Discuss lifestyle to determine extent of learning.

INTERVENTION/EVALUATION:

Monitor blood glucose levels, food intake. Be alert for conditions altering glucose (fever, stress, surgical procedures).

PATIENT/FAMILY TEACHING:

Discuss diet. Wear medical alert identification. Check with physician when glucose demands are altered (e.g., fever, stress).

---

milrinone lactate

mill-rih-known
(Primacor)

▶ CLASSIFICATION

PHARMACOTHERAPEUTIC: Cardiac inotropic agent. ***CLINICAL:*** Vasodilator (see p. 76C).

ACTION/THERAPEUTIC EFFECT

Possesses positive inotropic effect (increases force of myocardial contraction), direct arterial vasodilation. Reduces preload and afterload by direct effect on vascular smooth muscle. *Increases cardiac output, decreases pulmonary capillary wedge pressure and vascular resistance.*

PHARMACOKINETICS

	Onset	Peak	Duration
IV	5–15 min	—	—

Protein binding: 70%. Metabolized in liver; excreted in urine. Half-life: 2.4 hrs.

USES

Short-term management of congestive heart failure (CHF).

PRECAUTIONS

CONTRAINDICATIONS: Severe obstructive aortic or pulmonic valvular disease. ***CAUTIONS:*** Impaired renal, hepatic function.
▷***LIFESPAN CONSIDERATIONS:*** **Pregnancy/Lactation:** Unknown if drug crosses placenta or is distributed in breast milk. **Pregnancy Category C. Children:** Safety and efficacy not established. **Elderly:** Age-related renal impairment may require dosage adjustment.

INTERACTIONS

DRUG: Produces additive inotropic effects with **cardiac glycosides. HERBAL:** None known. ***FOOD:*** None known. ***LAB VALUES:*** None significant.

AVAILABILITY (Rx)

INJECTION: 1 mg/ml. ***INJECTION (premix):*** 200 mcg/ml.

ADMINISTRATION/HANDLING

IV 🔟

Storage:
• Store at room temperature.

Reconstitution:
• For IV infusion, dilute 20 mg (20 ml) vial with 80 or 180 ml diluent (0.9% NaCl, D₅W) to provide concentration of 200 or 100 mcg/ml, respectively. Maximum concentration: 100 mg/250 ml.

Rate of administration:
• For IV injection (loading dose), administer undiluted slowly over 10 min. • Monitor for arrhythmias, hypotension during IV therapy. Reduce or temporarily discontinue infusion until condition stabilizes.

IV INCOMPATIBILITY ⊘

Furosemide (Lasix).

IV COMPATIBILITIES

Calcium gluconate, digoxin (Lanoxin), diltiazem (Cardizem), dobutamine (Dobutrex), dopamine (Intropin), heparin, lidocaine, magnesium, midazolam (Versed), nitroglycerin, potassium, propofol (Diprivan).

INDICATIONS/ROUTES/DOSAGE

Congestive heart failure:

IV: Adults: Initially, 50 mcg/kg over 10 min. Continue with maintenance infusion rate of 0.375–0.75 mcg/kg/min based on hemodynamic and clinical response (total daily dose: 0.59–1.13 mg/kg). Reduce dose to 0.2–0.43 mcg/kg/min in pts with severe renal impairment.

SIDE EFFECTS

OCCASIONAL (1–3%): Headache, hypotension. ***RARE*** (<1%): Angina, chest pain.

ADVERSE REACTIONS/TOXIC EFFECTS

Supraventricular and ventricular arrhythmias occur in 12%; nonsustained ventricular tachycardia occurs in 2%, sustained ventricular tachycardia in 1% of those treated.

NURSING IMPLICATIONS

BASELINE ASSESSMENT:

Offer emotional support (difficulty breathing may produce anxiety). Assess B/P, apical pulse rate before treatment begins and during IV therapy. Assess lung sounds, check edema.

INTERVENTION/EVALUATION:

Monitor for hypotension during administration (discontinue or slow IV rate until condition stabilizes). Assess heart rate, serum electrolytes, I&O, renal function studies.

minocycline hydrochloride

min-know-**sigh**-clean
(Arestin, Dynacin, Minocin, Novo Minocycline✦)
Do not confuse with Dynabac, Mithracin.

▶CLASSIFICATION

PHARMACOTHERAPEUTIC: Tetracycline. ***CLINICAL:*** Antibiotic

M

ACTION/THERAPEUTIC EFFECT

Binds to ribosomes, *inhibiting protein synthesis. Bacteriostatic.*

USES/UNLABELED

Treatment of prostate, urinary tract, CNS infections (not meningitis), uncomplicated gonorrhea, inflammatory acne, brucellosis, skin granulomas, cholera, trachoma, nocardiasis, yaws, and syphilis when penicillins are contraindicated. *Treatment of atypical mycobacterial infections, rheumatoid arthritis, scleroderma.*

PRECAUTIONS

CONTRAINDICATIONS: Hypersensitivity to tetracyclines, last half of pregnancy, children <8 yrs. ***CAUTIONS:*** Renal impairment, sun or ultraviolet exposure (severe photosensitivity reaction).

INTERACTIONS

***DRUG: Cholestyramine, colestipol** may decrease absorption. May decrease effect of **oral contraceptives. Carbamazepine,*

phenytoin may decrease concentration. **HERBAL: St. John's wort** may increase risk of photosensitivity. **FOOD:** None known. **LAB VALUES:** May increase SGOT (AST), SGPT (ALT), alkaline phosphatase, amylase, bilirubin concentrations.

AVAILABILITY (Rx)

CAPSULES: 50 mg, 75 mg, 100 mg. **TABLETS:** 50 mg, 100 mg. **ORAL SUSPENSION:** 50 mg/5 ml. **POWDER FOR INJECTION:** 100 mg.

ADMINISTRATION/HANDLING

PO:

• Store at room temperature. • Give capsules, tablets with full glass of water.

IV 💉

Storage:

• IV solution is stable for 24 hrs at room temperature. • Use IV infusion (piggyback) immediately after reconstitution. • Discard if precipitate forms.

Reconstitution:

• For intermittent IV infusion (piggyback), reconstitute each 100 mg vial with 5–10 ml Sterile Water for Injection to provide concentration of 20 or 10 mg/ml, respectively. • Further dilute with 500–1,000 ml D$_5$W or 0.9% NaCl.

Rate of administration:

• Infuse over 6 hrs.

IV INCOMPATIBILITY ⊘

Piperacillin/tazobactam (Zosyn).

IV COMPATIBILITIES

Heparin, magnesium, potassium.

INDICATIONS/ROUTES/DOSAGE

Note: Space doses evenly around the clock.

Mild to moderate to severe infections:

PO: Adults, elderly: Initially, 100–200 mg, then 100 mg q12h or 50 mg q6h.

IV: Adults, elderly: Initially, 200 mg, then 100 mg q12h up to 400 mg/day.

PO/IV: Children >8 yrs: Initially, 4 mg/kg, then 2 mg/kg q12h.

SIDE EFFECTS

FREQUENT: Dizziness, lightheadedness, diarrhea, nausea, vomiting, stomach cramps, photosensitivity (may be severe). **OCCASIONAL:** Pigmentation of skin, mucous membranes, itching in rectal/genital area, sore mouth/tongue.

ADVERSE REACTIONS/TOXIC EFFECTS

Superinfection (esp. fungal), anaphylaxis, increased intracranial pressure, bulging fontanelles occur rarely in infants.

NURSING IMPLICATIONS

BASELINE ASSESSMENT:

Question for history of allergies, esp. tetracyclines, sulfite.

INTERVENTION/EVALUATION:

Assess ability to ambulate: drowsiness, vertigo, dizziness. Determine pattern of bowel activity and stool consistency. Assess skin for rash. Check B/P and LOC for increased intracranial pressure. Be alert for superinfection: diarrhea, ulceration or changes of oral mucosa, anal/genital pruritus.

PATIENT/FAMILY TEACHING:

Continue antibiotic for full length of treatment. Space doses evenly. Drink full glass of water with capsules, tablets and avoid bedtime doses. Avoid tasks that require alertness, motor skills until response to drug is established. Notify physician if diarrhea, rash, other new symptom occurs. Protect skin from sun exposure.

minoxidil

min-**ox**-ih-dill
(Loniten, Rogaine, Rogaine Extra Strength)
Do not confuse with Lotensin.

▶CLASSIFICATION

CLINICAL: Antihypertensive, hair growth stimulant (see p. 52C)

ACTION/*THERAPEUTIC EFFECT*

Direct action of vascular smooth muscle, producing vasodilation of arterioles, *decreasing peripheral vascular resistance, B/P.* **Topical:** Vasodilatory action *increases cutaneous blood flow, stimulates hair follicle epithelium, hair follicle growth.*

PHARMACOKINETICS

	Onset	Peak	Duration
PO	0.5 hrs	2–8 hrs	2–5 days

Well absorbed from GI tract, minimal absorption after topical application. Protein binding: None. Widely distributed. Metabolized in liver to active metabolite. Primarily excreted in urine. Removed by hemodialysis. Half-life: 4.2 hrs.

USES

Treatment of severe symptomatic hypertension, or hypertension associated with organ damage. Used for those who fail to respond to maximal therapeutic dosages of diuretic and two other antihypertensive agents. Treatment of alopecia androgenetica (males: baldness of vertex of scalp; females: diffuse hair loss or thinning of frontoparietal areas).

PRECAUTIONS

CONTRAINDICATIONS: Pheochromocytoma. ***CAUTIONS:*** Severe renal impairment, chronic CHF, coronary artery disease, recent MI (1 mo).
▷***LIFESPAN CONSIDERATIONS:***
Pregnancy/Lactation: Crosses placenta; distributed in breast milk. **Pregnancy Category C. Children:** No age-related precautions noted. **Elderly:** More sensitive to hypotensive effects. Age-related renal impairment may require dosage adjustment.

INTERACTIONS

DRUG:* Parenteral antihypertensives** may increase hypotensive effect. **NSAIDs** may decrease effect. ***HERBAL: None known. ***FOOD:*** None known. ***LAB VALUES:*** May increase BUN, creatinine, plasma renin activity, alkaline phosphatase, sodium. May decrease hemoglobin, hematocrit, erythrocyte count.

AVAILABILITY (Rx)

TABLETS: 2.5 mg, 10 mg. ***TOPICAL SOLUTION (OTC):*** 20 mg/ml, 50 mg/ml.

ADMINISTRATION/HANDLING

PO:

• Give without regard to food (with food if GI upset occurs). • Tablets may be crushed.

Topical:

• Shampoo and dry hair before applying medication. • Wash hands

M

immediately after application. • Do not use hair dryer after application (reduces effectiveness).

INDICATIONS/ROUTES/DOSAGE

Hypertension:

PO: Adults: Initially, 5 mg/day. Increase with at least 3 day intervals to 10 mg, 20 mg, up to 40 mg/day in 1–2 doses. **Elderly:** Initially, 2.5 mg/day. May increase gradually. **Maintenance:** 10–40 mg/day. **Maximum:** 100 mg/day. **Children:** Initially, 0.1–0.2 mg/kg (5 mg maximum) daily. Gradually increase at minimum 3 day intervals of 0.1–2 mg/kg. **Maintenance:** 0.25–1 mg/kg/day in 1–2 doses. **Maximum:** 50 mg/day.

Hair regrowth:

TOPICAL: Adults: 1 ml to total affected areas of scalp 2 times/day. Total daily dose not to exceed 2 ml.

SIDE EFFECTS

FREQUENT: PO: Edema with concurrent weight gain, hypertrichosis (elongation, thickening, increased pigmentation of fine body hair) develops in 80% of pts within 3–6 wks after beginning therapy. **OCCASIONAL:** T wave changes but usually these revert to pretreatment state with continued therapy or drug withdrawal. **Topical:** Itching, skin rash, dry/flaking skin, erythema. **RARE:** Rash, pruritus, breast tenderness in male and female, headache. **Topical:** Allergic reaction, alopecia, burning scalp, soreness at hair root, headache, visual disturbances.

ADVERSE REACTIONS/TOXIC EFFECTS

Tachycardia and angina pectoris may occur because of increased O_2 demands associated with increased heart rate, cardiac output. Fluid and electrolyte imbalance, CHF may be observed (esp. if diuretic is not given concurrently). Too-rapid reduction in B/P may result in syncope, cerebral vascular accident, MI, ischemia of special sense organs (vision, hearing). Pericardial effusion and tamponade may be seen in those with impaired renal function not on dialysis.

NURSING IMPLICATIONS

BASELINE ASSESSMENT:

Assess B/P on both arms and take pulse for 1 full min immediately before giving medication. If pulse increases 20 beats/min or more over baseline, or systolic or diastolic B/P decreases more than 20 mm Hg, withhold drug, contact physician.

INTERVENTION/EVALUATION:

Assess for peripheral edema of hands, feet (usually, first area of low extremity swelling is behind medial malleolus in ambulatory, sacral area in bedridden). Assess for signs of CHF (cough, rales at base of lungs, cool extremities, dyspnea on exertion). Monitor fluid and electrolyte serum levels. Assess for distant or muffled heart sounds by auscultation (pericardial effusion, tamponade).

PATIENT/FAMILY TEACHING:

Maximum B/P response occurs in 3–7 days. Reversible growth of fine body hair may begin 3–6 wks after treatment is initiated. When used topically for stimulation of hair growth, treatment must continue on a permanent basis—cessation of treatment will begin reversal of new hair growth.

mirtazapine

murr-**taz**-ah-peen
(Remeron, Remeron Soltab)
Do not confuse with Premarin.

▶CLASSIFICATION

PHARMACOTHERAPEUTIC:
Tetracyclic compound. **CLINI-CAL:** Antidepressant (see p. 36C).

ACTION/*THERAPEUTIC EFFECT*

Acts as antagonist at presynaptic alpha$_2$-adrenergic receptors, increasing both norepinephrine and serotonin neurotransmission. *Produces antidepressant effect.* Prominent sedative effects, low anticholinergic activity.

PHARMACOKINETICS

Rapidly, completely absorbed following PO administration (not affected by food). Protein binding: 85%. Metabolized in liver. Primarily excreted in urine. Unknown if removed by hemodialysis. Half-life: 20–40 hrs (longer in males than females [37 hrs vs. 26 hrs]).

USES

Treatment of various forms of depression, exhibited as persistent, prominent dysphoria (occurring nearly every day for at least 2 wks) manifested by 4 of 8 symptoms: appetite change, sleep pattern change, increased fatigue, impaired concentration, feelings of guilt or worthlessness, loss of interest in usual activities, psychomotor agitation or retardation, suicidal tendencies.

PRECAUTIONS

CONTRAINDICATIONS: Within 14 days of MAO inhibitor ingestion. **CAUTIONS:** History of MI, angina, hypotensive episodes, history of mania/hypomania, hepatic/renal function impairment, elderly.

▷**LIFESPAN CONSIDERATIONS:**
Pregnancy/Lactation: Unknown if distributed in breast milk. **Pregnancy Category C. Children:** Safety and efficacy not established. **Elderly:** Age-related renal impairment may require cautious use.

INTERACTIONS

DRUG: Alcohol, diazepam may increase impairment of cognition, motor skills. **MAO inhibitors** may increase risk of hypertensive crisis, severe convulsions. **HERBAL:** None known. **FOOD:** None known. **LAB VALUES:** May increase cholesterol, triglycerides, SGOT (ALT), SGPT (AST).

AVAILABILITY (Rx)

TABLETS: 15 mg, 30 mg. **ORAL DISINTEGRATING TABLETS.**

ADMINISTRATION/HANDLING

PO:

• Give without regard to food. • May crush or break scored tablets.

INDICATIONS/ROUTES/DOSAGE

Note: At least 14 days should elapse between discontinuing MAO inhibitors and instituting mirtazapine therapy. Also, allow at least 14 days after discontinuing mirtazapine and instituting MAO inhibitor therapy.

Depression:

PO: Adults, elderly: 15 mg/day as single dose, preferably in evening prior to sleep (high sedative effect). **Range:** 15–45 mg/day. Dose adjustment should be no sooner than at 1–2 wk intervals.

SIDE EFFECTS

FREQUENT: Somnolence (54%), dry mouth (25%), increase in appetite (17%), constipation (13%), weight gain (12%). **OCCASIONAL:** Asthenia (8%), dizziness (7%), flu syndrome (5%), abnormal dreams (4%). **RARE:** Abdominal discomfort, vasodilation, paresthesia, acne, dry skin, thirst, arthralgia.

ADVERSE REACTIONS/TOXIC EFFECTS

Higher incidence of seizures than with tricyclic antidepressants (esp. in those with no previous history of seizures). High dosage may produce cardiovascular effects (severe postural hypotension, dizziness, tachycardia, palpitations, arrhythmias). Abrupt withdrawal from prolonged therapy may produce headache, malaise, nausea, vomiting, vivid dreams. Agranulocytosis occurs rarely.

NURSING IMPLICATIONS

BASELINE ASSESSMENT:

For those on long-term therapy, liver/renal function tests, blood counts should be performed periodically.

INTERVENTION/EVALUATION:

Supervise suicidal risk pt closely during early therapy (as depression lessens, energy level improves, increasing suicide potential). Assess appearance, behavior, speech pattern, level of interest, mood. Monitor B/P, pulse for hypotension, arrhythmias.

PATIENT/FAMILY TEACHING:

Avoid tasks that require alertness, motor skills until response to drug is established. Change positions slowly to avoid hypotensive effect. Tolerance to sedative effects usually develops during early therapy. Do not abruptly discontinue medication. Notify physician if pregnancy is planned or if pregnancy occurs.

misoprostol

mis-oh-**pros**-toll
(Cytotec)

FIXED-COMBINATION(S)

With diclofenac, a NSAID **(Arthrotec)**
Do not confuse with Cytoxan.

▶**CLASSIFICATION**

PHARMACOTHERAPEUTIC: Prostaglandin. **CLINICAL:** Antisecretory, gastric protectant

ACTION/*THERAPEUTIC EFFECT*

Inhibits basal, nocturnal gastric acid secretion via direct action on parietal cells. *Increases production of protective gastric mucus.*

PHARMACOKINETICS

	Onset	Peak	Duration
PO	30 min	—	3–6 hrs

Rapidly absorbed from GI tract. Protein binding: 80–90%. Rapidly converted to active metabolite. Primarily excreted in urine. Unknown if removed by hemodialysis. Half-life: 20–40 min.

USES/*UNLABELED*

Prevention of NSAID-induced gastric ulcers and in those at high risk of developing gastric ulcer or gastric ulcer complication. *Treatment of duodenal or gastric ulcer, improvement of fat absorption in cystic fibrosis pts.*

PRECAUTIONS

CONTRAINDICATIONS: Pregnancy (produces uterine contractions). ***CAUTIONS:*** Impaired renal function.

▷***LIFESPAN CONSIDERATIONS:***
Pregnancy/Lactation: Unknown whether distributed in breast milk. Produces uterine contractions, uterine bleeding, expulsion of products of conception (abortifacient property). **Pregnancy Category X. Children:** Safety and efficacy not established. **Elderly:** No age-related precautions noted.

INTERACTIONS

DRUG: None significant. ***HERBAL:*** None known. ***FOOD:*** None known. ***LAB VALUES:*** None significant.

AVAILABILITY (Rx)

TABLETS: 100 mcg, 200 mcg.

ADMINISTRATION/HANDLING

PO:

• Give with or after meals (minimizes diarrhea).

INDICATIONS/ROUTES/DOSAGE

Prevention of NSAID-induced gastric ulcer:

PO: Adults: 200 mcg 4 times/day with food (last dose at bedtime). Continue for duration of NSAID therapy. May reduce dosage to 100 mcg if 200 mcg dose is not tolerable. **Elderly:** 100–200 mcg 4 times/day with food.

SIDE EFFECTS

FREQUENT (20–40%): Abdominal pain, diarrhea. ***OCCASIONAL*** (2–3%): Nausea, flatulence, dyspepsia, headache. ***RARE*** (1%): Vomiting, constipation.

ADVERSE REACTIONS/TOXIC EFFECTS

Overdosage may produce sedation, tremor, convulsions, dyspnea, palpitations, hypotension, bradycardia.

NURSING IMPLICATIONS

BASELINE ASSESSMENT:

Question for possibility of pregnancy before initiating therapy (Pregnancy Category X).

PATIENT/FAMILY TEACHING:

Avoid magnesium-containing antacids (minimizes potential for diarrhea). Women of childbearing potential must not be pregnant before or during medication therapy (may result in hospitalization, surgery, infertility, fetal death).

M

mitomycin

my-toe-**my**-sin
(Mutamycin)

▶**CLASSIFICATION**

PHARMACOTHERAPEUTIC: Antibiotic. ***CLINICAL:*** Antineoplastic (see p. 72C)

ACTION/*THERAPEUTIC EFFECT*

Causes cross-linking of DNA strands, inhibiting DNA synthesis and, to a lesser extent, RNA and protein synthesis, *preventing cellular division.* Cell cycle-phase nonspecific (most active in G and S phase of cell division).

PHARMACOKINETICS

Widely distributed. Does not cross blood-brain barrier. Primarily me-

---

tabolized in liver and excreted in urine. Half-life: 50 min.

Treatment of disseminated adenocarcinoma of stomach, pancreas. *Treatment of colorectal, breast, head/neck, bladder, lung, biliary, cervical carcinoma, chronic myelocytic leukemia.*

PRECAUTIONS

CONTRAINDICATIONS: Platelet count less than 75,000/mm^3, WBC less than 3,000/mm^3, serum creatinine greater than 1.7 mg/dl, coagulation disorders/bleeding tendencies, serious infection.

▷***LIFESPAN CONSIDERATIONS:*** **Pregnancy/Lactation:** If possible, avoid use during pregnancy, esp. first trimester. Breast feeding not recommended. Safety in pregnancy not established. **Children:** No age-related precautions noted. **Elderly:** Age-related renal impairment may require cautious use.

INTERACTIONS

DRUG: **Bone marrow depressants** may increase bone marrow depression. **Live virus vaccines** may potentiate virus replication, increase vaccine side effects, decrease pt's antibody response to vaccine. ***HERBAL:*** None known. ***FOOD:*** None known. ***LAB VALUES:*** May increase BUN, creatinine.

AVAILABILITY (Rx)

POWDER FOR INJECTION: 5 mg, 20 mg, 40 mg.

ADMINISTRATION/HANDLING

Note: May be carcinogenic, mutagenic, or teratogenic. Handle with extreme care during preparation/administration. Give IV via IV catheter, IV infusion. Extremely irritating to vein. May produce pain on injection, with induration, thrombophlebitis, paresthesia.

IV 🏥

Storage:
• Use only clear, blue-gray solutions. • Concentration of 0.5 mg/ml is stable for 7 days at room temperature or 2 wks if refrigerated. Further diluted solution with D_5W is stable for 3 hrs, 24 hrs if diluted with 0.9% NaCl.

Reconstitution:
• Reconstitute 5 mg vial with 10 ml Sterile Water for Injection (40 ml for 20 mg vial) to provide solution containing 0.5 mg/ml. • Do not shake vial to dissolve. Allow vial to stand at room temperature until complete dissolution occurs. • For IV infusion, further dilute with 50–100 ml D_5W or 0.9% NaCl.

Rate of administration:
• Give IV push given over 5–10 min. • Give IV through tubing of functional IV catheter or running IV infusion. • Extravasation may produce cellulitis, ulceration, tissue sloughing. Terminate immediately, inject ordered antidote. Apply ice intermittently for up to 72 hrs; keep area elevated.

IV INCOMPATIBILITY ⊘

Do not mix with any other medications.

IV COMPATIBILITIES

Cyclophosphamide (Cytoxan), dexamethasone (Decadron), doxorubicin (Adriamycin), granisetron (Kytril), ondansetron (Zofran).

INDICATIONS/ROUTES/DOSAGE

Note: Dosage individualized based on clinical response, tolerance to adverse effects. When used in combination therapy, consult specific protocols for optimum dosage, sequence of drug administration.

Initial dosage:

IV: **Adults, elderly:** 10–20 mg/m^2 as single dose. Repeat q6–8wks. Give additional courses only after circulating blood elements (platelets, WBC) are within acceptable levels.

SIDE EFFECTS

FREQUENT (>10%): Fever, anorexia, nausea, vomiting. **OCCASIONAL** (2–10%): Stomatitis, numbness of fingers/toes, purple color bands on nails, skin rash, alopecia, unusual tiredness. **RARE** (<1%): Thrombophlebitis, cellulitis, extravasation.

ADVERSE REACTIONS/TOXIC EFFECTS

Marked bone marrow depression results in hematologic toxicity manifested as leukopenia, thrombocytopenia and, to a lesser extent, anemia (generally occurs within 2–4 wks after initial therapy). Renal toxicity may be evidenced by rise in BUN and/or serum creatinine. Pulmonary toxicity manifested as dyspnea, cough, hemoptysis, pneumonia. Long-term therapy may produce hemolytic-uremic syndrome (HUS), characterized by hemolytic anemia, thrombocytopenia, renal failure, hypertension.

NURSING IMPLICATIONS

BASELINE ASSESSMENT:

Obtain WBC, platelet, differential, prothrombin, bleeding time, hemoglobin before and periodically during therapy. Antiemetics before and during therapy may alleviate nausea/vomiting.

INTERVENTION/EVALUATION:

Monitor hematologic status, BUN, serum creatinine, kidney function studies. Assess IV site for phlebitis, extravasation. Monitor for hematologic toxicity (fever, sore throat, signs of local infection, easy bruising, unusual bleeding from any site), symptoms of anemia (excessive tiredness, weakness). Assess for renal toxicity (foul odor, rise in BUN, serum creatinine).

PATIENT/FAMILY TEACHING:

Maintain fastidious oral hygiene. Immediately report any stinging, burning at injection site. Do not have immunizations without physician's approval (drug lowers body's resistance). Avoid contact with those who have recently received live virus vaccine. Promptly report fever, sore throat, signs of local infection, easy bruising, unusual bleeding from any site, burning on urination, increased frequency. Alopecia is reversible, but new hair growth may have different color or texture. Contact physician if nausea/vomiting continues at home.

M

mitotane

(Lysodren)

See Classification section under: Antineoplastics (p. 73C)

mitoxantrone

my-toe-**zan**-trone
(Novantrone)

►CLASSIFICATION

PHARMACOTHERAPEUTIC:
Anthracenedione. **CLINICAL:**
Antineoplastic (see p. 73C)

ACTION/*THERAPEUTIC EFFECT*

Inhibits DNA synthesis, *resulting in cell death.* Cell cycle-phase nonspecific. Most active in late S phase of cell division.

PHARMACOKINETICS

Protein binding: 78%. Widely distributed. Metabolized in liver. Primarily eliminated in feces via biliary system. Not removed by hemodialysis. Half-life: 2.3–13 days.

USES/*UNLABELED*

Treatment of acute, nonlymphocytic leukemia (monocytic, myelogenous, promyelocytic), late-stage hormone-resistant prostate cancer. Treatment of multiple sclerosis. *Treatment of breast, liver carcinoma, non-Hodgkin's lymphoma.*

PRECAUTIONS

CONTRAINDICATIONS: None significant. **CAUTIONS:** None significant.

▷**LIFESPAN CONSIDERATIONS:**
Pregnancy/Lactation: If possible, avoid use during pregnancy, esp. first trimester. May cause fetal harm. Breast feeding not recommended. **Pregnancy Category D. Children:** Safety and efficacy not established. **Elderly:** No age-related precautions noted.

INTERACTIONS

DRUG: May decrease effect of **antigout medications. Bone marrow depressants** may increase bone marrow depression. **Live virus vaccines** may potentiate virus replication, increase vaccine side effects, decrease pt's antibody response to vaccine. **HERBAL:** None known. **FOOD:** None known. **LAB VALUES:** May increase SGOT (AST), SGPT (ALT), bilirubin, uric acid.

AVAILABILITY (Rx)

INJECTION: 2 mg/ml.

ADMINISTRATION/HANDLING

Note: May be carcinogenic, mutagenic, or teratogenic. Handle with extreme care during preparation/administration. Give by IV injection, IV infusion. Must dilute before administration.

IV 🎢

Storage:
• Store vials at room temperature.

Reconstitution:
• Dilute with at least 50 ml D_5W or 0.9% NaCl.

Rate of administration:
• Infuse into freely running IV over at least 3 min. • IV infusion given over 15–30 min. • Do not mix with heparin in same infusion; may cause precipitate.

IV INCOMPATIBILITIES ⊘

Paclitaxel (Taxol), piperacillin/tazobactam (Zosyn).

IV COMPATIBILITIES

Allopurinol (Aloprim), etoposide (VP-16, Vepesid), granisetron (Kytril), ondansetron (Zofran).

INDICATIONS/ROUTES/DOSAGE
Leukemias:

IV: Adults, elderly, children >12 yrs: 12 mg/m²/day once daily for 2–3 days. *Acute leukemia in relapse:* 8–12 mg/m²/day once daily for 4–5 days. *ANLL:*10 mg/m²/day once daily for 3–5 days. **Children**

<2 yrs: 0.4 mg/kg/day once daily for 3–5 days.

Solid tumors:

IV: **Adults, elderly:** 12–14 mg/m² once q3–4wks. **Children:** 18–20 mg/m² once q3–4wks.

Multiple sclerosis:

IV: **Adults, elderly:** 12 mg/m²/dose q3mos.

SIDE EFFECTS

FREQUENT (>10%): Nausea, vomiting, diarrhea, cough, headache, stomatitis, abdominal discomfort, fever, alopecia. ***OCCASIONAL*** (4–9%): Easy bruising, fungal infection, conjunctivitis, urinary tract infection. ***RARE*** (3%): Arrhythmias.

ADVERSE REACTIONS/TOXIC EFFECTS

Bone marrow suppression may be severe, resulting in GI bleeding, sepsis, pneumonia. Renal failure, seizures, jaundice, CHF may occur.

NURSING IMPLICATIONS

BASELINE ASSESSMENT:

Offer emotional support. Establish baseline for CBC, temperature, rate and quality of pulse, lung status.

INTERVENTION/EVALUATION:

Monitor hematologic status, pulmonary function studies, hepatic and renal function tests. Monitor for stomatitis (burning/erythema of oral mucosa, ulceration, sore throat, difficulty swallowing), fever, signs of local infection, easy bruising, or unusual bleeding from any site.

PATIENT/FAMILY TEACHING:

Urine will appear blue/green 24 hrs after administration. Blue tint to sclera may also appear. Maintain adequate daily fluid intake (may protect against renal impairment). Do not have immunizations without physician's approval (drug lowers body's resistance). Avoid crowds, those with infection.

mivacurium chloride

(Mivacron)

See Classification section under: Neuromuscular blocking agents (p. 102C)

modafinil

mode-ah-**feen**-awl
(Provigil)

►CLASSIFICATION

PHARMACOTHERAPEUTIC: Alpha₁ agonist. ***CLINICAL:*** Wakefulness-promoting agent

ACTION/THERAPEUTIC EFFECT

Binds to dopamine reuptake carrier site, increasing alpha activity, decreasing delta, theta, and beta activity, *reducing the number of sleepiness episodes and duration of daytime total sleep time.*

PHARMACOKINETICS

Well absorbed. Protein binding: 60%. Widely distributed. Metabolized in lever. Excreted in the kidney. Unknown if removed by hemodialysis. Half-life: 8–10 hrs.

USES/UNLABELED

Treatment of excessive daytime

sleepiness associated with narcolepsy and other sleep disorders. *Depression.*

PRECAUTIONS

CONTRAINDICATIONS: None significant. ***CAUTIONS:*** None significant.

▷***LIFESPAN CONSIDERATIONS:*** **Pregnancy/Lactation:** Unknown if excreted in breast milk. Use caution if given to pregnant women. **Children:** Safety and efficacy in those <16 yrs of age not established. **Elderly:** Age-related renal or liver impairment in the elderly may require decreased dosage.

INTERACTIONS

DRUG: May increase effect of **warfarin.** ***HERBAL:*** None known. ***FOOD:*** None known. ***LAB VALUES:*** None significant.

AVAILABILITY (Rx)

TABLETS: 100 mg, 200 mg.

ADMINISTRATION/HANDLING

• Give without regard to meals.

INDICATIONS/ROUTES/DOSAGE

Narcolepsy, sleep disorders:
PO: Adults, elderly: 200–400 mg/day.

SIDE EFFECTS

Appears dose-related: Dry mouth, dry eyes, nausea, poor sleep, sweating, headache, dizziness, hot flushes, hypersalivation, anorexia, anxiety, bad temper, choking, dysphoria/euphoria, increased B/P, fatigue, weight gain, sexual hyperactivity.

ADVERSE REACTIONS/TOXIC EFFECTS

Overdosage may produce tachycardia, excitation, insomnia.

BASELINE ASSESSMENT:

Obtain baseline evidence of narcolepsy or other sleep disorders, including pattern, environmental situations, lengths of time of sleep episodes. Question for sudden loss of muscle tone (cataplexy) precipitated by strong emotion such as laughter prior to sleep episode. Assess frequency and severity of sleep episodes prior to drug therapy.

INTERVENTION/EVALUATION

Monitor sleep pattern, evidence of restlessness during sleep, length of insomnia episodes during night. Assess for dizziness, anxiety; initiate fall precautions. Sugarless gum, sips of tepid water may relieve dry mouth.

PATIENT/FAMILY TEACHING:

Avoid tasks that require alertness, motor skills until response to drug is established.

moexipril hydrochloride

mow-**ex**-ih-prill
(Univasc)

FIXED-COMBINATION(S)

With hydrochlorothiazide, a diuretic **(Uniretic)**

▶CLASSIFICATION

PHARMACOTHERAPEUTIC: Angiotensin-converting enzyme (ACE) inhibitor. ***CLINICAL:*** Antihypertensive (see p. 6C)

ACTION/*THERAPEUTIC EFFECT*

Suppresses renin-angiotensin-aldosterone system (prevents conversion of angiotensin I to angiotensin II, a potent vasoconstrictor; may also inhibit angiotensin II at local vascular and renal sites). *Reduces peripheral arterial resistance, B/P.*

PHARMACOKINETICS

	Onset	Peak	Duration
PO	1 hr	3–6 hrs	24 hrs

Incompletely absorbed from GI tract (food decreases absorption). Rapidly converted to active metabolite. Protein binding: 50%. Primarily recovered in feces, partially excreted in urine. Unknown if removed by dialysis. Half-life: 1 hr (metabolite 2–9 hrs).

USES

Treatment of hypertension. Used alone or in combination with thiazide diuretics.

PRECAUTIONS

CONTRAINDICATIONS: History of angioedema with previous treatment with ACE inhibitors. ***CAUTIONS:*** Renal impairment, those with sodium depletion or on diuretic therapy, dialysis, hypovolemia, coronary or cerebrovascular insufficiency, hyperkalemia, aortic stenosis, ischemic heart disease, angina, severe CHF, cerebrovascular disease.

▷*LIFESPAN CONSIDERATIONS:*
Pregnancy/Lactation: Crosses placenta; unknown if distributed in breast milk. **Pregnancy Category C:** First trimester. **Pregnancy Category D:** Second and third trimesters. Has caused fetal/neonatal mortality, morbidity. **Children:** Safety and efficacy not established. **Elderly:** No age-related precautions noted.

INTERACTIONS

DRUG: **Alcohol, diuretics, hypotensive agents** may increase effects. **NSAIDs** may decrease effect. **Potassium-sparing diuretics, potassium supplements** may cause hyperkalemia. May increase **lithium** concentration, toxicity. ***HERBAL:*** None known. ***FOOD:*** None known. ***LAB VALUES:*** May increase potassium, SGOT (AST), SGPT (ALT), alkaline phosphatase, bilirubin, BUN, creatinine. May decrease sodium. May cause positive ANA titer.

AVAILABILITY (Rx)

TABLETS: 7.5 mg, 15 mg.

ADMINISTRATION/HANDLING

PO:
• Give 1 hr before meals. • Tablets may be crushed.

INDICATIONS/ROUTES/DOSAGE

Hypertension (used alone):

PO: **Adults, elderly:** Initially, 7.5 mg once daily 1 hr before meals. Adjust according to B/P effect. **Maintenance:** 7.5–30 mg/daily in 1–2 divided doses 1 hr before meals.

Hypertension (concurrent diuretic therapy):

Note: To reduce risk of hypotension, discontinue diuretic 2–3 days before initiating moexipril therapy. If B/P not controlled, resume diuretic. If diuretic cannot be discontinued, give initial dose of 3.75 mg moexipril.

Renal function impairment:

PO: **Adults, elderly:** 3.75 mg once daily in pts with creatinine clearance of 40 ml/min/1.73m^2. **Maximum:** May titrate up to 15 mg/day.

M

SIDE EFFECTS

OCCASIONAL: Cough, headache (6%), dizziness (4%), nausea, fatigue (3%). **RARE:** Flushing, rash, myalgia, nausea, vomiting.

ADVERSE REACTIONS/TOXIC EFFECTS

Excessive hypotension ("first-dose syncope") may occur in those with CHF, severely salt/volume depleted. Angioedema (swelling of face/lips), hyperkalemia occur rarely. Agranulocytosis, neutropenia may be noted in those with impaired renal function or collagen vascular disease (systemic lupus erythematosus, scleroderma). Nephrotic syndrome may be noted in those with history of renal disease.

NURSING IMPLICATIONS

BASELINE ASSESSMENT:

Obtain B/P and apical pulse immediately before each dose, in addition to regular monitoring (be alert to fluctuations). If excessive reduction in B/P occurs, place pt in supine position, feet slightly elevated. Renal function tests should be performed before therapy begins. In those with renal impairment, autoimmune disease, or taking drugs that affect leukocytes or immune response, CBC and differential count should be performed before therapy begins and q2wks for 3 mos, then periodically thereafter.

INTERVENTION/EVALUATION:

Monitor B/P, WBC count, serum potassium. Monitor for cough, question for headache. Assist with ambulation if dizziness occurs.

PATIENT/FAMILY TEACHING:

To reduce hypotensive effect, rise slowly from lying to sitting position and permit legs to dangle from bed momentarily before standing. Full therapeutic effect may take 2–4 wks. Report any sign of infection (sore throat, fever), swelling of hands or feet or face, chest pain, difficulty breathing or swallowing. Skipping doses or voluntarily discontinuing drug may produce severe, rebound hypertension. Do not take cold preparations, nasal decongestants. Restrict sodium and alcohol as ordered.

molindone hydrochloride

(Moban)

See Classification section under: Antipsychotics

mometasone

(Elocon)

See Classification section under: Corticosteroids: topical (p. 82C)

montelukast

mon-**tee**-leu-cast
(Singulair)

▶CLASSIFICATION

PHARMACOTHERAPEUTIC: Leukotriene receptor inhibitor. **CLINICAL:** Antiasthmatic (see p. 64C)

ACTION/*THERAPEUTIC EFFECT*

Inhibits airway edema, smooth muscle contraction, altered cellular activity associated with the inflammatory process, *relieving signs and symptoms of bronchial asthma.*

PHARMACOKINETICS

	Onset	Peak	Duration
PO			
	—	—	24 hrs
PO, chewable			
	—	—	24 hrs

Rapidly absorbed from GI tract. Protein binding: 99%. Extensively metabolized in the liver. Excreted almost exclusively in the feces. Half-life: 2.7–5.5 hrs. Half-life slightly longer in the elderly.

USES

Prophylaxis and chronic treatment of asthma. Not for use in reversal of bronchospasm in acute asthma attacks, status asthmaticus, exercise-induced bronchospasm.

PRECAUTIONS

CONTRAINDICATIONS: None significant. ***CAUTIONS:*** Systemic corticosteroid treatment reduction during montelukast therapy, impaired liver function.
▷*LIFESPAN CONSIDERATIONS:*
Pregnancy/Lactation: Unknown if excreted in breast milk. Use during pregnancy only if necessary. **Pregnancy Category B. Children/Elderly:** No age-related precautions noted in those >6 yrs of age or the elderly.

INTERACTIONS

DRUG: **Phenobarbital, rifampin** may reduce duration of action of montelukast. ***HERBAL:*** None known. ***FOOD:*** None known.

LAB VALUES: May increase SGOT (AST), SGPT (ALT).

AVAILABILITY (Rx)

TABLETS: 10 mg. ***TABLETS (chewable):*** 4 mg, 5 mg.

ADMINISTRATION/HANDLING

PO:

• Administer in the evening without regard to food ingestion.

INDICATIONS/ROUTES/DOSAGE

Bronchial asthma:

PO: **Adults, elderly, adolescents >15 yrs:** One 10 mg tablet daily, taken in the evening. **Children 6–14 yrs:** One 5 mg chewable tablet daily, taken in the evening. **Children 2–5 yrs:** One 4 mg chewable tablet daily, taken in the evening.

SIDE EFFECTS

Adults, adolescents >15 yrs: ***FREQUENT*** (18%): Headache. ***OCCASIONAL*** (4%): Influenza. ***RARE*** (2–3%): Abdominal pain, cough, dyspepsia, dizziness, fatigue, dental pain. **Children 6–14 yrs: *RARE*** (< 2%): Diarrhea, laryngitis, pharyngitis, nausea, otitis media, sinusitis, viral infection.

ADVERSE REACTIONS/TOXIC EFFECTS

None significant.

NURSING IMPLICATIONS

BASELINE ASSESSMENT:

Chewable tablet contains phenylalanine (a component of aspartame); parents of phenylketonuric pts should be so informed. Montelukast should not be abruptly substituted for inhaled or oral corticosteroids.

M

INTERVENTION/EVALUATION:

Monitor rate, depth, rhythm, type of respirations, quality and rate of pulse. Assess lung sounds for rhonchi, wheezing, rales. Observe lips, fingernails for blue or dusky color in light-skinned pts, gray in dark-skinned pts.

PATIENT/FAMILY TEACHING:

Increase fluid intake (decreases lung secretion viscosity). Take as prescribed, even during symptom-free periods as well as during worsening asthma. Do not alter/stop other asthma medications. Drug is not for the treatment of acute asthma attacks. Pts sensitive to aspirin should avoid aspirin, NSAIDs while taking montelukast.

moricizine hydrochloride

(Ethmozine)

See Classification section under: Antiarrhythmics (p. 13C)

morphine sulfate

(Astramorph, Duramorph, Kadian, Kadian MSIR✦, M.O.S.✦, MS Contin, MSIR, Oramorph✦, RMS, Roxanol, Roxanol-T)

Do not confuse with hydromorphone, Roxicet.

▶CLASSIFICATION

PHARMACOTHERAPEUTIC: Narcotic agonist. *CLINICAL:* Opiate analgesic **(Schedule II)** (see p. 116C)

ACTION/*THERAPEUTIC EFFECT*

Binds with opioid receptors within CNS, *altering processes affecting pain perception, emotional response to pain. Decreases intestinal motility* by local, central actions.

PHARMACOKINETICS

Onset	Peak	Duration
PO		
Variable	60–120 min	4–5 hrs
Extended-release		
—	60–120 min	8–12 hrs
IM		
5–30 min	30–60 min	3–7 hrs
IV		
Rapid	20 min	4–5 hrs
Rectal		
20–60 min	—	4–5 hrs
Epidural		
15–60 min	—	16–24 hrs
Intrathecal		
15–60 min	—	16–24 hrs

Variably absorbed from GI tract. Readily absorbed after SubQ, IM administration. Protein binding: 20–35%. Widely distributed. Metabolized in liver. Primarily excreted in urine. Removed by hemodialysis. Half-life: 2–3 hrs.

USES

Relief of severe, acute, chronic pain, preop sedation, anesthesia supplement, analgesia during labor. Drug of choice for pain due to myocardial infarction, dyspnea from pulmonary edema not resulting from chemical respiratory irritant.

PRECAUTIONS

CONTRAINDICATIONS: Postop biliary tract surgery, surgical anastomosis. *EXTREME CAUTION:* CNS depression, anoxia, hypercapnia, respiratory depression, seizures, acute alcoholism, shock, untreated myxedema, respiratory dysfunction. **CAUTIONS:** Toxic psychoses, increased intracranial pressure, impaired hepatic function, acute abdominal conditions, hypothyroidism, prostatic hypertrophy, Addison's disease, urethral stricture, COPD.

▷**LIFESPAN CONSIDERATIONS:**
Pregnancy/Lactation: Crosses placenta; distributed in breast milk. May prolong labor if administered in latent phase of first stage of labor or before cervical dilation of 4–5 cm has occurred. Respiratory depression may occur in neonate if mother received opiates during labor. Regular use of opiates during pregnancy may produce withdrawal symptoms in neonate (irritability, excessive crying, tremors, hyperactive reflexes, fever, vomiting, diarrhea, yawning, sneezing, seizures). **Pregnancy Category B** (Category D if used for prolonged periods or in high doses at term). **Children:** Paradoxical excitement may occur; those <2 yrs of age more susceptible to respiratory depressant effects. **Elderly:** Paradoxical excitement may occur; age-related renal impairment may increase risk of urinary retention.

INTERACTIONS

DRUG: Alcohol, CNS depressants may increase CNS or respiratory depression, hypotension. **MAO inhibitors** may produce severe, fatal reaction (reduce dose $\frac{1}{4}$ usual dose). **HERBAL:** None known. **FOOD:** None known. **LAB VALUES:** May increase amylase, lipase.

AVAILABILITY (Rx)

CAPSULES (MSIR): 15 mg, 30 mg. **CAPSULES (sustained-release): (Kadian):** 20 mg, 30 mg, 50 mg, 60 mg, 100 mg. **SOLUTION FOR INJECTION:** 0.5 mg/ml, 1 mg/ml, 2 mg/ml, 4 mg/ml, 5 mg/ml, 8 mg/ml, 10 mg/ml, 15 mg/ml, 25 mg/ml, 50 mg/ml. **(Preservative-free):** 0.5 mg/ml, 1 mg/ml, 10 mg/ml, 25 mg/ml, 50 mg/ml. **EPIDURAL/INTRATHECAL VIA INFUSION DEVICE:** (Infumorph): 10 mg/ml, 25 mg/ml. **EPIDURAL, INTRATHECAL, IV INFUSION:** (Astramorph, Duramorph): 0.5 mg/ml, 1 mg/ml. **IV INFUSION (via PCA):** 1 mg/ml, 5 mg/ml. **ORAL SOLUTION:** 10 mg/5 ml, 20 mg/5 ml, 20 mg/ml, 100 mg/5 mg. **SUPPOSITORY (RMS):** 5 mg, 10 mg, 20 mg, 30 mg. **TABLETS (MSIR):** 15 mg/30 mg. **TABLETS (extended-release):** 15 mg, 30 mg, 60 mg, 100 mg, 200 mg.

ADMINISTRATION/HANDLING

Note: Give by IM injection if repeated doses necessary (repeated SubQ may produce local tissue irritation, induration). May also be given slow IV injection or IV infusion.

M

PO:

• Mix liquid form with fruit juice to improve taste. • Do not crush or break extended-release capsule. • **Kadian**: May mix with applesauce immediately prior to administration.

SubQ/IM:

• Administer slowly, rotating injection sites. • Pts with circulatory impairment experience higher risk of overdosage due to delayed absorption of repeated administration.

IV ▥

Storage:
• Store at room temperature.

Reconstitution:
• May give undiluted. • For IV in-

jection, may dilute 2.5–15 mg morphine in 4–5 ml Sterile Water for Injection. • For continuous IV infusion, dilute to concentration of 0.1–1 mg/ml in D_5W and give through controlled infusion device.

Rate of administration:

• Always administer very slowly, over 4–5 min. Rapid IV increases risk of severe adverse reactions (apnea, chest wall rigidity, peripheral circulatory collapse, cardiac arrest, anaphylactoid effects).

Rectal:

• If suppository is too soft, chill for 30 min in refrigerator or run cold water over foil wrapper. • Moisten suppository with cold water before inserting well up into rectum.

IV INCOMPATIBILITIES ⃠

Amphotericin B complex (Abelcet, Ambisome, Amphotec), cefepime (Maxipime), doxorubicin liposome (Doxil), thiopental.

IV COMPATIBILITIES

Amiodarone (Cordarone), bumetanide (Bumex), bupivacaine (Marcaine, Sensorcaine), diltiazem (Cardizem), dobutamine (Dobutrex), dopamine (Intropin), heparin, lidocaine, lorazepam (Ativan), magnesium, midazolam (Versed), milrinone (Primacor), nitroglycerin, potassium, propofol (Diprivan).

INDICATIONS/ROUTES/DOSAGE

Note: Reduce dosage in elderly/debilitated, those on concurrent CNS depressants.

Pain:

***PO:* Adults, elderly: (prompt-release):** 10–30 mg q4h as needed. **Children:** 0.2–0.5 mg/kg/dose q4–6h. **(Sustained-release):** 15–30 mg q8–12h. **Children:** 0.3–0.6 mg/kg/dose q12h.

***IV/IM/SuBQ:* Adults, elderly:** 2.5–20 mg/dose q2–6h. **Children:** 0.1–0.2 mg/kg/dose q2–4h. **Maximum:** 15 mg/dose.

***IV CONTINUOUS INFUSION:* Adults, elderly:** 0.8–10 mg/hr. **Range:** Up to 80 mg/hr. **Children:** 0.025–2.6 mg/kg/hr.

***EPIDURAL:* Adults, elderly:** Initially, 5 mg. May give 1–2 mg in 1 hr if no relief. **Maximum:** 10 mg/24 hrs.

***INTRATHECAL:* Adults, elderly:** 1/10 epidural dose: 0.2–1 mg/dose.

***PCA:* Loading dose:** 5–10 mg; **Intermittent bolus:** 0.5–3 mg. **Lockout interval:** 5–12 min. **Continuous infusion:** 1–10 mg/hr. **(4-hr limit):** 20–30 mg..

SIDE EFFECTS

Note: Effects dependent on dosage amount, route of administration. Ambulatory pts, those not in severe pain may experience dizziness, nausea, vomiting, hypotension more frequently than those in supine position or who have severe pain.

FREQUENT: Sedation, decreased B/P, increased sweating, flushed face, constipation, dizziness, drowsiness, nausea, vomiting. ***OCCASIONAL:*** Allergic reaction (rash, itching), difficulty breathing, confusion, pounding heartbeat, tremors, decreased urination, stomach cramps, vision changes, dry mouth, headache, decreased appetite, pain/burning at injection site. ***RARE:*** Paralytic ileus.

ADVERSE REACTIONS/TOXIC EFFECTS

Overdosage results in respiratory depression, skeletal muscle flaccidity, cold clammy skin, cyanosis, extreme somnolence progressing to convulsions, stupor, coma. Tolerance to analgesic effect, physical dependence may occur with repeated use. Prolonged duration of action, cumulative effect may occur in those with impaired hepatic, renal function.

dependence may occur with prolonged use of high doses.

NURSING IMPLICATIONS

BASELINE ASSESSMENT:

Pt should be in a recumbent position before drug is given by parenteral route. Assess onset, type, location, and duration of pain. Obtain vital signs before giving medication. If respirations are 12/min or lower (20/min or lower in children), withhold medication, contact physician. Effect of medication is reduced if full pain recurs before next dose.

INTERVENTION/EVALUATION:

Monitor vital signs 5–10 min after IV administration, 15–30 min after SubQ or IM. Be alert for decreased respirations or B/P. Check for adequate voiding; palpate bladder if output questionable. Monitor stools; avoid constipation. Initiate deep breathing and coughing exercises, particularly in those with impaired pulmonary function. Assess for clinical improvement and record onset of pain relief. Consult physician if pain relief is not adequate.

PATIENT/FAMILY TEACHING:

Discomfort may occur with injection. Change positions slowly to avoid orthostatic hypotension. Avoid tasks that require alertness, motor skills until response to drug is established. Avoid alcohol and CNS depressants. Tolerance/

moxifloxacin hydrochloride

mox-ih-**flocks**-ah-sin
(Avelox, Avelox IV)
Do not confuse with Avonex.

▶CLASSIFICATION

PHARMACOTHERAPEUTIC:
Fluoroquinolone. **CLINICAL:**
Antibacterial (see p. 22C)

ACTION/*THERAPEUTIC EFFECT*

Inhibits two enzymes, topoisomerase II and IV, in susceptible microorganisms, *interfering with bacterial DNA replication.* Prevents or delays resistance emergence. Bactericidal.

PHARMACOKINETICS

Well absorbed from GI tract following PO administration. Protein binding: 50%. Widely distributed throughout body with tissue concentration often exceeding plasma concentration. Metabolized in liver. Primarily excreted in urine with a lesser amount in feces. Half-life: 10.7–13.3 hrs.

USES

Treatment of acute bacterial exacerbation of chronic bronchitis, acute bacterial sinusitis, community-acquired pneumonia. Uncomplicated skin and skin structure infections.

PRECAUTIONS

CONTRAINDICATIONS: Hypersensitivity to quinolones. **CAUTIONS:** Renal/hepatic impairment, CNS disorders, cerebral

M

arthrosclerosis, seizures, those with prolonged QT interval, uncorrected hypokalemia, those receiving quinidine, procainamide, amiodarone, sotalol.

▷*LIFESPAN CONSIDERATIONS:*
Pregnancy/Lactation: May be distributed in breast milk. May produce teratogenic effects. **Pregnancy Category C. Children:** Safety and efficacy not established. **Elderly:** No age-related precautions noted.

INTERACTIONS

DRUG: **Antacids, iron preparations, sucralfate,** or **didanosine** chewable/buffered tablets or pediatric powder for oral solution may decrease moxifloxacin absorption. *HERBAL:* None known. *FOOD:* None significant. *LAB VALUES:* None significant.

AVAILABILITY (Rx)

TABLETS: 400 mg. *INJECTION:* 400 mg.

ADMINISTRATION/HANDLING
PO:

• Give without regard to meals. • Oral moxifloxacin should be administered 4 hrs before or 8 hrs after antacids, multivitamins, iron preparations, sucralfate, or didanosine chewable/buffered tablets or pediatric powder for oral solution.

INDICATIONS/ROUTES/DOSAGE

Note: Infuse IV over 60 min.

Acute bacterial sinusitis, community-acquired pneumonia:
IV/PO: **Adults >18 yrs, elderly:** 400 mg q24h for 10 days.

Acute bacterial exacerbation of chronic bronchitis:
IV/PO: **Adults >18 yrs, elderly:** 400 mg q24h for 5 days.

Skin/skin structure:
IV/PO: **Adults, elderly:** 400 mg once daily for 7 days.

SIDE EFFECTS

FREQUENT (6–8%): Nausea, diarrhea. *OCCASIONAL* (2–3%): Dizziness, headache, abdominal pain, vomiting. *RARE* (1%): Change in sense of taste, dyspepsia (heartburn, indigestion).

ADVERSE REACTIONS/TOXIC EFFECTS

Pseudomembranous colitis (severe abdominal pain/cramps, severe watery diarrhea, fever) may occur. Superinfection (genital-anal pruritus, ulceration or changes in oral mucosa, moderate to severe diarrhea) may occur.

NURSING IMPLICATIONS

BASELINE ASSESSMENT:

Question for history of hypersensitivity to moxifloxacin, quinolones.

INTERVENTION/EVALUATION:

Determine pattern of bowel activity. Assist with ambulation if dizziness occurs. Assess for headache, abdominal pain, vomiting, change in sense of taste, dyspepsia (heartburn, indigestion).

PATIENT/FAMILY TEACHING:

Do not skip dose; take full course of therapy. Take with 8 oz water; drink several glasses of water between meals. Moxifloxacin should not be taken at least 4 hrs before or 8 hrs after taking antacids, multivitamins, sucralfate, or Videx (didanosine chewable/buffered tablets or pediatric powder for oral solution) (reduces/destroys effectiveness).

mupirocin

mew-pie-ro-sin
(Bactroban)
Do not confuse with bacitracin.
baclofen.

▶CLASSIFICATION

PHARMACOTHERAPEUTIC:
Anti-infective. ***CLINICAL:*** Topical antibacterial

ACTION/*THERAPEUTIC EFFECT*

Inhibits bacterial protein, RNA synthesis. Less effective on DNA synthesis. **Nasal:** Eradicates nasal colonization of MRSA. *Prevents bacterial growth and replication. Bacteriostatic.*

PHARMACOKINETICS

Metabolized in skin to inactive metabolite. Transported to skin surface; removed by normal skin desquamation.

USES/*UNLABELED*

Topical treatment of impetigo, infected traumatic skin lesions. **Nasal:** Reduces spread of MRSA (methicillin-resistant *S. aureus*). *Treatment of infected eczema, folliculitis, minor bacterial skin infections.*

PRECAUTIONS

CONTRAINDICATIONS: None significant. ***CAUTIONS:*** Impaired renal function. Safety of nasal preparation not established in children <12 yrs.

▷*LIFESPAN CONSIDERATIONS:*
Pregnancy/Lactation: Unknown if present in breast milk; temporarily discontinue nursing while using mupirocin. **Pregnancy Category B. Children:** Safety and efficacy not established. **Elderly:** No information available.

INTERACTIONS

DRUG: None significant. ***HERBAL:*** None known. ***FOOD:*** None known. ***LAB VALUES:*** None significant.

AVAILABILITY (Rx)

OINTMENT: 2%. ***NASAL OINTMENT:*** 2%.

ADMINISTRATION/HANDLING
Topical:

• Gown and gloves are to be worn until 24 hrs after therapy is effective. Disease is spread by direct contact with moist discharges. • Apply small amount to affected areas. Cover affected areas with gauze dressing if desired.

INDICATIONS/ROUTES/DOSAGE
Usual topical dosage:

***TOPICAL:* Adults, elderly, children:** Apply 3 times/day (may cover with gauze).

Usual nasal dosage:

***INTRANASAL:* Adults, elderly, children:** Apply 2 times/day for 5 days.

SIDE EFFECTS

FREQUENT: Nasal (3–9%): Headache, rhinitis, upper respiratory congestion, pharyngitis, altered taste. ***OCCASIONAL: Nasal*** (2%): Burning, stinging, cough. ***Topical*** (1–2%): Pain, burning, stinging, itching. ***RARE: Nasal*** (<1%): Pruritis, diarrhea, dry mouth, epistaxis, nausea, rash. ***Topical*** (<1%): Rash, nausea, dry skin, contact dermatitis.

ADVERSE REACTIONS/TOXIC EFFECTS

Superinfection may result in bac-

M

terial or fungal infections, esp. with prolonged or repeated therapy.

NURSING IMPLICATIONS

BASELINE ASSESSMENT:

Assess skin for type and extent of lesions.

INTERVENTION/EVALUATION:

Keep neonates or pts with poor hygiene isolated. Wear gloves and gown if necessary when contact with discharges is likely; continue until 24 hrs after therapy is effective. Cleanse/dispose of articles soiled with discharge according to institutional guidelines. In event of skin reaction, stop applications, cleanse area gently, and notify physician.

PATIENT/FAMILY TEACHING:

For external use only. Avoid contact with eyes. Explain precautions to avoid spread of infection; teach how to apply medication. If skin reaction, irritation develops, notify physician. If there is no improvement in 3–5 days, pt should be reevaluated.

muromonab-CD3

meur-oh-**mon**-ab
(Orthoclone, OKT3)

►CLASSIFICATION

PHARMACOTHERAPEUTIC:
Murine monoclonal antibody.
CLINICAL: Immunosuppressant

ACTION/*THERAPEUTIC EFFECT*

Antibody (purified IgG$_2$ immune globulin) that reacts with T3 (CD3) antigen of human T-cell membranes. Blocks function of T-cells (has major role in acute renal rejection). *Reverses graft rejection.*

USES

Treatment of acute allograft rejection in renal transplant pts, steroid-resistant acute allograft rejection in cardiac, hepatic transplant pts.

PRECAUTIONS

CONTRAINDICATIONS: History of hypersensitivity to muromonab-CD3 or any murine origin product, those in fluid overload evidenced by chest x-ray or >3% weight gain within the week before initial treatment. **CAUTIONS:** Impaired hepatic, renal, cardiac function.

AVAILABILITY (Rx)

INJECTION: 1 mg/ml.

ADMINISTRATION/HANDLING

IV 🕮

Storage:
• Refrigerate ampule. • Do not shake ampule before using. • Fine translucent particles may develop; does not affect potency.

Reconstitution:
• Draw solution into syringe through 0.22 micron filter. Discard filter; use needle for IV administration.

Rate of administration:
• Administer IV push over <1 min. • Give methylprednisolone 1 mg/kg before and 100 mg hydrocortisone 30 min after dose (decreases adverse reaction to first dose).

IV INCOMPATIBILITY ⊘

Do not mix with any other medications.

INDICATIONS/ROUTES/DOSAGE

Prevention of allograft rejection:

IV: **Adults, elderly, children >30 kg:** 5 mg/day for 10–14 days. Begin when acute renal rejection is diagnosed. **Children <12 yrs:** 0.1 mg/kg/day for 10–14 days.

INTERACTIONS

DRUG: **Other immunosuppressants** may increase risk of infection or development of lymphoproliferative disorders. **Live virus vaccines** may potentiate virus replication, increase vaccine side effects, decrease pt's antibody response to vaccine. *HERBAL:* **Echinacea** may decrease effect. *FOOD:* None known. *LAB VALUES:* None significant.

SIDE EFFECTS

FREQUENT: First-dose reaction: Fever, chills, dyspnea, malaise occurs 30 min to 6 hrs after first dose (reaction markedly reduced with subsequent dosing after first 2 days of treatment). *OCCASIONAL:* Chest pain, nausea, vomiting, diarrhea, tremor.

ADVERSE REACTIONS/TOXIC EFFECTS

Cytokine release syndrome (CRS) may range from flulike illness to life-threatening shocklike reaction. Occasionally fatal hypersensitivity reactions. Severe pulmonary edema occurs in <2% of those treated with muromonab-CD3. Infection (due to immunosuppression) generally occurs within 45 days after initial treatment; cytomegalovirus occurs in 19%, herpes simplex in 27%. Severe and life-threatening infection occurs in <4.8%.

NURSING IMPLICATIONS

BASELINE ASSESSMENT:

Chest x-ray must be taken within 24 hrs of initiation of therapy and be clear of fluid. Weight should be ≤3% above minimum weight the week before treatment begins (pulmonary edema occurs where fluid overload is present before treatment). Have resuscitative drugs and equipment immediately available.

INTERVENTION/EVALUATION:

Monitor WBC, differential, platelet count, renal and hepatic function tests, and immunologic tests (plasma levels or quantitative T lymphocyte surface phenotyping) before and during therapy. If fever exceeds 100°F, antipyretics should be instituted. Monitor for fluid overload by chest x-ray and weight gain of >3% over weight before treatment began. Assess lung sounds for evidence of fluid overload. Monitor I&O. Assess stool frequency and consistency.

PATIENT/FAMILY TEACHING:

Inform pt of first-dose reaction prior to treatment; headache, tremor may occur as a response to medication. Avoid crowds, those with infections. Do not receive immunizations.

M

mycophenolate mofetil

my-koe-**phen**-oh-late
(CellCept)

▶CLASSIFICATION

PHARMACOTHERAPEUTIC: Immunologic agent. *CLINICAL:* Immunosuppressant

♣ - Canadian trade name ✳ - see also www.wbsaunders.com/SIMON/SaundersNDH

ACTION/*THERAPEUTIC EFFECT*

Inhibits inosine monophosphate dehydrogenase, an enzyme that deprives lymphocytes of nucleotides necessary for DNA and RNA synthesis. Inhibits proliferation of T- and B-lymphocytes. Suppresses immunologically mediated inflammatory response. *Prevents renal transplant rejection.*

PHARMACOKINETICS

Rapidly, extensively absorbed following PO administration (food does not alter the extent of absorption but plasma concentration decreased in presence of food). Protein binding: 97%. Completely hydrolyzed to active metabolite mycophenolic acid (MPA). Primarily excreted in urine. Not removed by hemodialysis. Half-life: 17.9 hrs.

USES

Prophylaxis of organ rejection in pts receiving allogeneic liver/renal/cardiac transplants. Should be used concurrently with cyclosporine and corticosteroids. *Prevents organ rejection in pts undergoing heart transplant.*

PRECAUTIONS

CONTRAINDICATIONS: Mycophenolic acid. ***CAUTIONS:*** Immunosuppressed pts, active, serious digestive system disease, renal function impairment.
▷***LIFESPAN CONSIDERATIONS:***
Pregnancy/Lactation: Unknown if drug crosses placenta or is distributed in breast milk. Avoid nursing. **Pregnancy Category C. Children:** Safety and efficacy not established. **Elderly:** No information available.

INTERACTIONS

DRUG: **Acyclovir, ganciclovir** competes with MPA (active metabolite for renal excretion); may increase plasma concentration of each in presence of renal impairment. **Antacids (magnesium, aluminum-containing), cholestyramine** may decrease absorption. **Other immunosuppressants** may increase risk of infection of development of lymphomas. **Live virus vaccines** may potentiate virus replication, increase vaccine side effects, decrease pt's antibody response to vaccine. **Probenecid** may increase concentration. ***HERBAL:*** **Echinacea** may decrease effect. ***FOOD:*** None known. ***LAB VALUES:*** May increase alkaline phosphatase, creatinine, SGOT (AST), SGPT (ALT), cholesterol, phosphate. Alters calcium, glucose, potassium, uric acid, lipid level.

AVAILABILITY (Rx)

CAPSULES: 250 mg. ***TABLETS:*** 500 mg. ***ORAL SUSPENSION:*** 200 mg/ml. ***INJECTION:*** 500 mg.

ADMINISTRATION/HANDLING

PO:
• Give on an empty stomach. • Do not open or crush capsules. Avoid inhalation of powder in capsules and avoid direct contact of powder on skin or mucous membranes. If contact occurs, wash thoroughly with soap and water, rinse eyes profusely with plain water.

IV 🜄

Storage:
• Store at room temperature. • Once reconstituted, is stable for 6 hrs.

Reconstitution:
• Reconstitute each 500 mg vial with 14 ml D_5W. Gently agitate. • For 1 g dose, further dilute with

140 ml D$_5$W; for 1.5 g dose further dilute with 210 ml D$_5$W, providing a concentration of 6 mg/ml.

Rate of administration:
• Infuse over at least 2 hrs.

IV INCOMPATIBILITIES ⊘
Compatible only with D$_5$W. Do not infuse concurrently with other drugs or IV solutions.

INDICATIONS/ROUTES/DOSAGE
Kidney transplant:

PO/IV INFUSION: Adults, elderly: 1 g twice/day (2 g/day). Give in combination with corticosteroids and cyclosporine.

Cardiac/liver transplant:

PO/IV INFUSION: Adults, elderly: 1.5 g twice/day.

Usual dosage for children:
PO: 600 mg/m^2/dose 2 times/day.
Maximum: 2 g/dose.

SIDE EFFECTS
FREQUENT (20–37%): UTI, hypertension, peripheral edema, diarrhea, constipation, fever, headache, nausea. **OCCASIONAL** (10–18%): Dyspepsia (heartburn, indigestion, epigastric pain), dyspnea, cough, hematuria, asthenia (loss of strength, energy), vomiting, edema, tremor, abdominal/chest/back pain, oral moniliasis, acne. **RARE** (6–9%): Insomnia, respiratory infection, rash, dizziness.

ADVERSE REACTIONS/TOXIC EFFECTS
Significant anemia, leukopenia, thrombocytopenia, neutropenia, leukocytosis may occur, particularly in those undergoing kidney rejection. Sepsis, infection occur occasionally, GI tract hemorrhage rarely. There is an increased risk of neoplasia (new, abnormal growth tumor).

NURSING IMPLICATIONS

BASELINE ASSESSMENT:
Women of childbearing potential should have a negative serum or urine pregnancy test within 1 wk prior to initiation of drug therapy. A negative pregnancy test report should be obtained before therapy is initiated. Assess medical history, esp. renal function, existence of active digestive system disease, drug history, esp. other immunosuppressants.

INTERVENTION/EVALUATION:
CBC should be performed weekly during first month of therapy, twice monthly during second and third months of treatment, then monthly throughout the first yr. If rapid fall in WBC occurs, dosage should be reduced or discontinued. Assess particularly for delayed bone marrow suppression. Report any major change in assessment of pt. Routinely watch for any change from normal.

PATIENT/FAMILY TEACHING:
Effective contraception should be used before, during, and for 6 wks after discontinuing therapy, even if there has been a history of infertility, other than hysterectomy. Two forms of contraception must be used concurrently unless abstinence is absolute. Contact physician if unusual bleeding or bruising, sore throat, mouth sores, abdominal pain, or fever occurs. Inform pts of need for laboratory tests while taking medication. Inform pts of risk of malignancies that may occur.

M

nabumetone ✳

nah-**byew**-meh-tone
(<u>Relafen</u>)

▶CLASSIFICATION

PHARMACOTHERAPEUTIC:
Nonsteroidal anti-inflammatory.
CLINICAL: Analgesic, anti-inflammatory (see p. 107C)

ACTION/THERAPEUTIC EFFECT

Produces analgesic and anti-inflammatory effect by inhibiting prostaglandin synthesis, *reducing inflammatory response and intensity of pain stimulus reaching sensory nerve endings.*

PHARMACOKINETICS

Readily absorbed from GI tract. Protein binding: >99%. Widely distributed. Metabolized in liver to active metabolite. Primarily excreted in urine. Not removed by hemodiaylsis. Half-life: 22–30 hrs.

USES

Acute and chronic treatment of osteoarthritis, rheumatoid arthritis.

PRECAUTIONS

CONTRAINDICATIONS: Active peptic ulcer, GI ulceration, chronic inflammation of GI tract, GI bleeding disorders, history of hypersensitivity to aspirin or NSAIDs, history of significantly impaired renal function.
CAUTIONS: Impaired renal/hepatic function, history of GI tract disease, predisposition to fluid retention.

▷**LIFESPAN CONSIDERATIONS:**
Pregnancy/Lactation: Distributed in low concentration in breast milk. Avoid use during last trimester (may adversely affect fetal cardiovascular system: premature closing of ductus arteriosus).
Pregnancy Category C (Category D if used in third trimester or near delivery). **Children:** Safety and efficacy not established. **Elderly:** Age-related renal impairment may increase risk of liver/renal toxicity; reduced dosage recommended. More likely to have serious adverse effects with GI bleeding/ulceration.

INTERACTIONS

DRUG: May increase effects of **oral anticoagulants, heparin, thrombolytics.** May decrease effect of **antihypertensives, diuretics. Salicylates, aspirin** may increase risk of GI side effects, bleeding. **Bone marrow depressants** may increase risk of hematologic reactions. May increase concentration, toxicity of **lithium.** May increase **methotrexate** toxicity. **Probenecid** may increase concentration. **HERBAL: Feverfew** effects may be decreased. **Ginkgo biloba** may increase risk of bleeding. **FOOD:** None known. **LAB VALUES:** May increase alkaline phosphatase, LDH, serum transaminase, potassium, urine protein, BUN, serum creatinine. May decrease uric acid.

AVAILABILITY (Rx)

TABLETS: 500 mg, 750 mg.

ADMINISTRATION/HANDLING

PO:

• Give with food, milk, or antacids if GI distress occurs. • Do not crush; swallow whole.

INDICATIONS/ROUTES/DOSAGE

Rheumatoid arthritis, osteoarthritis:

PO: Adults, elderly: Initially, 1,000 mg as single dose or in 2 divided doses. May increase up to

---

2,000 mg/day as single or in 2 divided doses.

SIDE EFFECTS

FREQUENT (12–14%): Diarrhea, abdominal cramping/pain, dyspepsia (heartburn, indigestion, epigastric pain). **OCCASIONAL** (3–9%): Nausea, constipation, flatulence, dizziness, headache. **RARE** (1–3%): Vomiting, stomatitis.

ADVERSE REACTIONS/TOXIC EFFECTS

Overdose may result in acute hypotension, tachycardia. Peptic ulcer, GI bleeding, nephrotoxicity (dysuria, cystitis, hematuria, proteinuria, nephrotic syndrome), gastritis, severe hepatic reaction (cholestasis, jaundice), severe hypersensitivity reaction (bronchospasm, angiofacial edema) occur rarely.

NURSING IMPLICATIONS

BASELINE ASSESSMENT:

Assess onset, type, location, and duration of pain or inflammation. Inspect appearance of affected joints for immobility, deformities, and skin condition.

INTERVENTION/EVALUATION:

Assist with ambulation if somnolence/drowsiness/dizziness occurs. Monitor for evidence of dyspepsia. Monitor pattern of daily bowel activity and stool consistency. Evaluate for therapeutic response: relief of pain, stiffness, swelling, increase in joint mobility, reduced joint tenderness, improved grip strength.

PATIENT/FAMILY TEACHING:

Avoid tasks that require alertness, motor skills until response to drug is established. If GI upset occurs, take with food, milk. Avoid aspirin, alcohol during therapy (increases risk of GI bleeding). Report headaches, GI distress.

nadolol

nay-**doe**-lol
(Apo-Nadol✦, Corgard, Novo-Nadolol✦)

FIXED-COMBINATION(S)

With bendroflumethiazide, a diuretic **(Corzide)**

▶ CLASSIFICATION

PHARMACOTHERAPEUTIC: Beta-adrenergic blocker. **CLINICAL:** Antianginal, antihypertensive (see p. 61C)

ACTION/THERAPEUTIC EFFECT

Nonselective beta-blocker. Blocks beta$_1$-adrenergic receptors, *slowing sinus heart rate, decreasing cardiac output, decreasing B/P.* Blocks beta$_2$-adrenergic receptors, *increasing airway resistance. Decreases myocardial ischemia severity* by decreasing O_2 requirements.

PHARMACOKINETICS

	Onset	Peak	Duration
PO	—	—	24 hrs

Partially absorbed from GI tract. Protein binding: 28%. Primarily excreted unchanged in urine. Moderately removed by hemodialysis. Half-life: 20–24 hrs (half-life increased with impaired renal function).

USES/UNLABELED

Management of mild to moderate hypertension. Used alone or in combination with diuretics, esp. thiazide type. Management of chronic stable angina pectoris. *Treatment of cardiac arrhythmias, hypertrophic cardiomyopathy, myocardial infarction, pheochromocytoma, vascular headaches, tremors, thyrotoxicosis, mitral valve prolapse syndrome, neuroleptic-induced akathisia.*

PRECAUTIONS

CONTRAINDICATIONS: Bronchial asthma, COPD, uncontrolled cardiac failure, sinus bradycardia, heart block greater than first degree, cardiogenic shock, CHF unless secondary to tachyarrhythmias, those on MAO inhibitors. ***CAUTIONS:*** Inadequate cardiac function, impaired renal/hepatic function, diabetes mellitus, hyperthyroidism.

▷***LIFESPAN CONSIDERATIONS:*** **Pregnancy/Lactation:** Crosses placenta; distributed in breast milk. Avoid use during first trimester. May produce bradycardia, apnea, hypoglycemia, hypothermia during delivery, small birth weight infants. **Pregnancy Category C** (Category D if used in second or third trimester). **Children:** Safety and efficacy not established. **Elderly:** Age-related peripheral vascular disease may require cautious use; risk of beta-blocker–induced hypoglycemia may be increased.

INTERACTIONS

DRUG: **Diuretics, other hypotensives** may increase hypotensive effect; **sympathomimetics, xanthines** may mutually inhibit effects; may mask symptoms of hypoglycemia, prolong hypoglycemic effect of **insulin, oral hypoglycemics; NSAIDs** may decrease antihypertensive effect; **cimetidine** may increase concentration. ***HERBAL:*** None known. ***FOOD:*** None known. ***LAB VALUES:*** May increase ANA titer, SGOT (AST), SGPT (ALT), alkaline phosphatase, LDH, bilirubin, BUN, creatinine, potassium, uric acid, lipoproteins, triglycerides.

AVAILABILITY (Rx)

TABLETS: 20 mg, 40 mg, 80 mg, 120 mg, 160 mg.

ADMINISTRATION/HANDLING

PO:
* Give without regard to meals. * Tablets may be crushed.

INDICATIONS/ROUTES/DOSAGE

Hypertension:

***PO:* Adults:** Initially, 40 mg/day. Increase by 40–80 mg/day at 7 day intervals. **Maintenance:** 40–80 mg/day up to 240–320 mg/day.

Angina pectoris:

***PO:* Adults:** Initially, 40 mg/day. Increase by 40–80 mg/day at 3–7 day intervals. **Maintenance:** 40–80 mg/day up to 160–240 mg/day.

Usual elderly dosage:

PO: Initially, 20 mg/day for angina/hypertension.

Dosage in renal impairment:

Dose is modified based on creatinine clearance.

Creatinine Clearance	% Normal Dose
10–50 ml/min	50
<10 ml/min	25

SIDE EFFECTS

Generally well tolerated, with transient and mild side effects. ***FREQUENT:*** Decreased sexual ability, drowsiness, unusual tiredness/

weakness. ***OCCASIONAL:*** Brady-cardia, difficulty breathing, de-pression, cold hands/feet, diar-rhea, constipation, anxiety, nasal congestion, nausea, vomiting. ***RARE:*** Altered taste, dry eyes, itching.

ADVERSE REACTIONS/TOXIC EFFECTS

Excessive dosage may produce profound bradycardia, hypoten-sion. Abrupt withdrawal may result in sweating, palpitations, head-ache, tremulousness, exacerba-tion of angina, MI, ventricular ar-rhythmias. May precipitate CHF, MI in those with cardiac disease, thyroid storm in those with thyro-toxicosis, peripheral ischemia in those with existing peripheral vas-cular disease. Hypoglycemia may occur in previously controlled dia-betics.

NURSING IMPLICATIONS

BASELINE ASSESSMENT:

Assess baseline renal/liver func-tion tests. Assess B/P, apical pulse immediately before drug is ad-ministered (if pulse is 60/min or below, or systolic B/P is below 90 mm Hg, withhold medication, contact physician). ***Antianginal:*** Record onset, type (sharp, dull, squeezing), radiation, location, intensity, and duration of anginal pain, and precipitating factors (exertion, emotional stress).

INTERVENTION/EVALUATION:

Monitor B/P for hypotension, res-piration for shortness of breath. Assess pulse for strength/weak-ness, irregular rate, bradycardia. Assess fingers for color, numb-ness (Raynaud's). Assess for evi-dence of CHF: dyspnea (particu-larly on exertion or lying down), night cough, peripheral edema, distended neck veins. Monitor I&O (increase in weight, decrease in urine output may in-dicate CHF).

PATIENT/FAMILY TEACHING:

Do not abruptly discontinue medication. Compliance with therapy regimen is essential to control hypertension, arrhyth-mias. To avoid hypotensive ef-fect, rise slowly from lying to sit-ting position; wait momentarily before standing. Avoid tasks that require alertness, motor skills until response to drug is estab-lished. Do not use nasal decon-gestants, OTC cold preparations (stimulants) without physician approval. Restrict salt, alcohol in-take.

nafarelin acetate

naf-ah-**rell**-in
(Synarel)

▶CLASSIFICATION

PHARMACOTHERAPEUTIC: Gonadotropin inhibitor. ***CLINI-CAL:*** Hormone agonist (see p. 87C)

ACTION/*THERAPEUTIC EFFECT*

Initially stimulates the release of the pituitary gonadotropins, luteinizing hormone and follicle-stimulating hormone, *resulting in temporary in-crease of ovarian steroidogenesis.* Continued dosing *abolishes the stimulatory effect on the pituitary gland* and, after about 4 wks, leads to *decreased secretion of gonadal steroids.*

USES

Management of endometriosis, including dysmenorrhea, dyspareunia, pelvic pain. Treatment of central precocious puberty.

PRECAUTIONS
CONTRAINDICATIONS: Hypersensitivity to nafarelin, other agonist analogues; undiagnosed abnormal vaginal bleeding. **CAUTIONS:** History of osteoporosis, chronic alcohol or tobacco use, intercurrent rhinitis.

AVAILABILITY (Rx)
NASAL SOLUTION: 2 mg/ml (each spray delivers 200 mcg).

INTERACTIONS
DRUG: None significant. **HERBAL:** None known. **FOOD:** None known. **LAB VALUES:** None significant.

INDICATIONS/ROUTES/DOSAGE
Endometriosis:

Note: Initiate treatment between days 2 and 4 of menstrual cycle. Duration of therapy is 6 mos.

INTRANASAL: Adults: 400 mcg/day: 200 mcg (1 spray) into 1 nostril in morning, 1 spray into other nostril in evening. For pts with persistent regular menstruation after mos of treatment, increase dose to 800 mcg/day (1 spray into each nostril in morning and evening).

Central precocious puberty:

INTRANASAL: Children: 1,600 mcg/day: 400 mcg (2 sprays into each nostril in morning and evening; total 8 sprays).

SIDE EFFECTS
FREQUENT (90%): Hot flashes. muscle pain, decreased breast size, myalgia, nasal irritation (10%). **OCCASIONAL** (13–22%): Decreased libido, vaginal dryness, headache, emotional lability,

acne. **RARE** (2–8%): Insomnia, edema, weight gain, seborrhea, depression.

ADVERSE REACTIONS/TOXIC EFFECTS
None significant.

NURSING IMPLICATIONS

BASELINE ASSESSMENT:
Inquire about menstrual cycle; therapy should begin between days 2 and 4 of cycle.

INTERVENTION/EVALUATION:
Check for pain relief as result of therapy. Inquire about menstrual cessation and other decreased estrogen effects.

PATIENT/FAMILY TEACHING:
Pt should use nonhormonal contraceptive during therapy. Do not take drug if pregnancy is suspected (risk to fetus). Importance of full length of therapy, regular visits to physician's office. Notify physician if regular menstruation continues (menstruation should stop with therapy).

---

nafcillin sodium

naph-**sill**-in
(Nafcil, Nallpen, Unipen)
Do not confuse with Unicap.

▶CLASSIFICATION

PHARMACOTHERAPEUTIC: Penicillinase-resistant penicillin. **CLINICAL:** Antibiotic (see p. 26C)

ACTION/THERAPEUTIC EFFECT
Binds to bacterial membranes, *in-*

hibiting cell wall synthesis. Bactericidal.

USES

Treatment of respiratory tract, skin/skin structure infections, osteomyelitis, endocarditis, meningitis; perioperatively, esp. in cardiovascular, orthopedic procedures. Predominantly treatment of infections caused by penicillinase-producing staphylococci.

PRECAUTIONS

CONTRAINDICATIONS: Hypersensitivity to any penicillin. ***CAUTIONS:*** History of allergies, particularly cephalosporins.

INTERACTIONS

DRUG: **Probenecid** may increase concentration, toxicity risk. ***HERBAL:*** None known. ***FOOD:*** None known. ***LAB VALUES:*** May cause positive Coombs test.

AVAILABILITY (Rx)

TABLETS: 500 mg. ***CAPSULES:*** 250 mg. ***POWDER FOR INJECTION:*** 500 mg, 1 g, 2 g.

ADMINISTRATION/HANDLING

Note: Space doses evenly around the clock.

PO:

• Give 1 hr before or 2 hrs after food/beverages. • ***PO solution:*** After reconstitution, is stable for 7 days if refrigerated.

IM:

• Reconstitute each 500 mg with 1.7 ml Sterile Water for Injection or 0.9% NaCl to provide concentration of 250 mg/ml. • Inject IM into large muscle mass.

IV 🏥

Storage:

• *IV infusion (piggyback):* Stable

for 24 hrs at room temperature, 96 hrs if refrigerated. Discard if precipitate forms.

Reconstitution:

• *For IV push,* reconstitute as above, then further dilute each vial with 15–30 ml Sterile Water for Injection or 0.9% NaCl. Administer over 5–10 min. • *For intermittent IV infusion (piggyback),* further dilute with 50–100 ml D_5W, $D_{10}W$, 0.9% NaCl, 0.45% NaCl, 0.2% NaCl, Ringer's, lactated Ringer's, or any combination thereof.

Rate of administration:

• Infuse over 30–60 min. • Because of potential for hypersensitivity/anaphylaxis, start initial dose at few drops per min, increase slowly to ordered rate; stay with pt first 10–15 min, then check q10min. • Limit IV therapy to <48 hrs, if possible. Stop infusion if pt complains of pain.

IV INCOMPATIBILITIES 🚫

Ditiazem (Cardizem), droperidol (Inapsine), fentanyl, insulin, labetalol (Normodyne, Trandate), midazolam (Versed), nalbuphine (Nubain), vancomycin (Vancocin), verapamil (Isoptin).

IV COMPATIBILITIES

Heparin, lidocaine, magnesium, potassium chloride, propofol (Diprivan).

INDICATIONS/ROUTES/DOSAGE

Usual dosage:

IV: **Adults, elderly:** 0.5–2 g q4–6h. **Children:** 50–200 mg/kg/day in divided doses q4–6h. **Maximum:** 12 g/day. **Neonates:** 50–100 mg/kg/day in divided doses q6–12h.

IM: **Adults, elderly:** 500 mg q4–6h. **Children:** 50–200 mg/kg/day in divided doses q4–6h. **Maximum:** 12 g/day.

PO: Adults, elderly: 250 mg–1 g q4–6h. **Children:** 50–100 mg/kg/day in divided doses q6h.

SIDE EFFECTS

FREQUENT: Mild hypersensitivity reaction (fever, rash, pruritus), GI effects (nausea, vomiting, diarrhea) more frequent with PO administration. **OCCASIONAL:** Hypokalemia with high IV doses, phlebitis, thrombophlebitis (more common in elderly). **RARE:** Extravasation with IV administration.

ADVERSE REACTIONS/TOXIC EFFECTS

Superinfections, potentially fatal antibiotic-associated colitis may result from altered bacterial balance. Hematologic effects (esp. involving platelets, WBCs), severe hypersensitivity reactions, anaphylaxis occur rarely.

NURSING IMPLICATIONS

BASELINE ASSESSMENT:
Question for history of allergies, esp. penicillins, cephalosporins.

INTERVENTION/EVALUATION:
Hold medication and promptly report rash (possible hypersensitivity) or diarrhea (with fever, abdominal pain, mucus and blood in stool may indicate antibiotic-associated colitis). Evaluate IV site frequently for phlebitis (heat, pain, red streaking over vein) and infiltration (potential extravasation). Check IM injection sites for pain, induration. Monitor potassium. Be alert for superinfection: increased fever, onset sore throat, vomiting, diarrhea, ulceration/changes of oral mucosa, anal/genital pruritus. Check hematology reports (esp. WBCs), periodic renal or hepatic reports in prolonged therapy.

PATIENT/FAMILY TEACHING:
Continue antibiotic for full length of treatment. Doses should be evenly spaced. Discomfort may occur with IM injection. Report IV discomfort immediately. Notify physician in event of diarrhea, rash, other new symptom.

---

naftifine hydrochloride

(Naftin)

See Classification section under: Antifungals: topical

---

nalbuphine hydrochloride

nail-**byew**-phin
(Nubain)
Do not confuse with Navane.

▶CLASSIFICATION

PHARMACOTHERAPEUTIC: Narcotic agonist, antagonist. **CLINICAL:** Opioid analgesic (see p. 116C)

ACTION/THERAPEUTIC EFFECT

Binds with opioid receptors within CNS, *altering pain perception, emotional response to pain.* May displace opioid agonists and competitively inhibit their action (may precipitate withdrawal symptoms).

PHARMACOKINETICS

	Onset	Peak	Duration
SubQ	<15 min	—	3–6 hrs
IM	<15 min	60 min	3–6 hrs
IV	2–3 min	30 min	3–6 hrs

Well absorbed after SubQ, IM administration. Protein binding: 50%. Metabolized in liver. Primarily eliminated in feces via biliary secretion. Half-life: 3.5–5 hrs.

USES

Relief of moderate to severe pain, preop sedation, obstetrical analgesia, adjunct to anesthesia.

PRECAUTIONS

CONTRAINDICATIONS: Respirations <12/min. ***CAUTIONS:*** Impaired hepatic/renal function, elderly, debilitated, head injury, increased intracranial pressure, MI with nausea, vomiting, respiratory disease, hypertension, before biliary tract surgery (produces spasm of sphincter of Oddi).

▷***LIFESPAN CONSIDERATIONS:*** **Pregnancy/Lactation:** Readily crosses placenta; distributed in breast milk (breast feeding not recommended). **Pregnancy Category B** (Category D if used for prolonged periods or in high doses at term). **Children:** Paradoxical excitement may occur. Those <2 yrs of age more susceptible to respiratory depression. **Elderly:** More susceptible to respiratory depression. Age-related impaired renal function may increase risk of urinary retention.

INTERACTIONS

DRUG: **Alcohol, CNS depressants** may increase CNS or respiratory depression, hypotension. **MAO inhibitors** may produce severe reaction (reduce dose to $1/4$ usual dose). Effects may be decreased with **buprenorphine.** ***HERBAL:*** None known. ***FOOD:*** None known. ***LAB VALUES:*** May increase amylase, lipase, serum levels.

AVAILABILITY (Rx)

INJECTION: 10 mg/ml, 20 mg/ml.

ADMINISTRATION/HANDLING

Note: Store parenteral form at room temperature.

IM:
• Rotate IM injection sites.

IV 🔟

Storage:
• Store at room temperature.

Reconstitution:
• May give undiluted.

Rate of administration:
• For IV push, administer each 10 mg >3–5 min.

IV INCOMPATIBILITIES ⊘

Amphotericin B complex (Abelcet, Ambisome, Amphotec), cefepime (Maxipime), docetaxel (Doxil), methotrexate, nafcillin (Nafcil), piperacillin/tazobactam (Zosyn), sargramostim (Leukine, Prokine), sodium bicarbonate.

IV COMPATIBILITIES

Lidocaine, midazolam (Versed), propofol (Diprivan).

INDICATIONS/ROUTES/DOSAGE

Note: Dosage based on severity of pain, physical condition of pt, concurrent use of other medications.

Analgesia:
SubQ/IM/IV: Adults, elderly: 10

mg q3–6h, as necessary. Do not exceed maximum single dose of 20 mg, maximum daily dose of 160 mg. In pts chronically receiving narcotic analgesics of similar duration of action, give 25% of usual dosage. **Children:** 0.1–0.15 mg/kg q3–6h as needed.

Supplement to anesthesia:

IV: **Adults, elderly:** Induction: 0.3–3 mg/kg over 10–15 min. **Maintenance:** 0.25–0.5 mg/kg as necessary.

SIDE EFFECTS

FREQUENT (35%): Sedation. *OCCASIONAL* (3–9%): Sweaty/clammy feeling, nausea, vomiting, dizziness, vertigo, dry mouth, headache. *RARE* (≤1%): Restlessness, crying, euphoria, hostility, confusion, numbness, tingling, flushing, paradoxical reaction.

ADVERSE REACTIONS/TOXIC EFFECTS

Abrupt withdrawal after prolonged use may produce symptoms of narcotic withdrawal (abdominal cramping, rhinorrhea, lacrimation, anxiety, increased temperature, piloerection [goose bumps]). Overdose results in severe respiratory depression, skeletal muscle flaccidity, cyanosis, extreme somnolence progressing to convulsions, stupor, coma. Tolerance to analgesic effect, physical dependence may occur with chronic use.

NURSING IMPLICATIONS

BASELINE ASSESSMENT:

Raise bed rails. Obtain vital signs before giving medication. If respirations are 12/min or lower (20/min or lower in children), withhold medication, contact physician. Assess onset, type, location, and duration of pain. Effect of medication is reduced if full pain recurs before next dose. Low abuse potential.

INTERVENTION/EVALUATION:

Monitor for change in respirations, B/P, change in rate or quality of pulse. Monitor pattern of daily bowel activity and stool consistency. Initiate deep breathing and coughing exercises, particularly in those with impaired pulmonary function. Assess for clinical improvement and record onset of relief of pain. Consult physician if pain relief is not adequate.

PATIENT/FAMILY TEACHING:

Change positions slowly to avoid dizziness. Avoid tasks that require alertness, motor skills until response to drug is established. Avoid alcohol and CNS depressants.

nalmefene

nal-meh-feen
(Revex)
Do not confuse with ReVia.

▶CLASSIFICATION

PHARMACOTHERAPEUTIC: Narcotic antagonist. *CLINICAL:* Antidote (see p. 117C)

ACTION/THERAPEUTIC EFFECT

An opioid antagonist, *prevents/reverses effects of opioids (respiratory depression, sedation, hypotension).*

USES

Complete/partial reversal of opioid drug effects; management of known or suspected opioid overdose.

PRECAUTIONS

CONTRAINDICATIONS: History of hypersensitivity to nalmefene. **CAUTIONS:** Current opioid dependence or addiction, cardiac disease, renal function impairment.

INTERACTIONS

DRUG: None significant. **HERBAL:** None significant. **FOOD:** None significant. **LAB VALUES:** May increase AST, creatinine kinase.

AVAILABILITY (Rx)

INJECTION: 100 mcg/ml, 1 mg/ml.

INDICATIONS/ROUTES/DOSAGE

Postop pts:

IV/IM/SubQ: Adults: Initially, 0.25 mcg/kg followed by additional 0.25 mcg doses at 2 to 5 min intervals until desired response. Cumulative doses >1 mcg/kg do not provide additional therapeutic effect.

Known/suspected overdose:

IV/IM/SubQ: Adults: Initially, 0.5 mg/70 kg. May give 1 mg/70 kg in 2–5 min. If physical opioid dependence suspected, initial dose is 0.1 mg/70 kg.

SIDE EFFECTS

FREQUENT (5–20%): Nausea, vomiting, tachycardia, hypertension. **OCCASIONAL** (1–5%): Postop pain, fever, dizziness, headache, chills, hypotension, vasodilation.

ADVERSE REACTIONS/TOXIC EFFECTS

None significant.

NURSING IMPLICATIONS

BASELINE ASSESSMENT:
Assess for sensitivity to nalmefene.

INTERVENTION/EVALUATION:
Monitor pt alertness, B/P, heart rate, respiratory rate.

PATIENT/FAMILY TEACHING:
N/A (used in treatment of overdose).

---

naloxone hydrochloride

nay-**lox**-own
(Narcan)
Do not confuse with Norcuron.

▶CLASSIFICATION

PHARMACOTHERAPEUTIC: Narcotic antagonist. **CLINICAL:** Antidote (see p. 117C)

ACTION/THERAPEUTIC EFFECT

Displaces opiates at opiate-occupied receptor sites in CNS, *blocking narcotic effects. Reverses opiate-induced sleep or sedation. Increases respiratory rate, returns depressed B/P to normal rate.*

PHARMACOKINETICS

	Onset	Peak	Duration
SubQ	2–5 min	—	1–4 hrs
IM	2–5 min	—	1–4 hrs
IV	1–2 min	—	1–4 hrs

Well absorbed after SubQ, IM administration. Metabolized in liver. Primarily excreted in urine. Half-life: 60–100 min.

USES

Diagnosis and treatment of opioid toxicity, treatment of opioid-induced respiratory depression and other effects (e.g., sedation, coma, convulsions). Used in neonates to reverse respiratory depression caused by opioids given to mother during labor and delivery. Adjunctive therapy to treat hypotension in management of septic shock.

PRECAUTIONS

CONTRAINDICATIONS: Respiratory depression due to nonopiate drugs. **CAUTIONS:** Opiate-dependent pt, cardiovascular disorders.

▷**LIFESPAN CONSIDERATIONS:** **Pregnancy/Lactation:** Unknown whether drug crosses placenta or is distributed in breast milk. **Pregnancy Category B. Children/Elderly:** No age-related precautions noted.

INTERACTIONS

DRUG: Reverses analgesic/side effects, may precipitate withdrawal symptoms of **butorphanol, nalbuphine, pentazocine, opioid agonist analgesics. HERBAL:** None known. **FOOD:** None known. **LAB VALUES:** None significant.

AVAILABILITY (Rx)

INJECTION: 0.02 mg/ml, 0.4 mg/ml, 1 mg/ml.

ADMINISTRATION/HANDLING

IM:

• Give in upper, outer quadrant of buttock.

IV ▥

Storage:

• Store parenteral form at room temperature. • Use mixture within 24 hrs; discard unused solution.

Reconstitution:

• May dilute 1 mg/ml with 50 ml Sterile Water for Injection to provide a concentration of 0.02 mg/ml. • For continuous IV infusion, dilute each 2 mg of naloxone with 500 ml of D_5W in water or 0.9% NaCl, producing solution containing 0.004 mg/ml.

Rate of administration:

• May administer undiluted. • Give each 0.4 mg as IV push over 15 sec. • Use the 0.4 mg/ml and 1 mg/ml for injection for adults, the 0.02 mg/ml concentration for neonates.

IV INCOMPATIBILITIES ⊘

Amphotericin B complex (Abelcet, Ambisome, Amphotec).

IV COMPATIBILITY

Propofol (Diprivan).

INDICATIONS/ROUTES/DOSAGE

Opioid toxicity (IV route preferred):

IM/IV/SubQ: Adults: 0.4–2 mg as single dose. May repeat at 2–3 min intervals. **Children:** 0.01 mg/kg. May repeat with 0.1 mg/kg.

Note: AAP recommends initial dose of 0.1 mg/kg for infants and children up to 5 yrs and weighing <20 kg. Children >5 yrs or >20 kg recommended initial dose is 2 mg.

Opioid respiratory depression:

IV: Adults: 0.1–0.2 mg q2–3min until adequate ventilation and alertness without pain are obtained. May repeat dose at 1–2 hr intervals. **Children:** 5–10 mcg (0.005–0.01 mg) q2–3min. **Neonates:** 10 mcg (0.01 mg)/kg. May repeat q2–3min.

Septic shock:

IV: Adults: 0.03–0.2 mg/kg initially, then IV infusion of 0.03–0.3 mg/kg/hr for 1–20 hrs.

SIDE EFFECTS

None significant (little or no pharmacologic effect in absence of narcotics).

ADVERSE REACTIONS/TOXIC EFFECTS

Too-rapid reversal of narcotic depression may result in nausea, vomiting, tremulousness, sweating, increased B/P, tachycardia. Excessive dosage in postop pts may produce significant reversal of analgesia, excitement, tremulousness. Hypotension or hypertension, ventricular tachycardia and fibrillation, pulmonary edema may occur in those with cardiovascular disease.

NURSING IMPLICATIONS

BASELINE ASSESSMENT:

Maintain clear airway. Obtain weight of children to calculate drug dosage.

INTERVENTION/EVALUATION:

Monitor vital signs esp. rate, depth, and rhythm of respiration during and frequently after administration. Carefully observe pt after satisfactory response (duration of opiate may exceed duration of naloxone, resulting in recurrence of respiratory depression). Assess for increased pain with reversal of opiate.

---

naltrexone hydrochloride

nal-**trex**-own
(ReVia)
Do not confuse with Revex.

▶CLASSIFICATION

PHARMACOTHERAPEUTIC:
Narcotic antagonist. **CLINICAL:**
Antidote (see p. 117C)

ACTION/*THERAPEUTIC EFFECT*

Binds to opioid receptors, *blocking physical effects of morphine, heroin, other opioids.* **Alcohol deterrent:** Exact mechanism unknown. *Decreases craving, drinking days, relapse rate.*

PHARMACOKINETICS

	Onset	Peak	Duration
PO	—	—	24–72 hrs

Rapid, complete absorption following oral administration. Protein binding: 21%. Undergoes extensive first-pass hepatic metabolism. Metabolized in liver to active metabolite. Excreted in urine. Half-life: 4–13 hrs.

USES/*UNLABELED*

Blockade of effects of exogenously administered opioids. Treatment of alcohol dependence. *Treatment of postconcussional syndrome unresponsive to other treatments; eating disorders.*

PRECAUTIONS

CONTRAINDICATIONS: Pts experiencing opiate withdrawal, opioid dependent, acute opioid withdrawal, failed naloxone challenge, positive urine screen for opioids, history of sensitivity to naltrexone,

N

---

acute hepatitis, liver failure. **CAUTIONS:** Active liver disease.

▷**LIFESPAN CONSIDERATIONS:**
Pregnancy/Lactation: Unknown whether drug crosses placenta or is distributed in breast milk. **Pregnancy Category C. Children/Elderly:** No age-related precautions noted.

INTERACTIONS

DRUG: Concurrent use with **thioridazine** may produce lethargy, somnolence. Benefits of opioid-containing products (**cough and cold preparations, antidiarrheal preparations, opioid analgesics**) are negated. **HERBAL:** None known. **FOOD:** None known. **LAB VALUES:** May increase serum transaminase, SGOT (AST), SGPT (ALT).

AVAILABILITY (Rx)
TABLETS: 50 mg.

ADMINISTRATION/HANDLING
IV/SubQ:

• In those with narcotic dependence, do not attempt treatment until pt has remained opioid free for 7–10 days. Test urine for opioids for verification. Pt should not be experiencing withdrawal symptoms. • Administer a naloxone challenge test (see Indications/Routes/Dosage). If pt experiences any signs/symptoms of withdrawal, withhold treatment (challenge test can be repeated in 24 hrs). Naloxone challenge test must be negative before naltrexone therapy is initiated.

INDICATIONS/ROUTES/DOSAGE
Naloxone challenge test:

IV: Adults, elderly: Draw 2 ampules naloxone, 2 ml (0.8 mg) into syringe. Inject 0.5 ml (0.2 mg); while needle is still in vein, observe for 30 sec for withdrawal signs/symptoms (see Adverse Reactions/Toxic Effects). If no evidence of withdrawal, inject remaining 1.5 ml (0.6 mg); observe for additional 20 min for withdrawal signs/symptoms.

SubQ: Adults, elderly: Give 2 ml (0.8 mg); observe for 45 min for withdrawal signs/symptoms.

Opioid-free state:

PO: Adults, elderly: Initially, 25 mg. Observe pt for 1 hr. If no withdrawal signs appear, give another 25 mg. May be given as 100 mg every other day or 150 mg q3days.

Adjunct in treatment of alcohol dependence:

PO: Adults, elderly: 50 mg once daily.

SIDE EFFECTS

FREQUENT: Alcoholism (7–10%): Nausea, headache, depression. **Narcotic addiction** (5–10%): Insomnia, anxiety, nervousness, headache, low energy, abdominal cramps, nausea, vomiting, joint/muscle pain. **OCCASIONAL: Alcoholism** (2–4%): Dizziness, nervousness, fatigue, insomnia, vomiting, anxiety, suicidal ideation. **Narcotic addiction** (10%): Irritability, increased energy, dizziness, anorexia, diarrhea or constipation, rash, chills, increased thirst.

ADVERSE REACTIONS/TOXIC EFFECTS

Signs and symptoms of opioid withdrawal include stuffy or runny nose, tearing, yawning, sweating, tremor, vomiting, piloerection (goose bumps), feeling of temperature change, joint/bone/muscle

---

pain, abdominal cramps, feeling of skin crawling. May cause hepatocellular injury if given in large doses. Accidental naltrexone overdosage produces withdrawal symptoms within 5 min of ingestion, lasts up to 48 hrs. Symptoms present as confusion, visual hallucinations, somnolence, significant vomiting and diarrhea.

NURSING IMPLICATIONS

BASELINE ASSESSMENT:

If there is any question of opioid dependence, a naloxone challenge test (see Indications/ Dosage/Routes) should be performed. Treatment with naltrexone should not be instituted unless pt is opioid free for 7–10 days before therapy begins. Obtain medication history (esp. opioids), other medical conditions (esp. hepatitis, other liver disease).

INTERVENTION/EVALUATION:

Monitor closely for evidence of hepatotoxicity (abdominal pain that lasts longer than a few days, white bowel movements, dark urine, jaundice), SGOT, SGPT, bilirubin, creatinine clearance lab values.

PATIENT/FAMILY TEACHING:

If heroin or other opiates are self-administered, there will be no effect. However, any attempt to overcome naltrexone's prolonged 24–72 hr blockade of opioid effect by taking large amounts of opioids is very dangerous and may result in coma, serious injury, or fatal overdose. Naltrexone also blocks effects of opioid-containing medicine (cough and cold preparations,

antidiarrheal preparations, opioid analgesics). Contact physician if abdominal pain that lasts longer than 3 days, white bowel movements, dark-colored urine, yellow eyes occurs.

naphazoline

na-**faz**-oh-leen
(Albalon, AK-Con, Clear Eyes, Naphcon, Privine, Vasocon)

FIXED-COMBINATION(S)

With pheniramine maleate, an antihistamine **(Naphcon-A)**

▶CLASSIFICATION

PHARMACOTHERAPEUTIC: Sympathomimetic. **CLINICAL:** Decongestant

ACTION/*THERAPEUTIC EFFECT*

Directly acts on alpha-adrenergic receptors in arterioles of conjunctiva, *causing vasoconstriction, with subsequent decreased congestion to area.*

USES

Ophthalmic: Relief of itching, congestion, and minor irritation; to control hyperemia in pts with superficial corneal vascularity. Occasionally may be used during some ocular diagnostic procedures. ***Intranasal:*** Relief of nasal congestion due to common cold, acute or chronic rhinitis, hay fever or other allergies.

PRECAUTIONS

CONTRAINDICATIONS: Narrow-angle glaucoma or those with a narrow angle who do not have glaucoma; before peripheral iri-

N

dectomy; eyes capable of angle closure. **CAUTIONS:** Hypertension, diabetes, hyperthyroidism, heart disease, hypertensive cardiovascular disease, coronary artery disease, cerebral arteriosclerosis, long-standing bronchial asthma.

INTERACTIONS

DRUG: Tricyclic antidepressants, maprotiline may increase effect. **HERBAL: Ma Huang (Ephedra)** may increase CNS effects. **FOOD:** None known. **LAB VALUES:** None significant.

AVAILABILITY (Rx)

OPHTHALMIC SOLUTION: 0.012%, 0.02%, 0.03%, 0.1%. **NASAL DROPS:** 0.05%. **NASAL SPRAY:** 0.05%.

INDICATIONS/ROUTES/DOSAGE

Usual nasal dosage:

INTRANASAL: Adults, elderly, children >12 yrs: 2 drops/sprays (0.05%) in each nostril q3–6h. **Children 6–12 yrs:** 1 spray/drop q6h as needed.

Usual ophthalmic dosage:

OPHTHALMIC: Adults, elderly, children >6 yrs: 1–2 drops q3–4h for 3–4 days.

SIDE EFFECTS

OCCASIONAL: Nasal: Burning, stinging, drying nasal mucosa, sneezing, rebound congestion. **Ophthalmic:** Blurred vision, large pupils, increased eye irritation. **Note: Systemic absorption:** Fast/irregular/pounding heartbeat, headache, lightheadedness, nervousness, trembling, insomnia, nausea.

ADVERSE REACTIONS/TOXIC EFFECTS

Large doses may produce tachy-cardia, palpitations, lightheadedness, nausea, vomiting. Overdosage in pts >60 yrs: hallucinations, CNS depression, seizures.

NURSING IMPLICATIONS

PATIENT/FAMILY TEACHING:
Do not use beyond 72 hrs without consulting a physician. Use caution with activities that require visual acuity. Discontinue and consult physician if the following occur: vision changes, headache, eye pain, floating spots, pain with light exposure, acute eye redness, insomnia, dizziness, weakness, tremor, irregular heartbeat. Too frequent use may result in rebound effect.

---

naproxen

nah-**prox**-en
(EC-Naprosyn, Naprelan, Naprosyn, Naxem✚)

naproxen sodium

(Aleve, Anaprox, Apo-Napro✚, Novonaprox✚, Synflex✚)

▶CLASSIFICATION
PHARMACOTHERAPEUTIC: Nonsteroidal anti-inflammatory. **CLINICAL:** Analgesic, anti-inflammatory (see p. 107C)

ACTION/*THERAPEUTIC EFFECT*
Produces analgesic and anti-inflammatory effect by inhibiting prostaglandin synthesis, *reducing inflammatory response and intensity of pain stimulus reaching sensory nerve endings.*

PHARMACOKINETICS

Onset	Peak	Duration
PO (analgesic)		
<1 hr	—	Up to 7 hrs
PO (antirheumatic)		
Up to 14 days	2–4 wks	—

Completely absorbed from GI tract. Protein binding: 99%. Metabolized in liver. Primarily excreted in urine. Not removed by hemodialysis. Half-life: 13 hrs.

USES/*UNLABELED*

Treatment of acute or long-term mild to moderate pain, primary dysmenorrhea, mild to moderately severe pain, rheumatoid arthritis, juvenile rheumatoid arthritis, osteoarthritis, ankylosing spondylitis, acute gouty arthritis, bursitis, tendinitis. *Treatment of vascular headaches.*

PRECAUTIONS

CONTRAINDICATIONS: GI ulceration, chronic inflammation of GI tract, bleeding disorders, history of hypersensitivity to aspirin or NSAIDs. **CAUTIONS:** Impaired renal/hepatic function, history of GI tract disease, predisposition to fluid retention.

▷**LIFESPAN CONSIDERATIONS:**
Pregnancy/Lactation: Crosses placenta; distributed in breast milk. Avoid use during third trimester (may adversely affect fetal cardiovascular system: premature closing of ductus arteriosus). **Pregnancy Category B** (Category D if used in third trimester or near delivery). **Children:** Safety and efficacy not established in those <2 yrs of age. Children >2 yrs at increased risk of skin rash.

Elderly: Age-related renal impairment may increase risk of liver and renal toxicity; reduced dosage recommended. More likely to have serious adverse effects with GI bleeding/ulceration.

INTERACTIONS

DRUG: May increase effects of **oral anticoagulants, heparin, thrombolytics.** May decrease effect of **antihypertensives, diuretics. Salicylates, aspirin** may increase risk of GI side effects, bleeding. **Bone marrow depressants** may increase risk of hematologic reactions. May increase concentration, toxicity of **lithium.** May increase **methotrexate** toxicity. **Probenecid** may increase concentration. **HERBAL:** Feverfew effects may be decreased. **Ginkgo biloba** may increase risk of bleeding. **FOOD:** None known. **LAB VALUES:** May prolong bleeding time, alter blood glucose levels. May increase liver function tests. May decrease sodium, uric acid.

AVAILABILITY (Rx)

GELCAP: 220 mg **(OTC). TABLETS:** 200 mg **(OTC),** 250 mg, 375 mg, 500 mg. **TABLETS (delayed-release):** 375 mg, 500 mg. **ORAL SUSPENSION:** 125 mg/5 ml.

ADMINISTRATION/HANDLING

PO:
• Swallow enteric-coated form whole; scored tablets may be broken or crushed. • May give with food, milk, or antacids if GI distress occurs.

INDICATIONS/ROUTES/DOSAGE

Note: Each 275 or 550 mg tablet of naproxen sodium equals 250 or 500 mg naproxen, respectively.

Rheumatoid arthritis, osteoarthritis, ankylosing spondylitis:

PO: Adults, elderly: 250–500 mg (275–550 mg) 2 times/day or 250 mg (275 mg) in morning and 500 mg (550 mg) in evening. *Naprelan:* 750–1,000 mg daily as single dose.

Juvenile rheumatoid arthritis (naproxen only):

PO: Children: 10–15 mg/kg/day in 2 divided doses. **Maximum:** 1,000 mg/day.

Acute gouty arthritis:

PO: Adults, elderly: Initially, 750 (825) mg, then 250 (275) mg q8h until attack subsides. *Naprelan:* Initially, 1,000–1,500 mg, then 1,000 mg/day as single dose until attack subsides.

Mild to moderate pain, dysmenorrhea, bursitis, tendinitis:

PO: Adults, elderly: Initially, 500 (550) mg, then 250 (275) mg q6–8h as needed. Total daily dose not to exceed 1.25 (1.375) g. *Naprelan:* 1,000 mg/day as single dose.

SIDE EFFECTS

FREQUENT (3–9%): Nausea, constipation, abdominal cramps/pain, heartburn, dizziness, headache, drowsiness. ***OCCASIONAL*** (1–3%): Stomatitis, diarrhea, indigestion. ***RARE*** (<1%): Vomiting, confusion.

ADVERSE REACTIONS/TOXIC EFFECTS

Peptic ulcer, GI bleeding, gastritis, severe hepatic reaction (cholestasis, jaundice) occur rarely. Nephrotoxicity (dysuria, hematuria, proteinuria, nephrotic syndrome) and severe hypersensitivity reaction (fever, chills, bronchospasm) occur rarely.

NURSING IMPLICATIONS

BASELINE ASSESSMENT:

Assess onset, type, location, and duration of pain or inflammation. Inspect appearance of affected joints for immobility, deformities, and skin condition.

INTERVENTION/EVALUATION:

Assist with ambulation if dizziness occurs. Monitor pattern of daily bowel activity and stool consistency. Evaluate for therapeutic response: relief of pain, stiffness, swelling, increase in joint mobility, reduced joint tenderness, improved grip strength.

PATIENT/FAMILY TEACHING:

Avoid tasks that require alertness, motor skills until response to drug is established. If GI upset occurs, take with food, milk. Avoid aspirin, alcohol during therapy (increases risk of GI bleeding). Report headache, rash, visual disturbances, weight gain, black stools, persistent headache.

---

naratriptan

nar-ah-**trip**-tan
(Amerge)
Do not confuse with Amaryl.

▶CLASSIFICATION

PHARMACOTHERAPEUTIC: Serotonin receptor agonist. ***CLINICAL:*** Antimigraine (see p. 53C).

ACTION/*THERAPEUTIC EFFECT*

Binds selectively to vascular receptors producing a vasoconstrictive effect on cranial blood vessels, *producing relief of migraine headache.*

PHARMACOKINETICS

Well absorbed following PO administration. Protein binding: 28–31%. Metabolized by the liver to inactive metabolite. Eliminated primarily in the urine with lesser amount excreted in the feces. Half-life: 6 hrs (half-life increased in renal/hepatic impairment).

USES

Treatment of acute migraine attack with or without aura in adults.

PRECAUTIONS

CONTRAINDICATIONS: Coronary artery disease, uncontrolled hypertension, severe renal impairment (Ccr <15 ml/min), severe hepatic impairment (Child-Pugh grade C), cerebrovascular or peripheral vascular syndromes, ischemic heart disease (angina pectoris, history of MI, silent ischemia), Prinzmetal's angina, concurrent use (or within 24 hrs) of ergotamine-containing preparations, concurrent (or within 2 wks) of MAO therapy, hemiplegic or basilar migraine, within 24 hrs of another serotonin receptor agonist. **CAUTIONS:** Mild-to-moderate renal/hepatic impairment, pt profile suggesting cardiovascular risks.
▷**LIFESPAN CONSIDERATIONS:** **Pregnancy/Lactation:** Unknown if excreted in human breast milk. **Pregnancy Category C. Children:** Safety and efficacy not established. **Elderly:** Not recommended in the elderly.

INTERACTIONS

DRUG: Ergotamine-containing drugs may produce vasospastic reaction. Oral contraceptives reduce naratriptan's clearance, volume of distribution. Combined use of **fluoxetine, fluvoxamine, paroxetine, sertraline** may produce weakness, hyperreflexia, uncoordination. **HERBAL:** None known. **FOOD:** None known. **LAB VALUES:** None significant.

AVAILABILITY (Rx)

TABLETS: 1 mg, 2.5 mg.

ADMINISTRATION/HANDLING

PO:

• Give without regard to food.

INDICATIONS/ROUTES/DOSAGE

Migraine:

PO: Adults: Give 1 or 2.5 mg. If headache returns or pt received only a partial response to initial dose, may repeat dose once after 4 hrs. **Maximum:** 5 mg per 24 hr period.

Mild-to-moderate renal/hepatic impairment:

PO: Adults: Consider with low starting dose. Do not exceed 2.5 mg over a 24 hr period.

SIDE EFFECTS

OCCASIONAL (5%): Nausea. **RARE** (2%): Paresthesia, dizziness, fatigue, drowsiness, neck/throat/jaw pressure.

ADVERSE REACTIONS/TOXIC EFFECTS

May produce corneal opacities and defects. Cardiac events (ischemia, coronary artery vasospasm, MI), noncardiac vasospasm-related reactions (hemorrhage, stroke) occur rarely but particularly in those with hypertension, obesity, smokers, diabetics, strong family history of coronary artery disease, male >40 yrs, postmenopausal women.

NURSING IMPLICATIONS

BASELINE ASSESSMENT:
Question regarding history of

N

peripheral vascular disease, renal/hepatic impairment, possibility of pregnancy. Question pt regarding onset, location, and duration of migraine and possible precipitating symptoms.

INTERVENTION/EVALUATION:

Assess for relief of migraine headache and potential for photophobia, phonophobia (sound sensitivity, nausea, vomiting).

PATIENT/FAMILY TEACHING:

Take a single dose as soon as symptoms of an actual migraine attack appear. Medication is intended to relieve migraine headaches, not to prevent or reduce number of attacks. If heart throbbing, pain/tightness in chest or throat, sudden or severe abdominal pain, or pain or weakness of extremities occurs, contact physician immediately.

---

natamycin

(Natacyn)

See Classification section under: Antifungals: topical

---

nateglinide

nah-**teg**-glih-nide
(Starlix)

▶CLASSIFICATION

PHARMACOTHERAPEUTIC:
Antihyperglycemic. ***CLINICAL:***
Antidiabetic (see p. 40C)

ACTION/*THERAPEUTIC EFFECT*

Stimulates release of insulin from beta cells of the pancreas by depolarizing beta cells, leading to an opening of calcium channels. Resulting calcium influx induces insulin secretion, *lowering glucose concentration.*

USES

Treatment of type 2 diabetes mellitus in pts who cannot be adequately controlled by diet and exercise and who have not been chronically treated with other antidiabetic agents. Used as monotherapy or in combination with metformin (Glucophage).

PRECAUTIONS

CONTRAINDICATIONS: Diabetic ketoacidosis, type 1 diabetes mellitus. ***CAUTIONS:*** Hepatic/renal function impairment.

INTERACTIONS

DRUG: **NSAIDs, salicylates, MAOIs, beta blockers** may increase hypoglycemic effect. **Thiazide diuretics, corticosteroids, thyroid medication, sympathomimetics** may decrease hypoglycemic effect. ***HERBAL:*** None significant. ***FOOD:*** Peak plasma levels may be significantly reduced if administered 10 min before a liquid meal. ***LAB VALUES:*** None significant.

AVAILABILITY (Rx)

TABLETS: 60 mg, 120 mg.

ADMINISTRATION/HANDLING
PO:

• Ideally, give within 15 min of a meal, but may be given immediately before a meal to as long as 30 min before a meal.

INDICATIONS/ROUTES/DOSAGE
Diabetes mellitus:

PO: Adults, elderly: 120 mg 3

---

times/day before meals. Initially, 60 mg may be given.

SIDE EFFECTS

FREQUENT (10%): Upper respiratory tract infection. ***OCCASIONAL*** (3–4%): Back pain, flu symptoms, dizziness, arthropathy, diarrhea. ***RARE*** (≤2%): Bronchitis, cough.

ADVERSE REACTIONS/TOXIC EFFECTS

Hypoglycemia occurs in <2%.

NURSING IMPLICATIONS

BASELINE ASSESSMENT:

Check fasting blood glucose and glycosylated Hgb (HbA$_1$C) periodically to determine minimum effective dose. Discuss lifestyle to determine extent of learning, emotional needs. Assure follow-up instruction if pt/family do not thoroughly understand diabetes management or glucose-testing technique. At least 1 wk should elapse to assess response to drug before new dose adjustment is made.

INTERVENTION/EVALUATION:

Monitor blood glucose and food intake. Assess for hypoglycemia (cool wet skin, tremors, dizziness, anxiety, headache, tachycardia, numbness in mouth, hunger, diplopia) or hyperglycemia (polyuria, polyphagia, polydipsia, nausea, vomiting, dim vision, fatigue, deep rapid breathing). Be alert to conditions that alter glucose requirements: fever, increased activity or stress, surgical procedures.

PATIENT/FAMILY TEACHING:

Diabetes mellitus requires lifelong control. Prescribed diet and exercise are principal parts of treatment; do not skip or delay meals. Continue to adhere to dietary instructions, a regular exercise program, and regular testing of blood glucose.

---

nedocromil sodium

ned-oh-**crow**-mul
(Alocril, Mireze✦, Tilade)

▶CLASSIFICATION

PHARMACOTHERAPEUTIC:
Mast cell stabilizer. ***CLINICAL:***
Respiratory inhalant anti-inflammatory (see p. 64C)

ACTION/*THERAPEUTIC EFFECT*

Prevents activation, release of mediators of inflammation (e.g., histamine, leukotrienes, mast cells, eosinophils, monocytes). *Prevents both early and late asthmatic responses.*

USES/*UNLABELED*

Maintenance therapy for preventing airway inflammation, bronchoconstriction in pts with mild to moderate bronchial asthma. ***Ophthalmic:*** Treatment of itching associated with allergic conjunctivitis. *Prevents bronchospasm in pts with reversible obstructive airway disease.*

PRECAUTIONS

CONTRAINDICATIONS: None significant. ***CAUTIONS:*** Not used for reversing acute bronchospasm.

INTERACTIONS

DRUG: None significant. ***HERBAL:*** None known. ***FOOD:*** None known. ***LAB VALUES:*** None significant.

N

AVAILABILITY (Rx)

AEROSOL. OPHTHALMIC SOLUTION: 2%.

INDICATIONS/ROUTES/DOSAGE

Asthma:

ORAL INHALATION: Adults, elderly, children >6 yrs: Two inhalations (4 mg) 4 times/day. May decrease to 3 times/day then 2 times/day as control of asthma occurs. **Maximum:** 16 mg/24 hrs.

Allergic conjunctivitis:

OPHTHALMIC: Adults, elderly, children: 1–2 drops in each eye 2 times/day.

SIDE EFFECTS

FREQUENT (5–10%): Cough, pharyngitis, bronchospasm, headache, unpleasant taste. ***OCCASIONAL*** (1–5%): Rhinitis, upper respiratory tract infection, abdominal pain, fatigue. ***RARE*** (<1%): Diarrhea, dizziness.

ADVERSE REACTIONS/TOXIC EFFECTS

None significant.

NURSING IMPLICATIONS

INTERVENTION/EVALUATION:

Evaluate therapeutic response: reduced dependence on antihistamine, less frequent/less severe asthmatic attacks.

PATIENT/FAMILY TEACHING:

Increase fluid intake (decreases lung secretion viscosity). Must be administered at regular intervals (even when symptom free) to achieve optimal results of therapy. Unpleasant taste after inhalation may be relieved by rinsing mouth with water immediately.

nefazodone hydrochloride

nef-**ah**-zoh-doan
(<u>Serzone</u>)

▶CLASSIFICATION

CLINICAL: Antidepressant (see p. 36C)

ACTION/*THERAPEUTIC EFFECT*

Exact mechanism unknown. Appears to inhibit neuronal uptake of serotonin and norepinephrine, antagonize alpha$_1$-adrenergic receptors, *producing antidepressant effect.*

PHARMACOKINETICS

Rapidly, completely absorbed from GI tract. Protein binding: >99%. Food delays absorption. Widely distributed in body tissues, including CNS. Extensively metabolized to active metabolites. Excreted in urine and eliminated in feces. Unknown if removed by hemodialysis. Half-life: 2–4 hrs.

USES

Treatment of depression exhibited as persistent, prominent dysphoria (occurring nearly every day for at least 2 wks) manifested by 4 of 8 symptoms: change in appetite, change in sleep pattern, increased fatigue, impaired concentration, feelings of guilt or worthlessness, loss of interest in usual activities, psychomotor agitation or retardation, or suicidal tendencies. Maintenance treatment for prevention of relapse of acute depressive episode.

PRECAUTIONS

CONTRAINDICATIONS: Within 14 days of MAO inhibitor ingestion, coadministration with astemizole, cisapride, or terfenadine therapy. **CAUTIONS:** Recent MI, unstable heart disease, hepatic cirrhosis, dehydration, hypovolemia, cerebrovascular disease, history of mania/hypomania, history of seizures.

▷**LIFESPAN CONSIDERATIONS:**
Pregnancy/Lactation: Unknown if drug crosses placenta or is distributed in breast milk. **Pregnancy Category C. Children:** Safety and efficacy not established. **Elderly:** No age-related precautions noted; lower dosage recommended.

INTERACTIONS

DRUG: May increase concentration, toxicity of **alprazolam triazolam** (dosage reduction advised). **MAOIs** may produce severe reactions (see Adverse Reactions/Toxic Effects). At least 14 days should elapse between discontinuing MAO inhibitors and initiation of nefazodone therapy. At least 7 days should elapse after discontinuing nefazodone and initiation of MAO inhibitor therapy. **HERBAL:** St. John's **wort** may increase risk of adverse effects. **FOOD:** None known. **LAB VALUES:** None significant.

AVAILABILITY (Rx)

TABLETS: 100 mg, 150 mg, 200 mg, 250 mg.

ADMINISTRATION/HANDLING
PO:

• Give without regard to meals.

INDICATIONS/ROUTES/DOSAGE
Note: At least 14 days should elapse between discontinuing MAO inhibitors and initiation of nefazodone therapy. At least 7 days should elapse after discontinuing nefazodone and initiation of MAO inhibitor therapy.

Depression, prevention of relapse of acute episode:

PO: Adults: Initially, 200 mg/day, given in two divided doses. Gradually increase dose in increments of 100–200 mg/day on a twice daily schedule, at intervals of at least 1 wk. **Elderly:** Initially, 100 mg/day on a twice daily schedule. Adjust the rate of subsequent dose titration based on clinical response. **Range:** 300–600 mg/day.

SIDE EFFECTS

Elderly/debilitated experience increased susceptibility to side effects. **FREQUENT:** Headache (36%), dry mouth, somnolence (25%), nausea (22%), dizziness (17%), constipation (14%), insomnia, asthenia (loss of strength, energy), lightheadedness (10%). **OCCASIONAL:** Dyspepsia, blurred vision (9%), diarrhea, infection (8%), confusion, abnormal vision (7%), pharyngitis (6%), increased appetite (5%), postural hypotension, vasodilation (flushing, feeling of warmth) (4%), peripheral edema, cough, flu syndrome (3%).

ADVERSE REACTIONS/TOXIC EFFECTS

Concurrent MAO inhibitor administration or if time frame between discontinuation and initiation of drug therapy (see Indications/Routes/Dosage) is not followed, serious reactions (hyperthermia, rigidity, myoclonus, extreme agitation, delirium, coma) occur. Coadministration with astemizole or terfenadine therapy may produce serious cardiovascular abnormalities.

NURSING IMPLICATIONS

BASELINE ASSESSMENT:
Question for history of sensitivity to nefazodone or trazodone, other

N

medication (esp. alprazolam, MAOIs, terfenadine, triazolam). Obtain history of cardiovascular or cerebrovascular disease, mania/hypomania, seizures.

INTERVENTION/EVALUATION:

Supervise suicidal risk pt closely during early therapy (as energy level improves, suicide potential increases). Assess appearance, behavior, speech pattern, level of interest, mood. Assist with ambulation if dizziness, lightheadedness occurs. Monitor stool frequency and consistency.

PATIENT/FAMILY TEACHING:

Maximum therapeutic response may require several wks of therapy. Dry mouth may be relieved by sugarless gum, sips of tepid water. Report headache, nausea, visual disturbances. Avoid tasks that require alertness, motor skills until response to drug is established. Avoid alcohol.

nelfinavir

nell-**fine**-ah-veer
(Viracept)

▶CLASSIFICATION

PHARMACOTHERAPEUTIC:
Protease inhibitor. ***CLINICAL:***
Antiviral (see pp. 58C, 96C)

ACTION/*THERAPEUTIC EFFECT*

Inhibits activity of HIV-1 protease, the enzyme necessary for the formation of infectious HIV, resulting in formation of immature noninfectious viral particles rather than HIV replication.

PHARMACOKINETICS

Well absorbed following PO admin-istration. Protein binding: >98%. Absorption increased with food. Metabolized by the liver. Highly bound to plasma proteins. Eliminated primarily in feces. Unknown if removed by hemodialysis. Half-life: 3.5–5 hrs.

USES

Treatment of HIV infection when antiretoviral therapy is warranted.

PRECAUTIONS

CONTRAINDICATIONS: Concurrent administration with midazolam, triazolam, rifampin. ***CAUTIONS:*** Hepatic function impairment.
▷***LIFESPAN CONSIDERATIONS:***
Pregnancy/Lactation: Unknown if distributed in breast milk. **Pregnancy Category B. Children:** No age-related precautions noted in those >2 yrs of age. **Elderly:** No information available.

INTERACTIONS

DRUG: **Alcohol, psychoactive drugs** may produce additive CNS effects. **Anticonvulsants, rifampin, rifabutin** lower nelfinavir plasma concentration. Increase **indinavir, saquinavir** plasma concentration. **Ritonavir** increases nelfinavir plasma concentration. Decreases effects of **oral contraceptives.** ***HERBAL:*** **St. John's wort** may decrease concentrations, effect. ***FOOD:*** **Food** increases plasma concentration. ***LAB VALUES:*** May decrease hemoglobin, WBCs, neutrophils; increase SGOT (AST), SGPT (ALT), creatine kinase.

AVAILABILITY (Rx)

TABLETS: 250 mg. ***POWDER:*** 50 mg/g.

ADMINISTRATION/HANDLING
PO:

• Give with food (light meal or

snack). • Mix oral powder with small amount of water, milk, formula, soy formula, soy milk, or dietary supplement. • Entire contents must be consumed in order to ingest full dose. • Do not mix with acidic food, orange juice, apple juice or applesauce (bitter taste), or with water in its original container.

INDICATIONS/ROUTES/DOSAGE
HIV infection:
PO: **Adults:** 750 mg (three 250 mg tablets) 3 times/day, or 1,250 mg 2 times/day in combination with nucleoside analogues (enhances antiviral activity). **Children 2–13 yrs:** 20–30 mg/kg/dose, 3 times daily. **Maximum:** 750 mg q8h.

SIDE EFFECTS
FREQUENT (20%): Diarrhea. *OC-CASIONAL* (3–7%): Nausea, rash. *RARE* (1–2%): Flatulence, asthenia.

ADVERSE REACTIONS/TOXIC EFFECTS
None significant.

NURSING IMPLICATIONS

BASELINE ASSESSMENT:
Check hematology, liver function tests for accurate baseline.

INTERVENTION/EVALUATION:
Determine pattern of bowel activity and stool consistency. Monitor liver enzyme studies for abnormalities. Be alert to development of opportunistic infections, (e.g., fever, chills, cough, myalgia).

PATIENT/FAMILY TEACHING:
Take with food (optimizes absorption). Take medication every day as prescribed. Doses should be evenly spaced around the clock. Do not alter dose or

discontinue medication without informing physician. Medication is not a cure for HIV infection, and pt may continue to experience illnesses, including opportunistic infections, nor does it reduce risk of transmission to others. Diarrhea can be controlled with OTC medication.

neomycin sulfate

nee-oh-**my**-sin
(Mycifradin, Myciguent)

FIXED-COMBINATION(S)
With polymyxin B, an anti-infective **(Neosporin, Neosporin G.U. Irrigant);** with polymyxin B and bacitracin, an antibiotic **(Mycitracin, Neosporin, Neo-Polycin);** with polymyxin B and hydrocortisone, a steroid **(Cortisporin);** with gicidin, an anti-infective **(Spectrocin)**

▶CLASSIFICATION

PHARMACOTHERAPEUTIC: Aminoglycoside. *CLINICAL:* Antibiotic (see p. 17C)

ACTION/*THERAPEUTIC EFFECT*
Binds to bacterial microorganisms by *interfering with protein synthesis.*

USES
Preparation of GI tract for surgery. Treatment of minor skin infections, diarrhea caused by *E. coli.* Adjunct in treatment of hepatic encephalopathy.

PRECAUTIONS
CONTRAINDICATIONS: Hypersensitivity to aminoglycosides. *CAUTIONS:* Elderly, infants with renal insufficiency/immaturity; neu-

N

romuscular disorders, prior hearing loss, vertigo, renal impairment.

INTERACTIONS

DRUG: If significant systemic absorption occurs, may increase nephrotoxicity, ototoxicity with aminoglycosides, other nephrotoxic, ototoxic medications. **HERBAL:** None known. **FOOD:** None known. **LAB VALUES:** None significant.

INDICATIONS/ROUTES/DOSAGE

Preop bowel antisepsis:

PO: Adults, elderly: 1 g each hr for 4 h doses; then 1 g q4h for 5 doses or 1 g at 1 PM, 2 PM, 10 PM (with erythromycin) on day prior to surgery. **Children:** 90 mg/kg/day in divided doses q4h for 2 days or 25 mg/kg at 1 PM, 2 PM, 10 PM on day prior to surgery.

Hepatic encephalopathy:

PO: Adults, elderly: 4–12 g/day in divided doses q4–6h. **Children:** 2.5–7 g/m^2/day in divided doses q4–6h.

Diarrhea caused by *E. coli:*

PO: Adults, elderly: 3 g/day in divided doses q6h. **Children:** 50 mg/kg/day in divided doses q6h.

Usual topical dosage:

Adults, elderly, children: Apply 1–3 times/day.

SIDE EFFECTS

FREQUENT: Systemic: Nausea, vomiting, diarrhea, irritation of mouth/rectal area. **Ophthalmic:** Hypersensitivity (itching, rash, redness, swelling). **Ophthalmic/Topical:** Itching, redness, swelling, rash. **OCCASIONAL: Ophthalmic:** Itching, burning, redness. **RARE: Systemic:** Malabsorption syndrome, neuromuscular blockade (drowsiness, weakness, difficulty breathing).

ADVERSE REACTIONS/TOXIC EFFECTS

Nephrotoxicity (evidenced by increased BUN and serum creatinine, decreased creatinine clearance) may be reversible if drug stopped at first sign of symptoms; irreversible ototoxicity (tinnitus, dizziness, ringing/roaring in ears, reduced hearing) and neurotoxicity (headache, dizziness, lethargy, tremors, visual disturbances) occur occasionally. Severe respiratory depression, anaphylaxis occur rarely. Superinfections, particularly with fungi, may occur.

NURSING IMPLICATIONS

BASELINE ASSESSMENT:

Dehydration must be treated before aminoglycoside therapy. Establish pt's baseline hearing acuity before beginning therapy.

INTERVENTION/EVALUATION:

Be alert to ototoxic and neurotoxic symptoms (see Adverse Reactions/Toxic Effects). Assess for hypersensitivity reaction (**ophthalmic**—assess for redness, burning, itching, tearing; **topical**—assess for rash, redness, itching). Be alert for superinfection, particularly genital/anal pruritus, changes of oral mucosa, diarrhea.

PATIENT/FAMILY TEACHING:

Continue antibiotic for full length of treatment. Space doses evenly. **Ophthalmic:** Blurred vision or tearing may occur briefly after application. **Topical:** Cleanse area gently before application; report redness, itching.

---

neostigmine bromide

nee-oh-**stig**-meen
(Prostigmin [oral])
Do not confuse with physostigmine.

neostigmine methylsulfate

(Prostigmin [parenteral])

▶CLASSIFICATION

PHARMACOTHERAPEUTIC:
Cholinergic. ***CLINICAL:*** Antimyasthenic, antidote (see p. 77C)

ACTION/*THERAPEUTIC EFFECT*
Prevents destruction of acetylcholine by attaching to enzyme, anticholinesterase. *Improves intestinal/skeletal muscle tone, increases secretions, salivation.*

USES
Improvement of muscle strength in control of myasthenia gravis, to diagnose myasthenia gravis, prevention/treatment of postop distention and urinary retention, as antidote for reversal of effects of nondepolarizing neuromuscular blocking agents after surgery.

PRECAUTIONS
CONTRAINDICATIONS: Concurrent use of high doses of halothane, cyclopropane, mechanical GI or GU obstruction, peritonitis, doubtful bowel viability. ***CAUTIONS:*** Bronchial asthma, bradycardia, epilepsy, coronary occlusion, vagotonia, hyperthyroidism, cardiac arrhythmias, peptic ulcer.

INTERACTIONS
DRUG: **Anticholinergics** reverse/prevent effects. **Cholinesterase in-** **hibitors** may increase toxicity. Antagonizes neuromuscular blocking agents. **Quinidine, procainamide** may antagonize action. ***HERBAL:*** None known. ***FOOD:*** None known. ***LAB VALUES:*** None significant.

INDICATIONS/ROUTES/DOSAGE
Myasthenia gravis:

PO: Adults, elderly: Initially, 15–30 mg 3–4 times/day. Increase as necessary. **Usual maintenance dose:** 150 mg/day (range of 15–375 mg). **Children:** 0.33 mg/kg/dose or 10 mg/m^2/dose 6 times/day

***SUBQ/IM/IV:* Adults:** 0.5–2.5 mg as needed. **Children:** 0.01–0.04 mg/kg q2–4h.

Diagnosis of myasthenia gravis:

Note: Discontinue all anticholinesterase therapy at least 8 hrs before testing. Give 0.011 mg/kg atropine sulfate IV simultaneously with neostigmine or IM 30 min before administering neostigmine (prevents adverse effects).

***IM:* Adults, elderly:** 0.022 mg/kg. If cholinergic reaction occurs, discontinue tests and administer 0.4–0.6 mg or more atropine sulfate IV. **Children:** 0.025–0.04 mg/kg IM preceded by atropine sulfate 0.011 mg/kg SubQ.

Prevention of postop urinary retention:

***SUBQ/IM:* Adults, elderly:** 0.25 mg q4–6h for 2–3 days.

Postop distention, urinary retention:

***SUBQ/IM:* Adults, elderly:** 0.5–1 mg. Catheterize if voiding does not occur within 1 hr. After voiding, continue 0.5 mg q3h for 5 injections.

Reversal of neuromuscular blockade:

***IV:* Adults, elderly:** 0.5–2.5 mg given slowly.

N

SIDE EFFECTS

FREQUENT: Muscarinic effects (diarrhea, increased sweating/watering of mouth, nausea, vomiting, stomach cramps/pain). **OCCASIONAL:** Muscarinic effects (increased frequency/urge to urinate, increased bronchial secretions, unusually small pupils/watering of eyes).

ADVERSE REACTIONS/TOXIC EFFECTS

Overdose produces a cholinergic reaction manifested as abdominal discomfort/cramping, nausea, vomiting, diarrhea, flushing, feeling of warmth/heat about face, excessive salivation and sweating, lacrimation, pallor, bradycardia/tachycardia, hypotension, urinary urgency, blurred vision, bronchospasm, pupillary contraction, involuntary muscular contraction visible under the skin (fasciculation).

NURSING IMPLICATIONS

BASELINE ASSESSMENT:
Larger doses should be given at time of greatest fatigue. Avoid large doses in those with megacolon or reduced GI motility.

INTERVENTION/EVALUATION:
Monitor for therapeutic response to medication (increased muscle strength, decreased fatigue, improved chewing, swallowing functions).

PATIENT/FAMILY TEACHING:
Report nausea, vomiting, diarrhea, sweating, increased salivary secretions, irregular heartbeat, muscle weakness, severe abdominal pain, or difficulty in breathing.

nesiritide

ness-**ear**-ih-tide
(Natrecor)

▶CLASSIFICATION
PHARMACOTHERAPEUTIC:
Brain natriuretic peptide. **CLINICAL:** Endogenous hormone

ACTION/*THERAPEUTIC EFFECT*

Facilitates cardiovascular homeostasis and fluid status through counter-regulation of the renin-angiotensin-aldosterone system, stimulating cyclic guanosine monophosphate, leading to smooth muscle cell relaxation and *promoting vasodilation, natriuresis, and diuresis, correcting CHF.*

PHARMACOKINETICS

	Onset	Peak	Duration
IV	15–30 min	1–2 hrs	4 hrs

Excreted primarily in the heart by the left ventricle. Metabolized by the natriuretic neutral endopeptidase enzymes on the vascular luminal surface. Half-life: 18–23 min.

USES

Treatment of acutely decompensated congestive heart failure (CHF) in pts who have dyspnea at rest or with minimal activity.

PRECAUTIONS

CONTRAINDICATIONS: Systolic B/P less than 90 mmHg, cardiogenic shock. **CAUTIONS:** Significant valvular stenosis, restrictive or obstructive cardiomyopathy, constrictive pericarditis, pericardial tamponade, suspected low cardiac filling pressures, atrial, ventricular arrhythmias/conduction defects, hypotension, hepatic/renal insufficiency.

▷*LIFESPAN CONSIDERATIONS:*
Pregnancy/Lactation: Unknown if drug crosses placenta or is distributed in breast milk. **Pregnancy Category C. Children:** Safety and efficacy not established. **Elderly:** No age-related precautions noted.

INTERACTIONS

DRUG: **IV nitroglycerin, angiotensin-converting enzyme (ACE) inhibitors, milrinone, nitroprusside** may increase risk of hypotension. *HERBAL:* None significant. *FOOD:* None significant. *LAB VALUES:* None significant.

AVAILABILITY (Rx)

POWDER FOR INJECTION: 1.5 mg/vial.

ADMINISTRATION/HANDLING

Note: Do not mix with other injections or infusions. Do not give IM.

IV 📷

Storage:
• Store vial at room temperature. Once reconstituted, use within 24 hrs at room temperature or refrigerated.

Reconstitution:
• Reconstitute one 1.5 mg vial with 5 ml D_5W or 0.9% NaCl, 0.2% NaCl or any combination thereof. Swirl or rock gently, and add to 250 ml bag ml D_5W or 0.9% NaCl, 0.2% NaCl or any combination thereof yielding a solution of 6 mcg/ml.

Rate of administration:
• Give as an IV bolus over approximately 60 seconds initially followed by continuous IV infusion.

IV INCOMPATIBILITIES ⊘

Sodium metabisulfite, bumetanide (Bumex), enalapril (Vasotec), ethacrynic acid (Edecrin), fusosemide (Lasix), heparin, hydralazine (Apresoline), insulin.

INDICATIONS/ROUTES/DOSAGE
CHF:

IV BOLUS: **Adults, elderly:** 2 mcg/kg followed by a continuous IV infusion of 0.01 mcg/kg/min. May be incrementally increased every 3 hrs to a maximum of 0.03 mcg/kg/min.

SIDE EFFECTS

FREQUENT (11–35%): Hypotension. *OCCASIONAL* (18–15%): Headache, nausea, bradycardia. *RARE* (≤1%): Confusion, paresthesia, somnolence, tremor.

ADVERSE REACTIONS/TOXIC EFFECTS

Ventricular arrhythmias (ventricular tachycardia, atrial fibrillation, atrial-ventricular node conduction abnormalities), angina pectoris occur rarely.

N

NURSING IMPLICATIONS

BASELINE ASSESSMENT:
Obtain B/P immediately before each dose, in addition to regular monitoring (be alert to fluctuations). If excessive reduction in B/P occurs, place pt in supine position with legs elevated.

INTERVENTION/EVALUATION:
B/P readings, pulse rate should be frequently monitored for hypotension during therapy. With physician, establish parameters for adjusting rate or stopping infusion. Maintain accurate I&O; measure urine output frequently.

Immediately notify physician of decreased urine output, cardiac arrhythmias, significant decrease in B/P or heart rate.

netilmicin sulfate

(Netromycin)

See Classification section under: Antibiotics: aminoglycosides (p. 17C)

nevirapine

neh-**vear**-ah-peen
(Viramune)

▶CLASSIFICATION

PHARMACOTHERAPEUTIC: Non-nucleoside reverse transcriptase inhibitor. **CLINICAL:** Antiviral (see pp. 58C, 96C)

ACTION/*THERAPEUTIC EFFECT*

Binds directly to virus type 1 (HIV-1) reverse transcriptase (RT), blocking RNA and DNA-dependent DNA polymerase activity (changes the shape of RT enzyme), *slowing HIV replication, reducing progression of HIV infection.*

PHARMACOKINETICS

Readily absorbed following PO administration (unaffected by food). Protein binding: 60%. Widely distributed. Extensively metabolized in liver; primarily excreted in urine.

USES/*UNLABELED*

Used in combination with nucleoside analogues or protease inhibitors for treatment of HIV-1 infected adults who have experienced clinical and immunologic deterioration. *Reduces risk of transmitting HIV from infected mother to newborn.*

PRECAUTIONS

CONTRAINDICATIONS: None significant. **CAUTIONS:** Renal or hepatic function impairment.

▷**LIFESPAN CONSIDERATIONS:** **Pregnancy/Lactation:** Crosses placenta, distributed in breast milk. Breast feeding not recommended (possibility of HIV transmission). **Pregnancy Category C. Children:** Granulocytopenia occurs more frequently. **Elderly:** No information available.

INTERACTIONS

DRUG: May decrease **ketoconazole, protease inhibitors, oral contraceptives,** plasma concentration. **Rifabutin, rifampin** may decrease concentration. **HERBAL: St. John's wort** may decrease concentrations, effects. **FOOD:** None known. **LAB VALUES:** May significantly increase SGPT (ALT), SGOT (AST), bilirubin, GGT. May significantly decrease hemoglobin, platelets, neutrophil count.

AVAILABILITY (Rx)

TABLETS: 200 mg. **ORAL SUSPENSION:** 50 mg/5 ml.

ADMINISTRATION/HANDLING
PO:

• Give without regard to meals.

INDICATIONS/ROUTES/DOSAGE

Note: Always administer nevirapine in combination with at least one additional antiretroviral agent (resistant HIV virus appears rapidly when nevirapine is given as monotherapy).

HIV-1 infection:

PO: Adults: 200 mg daily for 14 days (reduces risk of rash). **Maintenance:** 200 mg twice daily in combination with nucleoside analogue antiretroviral agents. **Children, 2 mos–8 yrs:** 4 mg/kg once daily for 14 days; then 7 mg/kg 2 times/day. **Children >8 yrs:** 4 mg/kg once daily for 14 days; then 4 mg/kg 2 times/day. **Maximum:** 400 mg/day.

SIDE EFFECTS

FREQUENT (3–8%): Rash, fever, headache, nausea. ***OCCASIONAL*** (1–3%): Stomatitis (burning/erythema of oral mucosa, mucosal ulceration, difficulty swallowing). ***RARE*** (<1%): Paresthesia, myalgia, abdominal pain.

ADVERSE REACTIONS/TOXIC EFFECTS

Rash may become severe and life threatening. Hepatitis occurs rarely.

NURSING IMPLICATIONS

BASELINE ASSESSMENT:

Establish baseline lab values, esp. liver function tests, prior to initiating therapy and at intervals during therapy. Obtain medication history (esp. use of oral contraceptives).

INTERVENTION/EVALUATION:

Closely monitor for evidence of rash (usually appears on trunk, face, and extremities; occurs within first 6 wks of drug initiation). Observe for rash accompanied by fever, blistering, oral lesions, conjunctivitis, swelling, muscle or joint aches, general malaise.

PATIENT/FAMILY TEACHING:

If nevirapine therapy is missed for more than 7 days, restart by using one 200 mg tablet daily for first 14 days, followed by one 200 mg tablet twice daily. Continue therapy for full length of treatment. Doses should be evenly spaced. Nevirapine is not a cure for HIV infection, nor does it reduce risk of transmission to others. If rash appears, contact physician before continuing therapy.

niacin, nicotinic acid

(Niacor, Niaspan, Nicobid, Nico-400, Nicotinex)
Do not confuse with Nitro-bid.

▶CLASSIFICATION

CLINICAL: Antihyperlipidemic, water-soluble vitamin (see pp. 50C, 128C)

N

ACTION/*THERAPEUTIC EFFECT*

Inhibits free fatty acid release in fat tissue, decreases rate of VLDL, LDL synthesis in liver, increases lipoprotein lipase activity. Component of coenzymes that are necessary for *lipid metabolism, tissue respiration, and glycogenolysis. Lowers serum cholesterol and triglycerides (decreases LDL, VLDL, increases HDL).*

PHARMACOKINETICS

Readily absorbed from GI tract. Widely distributed. Metabolized in liver. Primarily excreted in urine. Half-life: 45 min.

USES

Adjunct to diet therapy to decrease elevated serum cholesterol and triglyceride concentrations (elevated LDL, VLDL in treatment of Type II, III, IV, or V hyperlipoproteinemia). *Extended-release tablets:* Increases HDL cholesterol, prevention and treatment of vitamin B_3 deficiency states (i.e., pellagra).

PRECAUTIONS

CONTRAINDICATIONS: Hypersensitivity to niacin or tartrazine (frequently seen in pts sensitive to aspirin), active peptic ulcer, severe hypotension, hepatic dysfunction, arterial hemorrhaging. *CAUTIONS:* Diabetes mellitus, gallbladder disease, gout, history of jaundice or liver disease.

▷*LIFESPAN CONSIDERATIONS:* **Pregnancy/Lactation:** Not recommended for use during pregnancy/lactation. Distributed in breast milk. **Pregnancy Category A** (Category C if used in doses above RDA). **Children:** No age-related precautions noted. Not recommended in those <2 yrs of age. **Elderly:** No age-related precautions noted.

INTERACTIONS

DRUG: **Lovastatin, pravastatin, simvastatin** may increase risk of rhabdomyolysis and acute renal failure. *HERBAL:* None known. *FOOD:* None known. *LAB VALUES:* May increase uric acid.

AVAILABILITY (OTC)

TABLETS: 25 mg, 50 mg, 100 mg, 250 mg, 500 mg. *TABLETS (timed-release):* 250 mg, 500 mg, 750 mg, 1,000 mg. *CAPSULES (timed-release):* 125 mg, 250 mg, 300 mg, 400 mg, 500 mg. *ELIXIR:* 50 mg/5 ml. *INJECTION: (Rx):* 100 mg/ml.

ADMINISTRATION/HANDLING
PO:

• Give without regard to meals. • Take at bedtime, avoid alcohol.

INDICATIONS/ROUTES/DOSAGE
Hyperlipidemia:

PO: **Adults, elderly:** *(immediate-release):* Initially, 50–100 mg 2 times/day for 7 days. Increase gradually by doubling dose qwk up to 1–1.5 g/day in 2–3 doses. **Maximum:** 3 g/day. **Children:** Initially, 100–250 mg/day (**Maximum:** 10 mg/kg/day) in 3 divided doses. May increase by 100 mg/wk or 250 mg q2–3wks. **Maximum:** 2,250 mg/day.

(Extended-release): Initially, 500 mg/day in divided doses 2 times/day for 1 wk; then increase to 500 mg 2 times/day. **Maintenance:** 2 g/day.

Nutritional supplement:

PO: **Adults, elderly:** 10–20 mg/day.

SIDE EFFECTS

FREQUENT: Flushing (esp. of face, neck) occurring within 20 min of administration and lasting for 30–60 min, GI upset, pruritus. *OCCASIONAL:* Dizziness, hypotension, headache, blurred vision, burning or tingling of skin, flatulence, nausea, vomiting, diarrhea. *RARE:* Hyperglycemia, glycosuria, rash, hyperpigmentation, dry skin.

ADVERSE REACTIONS/TOXIC EFFECTS

Cardiac arrhythmias occur rarely.

NURSING IMPLICATIONS

BASELINE ASSESSMENT:

Question for history of hypersensitivity to niacin, tartrazine, or aspirin. Assess baselines: cholesterol, triglyceride, blood glucose, liver function tests.

INTERVENTION/EVALUATION:

Evaluate flushing and degree of discomfort. Check for headache, dizziness, blurred vision. Determine pattern of bowel activity. Monitor liver function, cholesterol, triglycerides. Check blood glucose levels carefully in those on insulin or oral antihyperglycemics. Assess skin for rash, dryness.

PATIENT/FAMILY TEACHING:

If dizziness occurs, avoid sudden posture changes and activities that require steady/alert response. Flushing may decrease with continued therapy; however, discuss considerable discomfort with physician.

nicardipine hydrochloride

nigh-**car**-dih-peen
(Cardene, Cardene SR)
Do not confuse with Cardizem SR, codeine, nifedipine.

▶CLASSIFICATION

PHARMACOTHERAPEUTIC: Calcium channel blocker. *CLINICAL:* Antianginal, antihypertensive (see p. 66C)

ACTION/THERAPEUTIC EFFECT

Inhibits calcium ion movement across cell membrane, depressing contraction of cardiac and vascular smooth muscle. *Increases heart rate, cardiac output. Decreases systemic vascular resistance, B/P.*

PHARMACOKINETICS

	Onset	Peak	Duration
PO	—	1–2 hrs	8 hrs

Rapidly, completely absorbed from GI tract. Protein binding: >95%. Undergoes first-pass metabolism in liver. Metabolized in liver. Primarily excreted in urine. Not removed by hemodialysis. Half-life: 8.6 hrs.

USES/*UNLABELED*

PO: Treatment of chronic stable (effort-associated) angina or essential hypertension. *Sustained-release:* Treatment of essential hypertension. *Parenteral:* Short-term treatment of hypertension when oral therapy not feasible or desirable. *Treatment of vasospastic angina, Raynaud's phenomena, subarachnoid hemorrhage, associated neurologic deficits.*

PRECAUTIONS

CONTRAINDICATIONS: Severe hypotension, advanced aortic stenosis. *CAUTIONS:* Impaired renal, hepatic function.
▷*LIFESPAN CONSIDERATIONS:* **Pregnancy/Lactation:** Unknown whether distributed in breast milk. **Pregnancy Category C. Children:** Safety and efficacy not established. **Elderly:** Age-related renal impairment may require cautious use.

INTERACTIONS

DRUG: **Beta-blockers** may have additive effect. May increase **digoxin** concentration. **Procainamide, quinidine** may increase risk of QT interval prolongation. **Hypokalemia-producing agents** may increase risk of arrhythmias. *HERBAL:* None known. *FOOD:* **Grapefruit/grapefruit juice** may alter absorption. *LAB VALUES:* None significant.

AVAILABILITY (Rx)

CAPSULES: 20 mg, 30 mg. *CAP-*

N

SULES (sustained-release): 30 mg, 45 mg, 60 mg. *INJECTION:* 2.5 mg/ml.

ADMINISTRATION/HANDLING

PO:

• Do not crush or break oral, sustained-release capsules. • Give without regard to food.

IV 🏶

Storage:

• Store at room temperature. • Diluted IV solution is stable for 24 hrs at room temperature.

Reconstitution:

• Dilute each 25 mg ampule with 250 ml D_5W, 0.9% NaCl, 0.45% NaCl, or any combination thereof to provide a concentration of 1 mg/10 ml.

Rate of administration:

• Give by slow IV infusion. • Change IV site q12h if administered peripherally.

IV INCOMPATIBILITIES ⊘

Furosemide (Lasix), heparin, thiopental (Pentothal).

IV COMPATIBILITIES

Dobutamine (Dobutrex), dopamine (Intropin), epinephrine, labetalol (Normodyne, Trandate), lorazepam (Ativan), midazolam (Versed), milrinone (Primacor), nitroglycerin, norepinephrine (Levophed), vecuronium (Norcuron).

INDICATIONS/ROUTES/DOSAGE

Chronic stable angina:

PO: **Adults, elderly:** Initially, 20 mg 3 times/day. **Range:** 20–40 mg 3 times/day.

Essential hypertension:

PO: **Adults, elderly:** Initially, 20 mg 3 times/day. **Range:** 20–40 mg 3 times/day.

SUSTAINED-RELEASE: **Adults, elderly:** Initially, 30 mg 2 times/day. **Range:** 30–60 mg 2 times/day.

Dosage in liver impairment:

Initially, 20 mg 2 times/day, then titrate.

Dosage in renal impairment:

Initially, 20 mg q8h (30 mg 2 times/day sustained-release), then titrate.

Usual parenteral dosage: Substitute for oral nicardipine:

IV: **Adults, elderly:** 0.5 mg/hr (20 mg q8h); 1.2 mg/hr (30 mg q8h); 2.2 mg/hr (40 mg q8h).

Drug-free pt:

IV: **Adults, elderly:** *(gradual B/P decrease):* Initially, 5 mg/hr. May increase by 2.5 mg/hr q15min. *(rapid B/P decrease):* Initially, 5 mg/hr. May increase by 2.5 mg/hr q5min. **Maximum:** 15 mg/hr until desired B/P attained.

Note: After B/P goal achieved, decrease rate to 3 mg/hr.

Changing to oral antihypertensive therapy:

Begin 1 hr after IV discontinued; for nicardipine, give first dose 1 hr before discontinuing IV.

SIDE EFFECTS

FREQUENT (7–10%): Headache, facial flushing, peripheral edema, lightheadedness, dizziness. *OCCASIONAL* (3–6%): Asthenia (loss of strength, energy), palpitations, angina, tachycardia. *RARE* (<2%): Nausea, abdominal cramps, dyspepsia, dry mouth, rash.

ADVERSE REACTIONS/TOXIC EFFECTS

Overdosage manifested as confusion, slurred speech, drowsiness, marked hypotension, bradycardia.

NURSING IMPLICATIONS

BASELINE ASSESSMENT:

Concurrent therapy of sublingual nitroglycerin may be used for relief of anginal pain. Record onset, type (sharp, dull, squeezing), radiation, location, intensity, and duration of anginal pain, and precipitating factors (exertion, emotional stress).

INTERVENTION/EVALUATION:

Monitor B/P during and after IV infusion. Assess for peripheral edema behind medial malleolus (sacral area in bedridden pts). Assess skin for facial flushing, dermatitis, rash. Question for asthenia, headache. Monitor liver enzyme results. Assess EKG, pulse for tachycardia, palpitations.

PATIENT/FAMILY TEACHING:

Do not abruptly discontinue medication. Compliance with therapy regimen is essential to control anginal pain. To avoid hypotensive effect, rise slowly from lying to sitting position; wait momentarily before standing. Avoid tasks that require alertness, motor skills until response to drug is established. Contact physician/nurse if irregular heartbeat, shortness of breath, pronounced dizziness, or nausea occurs.

nicotine polacrilex

nick-oh-teen
(Nicorette)

nicotine transdermal system

(Habitrol, Nicoderm, Nicotrol)
Do not confuse with Nitroderm.

▶CLASSIFICATION

PHARMACOTHERAPEUTIC: Cholinergic-receptor agonist. **CLINICAL:** Smoking deterrent

ACTION

Produces autonomic effects by binding to acetylcholine receptors. Produces both stimulating and depressant effects on peripheral and central nervous systems; respiratory stimulant; low amounts increase heart rate, B/P; high doses may decrease B/P; may increase motor activity of GI smooth muscle. Nicotine produces psychological and physical dependence.

PHARMACOKINETICS

Not absorbed from GI tract. Protein binding: <5%. Absorption increased from buccal mucosa, well absorbed after topical administration. Metabolized in liver. Primarily excreted in urine. Half-life: 1–2 hrs.

USES

An alternative, less potent form of nicotine (without tar, carbon monoxide, carcinogenic substances of tobacco) used as part of a smoking cessation program.

PRECAUTIONS

CONTRAINDICATIONS: During immediate post-MI period, life-threatening arrhythmias, severe or worsening angina. **CAUTIONS:** Hyperthyroidism, pheochromocytoma, insulin-dependent diabetes mellitus, severe renal impairment, eczematous dermatitis, oral or pharyngeal inflammation, esophagitis, peptic ulcer (delays healing in peptic ulcer disease).
▷**LIFESPAN CONSIDERATIONS:**
Pregnancy/Lactation: Passes freely into breast milk. Use of ciga-

N

rettes or nicotine gum associated with decrease in fetal breathing movements. **Pregnancy Category X:** Nicotine polacrilex; **Pregnancy Category D:** Transdermal nicotine. **Children:** Not recommended. **Elderly:** Age-related decrease in cardiac function may require cautious use.

INTERACTIONS

DRUG: Smoking cessation may increase effects of **beta-adrenergic blockers, bronchodilators (e.g., theophylline), insulin, propoxyphene.** ***HERBAL:*** None known. ***FOOD:*** None known. ***LAB VALUES:*** None significant.

AVAILABILITY (OTC)

TRANSDERMAL: Habitrol (Rx): 7 mg/day, 14 mg/day, 21 mg/day. ***Nicoderm (OTC):*** 7 mg/day, 14 mg/day, 21 mg/day. ***Nicotrol (Rx):*** 5 mg/day, 10 mg/day; ***(OTC):*** 15 mg/day. ***CHEWING GUM (OTC):*** 2 mg, 4 mg squares. ***NASAL SPRAY (Rx). INHALER (Rx).***

ADMINISTRATION/HANDLING

Transdermal:

• Apply promptly upon removal from protective pouch (prevents evaporation, loss of nicotine). Use only intact pouch. • Apply only once/day to hairless, clean, dry skin on upper body or outer arm. • Replace daily at different sites; do not use same site within 7 days; do not use same patch >24 hrs. • Wash hands after applying patch. Wash with water alone (soap may increase nicotine absorption). • Discard used patch by folding patch in half (sticky side together), placing in pouch of new patch, and throwing away in such a way as to prevent child/pet accessibility.

Gum:

• Do not swallow. • Chew 1 piece whenever urge to smoke present. • Chew slowly/intermittently for 30 min. • Chew until distinctive nicotine taste (peppery) or slight tingling in mouth perceived, then stop; when tingling almost gone (about 1 min) repeat chewing procedure (this allows constant slow buccal absorption). • Too-rapid chewing may cause excessive release of nicotine, resulting in adverse effects similar to oversmoking (e.g., nausea, throat irritation).

Inhaler:

• Insert cartridge into mouthpiece. • Vigorously puff for 20 min.

INDICATIONS/ROUTES/DOSAGE

Smoking deterrent:

Note: Individualize dose; stop smoking immediately.

TRANSDERMAL: Adults, elderly: (Habitrol/Nicoderm): 21 mg/day for 6 wks; then 14 mg/day for 2 wks; then 7 mg/day for 2 wks.

GUM: Adults, elderly: Usually, 10–12 pieces/day. **Maximum:** 30 pieces/day.

NASAL SPRAY: Adults, elderly: (1 dose = 2 sprays = 1 mg) 1–2 doses/hr up to 40 doses/day.

INHALER: Adults, elderly: Puff on nicotine cartridge mouthpiece for about 20 min as needed.

SIDE EFFECTS

FREQUENT: Hiccups, nausea. ***Gum:*** Mouth or throat soreness, nausea, hiccups. ***Transdermal:*** Erythema, pruritus, burning at application site. ***OCCASIONAL:*** Eructation, GI upset, dry mouth, insomnia, sweating, irritability. ***Gum:*** Hiccups, hoarseness. ***Inhaler:*** Mouth/throat irritation, cough. ***RARE:*** Dizziness, muscle/joint pain.

ADVERSE REACTIONS/TOXIC EFFECTS

Overdose produces palpitations, tachyarrhythmias, convulsions, depression, confusion, profuse diaphoresis, hypotension, rapid/weak pulse, difficulty breathing. Lethal dose, adults: 40–60 mg. Death results from respiratory paralysis.

NURSING IMPLICATIONS

BASELINE ASSESSMENT:

Screen, evaluate those with coronary heart disease (history of MI, angina pectoris), serious cardiac arrhythmias, Buerger's disease, Prinzmetal's variant angina.

INTERVENTION/EVALUATION:

If increase in cardiovascular symptoms occurs, discontinue use. Assess all symptoms carefully with regard to method of medication (see Side Effects).

PATIENT/FAMILY TEACHING:

Review proper application and disposal of transdermal system. Gradually withdraw or stop nicotine gum usage <3 mos, transdermal nicotine after 4–8 wks of use, progressively decreasing dose q2–4wks. Do not eat or drink anything during or immediately before nicotine gum use (reduces salivary pH).

---

nifedipine 🖉

nye-**fed**-ih-peen
(<u>Adalat</u>, Apo-Nifed ♣, Nifedicol XL, Novonifedin ♣, <u>Procardia</u>)
Do not confuse with nicardipine.

▶ **CLASSIFICATION**

PHARMACOTHERAPEUTIC: Calcium channel blocker. ***CLINICAL:*** Antianginal, antihypertensive (see p.66C)

ACTION/THERAPEUTIC EFFECT

Inhibits calcium ion movement across cell membrane, depressing contraction of cardiac and vascular smooth muscle. *Increases heart rate, cardiac output. Decreases systemic vascular resistance, B/P.*

PHARMACOKINETICS

Onset	Peak	Duration
PO		
20 min	30–60 min	—

Rapidly, completely absorbed from GI tract. Protein binding: 92–98%. Undergoes first-pass metabolism in liver. Metabolized in liver. Primarily excreted in urine. Not removed by hemodialysis. Half-life: 2–5 hrs.

USES/UNLABELED

Treatment of angina due to coronary artery spasm (Prinzmetal's variant angina), chronic stable angina (effort-associated angina). ***Extended-release:*** Treatment of essential hypertension. *Treatment of Raynaud's phenomena.*

PRECAUTIONS

CONTRAINDICATIONS: Severe hypotension, advanced aortic stenosis. ***CAUTIONS:*** Impaired renal/hepatic function.
▷***LIFESPAN CONSIDERATIONS:***
Pregnancy/Lactation: Insignificant amount distributed in breast milk. **Pregnancy Category C. Children:** Safety and efficacy not established. **Elderly:** Age-related

N

---

renal impairment may require cautious use.

INTERACTIONS

DRUG:* Beta-blockers** may have additive effect. May increase **digoxin** concentration. **Hypokalemia-producing agents** may increase risk of arrhythmias. ***HERBAL: None known. ***FOOD:* Grapefruit/grapefruit juice** may increase plasma concentration. ***LAB VALUES:*** May cause positive ANA, direct Coomb's' test.

AVAILABILITY (Rx)

CAPSULES: 10 mg, 20 mg. ***TABLETS (extended-release):*** 30 mg, 60 mg, 90 mg.

ADMINISTRATION/HANDLING

PO:

* Do not crush or break film-coated tablet or sustained-release capsule. * Give without regard to meals. * Grapefruit juice may alter absorption.

Sublingual:

* Capsule must be punctured, chewed, and/or squeezed to express liquid into mouth.

INDICATIONS/ROUTES/DOSAGE

Note: May give 10–20 mg sublingual as needed for acute attacks of angina.

Prinzmetal's variant angina, chronic stable angina:

***PO:* Adults, elderly:** Initially, 10 mg 3 times/day. Increase at 7–14 day intervals. **Maintenance:** 10 mg 3 times/day up to 30 mg 4 times/day.

***EXTENDED-RELEASE:* Adults, elderly:** Initially, 30–60 mg/day. **Maintenance:** Up to 120 mg/day.

Hypertension:

***EXTENDED-RELEASE:* Adults, elderly:** Initially, 30–60 mg/day. **Maintenance:** Up to 120 mg/day.

SIDE EFFECTS

FREQUENT (11–30%): Peripheral edema, headache, flushed skin, dizziness. ***OCCASIONAL*** (6–12%): Nausea, shakiness, muscle cramps/pain, drowsiness, palpitations, nasal congestion, cough, dyspnea, wheezing. ***RARE*** (3–5%): Hypotension, rash, pruritus, urticaria, constipation, abdominal discomfort, flatulence, sexual difficulties.

ADVERSE REACTIONS/TOXIC EFFECTS

May precipitate CHF, MI in those with cardiac disease, peripheral ischemia. Overdose produces nausea, drowsiness, confusion, slurred speech.

NURSING IMPLICATIONS

BASELINE ASSESSMENT:

Concurrent therapy of sublingual nitroglycerin may be used for relief of anginal pain. Record onset, type (sharp, dull, squeezing), radiation, location, intensity, and duration of anginal pain, and precipitating factors (exertion, emotional stress). Check B/P for hypotension immediately before giving medication.

INTERVENTION/EVALUATION:

Assist with ambulation if lightheadedness, dizziness occurs. Assess for peripheral edema behind medial malleolus (sacral area in bedridden pts). Assess skin for flushing. Monitor liver enzyme tests.

PATIENT/FAMILY TEACHING:

Rise slowly from lying to sitting position and permit legs to dangle from bed momentarily before standing to reduce hypotensive effect. Contact physician/

nurse if irregular heartbeat, shortness of breath, pronounced dizziness, or nausea occurs. Avoid concomitant grapefruit/ juice use.

nilutamide

nih-**lute**-ah-myd
(Anandron✦, Nilandron)

▶CLASSIFICATION

PHARMACOTHERAPEUTIC: Hormone. **CLINICAL:** Antineoplastic (see p. 73C)

ACTION/*THERAPEUTIC EFFECT*
Competitively inhibits androgen action by binding to androgen receptors in target tissue. *Decreases growth of prostatic carcinoma.*

PHARMACOKINETICS
Rapidly absorbed. Protein binding: 84%. Metabolized in liver. Primarily excreted in urine. Half-life: 41–49 hrs.

USES
Treatment of metastatic prostatic carcinoma (stage D_2) in combination with surgical castration. For maximum benefit, begin on same day or day after surgical castration.

PRECAUTIONS
CONTRAINDICATIONS: Severe liver impairment, severe respiratory insufficiency. **CAUTIONS:** Hepatitis, marked increase in liver enzymes.

INTERACTIONS
DRUG: None significant. **HERBAL:** None known. **FOOD:** None known.

LAB VALUES: May increase SGOT (AST), SGPT (ALT), bilirubin, creatinine.

INDICATIONS/ROUTES/DOSAGE
Prostatic carcinoma:

PO: Adults, elderly: 300 mg once a day for 30 days, then 150 mg once a day. Begin on same day or day after surgical castration.

SIDE EFFECTS
FREQUENT (>10%): Hot flashes, delay in recovering vision after bright illumination (sun, television, bright lights), loss of libido, sexual potency, mild nausea, gynecomastia, alcohol intolerance. **OCCASIONAL** (<10%): Constipation, hypertension, dizziness, dyspnea, urinary tract infections.

ADVERSE REACTIONS/TOXIC EFFECTS
Interstitial pneumonitis occurs rarely.

N

NURSING IMPLICATIONS

BASELINE ASSESSMENT:
Baseline chest x-ray, hepatic enzyme levels should be obtained before therapy begins.

INTERVENTION/EVALUATION:
Monitor B/P periodically and hepatic function tests in long-term therapy.

PATIENT/FAMILY TEACHING:
Contact physician if any side effects occur at home, esp. signs of liver toxicity (jaundice, dark urine, fatigue, abdominal pain). Caution about driving at night (tinted glasses may help).

nimodipine

nih-**moad**-ih-peen
(Nimotop)

►CLASSIFICATION

PHARMACOTHERAPEUTIC:
Calcium channel blocker. **CLINICAL:** Cerebral vasospasm
agent (see p. 66C)

ACTION/THERAPEUTIC EFFECT

Inhibits movement of calcium ions
across cellular membranes in vascular smooth muscle. *Produces
favorable effect on severity of neurologic deficits due to cerebral vasospasm. Greatest effect on cerebral arteries; may prevent cerebral spasm.*

PHARMACOKINETICS

Rapidly absorbed from GI tract.
Protein binding: >95%. Metabolized in liver. Excreted in urine,
eliminated in feces. Not removed
by hemodialysis. Half-life: (terminal): 8–9 hrs.

USES/UNLABELED

Improvement of neurologic deficits
due to spasm following subarachnoid hemorrhage from ruptured
congenital intracranial aneurysms
in pts in good neurologic condition. *Treatment of chronic and classic migraine, chronic cluster headaches.*

PRECAUTIONS

CONTRAINDICATIONS: Severe
hypotension. **CAUTIONS:** Impaired renal/hepatic function.
▷**LIFESPAN CONSIDERATIONS:**
Pregnancy/Lactation: Unknown
if drug crosses placenta or is distributed in breast milk. **Pregnancy Category C. Children:**
Safety and efficacy not established. **Elderly:** Age-related renal
impairment may require cautious
use.

INTERACTIONS

DRUG: None significant. **HERBAL:**
None known. **FOOD:** None known.
LAB VALUES: None significant.

AVAILABILITY (Rx)

CAPSULES: 30 mg.

ADMINISTRATION/HANDLING

PO:

• If pt unable to swallow, place
hole in both ends of capsule with
18 gauge needle to extract contents into syringe. • Empty into
NG tube; flush tube with 30 ml
normal saline.

INDICATIONS/ROUTES/DOSAGE

Subarachnoid hemorrhage:

PO: Adults, elderly: 60 mg q4h
for 21 days. Begin within 96 hrs of
subarachnoid hemorrhage.

SIDE EFFECTS

OCCASIONAL (2–6%): Hypotension, peripheral edema, diarrhea,
headache. **RARE** (<2%): Allergic
reaction (rash, hives), tachycardia,
flushing of skin.

ADVERSE REACTIONS/TOXIC EFFECTS

Overdosage produces nausea,
weakness, dizziness, drowsiness,
confusion, slurred speech.

NURSING IMPLICATIONS

BASELINE ASSESSMENT:

Assess LOC, neurologic response, initially and throughout
therapy. Monitor baseline liver

---

function tests. Assess B/P, apical pulse immediately before drug is administered (if pulse is 60/min or below, or systolic B/P is below 90 mm Hg, withhold medication, contact physician).

INTERVENTION/EVALUATION:

Monitor pulse rate for bradycardia. Assess skin for dermatitis, rash, flushing. Monitor daily bowel activity and stool consistency. Assess for headache.

PATIENT/FAMILY TEACHING:

To avoid hypotensive effect, rise slowly from lying to sitting position; wait momentarily before standing. Contact physician/nurse if irregular heartbeat, shortness of breath, pronounced dizziness, or nausea occurs.

nisoldipine

(Sular)

See Classification section under: Calcium channel blockers

nitrofurantoin sodium

ny-tro-feur-**an**-twon
(Apo-Nitrofurantoin✦,
Furadantin, Furalan,
Macrodantin)

▶CLASSIFICATION

PHARMACOTHERAPEUTIC: Antibacterial. **CLINICAL:** Urinary tract prophylaxis

ACTION/*THERAPEUTIC EFFECT*

Bactericidal. Inactivates or alters bacterial ribosomal proteins, *producing bacteriostatic activity; bactericidal at high concentrations.*

PHARMACOKINETICS

Microcrystalline: rapidly, completely absorbed; macrocrystalline: more slowly absorbed. Food increases absorption. Protein binding: 40%. Primarily concentrated in urine, kidneys. Metabolized in most body tissues. Primarily excreted in urine. Removed by hemodialysis. Half-life: 20–60 min.

USES/*UNLABELED*

Treatment of urinary tract infections, initial and chronic. *Prophylaxis of bacterial UTIs.*

PRECAUTIONS

CONTRAINDICATIONS: Infants <1 mo of age because of hemolytic anemia, anuria, oliguria, substantial renal impairment (creatinine clearance <40 ml/min). ***CAUTIONS:*** Renal impairment, diabetes mellitus, electrolyte imbalance, anemia, vitamin B deficiency, debilitated (greater risk of peripheral neuropathy), glucose 6-phosphate dehydrogenase (G-6-PD) deficiency (greater risk of hemolytic anemia).
▷*LIFESPAN CONSIDERATIONS:*
Pregnancy/Lactation: Readily crosses placenta; distributed in breast milk. Contraindicated at term and during lactation when infant suspected of having G-6-PD deficiency. **Pregnancy Category B. Children:** No age-related precations noted in those >1 mo of age. **Elderly:** More likely to develop acute pneumonitis and pe-

N

ripheral neuropathy. Age-related renal impairment may require dosage adjustment.

INTERACTIONS

DRUG: Hemolytics may increase risk of toxicity. **Neurotoxic medications** may increase risk of neurotoxicity. **Probenecid** may increase concentration, toxicity. **HERBAL:** None known. **FOOD:** None known. **LAB VALUES:** None significant.

AVAILABILITY (Rx)

CAPSULES: 25 mg, 50 mg, 100 mg. **CAPSULES:** 100 mg (25 mg as macrocrystals/75 mg as microcrystals). **ORAL SUSPENSION:** 25 mg/5 ml.

ADMINISTRATION/HANDLING

PO:
• Give with food, milk to enhance absorption, reduce GI upset.

INDICATIONS/ROUTES/DOSAGE

Initial or recurrent urinary tract infection (UTI):

PO: Adults, elderly: 50–100 mg 4 times/day. **Maximum:** 400 mg/day. **Children >1 mo:** 5–7 mg/kg in 4 divided doses. **Maximum:** 400 mg/day.

Long-term prophylactic therapy of UTI:

PO: Adults, elderly: 50–100 mg as single evening dose. **Children:** 1–2 mg/kg in 1–2 divided doses.

SIDE EFFECTS

FREQUENT: Anorexia, nausea, vomiting, dark yellow or brown urine. **OCCASIONAL:** Abdominal pain, diarrhea, rash, pruritus, urticaria, hypertension, headache, dizziness, drowsiness. **RARE:** Photosensitivity, transient alopecia, asthmatic attack in those with history of asthma.

ADVERSE REACTIONS/TOXIC EFFECTS

Superinfection, hepatotoxicity, peripheral neuropathy (may be irreversible), Stevens-Johnson syndrome, permanent pulmonary function impairment, anaphylaxis occur rarely.

NURSING IMPLICATIONS

BASELINE ASSESSMENT:
Question for history of asthma. Evaluate lab test results for renal and hepatic baselines.

INTERVENTION/EVALUATION:
Monitor I&O, renal function results. Determine pattern of bowel activity. Assess skin for rash, urticaria. Be alert for numbness or tingling, esp. of lower extremities (may signal onset of peripheral neuropathy). Watch for signs of hepatotoxicity: fever, rash, arthralgia, hepatomegaly. Perform respiratory assessment: Auscultate lungs, check for cough, chest pain, difficulty breathing.

PATIENT/FAMILY TEACHING:
Urine may become dark yellow or brown. Take with food or milk for best results and to reduce GI upset. Complete full course of therapy. Avoid sun and ultraviolet light; use sunscreens, wear protective clothing. Notify physician if cough, fever, chest pain, difficult breathing, numbness/tingling of fingers or toes occurs. Rare occurrence of alopecia is transient.

nitroglycerin

nigh-trow-**glih**-sir-in
(Deponit, Minitran, Nitrek, Nitro-Bid, Nitro-Dur, Nitrogard, Nitroglyn, Nitrolingual, NitroQucik, Nitrostat, Transderm-Nitro, Tridil)
Do not confuse with Hyperstat, Nicobid, Nicoderm, Nilstat, nitroprusside, Nizoral, Nystatin.

▶CLASSIFICATION

PHARMACOTHERAPEUTIC: Nitrate. **CLINICAL:** Antianginal, antihypertensive, coronary vasodilator (see p. 104C)

ACTION/*THERAPEUTIC EFFECT*

Decreases myocardial O_2 demand. Reduces left ventricular preload and afterload. *Dilates coronary arteries, improves collateral blood flow to ischemic areas within myocardium.* **IV:** *Produces peripheral vasodilation.*

PHARMACOKINETICS

Onset	Peak	Duration
Sublingual		
2–5 min	4–8 min	30–60 min
Transmucosal tablet		
2–5 min	4–10 min	3–5 hrs
Extended-release		
20–45 min	—	3–8 hrs
Topical		
15–60 min	0.5–2 hrs	3–8 hrs
Patch		
30–60 min	1–3 hrs	8–12 hrs
IV		
1–2 min	—	3–5 min

Well absorbed after PO, sublingual, topical administration. Undergoes extensive first-pass metabolism. Metabolized in liver, enzymes in bloodstream. Primarily excreted in urine. Not removed by hemodialysis. Half-life: 1–4 min.

USES

Lingual/sublingual/buccal dose used for acute relief of angina pectoris. Extended-release, topical forms used for prophylaxis, long-term angina management. IV form used in treatment of CHF associated with acute MI.

PRECAUTIONS

CONTRAINDICATIONS: Hypersensitivity to nitrates, severe anemia, closed-angle glaucoma, postural hypotension, head trauma, increased intracranial pressure. **Sublingual:** Early MI. **Transdermal:** Allergy to adhesives. **Extended-release:** GI hypermotility/malabsorption, severe anemia. **IV:** Uncorrected hypovolemia, hypotension, inadequate cerebral circulation, constrictive pericarditis, pericardial tamponade. **CAUTIONS:** Acute MI, hepatic/renal disease, glaucoma (contraindicated in closed-angle glaucoma), blood volume depletion from diuretic therapy, systolic B/P below 90 mm Hg.

▷**LIFESPAN CONSIDERATIONS: Pregnancy/Lactation:** Unknown whether drug crosses placenta or is distributed in breast milk. **Pregnancy Category B. Children:** Safety and efficacy not established. **Elderly:** More susceptible to hypotensive effects. Age-related renal imapirment may require cautious use.

INTERACTIONS

DRUG: Alcohol, antihypertensives, vasodilators may increase risk of orthostatic hypotension. **HERBAL:** None known. **FOOD:**

N

None known. *LAB VALUES:* May increase methemoglobin, urine catecholamines, urine VMA.

AVAILABILITY (Rx)

TABLETS (sublingual): 0.4 mg. **SPRAY:** 0.4 mg/dose. **TABLETS (buccal, controlled-release):** 1 mg, 2 mg, 3 mg. **CAPSULES (sustained-release):** 2.5 mg, 6.5 mg, 9 mg. **TRANSDERMAL:** 0.1 mg/hr, 0.2 mg/hr, 0.3 mg/hr, 0.4 mg/hr, 0.6 mg/hr, 0.8 mg/hr. **TOPICAL OINT-MENT:** 2%. **INJECTION:** 5 mg/ml. **INJECTION SOLUTION:** 100 mcg/ml, 200 mcg/ml.

ADMINISTRATION/HANDLING

PO:

* Do not chew extended-release form. * Do not shake oral aerosol canister before lingual spraying.

Sublingual:

* Do not swallow; dissolve under the tongue. * Administer while seated. * Slight burning sensation under tongue may be lessened by placing tablet in buccal pouch. * Keep sublingual tablets in original container.

Topical:

* Spread thin layer on clean/dry/hairless skin of upper arm or body (not below knee or elbow), using applicator or dose-measuring papers. Do not use fingers; do not rub or massage into skin.

Transdermal:

* Apply patch on clean/dry/hairless skin of upper arm or body (not below knee or elbow).

IV

Storage:

* Store at room temperature.

Reconstitution:

* Available in ready to use injectable containers. * Dilute vials in 250 or 500 ml of D_5W or 0.9% NaCl. Maximum concentration: 250 mg/250 ml.

Rate of administration:

* Use microdrop or infusion pump.

IV INCOMPATIBILITY ⊘

Alteplase (Activase).

IV COMPATIBILITIES

Amiodarone (Cordarone), diltiazem (Cardizem), dobutamine (Dobutrex), dopamine (Intropin), epinephrine, heparin, insulin, labetalol (Normodyne, Trandate), lidocaine, lorazepam (Ativan), midazolam (Versed), milrinone (Primacor), nicardipine (Cardene), norepinephrine (Levophed), propofol (Diprivan), sodium nitroprusside (Nipride).

INDICATIONS/ROUTES/DOSAGE

Acute angina, acute prophylaxis:

LINGUAL SPRAY: Adults, elderly: 1 spray onto or under tongue q3–5min until relief is noted (no more than 3 sprays in 15 min period).

SUBLINGUAL: Adults, elderly: 0.4 mg q5min until relief is noted (no more than 3 doses in 15 min period). Use prophylactically 5–10 min before activities that may cause an acute attack.

Long-term prophylaxis of angina:

PO (extended-release): Adults, elderly: 2.5–9 mg q8–12h.

TOPICAL: Adults, elderly: Initially, ½ inch q8h. Increase by ½ inch with each application. **Range:** 1–2 inches q8h up to 4–5 inches q4h.

TRANSDERMAL PATCH: **Adults, elderly:** Initially, 0.2–0.4 mg/hr. **Maintenance:** 0.4–0.8 mg/hr. Consider patch on 12–14 hrs, patch off 10–12 hrs (prevents tolerance).

Usual parenteral dosage:

IV: **Adults, elderly:** Initially, 5 mcg/min via infusion pump. Increase in 5 mcg/min increments at 3–5 min intervals until B/P response is noted or until dosage reaches 20 mcg/min; then increase as needed by 10 mcg/min. Dosage may be further titrated according to pt, therapeutic response up to 200 mcg/min. **Children:** Initially, 0.25–0.5 mcg/kg/min; titrate by 0.5–1 mcg/kg/min up tp 20 mcg/kg/min.

SIDE EFFECTS

FREQUENT: Headache (may be severe) occurs mostly in early therapy, diminishes rapidly in intensity, usually disappears during continued treatment; transient flushing of face and neck, dizziness (esp. if pt is standing immobile or is in a warm environment), weakness, postural hypotension. *Sublingual:* Burning, tingling sensation at oral point of dissolution. *Ointment:* Erythema, pruritus. *OCCASIONAL:* GI upset. *Transdermal:* Contact dermatitis.

ADVERSE REACTIONS/TOXIC EFFECTS

Drug should be discontinued if blurred vision, dry mouth occurs. Severe postural hypotension manifested by fainting, pulselessness, cold/clammy skin, profuse sweating. Tolerance may occur with repeated, prolonged therapy (minor tolerance with intermittent use of sublingual tablets). High dose tends to produce severe headache.

NURSING IMPLICATIONS

BASELINE ASSESSMENT:

Record onset, type (sharp, dull, squeezing), radiation, location, intensity, and duration of anginal pain, and precipitating factors (exertion, emotional stress). Assess B/P and apical pulse before administration and periodically after dose. Pt must have continuous EKG monitoring for IV administration.

INTERVENTION/EVALUATION:

Assess for facial/neck flushing. Cardioverter/defibrillator must not be discharged through paddle electrode overlying nitroglycerin system (may cause burns to pt or damage to paddle via arcing).

PATIENT/FAMILY TEACHING:

Rise slowly from lying to sitting position and dangle legs momentarily before standing. Take oral form on empty stomach (however, if headache occurs during therapy, take medication with meals). Use inhalants only when lying down. Dissolve sublingual tablet under tongue; do not swallow. Take at first sign of angina. If not relieved within 5 min, dissolve second tablet under tongue. Repeat if no relief in another 5 min. If pain continues, contact physician or go immediately to emergency room. Do not change brands. Keep container away from heat, moisture. Do not inhale lingual aerosol but spray onto or under tongue (avoid swallowing after spray is administered). Expel from mouth any remaining lingual/sublingual/intrabuccal tablet after pain is completely relieved. Place transmucosal tablets under upper lip or buccal pouch (between cheek and gum); do not chew or swallow tablet. Avoid alcohol (intensifies hypotensive effect). If alcohol is ingested soon after taking nitroglycerin, possible acute hypotensive episode (marked drop in B/P, vertigo, pallor) may occur.

nitroprusside sodium

night-troe-**pruss**-eyd
(Nipride, Nitropress)
Do not confuse with nitroglycerin.

▶CLASSIFICATION

PHARMACOTHERAPEUTIC:
Hypertensive emergency agent.
CLINICAL: Antihypertensive, vasodilator, CHF/MI adjunct, antidote

ACTION/*THERAPEUTIC EFFECT*

Direct vasodilating action on arterial, venous smooth muscle. Decreases peripheral vascular resistance, preload, afterload, improves cardiac output. *Dilates coronary arteries, decreases O_2 consumption, relieves persistent chest pain.*

PHARMACOKINETICS

	Onset	Peak	Duration
IV	1–2 min	Dependent on infusion rate	Dissipates rapidly after stopping IV

Reacts with hemoglobin in erythrocytes, producing cyanmethemoglobin, cyanide ions. Primarily excreted in urine. Half-life: 2 min.

USES/*UNLABELED*

Immediate reduction of B/P in hypertensive crisis. Produces controlled hypotension in surgical procedures to reduce bleeding. Treatment of acute CHF. *Controls paroxysmal hypertension prior to/during surgery for pheochromocytoma; treatment adjunct for myocardial infarction, valvular regurgitation, peripheral vasospasm caused by ergot alkaloid overdose.*

PRECAUTIONS

CONTRAINDICATIONS: Compensatory hypertension (arteriovenous shunt or coarctation of aorta), inadequate cerebral circulation, moribund pts. **CAUTIONS:** Severe hepatic, renal impairment, hypothyroidism, hyponatremia, elderly.
▷**LIFESPAN CONSIDERATIONS:**
Pregnancy/Lactation: Unknown whether drug crosses placenta or is distributed in breast milk. **Pregnancy Category C. Children:** Safety and efficacy not established. **Elderly:** More sensitive to hypotensive effect. Age-related renal impairment may require cautious use.

INTERACTIONS

DRUG: Dobutamine may increase cardiac output, decrease pulmonary wedge pressure. **Hypotensive-producing medications** may increase hypotensive effect. **HERBAL:** None known. **FOOD:** None known. **LAB VALUES:** None significant.

AVAILABILITY (Rx)

POWDER FOR INJECTION: 50 mg.

ADMINISTRATION/HANDLING
IV 🏥
Storage:

• Protect solution from light. • Solution should appear very faint brown in color. • Use only freshly prepared solution. Once prepared, do not keep or use longer than 24 hrs. • Deterioration evidenced by color change from brown to blue, green, or dark red. • Discard unused portion.

Reconstitution:

• Reconstitute 50 mg vial with 2–3 ml D_5W or Sterile Water for Injection without preservative. • Further dilute with 250–1,000 ml of D_5W to provide concentration of 200 mcg, 50 mcg/ml, respectively. Maximum concentration: 200 mg/250 ml. • Wrap infusion bottle in aluminum foil immediately after mixing.

Rate of administration:

• Give by IV infusion only using infusion rate chart provided by manufacturer or protocol. • Administer using IV infusion pump or microdrip (60 gtt/ml). • Be alert for extravasation (produces severe pain, sloughing).

IV INCOMPATIBILITY $\oslash$

Cisatracurium (Nimbex).

IV COMPATIBILITIES

Diltiazem (Cardizem), dobutamine (Dobutrex), dopamine (Intropin), enalapril (Vasotec), heparin, insulin, labetalol (Normodyne, Trandate), lidocaine, midazolam (Versed), milrinone (Primacor), nitroglycerin, propofol (Diprivan).

INDICATIONS/ROUTES/DOSAGE

Usual parenteral dosage:

***IV:* Adults, elderly, children:** Initially, 0.3 mcg/kg/min. **Range:** 0.5–10 mcg/kg/min. Do not exceed 10 mcg/kg/min (risk of precipitous drop in B/P).

SIDE EFFECTS

OCCASIONAL: Flushing of skin, increased intracranial pressure, rash, pain/redness at injection site.

ADVERSE REACTIONS/TOXIC EFFECTS

A too-rapid IV rate reduces B/P too quickly. Nausea, retching, diaphoresis (sweating), apprehension, headache, restlessness, muscle twitching, dizziness, palpitation, retrosternal pain, and abdominal pain may occur. Symptoms disappear rapidly if rate of administration is slowed or temporarily discontinued. Overdosage produces metabolic acidosis, tolerance to therapeutic effect.

NURSING IMPLICATIONS

BASELINE ASSESSMENT:

Pt must have continuous EKG monitoring and B/P. Check with physician for desired B/P level (B/P is normally maintained about 30–40% below pretreatment levels). Medication should be discontinued if therapeutic response is not achieved within 10 min following IV infusion at 10 mcg/kg/min.

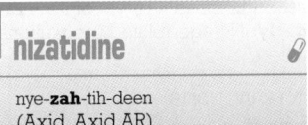

INTERVENTION/EVALUATION:

Monitor rate of infusion frequently. Monitor blood acid-base balance, electrolytes, laboratory results, I&O. Assess for metabolic acidosis (weakness, disorientation, headache, nausea, hyperventilation, vomiting). Assess for therapeutic response to medication. Monitor B/P for potential rebound hypertension after infusion is discontinued.

nizatidine

nye-**zah**-tih-deen
(Axid, Axid AR)

►CLASSIFICATION

PHARMACOTHERAPEUTIC:
H_2 receptor antagonist. ***CLINICAL:*** Antiulcer, gastric acid secretion inhibitor (see p. 88C)

ACTION/*THERAPEUTIC EFFECT*

Inhibits histamine action at H_2 receptors of parietal cells, *inhibiting basal and nocturnal gastric acid secretion.*

PHARMACOKINETICS

Rapidly, well absorbed from GI tract. Protein binding: 35%. Metabolized in liver. Primarily excreted in urine. Not removed by hemodialysis. Half-life: 1–2 hrs (half-life increased with renal function).

USES/*UNLABELED*

Short-term treatment of active duodenal ulcer, active benign gastric ulcer. Prevention of duodenal ulcer recurrence. Treatment of gastroesophageal reflux disease (GERD) including erosive esophagitis. *Treatment of gastric hypersecretory conditions, Zollinger-Ellison syndrome, multiple endocrine adenoma.*

PRECAUTIONS

CONTRAINDICATIONS: None significant. ***CAUTIONS:*** Impaired renal/hepatic function.
▷*LIFESPAN CONSIDERATIONS:*
Pregnancy/Lactation: Unknown whether drug crosses placenta or is distributed in breast milk. **Pregnancy Category B. Children:** Safety and efficacy not established in those <16 yrs of age. **Elderly:** No age-related precautions noted.

INTERACTIONS

DRUG: Antacids may decrease

absorption (do not give within 1 hr). May decrease absorption of **ketoconazole** (give at least 2 hrs after). ***HERBAL:*** None known. ***FOOD:*** None known. ***LAB VALUES:*** Interferes with skin tests using allergen extracts. May increase SGOT (AST), SGPT (ALT), alkaline phosphatase.

AVAILABILITY (Rx)

CAPSULES: 75 mg ***(OTC),*** 150 mg, 300 mg.

ADMINISTRATION/HANDLING

PO:

• Give without regard to meals. Best given after meals or at bedtime. • Do not administer within 1 hr of magnesium or aluminum-containing antacids (decreases absorption). • May give right before eating for heartburn prevention.

INDICATIONS/ROUTES/DOSAGE

Active duodenal ulcer:

***PO:* Adults, elderly:** 300 mg at bedtime or 150 mg 2 times/day.

Maintenance of healed ulcer:

***PO:* Adults, elderly:** 150 mg at bedtime.

GERD:

***PO:* Adults, elderly:** 150 mg 2 times/day.

Active benign gastric ulcer:

***PO:* Adults, elderly:** 150 mg 2 times/day or 300 mg at bedtime.

Usual OTC dosage:

***PO:* Adults, elderly:** 75 mg 30–60 min before meals; no more than 2 tablets/day..

Dosage in renal impairment:

Creatinine Clearance	Active Ulcer	Maintenance Therapy
20–50 ml/min	150 mg at bedtime	150 mg every other day

Creatinine Clearance	Active Ulcer	Maintenance Therapy
<20 ml/min	150 mg every other day	150 mg q3days

SIDE EFFECTS

OCCASIONAL (2%): Somnolence, fatigue. ***RARE*** (<1%): Sweating, rash.

ADVERSE REACTIONS/TOXIC EFFECTS

Asymptomatic ventricular tachycardia, hyperuricemia (not associated with gout), nephrolithiasis occur rarely.

NURSING IMPLICATIONS

INTERVENTION/EVALUATION:

Assess for abdominal pain, GI bleeding (overt blood in emesis or stool, tarry stools). Monitor blood tests for elevated SGOT (AST), SGPT (ALT), alkaline phosphatase (hepatocellular injury).

PATIENT/FAMILY TEACHING:

Avoid tasks that require alertness, motor skills until drug response is established. Avoid alcohol, aspirin, smoking.

norepinephrine bitartrate

nor-eh-pih-**nef**-rin
(Levophed)

▶CLASSIFICATION

PHARMACOTHERAPEUTIC:
Sympathomimetic. ***CLINICAL:***
Vasopressor (see p. 125C)

ACTION/*THERAPEUTIC EFFECT*

Stimulates beta$_1$-adrenergic receptors, *enhancing contractile myocardial force, increasing cardiac output.* Stimulates alpha-adrenergic receptors, *constricting resistance and capacitance vessels, resulting in increased systemic B/P, coronary artery blood flow.* Pressor effect primarily due to increased peripheral resistance.

PHARMACOKINETICS

	Onset	Peak	Duration
IV	Rapid	1–2 min	—

Localized in sympathetic tissue. Metabolized in liver. Primarily excreted in urine.

USES

Corrects hypotension unresponsive to adequate fluid volume replacement, as part of shock syndrome, caused by myocardial infarction, bacteremia, open heart surgery, renal failure.

PRECAUTIONS

CONTRAINDICATIONS: Hypovolemic states (unless an emergency measure), mesenteric/peripheral vascular thrombosis, profound hypoxia. ***CAUTIONS:*** Severe cardiac disease, hypertensive and hypothyroid pts, those on MAO inhibitors.

▷***LIFESPAN CONSIDERATIONS:***
Pregnancy/Lactation: Readily crosses placenta. May produce fetal anoxia due to uterine contraction, constriction of uterine blood vessels. **Pregnancy Category C. Children/Elderly:** No age-related precautions noted.

INTERACTIONS

DRUG: **Tricyclic antidepressants, maprotiline** may increase

---

cardiovascular effects. May decrease effect of **methyldopa.** May have mutually inhibitory effects with **beta-blockers.** May increase risk of arrhythmias with **digoxin. Ergonovine, oxytocin** may increase vasoconstriction. **HERBAL:** None known. **FOOD:** None known. **LAB VALUES:** None significant.

AVAILABILITY (Rx)
INJECTION: 1 mg/ml.

ADMINISTRATION/HANDLING
Note: Blood, fluid volume depletion should be corrected before drug is administered.

IV 🖳
Storage:
• Do not use if brown in color or contains precipitate. • Store amps at room temperature.

Reconstitution:
• Add 4 ml to 250 ml (16 mcg base/ml) or 1,000 ml (4 mcg base/ml) of D$_5$W. Maximum concentration: 32 mg/250 ml.

Rate of administration:
• Avoid catheter tie-in technique (encourages stasis, increases local drug concentration). • Closely monitor IV infusion flow rate (use microdrip or infusion pump). • Monitor B/P q2min during IV infusion until desired therapeutic response is achieved, then q5min during remaining IV infusion. Never leave pt unattended. • Maintain B/P at 80–100 mm Hg in previously normotensive pts, and 30–40 mm Hg below preexisting B/P in previously hypertensive pts. • Reduce IV infusion gradually. Avoid abrupt withdrawal. • If using peripherally inserted catheter, it is imperative to check the IV site frequently for free flow and infused vein for blanching, hardness to

vein, coldness, pallor to extremity. • If extravasation occurs, area should be infiltrated with 10–15 ml sterile saline containing 5–10 mg phentolamine (does not alter pressor effects of norepinephrine).

IV INCOMPATIBILITY ⊘
Insulin (Regular).

IV COMPATIBILITIES
Calcium gluconate, diltiazem (Cardizem), dobutamine (Dobutrex), dopamine (Intropin), epinephrine, heparin, labetalol (Normodyne, Trandate), lorazepam (Ativan), magnesium, midazolam (Versed), milrinone (Primacor), nicardipine (Cardene), nitroglycerin, potassium chloride, propofol (Diprivan).

INDICATIONS/ROUTES/DOSAGE
Acute hypotension:
IV: Adults, elderly: Initially, administer at 0.5–1 mcg/min. Adjust rate of flow to establish, maintain desired B/P (40 mm Hg below preexisting systolic pressure). **Average maintenance dose:** 8–12 mcg/min. **Children:** Administer at rate of 0.1 mcg. Adjust rate of flow to establish, maintain desired B/P, up to 2 mcg/kg/min.

SIDE EFFECTS
Norepinephrine produces less pronounced and less frequent side effects than epinephrine. **OCCASIONAL** (3–5%): Anxiety, bradycardia, awareness of slow, forceful heartbeat. **RARE** (1–2%): Nausea, anginal pain, shortness of breath, fever.

ADVERSE REACTIONS/TOXIC EFFECTS
Extravasation may produce tissue necrosis, sloughing. Overdosage

manifested as severe hypertension with violent headache (may be first clinical sign of overdosage), arrhythmias, photophobia, retrosternal/pharyngeal pain, pallor, excessive sweating, vomiting. Prolonged therapy may result in plasma volume depletion. Hypotension may recur if plasma volume is not maintained.

NURSING IMPLICATIONS

BASELINE ASSESSMENT:
Assess EKG and B/P continuously (be alert to precipitous B/P drop). Never leave pt alone during IV infusion. Be alert to pt complaint of headache.

INTERVENTION/EVALUATION:
Monitor IV flow rate diligently. Assess for extravasation characterized by blanching of skin over vein, coolness (results from local vasoconstriction); color and temperature of IV site extremity (pallor, cyanosis, mottling). Assess nailbed capillary refill. Monitor I&O; measure output hourly and report <30 cc. IV should not be reinstated unless systolic B/P falls below 70–80 mm Hg.

norfloxacin

nor-**flocks**-ah-sin
(Chibroxin, Noroxin)

▶CLASSIFICATION
PHARMACOTHERAPEUTIC:
Quinolone. **CLINICAL:** Anti-infective (see p. 22C)

ACTION/*THERAPEUTIC EFFECT*
Inhibits DNA replication and repair by interfering with DNA-gyrase in susceptible microorganisms, *producing bactericidal activity.*

USES
Treatment of complicated and uncomplicated urinary tract infections, uncomplicated gonococcal infections, acute/chronic prostatitis. **Ophthalmic:** Conjunctival keratitis, keratoconjunctivitis, corneal ulcers, blepharitis, blepharoconjunctivitis, acute meibomianitis, dacryocystitis.

PRECAUTIONS
CONTRAINDICATIONS: Hypersensitivity to norfloxacin, quinolones, or any component of preparation. Do not use in children <18 yrs of age (may produce arthropathy). **Ophthalmic:** Epithelial herpes simplex, keratitis, vaccinia, varicella, mycobacterial infection, fungal disease of ocular structure. Do not use after uncomplicated removal of foreign body. **CAUTIONS:** Impaired renal function; any predisposition to seizures.

INTERACTIONS
DRUG: Antacids, sucralfate may decrease absorption. Decrease clearance, may increase concentration, toxicity of **theophylline.** May increase effects of **oral anticoagulants. HERBAL:** None known. **FOOD:** None known. **LAB VALUES:** May increase SGOT (AST), SGPT (ALT), alkaline phosphatase, LDH, bilirubin, BUN, creatinine.

AVAILABILITY (Rx)
TABLETS: 400 mg. **OPHTHAL-MIC SOLUTION 0.3%:** 3 mg/ml.

ADMINISTRATION/HANDLING
PO:
• Give 1 hr before or 2 hrs after

N

meals, with 8 oz water. • Encourage additional glasses of water between meals. • Do not administer antacids with or within 2 hrs of norfloxacin dose. • Encourage cranberry juice, citrus fruits (to acidify urine).

Ophthalmic:

• Place finger on lower eyelid and pull out until a pocket is formed between eye and lower lid. • Hold dropper above pocket and place correct number of drops ($1/4$–$1/2$ inch ointment) into pocket. Close eye gently. • *Solution:* Apply digital pressure to lacrimal sac for 1–2 min (minimizes drainage into nose and throat, reducing risk of systemic effects). *Ointment:* Close eye for 1–2 min, rolling eyeball (increases contact area of drug to eye). • Remove excess solution or ointment around eye with tissue.

INDICATIONS/ROUTES/DOSAGE

Complicated or uncomplicated urinary tract infections:

PO: **Adults, elderly:** 400 mg 2 times/day for 7–21 days.

Prostatitis:

PO: **Adults:** 400 mg 2 times/day for 28 days.

Uncomplicated gonococcal infections:

PO: **Adults:** 800 mg as single dose.

Dosage in renal impairment:

The dose and/or frequency is modified based on degree of renal impairment.

Creatinine Clearance	Dosage
>30 ml/min	400 mg 2 times/day
<30 ml/min	400 mg once daily

Usual ophthalmic dosage:

OPHTHALMIC: **Adults, elderly:** 1–2 drops 4 times/day up to 7 days. For severe infections, may give 1–2 drops q2h while awake the first day.

SIDE EFFECTS

FREQUENT: Nausea, headache, dizziness. **Ophthalmic:** Bad taste in mouth. **OCCASIONAL: Ophthalmic:** Temporary blurring of vision, irritation, burning, stinging, itching. **RARE:** Vomiting, diarrhea, dry mouth, bitter taste, nervousness, drowsiness, insomnia, photosensitivity, tinnitus, crystalluria, rash, fever, seizures. **Ophthalmic:** Conjunctival hyperemia, photophobia, decreased vision, pain.

ADVERSE REACTIONS/TOXIC EFFECTS

Superinfection, anaphylaxis, Stevens-Johnson syndrome, arthropathy (joint disease) occurs rarely.

NURSING IMPLICATIONS

BASELINE ASSESSMENT:

Question for history of hypersensitivity to norfloxacin, quinolones.

INTERVENTION/EVALUATION:

Assess for nausea, headache, dizziness. Evaluate food tolerance. Assess for chest, joint pain. **Ophthalmic:** Check for therapeutic response.

PATIENT/FAMILY TEACHING:

Take 1 hr before or 2 hrs after meals. Complete full course of therapy. Take with 8 oz of water; drink several glasses of water between meals. Eat/drink high sources of ascorbic acid, e.g., cranberry juice, citrus fruits. Do not take antacids with or within 2 hrs of norfloxacin dose (reduces/destroys effectiveness).

Sugarless gum or hard candy may relieve bad taste. Report inflammation or tendon pain.

nortriptyline hydrochloride

nor-**trip**-teh-leen
(Aventyl, Pamelor)
Do not confuse with Ambenyl, amitriptyline, Bentyl.

▶CLASSIFICATION

PHARMACOTHERAPEUTIC: Tricyclic compound. *CLINICAL:* Antidepressant (see p. 35C)

ACTION/*THERAPEUTIC EFFECT*

Blocks reuptake of neurotransmitters (norepinephrine, serotonic) at neuronal presynaptic membranes, increasing availability at postsynaptic receptor sites. *Resulting enhancements of synaptic activity produces antidepressant effect.*

USES/*UNLABELED*

Treatment of various forms of depression, often in conjunction with psychotherapy. *Treatment of panic disorder, neurogenic pain, prophylaxis of migraine headache.*

PRECAUTIONS

CONTRAINDICATIONS: Acute recovery period following MI, within 14 days of MAO inhibitor ingestion. *CAUTIONS:* Prostatic hypertrophy, history of urinary retention or obstruction, glaucoma, diabetes mellitus, history of seizures, hyperthyroidism, cardiac/hepatic/renal disease, schizophrenia, increased intraocular pressure, hiatal hernia.

INTERACTIONS

DRUG: **Alcohol, CNS depressants** may increase CNS, respiratory depression, hypotensive effects. **Antithyroid agents** may increase risk of agranulocytosis. **Phenothiazines** may increase sedative, anticholinergic effects. **Cimetidine** may increase concentration, toxicity. May decrease effects of **clonidine, guanadrel.** May increase cardiac effects with **sympathomimetics.** May increase risk of hypertensive crisis, hyperpyretic convulsions with **MAO inhibitors. *HERBAL:*** None known. *FOOD:* None known. *LAB VALUES:* May alter EKG readings, glucose. Therapeutic blood serum level: Peak: 6–10 mcg/ml; trough: 0.5–2 mcg/ml. Toxic blood serum level: Peak: >12 mcg/ml; trough: >2 mcg/ml.

AVAILABILITY (Rx)

CAPSULES: 10 mg, 25 mg, 50 mg, 75 mg. *ORAL SOLUTION:* 10 mg/5 ml.

ADMINISTRATION/HANDLING
PO:

• Give with food or milk if GI distress occurs.

INDICATIONS/ROUTES/DOSAGE

PO: **Adults:** 75–100 mg/day in 1–4 divided doses until therapeutic response achieved. Reduce dosage gradually to effective maintenance level. **Elderly:** Initially, 10–25 mg at bedtime. May increase by 25 mg q3–7days. **Maximum:** 150 mg/day. **Children >12 yrs:** 30–50 mg/day in 3–4 divided doses. **Children 6–12 yrs:** 10–20 mg/day in 3–4 divided doses.

Enuresis:

PO: **Children >11 yrs:** 25–35 mg/day; **Children 8–11 yrs:** 10–20

N

mg/day; **Children 6–7 yrs:** 10 mg/day.

SIDE EFFECTS

FREQUENT: Drowsiness, fatigue, dry mouth, blurred vision, constipation, delayed micturition, postural hypotension, excessive sweating, disturbed concentration, increased appetite, urinary retention. ***OCCASIONAL:*** GI disturbances (nausea, GI distress, metallic taste sensation), photosensitivity. ***RARE:*** Paradoxical reaction (agitation, restlessness, nightmares, insomnia), extrapyramidal symptoms (particularly fine hand tremor).

ADVERSE REACTIONS/TOXIC EFFECTS

High dosage may produce cardiovascular effects (severe postural hypotension, dizziness, tachycardia, palpitations, arrhythmias) and seizures. May also result in altered temperature regulation (hyperpyrexia or hypothermia). Abrupt withdrawal from prolonged therapy may produce headache, malaise, nausea, vomiting, vivid dreams.

NURSING IMPLICATIONS

BASELINE ASSESSMENT:

For those on long-term therapy, liver/renal function tests, blood counts should be performed periodically.

INTERVENTION/EVALUATION:

Supervise suicidal risk pt closely during early therapy (as depression lessens, energy level improves, increasing suicide potential). Assess appearance, behavior, speech pattern, level of interest, mood. Monitor stool consistency; avoid constipation with increased fluids, bulky foods. Monitor B/P, pulse for hypotension, arrhythmias. Assess for urinary retention including output estimate and bladder palpation if indicated. Therapeutic blood serum level: Peak: 6–10 mcg/ml; trough: 0.5–2 mcg/ml. Toxic blood serum level: Peak: >12 mcg/ml; trough: >2 mcg/ml.

PATIENT/FAMILY TEACHING:

Change positions slowly to avoid hypotensive effect. Tolerance to postural hypotension, sedative, and anticholinergic effects usually develops during early therapy. Therapeutic effect may be noted in 2 or more wks. Photosensitivity to sun may occur. Use sunscreens, protective clothing. Dry mouth may be relieved by sugarless gum, sips of tepid water. Report visual disturbances. Do not abruptly discontinue medication. Avoid tasks that require alertness, motor skills until response to drug is established.

nystatin

nigh-**stat**-in
(Mycostatin, Nadostine✺, Nilstat, Nystop)
Do not confuse with Nilstat, Nitrostat.

FIXED-COMBINATION(S)

With triamcinolone, a steroid **(Mycolog II, Myco-Triacet II, Mykacet, Mytrex F)**

▶ CLASSIFICATION
CLINICAL: Antifungal (see p. 43C)

ACTION/*THERAPEUTIC EFFECT*

Binds to sterols in cell membrane

increasing permeability, permitting loss of potassium, other cell components. *Fungistatic.*

PHARMACOKINETICS

PO: Poorly absorbed from GI tract. Eliminated unchanged in feces. *Topical:* Not absorbed systemically from intact skin.

USES/*UNLABELED*

Treatment of intestinal and oral candidiasis, cutaneous/mucocutaneous mycotic infections caused by *Candida albicans* (oral thrush, paronychia, vulvovaginal candidiasis, diaper rash, perleche). *Prophylaxis/treatment of oropharyngeal candidiasis, tinea barbae, capitis.*

PRECAUTIONS

CONTRAINDICATIONS: None significant.
▷*LIFESPAN CONSIDERATIONS:*
Pregnancy/Lactation: Unknown if distributed in breast milk. Vaginal applicators may be contraindicated, requiring manual insertion of tablets during pregnancy. **Pregnancy Category A. Children:** No age-related precautions noted for suspension or topical use. Lozenges not recommended in those <5 yrs of age. **Elderly:** No age-related precautions noted.

INTERACTIONS

DRUG: None significant. ***HERBAL:*** None known. ***FOOD:*** None known. ***LAB VALUES:*** None significant.

AVAILABILITY (Rx)

TABLETS: 500,000 units. ***ORAL SUSPENSION:*** 100,000 units/ml. ***TROCHES:*** 200,000 units. ***VAGINAL TABLETS:*** 100,000 units. ***CREAM. OINTMENT. POWDER.***

ADMINISTRATION/HANDLING
PO:

• Dissolve lozenges (troches) slowly/completely in mouth (optimal therapeutic effect). Do not chew or swallow lozenges whole. • Shake suspension well before administration. • Place and hold suspension in mouth or swish throughout mouth as long as possible before swallowing.

INDICATIONS/ROUTES/DOSAGE
Intestinal candidiasis:

PO: **Adults, elderly:** 500,000–1,000,000 units 3 times/day. **Children:** 500,000 units 4 times/day.

Oral candidiasis:

PO: **Adults, elderly, children:** Oral suspension: 400,000–600,000 units 4 times/day. **Infants:** 100,000–200,000 units 4 times/day.

PO: **Adults, elderly, children:** Troches: 200,000–400,000 units 4–5 times/day up to 14 days.

Vulvovaginal candidiasis:

INTRAVAGINAL: **Adults, elderly:** 1 tablet high in vagina 1–2 times/day for 14 days.

Topical fungal infections:

TOPICAL: **Adults, elderly:** Apply 2–4 times/day.

SIDE EFFECTS

OCCASIONAL: PO: None significant. *Topical:* Skin irritation. *Vaginal:* Vaginal irritation.

ADVERSE REACTIONS/TOXIC EFFECTS

High dosage with oral form may produce nausea, vomiting, diarrhea, GI distress.

NURSING IMPLICATIONS

BASELINE ASSESSMENT:

Confirm that cultures or histologic tests were done for accurate diagnosis.

INTERVENTION/EVALUATION:

Assess for increased irritation with topical, increased vaginal discharge with vaginal application.

PATIENT/FAMILY TEACHING:

Do not miss dose; complete full length of treatment (continue vaginal use during menses). Notify physician if nausea, vomiting, diarrhea, stomach pain develop. **Vaginal:** Insert high in vagina. Check with physician regarding douching, sexual intercourse. **Topical:** Rub well into affected areas. Must not contact eyes. Use cream (sparingly)/powder on erythematous areas. Keep areas clean, dry; wear light clothing for ventilation. Separate personal items in contact with affected areas.

octreotide acetate

ock-**tree**-oh-tide
(Depot, Sandostatin, Sandostatin LAR)
Do not confuse with
OctreoScan, Sandimmune, Sandoglobulin.

▶CLASSIFICATION

CLINICAL: Secretory inhibitory, growth hormone suppressant

ACTION/*THERAPEUTIC EFFECT*

Suppresses secretion of serotonin, gastroenteropancreatic peptides.

Enhances fluid/electrolyte absorption from GI tract; *prolongs intestinal transit time.*

PHARMACOKINETICS

	Onset	Peak	Duration
SubQ	—	—	Up to 12 hrs

Rapidly, completely absorbed from injection site. Excreted in urine. Removed by hemodialysis. Half-life: 1.5 hrs.

USES/*UNLABELED*

Controls symptoms in pts with metastatic carcinoid tumors, vasoactive intestinal peptic-secreting tumors (VIPomas), secretory diarrhea, acromegaly. *AIDS-associated secretory diarrhea, control of bleeding of esophageal varices, insulinomas, small bowel fistulas, chemotherapy-induced diarrhea.*

PRECAUTIONS

CONTRAINDICATIONS: None significant. **CAUTIONS:** Insulin-dependent diabetes, renal failure.

▷**LIFESPAN CONSIDERATIONS:**
Pregnancy/Lactation: Excretion in breast milk unknown. **Pregnancy Category B. Children:** Dosage not established in children. **Elderly:** No age-related precautions noted.

INTERACTIONS

DRUG: May alter glucose concentrations with **insulin, oral hypoglycemics, glucagon, growth hormone. HERBAL:** None known. **FOOD:** None known. **LAB VALUES:** May decrease T_4 concentration.

AVAILABILITY (Rx)

INJECTION: 0.05 mg/ml, 0.1 mg/ml, 0.2 mg/ml, 0.5 mg/ml, 1 mg/ml. **SUSPENSION FOR INJECTION:** 10 mg, 20 mg, 30 mg vials.

ADMINISTRATION/HANDLING

Note: Sandostatin may be given IV, IM, SubQ. Sandostatin LAR may be givein only IM.

SubQ:

• Do not use if particulates and/or discoloration are noted. • Avoid multiple injections at the same site within short periods.

IM:

• Give immediately after mixing. • Administer intragluteally at 4 wk intervals. • Avoid deltoid injections.

INDICATIONS/ROUTES/DOSAGE

SANDOSTATIN:

Diarrhea:

SubQ: **Adults, elderly:** 50 mcg 1–2 times/day.

IV: **Adults, elderly:** Initially, 50–100 mcg q8h. May increase by 100 mcg/dose q48h. **Maximum:** 500 mcg q8h.

SubQ/IV: **Children:** 1–10 mcg/kg q12h.

Carcinoid tumors:

SubQ/IV: **Adults, elderly:** 100–600 mcg/day in 2–4 divided doses.

VIPomas:

SubQ/IV: **Adults, elderly:** 200–300 mcg/day in 2–4 divided doses.

Esophageal varices:

IV: **Adults, elderly:** Bolus of 25–50 mcg followed by IV infusion of 25–50 mcg/hr.

Acromegaly:

SubQ/IV: **Adults, elderly:** 50 mcg 3 times/day. Increase as needed. **Maximum:** 500 mcg 3 times/day.

SANDOSTATIN LAR:

Acromegaly:

IM: **Adults, elderly:** 20 mg q4wks for 3 mos. **Maximum:** 40 mg q4wks.

VIPomas, carcinoid tumors:

IM: **Adults, elderly:** 20 mg q4wks.

SIDE EFFECTS

FREQUENT (6–10%; 30–58% in acromegalics): Diarrhea, nausea, abdominal discomfort, headache, pain at injection site. ***OCCASIONAL*** (1–5%): Vomiting, flatulence, constipation, alopecia, flushing, itching, dizziness, fatigue, arrhythmias, bruising, blurred vision. ***RARE*** (<1%): Depression, decreased libido, vertigo, palpitations, shortness of breath.

ADVERSE REACTIONS/TOXIC EFFECTS

Increased risk of cholelithiasis. Potential for hypothyroidism with prolonged high therapy. Hepatitis, GI bleeding, seizures occur rarely.

NURSING IMPLICATIONS

BASELINE ASSESSMENT:

Establish baseline B/P, weight, blood glucose, electrolytes.

INTERVENTION/EVALUATION:

Evaluate blood glucose levels (esp. with diabetics), electrolytes (therapy generally reduces abnormalities). Weigh every 2–3 days, report >5 lbs gain/week. Monitor B/P, pulse, respirations periodically during treatment. Be alert for decreased urinary output, swelling of ankles, fingers. Monitor stools for frequency, consistency.

PATIENT/FAMILY TEACHING:

Therapy should provide significant improvement of symptoms.

ocular lubricant

ock-you-lar **lube**-rih-cant
(Hypotears, Lacrilube, Tears
Naturale♣)

►CLASSIFICATION

PHARMACOTHERAPEUTIC:
Topical ophthalmic. ***CLINICAL:***
Lubricant, toner, buffer, viscosity
agent

ACTION/*THERAPEUTIC EFFECT*

Maintains ocular tonicity (0.9%
NaCl equivalent); buffers to adjust
pH, viscosity agents to prolong
eye contact time. *Protects and lubricates eye.*

USES

Protection and lubrication of the
eye in exposure keratitis, decreased corneal sensitivity, recurrent corneal erosions, keratitis
sicca (particularly for nighttime
use), after removal of a foreign
body, during and following
surgery.

PRECAUTIONS

CONTRAINDICATIONS: None
significant. ***CAUTIONS:*** None significant.

▷***LIFESPAN CONSIDERATIONS:***
Pregnancy/Lactation: Pregnancy Category unknown. **Children/
Elderly:** No age-related precautions noted.

INTERACTIONS

DRUG: None significant. ***HERBAL:***
None known. ***FOOD:*** None known.
LAB VALUES: None significant.

AVAILABILITY (OTC)

***OPHTHALMIC OINTMENT. SO-
LUTION.***

ADMINISTRATION/HANDLING
Ophthalmic:

• Do not use with contact lenses. •
Ointment: Hold tube in hand for a
few mins to warm ointment. •
Avoid touching tip of tube or
dropper to any surface. • Gently
pull lower lid down to form pouch
between eye and lower lid (conjunctival sac). • Place ordered
amount of ointment into pouch
with a sweeping motion. Instruct
pt to close the eye for 1–2 min and
roll the eyeball around in all directions. • Inform pt of temporary
blurred vision. If possible, apply
just before bedtime. • ***Drops:*** Instruct pt to lie down or tilt head
backward and look up. • Gently
pull lower lid down to form pouch
between eye and lower lid (conjunctival sac). • Hold dropper
above pouch. Instill drop(s); have
pt close eye gently for 1–2 min
(placing drop(s) directly onto eye
may cause a sudden squeezing of
eyelid, with subsequent loss of solution). • Apply gentle pressure
with fingers to bridge of nose (inside corner of eye) for 1–2 min
(promotes absorption, minimizes
drainage into nose and throat)

INDICATIONS/ROUTES/DOSAGE
Usual ophthalmic dosage:

OPHTHALMIC: Adults, elderly:
Small amount in conjunctival cul-
de-sac.

SIDE EFFECTS

FREQUENT: Temporary blurring
after administration, esp. with ointment.

ADVERSE REACTIONS/TOXIC
EFFECTS

None significant.

NURSING IMPLICATIONS

PATIENT/FAMILY TEACHING:

Teach proper application. Do not use contact lenses. Temporary blurring will occur esp. with administration of ointment. Avoid activities requiring visual acuity until blurring clears. If eye pain, change of vision, or worsening of condition occurs, or if condition is unchanged after 72 hrs, notify physician. Do not touch to any surface (may contaminate).

ofloxacin

oh-**flocks**-ah-sin
(Apo-Oflox✤, Floxin, Floxin Otic, Ocuflox)
Do not confuse with Flexeril, Flexon, Ocufen.

▶CLASSIFICATION

PHARMACOTHERAPEUTIC:
Fluoroquinolone. **CLINICAL:**
Anti-infective (see p. 22C)

ACTION/*THERAPEUTIC EFFECT*

Inhibits DNA-gyrase in susceptible microorganisms, *interfering with bacterial DNA replication and repair.* Bactericidal.

PHARMACOKINETICS

Rapidly, well absorbed from GI tract. Protein binding: 20–25%. Widely distributed (penetrates CSF). Metabolized in liver. Primarily excreted in urine. Removed by hemodialysis. Half-life: 4.7–7 hrs (half-life increased with impaired renal function, elderly, cirrhosis).

USES

Treatment of infections of urinary tract, skin/skin structure, sexually transmitted diseases, lower respiratory tract, prostatitis due to *Escherichia coli,* PID. **Ophthalmic:** Bacterial conjunctivitis, corneal ulcers. **Otic:** Otitis externa, acute/chronic otitis media.

PRECAUTIONS

CONTRAINDICATIONS: Syphilis, hypersensitivity to any quinolones. Children <18 yrs. ***CAUTIONS:*** Renal impairment, CNS disorders, seizures, those taking theophylline or caffeine. May mask or delay symptoms of syphilis; serologic test for syphilis should be done at diagnosis and 3 mos after treatment.
▷*LIFESPAN CONSIDERATIONS:*
Pregnancy/Lactation: Distributed in breast milk; potentially serious adverse reactions in nursing infants. Risk of arthropathy to fetus. **Pregnancy Category C. Children:** Safety and efficacy not established (otic not established in those <1 yr). **Elderly:** No age-related precautions for otic. Age-related renal impairment may require dosage adjustment.

INTERACTIONS

DRUG: **Antacids, sucralfate** may decrease absorption, effect of ofloxacin. May increase **theophylline** concentrations, toxicity. **HERBAL:** None known. ***FOOD:*** None known. **LAB VALUES:** None significant.

AVAILABILITY (Rx)

TABLETS: 200 mg, 300 mg, 400 mg. ***INJECTION:*** 200 mg, 400 mg. ***OPHTHALMIC SOLUTION:*** 3 mg/ml. ***OTIC SOLUTION:*** 0.3%.

ADMINISTRATION/HANDLING

PO:
• Do not give with food; preferred

O

dosing time: 1 hr before or 2 hrs after meals. • Do not administer antacids (aluminum, magnesium) or iron-/zinc-containing products within 2 hrs of ofloxacin. • Encourage cranberry juice, citrus fruits (to acidify urine). • Give with 8 oz water and encourage fluid intake.

Ophthalmic:

• Tilt pt's head back; place solution in conjunctival sac. • Have pt close eyes; press gently on lacrimal sac for 1 min. • Do not use ophthalmic solutions for injection. • Unless infection very superficial, systemic administration generally accompanies ophthalmic.

Otic:

• Instruct pt to lie down with head turned so affected ear is upright. • Instill toward canal wall, not directly on eardrum. • Pull the auricle down and posterior in children; up and posterior in adults.

IV 🕮

Storage:

• Store at room temperature. • After dilution, IV is stable for 72 hrs at room temperature; 14 days if refrigerated. • Discard unused portions.

Reconstitution:

• Must dilute each 200 mg with 50 ml D_5W or 0.9% NaCl (400 mg with 100 ml) to provide concentration of 4 mg/ml.

Rate of administration:

• Give only by IV infusion over at least 60 min; avoid rapid or bolus IV administration. • Do not add or infuse other medication through same IV line at same time.

IV INCOMPATIBILITIES ⊘

Amphotericin B complex (Abelcet, Ambisome, Amphotec), ce-

fepime (Maxipime), doxorubicin liposome (Doxil).

IV COMPATIBILITY

Propofol (Diprivan).

INDICATIONS/ROUTES/DOSAGE

Urinary tract infection:

PO/IV INFUSION: Adults: 200 mg q12h.

Lower respiratory tract, skin/skin structure infections:

PO/IV INFUSION: Adults: 400 mg q12h for 10 days.

Prostatitis, sexually transmitted diseases (cervicitis, urethritis):

PO: Adults: 300 mg q12h.

PID:

PO: Adults: 400 mg q12h for 10–14 days.

Prostatitis:

IV INFUSION: Adults: 300 mg q12h.

Sexually transmitted diseases:

IV INFUSION: Adults: 400 mg as single dose.

Acute, uncomplicated gonorrhea:

PO: Adults: 400 mg 1 time.

Usual elderly dosage:

PO: 200–400 mg q12–24h for 7 days up to 6 wks.

Dosage in renal impairment:

After a normal initial dose, dosage/interval based on creatinine clearance.

Creatinine Clearance	Adjusted Dosage	Dose Interval
>50 ml/min	None	12 hrs
10–50 ml/min	None	24 hrs
<10 ml/min	½	24 hrs

Bacterial conjunctivitis:

OPHTHALMIC: Adults, elderly:

1–2 drops q2–4h for 2 days, then 4 times/day for 5 days.

Corneal ulcers:

OPHTHALMIC: **Adults:** 1–2 drops q30min while awake for 2 days, then q60min while awake for 5–7 days, then 4 times/day.

Usual otic dosage:

Adults, elderly, children: Twice daily. Ear drops should be at body temperature (wrap hand around bottle).

SIDE EFFECTS

FREQUENT (7–10%): Nausea, headache, insomnia. *OCCASIONAL* (3–5%): Abdominal pain, diarrhea, vomiting, dry mouth, flatulence, dizziness, fatigue, drowsiness, rash, pruritis, fever. *RARE* (<1%): Constipation, numbness of hands/feet.

ADVERSE REACTIONS/TOXIC EFFECTS

Superinfection, severe hypersensitivity reaction occur rarely. Arthropathy (joint disease with swelling, pain, clubbing of fingers and toes, degeneration of stress-bearing portion of a joint) may occur if given to children.

NURSING IMPLICATIONS

BASELINE ASSESSMENT:

Question for history of hypersensitivity to ofloxacin or any quinolones.

INTERVENTION/EVALUATION:

Assess skin and discontinue medication at first sign of rash or other allergic reaction. Determine pattern of bowel activity, stool consistency. Assess during the night for insomnia. Check for dizziness, headache, visual difficulties, tremors; provide ambulation assistance as needed. Be alert for superinfection, e.g., genital pruritus, vaginitis, fever, sores, and discomfort in mouth.

PATIENT/FAMILY TEACHING:

Do not skip dose; take full course of therapy. Take with 8 oz water; drink several glasses of water between meals. Eat/drink high sources of ascorbic acid (cranberry juice, citrus fruits). Do not take antacids (reduces/destroys effectiveness). Avoid tasks that require alertness, motor skills until response to drug is established.

olanzapine

oh-**lan**-sah-peen
(Zyprexa)
Do not confuse with
olanzapine, olsalazine, Zyrtec.

▶CLASSIFICATION

PHARMACOTHERAPEUTIC: Dibenzapine derivative. *CLINICAL:* Antipsychotic (see p. 55C)

ACTION/THERAPEUTIC EFFECT

Antagonizes dopamine, serotonin, muscarinic, histamine, and alpha$_1$-adrenergic receptors, *diminishing psychotic disorders.* Produces anticholinergic, histaminic, CNS depressant effects.

PHARMACOKINETICS

Well absorbed following PO administration. Protein binding: 93%. Extensively distributed throughout body. Extensively metabolized by first-pass liver metabolism. Excreted in urine, with lesser amount eliminated in feces. Not removed by dialysis. Half-life: 21–54 hrs.

O

Management of manifestations of psychotic disorders. Treatment of acute mania associated with bipolar disorder. *Anorexia, maintenance of treatment response in schizophrenic pts.*

PRECAUTIONS

CONTRAINDICATIONS: None significant. ***CAUTIONS:*** Hypersensitivity to clozapine, pts who should avoid anticholinergics (e.g., pts with benign prostatic hypertrophy), hepatic function impairment, elderly, concurrent potentially hepatotoxic drugs, dose escalation, known cardiovascular disease (history of MI or ischemia, heart failure, conduction abnormalities), cerebrovascular disease, conditions predisposing pts to hypotension (dehydration, hypovolemia, hypertensive medications), history of seizures, conditions lowering seizure threshold (e.g., Alzheimer's dementia), those at risk of aspiration pneumonia.
▷*LIFESPAN CONSIDERATIONS:*
Pregnancy/Lactation: Unknown if drug crosses placenta or is distributed in breast milk. **Pregnancy Category C. Children:** Safety and efficacy not established. **Elderly:** No age-related precautions noted.

INTERACTIONS

DRUG: **Alcohol, CNS depressants** may increase CNS depressant effects. **Antihypertensive agents** increase risk of hypotensive effect. May inhibit metabolism of **theophylline, imipramine. Fluvoxamine; ciprofloxacin (quinolone)** may increase olanzapine blood levels. Antagonizes effects of **levodopa, dopamine agonists.**

Carbamazepine increases olanzapine clearance. ***HERBAL:*** None known. ***FOOD:*** None known. ***LAB VALUES:*** May significantly increase SGPT (ALT), SGOT (AST), GGT levels, prolactin levels.

AVAILABILITY (Rx)

TABLETS: 2.5 mg, 5 mg, 7.5 mg, 10 mg, 15 mg, 20 mg. ***ORAL DISINTEGRATING TABLETS:*** 5 mg, 10 mg.

ADMINISTRATION/HANDLING
PO:
• Give without regard to meals.

INDICATIONS/ROUTES/DOSAGE
Psychotic disorders:
PO: **Adults, elderly:** Initially, 5–10 mg once daily with target dose of 10 mg/day within several days after initiation. If needed, dose increments/decrements of 5 mg once daily but not less than 1 wk intervals.

Debilitated, predisposition to hypotensive reactions, elderly >65 yrs:
PO: **Adults, elderly:** Initially, 5 mg/day.

SIDE EFFECTS

FREQUENT: Somnolence (26%), agitation (23%), insomnia (20%), headache (17%), nervousness (16%), hostility (15%), dizziness (11%), rhinitis (10%). ***OCCASIONAL:*** Anxiety, constipation (9%), nonaggressive objectionable behavior (8%), dry mouth (7%), weight gain (6%), postural hypotension, fever, joint pain, restlessness, cough, pharyngitis, dimness of vision (5%). ***RARE:*** Tachycardia, back/chest/abdominal pain, tremor, extremity pain.

ADVERSE REACTIONS/TOXIC EFFECTS

Seizures occur rarely. Neuroleptic malignant syndrome (NMS), a potentially fatal syndrome, occurs rarely and may present as hyperpyrexia, muscle rigidity, irregular pulse or B/P, tachycardia, diaphoresis, cardiac dysrhythmias. Extrapyramidal symptoms may occur. Dysphagia (esophageal dysmotility, aspiration) may be noted. Overdosage (300 mg) produces drowsiness, slurred speech.

NURSING IMPLICATIONS

BASELINE ASSESSMENT:

Obtain baseline hepatic function lab values before initiating treatment. Assess behavior, appearance, emotional status, response to environment, speech pattern, thought content.

INTERVENTION/EVALUATION:

Supervise suicidal risk pt closely during early therapy (as depression lessens, energy level improves, increasing suicide potential). Assess for therapeutic response (interest in surroundings, improvement in self-care, increased ability to concentrate, relaxed facial expression). Assist with ambulation if dizziness occurs. Assess sleep pattern. Notify physician if extrapyramidal symptoms occur.

PATIENT/FAMILY TEACHING:

Avoid dehydration, particularly during exercise, exposure to extreme heat, concurrent medication causing dry mouth, other drying effects. Notify physician if pregnancy occurs or if there is intention to become pregnant during olanzapine therapy. Take medication as ordered; do not stop taking or increase dosage. Sugarless gum, sips of tepid water may relieve dry mouth. Drowsiness generally subsides during continued therapy. Avoid driving or performing tasks that require alertness, motor skills until response to drug is established.

olsalazine sodium

ol-**sal**-ah-zeen
(Dipentum)

▶CLASSIFICATION

PHARMACOTHERAPEUTIC: Salicylic acid derivative. ***CLINICAL:*** Anti-inflammatory

ACTION/*THERAPEUTIC EFFECT*

Converted in colon by bacterial action to mesalamine, *reducing colonic inflammation* by blocking prostaglandin production in bowel mucosa.

PHARMACOKINETICS

Minimally absorbed from GI tract (99% reaches colon). Protein binding: 99%. Converted to mesalamine in colon. Primarily eliminated in feces. Unknown if removed by hemodialysis. Half-life: 0.9 hrs.

USES/*UNLABELED*

Maintenance of remission of ulcerative colitis in those intolerant of sulfasalazine medication. *Treatment of inflammatory bowel disease.*

PRECAUTIONS

CONTRAINDICATIONS: History of hypersensitivity to salicylates. ***CAUTIONS:*** Preexisting renal disease.

O

▷**LIFESPAN CONSIDERATIONS:**
Pregnancy/Lactation: Unknown if drug crosses placenta or is distributed in breast milk. **Pregnancy Category C. Children:** Safety and efficacy not established. **Elderly:** No age-related precautions noted.

INTERACTIONS

DRUG: None significant. **HERBAL:** None known. **FOOD:** None known. **LAB VALUES:** May increase SGOT (AST), SGPT (ALT).

AVAILABILITY (Rx)
CAPSULES: 250 mg.

ADMINISTRATION/HANDLING
PO:

• Give with food in evenly divided doses.

INDICATIONS/ROUTES/DOSAGE
Maintenance of controlled ulcerative colitis:

PO: Adults, elderly: 1 g/day in 2 divided doses (preferably q12h).

SIDE EFFECTS

FREQUENT (5–10%): Headache, diarrhea, abdominal pain/cramps, nausea. **OCCASIONAL** (1–5%): Depression, fatigue, dyspepsia, upper respiratory infection, decreased appetite, rash, itching, arthralgia. **RARE** (<1%): Dizziness, vomiting, stomatitis.

ADVERSE REACTIONS/TOXIC EFFECTS

Sulfite sensitivity in susceptible pts noted as cramping, headache, diarrhea, fever, rash, hives, itching, wheezing. Discontinue drug immediately. Excessive diarrhea associated with extreme fatigue noted rarely.

NURSING IMPLICATIONS

INTERVENTION/EVALUATION:

Encourage adequate fluid intake. Assess bowel sounds for peristalsis. Monitor daily bowel activity and stool consistency (watery, loose, soft, semisolid, solid) and record time of evacuation. Assess for abdominal disturbances. Assess skin for rash, hives. Medication should be discontinued if rash, fever, cramping, or diarrhea occurs.

PATIENT/FAMILY TEACHING:

Notify physician if diarrhea or cramping continues or increases, rash, fever, or pruritus occurs.

omeprazole

oh-**mep**-rah-zole
(Losec✦, <u>Prilosec</u>)
Do not confuse with prilocaine, Prinivil, Prozac.

▶**CLASSIFICATION**

PHARMACOTHERAPEUTIC: Benzimidazole. **CLINICAL:** Gastric acid pump inhibitor (see p. 122C)

ACTION/THERAPEUTIC EFFECT

Converted to active metabolites that irreversibly bind to and inhibit H+/K+ ATPase (an enzyme on surface of gastric parietal cells). Inhibits hydrogen ion transport into gastric lumen, _increasing gastric pH, reducing gastric acid production._

PHARMACOKINETICS

Rapidly absorbed from GI tract. Protein binding: 99%. Primarily distributed into gastric parietal cells. Metabolized extensively in liver. Primarily excreted in urine. Unknown if removed by hemodialysis. Half-life: 0.5–1 hr (increased in decreased liver function).

USES

Short-term treatment (4–8 wks) of erosive esophagitis (diagnosed by endoscopy); symptomatic gastroesophageal reflux disease (GERD) poorly responsive to other treatment. Long-term treatment of pathologic hypersecretory conditions; treatment of active duodenal ulcer. Maintenance healing of erosive esophagitis. Treatment of *H. pylori*-associated duodenal ulcer (with amoxicillin, clarithromycin), active benign gastric ulcers. Prevention/treatment of NSAID-induced ulcers.

PRECAUTIONS

CONTRAINDICATIONS: None significant. **CAUTIONS:** None significant.

▷**LIFESPAN CONSIDERATIONS:** **Pregnancy/Lactation:** Unknown if drug crosses placenta or is distributed in breast milk. **Pregnancy Category C. Children:** Safety and efficacy not established. **Elderly:** No age-related precautions noted.

INTERACTIONS

DRUG: May increase concentration of **oral anticoagulants, diazepam, phenytoin**. **HERBAL:** None known. **FOOD:** None known. **LAB VALUES:** May increase SGOT (AST), SGPT (ALT), alkaline phosphatase.

AVAILABILITY (Rx)

CAPSULES (delayed-release): 10 mg, 20 mg, 40 mg.

ADMINISTRATION/HANDLING

PO:

• Give before meals. • Do not crush or chew capsule; swallow whole.

INDICATIONS/ROUTES/DOSAGE

Erosive esophagitis, poorly responsive GERD, active duodenal ulcer, prevention/treatment of NSAID-induced ulcers:

PO: Adults, elderly: 20 mg/day.

Maintenance healing of erosive esophagitis:

PO: Adults, elderly: 20 mg/day.

Pathologic hypersecretory conditions:

PO: Adults, elderly: Initially, 60 mg/day up to 120 mg, 3 times/day.

H. pylori duodenal ulcer:

PO: Adults, elderly: 20 mg 2 times/day for 10 days.

Active benign gastric ulcer:

PO: Adults, elderly: 40 mg/day for 4–8 wks.

Usual dosage for children:

PO: 0.6–0.7 mg/kg/day..

SIDE EFFECTS

FREQUENT (7%): Headache. **OCCASIONAL** (2–3%): Diarrhea, abdominal pain, nausea. **RARE** (<2%): Dizziness, asthenia (loss of strength), vomiting, constipation, upper respiratory infection, back pain, rash, cough.

ADVERSE REACTIONS/TOXIC EFFECTS

None significant.

NURSING IMPLICATIONS

INTERVENTION/EVALUATION:

Evaluate for therapeutic response, i.e., relief of GI symptoms. Question if GI discomfort, nausea, diarrhea occur.

PATIENT/FAMILY TEACHING: Report headache. Swallow capsules whole; do not chew or crush. Take prior to eating.

ondansetron hydrochloride

on-**dan**-sah-tron
(Zofran)
Do not confuse with Zantac, Zosyn.

▶CLASSIFICATION

PHARMACOTHERAPEUTIC: Selective receptor antagonist. *CLINICAL:* Antinausea, antiemetic

ACTION/*THERAPEUTIC EFFECT*
Action may be central (CTZ) or peripheral (vagus nerve terminal), *preventing nausea/vomiting associated with cancer chemotherapy.*

PHARMACOKINETICS
Readily absorbed from GI tract. Protein binding: 70–76%. Metabolized in liver. Primarily excreted in urine. Unknown if removed by hemodialysis. Half-life: 4 hrs.

USES/*UNLABELED*
Prevention, treatment of nausea and vomiting due to cancer chemotherapy, including high-dose cisplatin. Prevention of postop nausea, vomiting. Prevention of radiation-induced nausea, vomiting. *Treatment of postop nausea/vomiting.*

PRECAUTIONS
CONTRAINDICATIONS: None significant. *CAUTIONS:* None significant.
▷*LIFESPAN CONSIDERATIONS:*
Pregnancy/Lactation: Unknown if drug crosses placenta or is distributed in breast milk. **Pregnancy Category B. Children:** Safety and efficacy not established. **Elderly:** No age-related precautions noted.

INTERACTIONS
DRUG: None significant. *HERBAL:* None known. *FOOD:* None known. *LAB VALUES:* May transiently increase SGOT (AST), SGPT (ALT), bilirubin.

AVAILABILITY (Rx)
TABLETS: 4 mg, 8 mg, 24 mg. *ORAL DISINTEGRATING TABLETS:* 4 mg, 8 mg. *ORAL SOLUTION:* 4 mg/5 ml. *INJECTION:* 2 mg/ml. *INJECTION (Premix):* 32 mg/50 ml.

ADMINISTRATION/HANDLING
PO:
• Give without regard to food.
IM:
• Inject into large muscle mass.
IV 🕱
Storage:
• Store at room temperature. • Stable for 48 hrs after dilution.
Reconstitution:
• May give undiluted. • For IV infusion, dilute with 50 ml D_5W or 0.9% NaCl before administration.
Rate of administration:
• Give IV push over 2–5 min. • Give IV infusion over 15 min.

IV INCOMPATIBILITIES ⊘
Acyclovir (Zovirax), allopurinol

(Aloprim), aminophylline, amphotericin B (Fungizone), amphotericin B complex (Abelcet, Ambisome, Amphotec), ampicillin (Polycillin), ampicillin/sulbactam (Unasyn), cefepime (Maxipime), cefoperazone (Cefobid), fluorouracil, lorazepam (Ativan), meropenem (Merrem IV), methylprednisolone (Solu-Medrol).

IV COMPATIBILITIES

Cisplatin (Platinol), cyclophosphamide (Cytoxan), cytarabine (Ara-C, Cytosar), dopamine (Intropin), doxorubicin (Adriamycin), etoposide (Vepesid), heparin, methotrexate, paclitaxel (Taxol), potassium chloride.

INDICATIONS/ROUTES/DOSAGE

Nausea, vomiting: chemotherapy:

Note: All oral doses given 30 min before chemotherapy and repeated at 8 hr intervals.

PO: Adults, elderly: 24 mg once a day or 8 mg 3 times/day. **Children 4–11 yrs:** 4 mg 3 times/day.

IV: Adults, elderly, children 4–18 yrs: 3 doses 0.15 mg/kg. First dose given 30 min before chemotherapy; then 4 and 8 hrs after first dose of ondansetron.

Nausea, vomiting: postop:

IM/IV: Adults, elderly: 4 mg undiluted over 2–5 min. **Children <40 kg:** 0.1 mg/kg. **>40 kg:** 4 mg.

Nausea, vomiting: radiation therapy:

PO: Adults, elderly: 8 mg 3 times/day.

SIDE EFFECTS

FREQUENT (5–13%): Anxiety, dizziness, drowsiness, headache, fatigue, constipation, diarrhea, hypoxia, urinary retention. *OCCASIONAL* (2–4%): Abdominal pain, xerostomia (diminished saliva secretion), fever, feeling of cold, redness/pain at injection site, paresthesia, weakness. *RARE* (<1%): Hypersensitivity reaction (rash, itching), blurred vision.

ADVERSE REACTIONS/TOXIC EFFECTS

Overdose may produce combination of CNS stimulation and depressant effects.

NURSING IMPLICATIONS

BASELINE ASSESSMENT:

Assess for dehydration if excessive vomiting occurs (poor skin turgor, dry mucous membranes, longitudinal furrows in tongue). Provide emotional support.

INTERVENTION/EVALUATION:

Monitor pt in environment. Assess bowel sounds for peristalsis. Provide supportive measures. Assess mental status. Monitor daily bowel activity and stool consistency (watery, loose, soft, semisolid, solid) and record time of evacuation.

PATIENT/FAMILY TEACHING:

Relief from nausea/vomiting generally occurs shortly after drug administration. Avoid alcohol, barbiturates. Report persistent vomiting.

oprelvekin (interleukin 11, IL-11)

oh-**prel**-vee-kinn
(Neumega)
Do not confuse with Neupogen.

▶CLASSIFICATION

PHARMACOTHERAPEUTIC:
Hematopoietic. **CLINICAL:** Platelet growth factor

ACTION/THERAPEUTIC EFFECT

Stimulates production of blood platelets (essential in the blood-clotting process), *resulting in increased platelet production.*

USES

Prevents severe thrombocytopenia; reduces need for platelet transfusions following myelosuppressive chemotherapy in pts with nonmyeloid malignancies.

PRECAUTIONS

CONTRAINDICATIONS: None significant. **CAUTIONS:** CHF, those susceptible to developing CHF, history of heart failure, history of atrial arrhythmia.

INTERACTIONS

DRUG: None significant. **HERBAL:** None known. **FOOD:** None known. **LAB VALUES:** May decrease hemoglobin, hematocrit (usually begins 3–5 days of initiation of therapy, reverses about 1 wk following discontinuance of therapy).

AVAILABILITY (Rx)
INJECTION: 5 mg.

ADMINISTRATION/HANDLING
SubQ:
Storage:
• Store in refrigerator. Once reconstituted, use within 3 hrs. Give single injection in abdomen, thigh or hip, upper arm.
Reconstitution:
Add 1 ml Sterile Water for Injection on side of vial and swirl con-

tents gently (avoid excessive agitation) to provide concentration of 5 mg/ml oprelvekin).
• Discard unused portion.

INDICATIONS/ROUTES/DOSAGE
Note: Dosing should begin 6–24 hrs following completion of chemotherapy dosing.
Prevention of thrombocytopenia:
SubQ: **Adults:** 50 mcg/kg once daily. **Children:** 75–100 mcg/kg once daily. Continue for 14–28 days or until platelet count reaches 50,000 cell/mcl after its nadir.

SIDE EFFECTS
FREQUENT: Nausea/vomiting (77%), fluid retention (59%), neutropenic fever (48%), diarrhea (43%), rhinitis (42%), headache (41%), dizziness (38%), fever (36%), insomnia (33%), cough (29%), rash, pharyngitis (25%), tachycardia (20%), vasodilation (19%).

ADVERSE REACTIONS/TOXIC EFFECTS
Transient atrial fibrillation or flutter occur in 10% of pts (may be due to increased plasma volume; drug is not directly arrhythmogenic). Arrhythmias usually are brief in duration and convert to normal sinus rhythm spontaneously. Papilledema in children.

NURSING IMPLICATIONS

BASELINE ASSESSMENT:
Obtain CBC prior to chemotherapy and at regular intervals thereafter.

INTERVENTION/EVALUATION:
Monitor platelet counts. Closely monitor fluid and electrolye sta-

tus, particularly those receiving diuretic therapy. Assess for fluid retention evidenced by peripheral edema, dyspnea on exertion (generally occurs during first week of therapy and continues for duration of treatment). Monitor platelet count periodically to assess therapeutic duration of therapy. Dosing should continue until postnadir platelet count is >50,000 cell/mcl. Treatment should be stopped >2 days before starting next round of chemotherapy.

orlistat

ore-leh-stat
(Xenical)

▶CLASSIFICATION

PHARMACOTHERAPEUTIC: Gastric/pancreatic lipase inhibitor. ***CLINICAL:*** Obesity management agent

ACTION/*THERAPEUTIC EFFECT*

Inhibits absorption of dietary fats by inactivating gastric and pancreatic enzymes *resulting in a caloric deficit that may have a positive effect on weight control.*

PHARMACOKINETICS

Minimal absorption following administration. Protein binding: >99%. Bound to plasma proteins. Primarily eliminated unchanged in feces. Unknown if removed by hemodialysis.

USES

Management of obesity including weight loss and weight maintenance when used in conjunction with a reduced-calorie diet.

PRECAUTIONS

CONTRAINDICATIONS: Chronic malabsorption syndrome, cholestasis. ***CAUTIONS:*** None significant.

▷***LIFESPAN CONSIDERATIONS:*** **Pregnancy/Lactation:** Unknown if excreted in breast milk. Not recommended during pregnancy or in nursing women. **Pregnancy Category B. Children:** Safety and efficacy not established. **Elderly:** No age-related precautions noted.

INTERACTIONS

DRUG: May increase concentration, risk of rhabdomyolysis with **pravastatin.** ***HERBAL:*** None known. ***FOOD:*** None significant. ***LAB VALUES:*** Decreases total cholesterol, LDL, glucose. Decreases absorption/levels of vitamins A and E.

AVAILABILITY (Rx)

TABLETS: 120 mg.

ADMINISTRATION/HANDLING

PO:

• Give without regard to food.

INDICATIONS/ROUTES/DOSAGE

Weight reduction:

PO: Adults, elderly: 120 mg three times/day.

SIDE EFFECTS

Note: Side effects tend to be mild and transient in nature, gradually diminishing during treatment.

FREQUENT (20–30%): Headache, abdominal discomfort, flatulence, fecal urgency, fatty/oily stool. ***OCCASIONAL*** (5–14%): Back pain, menstrual irregularity, nausea, fatigue, diarrhea, dizziness. ***RARE*** (<4%): Anxiety, rash, myalgia, dry skin, vomiting.

ADVERSE REACTIONS/TOXIC
EFFECTS
None significant.

NURSING IMPLICATIONS

INTERVENTION/EVALUATION:
Monitor cholesterol, LDL, glucose.

PATIENT/FAMILY TEACHING:
High-fiber, low-fat diet decreases fat evacuation.

orphenadrine citrate

(Norflex)

FIXED-COMBINATION(S)
With aspirin, non-narcotic analgesic and caffeine, a stimulant **(Norgesic)**

See Classification section under: Skeletal Muscle Relaxants

oseltamivir

oh-sell-**tam**-ih-veer
(Tamiflu)

▶CLASSIFICATION
PHARMACOTHERAPEUTIC:
Neuraminidase inhibitor. *CLINI-CAL:* Antiviral (see p. 59C)

ACTION/*THERAPEUTIC EFFECT*
Selective inhibitor of influenza virus neuraminidase, an enzyme essential for viral replication. Acts against both influenza A and B viruses. *Suppresses spread of infection within respiratory system, reduces duration of clinical symptoms.*

PHARMACOKINETICS
Readily absorbed. Protein binding: 3%. Extensively converted to active drug in the liver. Primarily excreted in urine. Half-life: 6–10 hrs.

USES
Symptomatic treatment of uncomplicated acute illness caused by influenza A or B virus in adults and children >1 yr of age who are symptomatic no longer than 2 days. Prevention of influenza in adults, children >13 yrs of age.

PRECAUTIONS
CONTRAINDICATIONS: None significant. *CAUTIONS:* Renal function impairment.

▷*LIFESPAN CONSIDERATIONS:*
Pregnancy/Lactation: Unknown if excreted in breast milk. **Pregnancy Category C. Children:** Safety and efficacy not established in those <1 yr of age. **Elderly:** No age-related precautions noted.

INTERACTIONS
DRUG: None significant. *HERBAL:* None known. *FOOD:* None known. *LAB VALUES:* None significant.

AVAILABILITY (Rx)
CAPSULES: 75 mg. *ORAL SUSPENSION:* 12 mg/ml.

ADMINISTRATION/HANDLING
PO:
• Give without regard to food.

INDICATIONS/ROUTES/DOSAGE
Influenza:

PO: Adults, elderly: 75 mg 2 times/day for 5 days. **Children (<15 kg):** 30 mg twice daily, **(15–23 kg):** 45 mg twice daily,

(23–40 kg): 60 mg twice daily, **(>40 kg):** 75 mg twice daily.

Dosage in renal impairment:

PO: **Adults, elderly:** 75 mg once daily for at least 7 days up to 6 wks.

Prophylaxis against influenza:

PO: **Adults, elderly:** 75 mg once daily.

SIDE EFFECTS

FREQUENT (>5%): Nausea, vomiting, diarrhea. ***OCCASIONAL*** (1–5%): Abdominal pain, bronchitis, dizziness, headache, cough, insomnia, fatigue, vertigo.

ADVERSE REACTIONS/TOXIC EFFECTS

Colitis, pneumonia, pyrexia occur rarely.

NURSING IMPLICATIONS

PATIENT/FAMILY TEACHING:

Begin as soon as possible from first appearance of flu symptoms. Avoid contact with those who are at high risk for influenza. Not a substitute for flu shot.

oxacillin

(Prostaphlin)

See Classification section under: Antibiotic: penicillins (p. 26C)

oxaprozin

ox-ah-**pro**-zin
(Daypro)
Do not confuse with oxazepam.

▶CLASSIFICATION

PHARMACOTHERAPEUTIC: Nonsteroidal anti-inflammatory ***CLINICAL:*** Analgesic, anti-inflammatory (see p. 107C)

ACTION/*THERAPEUTIC EFFECT*

Produces analgesic and anti-inflammatory effect by inhibiting prostaglandin synthesis, *reducing inflammatory response and intensity of pain stimulus reaching sensory nerve endings.*

PHARMACOKINETICS

Well absorbed from GI tract. Protein binding: >99%. Widely distributed. Metabolized in liver. Primarily excreted in urine; partially eliminated in feces. Not removed by hemodialysis. Half-life: 42–50 hrs.

USES

Acute and chronic treatment of osteoarthritis, rheumatoid arthritis.

PRECAUTIONS

CONTRAINDICATIONS: Active peptic ulcer, GI ulceration, chronic inflammation of GI tract, GI bleeding disorders, history of hypersensitivity to aspirin or NSAIDs. ***CAUTIONS:*** Impaired renal/hepatic function, history of GI tract disease, predisposition to fluid retention.
▷***LIFESPAN CONSIDERATIONS:***
Pregnancy/Lactation: Unknown whether drug is excreted in breast milk. Avoid use during third trimester (may adversely affect fetal cardiovascular system: premature closure of ductus arteriosus). **Pregnancy Category C** (Category D if used third trimester or near delivery). **Children:** Safety and efficacy not established. **Elderly:** Age-related renal impariment may increase

O

risk of liver or renal toxicity; decreased dosage recommended. GI bleeding or ulceration more likely to cause serious adverse effects.

INTERACTIONS

DRUG: May increase effects of **oral anticoagulants, heparin, thrombolytics.** May decrease effect of **antihypertensives, diuretics. Salicylates, aspirin** may increase risk of GI side effects, bleeding. **Bone marrow depressants** may increase risk of hematologic reactions. May increase concentration, toxicity of **lithium.** May increase **methotrexate** toxicity. **Probenecid** may increase concentration. **HERBAL:** Ginkgo **biloba** may increase risk of bleeding. May decrease **feverfew** effect. **FOOD:** None known. **LAB VALUES:** May increase SGOT (AST), SGPT (ALT), serum creatinine, BUN.

AVAILABILITY (Rx)

TABLETS: 600 mg.

ADMINISTRATION/HANDLING
PO:

• May give with food, milk, or antacids if GI distress occurs.

INDICATIONS/ROUTES/DOSAGE
Osteoarthritis:

PO: Adults, elderly: 1,200 mg once daily; 600 mg in pts with low body weight, mild disease. **Maximum:** 1,800 mg/day.

Rheumatoid arthritis:

PO: Adults, elderly: 1,200 mg once daily. **Range:** 600–1,800 mg/day.

SIDE EFFECTS

OCCASIONAL (3–9%): Nausea, diarrhea, constipation, dyspepsia (heartburn, indigestion, epigastric pain). **RARE** (<3%): Vomiting, abdominal cramping/pain, flatulence, anorexia, confusion, ringing in ears, insomnia, drowsiness.

ADVERSE REACTIONS/TOXIC EFFECTS

GI bleeding, coma may occur. Hypertension, acute renal failure, respiratory depression occur rarely.

NURSING IMPLICATIONS

BASELINE ASSESSMENT:
Assess onset, type, location, and duration of pain or inflammation.

INTERVENTION/EVALUATION:
Assist with ambulation if dizziness occurs. Monitor stools; avoid constipation through high-fiber diet, appropriate exercise, and increased fluids. Check for rash. Evaluate for therapeutic response: relief of pain, stiffness, swelling, increase in joint mobility, reduced joint tenderness, improved grip strength.

PATIENT/FAMILY TEACHING:
Avoid aspirin, alcohol during therapy (increases risk of GI bleeding). Report tarry stools. If GI upset occurs, take with food, milk. Avoid tasks that require alertness, motor skills until response to drug is established.

oxazepam ✳

ox-**az**-eh-pam
(Apo-Oxazepam ✿, Serax)
Do not confuse with Eurax, oxaprozin, Xerac.

►CLASSIFICATION

PHARMACOTHERAPEUTIC:
Benzodiazepine **(Schedule IV).**
CLINICAL: Antianxiety (see p. 11C)

ACTION/*THERAPEUTIC EFFECT*

Enhances inhibitory gamma-aminobutyric acid (GABA) neurotransmission at CNS, *producing anxiolytic effect.* Inhibits spinal afferent pathways, *producing skeletal muscle relaxation.* Depressant effects occur at all levels of CNS. Directly depresses motor nerve, muscle function.

PHARMACOKINETICS

Well absorbed from GI tract. Protein binding: >97%. Metabolized in liver. Primarily excreted in urine. Not removed by hemodialysis.

USES

Management of acute alcohol withdrawal symptoms (tremulousness, anxiety on withdrawal). Treatment of anxiety associated with depressive symptoms.

PRECAUTIONS

CONTRAINDICATIONS: Acute narrow-angle glaucoma. *CAUTIONS:* Impaired renal/hepatic function.

INTERACTIONS

DRUG: Potentiated effects when used with other **CNS depressants, including alcohol. HERBAL: Kava kava, valerian** may increase CNS depression. *FOOD:* None known. *LAB VALUES:* May produce abnormal renal function tests, elevate SGOT (AST), SGPT (ALT), LDH, alkaline phosphatase, serum bilirubin. Therapeutic blood serum level:

0.2–1.4 mcg/ml; toxic blood serum level: Not established.

AVAILABILITY (Rx)

CAPSULES: 10 mg, 15 mg, 30 mg.

INDICATIONS/ROUTES/DOSAGE

Note: Use smallest effective dose in elderly, debilitated, those with liver disease, low serum albumin.

Mild to moderate anxiety:
PO: **Adults:** 10–15 mg 3–4 times/day.

Severe anxiety:
PO: **Adults:** 15–30 mg 3–4 times/day.

Alcohol withdrawal:
PO: **Adults:** 15–30 mg 3–4 times/day.

Usual elderly dosage:
PO: Initially, 10–20 mg 3 times/day. May gradually increase up to 30–45 mg/day.

SIDE EFFECTS

FREQUENT: Mild, transient drowsiness at beginning of therapy. *OCCASIONAL:* Dizziness, headache. *RARE:* Paradoxical CNS hyperactivity/nervousness in children, excitement/restlessness in elderly/debilitated (generally noted during first 2 wks of therapy).

ADVERSE REACTIONS/TOXIC EFFECTS

Abrupt or too-rapid withdrawal may result in pronounced restlessness, irritability, insomnia, hand tremors, abdominal/muscle cramps, sweating, vomiting, seizures. Overdose results in somnolence, confusion, diminished reflexes, coma.

NURSING IMPLICATIONS

BASELINE ASSESSMENT:
Offer emotional support to anxious pt. Assess motor responses (agitation, trembling, tension)

and autonomic responses (cold, clammy hands, sweating).

INTERVENTION/EVALUATION:

For those on long-term therapy, liver/renal function tests, blood counts should be performed periodically. Assess for paradoxical reaction, particularly during early therapy. Assist with ambulation if drowsiness, lightheadedness occur. Evaluate for therapeutic response: a calm facial expression, decreased restlessness, and/or insomnia. Therapeutic blood serum level: 0.2–1.4 mcg/ml; toxic blood serum level: Not established.

PATIENT/FAMILY TEACHING:

Drowsiness usually disappears during continued therapy. If dizziness occurs, change positions slowly from recumbent to sitting position before standing. Avoid tasks that require alertness, motor skills until response to drug is established. Smoking reduces drug effectiveness. Do not abruptly withdraw medication after long-term therapy.

oxcarbazepine

ox-car-**bah**-zeh-peen
(Trileptal)

▶CLASSIFICATION

CLINICAL: Anticonvulsant (see p. 33C)

ACTION/*THERAPEUTIC EFFECT*

Produces blockade of sodium channels, resulting in stabilization of hyperexcited neural membranes, inhibiting repetitive neuronal firing, diminishing synaptic impulses, *preventing seizures.*

PHARMACOKINETICS

Completely absorbed and extensively metabolized to active metabolite in the liver. Protein binding: 40%. Primarily excreted in urine. Half-life: 2 hrs (metabolite: 6–10 hrs).

USES/*UNLABELED*

Monotherapy and adjunctive therapy in adults and adjunctive therapy in children 4–16 yrs of age in treatment of partial seizures. *Atypical panic disorder.*

PRECAUTIONS

CONTRAINDICATIONS: None significant. ***CAUTIONS:*** Renal function impairment, sensitivity to carbamazepine.
▷***LIFESPAN CONSIDERATIONS:***
Pregnancy/Lactation: Crosses placenta; distributed in breast milk. **Pregnancy Category C. Children:** No age-related precautions in those >4 yrs of age. **Elderly:** Age-related renal impairment may require dosage adjustment.

INTERACTIONS

DRUG: **Carbamazepine, phenobarbital, phenytoin, valproic acid, verapamil** may decrease concentration, effect. May decrease concentration, effect of **felodipine, oral contraceptives.** May increase concentration, toxicity of **phenobarbital, phenytoin.** ***HERBAL:*** None known. ***FOOD:*** None known. ***LAB VALUES:*** May increase gamma G-T, increase or decrease blood glucose, increase liver function tests, decrease calcium, potassium, sodium.

AVAILABILITY (Rx)
TABLETS: 150 mg, 300 mg, 600 mg. **ORAL SUSPENSION.**

ADMINISTRATION/HANDLING
PO:
• Give without regard to food.

INDICATIONS/ROUTES/DOSAGE
Note: Give all doses in a twice daily regimen.

Adjunctive therapy:
PO: Adults, elderly: Initially 600 mg/day in 2 divided doses. May increase by a maximum of 600 mg/day at weekly intervals. **Maximum:** 2,400 mg/day. **Children, 4–16 yrs:** 8–10 mg/kg. **Maximum:** 600 mg/day. Achieve maintenance dose over 2 wks based on pt's weight. **20–29 kg:** 900 mg/day; **29.1–39 kg:** 1,200 mg/day; **>39 kg:** 1,800 mg/day.

Conversion to monotherapy:
PO: Adults, elderly: 600 mg/day in 2 divided doses (while decreasing concomitant antiepilepsy drug over 3–6 wks) increasing up to 2,400 mg/day over 2–4 wks (see above for guideline to increasing dosage).

Initiation of monotherapy:
PO: Adults, elderly: 600 mg/day in 2 divided doses. May increase by 300 mg/day q3days up to 1,200 mg/day.

SIDE EFFECTS
FREQUENT (13–22%): Dizziness, nausea, headache. **OCCASIONAL** (5–7%): Vomiting, diarrhea, ataxia (muscular incoordination), nervousness, dyspepsia (heartburn, indigestion, epigastric pain), constipation. **RARE** (4%): Tremor, rash, back pain, nosebleed, sinusitis, diplopia (double vision).

ADVERSE REACTIONS/TOXIC EFFECTS
May produce clinically significant hyponatremia.

NURSING IMPLICATIONS

BASELINE ASSESSMENT:
Review history of seizure disorder (type, onset, intensity, frequency, duration, LOC), drug history (esp. other anticonvulsants). Provide safety precautions, quiet, dark environment. Initiate seizure precautions.

INTERVENTION/EVALUATION:
Assist with ambulation if dizziness, ataxia occurs. Assess for visual abnormalities, headache. Monitor serum sodium levels. Assess for signs of hyponatremia (nausea, malaise, headache, lethargy, confusion). Assess for clinical improvement (decrease in intensity/frequency of seizures).

PATIENT/FAMILY TEACHING:
Strict maintenance of drug therapy is essential for seizure control. If dizziness occurs, change positions slowly from recumbent to sitting position before standing. Avoid alcohol. Avoid tasks that require alertness, motor skills until response to drug is established.

---

oxiconazole

(Oxistat)

See Classification section under: Antifungals: topical (p. 43C)

---

oxybutynin chloride

ox-ee-**byoo**-tih-nin
(Ditropan)
Do not confuse with diazepam,
Oxycontin.

▶CLASSIFICATION

PHARMACOTHERAPEUTIC:
Anticholinergic. ***CLINICAL:*** Antispasmodic

ACTION/*THERAPEUTIC EFFECT*

Exerts antispasmodic (papaver-
ine-like) and antimuscarinic (at-
ropine-like) action on detrusor
smooth muscle of bladder. *Increases bladder capacity, diminishes frequency of uninhibited detrusor muscle contraction, delays
desire to void.*

PHARMACOKINETICS

	Onset	Peak	Duration
PO	0.5–1 hr	3–6 hrs	6–10 hrs

Rapid absorption from GI tract.
Metabolized in liver. Primarily excreted in urine. Unknown if removed by hemodialysis. Half-life:
1–2.3 hrs.

USES

Relief of symptoms (urgency, incontinence, frequency, nocturia,
urge incontinence) associated
with uninhibited neurogenic bladder or reflex neurogenic bladder.

PRECAUTIONS

CONTRAINDICATIONS: Angle-
closure glaucoma, GI obstruction,
myasthenia gravis, paralytic ileus,
megacolon, ulcerative colitis, intestinal atony, unstable cardiovascular disease. ***CAUTIONS:*** Impaired renal or hepatic function,
elderly, autonomic neuropathy.

▷*LIFESPAN CONSIDERATIONS:*
Pregnancy/Lactation: Unknown if
drug crosses placenta or is distributed in breast milk. **Pregnancy
Category B. Children:** No age-related precautions noted in those >5
yrs of age. **Elderly:** May be more
sensitive to anticholinergic effects
(e.g., dry mouth, urinary retention).

INTERACTIONS

DRUG: Medication with **anticholinergic effects (e.g., antihistamines)** may increase effects.
HERBAL: None known. ***FOOD:***
None known. ***LAB VALUES:*** None
significant.

AVAILABILITY (Rx)

TABLETS: 5 mg. ***SYRUP:*** 5 mg/5
ml. ***EXTENDED-RELEASE TAB-
LETS:*** 5 mg, 10 mg, 15 mg.

ADMINISTRATION/HANDLING
PO:

• Give without regard to meals.

INDICATIONS/ROUTES/DOSAGE
Neurogenic bladder:

PO: **Adults:** 5 mg 2–3 times/day.
Maximum: 5 mg 4 times/day.
Children >5 yrs: 5 mg 2 times/
day. **Maximum:** 5 mg 3 times/day.
Children 1–5 yrs: 0.2 mg/kg/dose
2–4 times/day.

Usual elderly dosage:

PO: Initially, 2.5–5 mg/day. May increase by 2.5 mg q1–2days.

Usual dosage extended-release:

PO: **Adults, elderly:** 5–30 mg/day
as single daily dose.

SIDE EFFECTS

FREQUENT: Constipation, dry
mouth, drowsiness, decreased sweating. ***OCCASIONAL:*** Decreased lacrimation, salivary/sweat gland secretion, sexual ability. Urinary hesitancy/

retention, suppressed lactation, blurred vision, mydriasis, nausea or vomiting, insomnia.

ADVERSE REACTIONS/TOXIC EFFECTS

Overdosage produces CNS excitation (nervousness, restlessness, hallucinations, irritability), hypo/hypertension, confusion, fast heartbeat or tachycardia, flushed or red face, respiratory depression (shortness of breath or troubled breathing).

NURSING IMPLICATIONS

BASELINE ASSESSMENT:

Assess dysuria, urgency, frequency, incontinence.

INTERVENTION/EVALUATION:

Monitor for symptomatic relief. Monitor I&O; palpate bladder for retention. Monitor bowel activity and stool consistency.

PATIENT/FAMILY TEACHING:

Avoid driving or other tasks requiring alertness, coordination, or manual dexterity until response to drug is established.

oxycodone

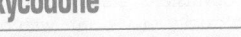

ox-ih-**koe**-doan
(Intensol, Oxycontin, OxyFast, OxyIR, Perolone, Roxicodone, Supeudol♣)
Do not confuse with oxybutynin.

FIXED-COMBINATION(S)

With acetaminophen, a non-narcotic analgesic **(Percocet, Roxicet, Tylox)**; with aspirin, a nonnarcotic analgesic **(Percodan, Roxiprin)**

► CLASSIFICATION
PHARMACOTHERAPEUTIC:
Opioid agonist **(Schedule II).**
CLINICAL: Narcotic analgesic
(see p. 117C)

ACTION/*THERAPEUTIC EFFECT*

Binds with opioid receptors within CNS, *altering processes affecting pain perception, emotional response to pain.*

PHARMACOKINETICS

	Onset	Peak	Duration
PO	10–15 min	30–60 min	3–6 hrs

Moderately absorbed from GI tract. Protein binding: 38–45%. Widely distributed. Metabolized in liver. Excreted in urine. Unknown if removed by hemodialysis. Half-life: 2–3 hrs.

USES

Relief of mild to moderately severe pain.

PRECAUTIONS

CONTRAINDICATIONS: None significant. ***EXTREME CAUTION:*** CNS depression, anoxia, hypercapnia, respiratory depression, seizures, acute alcoholism, shock, untreated myxedema, respiratory dysfunction. ***CAUTIONS:*** Increased intracranial pressure, impaired hepatic function, acute abdominal conditions, hypothyroidism, prostatic hypertrophy, Addison's disease, urethral stricture, COPD.

▷*LIFESPAN CONSIDERATIONS:*
Pregnancy/Lactation: Readily crosses placenta; distributed in breast milk. Respiratory depression may occur in neonate if mother received opiates during labor. Regular use of opiates during pregnancy may produce with-

O

drawal symptoms in neonate (irritability, excessive crying, tremors, hyperactive reflexes, fever, vomiting, diarrhea, yawning, sneezing, seizures). **Pregnancy Category B** (Category D if used for prolonged periods or in high doses at term). **Children:** Paradoxical excitement may occur. Those <2 yrs of age more susceptible to respiratory depressant effects. **Elderly:** Age-related renal impairment may increase risk of urinary retention. May be more susceptible to respiratory depressant effects.

INTERACTIONS

DRUG: **Alcohol, CNS depressants** may increase CNS or respiratory depression, hypotension. **MAO inhibitors** may produce severe, fatal reaction (reduce dose to ¼ usual dose). **HERBAL:** None known. **FOOD:** None known. **LAB VALUES:** May increase amylase, lipase.

AVAILABILITY (Rx)

CAPSULES (immediate-release) *(OxyIR):* 5 mg. **ORAL CONCENTRATE** *(OxyFast, Roxicodone, Intensol):* 20 mg/ml. **ORAL SOLUTION** *(Roxicodone):* 5 mg/ml. **TABLETS (immediate-release)** *(Percolone, Roxicodone):* 5 mg, 15 mg, 30 mg. **TABLETS (controlled-release)** *(Oxycontin):* 10 mg, 20 mg, 40 mg, 80 mg, 160 mg.

ADMINISTRATION/HANDLING
PO:

• Give without regard to meals. • Tablets may be crushed. • **Controlled-Release:** Swallow whole; do not crush, break, chew.

INDICATIONS/ROUTES/DOSAGE
Analgesia:

PO: Adults, elderly (immediate-release): Initially, 5 mg q6h as needed. May increase up to 30 mg q4h. **Usual:** 10–30 mg q4h as needed. **Children:** 0.05–0.15 mg/kg/dose q4–6h.

PO: Adults, elderly (controlled-release): Initially, 10 mg q12h. May increase q1–2days by 25–50%. **Usual:** 40 mg/day (*Cancer pain:* 100 mg/day).

SIDE EFFECTS

Note: Effects are dependent on dosage amount. Ambulatory pts and those not in severe pain may experience dizziness, nausea, vomiting, hypotension more frequently than those in supine position or having severe pain.

FREQUENT: Drowsiness, dizziness, hypotension, anorexia. **OCCASIONAL:** Confusion, diaphoresis, facial flushing, urinary retention, constipation, dry mouth, nausea, vomiting, headache. **RARE:** Allergic reaction, depression, paradoxical CNS hyperactivity/nervousness in children, excitement/restlessness in elderly/debilitated pts.

ADVERSE REACTIONS/TOXIC EFFECTS

Overdose results in respiratory depression, skeletal muscle flaccidity, cold, clammy skin, cyanosis, extreme somnolence progressing to convulsions, stupor, coma. Hepatotoxicity may occur with overdosage of acetaminophen component. Tolerance to analgesic effect, physical dependence may occur with repeated use.

NURSING IMPLICATIONS

BASELINE ASSESSMENT:

Assess onset, type, location, and duration of pain. Effect of medication is reduced if full pain recurs before next dose. Obtain vital signs before giving medication. If respirations are 12/min or lower (20/min or lower in children), withhold medication, contact physician.

INTERVENTION/EVALUATION:

Palpate bladder for urinary retention. Monitor pattern of daily bowel activity and stool consistency. Initiate deep breathing and coughing exercises, particularly in those with impaired pulmonary function. Assess for clinical improvement and record onset of relief of pain.

PATIENT/FAMILY TEACHING:

Change positions slowly to avoid orthostatic hypotension. Avoid tasks that require alertness, motor skills until response to drug is established. Tolerance/dependence may occur with prolonged use of high doses.

oxytocin

ox-ih-**toe**-sin
(Pitocin)
Do not confuse with Pitressin.

▶CLASSIFICATION

PHARMACOTHERAPEUTIC:
Uterine smooth muscle stimulant.
CLINICAL: Oxytocic

ACTION/THERAPEUTIC EFFECT

Acts on uterine myofibril activity, *stimulates contraction of uterine smooth muscle* (augments number of contracting myofibrils). Stimulates mammary smooth muscle to *enhance milk ejection from breasts.*

PHARMACOKINETICS

	Onset	Peak	Duration
IM	3–5 min	—	2–3 hrs
IV	Immediate	—	1 hr
Intranasal	Few min	—	20 min

Rapidly absorbed through nasal mucous membranes. Protein binding: 30%. Distributed in extracellular fluid. Metabolized in liver, kidney. Primarily excreted in urine.

USES

Parenteral (Antepartum): Initiates or improves uterine contraction to achieve early vaginal delivery; stimulate or reinforce labor; management of incomplete or inevitable abortion. **(Postpartum):** Produces uterine contractions during third stage of labor; controls uterine bleeding. **Nasal:** To promote breast milk ejection.

PRECAUTIONS

CONTRAINDICATIONS: Cephalopelvic disproportion, unfavorable fetal position or presentation, unengaged fetal head, fetal distress without imminent delivery, prematurity, when vaginal delivery is contraindicated (e.g., active genital herpes infection, placenta previa, cord presentation), obstetric emergencies that favor surgical intervention, grand multiparity, hypertonic or hyperactive uterus, adequate uterine activity that fails to progress. Nasal spray during pregnancy. **CAUTIONS:** Induction should be for medical, not elective reasons.

▷**LIFESPAN CONSIDERATIONS:**
Pregnancy/Lactation: Used as indicated, not expected to present risk of fetal abnormalities. Small amounts in breast milk; nursing not

recommended. **Children/Elderly:** Not used in these pt populations.

INTERACTIONS

DRUG: Caudal block anesthetics, vasopressors may increase pressor effects. **Other oxytocics** may cause uterine hypertonus, uterine rupture, or cervical lacerations. **HERBAL:** None known. **FOOD:** None known. **LAB VALUES:** None significant.

AVAILABILITY (Rx)

INJECTION: 10 units/ml. **NASAL SPRAY:** 40 units/ml.

ADMINISTRATION/HANDLING

Intranasal:

• With pt in sitting position, spray in one or both nostrils. • Give 2–3 min before nursing or pumping breasts.

IV 🔟

Storage:

• Store at room temperature.

Reconstitution:

• Dilute 10–40 units (1–4 ml) in 1,000 ml of 0.9% NaCl, lactated Ringer's, or D_5W to provide a concentration of 10–40 milliunits/ml solution.

Rate of administration:

• Give by IV infusion (use infusion device to carefully control rate of flow as ordered by physician).

IV INCOMPATIBILITY ⊘

No known incompatibilities via Y-site administration.

IV COMPATIBILITIES

Heparin, insulin, multivitamins, potassium chloride.

INDICATIONS/ROUTES/DOSAGE

Induction/stimulation of labor:

IV INFUSION: Adults: Initially, 0.5–2 milliunits/min; gradually increase in increments of 1–2 milliunits/min q15–30min (until contraction pattern similar to spontaneous labor reached). **Maximum:** Rarely >20 milliunits/min.

Incomplete/inevitable abortion:

IV INFUSION: Adults: 10 units in 500 ml (20 milliunits/ml) D_5W or 0.9% NaCl infused at 20–40 milliunits/min.

Control of postpartum bleeding:

IV INFUSION: Adults: 10–40 units (**maximum:** 40 units/1,000 ml) infused at rate of 20–40 milliunits/min after delivery of infant.

IM: Adults: 10 units after delivery of placenta.

Postabortion hemorrhage:

IV INFUSION: Adults: 10 units infused at rate of 20–100 milliunits/min.

Promote milk ejection:

NASAL: Adults: 1 spray to one or both nostrils 2–3 min before nursing or pumping breasts.

SIDE EFFECTS

OCCASIONAL: Tachycardia, PVCs, hypotension, nausea, vomiting. **RARE: Nasal:** Lacrimation (tearing), nasal irritation, rhinorrhea, unexpected uterine bleeding or contractions.

ADVERSE REACTIONS/TOXIC EFFECTS

Hypertonicity with tearing of uterus, increased bleeding, abruptio placenta, cervical and vaginal lacerations. **Fetal:** Bradycardia, CNS or brain damage, trauma due to rapid propulsion, low Apgar at 5 min, retinal hemorrhage occur rarely. Prolonged IV infusion of oxytocin with excessive fluid volume has caused severe water intoxication with seizures, coma, and death.

NURSING IMPLICATIONS

BASELINE ASSESSMENT:

Assess baselines for vital signs, B/P, and fetal heart rate. Determine frequency, duration, and strength of contractions.

INTERVENTION/EVALUATION:

Monitor B/P, pulse, respirations, fetal heart rate, intrauterine pressure, contractions (duration, strength, frequency) q15min. Notify physician of contractions that last >1 min, occur more frequently than every 2 min, or stop. Maintain careful I/O; be alert to potential water intoxication. Check for blood loss.

PATIENT/FAMILY TEACHING:

Keep pt, family informed of labor progress. ***Nasal spray:*** Teach proper use.

paclitaxel

pass-leh-**tax**-ell
(Paxene, Taxol)
Do not confuse with Paxil, Taxotere.

▶**CLASSIFICATION**

PHARMACOTHERAPEUTIC:
Taxoid, antimitotic agent. ***CLINICAL:*** Antineoplastic (see p. 73C)

ACTION/*THERAPEUTIC EFFECT***

Binds to fully assembled microtubules, stabilizes microtubules, prevents depolymerization, *resulting in halting mitosis and cell death.* May also interrupt mitosis by distorting mitotic spindles. Cell cycle-specific for G_2, M phases.

PHARMACOKINETICS

Does not readily cross blood-brain barrier. Protein binding: 89–98%. Metabolized in liver (active metabolites); eliminated via bile. Not removed by hemodialysis. Half-life: 1.3–8.6 hrs.

USES/*UNLABELED***

First-line treatment of advanced ovarian cancer, treatment for metastatic ovarian cancer following failure of first-line or subsequent chemotherapy. Treatment of breast cancer, AIDS-related Kaposi's sarcoma, non small cell lung cancer. *Treatment of head and neck, cancer, small cell lung cancer, adenocarcinoma of upper GI tract, hormone-refractory prostate cancer, non-Hodgkin's lymphona, transitional cell cancer of urothelium.*

PRECAUTIONS

CONTRAINDICATIONS: Baseline neutropenia <1,500 cells/mm^3, hypersensitivity to drugs developed with Cremophor EL (polyoxyethylated castor oil). ***CAUTIONS:*** History of CHF, cardiac conduction abnormalities, existing/recent chickenpox, infection, herpes zoster.

▷***LIFESPAN CONSIDERATIONS:***
Pregnancy/Lactation: May produce fetal harm. Unknown if distributed in breast milk. Avoid pregnancy. **Pregnancy Category D. Children:** Safety and efficacy not established. **Elderly:** No age-related precautions noted.

INTERACTIONS

***DRUG:* Bone marrow depressants** may increase bone marrow depression. **Live virus vaccines** may potentiate virus replication, increase vaccine side effects, decrease pt's antibody response to

P

vaccine. **HERBAL:** None known. **FOOD:** None known. **LAB VALUES:** May elevate alkaline phosphatase, SGOT (AST), SGPT (ALT), bilirubin. Decreases WBCs, RBCs, hemoglobin, hematocrit, platelets.

AVAILABILITY (Rx)

INJECTION: 30 mg, 100 mg.

ADMINISTRATION/HANDLING

IV 💊

Note: Wear gloves during handling; if contact with skin, wash hands thoroughly with soap and water. If in contact with mucous membranes, flush with water.

Storage:

• Refrigerate unopened vials. • Prepared solution is stable at room temperature for 24 hrs. • Store diluted solutions in bottles or plastic bags and administer through polyethylene-lined administration sets (avoid plasticized PVC equipment or devices).

Reconstitution:

• Dilute with 0.9% NaCl, D_5W, D_5W/0.9% NaCl, or D_5W/lactated Ringer's to final concentration of 0.3–1.2 mg/ml.

Rate of administration:

• Administer at rate as ordered by physician through in-line filter not greater than 0.22 microns. • Monitor vital signs during infusion, esp. during first hr. • Discontinue administration if severe hypersensitivity reaction occurs.

IV INCOMPATIBILITIES ⊘

Amphotericin B complex (Abelcet, Ambisome, Amphotec), chlorpromazine (Thorazine), doxorubicin liposome (Doxil), hydroxyzine (Vistaril), methylprednisolone (Solu-Medrol), mitoxantrone (Novantrone).

IV COMPATIBILITIES

Carboplatin (Paraplatin), cisplatin (Platinol), dexamethasone (Decadron), granisetron (Kytril), magnesium, mannitol, ondansetron (Zofran), potassium chloride.

INDICATIONS/ROUTES/DOSAGE

Note: Pretreat with corticosteroids, diphenhydramine, and H_2 antagonists.

Ovarian cancer:

IV INFUSION: **Adults:** 135–175 mg/m²/dose over 1–24 hrs q3wks.

Breast carcinoma:

IV INFUSION: **Adults, elderly:** 175 mg/m² over 3 hrs q3wks.

Kaposi's sarcoma:

IV INFUSION: 135 mg/m²/dose over 3 hrs q3wks or 100 mg/m²/dose over 3 hrs q2wks.

SIDE EFFECTS

COMMON (70–90%): Diarrhea, alopecia, nausea, vomiting. **FREQUENT** (46–48%): Myalgia/arthralgia, peripheral neuropathy. **OCCASIONAL** (13–20%): Mucositis, hypotension (during infusion), pain/redness at injection site. **RARE** (3%): Bradycardia.

ADVERSE REACTIONS/TOXIC EFFECTS

Neutropenic nadir occurs at median of 11 days. Anemia, leukopenia occur commonly, thrombocytopenia occurs occasionally. Severe hypersensitivity reaction (dyspnea, severe hypotension, angioedema, generalized urticaria) occurs rarely.

NURSING IMPLICATIONS

BASELINE ASSESSMENT:

Give emotional support to pt and family. Use strict asepsis and protect pt from infection. Check blood counts, particularly neutrophil, platelet count before each course of therapy, moly, or as clinically indicated.

INTERVENTION/EVALUATION:

Monitor for hematologic toxicity (fever, sore throat, signs of local infections, easy bruising, unusual bleeding), symptoms of anemia (excessive tiredness, weakness). Assess response to medication; monitor and report for diarrhea. Avoid IM injections, rectal temperatures, other traumas that may induce bleeding. Put pressure to injection sites for full 5 min.

PATIENT/FAMILY TEACHING:

Explain that alopecia is reversible, but new hair may have different color, texture. Do not have immunizations without physician's approval (drug lowers body's resistance). Avoid crowds, persons with known infections. Report signs of infection at once (fever, flulike symptoms). Contact physician if nausea/vomiting continue at home. Teach signs of peripheral neuropathy. Avoid pregnancy during therapy.

palivizumab

pal-**iv**-ih-zoo-mab
(Synagis)
Do not confuse with Synalgos-DC.

▶CLASSIFICATION

PHARMACOTHERAPEUTIC: Monoclonal antibody. **CLINICAL:** Pediatric lower respiratory tract infection agent

ACTION/*THERAPEUTIC EFFECT*

Exhibits neutralizing activity against respiratory syncytial virus (RSV) in infants, *inhibiting RSV replication in the lower respiratory tract.*

USES

Prevention of serious lower respiratory tract disease caused by RSV in pediatric pts at high risk for RSV disease.

PRECAUTIONS

CONTRAINDICATIONS: Hypersensitivity to palivizumab. **CAUTIONS:** None sigificant.

INTERACTIONS

DRUG: None known. **HERBAL:** None sigificant. **FOOD:** None sigificant. **LAB VALUES:** None known.

AVAILABILITY (Rx)

LYOPHILIZED INJECTION: 100 mg.

INDICATIONS/ROUTES/DOSAGE

Respiratory syncytial virus (RSV) prevention:

IM: Children: 15 mg/kg once a month.

SIDE EFFECTS

FREQUENT (22–49%): Upper respiratory tract infection, otitis media, rhinitis, rash. **OCCASIONAL** (2–10%): Pain, pharyngitis. **RARE** (<2%): Cough, diarrhea, vomiting, injection site reaction.

ADVERSE REACTIONS/TOXIC EFFECTS

None significant.

NURSING IMPLICATIONS

BASELINE ASSESSMENT:

Assess for sensitivity to palivizumab.

INTERVENTION/EVALUATION:

Monitor potential side effects, esp. otitis media, rhinitis, skin rash, upper respiratory tract infection.

PATIENT/FAMILY TEACHING:

Discuss with family the purpose and potential side effects.

pamidronate disodium

pam-ih-**drow**-nate
(Aredia)

▶CLASSIFICATION

PHARMACOTHERAPEUTIC: Biphosphate. ***CLINICAL:*** Hypocalcemic

ACTION/*THERAPEUTIC EFFECT*

Decreases release of phosphates, calcium from bone and increases renal excretion as parathyroid levels (usually suppressed in hypercalcemia in malignancy) return to normal levels. *Inhibits accelerated bone resorption* (bone formation and mineralization not inhibited).

PHARMACOKINETICS

After IV administration, rapidly absorbed by bone. Slowly excreted unchanged in urine. Unknown if removed by hemodialysis.

USES

Treatment of moderate to severe hypercalcemia associated with malignancy (with or without bone metastases). Treatment of moderate to severe Paget's disease, osteolytic bone lesions of multiple myeloma, breast cancer.

PRECAUTIONS

CONTRAINDICATIONS: Hypersensitivity to other biphosphonates (etidronate, tiludronate, risedronate, alendronate). ***CAUTIONS:*** Cardiac failure, renal function impairment.

▷***LIFESPAN CONSIDERATIONS:***
Pregnancy/Lactation: There are no adequate and well-controlled studies in pregnant women; unknown if fetal harm can occur. Excretion in breast milk unknown. **Pregnancy Category C. Children:** Safety and efficacy not established. **Elderly:** May become overhydrated. Careful monitoring of fluid and electrolytes; recommend diluted in smaller volume.

INTERACTIONS

DRUG: **Calcium-containing medications, vitamin D** may antagonize effects in treatment of hypercalcemia. ***HERBAL:*** None known. ***FOOD:*** None known. ***LAB VALUES:*** May decrease phosphate, potassium, magnesium, calcium levels.

AVAILABILITY (Rx)

POWDER FOR INJECTION: 30 mg, 60 mg, 90 mg.

ADMINISTRATION/HANDLING

IV 🕎

Storage:

• Store parenteral form at room temperature. • Reconstituted vial is stable for 24 hrs refrigerated; IV solution is stable for 24 hrs after dilution.

Reconstitution:

• Reconstitute each 30 mg vial with 10 ml Sterile Water for Injection to provide concentration of 3 mg/ml. • Allow drug to dissolve before withdrawing. • Further dilute with 1,000 ml sterile 0.45% or 0.9% NaCl or D_5W.

Rate of administration:

• Adequate hydration is essential in conjunction with pamidronate therapy (avoid overhydration in pts with potential for cardiac failure). • Administer as IV infusion over 2–24 hrs for treatment of hypercalcemia; over 2–4 hrs for other indications.

IV INCOMPATIBILITY ⊘

Do not mix with any other medications.

INDICATIONS/ROUTES/DOSAGE

Hypercalcemia:

***IV INFUSION:* Adults, elderly:** Moderate (corrected serum calcium 12–13.5 mg/dl): 60–90 mg. Severe (corrected serum calcium >13.5 mg/dl): 90 mg.

Paget's disease:

***IV INFUSION:* Adults, elderly:** 30 mg/day for 3 days.

Osteolytic bone lesion:

***IV INFUSION:* Adults, elderly:** 90 mg over 2–4 hrs.

SIDE EFFECTS

FREQUENT (>10%): 27% of pts have temperature elevation (at least 1° C) 24–48 hrs after administration. Drug-related redness, swelling, induration, pain at catheter site (18% of pts receiving 90 mg). Anorexia, nausea, fatigue. ***OCCASIONAL*** (1–10%): Constipation, rhinitis.

ADVERSE REACTIONS/TOXIC EFFECTS

Hypophosphatemia, hypokalemia, hypomagnesemia, hypocalcemia occur more frequently with higher dosage. Anemia, hypertension, tachycardia, atrial fibrillation, somnolence occur more often with 90 mg dosages. GI hemorrhage occurs rarely.

NURSING IMPLICATIONS

INTERVENTION/EVALUATION:

Provide adequate hydration; avoid overhydration. Monitor I&O carefully; check lungs for rales, dependent body parts for edema. Monitor B/P, temperature, pulse. Assess catheter site for redness, swelling, pain. Check electrolytes (esp. calcium and potassium) and CBC results. Monitor food intake and stool frequency. Be alert for potential GI hemorrhage with 90 mg dosage.

pancreatin ✳

pan-kree-**ah**-tin
(Pancreatin)

pancrelipase

pan-kree-**lie**-pace
(Cotazym, Creon, Ilozyme, Pancrease ♣, Pancrease MT, Ultrase, Viokase)

P

►CLASSIFICATION

PHARMACOTHERAPEUTIC: Digestive enzyme. ***CLINICAL:*** Pancreatic enzyme replenisher

ACTION/*THERAPEUTIC EFFECT*

Hydrolyzes fat to glycerol and fatty acids, converts starch into destrins and sugars, reduces fat and nitrogen content in stool, *aiding in digestion of protein, carbohydrate, fat in GI tract* (primarily in duodenum, upper jejunum).

USES

Pancreatic enzyme replacement/supplement when enzymes are absent or deficient (i.e., chronic pancreatitis, cystic fibrosis, ductal obstruction from pancreatic cancer, common bile duct). Treatment of steatorrhea associated with postgastrectomy syndrome, bowel resection; reduces malabsorption.

PRECAUTIONS

CONTRAINDICATIONS: Hypersensitivity to pork protein. **CAUTIONS:** None significant.
▷**LIFESPAN CONSIDERATIONS:** **Pregnancy/Lactation:** Unknown if drug crosses placenta or is distributed in breast milk. **Pregnancy Category C. Children:** Information not available. **Elderly:** No age-related precautions noted.

INTERACTIONS

DRUG: Antacids may decrease effect. May decrease absorption of **iron supplements. HERBAL:** None known. **FOOD:** None known. **LAB VALUES:** May increase uric acid.

AVAILABILITY (Rx)

TABLETS. CAPSULES.

ADMINISTRATION/HANDLING
PO:

• Give before or with meals. • Tablets may be crushed. Do not crush enteric-coated form. • Instruct pt not to chew (minimizes irritation to mouth, lips, tongue). May open capsule and spread over applesauce, mashed fruit, or rice cereal.

INDICATIONS/ROUTES/DOSAGE
Usual oral dosage:

PO: Adults, elderly: 1–3 capsules or tablets before or with meals, snacks. May increase up to 8 tablets/dose. **Children:** 1–2 tablets with meals.

SIDE EFFECTS

RARE: Allergic reaction, mouth irritation, shortness of breath, wheezing.

ADVERSE REACTIONS/TOXIC EFFECTS

Excessive dosage may produce nausea, cramping, and/or diarrhea. Hyperuricosuria, hyperuricemia reported with extremely high doses.

NURSING IMPLICATIONS

BASELINE ASSESSMENT:

Spilling powder on hands (Viokase) may irritate skin. Inhaling powder may irritate mucous membranes, produce bronchospasm.

INTERVENTION/EVALUATION:

Question for therapeutic relief from GI symptoms. Do not change brands without consulting physician.

pancuronium bromide

(Pavulon)
See Classification section under: Neuromuscular blockers (p. 103C)

pantoprazole

pan-tow-**pray**-zoll
(Protonix)
Do not confuse with Lotronix.

▶CLASSIFICATION

PHARMACOTHERAPEUTIC:
Benzimidazole. ***CLINICAL:*** Gastric acid pump inhibitor (see p. 122C)

ACTION/*THERAPEUTIC EFFECT*

Converted to active metabolites that irreversibly bind to and inhibit H^+/K^+ ATPase (an enzyme on surface of gastric parietal cells). Inhibits hydrogen ion transport into gastric lumen, *increasing gastric pH, reducing gastric acid production.*

PHARMACOKINETICS

	Onset	Peak	Duration
PO	—	—	24 hrs

Rapidly absorbed from GI tract. Protein binding; >98%. Primarily distributed into gastric parietal cells. Metabolized extensively in liver. Primarily excreted in urine. Not removed by hemodialysis. Half-life: 1 hr.

USES

Treatment of erosive esophagitis associated with gastroesophageal reflux disease (GERD). Maintenance treating of erosive esophagitis. *IV:* Short-term treatment of GERD, hypersecretion due to Zollinger-Ellison syndrome.

PRECAUTIONS

CONTRAINDICATIONS: None significant. ***CAUTIONS:*** History of chronic or current hepatic disease.
▷***LIFESPAN CONSIDERATIONS:***
Pregnancy/Lactation: Unknown if drug crosses placenta or is distributed in breast milk. **Pregnancy Category B. Children:** Safety and efficacy not established. **Elderly:** No age-related precautions noted.

INTERACTIONS

DRUG: None significant. ***HERBAL:*** None known. ***FOOD:*** None known. ***LAB VALUES:*** May increase creatinine, cholesterol, uric acid.

AVAILABILITY (Rx)

POWDER FOR INJECTION: 40 mg. ***TABLETS (delayed-release):*** 40 mg.

ADMINISTRATION/HANDLING

PO:
• Give without regard to meals. • Tablet should not be crushed, chewed or split; swallow whole.

IV 🏵

Storage:
• Refrigerate vials, protect from light. • Do not freeze reconstituted vials. • Once diluted, stable for 12 hrs at room temperature.

Reconstitution:
• Mix 40 mg vial with 10 ml 0.9% NaCl injection. • Further dilute with 100 ml D_5W, 0.9% NaCl, or lactated Ringers to concentration of 0.4 mg/ml.

Rate of administration:
• Infuse over 15 min using in-line filter provided. • Must position filter below the Y-site that is closest to the pt.

IV INCOMPATIBILITIES ⊘

Do not mix with other medications. Flush IV with D_5W, 0.9% NaCl, or lactated Ringers before and after administration.

INDICATIONS/ROUTES/DOSAGE

Erosive esophagitis:

PO: Adults, elderly: 40 mg/day for up to 8 wks. If not healed after 8 wks, may continue an additional 8 wks.

P

IV INFUSION: **Adults, elderly:** 40 mg/day for 7–10 days.

Zollinger-Ellison syndrome:
IV: **Adults, elderly:** 80 mg q8–12h.

SIDE EFFECTS

RARE (<2%): Diarrhea, headache, dizziness, pruritus, skin rash.

ADVERSE REACTIONS/TOXIC EFFECTS

None significant.

NURSING IMPLICATIONS

BASELINE ASSESSMENT:

Obtain baseline lab values including serum creatinine, cholesterol.

INTERVENTION/EVALUATION:

Evaluate for therapeutic response, i.e., relief of GI symptoms. Question if GI discomfort, nausea occur.

PATIENT/FAMILY TEACHING:

Report headache. Swallow capsules whole; do not chew or crush. Take prior to eating.

paroxetine hydrochloride 💊

pear-**ox**-eh-teen
(Paxil, Paxil CR)
Do not confuse with pyridoxine, Doxil, Taxol.

▶CLASSIFICATION

PHARMACOTHERAPEUTIC: Serotonin uptake inhibitor. *CLINICAL:* Antidepressant, antiobsessive-compulsive, antianxiety (see p. 36C)

ACTION/*THERAPEUTIC EFFECT*

Selectively blocks uptake of neurotransmitter, serotonin, at CNS neuronal presynaptic membranes, thereby increasing availability at postsynaptic neuronal receptor sites. Resulting enhancement of synaptic activity *produces antidepressant effect, reduces obsessive-compulsive behavior, decreases anxiety.*

PHARMACOKINETICS

Well absorbed from GI tract. Protein binding: 95%. Widely distributed. Metabolized in liver; excreted in urine. Not removed by hemodialysis. Half-life: 24 hrs.

USES

Treatment of major depression exhibited as persistent, prominent dysphoria (occurring nearly every day for at least 2 wks) manifested by 4 of 8 symptoms: change in appetite, change in sleep pattern, increased fatigue, impaired concentration, feelings of guilt or worthlessness, loss of interest in usual activities, psychomotor agitation or retardation, or suicidal tendencies. Treatment of panic disorder, obsessive-compulsive disorder manifested as repetitive tasks producing marked distress, time-consuming, or significantly interfering with social or occupational behavior. Treatment of social anxiety disorder, generalized anxiety disorder (GAD).

PRECAUTIONS

CONTRAINDICATIONS: Within 14 days of MAO inhibitor therapy. *CAUTIONS:* Severe renal, hepatic impairment. History of mania, seizures, those with metabolic or hemodynamic disease, history of drug abuse.
▷*LIFESPAN CONSIDERATIONS:* **Pregnancy/Lactation:** May im-

pair reproductive function. Not distributed in breast milk. **Pregnancy Category B. Children:** Safety and efficacy not established. **Elderly:** Age-related renal impairment may require dosage adjustment.

INTERACTIONS

DRUG: MAO inhibitors may cause serotonergic syndrome (excitement, diaphoresis, rigidity, hyperthermia, autonomic hyperactivity, coma). **Cimetidine** may increase concentrations; phenytoin may decrease concentrations. **Paroxetine** can increase risperidone concentrations enough to cause extrapyramidal symptoms. **HERBAL: St. John's wort** may increase adverse effects. **FOOD:** None known. **LAB VALUES:** May increase liver enzymes. May decrease hemoglobin, hematocrit, WBC.

AVAILABILITY (Rx)

TABLETS: 10 mg, 20 mg, 30 mg, 40 mg. **CONTROLLED-RELEASE TABLETS:** 12.5 mg, 25 mg. **ORAL SUSPENSION:** 10 mg/5 ml.

ADMINISTRATION/HANDLING
PO:

• Give with food or milk if GI distress occurs. • Scored tablet may be crushed. • Best if given as single morning dose.

INDICATIONS/ROUTES/DOSAGE

Note: Reduce dosage in elderly, pts with severe renal, hepatic impairment. Dose changes should occur at 1 wk intervals.

Depression:

PO: Adults: Initially, 20 mg/day, usually in morning. Dosage may be gradually increased in 10 mg/day increments to 50 mg/day.

EXTENDED-RELEASE: Initially, 12.5 mg. **Maximum:** 60 mg/day. **Elderly, debilitated, those with severe hepatic, renal impairment:** Initially, 10 mg/day. Do not exceed maximum 40 mg/day.

Panic disorder:

PO: Adults: Initially, 10 mg/day; increase 10 mg/day at intervals of at least 1 wk up to 40 mg/day. **Maximum:** 60 mg/day. **Elderly:** Initially 10 mg/day. **Maximum:** 40 mg/day.

Obsessive-compulsive disorder:

PO: Adults: Initially, 20 mg/day; increase 10 mg/day at intervals of at least 1 wk. **Elderly:** Initially, 10 mg/day. **Maximum:** 40 mg/day.

Social anxiety disorder, GAD:

PO: Adults, elderly: 20 mg/day.

SIDE EFFECTS

FREQUENT: Nausea (26%), somnolence (23%), headache, dry mouth (18%), weakness (15%), constipation (15%), dizziness, insomnia (13%), diarrhea (12%), excessive sweating (11%), tremor (8%). **OCCASIONAL:** Decreased appetite, respiratory disturbance (6%), anxiety, nervousness (5%), flatulence, paresthesia, yawning (4%), decreased libido/sexual dysfunction, abdominal discomfort (3%). **RARE:** Palpitations, vomiting, blurred vision, taste change, confusion.

ADVERSE REACTIONS/TOXIC EFFECTS

None significant.

NURSING IMPLICATIONS

BASELINE ASSESSMENT:

Assess appearance, behavior, speech pattern, level of interest, mood.

INTERVENTION/EVALUATION:

For those on long-term therapy, liver/renal function tests, blood counts should be performed periodically. Supervise suicidal risk pt closely during early therapy (as depression lessens, energy level improves, increasing suicide potential). Assess appearance, behavior, speech pattern, level of interest, mood.

PATIENT/FAMILY TEACHING:

Therapeutic effect may be noted within 1–4 wks. Do not abruptly discontinue medication. Avoid tasks that require alertness, motor skills until response to drug is established. Inform physician if intention of pregnancy or if pregnancy occurs.

peginterferon alfa-2b

peg-inn-ter-**fear**-on
(PEG-Intron)

►CLASSIFICATION

PHARMACOTHERAPEUTIC: Immunomodulator. **CLINICAL:** Immunologic agent

ACTION/*THERAPEUTIC EFFECT*

Inhibits viral replication in virus-infected cells, suppresses cell proliferation by binding to specific membrane receptors on cell surface, *increasing phagocytic action of macrophages, augmenting specific cytotoxicity of lymphocytes.*

USES

As monotherapy or in combination with ribavirin for treatment of chronic hepatitis C in those not previously treated with interferon alpha who have compensated liver disease and are ≥18 yrs.

PRECAUTIONS

CONTRAINDICATIONS: Autoimmune hepatitis, decompensated liver disease. **EXTREME CAUTION:** History of psychiatric disorders. **CAUTIONS:** Renal impairment (creatinine clearance < 50 ml/min), elderly, pulmonary disorders, compromised CNS function, cardiac diseases, autoimmune disorders, endocrine abnormalities, ophthalmologic disorders, myelosuppression.

INTERACTIONS

DRUG: Bone marrow depressants may have additive effect. **HERBAL:** None significant. **FOOD:** None significant. **LAB VALUES:** May increase SGPT (ALT), blood glucose levels. May decrease neutrophil, platelet counts.

AVAILABILITY (Rx)

POWDER FOR INJECTION: 100 mcg/ml, 160 mcg/ml, 240 mcg/ml, 300 mcg/ml.

ADMINISTRATION/HANDLING
SubQ:
Storage:
• Store at room temperature.

Reconstitution:
• Reconstitute with supplied diluent (5 ml vial). Use immediately or after reconstituted; may be refrigerated for ≤24 hrs before use.

INDICATIONS/ROUTES/DOSAGE

Chronic hepatitis C:

SubQ: Adults ≥18 yrs, elderly: Administer once weekly for 1 yr on the same day each wk.

Note: If severe adverse reactions occur, modify dose or temporarily discontinue. Dosage based on weight:

Vial Strength (mcg/ml)	Weight (kg)	mcg of Peg-interfon to Administer	ml of Peg-interfon to Administer
100	37–45	40	0.4
	46–56	50	0.5
160	57–72	64	0.4
	73–88	80	0.5
240	89–106	96	0.4
	107–136	120	0.5
300	137–160	150	0.5

SIDE EFFECTS

Note: Dose-related effects.

FREQUENT (47–50%): Flulike symptoms (fever, headache, rigors, body ache, fatigue, nausea); may decrease in severity as treatment continues. Injection site disorders (inflammation, bruising, itchiness, irritation). **OCCASIONAL** (18–29%): Depression, anxiety, emotional lability, irritability, insomnia, alopecia, diarrhea. **RARE:** Rash, increased sweating, dry skin, dizziness, flushing, vomiting, dyspepsia (heartburn, epigastric pain).

ADVERSE REACTIONS/TOXIC EFFECTS

Serious, acute hypersensitivity reactions (urticaria, angioedema, bronchoconstriction, anaphylaxis), pancreatitis occur rarely. Ulcerative colitis may occur within 12 wks of initiation of treatment. Pulmonary disorders, hypo/hyperthryroidism may occur.

NURSING IMPLICATIONS

BASELINE ASSESSMENT:

CBC, platelet counts, blood chemistries, urinalysis, renal and liver function tests, EKG should be performed prior to initial therapy and routinely thereafter. Pts with diabetes or hypertension should have an ophthalmological exam before treatment begins.

INTERVENTION/EVALUATION:

Monitor for evidence of depression; offer emotional support. Monitor for abdominal pain, bloody diarrhea for evidence of colitis. Monitor chest x-ray for pulmonary infiltrates. Assess for pulmonary function impairment, hyperglycemia. Encourage ample fluid intake, particularly during early therapy. Assess serum hepatitis C virus RNA levels after 24 wks of treatment.

PATIENT/FAMILY TEACHING:

Clinical response occurs in 1–3 mos. Flulike symptoms tend to diminish with continued therapy. Immediately report symptoms of depression or suicidal ideation.

P

pemoline

pem-oh-leen
(Cylert)

►CLASSIFICATION

CLINICAL: CNS stimulant **(Schedule IV)**

ACTION/THERAPEUTIC EFFECT

Appears to act through dopaminergic receptor sites. In children, *appears to reduce motor restlessness, increases mental alertness, provides mood elevation, reduces sense of fatigue.*

USES

Treatment of attention deficit disorder in children with moderate to severe distraction, short attention span, hyperactivity, emotional impulsiveness.

PRECAUTIONS

CONTRAINDICATIONS: Impaired hepatic function, pts with motor tics, family history of Tourette's disorder. ***CAUTIONS:*** Impaired renal function.

INTERACTIONS

DRUG: **CNS-stimulating medications** may increase CNS stimulation. ***HERBAL:*** None known. ***FOOD:*** None known. ***LAB VALUES:*** May increase SGOT (AST), SGPT (ALT), LDH.

AVAILABILITY (Rx)

TABLETS: 18.75 mg, 37.5 mg, 75 mg. ***CHEWABLE TABLETS:*** 37.5 mg.

INDICATIONS/ROUTES/DOSAGE

Attention deficit disorder:

PO: Children >6 yrs: Initially, 37.5 mg/day given as single dose in morning. May increase by 18.75 mg at weekly intervals until therapeutic response is achieved. **Range:** 56.25–75 mg/day. **Maximum:** 112.5 mg/day.

SIDE EFFECTS

FREQUENT: Anorexia, insomnia. ***OCCASIONAL:*** Nausea, abdominal discomfort, diarrhea, headache, dizziness, drowsiness.

ADVERSE REACTIONS/TOXIC EFFECTS

Dyskinetic movements of tongue, lips, face, and extremities, and vi-sual disturbances, rash have occurred. Large doses may produce extreme nervousness, tachycardia. Hepatic effects (hepatitis, jaundice) appear to be reversible when drug is discontinued. Prolonged administration to children with attention deficit disorder may produce a temporary suppression of weight and/or height patterns.

NURSING IMPLICATIONS

BASELINE ASSESSMENT:

Liver function tests should be performed before therapy begins and periodically during therapy.

PATIENT/FAMILY TEACHING:

Therapeutic response to medication may take 3–4 wks. Insomnia, anorexia usually disappear during continued therapy. Anorexia usually accompanied by weight loss. Return to normal weight usually occurs within 3–6 mos.

penbutolol

(Levatol)

See Classification section under: Beta-adrenergic blockers (p. 61C)

penciclovir

pen-**sigh**-klo-vear
(Denavir)

▶CLASSIFICATION

PHARMACOTHERAPEUTIC: Anti-infective. ***CLINICAL:*** Topical antiviral

ACTION/*THERAPEUTIC EFFECT*

Inhibits antiviral activity against herpes simples virus (HSV). *DNA synthesis and, therefore, HSV replication, is prevented.*

PHARMACOKINETICS

Not detected in plasma or urine.

USES

Treatment of recurrent herpes labialis (cold sores).

PRECAUTIONS

CONTRAINDICATIONS: None significant. *CAUTIONS:* None significant.

▷*LIFESPAN CONSIDERATIONS:* **Pregnancy/Lactation:** Excreted in breast milk of animals. **Pregnancy Category B. Children:** Safety and efficacy not established. **Elderly:** No age-related precautions noted.

INTERACTIONS

DRUG: None significant. *HERBAL:* None known. *FOOD:* None known. *LAB VALUES:* None significant.

AVAILABILITY (Rx)

CREAM: 1%.

ADMINISTRATION/HANDLING

Topical:

• Store at room temperature. Do not freeze.

INDICATIONS/ROUTES/DOSAGE

Note: Begin treatment as soon as possible (as soon as symptom indicating immediate onset of virus is evident or when lesions appear).

Herpes labialis (cold sores):

TOPICAL: **Adults, elderly:** Apply q2h during waking hrs for 4 days.

SIDE EFFECTS

FREQUENT (>5%): Headache, mild erythema. *OCCASIONAL* (1–5%): Application site reaction. *RARE* (<1%): Altered taste, rash.

ADVERSE REACTIONS/TOXIC EFFECTS

None significant.

NURSING IMPLICATIONS

BASELINE ASSESSMENT:

Use only on lips or face. Do not apply to oral mucous membranes. Avoid application in or near eyes (produces irritation).

PATIENT/FAMILY TEACHING:

Observe precautions to avoid exposure of cold sores to direct sunlight.

penicillamine

pen-ih-**sill**-ah-mine
(Cuprimine, Depen)
Do not confuse with penicillin.

P

▶CLASSIFICATION

PHARMACOTHERAPEUTIC: Heavy metal antagonist. *CLINICAL:* Chelating agent, anti-inflammatory

ACTION/*THERAPEUTIC EFFECT*

Chelates copper, iron, mercury, lead to form complexes, *promoting excretion of copper.* Combines with cystine-forming complex, thus reducing concentration of cystine to below levels for formation of cystine stones. *Prevents renal calculi. May dissolve existing stones. Rheumatoid arthritis:* Exact mechanism unknown. May decrease cell-mediated immune response; *acts as anti-inflammatory drug;* may inhibit collagen formation.

USES/*UNLABELED*

Promotes excretion of copper in treatment of Wilson's disease; decreases excretion of cystine, prevents renal calculi in cystinuria associated with nephrolithiasis; treatment of active rheumatoid arthritis not controlled with conventional therapy. *Treatment of rheumatoid vasculitis, heavy metal toxicity.*

PRECAUTIONS

CONTRAINDICATIONS: History of penicillamine-related aplastic anemia or agranulocytosis, rheumatoid arthritis pts with history or evidence of renal insufficiency, pregnancy, breast feeding. ***CAUTIONS:*** Elderly, debilitated, impaired renal/hepatic function, penicillin allergy.

INTERACTIONS

DRUG: **Iron supplements, antacids, food** may decrease absorption. **Bone marrow depressants, gold compounds, immunosuppressants** may increase risk of hematologic, renal adverse effects. ***HERBAL:*** None known. ***FOOD:*** None known. ***LAB VALUES:*** None significant.

AVAILABILITY (Rx)

CAPSULES (Cuprimine): 125 mg, 250 mg. ***TABLETS (Depen):*** 250 mg.

INDICATIONS/ROUTES/DOSAGE

Rheumatoid arthritis:

PO: **Adults, elderly:** 125–250 mg/day. May increase at 1–3 mo intervals up to 1–1.5 g/day.

Note: Dose >500 mg/day in divided doses.

Children: Initially, 3 mg/kg/day (*Maximum:* 250 mg) for 3 mos, then 6 mg/kg/day (*Maximum:* 500 mg) in 2 divided doses for 3 mos. **Maximum:** 10 mg/kg/day (1–1.5 g/day) in 3–4 divided doses.

Wilson's disease:

PO: **Adults, elderly:** 1 g/day in 4 divided doses. **Maximum:** 2 g/day. **Children:** 20 mg/kg/day in 2–4 doses. **Maximum:** 1 g/day.

Note: Titrate to maintain urinary copper excretion >1 mg/day.

Cystinuria:

Note: Doses titrated to maintain urinary cystine excretion at 100–200 mg/day.

PO: **Adults, elderly:** Initially, 2 g/day in divided doses q6h. **Range:** 1–4 g/day. **Children:** 30 mg/kg/day in 4 divided doses. **Maximum:** 4 g/day.

SIDE EFFECTS

FREQUENT: Rash (pruritic, erythematous, maculopapular, morbilliform), reduced/altered sense of taste (hypogeusia), GI disturbances (anorexia, epigastric pain, nausea, vomiting, diarrhea), oral ulcers, glossitis. ***OCCASIONAL:*** Proteinuria, hematuria, hot flashes, drug fever. ***RARE:*** Alopecia, tinnitus, pemphigoid rash (water blisters).

ADVERSE REACTIONS/TOXIC EFFECTS

Aplastic anemia, agranulocytosis, thrombocytopenia, leukopenia, myasthenia gravis, bronchiolitis, erythematouslike syndrome, evening hypoglycemia, skin friability at sites of pressure/trauma producing extravasation or white papules at venipuncture, surgical sites reported. Iron deficiency (particularly children, menstruating women) may develop.

NURSING IMPLICATIONS

BASELINE ASSESSMENT:

Baseline WBC, differential, hemoglobin, platelet count should be performed before therapy begins, q2wks thereafter for first 6 mos, then moly during therapy. Liver function tests (GGT, SGOT, SGPT, LDH) and x-ray for renal stones should also be ordered. A 2 hr interval is necessary between iron and penicillamine therapy. In event of upcoming surgery, dosage should be reduced to 250 mg/day until wound healing is complete.

INTERVENTION/EVALUATION:

Encourage copious amounts of water in those with cystinuria. Monitor WBC, differential, platelet count. If WBC <3,500, neutrophils <2,000/mm^3, monocytes >500/mm^3, or platelet counts <100,000, or if a progressive fall in either platelet count or WBC in three successive determinations noted, inform physician (drug withdrawal necessary). Assess for evidence of hematuria. Monitor urinalysis for hematuria, proteinuria (if proteinuria exceeds 1 g/24 hrs, inform physician).

PATIENT/FAMILY TEACHING:

Promptly report any missed menstrual periods/other indications of pregnancy, fever, sore throat, chills, bruising, bleeding, difficulty breathing on exertion, unexplained cough or wheezing. Take medication 1 hr before or 2 hrs after meals or at least 1 hr from any other drug, food, or milk.

penicillin G benzathine

pen-ih-**sil**-lin G **benz**-ah-thene (Bicillin, Permapen)

FIXED-COMBINATION(S)

With penicillin G procaine, an antibiotic **(Bicillin CR)**

penicillin G potassium, sodium

(Crystapen♣, Pentids, Pfizerpen)

penicillin G procaine

(Crystacillin, Pfizerpen, Wycillin)
Do not confuse with penicillamine.

FIXED-COMBINATION(S)

With probenecid, a renal tubular blocking agent **(Wycillin & Probenecid)**; with penicillin G benzathine, an antibiotic **(Bicillin-CR)**

▶CLASSIFICATION

PHARMACOTHERAPEUTIC: Penicillin. **CLINICAL:** Antibiotic (see p. 25C)

P

ACTION/THERAPEUTIC EFFECT

Binds to bacterial membranes, *inhibiting cell wall synthesis. Bactericidal.*

PHARMACOKINETICS

Slowly absorbed after IM administration. Protein binding: 65%. Widely distributed. Metabolized in liver. Primarily excreted in urine. Moderately removed by hemodialysis. Half-life: 0.5–0.7 hrs (half-life increased with impaired renal function).

USES

Benzathine, procaine: Mild to

moderate infections of respiratory tract, skin and skin structure, rheumatic fever prophylaxis, early syphilis, yaws, bejel, pinta. Follow-up to IM/IV therapy with penicillin G potassium, sodium. **PCN-G:** Treatment of infections of respiratory tract, skin and skin structure, bone and joints; septicemia, meningitis, endocarditis, pericarditis, diphtheria, Listeria, clostridium, disseminated gonococcal infections, actinomycosis, rheumatic fever prophylaxis, syphilis, necrotizing ulcerative gingivitis, anthrax, Lyme disease.

PRECAUTIONS

CONTRAINDICATIONS: Hypersensitivity to any penicillin. ***CAUTIONS:*** Renal impairment, history of allergies, particularly cephalosporins, aspirin (tartrazine reaction may occur in those sensitive to aspirin).

▷***LIFESPAN CONSIDERATIONS:***
Pregnancy/Lactation: Readily crosses placenta, appears in cord blood, amniotic fluid. Distributed in breast milk in low concentrations. May lead to allergic sensitization, diarrhea, candidiasis, skin rash in infant. **Pregnancy Category B. Children:** Use caution in neonates/young infants (may delay renal elimination). **Elderly:** Age-related renal impairment may require dosage adjustment.

INTERACTIONS

DRUG: **Probenecid** may increase concentration, toxicity risk. **Angiotensin-converting enzyme inhibitors, potassium-sparing diuretics, potassium supplements** may increase risk of hyperkalemia. ***HERBAL:*** None known. ***FOOD:*** None known. ***LAB VALUES:*** May cause positive Coomb's' test.

AVAILABILITY (Rx)

Benzathine: 300,000 units/ml, 600,000 units/ml.

PCN-G Potassium: POWDER FOR INJECTION: 1 million units, 5 million units, 10 million units, 20 million units.

PCN-G Sodium: POWDER FOR INJECTION: 5 million units.

Procaine: 300,000 units/ml, 500,000 units/ml, 600,000 units/ml.

ADMINISTRATION/HANDLING

Note: ***Benzathine, procaine:*** Do not give IV, intra-arterially, intravascularly, or SubQ. Space doses evenly around the clock.

IM:

• ***Benzathine, procaine:*** Refrigerate. • Give IM injection deeply into gluteus maximus or midlateral thigh. • Do not administer if blood is aspirated; draw up new dose; select another site. • Avoid areas of nerves, repeated IM injections into anterolateral thigh. • Administer IM injection slowly; stop if pt complains of severe pain.

IV 🔳

Storage:
• IV infusion (piggyback) is stable for 24 hrs at room temperature, 7 days if refrigerated. • Discard if precipitate forms.

Reconstitution:
• Follow dilution guide per manufacturer (initial dilution must be mixed with Sterile Water for Injection). • After reconstitution, dilute with 50–100 ml D_5W, 0.9% NaCl.

Rate of administration:
• Infuse over 1–2 hrs in adults, 15–30 min in neonates, children. • Because of potential for hypersensitivity/anaphylaxis, start initial dose at few drops/min, increase

slowly to ordered rate; stay with pt first 10–15 min, then check q10min.

IV INCOMPATIBILITY ⊘

No known incompatibilities via Y-site administration.

IV COMPATIBILITIES

Amiodarone (Cordarone), calcium gluconate, diltiazem (Cardizem), heparin, magnesium, potassium chloride.

INDICATIONS/ROUTES/DOSAGE

BENZATHINE:

Group A strep

***IM:* Adults, elderly:** 1.2 million units as single dose. **Children:** 300,000–900,000 units as single dose.

Prophylaxxis for recurrent rheumatic fever:

***IM:* Adults, elderly:** 1.2 million units q3–4wks or 600,000 units 2 times/mo. **Children:** 25,000–50,000 units/kg q3–4wks. **Maximum:** 1.2 million units.

Congenital syphyllis:

***IM:* Children:** 50,000 units/kg qwk for 3 wks. **Maximum:** 2.4 million units/dose.

Syphyllis >1 yr duration:

***IM:* Adults, elderly:** 2.4 million units once a wk for 3 doses. **Children:** 50,000 units/kg once a wk for 3 doses. **Maximum:** 2.4 million units.

PENICILLIN G

Usual dosage:

***IM/IV:* Adults, elderly:** 2–24 million units/day in divided doses q4–6h. **Maximum:** 24 million units/day. **Children:** 100,000–400,000 units/kg/day in divided doses q4–6h. **Maximum:** 24 million units/day. **Neonates:** 50,000–450,000 units/kg/day in divided doses q6–12h.

PROCAINE:

Usual dosage:

***IM:* Adults, elderly:** 0.6–4.8 million units/day in divided doses q12–24h. **Children:** 25–50,000 units/kg/day in divided doses q12–24h. **Maximum:** 4.8 million units/day.

Neurosyphyllis:

***IM:* Adults, elderly:** 2.4 million units/day for 10 days (with probenecid 500 mg q6h).

Congenital syphyllis:

***IM:* Children, neonates:** 50,000 units/kg/day for 10 days.

SIDE EFFECTS

FREQUENT: GI reactions (nausea, vomiting, diarrhea). ***OCCASIONAL:*** Pain, induration at IM injection site. ***PCN-G potassium, sodium:*** High IV dosage may cause electrolyte imbalance, phlebitis, thrombophlebitis. ***RARE:*** Bleeding.

ADVERSE REACTIONS/TOXIC EFFECTS

Hypersensitivity reactions occur frequently, ranging from rash, fever/chills to anaphylaxis. Nephrotoxicity may occur with high parenteral dosages, preexisting renal disease. Superinfections, potentially fatal antibiotic-associated colitis may result from altered bacterial balance. Toxic reaction to procaine (confusion, combativeness, seizures) with large doses.

NURSING IMPLICATIONS

BASELINE ASSESSMENT:

Question for history of allergies, particularly penicillins, cephalosporins, aspirin, procaine.

INTERVENTION/EVALUATION:

Hold medication and promptly

P

report rash (hypersensitivity) or diarrhea (with fever, abdominal pain, mucus and blood in stool may indicate antibiotic-associated colitis). Assess for food tolerance. Check IM injection sites for induration, tenderness. Check for wheezing, respiratory difficulty due to tartrazine sensitivity. Monitor I&O, urinalysis, renal function tests for nephrotoxicity. Be alert for superinfection: increased fever, sore throat, nausea, vomiting, diarrhea, ulceration or changes of oral mucosa, vaginal discharge, anal/genital pruritus. Evaluate hemoglobin levels and assess for signs of bleeding: overt bleeding, bruising/swelling of tissue.

PATIENT/FAMILY TEACHING:

Discomfort may occur with IM injection. Notify physician in event of rash, diarrhea, bleeding, bruising, other new symptom. Sodium content of penicillin G sodium must be considered for those on sodium-restricted diets.

penicillin V potassium 🖋

(Apo-Pen VK✤, Nadopen-V✤, Novopen VK✤, Pen Vee K, V-Cillin-K, <u>Veetids</u>)

▶CLASSIFICATION

PHARMACOTHERAPEUTIC: Penicillin. **CLINICAL:** Antibiotic (see p. 25C)

ACTION/*THERAPEUTIC EFFECT*

Binds to bacterial membranes, *inhibiting cell wall synthesis*. Bactericidal.

PHARMACOKINETICS

Moderately absorbed from GI tract. Protein binding: 80%. Widely distributed. Metabolized in liver. Primarily excreted in urine. Half-life: 1 hr (half-life increased with impaired renal function).

USES

Treatment of mild to moderate infections of respiratory tract and skin/skin structure, otitis media, necrotizing ulcerative gingivitis, prophylaxis for rheumatic fever, dental procedures.

PRECAUTIONS

CONTRAINDICATIONS: Hypersensitivity to any penicillin. **CAUTIONS:** Renal impairment, history of allergies, particularly cephalosporins, aspirin.
▷**LIFESPAN CONSIDERATIONS:** **Pregnancy/Lactation:** Readily crosses placenta; appears in cord blood, amniotic fluid. Distributed in breast milk in low concentrations. May lead to allergic sensitization, diarrhea, candidiasis, skin rash in infant. **Pregnancy Category B. Children:** Use caution in neonates/young infants (may delay renal elimination). **Elderly:** Age-related renal impairment may require dosage adjustment.

INTERACTIONS

DRUG: Probenecid may increase concentration, toxicity risk. **HERBAL:** None known. **FOOD:** None known. **LAB VALUES:** May cause positive Coomb's' test.

AVAILABILITY (Rx)

TABLETS: 125 mg, 250 mg, 500 mg. **POWDER FOR ORAL SOLUTION:** 125 mg/5 ml, 250 mg/5 ml.

ADMINISTRATION/HANDLING
PO:
• Store tabs at room temperature. Oral solution, after reconstitution, is stable for 14 days if refrigerated. • Space doses evenly around the clock. • Give without regard to meals.

INDICATIONS/ROUTES/DOSAGE
Systemic infections:
PO: Adults, elderly, children >12 yrs: 125–500 mg q6–8h. **Children <12 yrs:** 25–50 mg/kg/day in divided doses q6–8h. **Maximum:** 3 g/day.

Primary prevention of rheumatic fever:
PO: Adults, elderly: 500 mg 2–3 times/day for 10 days. **Children:** 250 mg 2–3 times/day for 10 days.

Prophylaxis for recurrent rheumatic fever:
PO: Adults, elderly, children: 250 mg 2 times/day.

SIDE EFFECTS
FREQUENT: Mild hypersensitivity reaction (rash, fever/chills), nausea, vomiting, diarrhea. ***RARE:*** Bleeding, allergic reaction.

ADVERSE REACTIONS/TOXIC EFFECTS
Severe hypersensitivity reaction, including anaphylaxis, may occur. Nephrotoxicity, antibiotic-associated colitis (severe abdominal pain and tenderness, fever, watery and severe diarrhea), other superinfections may result from high dosages, prolonged therapy.

NURSING IMPLICATIONS

BASELINE ASSESSMENT:
Question for history of allergies, particularly penicillins, cephalosporins.

INTERVENTION/EVALUATION:
Hold medication and promptly report rash (hypersensitivity) or diarrhea (with fever, abdominal pain, mucus and blood in stool may indicate antibiotic-associated colitis). Monitor I&O, urinalysis, renal function tests for nephrotoxicity. Be alert for superinfection: increased fever, sore throat, nausea, vomiting, diarrhea, ulceration or changes of oral mucosa, vaginal discharge, anal/genital pruritus. Review hemoglobin levels; check for bleeding: overt bleeding, bruising or swelling of tissue.

PATIENT/FAMILY TEACHING:
Continue antibiotic for full length of treatment. Space doses evenly. Notify physician immediately in event of rash, diarrhea, bleeding, bruising, or other new symptom.

pentaerythritol tetranitrate (P.E.T.N.)

(Duotrate, Peritrate)
See Classification section under: Nitrates

pentamidine isethionate

pen-**tam**-ih-deen
(NebuPent, Pentacarinat✽, Pentam-300)

▶CLASSIFICATION
PHARMACOTHERAPEUTIC: Anti-infective. ***CLINICAL:*** Antiprotozoal

P

ACTION/*THERAPEUTIC EFFECT*

Interferes with nuclear metabolism, incorporation of nucleotides; *inhibits DNA, RNA, phospholipid, protein synthesis.*

PHARMACOKINETICS

Minimal absorption following inhalation, well absorbed after IM administration. Widely distributed. Primarily excreted in urine. Minimally removed by hemodialysis. Half-life: 6.5 hrs (half-life increased with impaired renal function).

USES/*UNLABELED*

Treatment of pneumonia caused by *Pneumocystis carinii* (PCP). Prevention of PCP in high-risk HIV-infected pts. *Treatment of visceral/cutaneous Leishmaniasis, African Trypanosomiasis.*

PRECAUTIONS

CONTRAINDICATIONS: When PCP has been firmly established, there are no absolute contraindications. Inhalation of drug is contraindicated in those with history of severe asthma or anaphylactic reaction to drug by any route. **CAUTIONS:** Hyper/hypotension, hepatic/renal dysfunction, hyper/hypoglycemia, hypocalcemia, thrombocytopenia, leukopenia, anemia.
▷**LIFESPAN CONSIDERATIONS:**
Pregnancy/Lactation: Unknown if crosses placenta or is distributed in breast milk. **Pregnancy Category C. Children:** No age-related precautions noted. **Elderly:** Information not available.

INTERACTIONS

DRUG: Blood dyscrasias–producing medication, bone marrow depressants may increase abnormal hematologic effects. **Didanosine** may increase risk of pancreatitis. **Foscarnet** may increase hypocalcemia, hypomagnesemia, nephrotoxicity. **Nephrotoxic medications** may increase risk of nephrotoxicity. **HERBAL:** None known. **FOOD:** None known. **LAB VALUES:** May increase SGOT (AST), SGPT (ALT), alkaline phosphatase, bilirubin, BUN, creatinine. May decrease calcium, magnesium. May alter glucose levels.

AVAILABILITY (Rx)

INJECTION: 300 mg. **AEROSOL:** 300 mg.

ADMINISTRATION/HANDLING

Note: Pt must be in supine position during administration with frequent B/P checks until stable (potential for life-threatening hypotensive reaction). Have resuscitative equipment nearby.

IM:

• Reconstitute 300 mg vial with 3 ml Sterile Water for Injection to provide concentration of 100 mg/ml.

IV 📺

Storage:

• Store vials at room temperature. • After reconstitution, IV solution is stable for 48 hrs at room temperature. Use freshly prepared aerosol solution. • Discard unused portion.

Reconstitution:

• For intermittent IV infusion (piggyback), reconstitute each vial with 3–5 ml D_5W or Sterile Water for Injection. • Withdraw desired dose and further dilute with 50–250 ml D_5W.

Rate of administration:

• Infuse over 60 min. • Do not give by IV injection or rapid IV infusion (increases potential for severe hypotension).

Aerosol (nebulizer):

• Aerosol stable for 48 hrs at room temperature. • Reconstitute 300 mg vial with 6 ml Sterile Water for Injection. Avoid NaCl (may cause precipitate). • Do not mix with other medication in nebulizer reservoir.

IV INCOMPATIBILITIES ⊘

Interleukin (Proleukin), cefazolin (Ancef), cefotaxime (Claforan), ceftazidime (Fortaz), ceftriaxone (Rocephin), fluconazole (Diflucan), foscarnet (Foscavir).

IV COMPATIBILITIES

Diltiazem (Cardizem), zidovudine (AZT, Retrovir).

INDICATIONS/ROUTES/DOSAGE

Pneumocystis carinii pneumonia:

IM/IV: Adults, elderly, children: 4 mg/kg/day once daily for 14 days.

Prevention of *P. carinii* pneumonia:

AEROSOL (Nebulizer): Adults, elderly, children ≥5 yrs: 300 mg once q4wks via nebulizer. **Children <5 yrs:** 8 mg/kg.

SIDE EFFECTS

FREQUENT: (*Injection* >10%): Abscess, pain at injection site. **(*Inhalation* >5%):** Fatigue, metallic taste, shortness of breath, decreased appetite, dizziness, rash, cough, nausea, vomiting, chills. **OCCASIONAL: (*Injection* 1–10%):** Nausea, decreased appetite, hypotension, fever, rash, bad taste, confusion. **(*Inhalation* 1–5%):** Di-

arrhea, headache, anemia, muscle pain. **RARE: (*Injection* <1%):** Neuralgia, thrombocytopenia, phlebitis, dizziness.

ADVERSE REACTIONS/TOXIC EFFECTS

Life-threatening/fatal hypotension, arrhythmias, hypoglycemia, or leukopenia; nephrotoxicity and renal failure; anaphylactic shock; Stevens-Johnson syndrome; toxic epidural necrolysis occur rarely. Hyperglycemia and insulin-dependent diabetes mellitus (often permanent) may occur even mos after therapy.

NURSING IMPLICATIONS

BASELINE ASSESSMENT:

Avoid concurrent use of nephrotoxic drugs. Establish baseline for B/P, blood glucose. Obtain specimens for diagnostic tests before giving first dose.

INTERVENTION/EVALUATION:

Monitor B/P during administration until stable for both IM and IV administration (pt should remain supine). Check glucose levels and clinical signs for hypo glycemia (sweating, nervousness, tremor, tachycardia, palpitation, lightheadedness, headache, numbness of lips, double vision, incoordination), hyperglycemia (polyuria, polyphagia, polydipsia, malaise, visual changes, abdominal pain, headache, nausea/vomiting). Evaluate IM sites for pain, redness, and induration; IV sites for phlebitis (heat, pain, red streaking over vein). Monitor renal, hepatic, and hematology test results. Assess skin for rash. Evaluate equilibrium during ambulation. Be alert

P

for respiratory difficulty when administering by inhalation route.

PATIENT/FAMILY TEACHING:
Remain flat in bed during administration of medication and get up slowly with assistance when B/P stable. Notify nurse immediately of sweating, shakiness, lightheadedness, palpitations. Even several mos after therapy stops, drowsiness, increased urination, thirst, anorexia may develop.

---

pentazocine

(Talwin)

See Classification section under: Opioid analgesics

---

pentobarbital

(Nembutal)

See Classification section under: Sedative-Hypnotics

---

pentostatin

pen-toe-**stat**-inn
(Nipent)
Do not confuse with pentosan.

▶**CLASSIFICATION**

PHARMACOTHERAPEUTIC:
Antimetabolite. ***CLINICAL:*** Antineoplastic (see p. 73C)

ACTION/*THERAPEUTIC EFFECT*
Inhibits the enzyme ADA (increases intracellular levels of adenine deoxynucleotide *leading to cell death*). Greatest activity in T cells of lymphoid system. Inhibits ADA and RNA synthesis. Produces DNA damage.

PHARMACOKINETICS

After IV administration, rapidly distributed to body tissues (poorly distributed to CSF). Protein binding: 4%. Excreted primarily in urine unchanged or as active metabolite. Half-life: 5.7 hrs (half-life increased with impaired renal function).

USES

Treatment of hairy cell leukemia refractory to, or poor response to, interferon alpha therapy.

PRECAUTIONS

CONTRAINDICATIONS: None significant. ***EXTREME CAUTION:*** Preexisting myelosuppression, cardiac disease, impaired hepatic/renal function. Current or recent chickenpox, infection, herpes zoster, history of gout.

▷***LIFESPAN CONSIDERATIONS:***
Pregnancy/Lactation: If possible, avoid use during pregnancy (may be embryotoxic). Unknown if drug is distributed in breast milk (advise to discontinue nursing before drug initiation). **Pregnancy Category D. Children:** Safety and efficacy not established. **Elderly:** Age-related renal impairment may require caution.

INTERACTIONS

DRUG: May increase pulmonary toxicity with **fludarabine.** May increase effects, toxicity of **vidarabine.** May decrease effect of antigout medications. **Bone marrow depressants** may increase bone marrow depression. **Live virus vaccines** may potentiate virus replication, increase vaccine side effects, decrease pt's antibody response to vaccine. **HERBAL:** None known. **FOOD:** None known. **LAB VALUES:** May increase SGOT (AST), SGPT (ALT), alkaline phosphatase, LDH, uric acid, creatinine.

AVAILABILITY (Rx)

POWDER FOR INJECTION: 10 mg vial.

ADMINISTRATION/HANDLING

IV

Note: Give by IV injection or IV infusion (*never* SubQ or IM). Gloves, gowns, eye goggles recommended during preparation and administration of medication. If powder or solution comes in contact with skin, wash thoroughly. Avoid small veins, swollen/edematous extremities, and areas overlying joints, tendons. Follow institutional procedures for handling antineoplastic medication. Use protective clothing/gloves when handling.

Storage:

• Refrigerate vial. • Contains no preservatives; after reconstitution or dilution, use within 8 hrs when given at room temperature, environmental light. Discard unused portion.

Reconstitution:

• Reconstitute each 10 mg vial with 5 ml 0.9% NaCl to provide a concentration of 2 mg/ml. • Shake thoroughly to ensure dissolution.

Rate of administration:

• Adequately hydrate pt before and immediately after (decreases risk of adverse renal effects). • For IV push, give over 5 min. • For IV

infusion, further dilute with 25–50 ml D_5W or 0.9% NaCl and give over 20–30 min.

IV INCOMPATIBILITY ⊘

Do not mix with any other medications.

IV COMPATIBILITIES

Fludarabine (Fludara), ondansetron (Zofran), paclitaxel (Taxol).

INDICATIONS/ROUTES/DOSAGE

Note: Dosage individualized based on clinical response, tolerance to adverse effects. When used in combination therapy, consult specific protocols for optimum dosage, sequence of drug administration.

Hairy cell leukemia:

IV: Adults, elderly: 4 mg/m^2 q2wks until complete response attained (without any major toxicity). Discontinue if no response in 6 mos; partial response in 12 mos.

Note: Withhold/discontinue in those with severe reaction to pentostatin, nervous system toxicity, active underlying infections, increased serum creatinine, in pt with neutrophil count <200/mm^3 with baseline count >500/mm^3.

Dosage in renal impairment:

Only when benefits justify risks, give 2–3 mg/m^2 in pt with Ccr 50–60 ml/min.

SIDE EFFECTS

FREQUENT: Nausea, vomiting (53%), fever (42%), rash (26%), fatigue (29%), pain (20%), cough (17%), upper respiratory infection, anorexia (16%), diarrhea (15%). **OCCASIONAL** (10–13%): Headache, pharyngitis, sinusitis, myalgia, chills, arthralgia, peripheral edema, anorexia, blurred vision, conjunctivitis, skin discoloration, sweating, anxiety, depression, dizziness, confusion.

ADVERSE REACTIONS/TOXIC EFFECTS

Bone marrow depression is manifested as hematologic toxicity (principally leukopenia, anemia, thrombocytopenia). Doses higher than recommended ($20–50$ mg/m^2 in divided doses >5 days) may produce severe renal, hepatic, pulmonary, or CNS toxicity.

NURSING IMPLICATIONS

BASELINE ASSESSMENT:

Provide emotional support to pt and family. Obtain CBC, differential count (particularly platelets, neutrophils, lymphocytes), liver function studies (esp. SGOT [AST], SGPT [ALT], LDH, GGT, alkaline phosphatase), creatinine before initiating therapy. Antiemetics may be effective in preventing, treating nausea.

INTERVENTION/EVALUATION:

Severe occurrence of rash, severe hematologic, blood chemistry values that have significantly changed from baseline or evidence of pulmonary or CNS toxicity may indicate need to terminate medication. Monitor closely for bone marrow suppression: evidence of infection (fever, sore throat), bleeding (easy bruising, unusual bleeding from any site), symptoms of anemia (excessive tiredness, weakness). Be alert for CNS toxicity (agitation, nervousness, confusion, anxiety, depression, insomnia).

PATIENT/FAMILY TEACHING:

Bone marrow aspiration and biopsy may be a necessary part of program at 2–3 mo intervals to assess treatment response. Do not have immunizations without physician's approval (drug lowers body's resistance). Avoid crowds, those with infection. Promptly report fever, sore throat, signs of local infection, easy bruising, or unusual bleeding from any site.

pentoxifylline

pen-tox-ih-**fill**-in
(Trental)
Do not confuse with Tegretol.

▶CLASSIFICATION

PHARMACOTHERAPEUTIC: Blood viscosity-reducing agent. **CLINICAL:** Hemorheologic

ACTION/*THERAPEUTIC EFFECT*

Improves erythrocyte flexibility, microcirculatory flow, tissue O$_2$ concentration; *reduces blood viscosity.*

PHARMACOKINETICS

Completely absorbed from GI tract. Bound to erythrocyte membrane. Metabolized in erythrocytes, liver to active metabolite. Primarily excreted in urine. Unknown if removed by hemodialysis. Half-life: 0.4–0.8 hrs; metabolite: 1–1.6 hrs.

USES

Symptomatic treatment of intermittent claudication associated with occlusive peripheral vascular disease, diabetic angiopathies.

PRECAUTIONS

CONTRAINDICATIONS: History

of intolerance to xanthine derivatives (caffeine, theophylline, theobromine). **CAUTIONS:** Coronary artery disease, cerebrovascular disease, impaired renal function.

▷**LIFESPAN CONSIDERATIONS: Pregnancy/Lactation:** Unknown whether drug crosses placenta; distributed in breast milk. **Pregnancy Category C. Children:** Safety and efficacy not established. **Elderly:** Age-related renal impairment may require cautious use.

INTERACTIONS

DRUG: May increase effect of **antihypertensives. HERBAL:** None known. **FOOD:** None known. **LAB VALUES:** None significant.

AVAILABILITY (Rx)

TABLETS (controlled-release): 400 mg.

ADMINISTRATION/HANDLING

PO:

• Do not crush or break film-coated tablets. • Give with meals to avoid GI upset.

INDICATIONS/ROUTES/DOSAGE

Intermittent claudication:

PO: Adults, elderly: 400 mg 3 times/day. Decrease to 400 mg 2 times/day if GI or CNS side effects occur. Continue for at least 8 wks.

SIDE EFFECTS

OCCASIONAL (2–5%): Dizziness, nausea, bad taste, dyspepsia (heartburn, gastric pain, indigestion). **RARE** (<2%): Rash, pruritus, anorexia, constipation, dry mouth, blurred vision, edema, nasal congestion, anxiety.

ADVERSE REACTIONS/TOXIC EFFECTS

Angina, chest pain occur rarely.

May be accompanied by palpitations, tachycardia, arrhythmias. Overdosage (flushing, hypotension, nervousness, agitation, hand tremor, fever, somnolence) noted 4–5 hrs after ingestion, lasts 12 hrs.

NURSING IMPLICATIONS

INTERVENTION/EVALUATION:

Assist with ambulation if dizziness occurs. Assess for hand tremor. Monitor for relief of symptoms of intermittent claudication (pain, aching, cramping in calf muscles, buttocks, thigh, feet). Symptoms generally occur while walking/exercising and not at rest or with weight bearing in absence of walking/exercising.

PATIENT/FAMILY TEACHING:

Therapeutic effect generally noted in 2–4 wks. Avoid driving, tasks requiring alert response until response to drug known. Do not smoke (causes constriction and occlusion of peripheral blood vessels).

P

pergolide mesylate

purr-go-lied
(Permax)
Do not confuse with Pentrax, Pernox.

▶**CLASSIFICATION**

PHARMACOTHERAPEUTIC: Dopamine agonist. **CLINICAL:** Antidyskinetic

ACTION/THERAPEUTIC EFFECT

Inhibits prolactin secretion; directly stimulates postsynaptic dopamine receptors, *assisting in reduction in tremor, improvement in akinesia (absence of movement), posture and equilibrium disorders, rigidity of parkinsonism.*

PHARMACOKINETICS

Well absorbed from GI tract. Protein binding: 90%. Metabolized in liver (undergoes extensive first-pass effect). Primarily excreted in urine. Unknown if removed by hemodialysis.

USES

Adjunctive treatment with levodopa/carbidopa in those with Parkinson's disease.

PRECAUTIONS

CONTRAINDICATIONS: None significant. ***CAUTIONS:*** Cardiac dysrhythmias.
▷*LIFESPAN CONSIDERATIONS:* **Pregnancy/Lactation:** Unknown whether drug crosses placenta or is distributed in breast milk. May interfere with lactation. **Pregnancy Category B. Children:** Safety and efficacy not established. **Elderly:** No age-related precautions noted.

INTERACTIONS

DRUG:* Haloperidol, loxapine, methyldopa, metoclopramide, phenothiazines** may decrease effect. **Hypotension-producing medications** may increase hypotensive effect. ***HERBAL: None known. ***FOOD:*** None known. ***LAB VALUES:*** May increase plasma growth hormone.

AVAILABILITY (Rx)

TABLETS: 0.05 mg, 0.25 mg, 1 mg.

ADMINISTRATION/HANDLING
PO:
• Scored tablets may be crushed.
• Give without regard to meals.

INDICATIONS/ROUTES/DOSAGE

Note: Daily doses usually given in 3 divided doses.

Parkinsonism:

PO: **Adults, elderly:** Initially, 0.05 mg/day for 2 days. Increase by 0.1–0.15 mg/day q3days over the following 12 days; then may increase by 0.25 mg/day q3days. **Maximum:** 5 mg/day. **Range:** 3–4.6 mg/day.

SIDE EFFECTS

FREQUENT (10–24%): Nausea, dizziness, hallucinations, constipation, rhinitis, dystonia (impaired muscle tone), confusion, somnolence. ***OCCASIONAL*** (3–9%): Postural hypotension, insomnia, dry mouth, peripheral edema, anxiety, diarrhea, dyspepsia, abdominal pain, headache, abnormal vision, anorexia, tremor, depression, rash. ***RARE*** (<2%): Urinary frequency, vivid dreams, neck pain, hypotension, vomiting.

ADVERSE REACTIONS/TOXIC EFFECTS

Overdosage may require supportive measures to maintain arterial B/P (monitor cardiac function, vital signs, blood gases, serum electrolytes). Activated charcoal may be more effective than emesis or lavage.

NURSING IMPLICATIONS

INTERVENTION/EVALUATION:

Be alert to neurologic effects: headache, lethargy, mental confusion, agitation. Monitor for evidence of dyskinesia (difficulty with movement). Assess for clinical reversal of Parkinson symptoms (improvement of tremor of head/hands at rest, masklike facial expression, shuffling gait, muscular rigidity).

PATIENT/FAMILY TEACHING:
Tolerance to feeling of light-headedness develops during therapy. To reduce hypotensive effect, rise slowly from lying to sitting position and permit legs to dangle momentarily before standing. Avoid tasks that require alertness, motor skills until response to drug is established. Dry mouth, drowsiness, dizziness may be expected responses of drug. Avoid alcoholic beverages during therapy.

perindopril erbumine

(Aceon)

See Classification section under: Angiotensin-converting enzyme (ACE) inhibitors (p. 6C)

perphenazine

(Trilafon)

See Classification section under: Antipsychotics

phenazopyridine hydrochloride

feen-ah-zoe-**peer**-ih-deen
(Phenazo✦, Pyridium, Urodine)
Do not confuse with pyridoxine.

▶**CLASSIFICATION**

PHARMACOTHERAPEUTIC:
Interstitial cystitis agent. ***CLINICAL:*** Urinary tract analgesic

ACTION/*THERAPEUTIC EFFECT*
Exerts topical analgesic effect on urinary tract mucosa, *providing relief of urinary pain, burning, urgency, frequency.*

PHARMACOKINETICS
Well absorbed from GI tract. Partially metabolized in liver. Primarily excreted in urine.

USES
Symptomatic relief of pain, burning, urgency, frequency resulting from lower urinary tract mucosa irritation (may be caused by infection, trauma, surgery).

PRECAUTIONS
CONTRAINDICATIONS: Renal insufficiency. ***CAUTIONS:*** None significant.
▷***LIFESPAN CONSIDERATIONS:***
Pregnancy/Lactation: Unknown whether drug crosses placenta or is distributed in breast milk. **Pregnancy Category B. Children:** No age-related precautions noted in those >6 yrs of age. **Elderly:** Age-related renal impairment may increase toxicity.

INTERACTIONS
DRUG: None significant. ***HERBAL:*** None known. ***FOOD:*** None known. ***LAB VALUES:*** May interfere with urinalysis color reactions, e.g., urinary glucose, ketone tests, urinary protein, or determination of urinary steroids.

AVAILABILITY (Rx)
TABLETS: 100 mg, 200 mg.

ADMINISTRATION/HANDLING
PO:
• Give after meals.

INDICATIONS/ROUTES/DOSAGE

Analgesic:

PO: Adults: 100–200 mg 3–4 times/day. **Children >6 yrs:** 12 mg/kg/day in 3 divided doses for 2 days.

Dose interval in renal impairment:

Creatinine Clearance	Interval
50–80 ml/min	q8–16h
<50 ml/min	avoid use

SIDE EFFECTS

OCCASIONAL: Headache, GI disturbance, rash, pruritus.

ADVERSE REACTIONS/TOXIC EFFECTS

Overdosage levels or those with impaired renal function or severe hypersensitivity may develop renal toxicity, hemolytic anemia, hepatic toxicity. Methemoglobinemia generally occurs as result of massive, acute overdosage.

NURSING IMPLICATIONS

INTERVENTION/EVALUATION:

Assess for therapeutic response: relief of pain, burning, urgency, frequency of urination.

PATIENT/FAMILY TEACHING:

A reddish-orange discoloration of urine should be expected. May stain fabric. Take after meals (reduces possibility of GI upset).

phenelzine sulfate ∗

fen-ell-zeen
(Nardil)

▶CLASSIFICATION

PHARMACOTHERAPEUTIC:
MAO inhibitor. ***CLINICAL:*** Antidepressant (see p. 35C)

ACTION/*THERAPEUTIC EFFECT*

Inhibits monoamine oxidase (MAO) enzyme system at CNS storage sites. The reduced MAO activity causes an increased concentration in epinephrine, norepinephrine, serotonin, dopamine at neuron receptor sites, *producing antidepressant effect.*

USES/*UNLABELED*

Management of atypical, nonendogenous, neurotic depression associated with anxiety, phobic, hypochondriacal features in those not responsive to other antidepressant therapy. *Treatment of panic disorder, vascular/tension headaches.*

PRECAUTIONS

CONTRAINDICATIONS: Pts >60 yrs, debilitated/hypertensive pts, cerebrovascular/cardiovascular disease, foods containing tryptophan/tyramine, within 10 days of elective surgery, pheochromocytoma, CHF, history of liver disease, abnormal liver function tests, severe renal impairment, history of severe/recurrent headache. ***CAUTIONS:*** Impaired renal function, history of seizures, parkinsonian syndrome, diabetic pts, hyperthyroidism.

INTERACTIONS

DRUG: **Alcohol, CNS depressants** may increase CNS depressant effects. **Tricyclic antidepressants, fluoxetine, trazodone** may cause serotonin syndrome. May increase effect of oral **hypoglycemics, insulin.** B/P may increase with **buspirone. Caffeine-containing medications** may increase cardiac arrhythmias, hypertension. May precipitate hypertensive crises with **carbamazepine, cyclobenzaprine,**

maprotiline, other **MAO inhibitors. Meperidine, other opioid analgesics** may produce immediate excitation, diaphoresis, rigidity, severe hypertension or hypotension, severe respiratory distress, coma, convulsions, vascular collapse, death. May increase CNS stimulant effects of **methylphenidate.** Sympathomimetics may increase cardiac stimulant, vasopressor effects. Tyramine, foods with pressor amines (e.g., aged cheese) may cause sudden, severe hypertension. **HERBAL:** None known. **FOOD:** None known. **LAB VALUES:** None significant.

INDICATIONS/ROUTES/DOSAGE
Depression:
PO: Adults, elderly: Initially, 1 mg/kg/day. **Maintenance:** 45 mg/day.

SIDE EFFECTS
FREQUENT: Postural hypotension, restlessness, GI upset, insomnia, dizziness, headache, lethargy, weakness, dry mouth, peripheral edema. **OCCASIONAL:** Flushing, increased perspiration, rash, urinary frequency, increased appetite, transient impotence. **RARE:** Visual disturbances.

ADVERSE REACTIONS/TOXIC EFFECTS
Hypertensive crisis may be noted by hypertension, occipital headache radiating frontally, neck stiffness/soreness, nausea, vomiting, sweating, fever/chilliness, clammy skin, dilated pupils, palpitations. Tachycardia or bradycardia, constricting chest pain may also be present. Antidote for hypertensive crisis: 5–10 mg phentolamine IV injection.

NURSING IMPLICATIONS
BASELINE ASSESSMENT:
Periodic liver function tests should be performed in those requiring high dosage undergoing prolonged therapy.

INTERVENTION/EVALUATION:
Assess appearance, behavior, speech pattern, level of interest, mood. Monitor for occipital headache radiating frontally and/or neck stiffness/soreness (may be first signal of impending hypertensive crisis). Monitor B/P diligently for hypertension.

PATIENT/FAMILY TEACHING:
Antidepressant relief may be noted during first week of therapy; maximum benefit noted in 2–6 wks. Report headache, neck stiffness/soreness immediately. Avoid foods that require bacteria or molds for their preparation or preservation or those that contain tyramine, e.g., cheese, sour cream, beer, wine, figs, raisins, bananas, avocados, soy sauce, yeast extracts, yogurt, papaya, broad beans, meat tenderizers, or excessive amounts of caffeine (coffee, tea, chocolate), or OTC preparations for hay fever, colds, weight reduction.

phenobarbital
feen-oh-**bar**-bih-tall
(Luminal)
FIXED-COMBINATION(S)
With phenytoin sodium, an anticonvulsant (**Dilantin with Phenobarbital Kapseals**); with belladonna, an anticholinergic and ergotamine (**Bellergal-S**)

►CLASSIFICATION

PHARMACOTHERAPEUTIC:
Barbiturate **(Schedule IV).**
CLINICAL: Anticonvulsant, hypnotic (see p. 31C)

ACTION/*THERAPEUTIC EFFECT*

Decreases motor activity to electrical/chemical stimulation, *producing anticonvulsant effect.* CNS depressant effect produces all levels from mild sedation, hypnosis to deep coma.

PHARMACOKINETICS

	Onset	Peak	Duration
PO	20–60 min	—	—
IM	10–15 min	—	4–6 hrs
IV	5 min	30 min	4–6 hrs

Well absorbed after PO, parenteral administration. Protein binding: 35–50%. Rapidly, widely distributed. Metabolized in liver. Primarily excreted in urine. Removed by hemodialysis. Half-life: 53–118 hrs.

USES/*UNLABELED*

Management of generalized tonic-clonic (grand mal) seizures, partial seizures, control of acute convulsive episodes (status epilepticus, eclampsia, febrile seizures). Relieves anxiety, provides preop sedation. *Prophylaxis/treatment of hyperbilirubinemia.*

PRECAUTIONS

CONTRAINDICATIONS: History of porphyria, bronchopneumonia. **EXTREME CAUTION:** Nephritis, renal insufficiency. **CAUTIONS:** Uncontrolled pain (may produce paradoxical reaction), impaired liver function.

▷*LIFESPAN CONSIDERATIONS:*
Pregnancy/Lactation: Readily crosses placenta; distributed in breast milk. Produces respiratory depression in neonates during labor. May cause postpartum hemorrhage, hemorrhagic disease in newborn. Withdrawal symptoms may appear in neonates born to women receiving barbiturates during last trimester of pregnancy. Lowers serum bilirubin concentration in neonates. **Pregnancy Category D. Children:** May cause paradoxical excitement. **Elderly:** May exhibit excitement, confusion, mental depression.

INTERACTIONS

DRUG: May decrease effects of **glucocorticoids, digoxin, metronidazole, oral anticoagulants, quinidine, tricyclic antidepressants. Alcohol, CNS depressants** may increase effect. May increase metabolism of **carbamazepine. Valproic acid** decreases metabolism, increases concentration, toxicity. **HERBAL:** None known. **FOOD:** None known. **LAB VALUES:** May decrease bilirubin. Therapeutic blood serum level: 10–40 mcg/ml; toxic blood serum level: >40 mcg/ml.

AVAILABILITY (Rx)

TABLETS: 15 mg, 30 mg, 60 mg, 100 mg. **ELIXIR:** 20 mg/5 ml. **INJECTION:** 30 mg/ml, 60 mg/ml, 130 mg/ml.

ADMINISTRATION/HANDLING
PO:

• Give without regard to meals. Tablets may be crushed. • Elixir may be mixed with water, milk, fruit juice.

IM:

• Do not inject more than 5 ml in any one IM injection site (produces tissue irritation). • Inject IM deep into gluteus maximus or lateral aspect of thigh.

IV 🈪

Storage:

• Store vials at room temperature.

Reconstitution:

• May give undiluted or may dilute with NaCl, D_5W, lactated Ringer's.

Rate of administration:

• Adequately hydrate pt before and immediately after (decreases risk of adverse renal effects). • Administer at rate not greater than 60 mg/min (too-rapid IV may produce severe hypotension, marked respiratory depression). • Inadvertent intra-arterial injection may result in arterial spasm with severe pain, tissue necrosis. Extravasation in SubQ tissue may produce redness, tenderness, tissue necrosis. If either occurs, treat with 0.5% procaine solution into affected area, apply moist heat.

IV INCOMPATIBILITIES ⊘

Amphotericin B complex (Abelcet, Ambisome, Amphotec), hydromorphone (Dilaudid).

IV COMPATIBILITIES

Heparin, fosphenytoin (Cerebyx), propofol (Diprivan).

INDICATIONS/ROUTES/DOSAGE

Status epilepticus:

***IV:* Adults, elderly, children, neonates:** *(Loading dose):* 15–20 mg/kg as single dose or in divided doses.

Anticonvulsant:

Note: Maintenance dose to begin 12 hrs after loading dose:

***IV/PO:* Adults, elderly, children >12 yrs:** 1–3 mg/kg/day. **Children 5–12 yrs:** 4–6 mg/kg/day. **Children 1–5 yrs:** 6–8 mg/kg/day. **Neonates:** 3–4 mg/kg/day.

Sedation:

***PO/IM:* Adults, elderly:** 30–120 mg/day in 2–3 divided doses. **Children:** 2 mg/kg 3 times/day.

Hypnotic:

***PO/IM/IV/SubQ:* Adults, elderly:** 100–320 mg at bedtime. **Children:** 3–5 mg/kg.

SIDE EFFECTS

OCCASIONAL (1–3%): Somnolence. ***RARE*** (<1%): Confusion, paradoxical CNS hyperactivity/nervousness in children, excitement/restlessness in elderly (generally noted during first 2 wks of therapy, particularly noted in presence of uncontrolled pain).

ADVERSE REACTIONS/TOXIC EFFECTS

Abrupt withdrawal after prolonged therapy may produce effects ranging from markedly increased dreaming, nightmares and/or insomnia, tremor, sweating, vomiting, to hallucinations, delirium, seizures, status epilepticus. Skin eruptions appear as hypersensitivity reaction. Blood dyscrasias, liver disease, hypocalcemia occur rarely. Overdosage produces cold, clammy skin, hypothermia, severe CNS depres-

P

sion, cyanosis, rapid pulse, Cheyne-Stokes respirations. Toxicity may result in severe renal impairment.

NURSING IMPLICATIONS

BASELINE ASSESSMENT:

Assess B/P, pulse, respirations immediately before administration. *Hypnotic:* Raise bed rails, provide environment conducive to sleep (back rub, quiet environment, low lighting). *Seizures:* Review history of seizure disorder (length, presence of auras, LOC). Observe frequently for recurrence of seizure activity. Initiate seizure precautions.

INTERVENTION/EVALUATION:

Assess elderly, debilitated, children for evidence of paradoxical reaction, particularly during early therapy. Evaluate for therapeutic response: decrease in length, number of seizures. Monitor for therapeutic serum level (10–30 mcg/ml). Therapeutic blood serum level: 10–40 mcg/ml; toxic blood serum level: >40 mcg/ml.

PATIENT/FAMILY TEACHING:

Drowsiness may gradually decrease/disappear with continued use. Do not abruptly withdraw medication following long-term use (may precipitate seizures). Avoid tasks that require alertness, motor skills until response to drug is established. Tolerance/dependence may occur with prolonged use of high doses. Strict maintenance of drug therapy is essential for seizure control.

phenoxybenzamine hydrochloride

fen-ox-ee-**bends**-ah-mean
(Dibenzyline)

▶CLASSIFICATION
PHARMACOTHERAPEUTIC:
Alpha-adrenergic blocking agent.
CLINICAL: Antihypertensive

ACTION/*THERAPEUTIC EFFECT*
Irreversibly combines with postganglionic alpha-adrenergic receptors, prevents or reverses effects of catecholamines in exocrine glands, smooth muscle. *Increases blood flow to skin, mucosa, and abdominal viscera; lowers both supine and standing B/P.*

USES/*UNLABELED*
Controls/prevents hypertension and sweating in pts with pheochromocytoma. *Treatment of benign prostatic hypertrophy.*

PRECAUTIONS
CONTRAINDICATIONS: Conditions when decrease in B/P is unwarranted. ***CAUTIONS:*** Compounds that produce further fall in B/P, marked cerebral/coronary arteriosclerosis, renal impairment/damage.

INTERACTIONS
DRUG: May decrease effects of sympathomimetics (e.g., dopamine, phenylephrine). ***HERBAL:*** None known. ***FOOD:*** None known. ***LAB VALUES:*** None significant.

AVAILABILITY (Rx)
CAPSULES: 10 mg.

INDICATIONS/ROUTES/DOSAGE

Pheochromocytoma:

PO: Adults, elderly: Initially, 10 mg 2 times/day. **Maintenance:** 20–40 mg 2–3 times/day. May increase dose every other day. **Children:** Initially, 0.2 mg/kg once daily. **Maximum:** 10 mg. **Maintenance:** 0.4–1.2 mg/kg/day in divided doses q6–8h.

SIDE EFFECTS

FREQUENT: Miosis, nasal stuffiness, reflex tachycardia. *OCCASIONAL:* Confusion, dry mouth, headache, inhibition of ejaculation, drowsiness, lack of energy.

ADVERSE REACTIONS/TOXIC EFFECTS

Severe hypotension occurs rarely.

NURSING IMPLICATIONS

INTERVENTION/EVALUATION:

Assist with ambulation if dizziness, drowsiness occurs. Monitor B/P.

PATIENT/FAMILY TEACHING:

Side effects tend to diminish as therapy continues. Avoid alcoholic beverages, OTC cough, cold medications. Avoid driving or tasks that require alert response until drug effects known.

phentolamine

fen-**toll**-ah-mean
(Regitine)
Do not confuse with phentermine.

▶CLASSIFICATION

PHARMACOTHERAPEUTIC: Alpha-adrenergic blocking agent. *CLINICAL:* Pheochromocytoma agent

ACTION/THERAPEUTIC EFFECT

Blocks presynaptic (alpha$_2$) and postsynaptic (alpha$_1$) adrenergic receptors, acting on both arterial tree and venous bed. *Decreases total peripheral resistance, diminishes venous return to heart.*

PHARMACOKINETICS

Metabolized in the liver. Excreted in urine. Half-life: 19 min.

USES/UNLABELED

Diagnosis of pheochromocytoma. Controls/prevents hypertensive episodes immediately before, during surgical excision. Prevents/treats dermal necrosis and sloughing following IV administration of norepinephrine/dopamine. *Treatment of CHF.*

PRECAUTIONS

CONTRAINDICATIONS: Epinephrine, myocardial infarction, coronary insufficiency, angina, coronary artery disease. *CAUTIONS:* Severe coronary insufficiency, recent MI, cerebrovascular disease, chronic renal failure, Raynaud's disease, thromboangitis obliterans.

▷*LIFESPAN CONSIDERATIONS:* **Pregnancy/Lactation:** Unknown if drug crosses placenta or is distributed in breast milk. **Pregnancy Category C. Children:** Safety and efficacy not established. **Elderly:** No age-related precautions noted.

INTERACTIONS

DRUG: May decrease effects of **sympathomimetics (e.g., dopamine, phenylephrine).** *HERBAL:* None known. *FOOD:* None known. *LAB VALUES:* None significant.

AVAILABILITY (Rx)

INJECTION: 5 mg vials.

ADMINISTRATION/HANDLING

Note: Maintain pt in supine position (preferably in quiet, darkened room) during pheochromocytoma testing. Decrease in B/P noted generally <2 min.

IV 🜀

Storage:
• Store vials at room temperature.
• After reconstitution, is stable for 48 hrs at room temperature or 1 wk if refrigerated.

Reconstitution:
• Reconstitute 5 mg vial with 1 ml Sterile Water for Injection to provide concentration of 5 mg/ml.

Rate of administration:
• Inject rapidly. Monitor B/P immediately after injection, q30sec for 3 min, then q60sec for 7 min.

IV INCOMPATIBILITY ⊘

Do not mix with any other medications.

IV COMPATIBILITIES

Amiodarone (Cordarone), dobutamine (Dobutrex).

INDICATIONS/ROUTES/DOSAGE

Diagnosis of pheochromocytoma:
***IM/IV:* Adults, elderly:** 2.5–5 mg.
Children: 0.05–0.1 mg/kg/dose.
Maximum: 5 mg.

Prevent/control hypertension in pheochromocytoma:
***IV:* Adults, elderly:** 5 mg 1–2 hrs before surgery. May repeat. **Children:** 0.05–0.1 mg/kg/dose 1–2 hrs before surgery. May repeat.

Prevent/treat necrosis/sloughing:
Infiltrate area with 1 ml of solution (reconstituted by diluting 5–10 mg in 0.9% NaCl) within 12 hrs of ex-

travasation. **Maximum:** 0.1–0.2 mg/kg or 5 mg total.

SIDE EFFECTS

OCCASIONAL: Weakness, dizziness, flushing, nausea, vomiting, diarrhea, orthostatic hypotension.

ADVERSE REACTIONS/TOXIC EFFECTS

Tachycardia, arrhythmias, acute/prolonged hypotension may occur. Do not use epinephrine (will produce further drop in B/P).

NURSING IMPLICATIONS

BASELINE ASSESSMENT:

Positive pheochromocytoma test indicated by decrease in B/P >35 mm Hg systolic, >25 mm Hg diastolic pressure. Negative test indicated by no B/P change, elevated B/P, or B/P elevated 35 mm Hg systolic and 25 mm Hg diastolic. Preinjection B/P generally occurs within 15–30 min after administration.

INTERVENTION/EVALUATION:

Monitor B/P continuously during therapy/tests.

phenylephrine hydrochloride

fen-ill-**eh**-frin
(AK-Dilate, Neo-Synephrine, Prefrin)

FIXED-COMBINATION[S]

With zinc sulfate, an astringent **(Zincfrin);** with pyrilamine maleate, an antihistamine **(Prefrin-A);** with sulfacetamide, an anti-infective **(Vasosulf);** with pheniramine maleate, an antihistamine **(Dristan)**; with naphazoline, a vasoconstrictor, and pyrilamine, an antihistamine **(4 Way Nasal Spray)**

▶CLASSIFICATION

PHARMACOTHERAPEUTIC: Sympathomimetic, alpha receptor stimulant. **CLINICAL:** Nasal decongestant, mydriatic, vasopressor (see p. 125C)

ACTION/*THERAPEUTIC EFFECT*

Acts on alpha-adrenergic receptors of vascular smooth muscle. *Increases systolic/diastolic B/P, produces constriction of blood vessels, conjunctival arterioles, nasal arterioles.*

PHARMACOKINETICS

Onset	Peak	Duration
Ophthalmic		
Immediate	—	0.5–4 hrs
Nasal		
Immediate	—	0.5–4 hrs
IV		
Immediate	—	15–20 min
IM		
10–15 min	—	0.5–2 hrs

Minimal absorption following intranasal, ophthalmic administration. Metabolized in liver, GI tract. Primarily excreted in urine. Half-life: 2.5 hrs.

USES

Nasal: Topical application to nasal mucosa reduces nasal secretion, promoting drainage of sinus secretions. **Ophthalmic:** Topical application to conjunctiva relieves congestion, itching, minor irritation; whitens sclera of eye. **Parenteral:** Vascular failure in shock, drug-induced hypotension.

PRECAUTIONS

CONTRAINDICATIONS: Idiosyncrasy to sympathomimetics manifested by insomnia, dizziness, weakness, tremor, arrhythmias, MAO inhibitor therapy. **Ophthalmic:** Angle-closure glaucoma, those with soft contact lenses, use of 10% solution in infants. **Nasal:** Those with insomnia, tremor, asthenia, dizziness, arrhythmias due to previous drug doses. **CAUTIONS:** Marked hypertension, cardiac disorders, advanced arteriosclerotic disease, type I (insulin-dependent) diabetes mellitus, hyperthyroidism, children with low body weight, elderly.

▷**LIFESPAN CONSIDERATIONS:** **Pregnancy/Lactation:** Crosses placenta; distributed in breast milk. **Pregnancy Category C. Children:** May exhibit increased absorption, toxicity with nasal preparation. No age-related precautions noted with systemic use. **Elderly:** No age-related precautions noted.

INTERACTIONS

DRUG: Tricyclic antidepressants, maprotiline may increase cardiovascular effects. May decrease effect of **methyldopa.** May have mutually inhibitory effects with **beta-blockers.** May increase risk of arrhythmias with **digoxin. Ergonovine, oxytocin** may increase vasoconstriction. **MAO inhibitors** may increase vasopressor effects. **HERBAL: Ma Huang (Ephedra)** may increase CNS stimulation. **FOOD:** None known. **LAB VALUES:** None significant.

AVAILABILITY (OTC)

INJECTION (Rx): 1% (10 mg/ml). **NASAL SOLUTION:** 0.25%, 0.5%,

P

✦ - Canadian trade name   ✳ - see also www.wbsaunders.com/SIMON/SaundersNDH

1%. ***OPHTHALMIC SOLUTION:*** 0.12%, 2.5% *(Rx)*, 10% *(Rx)*.

ADMINISTRATION/HANDLING
Nasal:

• Blow nose before medication is administered. With head tilted back, apply drops in 1 nostril. Remain in same position and wait 5 min before applying drops in other nostril. • Sprays should be administered into each nostril with head erect. Sniff briskly while squeezing container. Wait 3–5 min before blowing nose gently. Rinse tip of spray bottle.

Ophthalmic:

• Instruct pt to tilt head backward and look up. • Gently pull lower lid down to form pouch and instill medication. • Do not touch tip of applicator to lids or any surface. • When lower lid is released, have pt keep eye open without blinking for at least 30 sec. • Apply gentle finger pressure to lacrimal sac (bridge of the nose, inside corner of the eye) for 1–2 min. • Remove excess solution around eye with tissue. Wash hands immediately to remove medication on hands.

IV ▥

Storage:

• Store vials at room temperature.

Reconstitution:

• For IV push, dilute 1 ml of 10 mg/ml solution with 9 ml Sterile Water for Injection to provide a concentration of 1mg/ml. • For IV infusion, dilute 10 mg vial with 500 ml D_5W or 0.9% NaCl to provide a concentration of 2 mcg/ml. Maximum concentration: 500 mg/250 ml.

Rate of administration:

• For IV push, give over 20–30 sec. • For IV infusion, give as per physician order.

IV INCOMPATIBILITY ⊘
Thiopentothal (Pentothal).

IV COMPATIBILITIES
Amiodarone (Cordarone), dobutamine (Dobutrex), lidocaine, potassium chloride, propofol (Diprivan).

INDICATIONS/ROUTES/DOSAGE
Nasal decongestant:

PO: Adults, elderly, children >12 yrs: 2–3 drops, 1–2 sprays of 0.25–0.5% solution into each nostril. **Children 6–12 yrs:** 2–3 drops or 1–2 sprays of 0.25% solution in each nostril. **Children <6 yrs:** 2–3 drops of 0.125% solution in each nostril. Repeat q4h as needed. Do not use longer than 3 days.

Ophthalmic:

OPHTHALMIC: Adults, elderly, children >12 yrs: 1–2 drops of 0.125% solution q3–4h.

Hypotension/shock:

IM/SUBQ: Adults, elderly: 2–5 mg/dose q1–2h. **Children:** 0.1 mg/kg/dose q1–2h.

IV BOLUS: Adults, elderly: 0.1–0.5 mg/dose q10–15min as needed. **Children:** 5–20 mcg/kg/dose q10–15min.

IV INFUSION: Adults, elderly: 100–180 mcg/min. **Children:** 0.1–0.5 mcg/kg/min. Titrate to desired effect.

SIDE EFFECTS
FREQUENT: Nasal: Rebound nasal congestion due to overuse (longer than 3 days). ***OCCASIONAL:*** Mild CNS stimulation (restlessness, nervousness, tremors, headache, insomnia), particularly in those hypersensitive to sympathomimetics (generally, elderly pts). ***Nasal:*** Stinging, burning, drying of nasal mucosa. ***Ophthalmic:*** Transient burning/stinging, brow ache, blurred vision.

ADVERSE REACTIONS/TOXIC EFFECTS

Large doses may produce tachycardia, palpitations (particularly in those with cardiac disease), lightheadedness, nausea, vomiting. Overdosage in those >60 yrs may result in hallucinations, CNS depression, seizures. Prolonged nasal use may produce chronic swelling of nasal mucosa, rhinitis.

NURSING IMPLICATIONS

BASELINE ASSESSMENT:

If phenylephrine 10% ophthalmic is instilled into denuded or damaged corneal epithelium, corneal clouding may result.

PATIENT/FAMILY TEACHING:

Discontinue drug if adverse reactions occur. Do not use for nasal decongestion longer than 3–5 days (rebound congestion). Discontinue drug if insomnia, dizziness, weakness, tremor, or feeling of irregular heartbeat occurs. **Nasal:** Stinging/burning of inside nose may occur. **Ophthalmic:** Blurring of vision with eye instillation generally subsides with continued therapy. Discontinue medication if redness/swelling of eyelids, itching appears.

phenytoin

phen-ih-toyn
(Dilantin)
Do not confuse with Dilaudid, mephenytoin.

phenytoin sodium

(Dilantin)

FIXED-COMBINATION(S)

With phenobarbital, a barbiturate **(Dilantin with Phenobarbital)**

▶CLASSIFICATION

PHARMACOTHERAPEUTIC: Hydantoin. **CLINICAL:** Anticonvulsant, antiarrhythmic (see p. 32C)

ACTION/THERAPEUTIC EFFECT

Anticonvulsant: Stabilizes neuronal membranes in motor cortex, limits spread of seizure activity. Stabilizes threshhold against hyperexcitability. Decreases post-tetanic potentiation and repetitive discharge. **Antiarrhythmic:** Decreases abnormal ventricular automaticity (shortens refractory period, QT interval, action potential duration).

PHARMACOKINETICS

Slow, variably absorbed after PO administration; slow but complete absorption following IM administration. Protein binding: 90–95%. Widely distributed. Metabolized in liver. Primarily excreted in urine. Not removed by hemodialysis. Half-life: 22 hrs.

USES/UNLABELED

Management of generalized tonic-clonic seizures (grand mal), complex partial seizures (psychomotor), cortical focal seizures, status epilepticus. Ineffective in absence seizures, myoclonic seizures, atonic epilepsy when used alone. Treatment of cardiac arrhythmias due to digitalis intoxication. Treatment of digoxin-induced arrhythmias, trigeminal neuralgia; muscle relaxant in treatment of muscle hyperirritability; adjunct in treatment of tricyclic antidepressant toxicity.

P

PRECAUTIONS

CONTRAINDICATIONS: Seizures due to hypoglycemia, hydantoin hypersensitivity. ***IV route only:*** Sinus bradycardia, sinoatrial block, second-and third-degree heart block, Adam-Stokes syndrome. ***EXTREME CAUTION: IV route only:*** Respiratory depression, myocardial infarction, CHF, damaged myocardium. ***CAUTIONS:*** Impaired hepatic/renal function, severe myocardial insufficiency, hypotension, hyperglycemia.

▷***LIFESPAN CONSIDERATIONS:***
Pregnancy/Lactation: Crosses placenta; is distributed in small amount in breast milk. Fetal hydantoin syndrome (craniofacial abnormalities, nail/digital hypoplasia, prenatal growth deficiency) has been reported. There is increased frequency of seizures in pregnant women due to altered absorption of metabolism of phenytoin. May increase risk of hemorrhage in neonate, maternal bleeding during delivery. **Pregnancy Category D. Children:** More susceptible to gingival hyperplasia, coarsening of facial features, excess body hair. **Elderly:** No age-related precautions noted but lower doses recommended.

INTERACTIONS

DRUG: May decrease effect of **glucocorticoids. Alcohol, CNS depressants** may increase CNS depression. **Antacids** may decrease absorption. **Amiodarone, anticoagulants, cimetidine, disulfiram, fluoxetine, isoniazid, sulfonamides** may increase phenytoin concentration, effects, toxicity. **Fluconazole, ketoconazole, miconazole** may increase concentration. **Lidocaine, propranolol** may increase cardiac depressant effects.

Valproic acid may increase concentration, decrease metabolism. May increase **xanthine** metabolism. ***HERBAL:*** None known. ***FOOD:*** None known. ***LAB VALUES:*** May increase alkaline phosphatase, GGT, glucose. Therapeutic blood serum level: 10–20 mcg/ml; toxic blood serum level: >20 mcg/ml.

AVAILABILITY (Rx)

CAPSULES: 30 mg, 100 mg. ***TABLETS (chewable):*** 50 mg. ***ORAL SUSPENSION:*** 125 mg/5 ml. ***INJECTION:*** 50 mg/ml.

ADMINISTRATION/HANDLING
PO:
• Give with food if GI distress occurs. • Do not chewith break capsules. Tablets may be chewed. • Shake oral suspension well before using.

IV 🖫

Note: Give by IV push.

Storage:
• Precipitate may form if parenteral form is refrigerated (will dissolve at room temperature). • Slight yellow discoloration of parenteral form does not affect potency, but do not use if solution is not clear or if precipitate is present.

Reconstitution:
• May give undiluted or may dilute with 0.9% NaCl.

Rate of administration:
• Administer 50 mg >2–3 min for elderly. In neonates, administer at rate not exceeding 1–3 mg/kg/min. • Severe hypotension, cardiovascular collapse occurs if rate of IV injection exceeds 50 mg/min for adults. IV push very painful (chemical irritation of vein due to alkalinity of solution). To minimize effect,

flush vein with sterile saline solution through same IV needle/catheter following each IV push. • IV toxicity characterized by CNS depression, cardiovascular collapse.

IV INCOMPATIBILITIES ⊘

Amphotericin B complex (Abelcet, Ambisome, Amphotec), ciprofloxacin (Cipro), diltiazem (Cardizem), enalapril (Vasotec), heparin, hydromorphone (Dilaudid), potassium chloride, propofol (Diprivan), sufentanil (Sufenta), theophylline.

INDICATIONS/ROUTES/DOSAGE

Note: Maintenance dose usually 12 hrs after loading dose.

Status epilepticus:

IV: Adults, elderly, children: (Loading dose): 15–18 mg/kg. **Neonates:** 15–20 mg/kg. **Adults, elderly:** *(Maintenance dose):* 300 mg/day in 2–3 divided doses. **Children 10–16 yrs:** 6–7 mg/kg/day. **Children 7–9 yrs:** 7–8 mg/kg/day. **Children 4–6 yrs:** 7.5–9 mg/kg/day. **Children 0.5–3 yrs:** 8–10 mg/kg/day. **Neonates:** 5–8 mg/kg/day.

Anticonvulsant:

PO: Adults, elderly, children: (Loading dose): 15–20 mg/kg in 3 divided doses 2–4 hrs apart. *(Maintenance dose):* Same as above.

Arrhythmias:

IV: Adults, elderly, children: (Loading dose): 1.25 mg/kg q5min. May repeat up to toal dose of 15 mg/kg.

PO: Adults, elderly: (Maintenance dose): 250 mg 4 times/day for 1 day, then 250 mg 2 times/day for 2 days, then 300–400 mg/day in divided doses 1–4 times/day.

PO/IV: Children: (Maintenance dose): 5–10 mg/kg/day in 2–3 divided doses.

SIDE EFFECTS

FREQUENT: Drowsiness, lethargy, confusion, slurred speech, irritability, gingival hyperplasia, hypersensitivity reaction (fever, rash, lymphadenopathy), constipation, dizziness, nausea. **OCCASIONAL:** Headache, hair growth, insomnia, muscle twitching.

ADVERSE REACTIONS/TOXIC EFFECTS

Abrupt withdrawal may precipitate status epilepticus. Blood dyscrasias, lymphadenopathy, osteomalacia (due to interference of vitamin D metabolism) may occur. Phenytoin blood concentration of 25 mcg/ml (toxic) may produce ataxia (muscular incoordination), nystagmus (rhythmic oscillation of eyes), double vision. As level increases, extreme lethargy to comatose states occur.

NURSING IMPLICATIONS

BASELINE ASSESSMENT:

Anticonvulsant: Review history of seizure disorder (intensity, frequency, duration, LOC). Initiate seizure precautions. Liver function tests, CBC, platelet count should be performed before therapy begins and periodically during therapy. Repeat CBC, platelet count 2 wks after therapy begins and 2 wks after maintenance dose is given.

INTERVENTION/EVALUATION:

Observe frequently for recurrence of seizure activity. Assess for clinical improvement (decrease in intensity/frequency of seizures). Assist with ambulation

P

if drowsiness, lethargy occurs. Monitor for therapeutic serum level (10–20 mcg/ml). Therapeutic blood serum level: 10–20 mcg/ml; toxic blood serum level: >20 mcg/ml.

PATIENT/FAMILY TEACHING:

Pain may occur with IV injection. To prevent gingival hyperplasia (bleeding, tenderness, swelling of gums), encourage good oral hygiene care, gum massage, regular dental visits. CBC should be performed every mo for 1 yr after maintenance dose is established and q3mos thereafter. Urine may appear pink, red, or red-brown. Report sore throat, fever, glandular swelling, skin reaction (hematologic toxicity). Drowsiness usually diminishes with continued therapy. Do not abruptly withdraw medication following long-term use (may precipitate seizures). Strict maintenance of drug therapy is essential for seizure control, arrhythmias. Avoid tasks that require alertness, motor skills until response to drug is established. Avoid alcohol.

phosphates

(Fleet enema, Fleet Phosphosoda, K-Phosphate, Neutra-phos K, Uro KP)

▶**CLASSIFICATION**

PHARMACOTHERAPEUTIC: Electrolyte. ***CLINICAL:*** Mineral

ACTION/*THERAPEUTIC EFFECT*

Modifies calcium concentration and buffer effect on acid-base equilibrium; influences renal excretion of hydrogen.

PHARMACOKINETICS

Well absorbed from GI tract. Primarily excreted in urine.

USES/*UNLABELED*

Prophylactic treatment of hypophosphatemia. Short-term treatment of constipation, for evacuation of colon for exams; urinary acidifier for reduction of formation of calcium stones. *Prevents calcium renal calculi.*

PRECAUTIONS

CONTRAINDICATIONS: Addison's disease, hyperkalemia, acidification of urine in urinary stone disease, those with infected urolithiasis or struvite stone formation, severely impaired renal function (<30% of normal), hyperphosphatemia. ***CAUTIONS:*** Those on sodium/potassium-restricted diet, cardiac disease, dehydration, renal impairment, tissue breakdown, myotonia congenita (spasm/rigidity of muscle upon attempts at muscle movement), cardiac failure, cirrhosis/severe hepatic disease, peripheral and pulmonary edema, hypernatremia, hypertension, pre-eclampsia, hypoparathyroidism, osteomalacia, acute pancreatitis.

▷***LIFESPAN CONSIDERATIONS:*** **Pregnancy/Lactation:** Unknown if drug crosses placenta or is distributed in breast milk. **Pregnancy Category C. Children/Elderly:** No age-related precautions noted.

INTERACTIONS

DRUG: **Glucocorticoids** with sodium phosphate may cause edema. **Antacids** may decrease absorption. **Calcium-containing medications** may increase risk of calcium deposition in soft tissues, decrease phosphate absorption. **NSAIDs, ACE inhibitors, potassium-sparing diuretics, potas-**

sium-containing medications, salt substitutes with **potassium phosphate** may increase potassium concentration. **Digoxin** and **potassium phosphate** may increase risk of heart block (due to hyperkalemia). **Phosphate-containing medications** may increase risk of hyperphosphatemia. **Sodium-containing medication** with sodium phosphate may increase risk of edema. *HERBAL:* None known. *FOOD:* None known. *LAB VALUES:* None significant.

AVAILABILITY (Rx)

INJECTION: 3 mM/ml. *TABLETS. ORAL SOLUTION. ENEMA. POWDER.*

ADMINISTRATION/HANDLING
PO:

• Dissolve tablets in water. • Take after meals or with food (decreases GI upset). • Maintain high fluid intake (prevents kidney stones).

IV

Storage:

• Store at room temperature.

Reconstitution:

• Must be diluted. Soluble in all commonly used IV solutions.

Rate of administration:

• Infuse slowly with maximum infusion rate of 0.2 mM phosphate/kg/hr.

IV INCOMPATIBILITY ⊘

No incompatibilities via Y site noted.

INDICATIONS/ROUTES/DOSAGE
Hypophosphatemia:

IV: Adults, elderly: 50–70 mmol/day. **Children:** 0.5–1.5 mmol/day.

PO: Adults, elderly: 50–150 mmol/day. **Children:** 2–3 mmol/kg/day.

Laxative:

PO: Adults, elderly, children >4 yrs: 1–2 capsules/packets 4 times/day. **Children <4 yrs:** 1 capsule/packet 4 times/day.

RECTAL: Adults, elderly, children >12 yrs: 4.5 oz enema as single dose. May repeat. **Children <12 yrs:** 2.25 oz enema as single dose. May repeat.

Urinary acidification:

PO: Adults, elderly: 2 tablets 4 times/day.

SIDE EFFECTS

FREQUENT: Mild laxative effect first few days of therapy. *OCCASIONAL:* GI upset (diarrhea, nausea, abdominal pain, vomiting). *RARE:* Headache, dizziness, mental confusion, heaviness of legs, fatigue, muscle cramps, numbness/tingling of hands, feet, around lips, peripheral edema, irregular heartbeat, weight gain, thirst.

ADVERSE REACTIONS/TOXIC EFFECTS

High phosphate levels may produce extra skeletal calcification.

NURSING IMPLICATIONS

INTERVENTION/EVALUATION:
Monitor serum calcium, phosphorus, potassium, sodium levels routinely.

PATIENT/FAMILY TEACHING:
Report diarrhea, nausea, vomiting.

physostigmine

(Antilirium, Eserine Sulfate)
Do not confuse with
pyridostigmine, Prostigmin.

►CLASSIFICATION

PHARMACOTHERAPEUTIC:
Parasympathomimetic (cholinergic). **CLINICAL:** Anticholinesterase agent (see p. 44C)

ACTION/THERAPEUTIC EFFECT

Inhibits destruction of acetylcholine by enzyme acetylcholinesterase. *Improves skeletal muscle tone, stimulates salivary and sweat gland secretion.* Constricts iris sphincter and ciliary muscle, *producing miosis and increasing accommodation. Intraocular pressure (IOP) reduced by increasing aqueous humor outflow.*

USES/UNLABELED

Antidote for reversal of toxic CNS effects due to anticholinergic drugs, tricyclic antidepressants; reduces IOP in primary glaucoma. **Systemic:** *Treatment of hereditary ataxia.* **Ophthalmic:** *Treatment of secondary glaucoma, angle-closure glaucoma during/after iridectomy.*

PRECAUTIONS

CONTRAINDICATIONS: Asthma, gangrene, diabetes, cardiovascular disease, mechanical obstruction of intestinal/urogenital tract, vagotonic state, those receiving ganglionic blocking agents. Hypersensitivity to cholinesterase inhibitors or any component of the preparation; active uveal inflammation; angle-closure (narrow-angle) glaucoma before iridectomy; glaucoma associated with iridocyclitis. **CAUTIONS:** Bronchial asthma, GI disturbances, peptic ulcer, bradycardia, hypotension, recent myocardial infarction, epilepsy, parkinsonism, and other disorders that may respond adversely to vagotonic effects. Use ophthalmic physostigmine only when shorter acting miotics are not adequate, except in aphakics. Discontinue at least 3 wks before ophthalmic surgery.

INTERACTIONS

DRUG: May increase effects of **cholinesterases (e.g., bethanechol, carbachol).** May prolong action of **succinylcholine. HERBAL:** None known. **FOOD:** None known. **LAB VALUES:** None significant.

INDICATIONS/ROUTES/DOSAGE

Antidote:

IM/IV: Adults, elderly: Initially, 0.5–2 mg. If no response, repeat q20min until response occurs or adverse cholinergic effects occur. If initial response occurs, may give additional doses of 1–4 mg at 30–60 min intervals as life-threatening signs recur (arrhythmias, seizures, deep coma). **Children:** 0.01–0.3 mg/kg. May give additional doses at 5–10 min intervals until response occurs, adverse cholinergic effects occur, or total dose of 2 mg given.

Glaucoma:

OPHTHALMIC: Adults, elderly: *Ointment:* Apply small quantity 1–3 times/day.

SIDE EFFECTS

COMMON: Miosis, increased GI and skeletal muscle tone, reduced pulse rate, **Ophthalmic:** Stinging, burning, tearing, hypersensitivity reaction, painful ciliary/accommodative spasm, blurred vision/myopia, poor vision in dim light. **OCCASIONAL:** Hypertensive pts may react with marked fall in B/P. **Ophthalmic:** Increased visibility of floaters, headache, brow ache, photophobia, ocular pain. **RARE:** Allergic reaction.

ADVERSE REACTIONS/TOXIC EFFECTS

Parenteral overdosage produces a cholinergic reaction manifested as abdominal discomfort/cramping, nausea, vomiting, diarrhea, flushing, feeling of warmth/heat about face, excessive salivation and sweating, urinary urgency, blurred vision. Requires a withdrawal of all anticholinergic drugs and immediate use of 0.6–1.2 mg atropine sulfate IM/IV for adults, 0.01 mg/kg in infants and children under 12 yrs.

NURSING IMPLICATIONS

BASELINE ASSESSMENT:
Have tissues readily available at pt's bedside.

INTERVENTION/EVALUATION:
Parenteral: Assess vital signs immediately before and q15–30min following administration. Monitor diligently for cholinergic reaction (sweating, irregular heartbeat, muscle weakness, abdominal pain, dyspnea, hypotension). *Ophthalmic:* Be alert for systemic toxicity: severe nausea, vomiting, diarrhea, frequent urination, excessive salivation, bradycardia.

PATIENT/FAMILY TEACHING:
Adverse effects often subside after the first few days of therapy. Avoid night driving, activities requiring visual acuity in dim light.

pilocarpine

pie-low-**car**-pine
(Ocusert)

pilocarpine hydrochloride

(Adsorbocarpine, Akarpine, Carpine, Isopto, Ocu-Carpine, Pilocar, Pilopine, Piloptic, Pilostat, Salagen)

pilocarpine nitrate

(Liquifilm, Pilagan)

FIXED-COMBINATION(S)

With epinephrine bitartrate, a vasoconstrictor **(E-Pilo-1, 2, 3, 4 or 6)**; with physostigmine salicylate, a miotic **(Isopto P-ES)**

See Classification section under: Antiglaucoma agents (p. 44C)

pimecrolimus

(Elidel)
See new Drug Supplement.

pimozide

pim-oh-zied
(Orap)

▶**CLASSIFICATION**

PHARMACOTHERAPEUTIC: Diphenylbutylpiperidine. *CLINICAL:* Tourette's agent

ACTION/*THERAPEUTIC EFFECT*

Inhibits dopamine receptors in CNS, *interrupting impulse movement.* Produces strong extrapyramidal, moderate anticholinergic, sedative effects.

USES/*UNLABELED*

Suppression of severely compromising motor and phonic tics in those with Tourette's disorders who have failed to respond adequately to standard treatment. Sjögren's syndrome. *Treatment of psychotic disorders.*

PRECAUTIONS

CONTRAINDICATIONS: Congenital QT syndrome, history of cardiac arrhythmias, administra-

P

tion with other drugs that prolong QT interval (azithromycin, clarithromycin, dirithromycin, erythromycin), severe toxic CNS depression, comatose states. *CAUTIONS:* History of seizures, cardiovascular disease, impaired respiratory, hepatic/renal function, alcohol withdrawal, urinary retention, glaucoma, prostatic hypertrophy.

▷*LIFESPAN CONSIDERATIONS:*
Pregnancy/Lactation: Unknown if drug crosses placenta or is distributed in breast milk. **Pregnancy Category C.**

INTERACTIONS

DRUG: **Alcohol, CNS depressants** may increase CNS depressant effect. **Methylphenidate, pemoline** may mask signs of tics. **Anticholinergics** may increase anticholinergic effects. **Tricyclic antidepressants, phenothiazines, quinidine** may increase risk of cardiac arrhythmias. **Extrapyramidal symptom–producing medications** (EPS) may increase anticholinergic, CNS depressant, and EPS effects. **Clarithromycin** may inhibit metabolism. *HERBAL:* None known. *FOOD:* None known. *LAB VALUES:* None significant.

AVAILABILITY (Rx)

TABLETS: 1 mg, 2 mg, 4 mg, 10 mg.

INDICATIONS/ROUTES/DOSAGE

Tourette's disorder:
PO: **Adults:** Initially, 1–2 mg/day in divided doses. Increase every other day. **Maintenance:** 0.2 mg/kg/day or 10 mg/day, whichever is less. **Maximum:** 0.2 mg/kg/day or 10 mg/day.

Sjögren's syndrome:
PO: **Adults:** 5 mg 4 times/day.

SIDE EFFECTS

FREQUENT: Drowsiness, salivation, constipation, dizziness, tachycardia. *OCCASIONAL:* Nausea, sweating, dry mouth, headache, hypotension, GI upset, weight gain. *RARE:* Visual disturbances, diarrhea, rash, urinary abnormalities.

ADVERSE REACTIONS/TOXIC EFFECTS

Extrapyramidal reactions occur frequently but are usually mild and reversible (generally noted during first few days of therapy). Motor restlessness, dystonia, hyperreflexia occur much less frequently. Persistent tardive dyskinesia has occurred. Those on long-term maintenance may experience transient dyskinetic signs following abrupt withdrawal.

NURSING IMPLICATIONS

BASELINE ASSESSMENT:
Obtain baseline EKG. Potassium level should be checked and corrected if necessary.

INTERVENTION/EVALUATION:
EKG should be periodically monitored. Assess for extrapyramidal symptoms. Monitor WBC, differential count for blood dyscrasias. Monitor for fine tongue movement (may be early sign of tardive dyskinesia). Assess for therapeutic response (decreased tic activity).

PATIENT/FAMILY TEACHING:
Do not abruptly withdraw from long-term drug therapy. Report visual disturbances. Drowsiness generally subsides during con-

tinued therapy. Avoid tasks that require alertness, motor skills until response to drug is established. Avoid alcohol and CNS depressants.

pindolol

(Apo-Pindol✤, Visken)
Do not confuse with Panadol, Parlodel, Plendil.

FIXED-COMBINATION(S)

With hydrochlorothiazide, a diuretic **(Viskazide)**

See Classification section under: Beta-adrenergic blockers (p. 61C)

pioglitazone

pie-oh-**glit**-ah-zone
(Actos)

▶CLASSIFICATION

CLINICAL: Antidiabetic (see p. 40C)

ACTION/*THERAPEUTIC EFFECT*

Improves target cell response to insulin without increasing pancreatic insulin secretion. Decreases hepatic glucose output, increases insulin-dependent glucose utilization in skeletal muscle, *lowering blood glucose concentration.*

PHARMACOKINETICS

Rapidly absorbed. Highly protein bound (>99%), primarily to albumin. Metabolized in liver. Excreted in urine. Unknown if removed by hemodialysis. Half-life: 16–24 hrs.

USES

Adjunct to diet and exercise to lower blood glucose in those with Type II noninsulin-dependent diabetes mellitus (NIDDM). Used as monotherapy or in combination with a sulfonylurea or insulin to improve glycemic control.

PRECAUTIONS

CONTRAINDICATIONS: Diabetic ketoacidosis, Type 1 diabetes mellitus, active liver disease, or increased serum transaminase levels (ALT [SGPT] >2.5 times normal serum level). ***CAUTIONS:*** Hepatic function impairment, CHF, edematous pts.
▷***LIFESPAN CONSIDERATIONS:***
Pregnancy/Lactation: Unknown if drug crosses placenta or is distributed in breast milk. Not recommended in pregnant or nursing women. **Pregnancy Category C. Children:** Safety and efficacy not established. **Elderly:** No age-related precautions noted.

INTERACTIONS

DRUG: May alter effects of **oral contraceptives. Ketoconazole** may significantly inhibit metabolism of pioglitazone. ***FOOD:*** None known. ***HERBAL:*** None known. ***LAB VALUES:*** May decrease hemoglobin levels by 2–4%, bilirubin, AST (SGOT), alkaline phosphatase. Less than 1% experience ALT (SGPT) values = 3 times normal level. May increase CPK levels.

AVAILABILITY (Rx)

TABLETS: 15 mg, 30 mg, 45 mg.

ADMINISTRATION/HANDLING

PO:

• Give without regard to meals.

INDICATIONS/ROUTES/DOSAGE

Diabetes mellitus, combination therapy:

PO: Adults, elderly: Insulin: Initially, 15–30 mg once/day. Initially, continue current insulin dose, then decrease insulin dose by 10–25% if hypoglycemia or plasma glucose levels decrease to <100 mg/dl. **Maximum:** 45 mg/day.

SULFONYLUREAS: Initially, 15–30 mg/day. Decrease sulfonylurea if hypoglycemia occurs.

MONOTHERAPY: Monotherapy is not to be used if pt is well controlled with diet and exercise alone. Initially, 15–30 mg/day. May increase dosage in increments up to 45 mg/day.

SIDE EFFECTS

FREQUENT (9–13%): Headache, upper respiratory tract infection. *OCCASIONAL* (5–6%): Sinusitis, myalgia (muscle aches), pharyngitis, aggravated diabetes mellitus.

ADVERSE REACTIONS/TOXIC EFFECTS

None significant.

NURSING IMPLICATIONS

BASELINE ASSESSMENT:

Obtain liver enzyme levels prior to initiation of therapy and periodically thereafter. Assure follow-up instruction if pt/family do not thoroughly understand diabetes management or glucose-testing technique.

INTERVENTION/EVALUATION:

Monitor blood glucose, hemoglobin, liver function tests, esp. SGOT, SGPT. Assess for hypoglycemia (cool wet skin, tremors, dizziness, anxiety, headache, tachycardia, numbness in mouth, hunger, diplopia) or hyperglycemia (polyuria, polyphagia, polydipsia, nausea, vomiting, dim vision, fatigue, deep rapid breathing). Be alert to conditions that alter glucose requirements: fever, increased activity or stress, surgical procedures.

PATIENT/FAMILY TEACHING:

Diabetes mellitus requires lifelong control. Prescribed diet and exercise are principal parts of treatment; do not skip or delay meals. Wear medical alert identification. Continue to adhere to dietary instructions, a regular exercise program, and regular testing of urine or blood glucose.

pipecuronium

(Arduan)

See Classification section under: Neuromuscular blockers

piperacillin sodium

(Pipracil)

See Classification section under: Antibiotic: Penicillins

piperacillin sodium/ tazobactam sodium

pip-ur-ah-**sill**-in/tay-zoe-**back**-tam
(Tazocin♣, Zosyn)
Do not confuse with Zofran, Zyvox.

▶CLASSIFICATION

PHARMACOTHERAPEUTIC:
Penicillin. **CLINICAL:** Antibiotic
(see p. 27C)

ACTION/*THERAPEUTIC EFFECT*

Piperacillin: Binds to bacterial membranes, *inhibiting cell wall synthesis. Bactericidal.* **Tazobactam:** Inactivates bacterial beta-lactamase enzymes. *Protects piperacillin from inactivation by beta-lactamase-producing organisms, extends spectrum of activity, prevents bacterial overgrowth.*

PHARMACOKINETICS

Protein binding: 16–30%. Widely distributed. Primarily excreted unchanged in urine. Removed by hemodialysis. Half-life: 0.7–1.2 hrs (half-life increased with impaired renal function, hepatic cirrhosis).

USES

Treatment of appendicitis (complicated by rupture or abscess), peritonitis, uncomplicated and complicated skin and skin structure infections including cellulitis, cutaneous abscesses, ischemic/diabetic foot infections, postpartum endometritis, pelvic inflammatory disease, community-acquired pneumonia (moderate severity only), moderate to severe nosocomial pneumonia.

PRECAUTIONS

CONTRAINDICATIONS: Hypersensitivity to any penicillin. **CAUTIONS:** History of allergies, esp. cephalosporins, other drugs.

▷*LIFESPAN CONSIDERATIONS:*
Pregnancy/Lactation: Readily crosses placenta; appears in cord blood, amniotic fluid. Distributed in breast milk in low concentra-

tions. May lead to allergic sensitization, diarrhea, candidiasis, skin rash in infant. **Pregnancy Category B. Children:** Dosage not established for those <12 yrs of age. **Elderly:** Age-related renal impairment may require dosage adjustment.

INTERACTIONS

DRUG: Probenecid may increase concentration, risk of toxicity. **Hepatotoxic** medications may increase hepatotoxicity. **HERBAL:** None known. **FOOD:** None known. **LAB VALUES:** May increase SGOT (AST), SGPT (ALT), alkaline phosphatase, bilirubin, LDH, sodium. May cause positive Coomb's' test. May decrease potassium.

AVAILABILITY (Rx)

POWDER FOR INJECTION: 2.25 g, 3.375 g, 4.5 g.

ADMINISTRATION/HANDLING

IV ▨
Storage:
• Reconstituted vial is stable for 24 hrs at room temperature or 48 hrs if refrigerated. • After further dilution, is stable for 24 hrs at room temperature or 7 days if refrigerated.

Reconstitution:
• Reconstitute each 1 g with 5 ml D_5W or 0.9% NaCl. Shake vigorously to dissolve. • Further dilute with at least 50 ml D_5W, 0.9% NaCl, D_5With 0.9% NaCl, or lactated Ringer's.

Rate of administration:
• Infuse over 30 min.

IV INCOMPATIBILITIES ⊘

Amphotericin (Fungizone), amphotericin B complex (Abelcet, Ambisome, Amphotec), chlorpro-

P

mazine (Thorazine), dacarbazine (DTIC), daunorubicin (Cerubidine), dobutamine (Dobutrex), doxorubicin (Adriamycin), doxorubicin liposome (Doxil), droperidol (Inapsine), famotidine (Pepcid), haloperidol (Haldol), hydroxyzine (Vistaril), idarubicin (Idamycin), minocycline (Minocin), nalbuphine (Nubain), prochlorpromazine (Compazine), promethazine (Phenergan), vancomycin (Vancocin).

IV COMPATIBILITIES

Bumetanide (Bumex), calcium gluconate, dopamine (Intropin), heparin, lorazepam (Ativan), magnesium, methylprednisolone (Solu-Medrol), potassium chloride.

INDICATIONS/ROUTES/DOSAGE
Usual parenteral dosage:
IV: **Adults, elderly:** 12 g/1.5 g/day as 3.375 g q6hrs.

Dosage in renal impairment:
Dose and/or frequency based on creatinine clearance.

Creatinine Clearance	Dosage
20–40 ml/min	8 g/1 g/day (2.25 g q6h)
<20 ml/min	6 g/0.75 g/day (2.25 g q8h)

Hemodialysis:
IV: **Adults, elderly:** 2.25 g q8h with additional dose of 0.75 g after each dialysis.

SIDE EFFECTS

FREQUENT: Diarrhea, headache, constipation, nausea, insomnia, rash. *OCCASIONAL:* Vomiting, dyspepsia, pruritus, fever, agitation, pain, moniliasis, dizziness, abdominal pain, edema, anxiety, dyspnea, rhinitis.

ADVERSE REACTIONS/TOXIC EFFECTS

Antibiotic-associated colitis (severe abdominal pain and tenderness, fever, watery and severe diarrhea) may result from altered bacterial balance. Overdosage, more often with renal impairment, may produce seizures, neurologic reactions. Severe hypersensitivity reactions, including anaphylaxis, occur rarely.

NURSING IMPLICATIONS

BASELINE ASSESSMENT:

Question for history of allergies, esp. penicillins, cephalosporins.

INTERVENTION/EVALUATION:

Monitor bowel activity and stool consistency carefully; mild GI effects may be tolerable, but increasing severity may indicate onset of antibiotic-associated colitis. Monitor I&O, renal function reports for nephrotoxicity. Be alert for superinfection: severe genital/anal pruritus, abdominal pain, severe mouth soreness, moderate to severe diarrhea. Monitor I&O, urinalysis, renal function tests. Monitor electrolytes, esp. potassium.

PATIENT/FAMILY TEACHING:

Notify physician in event of rash, diarrhea, bleeding, bruising, other new symptom.

piroxicam

purr-**ox**-i-kam
(Apo-Piroxicam✦, Feldene, Fexicam✦, Novopirocam✦)

▶CLASSIFICATION

PHARMACOTHERAPEUTIC:
Nonsteroidal anti-inflammatory.
CLINICAL: Anti-inflammatory,
analgesic (see p. 107C)

ACTION/*THERAPEUTIC EFFECT*

Produces analgesic and anti-inflammatory effect by inhibiting
prostaglandin synthesis, *reducing
inflammatory response and intensity of pain stimulus reaching sensory nerve endings.*

USES/*UNLABELED*

Symptomatic treatment of acute/
chronic rheumatoid arthritis, osteoarthritis. *Treatment of ankylosing spondylitis, acute gouty arthritis, dysmenorrhea.*

PRECAUTIONS

CONTRAINDICATIONS: Active
peptic ulcer, GI ulceration, chronic
inflammation of GI tract, GI bleeding disorders, history of hypersensitivity to aspirin/NSAIDs. *CAU-
TIONS:* Impaired renal/hepatic
function, history of GI tract disease,
predisposition to fluid retention.

INTERACTIONS

DRUG: May increase effects of
**oral anticoagulants, heparin,
thrombolytics.** May decrease effect of **antihypertensives, diuretics. Salicylates, aspirin** may increase risk of GI side effects,
bleeding. **Bone marrow depressants** may increase risk of hematologic reactions. May increase
concentration, toxicity of **lithium.**
May increase **methotrexate** toxicity. **Probenecid** may increase concentration. **HERBAL: St. John's
wort** may increase risk of phototoxicity. May decrease effect of
feverfew. Ginkgo biloba may increase risk of bleeding. **FOOD:**
None known. **LAB VALUES:** May
increase serum transaminase activity. May decrease uric acid.

AVAILABILITY (Rx)
CAPSULES: 10 mg, 20 mg.

ADMINISTRATION/HANDLING
PO:
• Do not crush or break capsule
form. • May give with food, milk,
or antacids if GI distress occurs.

INDICATIONS/ROUTES/DOSAGE
**Acute/chronic rheumatoid
arthritis, osteoarthritis:**
PO: Adults, elderly: Initially, 10–20
mg/day as single/divided doses.
Some pts may require up to 30–40
mg/day. **Children:** 0.2–0.3 mg/kg/
day. **Maximum:** 15 mg/day.

SIDE EFFECTS
FREQUENT (3–9%): Dyspepsia,
nausea, dizziness. *OCCASIONAL*
(1–3%): Diarrhea, constipation,
abdominal cramping/pain, flatulence, stomatitis. *RARE* (<1%): Increased B/P, hives, painful/difficult
urination, ecchymosis, blurred vision, insomnia.

ADVERSE REACTIONS/TOXIC
EFFECTS
Peptic ulcer, GI bleeding, gastritis,
severe hepatic reaction (cholestasis, jaundice) occur rarely. Nephrotoxicity (dysuria, hematuria, proteinuria, nephrotic syndrome),
severe hypersensitivity reaction
(fever, chills, bronchospasm), hematologic toxicity (anemia, leukopenia, eosinophilia, thrombocytopenia) may occur rarely with
long-term treatment.

P

NURSING IMPLICATIONS

BASELINE ASSESSMENT:

Assess onset, type, location, duration of pain/inflammation. Inspect appearance of affected joints for immobility, deformities, and skin condition.

INTERVENTION/EVALUATION:

Monitor pattern of daily bowel activity, stool consistency. Monitor for evidence of nausea, GI distress. Evaluate for therapeutic response (relief of pain, stiffness, swelling, increase in joint mobility, reduced joint tenderness, improved grip strength).

PATIENT/FAMILY TEACHING:

Avoid aspirin, alcohol during therapy (increases risk of GI bleeding). If GI upset occurs, take with food, milk, or antacids. Avoid tasks that require alertness until response to drug is established.

plicamycin

ply-kah-**my**-sin
(Mithracin)
Do not confuse with Minocin.

▶CLASSIFICATION

PHARMACOTHERAPEUTIC:
Antibiotic. **CLINICAL:** Antineoplastic, antihypercalcemic (see p. 73C)

ACTION/*THERAPEUTIC EFFECT*

Protein binding: None. Forms complexes with DNA, inhibiting DNA-directed RNA synthesis. *Lowers serum calcium concentration. Blocks hypercalcemic action* of vitamin D and blocks action of parathyroid hormone. Decreases serum phosphate levels.

PHARMACOKINETICS

Protein binding: None. Localized in liver, kidney, formed bone surfaces. Crosses blood-brain barrier, enters CSF. Primarily excreted in urine.

USES/*UNLABELED*

Treatment of malignant testicular tumors, hypercalcemia, hypercalcuria associated with advanced neoplasms. *Treatment of Paget's disease refractory to other therapy.*

PRECAUTIONS

CONTRAINDICATIONS: Existing thrombocytopenia, thrombocytopathy, coagulation disorders, tendency to hemorrhage, impaired bone marrow function. **EXTREME CAUTION:** Renal/hepatic impairment. **CAUTIONS:** Electrolyte imbalance.

▷**LIFESPAN CONSIDERATIONS:**
Pregnancy/Lactation: Contraindicated during pregnancy. Breast feeding not recommended. **Pregnancy Category X. Children/Elderly:** No information available.

INTERACTIONS

DRUG: May increase effect of **oral anticoagulants, heparin, thrombolytics.** May increase risk of hemorrhage with **NSAIDs, aspirin, dipyridamole, sulfinpyrazone, valproic acid. Bone marrow depressants, hepatotoxic, nephrotoxic medications** may increase toxicity. **Calcium-containing medications, vitamin D** may decrease effect. **Live virus vaccines** may potentiate virus replication, increase vaccine side effects, decrease pt's antibody response to vaccine. **HERBAL:** None known. ***FOOD:*** None known. ***LAB VALUES:*** None significant.

AVAILABILITY (Rx)

POWDER FOR INJECTION: 2,500 mcg.

ADMINISTRATION/HANDLING

IV

Note: May be carcinogenic, mutagenic, or teratogenic. Handle with extreme care during preparation/administration.

Storage:

• Refrigerate vials. • Solution must be freshly prepared before use; discard unused portions.

Reconstitution:

• Reconstitute 2,500 mcg (2.5 mg) vial with 4.9 ml Sterile Water for Injection to provide concentration of 500 mcg/ml (0.5 mg/ml). • Dilute with 500–1,000 ml D_5W or 0.9% NaCl.

Rate of administration:

• Infuse over 4–6 hrs. • Extravasation produces painful inflammation, induration. Sloughing may occur. Aspirate as much drug as possible. Apply warm compresses.

IV INCOMPATIBILITY ⊘

Cefepime (Maxipime).

IV COMPATIBILITY

Granisetron (Kytril).

INDICATIONS/ROUTES/DOSAGE

Note: Dosage individualized based on clinical response, tolerance to adverse effects. Dose based on actual body weight. Use ideal body weight for obese or edematous pts. Do not exceed 30 mcg/kg/day or more than 10 daily doses (increases potential for hemorrhage).

Testicular tumors:

IV: Adults, elderly: 25–30 mcg/kg/day for 8–10 days. Repeat at monthly intervals.

Hypercalcemia/hyperuricemia:

IV: Adults, elderly: 15–25 mcg/kg/day for 3–4 days. Repeat at weekly or longer intervals until desired response achieved. Reduce dose to 12.5 mcg/kg in pts with renal or hepatic impairment.

Paget's disease:

IV: Adults, elderly: 15 mcg/kg/day for 10 days.

SIDE EFFECTS

FREQUENT: Nausea, vomiting, anorexia, diarrhea, stomatitis. ***OCCASIONAL:*** Fever, drowsiness, weakness, lethargy, malaise, headache, mental depression, nervousness, dizziness, rash, acne.

ADVERSE REACTIONS/TOXIC EFFECTS

Hematologic toxicity noted by marked facial flushing, persistent nosebleeds, hemoptysis, purpura, ecchymoses, leukopenia, thrombocytopenia. Risk of bleeding tendencies increases with higher doses and/or when more than 10 doses are given. May produce electrolyte imbalance.

P

NURSING IMPLICATIONS

BASELINE ASSESSMENT:

Question for possibility of pregnancy before initiating therapy (Pregnancy Category X). Antiemetics may be effective in preventing, treating nausea. Discontinue therapy if platelet count falls below 150,000/mm³, if WBC falls below 4,000/mm³, or if prothrombin time is 4 sec higher than control test. Renal/hepatic studies should be performed daily in those with impairment.

INTERVENTION/EVALUATION:

Monitor hematologic, renal, hepatic function studies; platelet count; prothrombin, bleeding times; serum calcium, phosphorus, potassium levels. Assess pattern of daily bowel activity, stool consistency. Monitor for stomatitis (burning/erythema of oral mucosa at inner margin of lips, sore throat, difficulty swallowing, oral ulceration). Monitor for thrombocytopenia (bleeding from gums, tarry stool, petechiae, small SubQ hemorrhages). Avoid IM injections, rectal temperatures, any trauma that may induce bleeding.

PATIENT/FAMILY TEACHING:

Maintain fastidious oral hygiene. Do not have immunizations without physician's approval (drug lowers body's resistance). Avoid crowds, those with infection. Promptly report fever, sore throat, signs of local infection, easy bruising, unusual bleeding from any site. Contact physician if nausea/vomiting continues at home. Use nonhormonal contraception.

polycarbophil

polly-**car**-bow-fill
(Fibercon, Mitrolan, Replens ✦)

▶CLASSIFICATION

CLINICAL: Bulk-forming laxative, antidiarrheal (see p. 100C)

ACTION/THERAPEUTIC EFFECT

Laxative: Retains water in intestine, opposes dehydrating forces of the bowel (promotes well-formed stools). **Antidiarrheal:** Absorbs free fecal water (forms gel, producing formed stool). *Restores normal moisture level, provides bulk.*

PHARMACOKINETICS

	Onset	Peak	Duration
PO	12–72 hrs	—	—

Acts in small/large intestine.

USES

Treatment of diarrhea associated with irritable bowel syndrome, diverticulosis, acute nonspecific diarrhea. Relieves constipation associated with irritable or spastic bowel.

PRECAUTIONS

CONTRAINDICATIONS: Abdominal pain, nausea, vomiting, symptoms of appendicitis, partial bowel obstruction, dysphagia. **CAUTIONS:** None significant.

▷**LIFESPAN CONSIDERATIONS:**
Pregnancy/Lactation: Safe for use in pregnancy. **Pregnancy Category C. Children:** Not recommended in those <6 yrs of age. **Elderly:** No age-related precautions noted.

INTERACTIONS

DRUG: May interfere with effects of **potassium-sparing diuretics, potassium supplements.** May decrease effect of **oral anticoagulants, digoxin, salicylates, tetracyclines** by decreasing absorption. **HERBAL:** None known. **FOOD:** None known. **LAB VALUES:** May increase glucose. May decrease potassium.

AVAILABILITY (OTC)

TABLETS: 500 mg, 1,000 mg. ***TABLETS (chewable):*** 500 mg.

INDICATIONS/ROUTES/DOSAGE

Note: For severe diarrhea, give every half hour up to maximum daily dosage; for laxative, give with 8 oz liquid.

Laxative, antidiarrheal:

PO: Adults, elderly, children >12 yrs: 1 g 1–4 times/day, or as needed. **Maximum:** 4 g/24 hrs. **Children 6–12 yrs:** 500 mg 1–4 times/day, or as needed. **Maximum:** 2 g/24 hrs. **Children <6 yrs:** Consult product labeling.

SIDE EFFECTS

RARE: Some degree of abdominal discomfort, nausea, mild cramps, griping, faintness.

ADVERSE REACTIONS/TOXIC EFFECTS

Esophageal/bowel obstruction may occur if administered with insufficient liquid (less than 250 ml or 1 full glass).

NURSING IMPLICATIONS

INTERVENTION/EVALUATION:
Encourage adequate fluid intake. Assess bowel sounds for peristalsis. Monitor daily bowel activity, stool consistency (watery, loose, soft, semisolid, solid) and record time of evacuation. Monitor serum electrolytes in those exposed to prolonged, frequent, or excessive use of medication.

PATIENT/FAMILY TEACHING:
Institute measures to promote defecation (increase fluid intake, exercise, high-fiber diet). Drink 6–8 glasses of water/day when used as laxative (aids stool softening).

---

polyethylene glycol-electrolyte solution (PEG-ES)

poly-**eth**-ah-leen
(CoLyte, GoLYTELY, Klean-Prep ♣, MiraLax, NuLytely, OCL, Peglyte ♣, Pro-Lax ♣)

▶CLASSIFICATION

PHARMACOTHERAPEUTIC:
Laxative. ***CLINICAL:*** Bowel evacuant (see p. 101C)

ACTION/*THERAPEUTIC EFFECT*

Osmotic effect. *Induces diarrhea, cleanses bowel* (electrolytes in solution prevent water/electrolyte imbalance).

PHARMACOKINETICS

	Onset	Peak	Duration
PO	30–60 min	—	Completed: 4 hrs

USES

Bowel cleansing before GI examination and colon surgery. ***MiraLax:*** Treatment of occasional constipation.

PRECAUTIONS

CONTRAINDICATIONS: GI obstruction, gastric retention, bowel perforation, toxic colitis, toxic megacolon, ileus. ***CAUTIONS:*** Ulcerative colitis.

▷*LIFESPAN CONSIDERATIONS:*
Pregnancy/Lactation: Unknown whether drug crosses placenta or is distributed in breast milk. **Pregnancy Category C. Children/Elderly:** No age-related precautions noted.

INTERACTIONS

DRUG: May decrease absorption of **oral medications** if given within 1 hr (may be flushed from GI tract). **HERBAL:** None known. **FOOD:** None known. **LAB VALUES:** None significant.

AVAILABILITY (Rx)

POWDER FOR ORAL SOLUTION. ORAL SOLUTION.

ADMINISTRATION/HANDLING

PO:

• Refrigerate reconstituted solutions; use within 48 hrs. • May use tap water to prepare solution. Shake vigorously several mins to ensure complete dissolution of powder. • Fasting should occur at least 3 hrs before ingestion of solution (solid food should always be avoided <2 hrs before administration). • Only clear liquids permitted after administration. • May give via NG tube. • Rapid drinking preferred.

INDICATIONS/ROUTES/DOSAGE

Bowel evacuant:

PO: Adults, elderly: 4 L prior to GI examination: 240 ml (8 oz) q10min until 4 L consumed or rectal effluent clear. NG tube: 20–30 ml/min until 4 L given. **Children:** 25–40 ml/kg/hr until rectal effluent clear.

Constipation:

PO: Adults (MiraLax): 17 g (or 1 heaping tbs) daily.

SIDE EFFECTS

FREQUENT (50%): Some degree of abdominal fullness, nausea, bloating. **OCCASIONAL** (1–10%): Abdominal cramping, vomiting, anal irritation. **RARE** (<1%): Urticaria, rhinorrhea, dermatitis.

ADVERSE REACTIONS/TOXIC EFFECTS

None significant.

NURSING IMPLICATIONS

BASELINE ASSESSMENT:

Do not give oral medication within 1 hr of start of therapy (may not adequately be absorbed before GI cleansing).

INTERVENTION/EVALUATION:

Assess bowel sounds for peristalsis. Monitor bowel activity, stool consistency (watery, loose, soft, semisolid, solid) and record time of evacuation. Assess for abdominal disturbances.

polymyxin B sulfate

polly-**mix**-in
(Aerosporin)

FIXED-COMBINATION(S)

Ophthalmic: With bacitracin, an anti-infective **(AK-Poly-Bac, Ocumycin, Polysporin Ophthalmic);** with neomycin, an aminoglycoside **(Statrol);** with neomycin and bacitracin, anti-infectives **(AK-Spore, Neosporin, Ocutricin);** with neomycin and bacitracin, anti-infectives, and hydrocortisone, a corticosteroid **(Coracin);** with dexamethasone, a corticosteroid, and neomycin, an aminoglycoside **(AK-Trol, Dexacidin, Dex-Ide, Maxitrol);** with chloramphenicol, an antibiotic **(Ophthocort).** *Misc:* With neomycin, an aminoglycoside **(Neosporin GU irrigant)**

►CLASSIFICATION

PHARMACOTHERAPEUTIC: Polypeptide. **CLINICAL:** Antibiotic

ACTION/*THERAPEUTIC EFFECT*

Alters cell membrane permeability in susceptible microorganisms, *producing bactericidal activity.*

USES

Topically for wound irrigation and bladder irrigation.

PRECAUTIONS

CONTRAINDICATIONS: None significant. ***CAUTIONS:*** Renal impairment, neuromuscular disorders.

INTERACTIONS

DRUG: May produce muscle paralysis, prolonged or increased skeletal muscle relaxation with **neuromuscular blocking agents** or **anesthetics. Aminoglycosides, other nephrotoxic drugs** may increase nephrotoxicity. ***HERBAL:*** None known. ***FOOD:*** None known. ***LAB VALUES:*** None significant.

AVAILABILITY (Rx)

INJECTION. OPHTHALMIC POWDER FOR SOLUTION.

INDICATIONS/ROUTES/DOSAGE

Usual irrigation dosage:
CONTINUOUS BLADDER IRRIGATION: **Adults, elderly:** 1 ml urogenital concentrate (contains 200,000 units polymyxin B, 57 mg neomycin) added to 1,000 ml 0.9% NaCl. Give each 1,000 ml >24 hrs for up to 10 days (may increase to 2,000 ml/day when urine output >2 L/day).

Usual ophthalmic dosage:
OPHTHALMIC: **Adults, elderly, children:** 1 drop q3–4h.

SIDE EFFECTS

OCCASIONAL: Fever, urticaria.

ADVERSE REACTIONS/TOXIC EFFECTS

Nephrotoxicity, esp. with concurrent/sequential use of other nephrotoxic drugs, renal impairment, concurrent/sequential use of muscle relaxants. Superinfection, esp. with fungi, may occur.

NURSING IMPLICATIONS

BASELINE ASSESSMENT:
Assess for hypersensitivity to polymyxin.

INTERVENTION/EVALUATION:
Monitor for fever, urticaria.

PATIENT/FAMILY TEACHING:
With ophthalmic therapy, report any increased irritation, inflammation, itching, burning.

poractant alfa

pour-**act**-tant
(Curosurf, Curosurg✤)

▶CLASSIFICATION

CLINICAL: Pulmonary surfactant

P

ACTION/*THERAPEUTIC EFFECT*

Reduces surface tension of alveoli during ventilation; stabilizes alveoli against collapse that may occur at resting transpulmonary pressures. *Replenishes surfactant, restores surface activity to lungs.*

USES

Treatment (rescue) of respiratory distress syndrome (RDS—hyaline membrane disease) in premature infants. *Prophylaxis for RDS; adult*

✤ - Canadian trade name   ✳ - see also www.wbsaunders.com/SIMON/SaundersNDH

RDS due to viral pneumonia, HIV-infected infants with Pneumocystis carinii pneumonia, treatment in adult RDS following near drowning.

PRECAUTIONS

CONTRAINDICATIONS: None significant. ***CAUTIONS:*** Those at risk for circulatory overload.
▷***LIFESPAN CONSIDERATIONS:***
Neonate: No age-related precautions noted for neonate.

INTERACTIONS

DRUG: None significant. ***HERBAL:*** None known. ***FOOD:*** None known. ***LAB VALUES:*** None significant.

AVAILABILITY (Rx)

INTRATRACHEAL SUSPENSION: 1.5 ml (120 mg), 3 ml (240 mg).

ADMINISTRATION/HANDLING

Intratracheal:

Storage:

• Refrigerate vials. • Warm by standing vial at room temperature for 20 min or warm in hand 8 min. • To obtain uniform suspension, turn upside down gently, swirl vial (do not shake). • After warming, may return to refrigerator one time only. • Withdraw entire contents of vial into a 3 or 5 ml plastic syringe through large-gauge needle (≥20 gauge).

Administration:

• Attach syringe to catheter and instill through catheter inserted into infant's endotracheal tube. Monitor for bradycardia, decreased O_2 saturation during administration. Stop dosing procedure if these effects occur; begin appropriate measures before re-instituting therapy.

INDICATIONS/ROUTES/DOSAGE

RDS:

ENDOTRACHEAL: **Infants:** Initially, 2.5 ml/kg birth weight (BW). Up to 2 subsequent doses of 1.25 ml/kg BW at 12 hr intervals. **Maximum:** 5 ml/kg.

SIDE EFFECTS

FREQUENT: Transient bradycardia, O_2 desaturation; increased CO_2 tension. ***OCCASIONAL:*** Endotracheal tube reflux. ***RARE:*** Apnea, endotracheal tube blockage, hypo/hypertension, pallor, vasoconstriction.

ADVERSE REACTIONS/TOXIC EFFECTS

Pneumonia (17%), septicemia (14%), bronchopulmonary dysplasia (18%), intracranial hemorrhage (51%), patent ductus arteriosus (60%), pneumothorax (21%), pulmonary interstitial emphysema (21%) may occur.

NURSING IMPLICATIONS

BASELINE ASSESSMENT:

Immediately before administration, change ventilator setting to 40–60 breaths/min, inspiratory time 0.5 sec, and supplemental O_2 sufficient to maintain SaO_2 >92%. Drug must be administered in highly supervised setting. Clinicians in care of neonate must be experienced with intubation, ventilator management. Offer emotional support to parents.

INTERVENTION/EVALUATION:

Monitor infant with arterial or transcutaneous measurement of systemic O_2 and CO_2. Assess lung sounds for rales and moist breath sounds.

porfimer

(Photofrin)

See Classification section under: Antineoplastics

potassium acetate

(Potassium acetate)

potassium bicarbonate/citrate

(K-Lyte)

potassium chloride 🔗

(Apo-K♣, Kaochlor, <u>K-Dur</u>, K-Lor, Klotrix, K-Lyte-Cl, Micro-K, Slow-K)

potassium gluconate

(Kaon)

potassium phosphate

(Potassium phosphate)
Do not confuse with Cardura, Slow-FE.

▶CLASSIFICATION

PHARMACOTHERAPEUTIC: Electrolyte. **CLINICAL:** Potassium replenisher

ACTION/*THERAPEUTIC EFFECT*
Necessary for multiple cellular metabolic processes. Primary action intracellular. Necessary *for nerve impulse conduction, contraction of cardiac, skeletal, smooth muscle; maintains normal renal function, acid-base balance.*

PHARMACOKINETICS
Well absorbed from GI tract. Enters cells via active transport from extracellular fluid. Primarily excreted in urine.

USES
Treatment of potassium deficiency found in severe vomiting, diarrhea, loss of GI fluid, malnutrition, prolonged diuresis, debilitated, poor GI absorption, metabolic alkalosis, prolonged parenteral alimentation; prevents hypokalemia in risk pts.

PRECAUTIONS
CONTRAINDICATIONS: Severe renal impairment, untreated Addison's disease, postop oliguria, shock with hemolytic reaction and/or dehydration, hyperkalemia, those receiving potassium-sparing diuretics, digitalis toxicity, heat cramps, severe burns. **CAUTIONS:** Cardiac disease, tartrazine sensitivity (mostly noted in those with aspirin hypersensitivity).

▷**LIFESPAN CONSIDERATIONS:**
Pregnancy/Lactation: Unknown if drug crosses placenta or is distributed in breast milk. **Pregnancy Category A. Children:** No age-related precautions noted. **Elderly:** May be at increased risk for hyperkalemia. Age-related ability to excrete potassium is reduced.

INTERACTIONS
DRUG: Angiotensin-converting enzyme (ACE) inhibitors, NSAIDs, beta-adrenergic blockers, potassium-sparing diuretics, heparin, potassium-containing medications, salt substitutes may increase potassium concentration. **Anticholinergics** may increase risk of GI lesions. **HERBAL:** None

P

known. **FOOD:** None known. **LAB VALUES:** None significant.

AVAILABILITY (Rx)

Acetate: INJECTION: 2 mEq/ml.

Bicarbonate/Citrate: EFFERVESCENT TABLETS: 25 mEq, 50 mEq

Chloride: TABLETS: 6.7 mEq, 8 mEq, 10 mEq, 20 mEq. **LIQUID:** 20 mEq/15 ml, 30 mEq/15 ml, 40 mEq/15 ml. **ORAL POWDER:** 20 mEq, 25 mEq. **INJECTION:** 2 mEq/ml.

Gluconate: LIQUID: 20 mEq/15 ml.

Phosphate: INJECTION: 3 mM/ml (mM = millimoles).

ADMINISTRATION/HANDLING

PO:

• Take with or after meals and with full glass of water (decreases GI upset). • Liquids, powder, or effervescent tablets: Mix, dissolve with juice, water before administering. • Do not chew, crush tablets; swallow whole.

IV [IV]

Storage:

• Store at room temperature.

Reconstitution:

• For IV infusion only, must dilute before administration, mixed well, infused slowly. • Avoid adding potassium to hanging IV.

Rate of administration:

• Give at rate no more than 40 mEq/L; no faster than 20 mEq/hr. (Higher concentrations/faster rates may sometimes be necessary.) • Check IV site closely during infusion for evidence of phlebitis (heat, pain, red streaking of skin over vein, hardness to vein), extravasation (swelling, pain, cool skin, little or no blood return).

IV INCOMPATIBILITIES ⊘

Amphotericin B complex (Abelcet, Ambisome, Amphotec), methylprednisolone (Solu-Medrol), phenytoin (Dilantin).

IV COMPATIBILITIES

POTASSIUM CHLORIDE

Amiodarone (Cordarone), aztreonam (Azactam), calcium gluconate, ciprofloxacin (Cipro), digoxin (Lanoxin), diltiazem (Cardizem), dobutamine (Dobutrex), dopamine (Intropin), heparin, insulin, lidocaine, lorazepam (Ativan), magnesium, midazolam (Versed), piperacillin/tazobactam (Zosyn), propofol (Diprivan).

POTASSIUM PHOSPHATE

Magnesium, diltiazem (Cardizem).

INDICATIONS/ROUTES/DOSAGE

Treatment/prevention of hypokalemia:

Note: Dosage is individualized.

PO: Adults, elderly: Prevention: 20 mEq/day. **Treatment:** 40–100 mEq/day. **Children:** No more than 3 mEq/kg/day. **Infants:** 2–6 mEq/kg/day. Give in 2–4 divided doses.

IV: Adults, elderly, children: Individualize based on EKG, serum potassium concentrations.

SIDE EFFECTS

OCCASIONAL: Nausea, vomiting, diarrhea, flatulence, abdominal discomfort with distention, phlebitis with IV administration (particularly when potassium concentration of >40 mEq/L is infused). **RARE:** Rash.

ADVERSE REACTIONS/TOXIC EFFECTS

Hyperkalemia (observed particularly in elderly or in those with impaired renal function) manifested as paresthesia of extremities, heaviness of legs, cold skin, grayish pallor, hypotension, mental confusion, irritability, flaccid paralysis, cardiac arrhythmias.

NURSING IMPLICATIONS

BASELINE ASSESSMENT:
Oral dose should be given with food or after meals with full glass of water or fruit juice (minimizes GI irritation).

INTERVENTION/EVALUATION:
Monitor serum potassium level (particularly in renal function impairment). If GI disturbance is noted, dilute preparation further or give with meals. Be alert to decrease in urinary output (may be indication of renal insufficiency). Monitor daily bowel activity, stool consistency. Assess I&O diligently during diuresis, IV site for extravasation, phlebitis. Be alert to evidence of hyperkalemia (skin pallor/coldness, complaints of paresthesia of extremities, feeling of heaviness of legs).

PATIENT/FAMILY TEACHING:
Foods rich in potassium include beef, veal, ham, chicken, turkey, fish, milk, bananas, dates, prunes, raisins, avocados, watermelon, cantaloupe, apricots, molasses, beans, yams, broccoli, brussel sprouts, lentils, potatoes, spinach. Report paresthesia of extremities, feeling of heaviness of legs.

pramipexole

pram-ih-**pecks**-all
(Mirapex)
Do not confuse with Mifeprex, MiraLax.

▶CLASSIFICATION

PHARMACOTHERAPEUTIC: Dopamine receptor agonist. ***CLINICAL:*** Antiparkinson agent

ACTION/*THERAPEUTIC EFFECT*
Stimulates dopamine receptors in the striatum, *relieving signs/symptoms of Parkinson's disease.*

PHARMACOKINETICS
Rapid, extensive absorption following PO administration. Protein binding: 15%. Widely distributed. Steady-state concentrations achieved within 2 days. Primarily eliminated in urine. Not removed by hemodialysis. Half-life: 8 hrs (12 hrs in those >65 yrs).

USES
Treatment of signs and symptoms of idiopathic Parkinson's disease.

PRECAUTIONS
CONTRAINDICATIONS: History of hypersensitivity to medication. ***CAUTIONS:*** History of orthostatic hypotension, syncope, hallucinations, renal function impairment, use of concomitant CNS depressants.
▷***LIFESPAN CONSIDERATIONS:*** **Pregnancy/Lactation:** Unknown if distributed in breast milk. **Pregnancy Category C. Children:** Safety and efficacy not established. **Elderly:** Increased risk of hallucinations.

INTERACTIONS
***DRUG:* Cimetidine** increases pramipexole's plasma concentration and increases its half-life. Combined use of **cimetidine, ranitidine, diltiatem, triamterene, verapamil, quinidine, quinine** may decrease pramipexole clearance. May increase plasma levels of **carbidopa** or **levodopa**

combinations. ***HERBAL:*** None known. ***FOOD:*** Time to maximum plasma levels is increased by 1 hr when taken with food (extent of absorption not affected). ***LAB VALUES:*** None significant.

AVAILABILITY (Rx)

TABLETS: 0.125 mg, 0.25 mg, 1 mg, 1.5 mg.

ADMINISTRATION/HANDLING
PO:

• Give without regard to food.

INDICATIONS/ROUTES/DOSAGE
Parkinson's disease:

PO: Adults, elderly: Initially, 0.375 mg/day in 3 divided doses. Do not increase dose more frequently than q5–7days. **Maintenance:** 1.5–4.5 mg/day in equally divided doses 3 times/day.

Renal function impairment:

PO: Adults, elderly, creatinine clearance >60 ml/min: Initially, 0.125 mg 3 times/day. **Maximum:** 1.5 mg 3 times/day. **Creatinine clearance 35–59 ml/min:** Initially, 0.125 mg 2 times/day. **Maximum:** 1.5 mg twice daily. **Creatinine clearance 15–34 ml/min:** Initially, 0.125 mg 1 time/day. **Maximum:** 1.5 mg once daily.

SIDE EFFECTS
Early Parkinson's disease:

FREQUENT (10–28%): Nausea, asthenia (weakness), dizziness, somnolence, insomnia, constipation. ***OCCASIONAL*** (2–5%): Edema, malaise, confusion, amnesia, akathisia (restlessness), anorexia, dysphagia, peripheral edema, altered vision, impotence.

Advanced Parkinson's disease:

FREQUENT (17–53%): Postural hypotension, dyskinesia, ex-trapyramidal signs, insomnia, dizziness, hallucinations. ***OCCASIONAL*** (7–10%): Asthenia, somnolence, confusion, constipation, gait abnormality, dry mouth. ***RARE*** (2–6%): General edema, malaise, chest pain, amnesia, tremors, urinary frequency/incontinence, dyspnea, rhinitis, vision changes.

ADVERSE REACTIONS/TOXIC EFFECTS

None significant.

NURSING IMPLICATIONS

INTERVENTION/EVALUATION:

Instruct pt to rise from lying to sitting or sitting to standing position slowly to prevent risk of postural hypotension. Assess for clinical improvement. Assist with ambulation if dizziness occurs. Assess for constipation; encourage fiber, fluids, and exercise.

PATIENT/FAMILY TEACHING:

Inform pt that hallucination may occur, more so in the elderly than in younger pts with Parkinson's disease. Postural hypotension may occur more frequently during initial therapy. Avoid tasks that require alertness, motor skills until response to drug is established. If nausea occurs, take medication with food. Avoid abrupt withdrawal.

pravastatin 🖉

pra-vah-sta-tin
(<u>Pravachol</u>)
Do not confuse with Prevacid, propranolol.

►CLASSIFICATION

PHARMACOTHERAPEUTIC:
HMG-CoA reductase inhibitor.
CLINICAL: Antihyperlipidemic
(see p. 50C)

ACTION/*THERAPEUTIC EFFECT*

Interferes with cholesterol biosynthesis by preventing the conversion of HMG-CoA reductase to mevalonate, a precursor to cholesterol. *Lowers LDL cholesterol, VLDL, plasma triglycerides; increases HDL concentration.*

PHARMACOKINETICS

Poorly absorbed from GI tract. Protein binding: 50%. Metabolized in liver (minimal active metabolites). Primarily excreted in feces via biliary system. Not removed by hemodialysis. Half-life: 2.7 hrs.

USES

Treatment of hypercholesterolemia by reducing total and LDL cholesterol, apo B, triglycerides, increasing HDL cholesterol. Preventive therapy to reduce risks of the following in pts with previous myocardial infarction (MI) and normal cholesterol levels: recurrent MI, undergoing myocardial revascularization procedures; stroke or transient ischemic attack. Prevents CV events in pts with elevated cholesterol levels.

PRECAUTIONS

CONTRAINDICATIONS: Active liver disease or unexplained, persistent elevations of liver function tests. Safety and efficacy in individuals <18 yrs of age has not been established. ***CAUTIONS:*** History of liver disease, substantial alcohol consumption. Withholding/discontinuing pravastatin

may be necessary when pt at risk for renal failure secondary to rhabdomyolysis. Severe metabolic, endocrine, or electrolyte disorders.

▷*LIFESPAN CONSIDERATIONS:*
Pregnancy/Lactation: Contraindicated in pregnancy (suppression of cholesterol biosynthesis may cause fetal toxicity) and lactation. Unknown if drug is distributed in breast milk, but there is risk of serious adverse reactions in nursing infants. **Pregnancy Category X. Children:** Safety and efficacy not established. **Elderly:** No age-related precautions noted.

INTERACTIONS

DRUG: Increased risk of rhabdomyolysis, acute renal failure with **cyclosporine, erythromycin, gemfibrozil, niacin, other immunosuppressants.** ***HERBAL:*** None known. ***FOOD:*** None known. ***LAB VALUES:*** May increase creatinine kinase, serum transaminase concentrations.

AVAILABILITY (Rx)

TABLETS: 10 mg, 20 mg, 40 mg.

ADMINISTRATION/HANDLING

PO:
• Give without regard to meals. • Administer in evening.

INDICATIONS/ROUTES/DOSAGE

Note: Before initiating therapy, pt should be on standard cholesterol-lowering diet for minimum of 3–6 mos. Continue diet throughout pravastatin therapy.

Usual dosage:

PO: Adults: Initially, 10–20 mg/day at bedtime. **Elderly:** Initially, 10 mg/day at bedtime. **Range:** 10–40 mg/day at bedtime.

SIDE EFFECTS

Generally well tolerated. Side effects usually mild and transient. **OCCASIONAL** (4–7%): Nausea, vomiting, diarrhea, constipation, abdominal pain, headache, rhinitis, rash, pruritus. **RARE** (2–3%): Heartburn, myalgia, dizziness, cough, fatigue, flulike symptoms.

ADVERSE REACTIONS/TOXIC EFFECTS

Potential for malignancy, cataracts. Hypersensitivity occurs rarely.

NURSING IMPLICATIONS

BASELINE ASSESSMENT:

Question for possibility of pregnancy before initiating therapy (Pregnancy Category X). Assess baseline lab results: cholesterol, triglycerides, liver function tests.

INTERVENTION/EVALUATION:

Monitor cholesterol and triglyceride lab results for therapeutic response. Monitor liver function tests. Determine pattern of bowel activity. Check for headache, dizziness (provide assistance as needed). Assess for rash, pruritus. Be alert for malaise, muscle cramping/weakness; if accompanied by fever, may require discontinuation of medication.

PATIENT/FAMILY TEACHING:

Follow special diet (important part of treatment). Periodic lab tests are essential part of therapy. Report promptly any muscle pain/weakness, esp. if accompanied by fever or malaise. Do not drive/perform activities that require alert response if dizziness occurs. Use nonhormonal contraception.

praziquantel

pray-zih-**kwon**-tel
(Biltricide)

▶CLASSIFICATION

PHARMACOTHERAPEUTIC:
Isoquinolone derivative. **CLINICAL:** Anthelmintic

ACTION/THERAPEUTIC EFFECT

Vermicidal. Increases cell permeability in susceptible helminths resulting in loss of intracellular calcium, massive contractions and paralysis of their musculature, followed by attachment of phagocytes to the parasites, *dislodging the dead and dying worms.*

USES

Treatment of all stages of schistosomiasis (bilharziasis or fluke infections), infections due to liver flukes, clonorchiasis and opisthorchiasis.

PRECAUTIONS

CONTRAINDICATIONS: Ocular cysticercosis. **CAUTIONS:** None significant.

INTERACTIONS

DRUG: None significant. **HERBAL:** None known. **FOOD:** None known. **LAB VALUES:** None significant.

AVAILABILITY (Rx)

TABLETS (tri-scored): 600 mg.

INDICATIONS/ROUTES/DOSAGE

Schistosomiasis:

PO: Adults, elderly, children: 20 mg/kg/dose 2–3 times/day for 1 day at 4–6 hr intervals.

Flukes:

PO: Adults, elderly, children: 25 mg/kg/dose q8h for 1–2 days.

Clonorchiasis/opisthorchiasis:

PO: Adults, elderly: 3 doses of 25 mg/kg as 1 day treatment.

SIDE EFFECTS

FREQUENT: Headache, dizziness, malaise, abdominal pain occur in 90% of pts. **OCCASIONAL:** Anorexia, vomiting, diarrhea. Severe cramping abdominal pain may occur within 1 hr of administration with fever, sweating, bloody stools. **RARE:** Giddiness, urticaria.

ADVERSE REACTIONS/TOXIC EFFECTS

Overdose should be treated with fast-acting laxative.

NURSING IMPLICATIONS

BASELINE ASSESSMENT:

Obtain stool, urine specimens to confirm diagnosis.

INTERVENTION/EVALUATION:

Collect stool, urine specimens as required to monitor effectiveness of therapy. Monitor CNS reactions, provide safety measures for ambulation. Check hematology results for anemia. Assess for urticaria.

PATIENT/FAMILY TEACHING:

Complete full course of therapy. If iron supplements are ordered, continue as directed (may be up to 6 mos post therapy). Notify physician if symptoms do not improve in a few days, or if they become worse. Follow-up office visits (several mos after therapy is complete) are essential to assure cure.

prazosin hydrochloride ✳

pray-zoe-sin
(Minipress)
FIXED-COMBINATION(S)
With polythiazide, a diuretic **(Minizide)**

▶CLASSIFICATION

PHARMACOTHERAPEUTIC: Alpha-adrenergic blocker. **CLINICAL:** Antihypertensive, antidote, vasodilator (see p. 52C)

ACTION/THERAPEUTIC EFFECT

Selectively blocks alpha$_1$ adrenergic receptors, decreasing peripheral vascular resistance. Resulting peripheral vasodilation lowers B/P, relaxes smooth muscle of bladder/prostate.

USES/UNLABELED

Treatment of mild to moderate hypertension. Used alone or in combination with other antihypertensives. Treatment of CHF, ergot alkaloid toxicity, pheochromocytoma, Raynaud's phenomena, benign prostate hypertrophy.

PRECAUTIONS

CONTRAINDICATIONS: None significant. **CAUTIONS:** Chronic renal failure, impaired hepatic function.

INTERACTIONS

DRUG: Estrogen, NSAIDs, sympathomimetics may decrease effect. **Hypotension-producing medications** may increase antihypertensive effect. **HERBAL:** None known. **FOOD:** None known. **LAB VALUES:** None significant.

P

AVAILABILITY (Rx)

CAPSULES: 1 mg, 2 mg, 5 mg.

ADMINISTRATION/HANDLING

PO:

• Give without regard to food. • Administer first dose at bedtime (minimizes risk of fainting due to "first-dose syncope").

INDICATIONS/ROUTES/DOSAGE

Hypertension:

PO: **Adults, elderly:** Initially, 1 mg 2–3 times/day. **Maintenance:** 3–15 mg/day in divided doses. **Maintenance:** 20 mg/day. **Children:** 5 mcg/kg/dose q6h. Gradually increase up to 25 mcg/kg/dose. **Maximum:** 15 mg or 400 mcg/kg/day.

SIDE EFFECTS

FREQUENT (7–10%): Dizziness, drowsiness, headache, asthenia (loss of strength, energy). ***OCCASIONAL*** (4–5%): Palpitations, nausea, dry mouth, nervousness. ***RARE*** (<1%): Angina, urinary urgency.

ADVERSE REACTIONS/TOXIC EFFECTS

"First-dose syncope" (hypotension with sudden loss of consciousness) generally occurs 30–90 min after giving initial dose of 2 mg or greater, a too rapid increase in dose, or addition of another hypotensive agent to therapy. May be preceded by tachycardia (120–160 beats/min).

NURSING IMPLICATIONS

BASELINE ASSESSMENT:

Give first dose at bedtime. If initial dose is given during daytime, pt must remain recumbent for 3–4 hrs. Assess B/P, pulse immediately before each dose and q15–30min until stabilized (be alert to B/P fluctuations).

INTERVENTION/EVALUATION:

Monitor pulse diligently (first-dose syncope may be preceded by tachycardia). Monitor pattern of daily bowel activity and stool consistency. Assist with ambulation if dizziness occurs.

PATIENT/FAMILY TEACHING:

Avoid driving for 12–24 hrs after first dose or increase in dosage. Use caution driving or operating machinery and when rising from sitting or lying position. Report dizziness or palpitations if bothersome.

prednicarbate

(Dermatop)

See Classification section under: Corticosteroids: topical (p. 82C)

prednisolone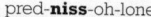

pred-**niss**-oh-lone
(AK-Pred, Econopred, Inflamase, Orapred, Pediapred, Pred Forte, Pred Mild, Prelone)

FIXED-COMBINATION(S)

Prednisolone acetate with sulfacetamide sodium, a sulfonamide **(Blephamide Liquifilm, Isopto Cetopred);** with atropine sulfate, a mydriatic **(Mydrapred);** with neomycin and polymyxin B, anti-infectives **(Poly-Pred Liquifilm).** Prednisolone sodium phosphate with sulfacetamide, a sulfonamide **(Optimyd, Vasocidin)**

▶CLASSIFICATION

PHARMACOTHERAPEUTIC: Adrenal corticosteroid. ***CLINICAL:*** Glucocorticoid (see p. 79C)

ACTION/*THERAPEUTIC EFFECT*

Inhibits accumulation of inflammatory cells at inflammation sites, phagocytosis, lysosomal enzyme release and synthesis, and/or release of mediators of inflammation. *Prevents/suppresses cell-mediated immune reactions. Decreases/prevents tissue response to inflammatory process.*

USES

Substitution therapy in deficiency states: Acute/chronic adrenal insufficiency, congenital adrenal hyperplasia, adrenal insufficiency secondary to pituitary insufficiency. ***Nonendocrine disorders:*** Arthritis, rheumatic carditis; allergic, collagen, intestinal tract, liver, ocular, renal, skin diseases; bronchial asthma, cerebral edema, malignancies.

PRECAUTIONS

CONTRAINDICATIONS: Hypersensitivity to any corticosteroid or tartrazine, systemic fungal infection, peptic ulcers (except life-threatening situations). Avoid live virus vaccine such as smallpox. ***CAUTIONS:*** Thromboembolic disorders, history of tuberculosis (may reactivate disease), hypothyroidism, cirrhosis, nonspecific ulcerative colitis, CHF, hypertension, psychosis, renal insufficiency, seizure disorders. Prolonged therapy should be discontinued slowly.

INTERACTIONS

DRUG:* Amphotericin** may increase hypokalemia. May decrease effect of oral **hypoglycemics, insulin, diuretics, potassium supplements.** May increase **digoxin** toxicity (due to hypokalemia). **Hepatic enzyme inducers** may decrease effect. **Live virus vaccines** may potentiate virus replication, increase vaccine side effects, decrease pt's antibody response to vaccine. ***HERBAL: None known. ***FOOD:*** None known. ***LAB VALUES:*** May decrease calcium, potassium, thyroxine. May increase cholesterol, lipids, glucose, sodium, amylase.

AVAILABILITY (Rx)

OPHTHALMIC SUSPENSION: 0.12%, 0.125%, 1%. ***OPHTHALMIC SOLUTION:*** 0.125%, 1%. ***ORAL SOLUTION:*** 5 mg/5 ml, 15 mg/5 ml. ***TABLETS:*** 5 mg.

INDICATIONS/ROUTES/DOSAGE

Usual adult dosage:

PO: 5–60 mg/day.

Acute asthma:

***PO:* Children:** 1–2 mg/kg/day in divided doses.

Anti-inflammation/ immunosuppression:

***PO:* Children:** 0.1–2 mg/kg/day in divided doses.

Usual ophthalmic dosage:

***OPHTHALMIC:* Adults, elderly:** *Solution:* 1–2 drops q1h during day; q2h during night; after response, decrease dose to 1 drop q4h, then 1 drop 3–4 times/day. *Ointment:* thin coat 3–4 times/day; after response, decrease to 2 times/day; then once daily.

SIDE EFFECTS

FREQUENT: Insomnia, heartburn, nervousness, abdominal disten-

P

tion, increased sweating, acne, mood swings, increased appetite, facial flushing, delayed wound healing, increased susceptibility to infection, diarrhea/constipation. ***OCCASIONAL:*** Headache, edema, change in skin color, frequent urination. ***RARE:*** Tachycardia, allergic reaction (rash, hives), psychic changes, hallucinations, depression. *Ophthalmic:* Stinging or burning, posterior subcapsular cataracts.

ADVERSE REACTIONS/TOXIC EFFECTS

Long-term therapy: Hypocalcemia, hypokalemia, muscle wasting (esp. arms, legs), osteoporosis, spontaneous fractures, amenorrhea, cataracts, glaucoma, peptic ulcer, CHF. ***Abrupt withdrawal following long-term therapy:*** Anorexia, nausea, fever, headache, sudden, severe joint pain, rebound inflammation, fatigue, weakness, lethargy, dizziness, orthostatic hypotension. Sudden discontinuance may be fatal.

NURSING IMPLICATIONS

BASELINE ASSESSMENT:

Obtain baselines for height, weight, B/P, glucose, electrolytes. Check results of initial tests, e.g., TB skin test, x-rays, EKG. Never give live virus vaccine (i.e., smallpox).

INTERVENTION/EVALUATION:

Monitor I&O, weight; assess for edema. Evaluate bowel activity; report hyperacidity promptly. Check vital signs at least 2 times/day. Be alert to infection (sore throat, fever, or vague symptoms); assess mouth daily for signs of candida infection (white patches, painful tongue and mucous membranes). Monitor electrolytes. Watch for hypocalcemia (muscle twitching, cramps, positive Trousseau's or Chvostek's signs) or hypokalemia (weakness and muscle cramps, numbness/tingling [esp. lower extremities], nausea and vomiting, irritability, EKG changes). Assess emotional status, ability to sleep.

PATIENT/FAMILY TEACHING:

Take oral dose with food or milk. Do not change dose/schedule or stop taking drug; must taper off gradually under medical supervision. Notify physician of fever, sore throat, muscle aches, sudden weight gain/swelling. Maintain careful personal hygiene, avoid exposure to disease or trauma. Severe stress (serious infection, surgery or trauma) may require increased dosage. Follow-up visits, lab tests are necessary; children must be assessed for growth retardation. Inform dentist or other physicians of methylprednisolone therapy now or within past 12 mos. Caution against overuse of joints injected for symptomatic relief.

prednisone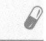

pred-nih-sewn
(Apo-Prednisone✤, Deltasone, Meticorten, Winpred✤)
Do not confuse with
prednisolone, Primidone.

▶CLASSIFICATION

PHARMACOTHERAPEUTIC:
Adrenal corticosteroid. ***CLINICAL:*** Glucocorticoid (see p. 79C)

ACTION/*THERAPEUTIC EFFECT*

Inhibits accumulation of inflammatory cells at inflammation sites, phagocytosis, lysosomal enzyme release and synthesis, and/or release of mediators of inflammation. *Prevents/suppresses cell-mediated immune reactions. Decreases/prevents tissue response to inflammatory process.*

PHARMACOKINETICS

Well absorbed from GI tract. Protein binding: 70–90%. Widely distributed. Metabolized in liver (converted to prednisolone). Primarily excreted in urine. Not removed by hemodialysis. Half-life: 3.4–3.8 hrs.

USES

Substitution therapy in deficiency states: Acute/chronic adrenal insufficiency, congenital adrenal hyperplasia, adrenal insufficiency secondary to pituitary insufficiency. *Nonendocrine disorders:* Arthritis, rheumatic carditis; allergic, collagen, intestinal tract, liver, ocular, renal, skin diseases; bronchial asthma, cerebral edema, malignancies.

PRECAUTIONS

CONTRAINDICATIONS: Hypersensitivity to any corticosteroid, systemic fungal infection, peptic ulcer (except life-threatening situations), breast feeding. *CAUTIONS:* Thromboembolic disorders, history of tuberculosis (may reactivate disease), hypothyroidism, cirrhosis, nonspecific ulcerative colitis, CHF, hypertension, psychosis, renal insufficiency, seizure disorders.

▷*LIFESPAN CONSIDERATIONS:*
Pregnancy/Lactation: Crosses placenta; distributed in breast milk. Cleft palate generally occurs with chronic use, first trimester. **Pregnancy Category B. Children:** Prolonged treatment or high doses may decrease short-term growth rate, cortisol secretion. **Elderly:** May be more susceptible to developing hypertension or osteoporosis.

INTERACTIONS

DRUG: **Amphotericin** may increase hypokalemia. May decrease effect **of oral hypoglycemics, insulin, diuretics, potassium supplements.** May increase **digoxin** toxicity (due to hypokalemia). **Hepatic enzyme inducers** may decrease effect. **Live virus vaccines** may potentiate virus replication, increase vaccine side effects, decrease pt's antibody response to vaccine. *HERBAL:* None known. *FOOD:* None known. *LAB VALUES:* May decrease calcium, potassium, thyroxine. May increase cholesterol, lipids, glucose, sodium, amylase.

AVAILABILITY (Rx)

TABLETS: 1 mg, 2.5 mg, 5 mg, 10 mg, 20 mg, 50 mg. *ORAL SOLUTION:* 5 mg/5 ml, 5 mg/ml. *SYRUP:* 5 mg/5 ml.

ADMINISTRATION/HANDLING
PO:

• Give without regard to meals (give with food if GI upset occurs).
• Give single doses before 9 AM, multiple doses at evenly spaced intervals.

INDICATIONS/ROUTES/DOSAGE
Usual adult dosage:
PO: 5–60 mg/day.

Acute asthma:
PO: **Children:** 1–2 mg/kg/day in divided doses.

Anti-inflammation/ immunosuppression:

PO: Children: 0.1–2 mg/kg/day in divided doses.

SIDE EFFECTS

FREQUENT: Insomnia, heartburn, nervousness, abdominal distention, increased sweating, acne, mood swings, increased appetite, facial flushing, delayed wound healing, increased susceptibility to infection, diarrhea/constipation. **OCCASIONAL:** Headache, edema, change in skin color, frequent urination. **RARE:** Tachycardia, allergic reaction (rash, hives), psychic changes, hallucinations, depression.

ADVERSE REACTIONS/TOXIC EFFECTS

Long-term therapy: Muscle wasting (esp. arms, legs), osteoporosis, spontaneous fractures, amenorrhea, cataracts, glaucoma, peptic ulcer, CHF. **Abrupt withdrawal following long-term therapy:** Anorexia, nausea, fever, headache, sudden or severe joint pain, rebound inflammation, fatigue, weakness, lethargy, dizziness, orthostatic hypotension. Sudden discontinuance may be fatal.

NURSING IMPLICATIONS

BASELINE ASSESSMENT:

Obtain baselines for height, weight, B/P, glucose, electrolytes. Check results of initial tests, e.g., TB skin test, x-rays, EKG. Never give live virus vaccine (i.e., smallpox).

INTERVENTION/EVALUATION:

Monitor I&O, weight; assess for edema. Evaluate bowel activity; report hyperacidity promptly.

Check vital signs at least 2 times/day. Be alert to infection (sore throat, fever, or vague symptoms); assess mouth daily for signs of candida infection (white patches, painful tongue and mucous membranes). Monitor electrolytes. Watch for hypocalcemia (muscle twitching, cramps, positive Trousseau's or Chvostek's signs) or hypokalemia (weakness and muscle cramps, numbness/tingling [esp. lower extremities], nausea and vomiting, irritability, EKG changes). Assess emotional status, ability to sleep.

PATIENT/FAMILY TEACHING:

Do not change dose/schedule or stop taking drug; must taper off gradually under medical supervision. Notify physician of fever, sore throat, muscle aches, sudden weight gain/swelling. Eat sodium low, high protein and potassium foods. Maintain careful personal hygiene, avoid exposure to disease or trauma. Severe stress (serious infection, surgery or trauma) may require increased dosage. Follow-up visits, lab tests are necessary; children must be assessed for growth retardation. Inform dentist or other physicians of prednisone therapy now or within past 12 mos.

---

primidone ✳

prih-mih-doan
(Apo-Primidone ♣, Mysoline)
Do not confuse with prednisone.

▶CLASSIFICATION

PHARMACOTHERAPEUTIC: Barbiturate. **CLINICAL:** Anticonvulsant (see p. 31C)

ACTION/*THERAPEUTIC EFFECT*

Decreases motor activity to electrical/chemical stimulation, stabilizes threshhold against hyperexcitability, *producing anticonvulsant effect.*

USES/*UNLABELED*

Management of partial seizures with complex symptomatology (psychomotor seizures), generalized tonic-clonic (grand mal) seizures. *Treatment of essential tremor.*

PRECAUTIONS

CONTRAINDICATIONS: History of porphyria, bronchopneumonia. ***EXTREME CAUTION:*** Nephritis, renal insufficiency. ***CAUTIONS:*** Uncontrolled pain (may produce paradoxical reaction), impaired liver function.

INTERACTIONS

DRUG: May decrease effects of **glucocorticoids, digoxin, metronidazole, oral anticoagulants, quinidine, tricyclic antidepressants. Alcohol, CNS depressants** may increase effect. May increase metabolism of **carbamazepine. Valproic acid** decreases metabolism, increases concentration, toxicity. ***HERBAL:*** None known. ***FOOD:*** None known. ***LAB VALUES:*** May decrease bilirubin. Therapeutic blood serum level: 4–12 mcg/ml; toxic blood serum level: >12 mcg/ml.

AVAILABILITY (Rx)

TABLETS: 50 mg, 250 mg. ***ORAL SUSPENSION:*** 250 mg/5 ml.

INDICATIONS/ROUTES/DOSAGE

Anticonvulsant:

PO: Adults, elderly, children >8 yrs: 125–150 mg/day at bedtime.
May increase by 125–250 mg/day q3–7days. **Maximum:** 2 g/day. **Children <8 yrs:** Initially, 50–125 mg/day at bedtime. May increase by 50–125 mg/day q3–7days. ***Usual dose:*** 10–25 mg/kg/day in divided doses. **Neonates:** 12–20 mg/kg/day in divided doses.

SIDE EFFECTS

FREQUENT: Ataxia, dizziness. ***OCCASIONAL:*** Loss of appetite, drowsiness, mental changes, nausea, vomiting, paradoxical excitement. ***RARE:*** Skin rash.

ADVERSE REACTIONS/TOXIC EFFECTS

Abrupt withdrawal after prolonged therapy may produce effects ranging from markedly increased dreaming, nightmares and/or insomnia, tremor, sweating, vomiting, to hallucinations, delirium, seizures, status epilepticus. Skin eruptions may appear as hypersensitivity reaction. Blood dyscrasias, liver disease, hypocalcemia occur rarely. Overdosage produces cold clammy skin, hypothermia, severe CNS depression followed by high fever, coma.

P

NURSING IMPLICATIONS

BASELINE ASSESSMENT:

Review history of seizure disorder (intensity, frequency, duration, LOC). Observe frequently for recurrence of seizure activity. Initiate seizure precautions.

INTERVENTION/EVALUATION:

For those on long-term therapy, liver/renal function tests, blood counts should be performed periodically. Assist with ambulation if dizziness, ataxia occurs. Assess children, elderly for paradoxical reaction (particularly during early therapy). Assess for clinical improvement (decrease in intensity/frequency of seizures). Monitor for therapeutic serum level (5–12 mcg/ml). Therapeutic blood serum level: 4–12 mcg/ml; toxic blood serum level: >12 mcg/ml.

PATIENT/FAMILY TEACHING:

Do not abruptly withdraw medication following long-term use (may precipitate seizures). Strict maintenance of drug therapy is essential for seizure control. Drowsiness usually disappears during continued therapy. If dizziness occurs, change positions slowly from recumbent to sitting position before standing. Avoid tasks that require alertness, motor skills until response to drug is established. Avoid alcohol.

probenecid

pro-**ben**-ah-sid
(Benemid, Benuryl✤, Probalan)

FIXED-COMBINATION(S)

With colchicine, antigout agent **(ColBenemid, Proben-C)**

▶CLASSIFICATION

PHARMACOTHERAPEUTIC: Uricosuric. ***CLINICAL:*** Antigout

ACTION/*THERAPEUTIC EFFECT*

Inhibits tubular reabsorption of urate at proximal renal tubule, *increasing urinary excretion of uric acid.*

USES

Treatment of hyperuricemia associated with gout or gouty arthritis.

Adjunctive therapy with penicillins or cephalosporins to elevate and prolong antibiotic plasma levels.

PRECAUTIONS

CONTRAINDICATIONS: Blood dyscrasias, uric acid kidney stones, concurrent use with penicillin in presence of renal impairment. ***CAUTIONS:*** Impaired renal function, history of peptic ulcer.

INTERACTIONS

DRUG: May increase concentrations of **cephalosporins, methotrexate, NSAIDs, nitrofurantoin, penicillins, zidovudine. Antineoplastics** may increase risk of uric acid nephropathy. **Salicylates** may decrease uricosuric effect. May increase, prolong effects of **heparin.** ***HERBAL:*** None known. ***FOOD:*** None known. ***LAB VALUES:*** May inhibit renal excretion of PSP (phenolsulfonphthalein), 17-ketosteroids, BSP (sulfobromophthalein) tests.

AVAILABILITY (Rx)
TABLETS: 500 mg.

ADMINISTRATION/HANDLING
PO:

• Give with or immediately after meals or milk. • Instruct pt to drink at least 6–8 glasses (8 oz) of water/day (prevents kidney stone development).

INDICATIONS/ROUTES/DOSAGE
Gout:

Note: Do not start until acute gout attack subsides; continue if acute attack occurs during therapy.

PO: Adults, elderly: Initially, 250 mg 2 times/day for 1 wk; then 500 mg 2 times/day. May increase by 500 mg q4wks. **Maximum:** 2–3 g/day. **Maintenance:** Dosage that maintains normal uric acid levels.

Penicillin/cephalosporin therapy:

Note: Do not use in presence of renal impairment.

PO: Adults, elderly: 2 g/day in divided doses. **Children (2–14 yrs):** Initially, 25 mg/kg. **Maintenance:** 40 mg/kg/day in 4 divided doses. **Children >50 kg:** Receive adult dosage.

Gonorrhea:

PO: Adults, elderly: 1 g 30 min prior to penicillin, ampicillin, or amoxicillin.

SIDE EFFECTS

FREQUENT (5–10%): Headache, anorexia, nausea, vomiting. **OCCASIONAL** (1–5%): Lower back/side pain, rash, hives, itching, dizziness, flushed face, frequent urge to urinate, gingivitis.

ADVERSE REACTIONS/TOXIC EFFECTS

Severe hypersensitivity reactions (including anaphylaxis) occur rarely (usually within a few hrs after readministration following previous use). Discontinue immediately, contact physician. Pruritic maculopapular rash should be considered a toxic reaction. May be accompanied by malaise, fever, chills, joint pain, nausea, vomiting, leukopenia, aplastic anemia.

NURSING IMPLICATIONS

BASELINE ASSESSMENT:

Do not initiate therapy until acute gouty attack has subsided. Question pt for hypersensitivity to probenecid or if taking penicillin or cephalosporin antibiotics. Instruct pt to drink 6–8 glasses (8 oz) of fluid daily while on medication.

INTERVENTION/EVALUATION:

If exacerbation of gout recurs following therapy, use other agents for gout. Discontinue medication immediately if rash or other evidence of allergic reaction appears. Encourage high fluid intake (3,000 ml/day). Monitor I&O (output should be at least 2,000 ml/day). Assess CBC, serum uric acid levels. Assess urine for cloudiness, unusual color, odor. Assess for therapeutic response (reduced joint tenderness, swelling, redness, limitation of motion).

PATIENT/FAMILY TEACHING:

Encourage low-purine food intake (reduce/omit meat, fowl, fish; use eggs, cheese, vegetables). Foods high in purine: kidneys, liver, sweetbreads, sardines, anchovies, meat extracts. May take 1 or more wks for full therapeutic effect. Drink 6–8 glasses (8 oz) of fluid daily while on medication.

P

procainamide hydrochloride

pro-**cane**-ah-myd
(ProcanBid, Procan-SR, Pronestyl)
Do not confuse with Ponstel, probenecid.

▶CLASSIFICATION

CLINICAL: Antiarrhythmic (see p. 12C)

ACTION/*THERAPEUTIC EFFECT*

Prolongs refractory period by direct effect, decreasing myocardial excitability and conduction velocity. *Depresses myocardial contractility.*

PHARMACOKINETICS

Rapidly, completely absorbed from GI tract. Protein binding: 15–20%. Widely distributed. Metabolized in liver to active metabolite. Primarily excreted in urine. Removed by hemodialysis. Half-life: 2.5–4.5 hrs; metabolite: 6 hrs.

USES/*UNLABELED*

Prophylactic therapy to maintain normal sinus rhythm after conversion of atrial fibrillation and/or flutter. Treatment of premature ventricular contractions, paroxysmal atrial tachycardia, atrial fibrillation, ventricular tachycardia. *Conversion/management of atrial fibrillation and PAT.*

PRECAUTIONS

CONTRAINDICATIONS: Complete AV block, second-and third-degree AV block without pacemaker, abnormal impulses/rhythms because of escape mechanism. ***CAUTIONS:*** Ventricular tachycardia during coronary occlusion, renal/hepatic disease, incomplete AV nodal block, digitalis intoxication, CHF, preexisting hypotension.

▷*LIFESPAN CONSIDERATIONS:* **Pregnancy/Lactation:** Crosses placenta; unknown if distributed in breast milk. **Pregnancy Category C. Children:** No age-related precautions noted. **Elderly:** More susceptible to hypotensive effect. Age-related renal impairment may require dosage adjustment.

INTERACTIONS

DRUG: **Pimozide, other antiar-**

rhythmics may increase cardiac effects. May increase effects of **antihypertensives (IV procainamide), neuromuscular blockers.** May decrease antimyasthenic effect on skeletal muscle. ***HERBAL:*** None known. ***FOOD:*** None known. ***LAB VALUES:*** May cause positive ANA, Coomb's' test, EKG changes. May increase SGOT (AST), SGPT (ALT), alkaline phosphatase, bilirubin, LDH. Therapeutic blood serum level: 4–8 mcg/ml; toxic blood serum level: >10 mcg/ml.

AVAILABILITY (Rx)

CAPSULES: 250 mg, 375 mg, 500 mg. ***TABLETS:*** 250 mg, 375 mg, 500 mg. ***TABLETS (sustained-release):*** 250 mg, 500 mg, 750 mg, 1,000 mg. ***INJECTION:*** 100 mg/ml, 500 mg/ml.

ADMINISTRATION/HANDLING

PO:

• Do not crush or break sustained-release tablets.

IM/IV 📷

Note: May give by IM, IV push or IV infusion.

Storage:

• Solution appears clear, colorless to light yellow. • Discard if solution darkens/appears discolored or if precipitate forms. • When diluted with D_5W, solution is stable for 24 hrs at room temperature or for 7 days if refrigerated.

Reconstitution:

• For IV push, dilute with 5–10 ml D_5W. • For initial loading IV infusion, add 1 g to 50 ml D_5W to provide a concentration of 20 mg/ml. • For IV infusion, add 1 g to 250–500 ml D_5W to provide concentration of 2–4 mg/ml. Maximum concentration: 4 g/250 ml.

Rate of administration:

• For IV push, with pt in supine position, administer at rate not exceeding 25–50 mg/min. • For initial loading infusion, infuse 1 ml/min for up to 25–30 min. • For IV infusion, infuse at 1–3 ml/min. • Check B/P q5–10min during infusion. If fall in B/P exceeds 15 mm Hg, discontinue drug, contact physician. • Monitor EKG for cardiac changes, particularly widening of QRS, prolongation of PR and QT interval. Notify physician of any significant interval changes. • B/P, EKG should be monitored continuously during IV administration and rate of infusion adjusted to eliminate arrhythmias.

IV INCOMPATIBILITY ⊘

Milrinone (Primacor).

IV COMPATIBILITIES

Amiodarone (Cordarone), dobutamine (Dobutrex), heparin, lidocaine, potassium chloride.

INDICATIONS/ROUTES/DOSAGE

Note: Dose, interval of administration individualized based on underlying myocardial disease, pt's age, renal function, clinical response. Extended-release capsules used for maintenance therapy.

Arrhythmias:

IV: **Adults, elderly:** *(Loading dose):* 50–100 mg/dose. May repeat q5–10min or 15–18 mg/kg. (*Maximum:* 1–1.5 g) then maintenance infusion of 3–4 mg/min. **Range:** 1–6 mg/min. **Children:** *(Loading dose):* 3–6 mg/kg/dose over 5 min (*Maximum:* 100 mg). May repeat q5–10min to maximum total dose of 15 mg/kg then maintenance dose of 20–80 mcg/kg/min. **Maximum:** 2 g/day.

PO: **Adults, elderly:** *(Immediate-release):* 250–500 mg q3–6h. *(Sustained-release):* 0.5–1 g q6h. *(Procanabid):* 1–2 g q12h. **Children:** *(Immediate-release):* 15–50 mg/kg/day in divided doses q3–6h. **Maximum:** 4 g/day.

Dosage in renal impairment:

Creatinine Clearance	Dosage Interval
10–50 ml/min	q6–12h
<10 ml/min	q8–24h

SIDE EFFECTS

FREQUENT: PO: Abdominal pain/cramping, nausea, diarrhea, vomiting. ***OCCASIONAL:*** Dizziness, giddiness, weakness, hypersensitivity reaction (rash, urticaria, pruritus, flushing). ***INFREQUENT: IV:*** Transient, but at times, marked hypotension. ***RARE:*** Confusion, mental depression, psychosis.

ADVERSE REACTIONS/TOXIC EFFECTS

Paradoxical, extremely rapid ventricular rate may occur during treatment of atrial fibrillation/flutter. Systemic lupus erythematosus–like syndrome (fever, joint pain, pleuritic chest pain) with prolonged therapy. Cardiotoxic effects occur most commonly with IV administration, observed as conduction changes (50% widening of QRS complex, frequent ventricular premature contractions, ventricular tachycardia, complete AV block). Prolonged PR and QT intervals, flattened T waves occur less frequently (discontinue drug immediately).

NURSING IMPLICATIONS

BASELINE ASSESSMENT:

Check B/P and pulse for 1 full min (unless pt is on continuous

P

monitor) before giving medication.

INTERVENTION/EVALUATION:

Monitor EKG for cardiac changes, particularly widening of QRS, prolongation of PR and QT interval. Assess pulse for strength/weakness, irregular rate. Monitor I&O, electrolyte serum level (potassium, chloride, sodium). Assess for complaints of GI upset, headache, dizziness, joint pain. Monitor pattern of daily bowel activity, stool consistency. Assess for dizziness. Monitor B/P for hypotension. Assess skin for evidence of hypersensitivity reaction (esp. in those on high-dose therapy). Monitor for therapeutic serum level (3–10 mcg/ml). Therapeutic blood serum level: 4–8 mcg/ml; toxic blood serum level: >10 mcg/ml.

PATIENT/FAMILY TEACHING:

Take medication at evenly spaced doses around the clock. Contact physician if fever, joint pain/stiffness, signs of upper respiratory infection occur. Do not abruptly discontinue medication. Compliance with therapy regimen is essential to control arrhythmias. Do not use nasal decongestants, OTC cold preparations (stimulants) without physician approval. Restrict salt, alcohol intake.

procaine hydrochloride

(Novocain)

See Classification section under: Anesthetics: local (p. 4C)

procarbazine hydrochloride

pro-**car**-bah-zeen
(Matulane)
Do not confuse with dacarbazine.

▶**CLASSIFICATION**

PHARMACOTHERAPEUTIC:
Methylhydrazine derivative. **CLIN-ICAL:** Antineoplastic (see p. 73C)

ACTION/*THERAPEUTIC EFFECT*

Inhibits DNA, RNA, protein synthesis. May also directly damage DNA. Cell cycle-specific for S phase of cell division.

USES/*UNLABELED*

Treatment of advanced Hodgkin's disease. *Treatment of non-Hodgkin's lymphoma, primary brain tumors, lung carcinoma, malignant melanoma, multiple myeloma, polycythemia vera.*

PRECAUTIONS

CONTRAINDICATIONS: Inadequate bone marrow reserve. **CAUTIONS:** Impaired renal/hepatic function.

INTERACTIONS

DRUG: Alcohol may cause disulfiram reaction. **Anticholinergics, antihistamines** may increase anticholinergic effects. **Tricyclic antidepressants** may increase anticholinergic effects, cause hyperpyretic crisis, convulsions. May increase effects of **oral hypoglycemics, insulin. Bone marrow depressants** may increase bone marrow depression. May increase B/P with **buspirone, caffeine-containing medications.** May cause hyperpyretic crisis, seizures, death with **carbamazepine, cyclobenzaprine, maprotiline, MAO inhibitors. CNS depressants** may increase CNS depression. **Meperidine** may produce immediate excitation, sweating, rigidity, severe hypertension or hypotension, severe respiratory distress, coma, convulsions, vascular collapse. **Sympathomimetics** may increase cardiac stimulant, vasopressor effects. **_HERBAL:_** None known. **_FOOD:_** None known. **_LAB VALUES:_** None significant.

AVAILABILITY (Rx)

CAPSULES: 50 mg.

INDICATIONS/ROUTES/DOSAGE

Hodgkin's disease:

_PO:_ Adults, elderly: Initially, 2–4 mg/kg daily as single or divided dose for 1 wk, then 4–6 mg/kg day. **Children:** 50 mg/m^2 daily for 1 wk, then 100 mg/m^2 daily. Continue until maximum response, leukocyte count falls below 4,000/mm^3, or platelets fall below 100,000/mm^3.

Maintenance:

_PO:_ Adults, elderly: 1–2 mg/kg/ day. **Children:** 50 mg/m^2 daily.

SIDE EFFECTS

FREQUENT: Severe nausea, vomiting, respiratory disorders (cough, effusion), myalgia, arthralgia, drowsiness, nervousness, insomnia, nightmares, sweating, hallucinations, seizures. **_OCCASIONAL:_** Hoarseness, tachycardia, nystagmus, retinal hemorrhage, photophobia, photosensitivity, urinary frequency, nocturia, hypotension, diarrhea, stomatitis, paresthesia, unsteadiness, confusion, decreased reflexes, foot drop. **_RARE:_** Hypersensitivity reaction (dermatitis, pruritus, rash, urticaria), hyperpigmentation, alopecia.

ADVERSE REACTIONS/TOXIC EFFECTS

Major toxic effects are bone marrow depression manifested as hematologic toxicity (principally leukopenia, thrombocytopenia, anemia) and hepatotoxicity manifested by jaundice, ascites. Urinary tract infection secondary to leukopenia may occur. Therapy should be discontinued if stomatitis, diarrhea, paresthesia, neuropathies, confusion, hypersensitivity reaction occurs.

NURSING IMPLICATIONS

BASELINE ASSESSMENT:

Obtain bone marrow tests, hemoglobin, hematocrit, leukocyte, differential, reticulocyte, platelet, urinalysis, serum transaminase, serum alkaline phosphatase, BUN results before therapy and periodically thereafter. Therapy should be interrupted if WBC falls below 4,000/mm^3 or platelet count falls below 100,000/mm^3.

INTERVENTION/EVALUATION:

Monitor hematologic status, renal, hepatic function studies. Assess for stomatitis (burning/ erythema of oral mucosa at inner margin of lips, sore throat, difficulty swallowing, oral ulceration). Monitor for hematologic toxicity (fever, sore throat, signs of local infection, easy bruising,

P

unusual bleeding from any site), symptoms of anemia (excessive tiredness, weakness).

PATIENT/FAMILY TEACHING:

Do not drink alcoholic beverages during or for 2 wks after therapy (Antabuse-like reaction: severe headache, tachycardia, chest pain, stiff neck). Avoid foods with high tyramine content (e.g., yogurt, ripe cheese, smoked meat, overripe fruit). Avoid crowds, those with infection. Promptly report fever, sore throat, signs of local infection, easy bruising, or unusual bleeding from any site. Wear protective clothing, sunscreens to protect from sun/ultraviolet light.

prochlorperazine

pro-klor-**pear**-ah-zeen
(Compazine, Stemetil✚)
Do not confuse with
chlorpromazine, Copaxone.

▶CLASSIFICATION

PHARMACOTHERAPEUTIC:
Phenothiazine. **CLINICAL:** Antiemetic, antipsychotic

ACTION/THERAPEUTIC EFFECT

Antiemetic: Acts centrally to inhibit/block dopamine receptors in chemoreceptor trigger zone and peripherally to block vagus nerve in GI tract. *Relieves nausea and vomiting.* **Antipsychotic:** Antagonizes dopamine neurotransmission at synapses by blocking postsynaptic dopaminergic receptors in brain. *Suppresses behavioral response in psychosis.*

PHARMACOKINETICS

(Antiemetic)	Onset	Peak	Duration
Tablets, syrup			
	30–40 min	—	3–4 hrs
Extended-Release			
	30–40 min	—	10–12 hrs
IM			
	10–20 min	—	3–4 hrs
Rectal			
	60 min	—	3–4 hrs

Variably absorbed after PO administration, well absorbed after IM administration. Widely distributed. Metabolized in liver, GI mucosa. Primarily excreted in urine. Unknown if removed by hemodialysis. Half-life: 23 hrs.

USES

Control of severe nausea and vomiting, management of psychotic disorders, moderate to severe anxiety and tension in psychoneurotic pts.

PRECAUTIONS

CONTRAINDICATIONS: Suspected Reye's syndrome, severe CNS depression, comatose states, severe cardiovascular disease, bone marrow depression, subcortical brain damage. **CAUTIONS:** Impaired respiratory/hepatic/renal/cardiac function, alcohol withdrawal, history of seizures, urinary retention, glaucoma, prostatic hypertrophy, hypocalcemia (increases susceptibility to dystonias).

▷**LIFESPAN CONSIDERATIONS:**
Pregnancy/Lactation: Crosses placenta; distributed in breast milk. **Pregnancy Category C. Children:** More prone to develop extrapyramidol symptoms (EPS) (e.g., dystonias). **Elderly:** More susceptible to orthostatic hypotension, anticholinergic effects

(e.g., dry mouth), sedation, EPS; lower dosage recommended.

INTERACTIONS

DRUG:* Alcohol, CNS depressants** may increase CNS, respiratory depression, hypotensive effects. **Tricyclic antidepressants, MAO inhibitors** may increase sedative, anticholinergic effects. **Antithyroid agents** may increase risk of agranulocytosis. Extrapyramidal symptoms (EPS) may increase with **EPS-producing medications. Hypotensives** may increase hypotension. May decrease **levodopa** effects. **Lithium** may decrease absorption, produce adverse neurologic effects. ***HERBAL: None known. ***FOOD:*** None known. ***LAB VALUES:*** None significant.

AVAILABILITY (Rx)

TABLETS: 5 mg, 10 mg, 25 mg. ***CAPSULES (sustained-release):*** 10 mg, 15 mg. ***SYRUP:*** 5 mg/5 ml. ***SUPPOSITORY:*** 2.5 mg, 5 mg, 25 mg. ***INJECTION:*** 5 mg/ml.

ADMINISTRATION/HANDLING
PO:

• Give without regard to meals.

Parenteral: Pt must remain recumbent for 30–60 min in head-low position with legs raised to minimize hypotensive effect.

IM:

• Inject slow, deep IM into upper outer quadrant of gluteus maximus. If irritation occurs, further injections may be diluted with 0.9% NaCl or 2% procaine hydrochloride. • Massage IM injection site to reduce discomfort.

IV 🏥

Note: Give by IV push or IV infusion.

Storage:

• Protect from light (darkens on exposure). • Slight yellow discoloration of solution does not affect potency, but discard if markedly discolored or precipitate forms. • Store suppository form at room temperature.

Reconstitution:

• For IV infusion, dilute 20 mg (4 ml) prochlorperazine with 0.9% NaCl.

Rate of administration:

• For IV push, administer each 5 mg >1 min. • For IV infusion, administer 5 mg/min rate of infusion. • Monitor B/P diligently for hypotension during IV administration.

Rectal:

• Moisten suppository with cold water before inserting well up into rectum.

IV INCOMPATIBILITIES ⊘

Aldesleukin (Interleukin, Proleukine), allopurinol (Aloprim), amifostine (Ethyol), cefepime (Maxipime), etoposide (Vepesid, VP-16), fludarabine (Fludara), foscarnet (Foscavir), filgrastim (Neupogen), gemcitabine (Gemzar), piperacillin/tazobactam (Zosyn).

IV COMPATIBILITIES

Calcium gluconate, heparin, potassium chloride, propofol (Diprivan).

INDICATIONS/ROUTES/DOSAGE
Antiemetic:

IV: Adults, elderly: 2.5–10 mg. May repeat q3–4h as needed.

IM: Adults, elderly: 5–10 mg q3–4h. **Maximum:** 40 mg/day. **Children:** 0.1–0.15 mg/kg/dose.

PO: Adults, elderly: 5–10 mg 3–4

P

times/day. **Children:** 0.4 mg/kg/day in 3–4 divided doses.

PO (extended-release): **Adults, elderly:** 10 mg 2 times/day or 15 mg once/day.

RECTAL: **Adults, elderly:** 25 mg 2 times/day. **Children:** 0.4 mg/kg/day in 3–4 divided doses.

Psychosis:

IM: **Adults, elderly:** 10–20 mg q4h as needed. **Children 2–12 yrs:** 0.13 mg/kg/dose.

PO: **Adults, elderly:** 5–10 mg 3–4 times/day. **Maximum:** 150 mg/day. **Children:** 2.5 mg 2–3 times/day. **Maximum:** 20 mg *(2–5 yrs)*, 25 mg *(6–12 yrs)*.

SIDE EFFECTS

FREQUENT: Drowsiness, hypotension, dizziness, fainting occur frequently after first dose, occasionally after subsequent dosing, and rarely with oral dosage. *OCCASIONAL:* Dry mouth, blurred vision, lethargy, constipation/diarrhea, muscular aches, nasal congestion, peripheral edema, urinary retention.

ADVERSE REACTIONS/TOXIC EFFECTS

Extrapyramidal symptoms appear dose related (particularly with high dosage) and are divided into 3 categories: akathisia (inability to sit still, tapping of feet, urge to move around), parkinsonian symptoms (masklike face, tremors, shuffling gait, hypersalivation), and acute dystonias: torticollis (neck muscle spasm), opisthotonos (rigidity of back muscles), and oculogyric crisis (rolling back of eyes). Dystonic reaction may also produce profuse sweating, pallor. Tardive dyskinesia (protrusion of tongue, puffing of cheeks, chewing/puckering of the mouth) occurs rarely (may be irreversible). Abrupt withdrawal following long-term therapy may precipitate nausea, vomiting, gastritis, dizziness, tremors. Blood dyscrasias, particularly agranulocytosis, mild leukopenia (sore mouth/gums/throat) may occur. May lower seizure threshold.

NURSING IMPLICATIONS

BASELINE ASSESSMENT:

Avoid skin contact with solution (contact dermatitis). *Antiemetic:* Assess for dehydration (poor skin turgor, dry mucous membranes, longitudinal furrows in tongue). *Antipsychotic:* Assess behavior, appearance, emotional status, response to environment, speech pattern, thought content.

INTERVENTION/EVALUATION:

Monitor B/P for hypotension. Assess for extrapyramidal symptoms. Monitor WBC, differential count for blood dyscrasias. Monitor for fine tongue movement (may be early sign of tardive dyskinesia). Supervise suicidal risk pt closely during early therapy (as depression lessens, energy level improves, increasing suicide potential). Assess for therapeutic response (interest in surroundings, improvement in self-care, increased ability to concentrate, relaxed facial expression).

PATIENT/FAMILY TEACHING:

Urine may turn pink or reddish brown. Do not abruptly withdraw from long-term drug therapy. Report visual disturbances. Sugarless gum, sips of tepid water may relieve dry mouth. Drowsiness generally subsides during continued therapy. Avoid tasks that require alertness, motor skills until response to drug is established. Avoid alcohol, CNS depressants. Use sunscreen, protective clothing in sun or ultraviolet light. Use caution in hot weather (possibility of heat stroke).

progesterone

proe-**jess**-ter-one
(Crinone, Gesterol, Prometrium)

▶CLASSIFICATION

PHARMACOTHERAPEUTIC:
Progestin. ***CLINICAL:*** Hormone

ACTION/*THERAPEUTIC EFFECT*

Transforms endometrium from proliferative to secretory (in an estrogen-primed endometrium); inhibits secretion of pituitary gonadotropins, preventing follicular maturation and ovulation. Stimulates the growth of mammary alveolar tissue; relaxes uterine smooth muscle. *Restores hormonal balance.*

USES/*UNLABELED*

Treatment of primary or secondary amenorrhea, abnormal uterine bleeding due to hormonal imbalance, endometriosis. Prevention of endometrial hyperplasia in estrogen recipients. ***Vaginal Gel*** (8%): Treatment of infertility. *Treatment of corpus luteum dysfunction.*

PRECAUTIONS

CONTRAINDICATIONS: Thrombophlebitis, thromboembolic disorders, cerebral apoplexy or history of these conditions; severe liver dysfunction; breast cancer; undiagnosed vaginal bleeding; missed abortion; use as a diagnostic test for pregnancy. ***CAUTIONS:*** Diabetes, conditions aggravated by fluid retention (e.g., asthma, epilepsy, migraine, cardiac/renal dysfunction), history of mental depression.

INTERACTIONS

DRUG: May interfere with effects of **bromocriptine. HERBAL:** None known. ***FOOD:*** None known. ***LAB VALUES:*** May increase alkaline phosphatase, LDL. May decrease HDL. May cause abnormal thyroid, metapyrone, liver, endocrine function tests, decrease glucose tolerance.

AVAILABILITY (Rx)

INJECTION: 50 mg/ml. ***CAPSULES:*** 100 mg. ***VAGINAL GEL:*** 4%, 8%.

INDICATIONS/ROUTES/DOSAGE

Amenorrhea:

***IM:* Adults:** 5–10 mg for 6–8 days. Withdrawal bleeding expected in 48–72 hrs if ovarian activity produced proliferative endometrium.

***VAGINAL:* Adults:** Apply every other day for up to 6 doses.

***PO:* Adults:** 400 mg daily in evening for 10 days.

Abnormal uterine bleeding:

***IM:* Adults:** 5–10 mg for 6 days. (When estrogen given concomitantly, begin progesterone after 2 wks of estrogen therapy; discontinue when menstrual flow begins.)

Prevention of endometrial hyperplasia:

***PO:* Adults:** 200 mg in evening for 12 days per 28 day cycle in combination with daily conjugated estrogen.

SIDE EFFECTS

FREQUENT: Breakthrough bleed-

P

---

ing or spotting at beginning of therapy. Amenorrhea, change in menstrual flow, breast tenderness. **OCCASIONAL:** Edema, weight gain or loss, rash, pruritus, photosensitivity, skin pigmentation. **RARE:** Pain/swelling at injection site, acne, mental depression, alopecia, hirsutism.

ADVERSE REACTIONS/TOXIC EFFECTS

Thrombophlebitis, cerebrovascular disorders, retinal thrombosis, pulmonary embolism occurs rarely.

NURSING IMPLICATIONS

BASELINE ASSESSMENT:

Question for possibility of pregnancy or hypersensitivity to progestins before initiating therapy. Obtain baseline weight, blood glucose level, B/P.

INTERVENTION/EVALUATION:

Check weight daily; report weekly gain of 5 lbs or more. Assess skin for rash, hives. Immediately report the development of chest pain, sudden shortness of breath, sudden decrease in vision, migraine headache, pain (esp. with swelling, warmth, and redness) in calves, numbness of an arm/leg (thrombotic disorders). Check B/P periodically. Note progesterone therapy on pathology specimens.

PATIENT/FAMILY TEACHING:

Use sunscreens, protective clothing to protect from sunlight/ultraviolet light until tolerance determined. Notify physician of abnormal vaginal bleeding or other symptoms. Stop taking medication and contact physician at once if pregnancy suspected.

promethazine hydrochloride

pro-**meth**-ah-zeen
(Phenergan)
Do not confuse with promazine.

FIXED-COMBINATION(S)

With codeine, a narcotic analgesic **(Phenergan with Codeine);** with dextromethorphan, an antitussive **(Phenergan with Dextromethorphan);** with meperidine, a narcotic analgesic **(Mepergan);** with phenylephrine, a nasal vasoconstrictor **(Phenergan VC);** with phenylephrine and codeine **(Phenergan VC with Codeine).**

►CLASSIFICATION

PHARMACOTHERAPEUTIC: Phenothiazine. **CLINICAL:** Antihistamine, antiemetic, sedative-hypnotic (see p. 48C)

ACTION/*THERAPEUTIC EFFECT*

Antihistamine: Inhibits histamine at histamine receptor sites, *preventing, antagonizing most allergic effects (e.g., urticaria, pruritus).* **Antiemetic:** Diminishes vestibular stimulation, depresses labyrinthine function, acts on chemoreceptor trigger zone, *producing antiemetic effect.* **Sedative-hypnotic:** Decreases stimulation to brain stem reticular formation, *producing CNS depression.*

PHARMACOKINETICS

	Onset	Peak	Duration
PO	20 min	—	2–8 hrs
IM	20 min	—	2–8 hrs
Rectal	20 min	—	2–8 hrs
IV	3–5 min	—	2–8 hrs

...m GI tract, after
...n. Widely distrib-
Well abs... in liver. Primar-
IM ac... urine.
...ute

...nptomatic relief of al-
...ptoms; sedative/anti-
...rgery/labor; decreases
...nausea/vomiting; adjunct to
...gesics in control of pain; management of motion sickness.

PRECAUTIONS

CONTRAINDICATIONS: Comatose, those receiving large
doses of other CNS depressants,
acutely ill/dehydrated children,
acute asthmatic attack, vomiting of
unknown etiology in children,
Reye's syndrome, those receiving
MAO inhibitors. ***EXTREME CAU-
TION:*** History of sleep apnea,
young children, family history of
sudden infant death syndrome
(SIDS), those difficult to arouse
from sleep. ***CAUTIONS:*** Narrow-
angle glaucoma, peptic ulcer, prostatic hypertrophy, pyloroduode-
nal/bladder neck obstruction,
asthma, COPD, increased intraocular pressure, cardiovascular disease, hyperthyroidism, hypertension, seizure disorders.

▷***LIFESPAN CONSIDERATIONS:***
Pregnancy/Lactation: Readily
crosses placenta; unknown if drug
is excreted in breast milk. May inhibit platelet aggregation in neonates if taken within 2 wks of birth.
May produce jaundice, extrapyramidal symptoms in neonates if
taken during pregnancy. **Pregnancy Category C. Children:**
May experience increased excitement. Not recommended for those
<2 yrs of age. **Elderly:** More sen-
sitive to dizziness, sedation, confusion, hypotension, hyperexcitabil-

ity, anticholinergic effects (e.g.,
dry mouth).

INTERACTIONS

***DRUG:* Alcohol, CNS depres-
sants** may increase CNS depressant effects. **Anticholinergics**
may increase anticholinergic effects. **MAO inhibitors** may prolong, intensify anticholinergic,
CNS depressant effects. ***HERBAL:***
None known. ***FOOD:*** None known.
LAB VALUES: May suppress wheal
and flare reactions to antigen skin
testing, unless discontinued 4
days before testing.

AVAILABILITY (Rx)

TABLETS: 12.5 mg, 25 mg, 50 mg.
SYRUP: 6.25 mg/5 ml. ***SUPPOSI-
TORY:*** 12.5 mg, 25 mg, 50 mg. ***IN-
JECTION:*** 25 mg/ml, 50 mg/ml.

ADMINISTRATION/HANDLING
PO:

• Give without regard to meals. •
Scored tablets may be crushed.

IM:

Note: Significant tissue necrosis
may occur if given SubQ. Inadvertent intra-arterial injection may
produce severe arteriospasm, resulting in severe circulation impairment.

• Inject deep IM.

IV
Storage:

• Store at room temperature.

Reconstitution:

• May be given undiluted or dilute
with 0.9% NaCl. Final dilution
should not exceed 25 mg/ml.

Rate of administration:

• Administer at 25 mg/min rate
through IV infusion tube. • A too-
rapid rate of infusion may result in
transient fall in B/P, producing or-

P

thostatic hypotension, reflex tachycardia. • If pt complains of pain at IV site, stop injection immediately (possibility of intra-arterial needle placement/perivascular extravasation).

Rectal:

• Refrigerate suppository. • Moisten suppository with cold water before inserting well up into rectum.

IV INCOMPATIBILITIES ⊘

Allopurinol (Aloprim), amphotericin B complex (Abelcet, Ambisome, Amphotec), piperacillin tazobactam (Zosyn).

INDICATIONS/ROUTES/DOSAGE

Allergic symptoms:

PO: **Adults, elderly:** 25 mg at bedtime or 12.5 mg 4 times/day. **Children:** 0.1 mg/kg/dose q6h and 0.5 mg/kg at bedtime.

RECTAL/IM/IV: **Adults, elderly:** 25 mg, may repeat in 2 hrs.

Motion sickness:

PO: **Adults, elderly:** 25 mg 30–60 min before departure; may repeat in 8–12 hrs, then every morning on arising and before evening meal. **Children:** 0.5 mg/kg (same regimen).

Prevention of nausea, vomiting:

PO/IM/IV/RECTAL: **Adults, elderly:** 12.5–25 mg q4–6h as needed. **Children:** 0.25–1 mg/kg q4–6h as needed.

Pre- and postop sedation; adjunct to analgesics:

IM/IV: **Adults, elderly:** 25–50 mg. **Children:** 12.5–25 mg.

SIDE EFFECTS

HIGH INCIDENCE: Drowsiness, disorientation. Hypotension, confusion, syncope more likely noted in elderly. ***FREQUENT:*** Dry mouth, urinary retention, t... bronchial secretions. ...
AL: Epigastric distress... visual disturbances, hea... turbances, wheezing, pare... sweating, chills. ***RARE:*** Dizz... urticaria, photosensitivity, n... mares. Fixed-combination fc... with pseudoephedrine may... duce mild CNS stimulation.

ADVERSE REACTIONS/TOXIC EFFECTS

Paradoxical reaction (particularly in children) manifested as excitation, nervousness, tremor, hyperactive reflexes, convulsions. CNS depression has occurred in infants and young children (respiratory depression, sleep apnea, SIDS). Long-term therapy may produce extrapyramidal symptoms noted as dystonia (abnormal movements), pronounced motor restlessness (most frequently occurs in children), and parkinsonian symptoms (esp. noted in elderly). Blood dyscrasias, particularly agranulocytosis, have occurred.

NURSING IMPLICATIONS

BASELINE ASSESSMENT:

Assess B/P and pulse for bradycardia/tachycardia if pt is given parenteral form. If used as an antiemetic, assess for dehydration (poor skin turgor, dry mucous membranes, longitudinal furrows in tongue).

INTERVENTION/EVALUATION:

Monitor serum electrolytes in pts with severe vomiting. Assist with ambulation if drowsiness, lightheadedness occurs.

PATIENT/FAMILY TEACHING:

Drowsiness, dry mouth may be an expected response to drug.

Sugarless gum, sips of tepid water may relieve dry mouth. Coffee/tea may help reduce drowsiness. Report visual disturbances. Avoid tasks that require alertness, motor skills until response to drug is established. Avoid alcohol and other CNS depressants.

propafenone hydrochloride

pro-**pah**-phen-own
(Rythmol)

►CLASSIFICATION

CLINICAL: Antiarrhythmic (see p. 13C)

ACTION/*THERAPEUTIC EFFECT*

Decreases the fast sodium current in Purkinje/myocardial cells. *Decreases excitability, automaticity; prolongs conduction velocity, refractory period.* Greatest effects on Purkinje system.

USES/*UNLABELED*

Treatment of documented, life-threatening ventricular arrhythmias (e.g., sustained ventricular tachycardias). Prolongs time to recurrence of paroxysmal supraventricular tachycardia (PSVT) and paroxysmal atrial fibrillation/flutter (PAF) associated with disabling symptoms. *Treatment of supraventricular arrhythmias.*

PRECAUTIONS

CONTRAINDICATIONS: Uncontrolled CHF, cardiogenic shock, sinoatrial, AV and intraventricular disorders of impulse/conduction (sick-sinus syndrome [bradycardia-tachycardia], AV block) without presence of pacemaker, bradycardia, marked hypotension, bronchospastic disorders, manifest electrolyte imbalance. **CAUTIONS:** Impaired renal/hepatic function, recent myocardial infarction, CHF, conduction disturbances.

INTERACTIONS

DRUG: May increase concentrations of **digoxin, propranolol.** May increase effects of **warfarin.** **HERBAL:** None known. **FOOD:** None known. **LAB VALUES:** May cause EKG changes (e.g., QRS widening, PR prolongation), positive ANA titers.

AVAILABILITY (Rx)

TABLETS: 150 mg, 300 mg.

INDICATIONS/ROUTES/DOSAGE

Usual dosage:

PO: Adults, elderly: Initially, 150 mg q8h, may increase at 3–4 day intervals to 225 mg q8h, then to 300 mg q8h. **Maximum:** 900 mg/day.

SIDE EFFECTS

FREQUENT (7–13%): Dizziness, nausea, vomiting, unusual taste, constipation. **OCCASIONAL** (3–6%): Headache, dyspnea, blurred vision, dyspepsia (heartburn, indigestion, epigastric pain). **RARE** (<2%): Rash, weakness, dry mouth, diarrhea, rash, edema, hot flashes.

ADVERSE REACTIONS/TOXIC EFFECTS

May produce/worsen existing arrhythmias. Overdosage may produce hypotension, somnolence, bradycardia, intra-atrial and intraventricular conduction disturbances.

P

NURSING IMPLICATIONS

BASELINE ASSESSMENT:
Correct electrolyte imbalance before administering medication.

INTERVENTION/EVALUATION:
Assess pulse for strength/weakness, irregular rate. Monitor EKG for cardiac performance/changes, particularly widening of QRS, prolongation of PR interval. Question for visual disturbances, headache, GI upset. Monitor fluid, electrolyte serum levels. Monitor pattern of daily bowel activity, stool consistency. Assess for dizziness, unsteadiness. Monitor liver enzymes results. Monitor for therapeutic serum level (0.06–1 μ/ml).

PATIENT/FAMILY TEACHING:
Compliance with therapy regimen is essential to control arrhythmias. Unusual taste sensation may occur. Report headache, blurred vision, fever.

proparacaine

(AK-Taine, Alcaine, I-Paracaine, Kainair, Ophthaine, Ophthetic)

FIXED-COMBINATION(S)

With fluorescein, a water-soluble dye **(Fluoracaine, Ocu-Flurcaine, Parascein)**

See Classification section under: Anesthetics: local

propofol

pro-**poe**-foal
(Diprivan)

𝒪 - see color pill atlas

▶CLASSIFICATION

PHARMACOTHERAPEUTIC:
Rapid-acting general anesthetic. ***CLINICAL:*** Sedative-hypnotic (see p. 3C)

ACTION/*THERAPEUTIC EFFECT*

Inhibits sympathetic vasoconstrictor nerve activity, decreases vascular resistance. *Produces hypnosis rapidly.*

PHARMACOKINETICS

	Onset	Peak	Duration
IV	40 sec	—	—

Protein binding: 97–99%. Rapidly, extensively distributed. Metabolized in liver. Primarily excreted in urine. Unknown if removed by hemodialysis. Half-life: 3–12 hrs.

USES

Induction and maintenance of anesthesia. Continuous sedation in intubated/respiratory controlled adult pts in ICU.

PRECAUTIONS

CONTRAINDICATIONS: Increased intracranial pressure, impaired cerebral circulation. ***CAUTIONS:*** Debilitated, impaired respiratory, circulatory, renal, hepatic, lipid metabolism disorders.

▷***LIFESPAN CONSIDERATIONS:***
Pregnancy/Lactation: Unknown if drug crosses placenta. Distributed in breast milk. Not recommended for obstetrics, nursing mothers. **Pregnancy Category B. Children:** Safety and efficacy not established. FDA approved for use in those >3 yrs of age. **Elderly:** No age-related precautions noted; lower doses recommended.

INTERACTIONS

DRUG: **Alcohol, CNS depressants** may increase CNS, respiratory, depression, hypotensive effect. ***HERBAL:*** None known. ***FOOD:*** None known. ***LAB VALUES:*** None significant.

AVAILABILITY (Rx)

INJECTION: 10 mg/ml.

ADMINISTRATION/HANDLING
IV 💉

Note: Do not give through same IV line with blood or plasma.

Storage:

• Store at room temperature. • Discard unused portions. • Do not use if emulsion separates. • Shake well before using.

Reconstitution:

• May give undiluted, or dilute only with D_5W. • Do not dilute to concentration <2 mg/ml (4 ml D_5W to 1 ml propofol yields 2 mg/ml).

Rate of administration:

• A too-rapid IV may produce marked severe hypotension, respiratory depression, irregular muscular movements. • Observe for signs of intra-arterial injection (pain, discolored skin patches, white/blue color to hand, delayed onset of drug action). • Inadvertent intra-arterial injection may result in arterial spasm with severe pain, thrombosis, gangrene.

IV INCOMPATIBILITIES ⊘

Amikacin (Amikin), amphotericin B complex (Abelcet, Ambisome, Amphotec), bretylium (Bretylol), caclium chloride, ciprofloxacin (Cipro), diazepam (Valium), digoxin (Lanoxin), doxorubicin (Adriamycin), gentamicin (Garamycin), methylprednisolone (Solu-Medrol), minocycline (Minocin), phenytoin (Dilantin), tobramycin (Nebcin), verapamil (Isoptin).

IV COMPATIBILITIES

Acyclovir (Zovirax), bumetanide (Bumex), calcium gluconate, ceftazidime (Fortaz), dobutamine (Dobutrex), dopamine (Intropin), enalapril (Vasotec), fentanyl, heparin, insulin, labetalol (Normodyne, Trandate), lidocaine, lorazepam (Ativan), magnesium, milrinone (Primacor), nitroglycerin, norepinephrine (Levophed), potassium chloride, vancomycin (Vancocin).

INDICATIONS/ROUTES/DOSAGE
ICU sedation:

IV: **Adults, elderly:** Initially, 5 mcg/kg/min for at least 5 min until onset of peak effect. May increase by increments of 5–10 mcg/kg/min over 5–10 min intervals. **Maintenance:** 5–50 mcg/kg/min (some pts may require higher dosage).

Anesthesia:

IV: **Adults ASA I & II:** 2–2.5 mg/kg (about 40 mg q10sec until onset of anesthesia). ***IV:*** **Elderly, debilitated, hypovolemic, or ASA III or IV:** 1–1.5 mg/kg q10sec until onset of anesthesia.

Maintenance:

IV: **Adults ASA I & II:** 0.1–0.2 mg/kg/min. ***IV:*** **Elderly, debilitated, hypovolemic, or ASA III or IV:** 0.05–0.1 mg/kg/min.

SIDE EFFECTS

FREQUENT: Involuntary muscular movement, apnea (common during induction; lasts >60 sec), hypotension, nausea, vomiting, burning/stinging at IV site. ***OCCASIONAL:*** Twitching, bucking, jerking, thrashing, headache, dizziness, bradycardia, hypertension, fever, abdominal cramping, tingling, numbness, coldness, cough, hiccups, facial flushing. ***RARE:*** Rash, dry mouth, agitation, confusion, myalgia, thrombophlebitis.

ADVERSE REACTIONS/TOXIC EFFECTS

Continuous/repeated intermittent infusion may result in extreme somnolence, respiratory/circulatory depression. A too rapid IV may produce marked severe hypotension, respiratory depression, irregular muscular movements. Acute allergic reaction (erythema, pruritus, urticaria, rhinitis, dyspnea, hypotension, restlessness, anxiety, abdominal pain) may occur.

NURSING IMPLICATIONS

BASELINE ASSESSMENT:
Resuscitative equipment, endotracheal tube, suction, O_2 must be available. Obtain vital signs before administration.

INTERVENTION/EVALUATION:
Monitor for hypotension, bradycardia q3–5min during and after administration until recovery is achieved. Assess diligently for apnea during administration. Monitor for involuntary skeletal muscle movement.

propoxyphene hydrochloride

pro-**pox**-ih-feen
(Darvon)

FIXED-COMBINATION(S)
With aspirin, caffeine **(Darvon Compound-65)**; with acetaminophen **(Wygesic)**

propoxyphene napsylate

(Darvon-N✦)

FIXED-COMBINATION(S)
With acetaminophen **(Darvocet-N)**

▶**CLASSIFICATION**
PHARMACOTHERAPEUTIC: Opioid agonist **(Schedule IV).** ***CLINICAL:*** Analgesic (see p. 117C)

ACTION/*THERAPEUTIC EFFECT*
Binds with opioid receptors within CNS, *altering processes affecting pain perception, emotional response to pain.*

PHARMACOKINETICS

	Onset	Peak	Duration
PO	15–60 min	—	4–6 hrs

Well absorbed from GI tract. Protein binding: High. Widely distributed. Metabolized in liver. Primarily excreted in urine. Not removed by hemodialysis. Half-life: 6–12 hrs; metabolite: 30–36 hrs.

USES
Relief of mild to moderate pain.

PRECAUTIONS
CONTRAINDICATIONS: None significant. ***EXTREME CAUTION:*** Severe CNS depression, anoxia, hypercapnia, respiratory depression, seizures, acute alcoholism, shock, untreated myxedema, respiratory dysfunction. ***CAUTIONS:*** Increased intracranial pressure, impaired hepatic function, acute abdominal conditions, hypothyroidism, prosta-

tic hypertrophy, Addison's disease, urethral stricture, COPD.

▷**LIFESPAN CONSIDERATIONS:**
Pregnancy/Lactation: Crosses placenta; minimal amount distributed in breast milk. Respiratory depression may occur in neonate if mother received opiates during labor. Regular use of opiates during pregnancy may produce withdrawal symptoms in neonate (irritability, excessive crying, tremors, hyperactive reflexes, fever, vomiting, diarrhea, yawning, sneezing, seizures). **Pregnancy Category C** (Category D if used for prolonged periods). **Children:** Dosage not established. **Elderly:** More susceptible to respiratory depressant effects. Age-related renal impairment may increase susceptibility to urinary retention.

INTERACTIONS

DRUG: Alcohol, CNS depressants may increase CNS or respiratory depression, risk of hypotension. May increase concentration, toxicity of **carbamazepine.** Effects may be decreased with **buprenorphine. MAO inhibitors** may produce severe, fatal reaction (reduce to ¼ usual dose). **HERBAL:** None known. **FOOD:** None known. **VALUES:** May increase amylase, SGOT (AST), SGPT (ALT), LDH, alkaline phosphatase, bilirubin. Therapeutic blood serum level: 100–400 ng/ml; toxic blood serum level: >500 ng/ml.

AV...
Hy...**Y (Rx)**
mode: **CAPSULES:** 32
Na...
SUBLETS: 100 mg.
0 mg/ml.
ADN...
PO: ./HANDLING
• Gi...
.ard to meals. •

Capsules may be emptied and mixed with food. • Shake oral suspension well. • Do not crush or break film-coated tablets.

INDICATIONS/ROUTES/DOSAGE

Note: Reduce initial dosage in those with hypothyroidism, concurrent CNS depressants, Addison's disease, renal insufficiency, elderly/debilitated.

Propoxyphene hydrochloride:
PO: Adults, elderly: 65 mg q4h, as needed. **Maximum:** 390 mg/day.

Propoxyphene napsylate:
PO: Adults, elderly: 100 mg q4h, as needed. **Maximum:** 600 mg/day.

SIDE EFFECTS

Note: Effects dependent on dosage amount. Ambulatory pts and those not in moderate pain may experience dizziness, nausea, vomiting, hypotension more frequently than those in supine position or having moderate pain.

FREQUENT: Dizziness, drowsiness, dry mouth, euphoria, hypotension, nausea, vomiting, unusual tiredness. **OCCASIONAL:** Histamine reaction (decreased B/P, increased sweating, flushing, wheezing), trembling, decreased urination, altered vision, constipation, headache. **RARE:** Confusion, increased B/P, depression, stomach cramps, anorexia.

ADVERSE REACTIONS/TOXIC EFFECTS

Overdosage results in respiratory depression, skeletal muscle flaccidity, cold clammy skin, cyanosis, extreme somnolence progressing to convulsions, stupor, coma. Hepatotoxicity may occur with overdosage of acetaminophen component. Tolerance to analgesic effect,

P

✳ - see also www.wbsaunders.com/SIMON/SaundersNDH

physical dependence may occur with repeated use.

NURSING IMPLICATIONS

BASELINE ASSESSMENT:

Obtain vital signs before giving medication. If respirations are 12/min or lower (20/min or lower in children), withhold medication, contact physician. Assess onset, type, location, and duration of pain. Effect of medication is reduced if full pain recurs before next dose.

INTERVENTION/EVALUATION:

Palpate bladder for urinary retention. Monitor pattern of daily bowel activity, stool consistency. Initiate deep breathing and coughing exercises, particularly in those with impaired pulmonary function. Assess for clinical improvement, record onset of relief of pain. Contact physician if pain is not adequately relieved. Therapeutic blood serum level: 100–400 ng/ml; toxic blood serum level: >500 ng/ml.

PATIENT/FAMILY TEACHING:

Change positions slowly to avoid orthostatic hypotension. Avoid tasks that require alertness, motor skills until response to drug is established. Tolerance/dependence may occur with prolonged use of high doses.

propranolol hydrochloride

pro-**pran**-oh-lol
(Apo-Propranolol ♣, Inderal)
Do not confuse with Adderall, Isordil, Pravachol.

FIXED-COMBINATION(S)

With hydrochlorothiazide, a diuretic **(Inderide)**

►CLASSIFICATION

PHARMACOTHERAPEUTIC:
Beta-adrenergic blocker. **CLINICAL:** Antihypertensive, antianginal, antiarrhythmic, antimigraine (see pp. 13C, 61C)

ACTION/THERAPEUTIC EFFECT

Blocks beta$_1$-adrenergic receptors, *slowing sinus heart rate, decreasing cardiac output, decreasing B/P.* Blocks beta$_2$-adrenergic receptors, *increasing airway resistance. Decreases myocardial ischemia severity* by decreasing O_2 requirements. Slows AV conduction, increases refractory period in AV node; *exhibits antiarrhythmic activity.*

PHARMACOKINETICS

Onset	Peak	Duration
PO		
—	60–90 min	—
PO (long-acting)		
—	6 hrs	—
IV		
Immediate	1 min	—

Almost completely absorbed fr[om] GI tract. Protein binding: 9[ ]. Widely distributed. Metabol[ized] in liver. Primarily excrete[d in] urine. Not removed by hemo[dialy]sis. Half-life: 3–5 hrs.

USES/UNLABELED

Treatment of hypertension[,] various cardiac arrhythm[ias,] pertrophic subaortic ster[osis, mi]graine headache, essenti[al tremor] and as an adjunct to al[pha-block]ing agents in the tre[atment of] pheochromocytoma. [To re]duce risk of cardiovasc[ular mortal]ity and reinfarction in [

previously suffered a myocardial infarction (MI). *Treatment of adjunct anxiety, thyrotoxicosis, mitral valve prolapse syndrome.*

PRECAUTIONS

CONTRAINDICATIONS: Bronchial asthma, COPD, uncontrolled cardiac failure, sinus bradycardia, heart block greater than first degree, cardiogenic shock, CHF, unless secondary to tachyarrhythmias, those on MAO inhibitors. ***CAUTIONS:*** Inadequate cardiac function, impaired renal/hepatic function, those with Wolff-Parkinson-White syndrome, diabetes mellitus, hyperthyroidism.

▷***LIFESPAN CONSIDERATIONS:*** **Pregnancy/Lactation:** Crosses placenta; is distributed in breast milk. Avoid use during first trimester. May produce bradycardia, apnea, hypoglycemia, hypothermia during delivery, small birth weight infants. **Pregnancy Category C** (Category D if used in second or third trimester). **Children:** No age-related precautions noted. **Elderly:** Age-related peripheral vascular disease may increase susceptibility to decreased peripheral circulation.

INTERACTIONS

DRUG: **Diuretics, other hypotensives** may increase hypotensive effect. **Sympathomimetics, xanthines** may mutually inhibit effects. May mask symptoms of hypoglycemia, prolong hypoglycemic effect of **insulin, oral hypoglycemics. NSAIDs** may decrease antihypertensive effect. May increase cardiac depressant effect with **IV phenytoin. HERBAL:** None known. ***FOOD:*** None known. ***LAB VALUES:*** May increase ANA titer, SGOT (AST), SGPT (ALT), alkaline phosphatase, LDH, bilirubin, BUN, creatinine, potassium, uric acid, lipoproteins, triglycerides.

AVAILABILITY (Rx)

TABLETS: 10 mg, 20 mg, 40 mg, 60 mg, 80 mg, 90 mg. ***CAPSULES (sustained-release):*** 60 mg, 80 mg, 120 mg, 160 mg. ***ORAL SOLUTION:*** 4 mg/ml, 8 mg/ml. ***SOLUTION (concentrate):*** 80 mg/ml. ***INJECTION:*** 1 mg/ml.

ADMINISTRATION/HANDLING

PO:
• May crush scored tablets. • Give at same time each day.

IV 🖥

Storage:
• Store at room temperature.

Reconstitution:
• Give undiluted for IV push. • For IV infusion, may dilute each 1 mg in 10 ml D_5W.

Rate of administration:
• Do not exceed 1 mg/min injection rate. • For IV infusion, give 1 mg over 10–15 min.

IV INCOMPATIBILITIES ⊘

Amphotericin B complex (Abelcet, Ambisome, Amphotec).

IV COMPATIBILITIES

Alteplase (Activase), heparin, milrinone (Primacor), potassium chloride, propofol (Diprivan).

INDICATIONS/ROUTES/DOSAGE

Hypertension:

PO: Adults, elderly: Initially, 40 mg 2 times/day or 80 mg daily as extended-release capsule. Increase at 3–7 day intervals. **Maintenance:** 120–240 mg/day as tablets or oral solution, 120–160 mg/day as extended-release capsules. **Maximum:** 640 mg/day.

Children: Initially, 0.5–1 mg/kg/day in 2–4 divided doses. Increase at 3–5 day intervals. **Maximum:** 8 mg/kg/day.

Angina pectoris:

PO: Adults, elderly: Initially, 80–320 mg/day in 2–4 divided doses or 80 mg/day (sustained-release). **Maximum:** 320 mg/day. **Maintenance:** 160 mg/day.

Cardiac arrhythmias:

PO: Adults, elderly: 10–30 mg 3–4 times/day.

Life-threatening arrhythmias:

IV: Adults, elderly: 0.5–3 mg. Repeat once in 2 min. Give additional doses at intervals of at least 4 hrs. **Children:** 0.01–0.1 mg/kg.

Hypertrophic subaortic stenosis:

PO: Adults, elderly: 20–40 mg in 3–4 divided doses or 80–160 mg/day as extended-release capsule.

Pheochromocytoma:

PO: Adults, elderly: 60 mg/day in divided doses with alpha-blocker for 3 days before surgery. **Maintenance (inoperable tumor):** 30 mg/day with alpha-blocker.

Migraine headache:

PO: Adults, elderly: 80 mg/day in divided doses or 80 mg once daily as extended-release capsule. Increase up to 160–240 mg/day in divided doses. **Children:** 0.6–1.5 mg/kg/day in divided doses q8h. **Maximum:** 4 mg/kg/day.

Myocardial infarction:

PO: Adults, elderly: 180–240 mg/day in divided doses beginning 5–21 days after MI.

Essential tremor:

PO: Adults, elderly: Initially, 40 mg 2 times/day increased up to 120–320 mg/day in 3 divided doses.

SIDE EFFECTS

FREQUENT: Decreased sexual ability, drowsiness, difficulty sleeping, unusual tiredness/weakness. **OCCASIONAL:** Bradycardia, depression, cold hands/feet, diarrhea, constipation, anxiety, nasal congestion, nausea, vomiting. **RARE:** Altered taste, dry eyes, itching, numbness of fingers, toes, scalp.

ADVERSE REACTIONS/TOXIC EFFECTS

May produce profound bradycardia, hypotension. Abrupt withdrawal may result in sweating, palpitations, headache, tremulousness. May precipitate CHF, MI in those with cardiac disease, thyroid storm in those with thyrotoxicosis, peripheral ischemia in those with existing peripheral vascular disease. Hypoglycemia may occur in previously controlled diabetics.

NURSING IMPLICATIONS

BASELINE ASSESSMENT:

Assess baseline renal/liver function tests. Assess B/P, apical pulse immediately before drug is administered (if pulse is 60/min or below or systolic B/P is below 90 mm Hg, withhold medication, contact physician). **Anginal:** Record onset, type (sharp, dull, squeezing), radiation, location, intensity, and duration of anginal pain and precipitating factors (exertion, emotional stress).

INTERVENTION/EVALUATION:

Assess pulse for strength/weakness, irregular rate, bradycardia. Monitor EKG for cardiac arrhythmias. Assess fingers for color, numbness (Raynaud's). Assess for evidence of CHF (dyspnea [particularly on exertion or lying down], night cough, peripheral edema, distended neck veins). Monitor I&O (increase in weight, decrease in urine output may indicate CHF). Assess for rash, fatigue, behavioral changes. Therapeutic response ranges from a few days to several wks. Measure B/P near end of dosing interval (determines if B/P is controlled throughout day).

PATIENT/FAMILY TEACHING:

Do not abruptly discontinue medication. Compliance with therapy regimen is essential to control hypertension, arrhythmia, anginal pain. To avoid hypotensive effect, rise slowly from lying to sitting position, wait momentarily before standing. Avoid tasks that require alertness, motor skills until response to drug is established. Report excessively slow pulse rate (<60 beats/min), peripheral numbness, dizziness. Do not use nasal decongestants, OTC cold preparations (stimulants) without physician approval. Restrict salt, alcohol intake.

propylthiouracil

pro-pill-thye-oh-**your**-ah-sill
(Propylthiouracil, Propyl-
Thyracil✤)

▶CLASSIFICATION

PHARMACOTHERAPEUTIC:
Thiourea derivative. ***CLINICAL:***
Antithyroid

ACTION/*THERAPEUTIC EFFECT*

In hyperthyroidism, *inhibits synthesis of thyroid hormone.* Diverts iodine from thyroid hormone synthesis.

USES

Palliative treatment of hyperthyroidism; adjunct to ameliorate hyperthyroidism in preparation for surgical treatment or radioactive iodine therapy.

PRECAUTIONS

CONTRAINDICATIONS: None significant. ***CAUTIONS:*** Pts >40 yrs of age or in combination with other agranulocytosis-inducing drugs.

INTERACTIONS

DRUG: Amiodarone, iodinated glycerol, iodine, potassium iodide may decrease response. May decrease effect of **oral anticoagulants.** May increase concentration of **digoxin** (as pt becomes euthyroid). May decrease thyroid uptake of I[131]. ***HERBAL:*** None known. ***FOOD:*** None known. ***LAB VALUES:*** May increase SGOT (AST), SGPT (ALT), alkaline phosphatase, LDH, bilirubin, prothrombin time.

AVAILABILTIY (Rx)

TABLETS: 50 mg.

INDICATIONS/ROUTES/DOSAGE

Hyperthyroidism:

PO: Adults, elderly: Initially: 300–400 mg/day. **Maintenance:** 100–150 mg/day. **Children (6–10 yrs):** Initially: 50–150 mg/day; **(>10 yrs):** 150–300 mg/day. **Maintenance:** Determined by pt response.

SIDE EFFECTS

FREQUENT: Urticaria, rash, pruritus, nausea, skin pigmentation, hair loss, headache, paresthesia. ***OCCASIONAL:*** Drowsiness, lymphadenopathy, vertigo. **RARE:** Drug fever, lupuslike syndrome.

ADVERSE REACTIONS/TOXIC EFFECTS

Agranulocytosis (may occur as long as 4 mos after therapy), pancytopenia, fatal hepatitis have occurred.

NURSING IMPLICATIONS

BASELINE ASSESSMENT:

Obtain baseline weight, pulse.

INTERVENTION/EVALUATION:

Monitor pulse, weight daily. Check for skin eruptions, itching, swollen lymph glands. Be alert to hepatitis (nausea, vomiting, drowsiness, jaundice). Monitor hematology results for bone marrow suppression; check for signs of infection/bleeding.

PATIENT/FAMILY TEACHING:

Space evenly around the clock. Take resting pulse daily (teach pt/family), report as directed. Seafood, iodine products may be restricted. Report illness, unusual bleeding/bruising immediately. Inform physician of sudden/continuous weight gain, cold intolerance, or depression.

protamine sulfate

pro-tah-meen
(Protamine ♣, Protamine sulfate)
Do not confuse with
ProAmatine, Protopam, Protripin.

▶ CLASSIFICATION

PHARMACOTHERAPEUTIC:
Protein. ***CLINICAL:*** Heparin antagonist

ACTION/*THERAPEUTIC EFFECT*

Complexes with heparin to form a stable salt, *resulting in reduction of anticoagulant activity of heparin.*

USES/*UNLABELED*

Treatment of severe heparin overdose (causing hemorrhage). Neutralizes effects of heparin administered during extracorporeal circulation. *Treatment of enoxaparin toxicity.*

PRECAUTIONS

CONTRAINDICATIONS: None significant. ***CAUTIONS:*** History of allergy to fish, vasectomized/infertile men, those on isophane (NPH) insulin or previous protamine therapy (propensity to hypersensitivity reaction).

INTERACTIONS

DRUG: None significant. ***HERBAL:*** None known. ***FOOD:*** None known. ***LAB VALUES:*** None significant.

AVAILABILTIY (Rx)

INJECTION: 10 mg/ml.

INDICATIONS/ROUTES/DOSAGE

Antidote:

IV: Adults, elderly: 1 mg protamine sulfate neutralizes 90–115 units of heparin. Heparin disappears rapidly from circulation, reducing the dosage demand for protamine as time elapses.

SIDE EFFECTS

FREQUENT: Decreased B/P, dyspnea. ***OCCASIONAL:*** Hypersensitivity reaction: urticaria, angioedema; nausea, vomiting (generally occurs in those sensitive to fish, vasectomized or infertile men, those on isophane [NPH], insulin, or previous protamine therapy). ***RARE:*** Back pain.

ADVERSE REACTIONS/TOXIC EFFECTS

A too-rapid IV administration may

produce acute hypotension, bradycardia, pulmonary hypertension, dyspnea, transient flushing, feeling of warmth. Heparin rebound may occur several hrs after heparin has been neutralized by protamine (usually evident 8–9 hrs after protamine administration). Occurs most often following arterial/cardiac surgery.

NURSING IMPLICATIONS

BASELINE ASSESSMENT:
Check prothrombin time, activated partial thromboplastin time (APTT), hematocrit; assess for bleeding.

INTERVENTION/EVALUATION:
Monitor pts closely after cardiac surgery for evidence of hyperheparinemia/bleeding. Monitor APTT or activated coagulation time (ACT) 5–15 min after protamine administration. Because of possibility of heparin rebound, repeat tests in 2–8 hrs. Assess hematocrit, platelet count, urine/stool culture for occult blood. Assess for decrease in B/P, increase in pulse rate, complaint of abdominal/back pain, severe headache (may be evidence of hemorrhage). Question for increase in amount of discharge during menses. Assess peripheral pulses; skin for bruises, petechiae. Check for excessive bleeding from minor cuts, scratches. Assess gums for erythema, gingival bleeding. Assess urine output for hematuria.

protriptyline hydrochloride

(Vivactil)

See Classification section under: Antidepressants (p. 35C)

pseudoephedrine hydrochloride

su-do-eh-**fed**-rin
(Eltor♣, Novafed, Sudafed)

pseudoephedrine sulfate

(Afrinol Repetabs)

FIXED-COMBINATION(S)

With acrivastine, an antihistamine **(Semprex-D);** with loratidine, an antihistamine **(Claritin-D);** with cetirizine, an antihistamine **(Zyrtec D 12 Hour);** with fexofenidine, an antihistamine **(Allegra-D)**

▶**CLASSIFICATION**

PHARMACOTHERAPEUTIC: Sympathomimetic. *CLINICAL:* Nasal decongestant

ACTION/*THERAPEUTIC EFFECT*

Acts directly on alpha-adrenergic receptors and, to lesser extent, on beta-adrenergic receptors, *producing vasoconstriction of respiratory tract mucosa, resulting in shrinkage of nasal mucous membranes, edema, nasal congestion.* Produces little, if any, rebound nasal congestion.

PHARMACOKINETICS

Onset	Peak	Duration
Tablets, syrup		
15–30 min	—	4–6 hrs
Extended-release		
—	—	8–12 hrs

Well absorbed from GI tract. Partially metabolized in liver. Primarily excreted in urine. Not removed by hemodialysis. Half-life: 9–16 hrs.

P

USES

For nasal congestion, treatment of obstructed eustachian ostia in those with otic inflammation, infection.

PRECAUTIONS

CONTRAINDICATIONS: Severe hypertension, coronary artery disease, lactating women, MAO inhibitor therapy. ***CAUTIONS:*** Elderly, hyperthyroidism, diabetes, ischemic heart disease, prostatic hypertrophy.

▷***LIFESPAN CONSIDERATIONS:***
Pregnancy/Lactation: Crosses placenta; is distributed in breast milk. **Pregnancy Category C. Children:** Safety and efficacy not established in those <2 yrs of age. **Elderly:** Age-related prostatic hypertrophy may require dosage adjustment.

INTERACTIONS

DRUG: May decrease effects of **antihypertensive, diuretics, beta-adrenergic blockers. MAO inhibitors** may increase cardiac stimulant, vasopressor effects. ***HERBAL:*** Ma Huang (Ephedra) may increase CNS stimulation. ***FOOD:*** None known. ***LAB VALUES:*** None significant.

AVAILABILITY (OTC)

TABLETS: 30 mg, 60 mg. ***TABLETS (extended-release):*** 120 mg, 240 mg. ***CAPSULES:*** 60 mg. ***CAPSULES (extended-release):*** 120 mg. ***LIQUID:*** 15 mg/5 ml, 30 mg/5 ml. ***DROPS:*** 7.5 mg/0.8 ml.

ADMINISTRATION/HANDLING
PO:

• Do not crush, chew extended-release tablets; swallow whole.

✐ - see color pill atlas

INDICATIONS/ROUTES/DOSAGE
Decongestant:

PO: Adults, children >12 yrs: 60 mg q4–6h. **Maximum:** 240 mg/day. **Children 6–12 yrs:** 30 mg q6h. **Maximum:** 120 mg/day. **Children 2–5 yrs:** 15 mg q6h. **Maximum:** 60 mg/day. **Children <2 yrs:** 4 mg/kg/day in divided doses q6h

Usual elderly dose:

PO: 30–60 mg q6h as needed.

Extended-release:

PO: Adults, children >12 yrs: 120 mg q12h.

SIDE EFFECTS

OCCASIONAL (5–10%): Nervousness, restlessness, insomnia, trembling, headache. ***RARE*** (1–4%): Increased sweating, weakness.

ADVERSE REACTIONS/TOXIC EFFECTS

Large doses may produce tachycardia, palpitations (particularly in those with cardiac disease), light-headedness, nausea, vomiting. Overdosage in those >60 yrs may result in hallucinations, CNS depression, seizures.

NURSING IMPLICATIONS

PATIENT/FAMILY TEACHING
Discontinue drug if adverse reactions occur. Report insomnia, dizziness, tremors, rapid or irregular heartbeat.

psyllium

sill-ee-um
(Fiberall, Hydrocil, Konsyl, Metamucil, Perdiem, Prodiem Plain✦)

►CLASSIFICATION

PHARMACOTHERAPEUTIC:
Bulk-forming laxative (see p. 99C)

ACTION/*THERAPEUTIC EFFECT*

Powder, wafer dissolves and swells in water (provides increased bulk, moisture content in stool). *Increased bulk promotes peristalsis, bowel motility.*

PHARMACOKINETICS

	Onset	Peak	Duration
PO	12–72 hrs	—	—

Acts in small/large intestine.

USES

Prophylaxis in those who should not strain during defecation. Facilitates defecation in those with diminished colonic motor response.

PRECAUTIONS

CONTRAINDICATIONS: Abdominal pain, nausea, vomiting, symptoms of appendicitis, partial bowel obstruction, dysphagia. *CAUTIONS:* None significant.

▷*LIFESPAN CONSIDERATIONS:* **Pregnancy/Lactation:** Safe for use in pregnancy. **Pregnancy Category C. Children:** Safety and efficacy not established for those <6 yrs of age. **Elderly:** No age-related precautions noted.

INTERACTIONS

DRUG: May interfere with effects of **potassium-sparing diuretics, potassium supplements.** May decrease effect of **oral anticoagulants, digoxin, salicylates** by decreasing absorption. *HERBAL:* None known. *FOOD:* None known.

LAB VALUES: May increase glucose. May decrease potassium.

AVAILABILITY (OTC)
POWDER. WAFER.

ADMINISTRATION/HANDLING

PO:

• Drink 6–8 glasses of water/day (aids stool softening). • Do not swallow in dry form; mix with at least 1 full glass (8 oz) liquid.

INDICATIONS/ROUTES/DOSAGE

Laxative:

PO: Adults, elderly: 1–2 rounded tsp, packet, or wafer in water 1–4 times/day. **Children 6–11 yrs:** ½–1 tsp in water 1–3 times/day

SIDE EFFECTS

RARE: Some degree of abdominal discomfort, nausea, mild cramps, griping, faintness.

ADVERSE REACTIONS/TOXIC EFFECTS

Esophageal/bowel obstruction may occur if administered with insufficient liquid (less than 250 ml or 1 full glass).

P

NURSING IMPLICATIONS

INTERVENTION/EVALUATION:

Encourage adequate fluid intake. Assess bowel sounds for peristalsis. Monitor daily bowel activity, stool consistency (watery, loose, soft, semisolid, solid). Monitor serum electrolytes in those exposed to prolonged, frequent, or excessive use of medication.

PATIENT/FAMILY TEACHING:

Institute measures to promote defecation (increase fluid intake, exercise, high-fiber diet).

pyrazinamide

peer-a-**zin**-a-mide
(Pyrazinamide, Tebrazid✦)

FIXED-COMBINATION(S)
With ioniazid and rifampin, anti-tuberculars **(Rifater)**

▶**CLASSIFICATION**
CLINICAL: Antitubercular

ACTION/THERAPEUTIC EFFECT
Exact mechanism unknown. *Either bacteriostatic or bactericidal, depending on its concentration at infection site and susceptibility of infecting bacteria.*

USES
In conjunction with at least one other antitubercular agent in treatment of clinical tuberculosis after failure of primary agents (isoniazid, rifampin).

PRECAUTIONS
CONTRAINDICATIONS: Severe hepatic dysfunction. **CAUTIONS:** Diabetes mellitus, renal impairment, history of gout, children (safety not established). Possible cross-sensitivity with isoniazid, ethionamide, niacin.

INTERACTIONS
DRUG: May decrease effects of **allopurinol, colchicine, probenecid, sulfinpyrazone. HERBAL:** None known. **FOOD:** None known. **LAB VALUES:** May increase SGOT (AST), SGPT (ALT), uric acid concentrations.

AVAILABILITY (Rx)
TABLETS: 500 mg.

𝒫 - see color pill atlas

INDICATIONS/ROUTES/DOSAGE
Tuberculosis:
PO: Adults: 15–30 mg/kg/day in 1–4 doses. **Maximum:** 3 g/day. **Children:** 20–40 mg/kg/day in 1 or 2 doses. **Maximum:** 2 g/day.

SIDE EFFECTS
FREQUENT: Arthralgia, myalgia (usually mild and self-limiting). **RARE:** Hypersensitivity (rash, urticaria, pruritus), photosensitivity.

ADVERSE REACTIONS/TOXIC EFFECTS
Hepatoxicity, thrombocytopenia, anemia occurs rarely.

NURSING IMPLICATIONS

BASELINE ASSESSMENT:
Question for hypersensitivity to pyrazinamide, isoniazid, ethionamide, niacin. Assure collection of specimens for culture, sensitivity. Evaluate results of initial CBC, hepatic function tests, uric acid levels.

INTERVENTION/EVALUATION:
Monitor hepatic function results and be alert for hepatic reactions: jaundice, malaise, fever, liver tenderness, anorexia/nausea/vomiting (stop drug, notify physician promptly). Check serum uric acid levels and assess for hot, painful, swollen joints, esp. big toe, ankle, or knee (gout). Evaluate blood sugars, diabetic status carefully (pyrazinamide makes management difficult). Assess for rash, skin eruptions. Monitor CBC for thrombocytopenia, anemia.

PATIENT/FAMILY TEACHING:
Do not skip doses; complete full length of therapy (may be mos,

yrs). Office visits, lab tests are essential part of treatment. Take with food to reduce GI upset. Avoid too much sun or ultraviolet light until photosensitivity is determined. Notify physician of any new symptom, immediately for yellow eyes or skin; unusual tiredness; fever; loss of appetite; hot, painful, or swollen joints.

pyridostigmine bromide

pier-id-oh-**stig**-meen
(Mestinon, Regonol)
Do not confuse with Mesantoin, Metatensin, physotigmine, Renagel, Reglan, Regroton.

▶CLASSIFICATION

PHARMACOTHERAPEUTIC:
Anticholinesterase. **CLINICAL:**
Cholinergic muscle stimulant (see p. 77C)

ACTION/THERAPEUTIC EFFECT

Prevents destruction of acetylcholine by enzyme, anticholinesterase. *Produces miosis, increases tone of intestinal and skeletal muscles, stimulates salivary, sweat gland secretions.*

USES

Improvement of muscle strength in control of myasthenia gravis, reversal of effects of nondepolarizing neuromuscular blocking agents after surgery.

PRECAUTIONS

CONTRAINDICATIONS: Mechanical GI, urinary obstruction. **CAUTIONS:** Bronchial asthma, bradycardia, epilepsy, recent coronary occlusion, vagotonia, hyperthy-

roidism, cardiac arrhythmias, peptic ulcer.

INTERACTIONS

DRUG: Anticholinergics reverse/prevent effects. **Cholinesterase inhibitors** may increase toxicity. Antagonizes **neuromuscular blocking agents. Quinidine, procainamide** may antagonize action. **HERBAL:** None known. **FOOD:** None known. **LAB VALUES:** None significant.

AVAILABILITY (Rx)

TABLETS: 60 mg. **TABLETS (sustained-release):** 180 mg. **SYRUP:** 60 mg/5 ml. **INJECTION:** 5 mg/ml.

ADMINISTRATION/HANDLING

PO:

• Give with food or milk. • Tablets may be crushed; do not chew, crush extended-release tablets (may be broken). • Give larger dose at times of increased fatigue (e.g., for those with difficulty in chewing, 30–45 min before meals).

IM/IV ▧

• Give large parenteral doses concurrently with 0.6–1.2 mg atropine sulfate IV to minimize side effects.

IV INCOMPATIBILITY ⊘

Do not mix with any other medications.

INDICATIONS/ROUTES/DOSAGE

Note: Dosage, frequency of administration dependent on daily clinical pt response (remissions, exacerbations, physical and emotional stress).

Myasthenia gravis:

PO: Adults, elderly: Initially, 60

P

mg 3 times/day. Increase dose at intervals of 48 hrs or more until therapeutic response is achieved. When increased dosage does not produce further increase in muscle strength, reduce dose to previous dosage level. **Maintenance:** 60–1,500 mg/day. **Children:** Initially, 7 mg/kg/day in 5–6 divided doses.

***EXTENDED-RELEASE:* Adults, elderly:** 180–540 mg 1–2 times/day (must maintain at least 6 hrs between doses).

***IM/IV:* Adults, elderly:** 2 mg q2–3h.

***PO:* Neonate:** 5 mg q4–6h.

***IM:* Neonate:** 0.05–0.15 mg/kg q4–6h.

Reversal of nondepolarizing muscle relaxants:

***IV:* Adults, elderly:** 10–20 mg with, or shortly after, 0.6–1.2 mg atropine sulfate or 0.3–0.6 mg glycopyrrolate.

SIDE EFFECTS

COMMON: Miosis, increased GI and skeletal muscle tone, reduced pulse rate, constriction of bronchi and ureters, salivary and sweat gland secretion. ***OCCASIONAL:*** Headache, rash, slight temporary decrease in diastolic B/P with mild reflex tachycardia, short periods of atrial fibrillation in hyperthyroid pts. Hypertensive pts may react with marked fall in B/P.

ADVERSE REACTIONS/TOXIC EFFECTS

Overdosage may produce a *cholinergic crisis,* manifested by increasingly severe muscle weakness (appears first in muscles involving chewing, swallowing, followed by muscular weakness of shoulder girdle and upper extremities), respiratory muscle paralysis followed by pelvis girdle and leg muscle paralysis. Requires withdrawal of all cholinergic drugs and immediate use of 1–4 mg atropine sulfate IV for adults, 0.01 mg/kg in infants and children <12 yrs.

NURSING IMPLICATIONS

BASELINE ASSESSMENT:

Larger doses should be given at time of greatest fatigue. Assess muscle strength before testing for diagnosis of myasthenia gravis and after drug administration. Avoid large doses in those with megacolon or reduced GI motility. Have tissues readily available at pt's bedside.

INTERVENTION/EVALUATION:

Monitor respirations closely during myasthenia gravis testing or if dosage is increased. Assess diligently for cholinergic reaction, as well as bradycardia in the myasthenic pt in crisis. Coordinate dosage time vs. periods of fatigue and increased/decreased muscle strength. Monitor for therapeutic response to medication (increased muscle strength, decreased fatigue, improved chewing, swallowing functions).

PATIENT/FAMILY TEACHING:

Report nausea, vomiting, diarrhea, sweating, increased salivary secretions, irregular heartbeat, muscle weakness, severe abdominal pain, or difficulty in breathing.

---

pyridoxine hydrochloride (vitamin B₆)

pie-rih-**docks**-in
(Hexa-Betalin✚, Pyridoxine)
Do not confuse with paroxetine, pralidoxime, Pyridium.

▶CLASSIFICATION

PHARMACOTHERAPEUTIC:
Coenzyme. ***CLINICAL:*** Vitamin (B₆) (see p. 128C)

ACTION/*THERAPEUTIC EFFECT*

Coenzyme for various metabolic functions *affecting protein, carbohydrate, lipid utilization.*

PHARMACOKINETICS

Readily absorbed primarily in jejunum. Stored in liver, muscle, brain. Metabolized in liver. Primarily excreted in urine. Removed by hemodialysis. Half-life: 15–20 days.

USES

Prevention, treatment of pyridoxine deficiency caused by inadequate diet, drug-induced (e.g., INH, penicillamine, cyclosporine) or inborn error of metabolism. Treatment of INH poisoning. Treatment of seizures in neonate unresponsive to conventional therapy. Treatment of sideroblastic anemia associated with increased serum iron concentrations.

PRECAUTIONS

CONTRAINDICATIONS: IV therapy in cardiac pts. ***CAUTIONS:*** Megadosage in pregnancy.
▷*LIFESPAN CONSIDERATIONS:*
Pregnancy/Lactation: Crosses placenta; is excreted in breast milk. High doses in utero may produce seizures in neonates. **Pregnancy Category A** (Category C if doses above RDA). **Children/Elderly:** No age-related precautions noted.

INTERACTIONS

DRUG:* Immunosuppressants, isoniazid, penicillamine** may antagonize pyridoxine (may cause anemia/peripheral neuritis). Reverses effects of **levodopa. *HERBAL: None known. ***FOOD:*** None known. ***LAB VALUES:*** None significant.

AVAILABILITY (OTC)

TABLETS: 25 mg, 50 mg, 100 mg.
TABLETS (time-release): 100 mg.
INJECTION (Rx): 100 mg/ml.

ADMINISTRATION/HANDLING

Note: Give orally unless nausea, vomiting, or malabsorption occurs. Avoid IV use in cardiac pts.

IV ▥

• Give undiluted or add to IV solutions and give as infusion.

IV INCOMPATIBILITY ⊘

Do not mix iwth any other medications.

INDICATIONS/ROUTES/DOSAGE

Pyridoxine deficiency:

PO: Adults, elderly: (Diet): 2.5–10 mg/day; after signs of deficiency decrease, 2.5–5 mg/day for several wks. ***(Drug-induced):*** 10–50 mg/day (INH, penicillamine); 100–300 mg/day (cyclosporine). ***(Error metabolism):*** 100–500 mg/day. **Children:** 5–25 mg/day for 3 wks, then 1.5–2.5 mg/day.

P

Seizures in neonates:

IM/IV: **Neonates:** 10–100 mg/day; then oral therapy of 2–100 mg/day for life.

Drug-induced neuritis:

PO: **Adults:** 100–300 mg/day in divided doses for 3 wks, then 25–100 mg/day. **Children:** 50–100 mg/day as treatment, then 1–2 mg/kg/day as prophylaxis.

Sideroblastic anemia:

PO: **Adults, elderly:** 200–600 mg/day. After adequate response, 30–50 mg/day for life.

SIDE EFFECTS

OCCASIONAL: Stinging at IM injection site. *RARE:* Headache, nausea, somnolence; high doses cause sensory neuropathy (paresthesia, unstable gait, clumsiness of hands).

ADVERSE REACTIONS/TOXIC EFFECTS

Long-term megadoses (2–6 g >2 mos) may produce sensory neuropathy (reduced deep tendon reflex, profound impairment of sense of position in distal limbs, gradual sensory ataxia). Toxic symptoms reverse with drug discontinuance. Seizures have occurred following IV megadoses.

NURSING IMPLICATIONS

INTERVENTION/EVALUATION:

Observe for improvement of deficiency symptoms, including nervous system abnormalities (anxiety, depression, insomnia, motor difficulty, peripheral numbness and tremors), skin lesions (glossitis, seborrhealike lesions around mouth, nose, eyes). Evaluate for nutritional adequacy.

PATIENT/FAMILY TEACHING:

Discomfort may occur with IM injection. Foods rich in pyridoxine include legumes, soybeans, eggs, sunflower seeds, hazelnuts, organ meats, tuna, shrimp, carrots, avocado, banana, wheat germ, bran.

quazepam

(Doral)

See Classification section under: Sedative-hypnotics (p. 123C)

quetiapine

kwe-**tie**-ah-peen
(Seroquel)

▶CLASSIFICATION

PHARMACOTHERAPEUTIC: Dibenzapine derivative. *CLINICAL:* Antipsychotic (see p. 56C)

ACTION/THERAPEUTIC EFFECT

Interacts with neurotransmitter receptors, including dopamine, serotonin, histamine, and alpha$_1$-adrenergic receptors, *diminishing psychotic disorders.* Produces moderate sedation, few extrapyramidal effects, no anticholinergic effects.

PHARMACOKINETICS

Well absorbed following PO administration. Protein binding: 83%. Highly bound to plasma proteins. Widely distributed in tissues; CNS concentration exceeds plasma concentration. Extensively metabolized by first-pass liver metabolism. Primarily excreted in the urine. Half-life: 6 hrs.

USES

Management of manifestations of psychotic disorders.

PRECAUTIONS

CONTRAINDICATIONS: None significant. ***CAUTIONS:*** Alzheimer's dementia, history of breast cancer, cardiovascular disease (e.g., CHF, history of myocardial infarction), cerebrovascular disease, impaired liver function, dehydration, hypovolemia, history of drug abuse or drug dependence, seizures, hypothyroidism.

▷*LIFESPAN CONSIDERATIONS:*
Pregnancy/Lactation: Unknown if distributed in breast milk. Not recommended for nursing mothers. **Pregnancy Category C. Children:** Safety and efficacy not established. **Elderly:** No age-related precautions noted, but lower initial and target doses may be necessary.

INTERACTIONS

DRUG: **Alcohol, CNS depressants** may increase CNS depression. May increase effects of **antihypertensives.** Hepatic enzyme induces (e.g., **phenytoin**), may increase drug clearance. ***HERBAL:*** None known. ***FOOD:*** None known. ***LAB VALUES:*** May produce false-positive pregnancy test. May decrease total and free thyroxine (T4) levels. May increase cholesterol, triglycerides, transaminase levels (e.g., ALT, AST).

AVAILABILITY (Rx)

TABLETS: 25 mg, 100 mg, 200 mg.

ADMINISTRATION/HANDLING

PO:

• Dosage adjustments should occur at 2 day intervals. • Initial dose and dose titration should occur at a lower dose in elderly, those with hepatic impairment, debilitated or those predisposed to hypotensive reactions. • When restarting pts who have been off quetiapine for <1 wk, titration is not required and maintenance dose can be reinstituted. • When restarting pts who have been off quetiapine for >1 wk, follow initial titration schedule. • Give without regard to food.

INDICATIONS/ROUTES/DOSAGE

Psychotic disorder:

PO: Adults: Initially, 25 mg 2 times/day, then 25–50 mg 2–3 times daily on second and third days, up to 300–400 mg/day by the fourth day, given 2–3 times daily. Further adjustments of 25–50 mg 2 times/day made at ≥2-day intervals.

SIDE EFFECTS

FREQUENT (10–19%): Headache, somnolence/drowsiness, dizziness. ***OCCASIONAL*** (3–9%): Constipation, postural hypotension, tachycardia, dry mouth, dyspepsia, rash, weakness, abdominal pain, rhinitis. ***RARE*** (2%): Back pain, fever, weight gain.

ADVERSE REACTIONS/TOXIC EFFECTS

Overdosage produces heart block (slow, irregular), decreased B/P, hypokalemia (weakness), tachycardia.

NURSING IMPLICATIONS

BASELINE ASSESSMENT:

Assess behavior, appearance, emotional status, response to environment, speech pattern, thought content. Obtain baseline CBC, hepatic function serum

Q

levels prior to initiation of treatment and periodically thereafter.

INTERVENTION/EVALUATION:

Assist with ambulation if dizziness occurs. Supervise suicidal risk pt closely during early therapy (as psychosis, depression lessens, energy level improves, increasing suicide potential). Monitor B/P for hypotension. Assess pulse for tachycardia (esp. with rapid increase in dosage). Monitor CBC for evidence of blood dyscrasias. Question bowel activity for evidence of constipation. Assess for therapeutic response (improved thought content, increased ability to concentrate, improvement in self-care).

PATIENT/FAMILY TEACHING:

Avoid exposure to extreme heat. Drink fluids often, esp. during physical activity. Take medication as ordered; do not stop taking or increase dosage. Drowsiness generally subsides during continued therapy. Avoid driving or performing tasks that require alertness, motor skills until response to drug is established. Avoid alcohol. Change positions slowly to reduce hypotensive effect.

quinapril hydrochloride 🖉

quin-ah-prill
(Accupril)
Do not confuse with Accolate, Accutane.

FIXED-COMBINATION(S)

With hydrochlorothiazide, a diuretic **(Accuretic)**

▶CLASSIFICATION

PHARMACOTHERAPEUTIC:
Angiotensin converting enzyme (ACE) inhibitor. ***CLINICAL:*** Antihypertensive (see p. 6C)

ACTION/*THERAPEUTIC EFFECT*

Suppresses renin-angiotensin-aldosterone system (prevents conversion of angiotensin I to angiotensin II, a potent vasoconstrictor; may also inhibit angiotensin II at local vascular and renal sites). *Reduces peripheral arterial resistance, B/P, pulmonary capillary wedge pressure; improves cardiac output.*

PHARMACOKINETICS

	Onset	Peak	Duration
PO	1 hr	2–4 hrs	—

Readily absorbed from GI tract. Protein binding: 97%. Metabolized in liver, GI tract, extravascular tissue to active metabolite. Primarily excreted in urine. Minimal removal by hemodialysis. Half-life: 1–2 hrs; metabolite: 3 hrs (half-life increased with impaired renal function).

USES/*UNLABELED*

Treatment of hypertension. Used alone or in combination with other antihypertensives. Adjunctive therapy in management of heart failure. *Treatment of hypertension/renal crisis in scleroderma.*

PRECAUTIONS

CONTRAINDICATIONS: MI, coronary insufficiency, angina, evidence of coronary artery disease, hypersensitivity to phentolamine, history of angioedema with previous treatment with ACE inhibitors. ***CAUTIONS:*** Renal impairment, those with sodium depletion or on diuretic therapy, dialysis, hypovolemia, coronary/cerebrovascular insufficiency.

▷*LIFESPAN CONSIDERATIONS:*
Pregnancy/Lactation: Crosses placenta; unknown if distributed in breast milk. May cause fetal-neonatal mortality/morbidity. **Pregnancy Category D. Children:** Safety and efficacy not established. **Elderly:** May be more sensitive to hypotensive effects.

INTERACTIONS

DRUG: **Alcohol, diuretics, hypotensive agents** may increase effects. **NSAIDs** may decrease effect. **Potassium-sparing diuretics, potassium supplements** may cause hyperkalemia. May increase **lithium** concentration, toxicity. **HERBAL:** None known. *FOOD:* None known. *LAB VALUES:* May increase potassium, SGOT (AST), SGPT (ALT), alkaline phosphatase, bilirubin, BUN, creatinine. May decrease sodium. May cause positive ANA titer.

AVAILABILITY (Rx)

TABLETS: 5 mg, 10 mg, 20 mg, 40 mg.

ADMINISTRATION/HANDLING
PO:

• Give without regard to food. • Tablets may be crushed.

INDICATIONS/ROUTES/DOSAGE
Hypertension (used alone):

PO: **Adults:** Initially, 10–20 mg/day. May adjust dose after at least 2 wk intervals. **Maintenance:** 20–80 mg/day as single or 2 divided doses. **Maximum:** 80 mg/day.

Hypertension (combination therapy):

Note: Discontinue diuretic 2–3 days before initiating quinapril therapy.

PO: **Adults:** Initially, 5 mg/day titrated to pt's needs.

Usual elderly dose:

PO: Initially, 2.5–5 mg/day. May increase by 2.5–5 mg q1–2wks.

Heart failure:

PO: **Adults, elderly:** Initially, 5 mg 2 times/day. **Range:** 20–40 mg/day.

Dosage in renal impairment:

Titrate to pt need after following initial doses:

Creatinine Clearance	Initial Dose
>60 ml/min	10 mg
30–60 ml/min	5 mg
10–30 ml/min	2.5 mg

SIDE EFFECTS

FREQUENT (5–7%): Headache, dizziness. *OCCASIONAL* (2–4%): Fatigue, vomiting, nausea, hypotension, chest pain, cough, syncope. *RARE* (<2%): Diarrhea, cough, dyspnea, rash, palpitations, impotence, insomnia, drowsiness, malaise.

ADVERSE REACTIONS/TOXIC EFFECTS

Excessive hypotension ("first-dose syncope") may occur in those with CHF, severely salt/volume depleted. Angioedema (swelling of face/lips), hyperkalemia occur rarely. Agranulocytosis, neutropenia may be noted in those with impaired renal function or collagen vascular disease (systemic lupus erythematosus, scleroderma). Nephrotic syndrome may be noted in those with history of renal disease.

Q

NURSING IMPLICATIONS

BASELINE ASSESSMENT:

Obtain B/P immediately before each dose in addition to regular monitoring (be alert to fluctuations). If excessive reduction in B/P occurs, place pt in supine position with legs slightly elevated. Renal function tests should be performed before therapy begins. In those with prior renal disease, urine test for protein by dipstick method should be made with first urine of day before therapy begins and periodically thereafter. In those with renal impairment, autoimmune disease or those taking drugs that affect leukocytes/immune response, CBC and differential count should be performed before therapy begins and q2wks for 3 mos, then periodically thereafter.

INTERVENTION/EVALUATION:

Assist with ambulation if dizziness occurs. Question for evidence of headache. Noncola carbonated beverage, unsalted crackers, dry toast may relieve nausea.

PATIENT/FAMILY TEACHING:

To reduce hypotensive effect, rise slowly from lying to sitting position and permit legs to dangle from bed momentarily before standing. Full therapeutic effect may take 1–2 wks. Report any sign of infection (sore throat, fever). Skipping doses or voluntarily discontinuing drug may produce severe rebound hypertension. Avoid driving and other tasks that require alert responses until reaction to drug is known.

quinidine

kwin-ih-deen
(Apo-Quinidine✦, Cardioquin, Cin-quin, Duraquin, Quinaglute, Quinate✦, Quinidex)
Do not confuse with clonidine, quinine.

▶CLASSIFICATION

CLINICAL: Antiarrhythmic (see p. 12C)

ACTION/*THERAPEUTIC EFFECT*

Direct cardiac effects. Suppresses automaticity of His-Purkinje system in myocardium. *Decreases myocardial excitability, conduction velocity, automaticity, membrane responsiveness; prolongs refractory period.*

USES/*UNLABELED*

Prophylactic therapy to maintain normal sinus rhythm after conversion of atrial fibrillation and/or flutter. Prevention of premature atrial, AV and ventricular contractions, paroxysmal atrial tachycardia, paroxysmal AV junctional rhythm, atrial fibrillation, atrial flutter, paroxysmal ventricular tachycardia not associated with complete heart block. *Treatment of malaria (IV only).*

PRECAUTIONS

CONTRAINDICATIONS: Complete AV block, intraventricular conduction defects, abnormal impulses and rhythms due to escape mechanism, myasthenia gravis. *EXTREME CAUTION:* Incomplete AV block, digitalis intoxication, CHF, preexisting hypotension. *CAUTIONS:* Preexisting asthma, muscle weakness, infection with fever, hepatic/renal insufficiency.

INTERACTIONS

DRUG: May increase concentration of **digoxin. Pimozide, other antiarrhythmics** may increase cardiac effects. **Urinary alkalizers (e.g., antacids)** may decrease excretion. May increase effects of **oral anticoagulants, neuromuscular blockers.** May decrease effects of **antimyasthenics** on skeletal muscle. **HERBAL:** None known. **FOOD:** None known. **LAB VALUES:** None significant. Therapeutic blood serum level: 2–5 mcg/ml; toxic blood serum level: >5 mcg/ml.

AVAILABILITY (Rx)

Gluconate: TABLETS (sustained-release): 324 mg. **INJECTION:** 80 mg/ml (50 mg/ml quinidine).

Polygalacturonate: TABLETS: 275 mg (200 mg quinidine).

Sulfate: TABLETS: 200 mg, 300 mg. **TABLETS (sustained-release):** 300 mg.

ADMINISTRATION/HANDLING

PO:

• Do not crush or chew sustained-release tablets. • GI upset can be reduced if given with food.

IV 🅦

Note: B/P, EKG should be monitored continuously during IV administration and rate of infusion adjusted to eliminate arrhythmias.

Storage:

• Use only clear, colorless solution. • Solution is stable for 24 hrs at room temperature when diluted with D_5W.

Reconstitution:

• For IV infusion, dilute 800 mg with 40 ml D_5W to provide concentration of 16 mg/ml.

Rate of administration:

• Administer with pt in supine position. • For IV infusion, give at rate of 1 ml (16 mg)/min (a too-rapid rate may markedly decrease arterial pressure). • Monitor EKG for cardiac changes, particularly prolongation of PR, QT interval, widening of QRS complex. Notify physician of any significant interval changes.

IV INCOMPATIBILITIES ⃠

Furosemide (Lasix), heparin.

IV COMPATIBILITY

Milrinone (Primacor).

INDICATIONS/ROUTES/DOSAGE

Usual dosage:

IV: Adults, elderly: 200–400 mg/dose. **Children:** 2–10 mg/kg/dose.

PO: Adults, elderly: 100–600 mg/dose q4–6h. **(Long-acting):** 324–972 mg q8–12h. **Children:** 30 mg/kg/day in divided doses q4–6h.

SIDE EFFECTS

FREQUENT: Abdominal pain/cramps, nausea, diarrhea, vomiting (can be immediate, intense). **OCCASIONAL:** Mild cinchonism (ringing in ears, blurred vision, hearing loss) or severe cinchonism (headache, vertigo, sweating, lightheadedness, photophobia, confusion, delirium). **RARE:** Hypotension (particularly with IV administration), hypersensitivity reaction (fever, anaphylaxis, thrombocytopenia).

ADVERSE REACTIONS/TOXIC EFFECTS

Cardiotoxic effects occur most commonly with IV administration, particularly at high concentration, observed as conduction changes

(50% widening of QRS complex, prolonged QT interval, flattened T waves, disappearance of P wave), ventricular tachycardia/flutter, frequent PVCs, complete AV block. Quinidine-induced syncope may occur with usual dosage (discontinue drug). Severe hypotension may result from high doses. Atrial flutter/fibrillation pts may experience a paradoxical, extremely rapid ventricular rate (may be prevented by prior digitalization). Hepatotoxicity with jaundice due to drug hypersensitivity.

NURSING IMPLICATIONS

BASELINE ASSESSMENT:

Check B/P and pulse for 1 full min (unless pt is on continuous monitor) before giving medication. For those on long-term therapy, CBC and liver/renal function tests should be performed periodically.

INTERVENTION/EVALUATION:

Monitor EKG for cardiac changes, particularly prolongation of PR, QT interval, widening of QRS complex. Monitor I&O, CBC, serum potassium, hepatic/renal function tests. Monitor pattern of daily bowel activity, stool consistency. Monitor B/P for hypotension (esp. in those on high-dose therapy). If cardiotoxic effect occurs (see Adverse Reactions/Toxic Effects), notify physician immediately. Therapeutic blood serum level: 2–5 mcg/ml; toxic blood serum level: >5 mcg/ml.

PATIENT/FAMILY TEACHING:

Report visual disturbances, ringing in ears, hearing loss. Teach pt/family to take pulse properly. Photophobia may occur—sunglasses will provide some relief.

quinine sulfate ✳

kwye-nine
(Quinine)
Do not confuse with quinidine.

FIXED-COMBINATION(S)

With vitamin E for nocturnal leg cramps **(M-KYA, Q-vel)**

▶CLASSIFICATION

PHARMACOTHERAPEUTIC:
Cinchone alkaloid. ***CLINICAL:***
Antimalarial, antimyotonic

ACTION/*THERAPEUTIC EFFECT*

Myotonia: *Relaxes skeletal muscle* by increasing the refractory period, decreasing excitability of motor end plates (curarelike), and affecting distribution of calcium with muscle fiber. ***Antimalaria:*** Depresses O_2 uptake, carbohydrate metabolism, elevates pH in intracellular organelles of parasites, *producing parasitic death.*

USES

Prevention, treatment of nocturnal recumbency leg cramps. Generally replaced by more effective, less toxic antimalarials. Used alone, with pyrimethamine and sulfonamide (or with oral tetracycline) for treatment of chloroquine-resistant falciparum malaria.

PRECAUTIONS

CONTRAINDICATIONS: Hypersensitivity to quinine (possible cross-sensitivity to quinidine), G-6-PD deficiency, tinnitus, optic neuritis, history of thrombocytopenia during previous quinine therapy, blackwater fever. ***CAUTIONS:*** Cardiovascular disease (as with quinidine), myasthenia gravis, asthma.

INTERACTIONS

DRUG: May increase concentration of **digoxin. Mefloquine** may increase seizures, EKG abnormalities. **HERBAL:** None known. **FOOD:** None known. **LAB VALUES:** May interfere with 17-OH steroid determinations.

AVAILABILITY (Rx)

CAPSULES: 65 mg, 200 mg, 300 mg. **TABLETS:** 160 mg, 260 mg.

INDICATIONS/ROUTES/DOSAGE

Nocturnal leg cramps:

PO: Adults, elderly: 260–300 mg at bedtime as needed.

Treatment of malaria:

PO: Adults, elderly: 260–650 mg 3 times a day for 6–12 days. **Children:** 10 mg/kg q8h for 5–7 days.

SIDE EFFECTS

FREQUENT: Nausea, headache, tinnitus, slight visual disturbances (mild cinchonism). **OCCASIONAL:** Extreme flushing of skin with intense generalized pruritus is most typical hypersensitivity reaction; also rash, wheezing, dyspnea, angioedema. Prolonged therapy: cardiac conduction disturbances, decreased hearing.

ADVERSE REACTIONS/TOXIC EFFECTS

Overdosage (severe cinchonism): cardiovascular effects, severe headache, intestinal cramps with vomiting and diarrhea, apprehension, confusion, seizures, blindness, respiratory depression. Hypoprothrombinemia, thrombocytopenic purpura, hemoglobinuria, asthma, agranulocytosis, hypoglycemia, deafness, optic atrophy occur rarely.

NURSING IMPLICATIONS

BASELINE ASSESSMENT:

Question for possibility of pregnancy before initiating therapy (Pregnancy Category X). Question for hypersensitivity to quinine, quinidine. Evaluate initial EKG, CBC results.

INTERVENTION/EVALUATION:

Check for hypersensitivity: flushing, rash/urticaria, itching, dyspnea, wheezing. Assess level of hearing, visual acuity, presence of headache/tinnitus, nausea and report adverse effects promptly (possible cinchonism). Monitor CBC results for blood dyscrasias; be alert to infection (fever, sore throat) and bleeding/bruising or unusual tiredness/weakness. Assess pulse, EKG for arrhythmias. Check FBS levels and watch for hypoglycemia (cold sweating, tremors, tachycardia, hunger, anxiety).

PATIENT/FAMILY TEACHING:

Use appropriate contraceptive measures (Pregnancy Category X). Use nonhormonal contraception. Report visual/hearing difficulties, shortness of breath, rash/itching, nausea. Periodic lab tests are part of therapy.

Q

quinupristin-dalfopristin

quin-you-pris-tin/**dal**-foh-pris-tin (Synercid)

►CLASSIFICATION

PHARMACOTHERAPEUTIC: Streptogramin. **CLINICAL:** Antimicrobial

---

✦ - Canadian trade name   ✳ - see also www.wbsaunders.com/SIMON/SaundersNDH

ACTION/*THERAPEUTIC EFFECT*

Bactericidal (in combination). Two chemically distinct compounds that, when given together, bind to different sites on bacterial ribosomes forming a drug-ribosome complex. Protein synthesis is interrupted, *resulting in bacterial cell death.*

PHARMACOKINETICS

After IV administration, both are extensively metabolized in the liver, with dalfopristin to active metabolite. Protein binding: *(quinupristin)* 23–32%, *(dalfopristin)* 50–56%. Primarily eliminated in feces. Half-life: 1–2 hrs.

USES

Treatment of intra-abdominal, skin/skin structure, urinary tract, central catheter, bone and joint, respiratory infections, endocarditis, bacteremia.

PRECAUTIONS

CONTRAINDICATIONS: None significant. ***CAUTIONS:*** Liver/renal dysfunction.
▷*LIFESPAN CONSIDERATIONS:*
Pregnancy/Lactation: Unknown if drug crosses placenta or is distributed in breast milk. **Pregnancy Category B. Children:** Safety and efficacy not established. **Elderly:** No age-related precautions noted.

INTERACTIONS

DRUG: None significant. ***HERBAL:*** None known. ***FOOD:*** None known. ***LAB VALUES:*** May increase SGOT (AST), SGPT (ALT), LDH, serum creatinine, bilirubin.

AVAILABILITY (Rx)

INJECTION: 500 mg vial (350 mg dalfopristin/150 mg quinupristin).

ADMINISTRATION/HANDLING

Note: Space doses evenly around the clock for full effectiveness.

IV 🍳

Storage:
• Refrigerate vials. • After reconstitution, is stable for 6 hrs at room temperature, 72 hrs refrigerated.

Reconstitution:
• Reconstitute with D_5W (compatibility with 0.9% NaCl unknown).

Rate of administration:
• For intermittent IV infusion (piggyback), infuse over 1 hr.

IV INCOMPATIBILITY ⊘

Do not mix with any other medications.

INDICATIONS/ROUTES/DOSAGE

Usual adult dosage:
IV INFUSION: Adults, elderly: 7.5 mg/kg q8–12h.

SIDE EFFECTS

Generally well tolerated. ***FREQUENT:*** Mild erythema, itching, pain, or burning at infusion site for doses of 7 mg/kg or higher. ***OCCASIONAL:*** Headache, diarrhea. ***RARE:*** Vomiting, arthralgia, myalgia.

ADVERSE REACTIONS/TOXIC EFFECTS

Superinfection, including antibiotic-associated colitis, may result from bacterial imbalance. Liver function abnormalities, peripheral venous intolerability may occur.

NURSING IMPLICATIONS

BASELINE ASSESSMENT:

Assess temperature, B/P, respiratory rate, pulse. Obtain baseline liver function tests, BUN, CBC, urinalysis.

INTERVENTION/EVALUATION:

Hold medication and promptly inform physician if diarrhea (with fever, abdominal pain, mucous and blood in stool may indicate antibiotic-associated colitis). Evaluate IV site for mild erythema, itching, pain, or burning. Be alert for superinfection: increased fever, onset sore throat, nausea, vomiting, diarrhea, ulceration or changes of oral mucosa, anal/genital pruritus. Check liver function studies. Assess cultures of infection site. Monitor temperature for sign of infection.

rabeprazole sodium

rah-**bep**-rah-zole
(Aciphex)
Do not confuse with Accupril, Aricept.

▶CLASSIFICATION

PHARMACOTHERAPEUTIC: Proton pump inhibitor. **CLINICAL:** Gastric acid inhibitor (see p. 122C)

ACTION/THERAPEUTIC EFFECT

Converts to active metabolites that irreversibly binds to and inhibits $H+/K+$ ATPase (an enzyme on surface of gastric parietal cells). Actively secretes hydrogen ions for potassium ions, resulting in an accumulation of $H+$ in gastric lumen, *increasing gastric pH, reducing gastric acid production.*

PHARMACOKINETICS

Rapidly absorbed from GI tract after passing through stomach rel-atively intact. Protein binding: 96%. Metabolized extensively in liver. Primarily excreted in urine. Unknown if removed by hemodialysis. Half-life: 1–2 hrs (half-life increased with impaired liver function).

USES

Short-term treatment (4–8 wks) in healing and maintenance of erosive or ulcerative gastroesophageal reflux disease (GERD). Short-term treatment (up to 4 wks) in healing and symptomatic relief of duodenal ulcers. Long-term treatment of pathologic hypersecretory conditions, including Zollinger-Ellison syndrome. Treatment of NSAID-induced ulcers.

PRECAUTIONS

CONTRAINDICATIONS: None significant. **CAUTIONS:** Impaired hepatic function.
▷**LIFESPAN CONSIDERATIONS:**
Pregnancy/Lactation: Unknown if drug crosses placenta or is distributed in breast milk. **Pregnancy Category B. Children:** Safety and efficacy not established. **Elderly:** No age-related precautions noted.

INTERACTIONS

DRUG: May decrease concentration of **ketoconazole.** May increase plasma concentration of **digoxin. HERBAL:** None known. **FOOD:** None known. **LAB VALUES:** May increase SGOT (AST), SGPT (ALT), alkaline phosphatase.

AVAILABILITY (Rx)

TABLETS (delayed-release): 20 mg.

ADMINISTRATION/HANDLING

PO:

• Give before meals. • Do not crush, chew, or split capsule; swallow whole.

R

INDICATIONS/ROUTES/DOSAGE

Gastroesophageal reflux disease (GERD):

PO: **Adults, elderly:** 20 mg/day.

Duodenal ulcer:

PO: **Adults, elderly:** 20 mg/day after morning meal.

Pathologic hypersecretory conditions:

PO: **Adults, elderly:** Initially, 60 mg/day. Divided doses may be needed.

SIDE EFFECTS

RARE (≤2%): Headache, nausea, dizziness, rash, diarrhea, malaise.

ADVERSE REACTIONS/TOXIC EFFECTS

Hyperglycemia, hypokalemia, hyponatremia, hyperlipemia occur rarely.

NURSING IMPLICATIONS

BASELINE ASSESSMENT:
Obtain baseline lab values.

INTERVENTION/EVALUATION:
Monitor ongoing laboratory results. Evaluate for therapeutic response, i.e., relief of GI symptoms. Question if GI discomfort, nausea, diarrhea, headache occurs. Assess skin for evidence of rash. Monitor for evidence of dizziness and utilize appropriate safety precautions.

PATIENT/FAMILY TEACHING:
Swallow tablets whole; do not chew, split, or crush tablets.

raloxifene

rah-**lock**-sih-feen
(Evista)

▶CLASSIFICATION

PHARMACOTHERAPEUTIC: Selective estrogen receptor modulator. ***CLINICAL:*** Osteoporosis preventative

ACTION/*THERAPEUTIC EFFECT*

Increases mineral bone density, lowers LDL and total cholesterol, *preventing bone loss and lowering cholesterol without stimulating the endometrium.*

PHARMACOKINETICS

Rapidly absorbed following PO administration. Highly bound to plasma proteins (>95%) and albumin. Undergoes extensive first-pass metabolism in liver. Excreted mainly in feces with a lesser amount in urine. Unknown if removed by hemodialysis. Half-life: 27.7 hrs.

USES/*UNLABELED*

Prevention and treatment of osteoporosis in postmenopausal women. *Prevents fractures, breast cancer in postmenopausal women.*

PRECAUTIONS

CONTRAINDICATIONS: Pregnancy, those who may become pregnant, active or history of venous thromboembolic events (deep vein thrombosis, pulmonary embolism, retinal vein thrombosis). ***CAUTIONS:*** Hepatic function impairment.

▷*LIFESPAN CONSIDERATIONS:* **Pregnancy/Lactation:** Unknown if distributed in breast milk. Not recommended for nursing mothers. **Pregnancy Category X. Children:** Not used in this population. **Elderly:** No age-related precautions noted.

INTERACTIONS

DRUG:* Cholestyramine, ampicillin** reduces raloxifene peak levels, extent of absorption. May decrease effect of **warfarin** (decreases prothrombin time). Do not use concurrently with systemic **estrogen or hormone replacement** therapy. ***HERBAL: None known. ***FOOD:*** None known. ***LAB VALUES:*** Lowers serum total and LDL cholesterol (does not affect HDL cholesterol or triglycerides). Slight decrease in serum total calcium, inorganic phosphate, total protein, albumin, platelet count.

AVAILABILITY (Rx)

TABLETS: 60 mg.

ADMINISTRATION/HANDLING

PO:

• Give at any time of day without regard to meals.

INDICATIONS/ROUTES/DOSAGE

Prevention/treatment of osteoporosis:

PO: Adults: 60 mg daily.

SIDE EFFECTS

FREQUENT (10–25%): Hot flashes, flu syndrome, arthralgia, sinusitis. ***OCCASIONAL*** (5–9%): Weight gain, nausea, myalgia, pharyngitis, cough, dyspepsia, leg cramps, rash, depression. ***RARE*** (3–4%): Vaginitis, urinary tract infection, peripheral edema, flatulence, vomiting, fever, migraine, sweating.

ADVERSE REACTIONS/TOXIC EFFECTS

Pneumonia, gastroenteritis, chest pain, vaginal bleeding, breast pain occur rarely.

NURSING IMPLICATIONS

BASELINE ASSESSMENT:

Question for possibility of pregnancy (Pregnancy Category X). Drug should be discontinued 72 hrs before and during prolonged immobilization (postop recovery, prolonged bed rest). Therapy may be resumed only after pt is fully ambulatory. Determine total and LDL cholesterol serum blood levels prior to therapy and routinely thereafter.

INTERVENTION/EVALUATION:

Monitor total and LDL cholesterol, total calcium, inorganic phosphate, total protein, albumin, and platelet count.

PATIENT/FAMILY TEACHING:

Avoid prolonged restriction of movement during travel (increased risk of venous thromboembolic events). Take supplemental calcium, vitamin D if daily dietary intake is inadequate. Weight-bearing exercise, decrease or modification of cigarette smoking, alcohol consumption is advised.

R

ramipril

ram-ih-prill
(Altace)
Do not confuse with Alteplase, Artane.

▶CLASSIFICATION

PHARMACOTHERAPEUTIC: Renin angiotensin system antagonist. ***CLINICAL:*** Antihypertensive (see p. 6C)

ACTION/*THERAPEUTIC EFFECT*

Suppresses renin-angiotensin-aldosterone system. Decreases plasma angiotensin II, increases plasma renin activity, decreases aldosterone secretion. *Reduces peripheral arterial resistance, decreasing B/P.*

PHARMACOKINETICS

	Onset	Peak	Duration
PO	1–2 hrs	3–6 hrs	24 hrs

Well absorbed from GI tract. Protein binding: 73%. Metabolized in liver to active metabolite. Primarily excreted in urine. Not removed by hemodialysis. Half-life: 5.1 hrs.

USES/*UNLABELED*

Treatment of hypertension. Used alone or in combination with other antihypertensives. Treatment of CHF. *Treatment of hypertension/renal crisis in scleroderma. Prevention of heart attacks, stroke.*

PRECAUTIONS

CONTRAINDICATIONS: History of angioedema with previous treatment with ACE inhibitors. ***CAUTIONS:*** Renal impairment, those with sodium depletion or on diuretic therapy, dialysis, hypovolemia, coronary/cerebrovascular insufficiency.

▷***LIFESPAN CONSIDERATIONS:*** **Pregnancy/Lactation:** Crosses placenta; distributed in breast milk. May cause fetal/neonatal mortality/morbidity. **Pregnancy Category D. Children:** Safety and efficacy not established. **Elderly:** May be more sensitive to hypotensive effects.

INTERACTIONS

DRUG:* Alcohol, diuretics, hypotensive agents** may increase effects. **NSAIDs** may decrease effect. **Potassium-sparing diuretics, potassium supplements** may cause hyperkalemia. May increase **lithium** concentration, toxicity. ***HERBAL: None known. ***FOOD:*** None known. ***LAB VALUES:*** May increase potassium, SGOT (AST), SGPT (ALT), alkaline phosphatase, bilirubin, BUN, creatinine. May decrease sodium. May cause positive ANA titer.

AVAILABILITY (Rx)

CAPSULES: 1.25 mg, 2.5 mg, 5 mg, 10 mg.

ADMINISTRATION/HANDLING

PO:

• Give without regard to food. • Do not chew or break capsules. • May mix with water, apple juice/sauce.

INDICATIONS/ROUTES/DOSAGE

Hypertension (used alone):

PO: Adults, elderly: Initially, 2.5 mg/day. **Maintenance:** 2.5–20 mg/day as single or in 2 divided doses.

Hypertension (combination therapy):

Note: Discontinue diuretic 2–3 days before initiating ramipril therapy.

PO: Adults, elderly: Initially, 1.25 mg/day titrated to pt's needs.

CHF:

PO: Adults, elderly: Initially, 1.25–2.5 mg 2 times/day. **Maximum:** 5 mg 2 times/day.

Dosage in renal impairment (creatinine <40 ml/min; serum creatinine >2.5 mg/dl):

Initially, 1.25 mg/day titrated up to maximum of 5 mg/day.

SIDE EFFECTS

FREQUENT (5–12%): Cough, headache. ***OCCASIONAL*** (2–4%): Dizziness, fatigue, nausea, asthenia (loss of strength). ***RARE*** (<2%): Palpitations, insomnia, nervousness, malaise, abdominal pain, myalgia.

ADVERSE REACTIONS/TOXIC EFFECTS

Excessive hypotension ("first-dose syncope)) may occur in those with CHF, severely salt/volume depleted. Angioedema (swelling of face/lips), hyperkalemia occur rarely. Agranulocytosis, neutropenia may be noted in those with impaired renal function or collagen vascular disease (systemic lupus erythematosus, scleroderma). Nephrotic syndrome may be noted in those with history of renal disease.

NURSING IMPLICATIONS

BASELINE ASSESSMENT:

Obtain B/P immediately before each dose, in addition to regular monitoring (be alert to fluctuations). If excessive reduction in B/P occurs, place pt in supine position with legs elevated. Renal function tests should be performed before therapy begins. In those with prior renal disease, urine test for protein by dipstick method should be made with first urine of day before therapy begins and periodically thereafter. In those with renal impairment, autoimmune disease, or taking drugs that affect leukocytes/immune response, CBC and differential count should be performed before therapy begins and q2wks for 3 mos, then periodically thereafter.

INTERVENTION/EVALUATION:

Assess for cough (frequent effect). Assist with ambulation if dizziness occurs. Assess lung sounds for rales, wheezing in those with CHF. Monitor urinalysis for proteinuria. Monitor serum potassium levels in those on concurrent diuretic therapy.

PATIENT/FAMILY TEACHING:

Several wks may be needed for full therapeutic effect of B/P reduction. Skipping doses or voluntarily discontinuing drug may produce severe, rebound hypertension.

---

ranitidine

rah-**nih**-tih-deen
(Apo-Ranitidine✤, Novo-Ranidine✤, Zantac)
Do not confuse with Xanax.

ranitidine bismuth citrate

(Tritec)

▶CLASSIFICATION

PHARMACOTHERAPEUTIC: Histamine H$_2$ receptor antagonist. ***CLINICAL:*** Antiulcer (see p. 88C)

ACTION/*THERAPEUTIC EFFECT*

Inhibits histamine action at H$_2$ receptors of gastric parietal cells, *inhibiting gastric acid secretion (fasting, nocturnal, or when stimulated by food, caffeine, insulin). Reduces volume, hydrogen ion concentration of gastric juice.*

PHARMACOKINETICS

Rapidly absorbed from GI tract.

R

Protein binding: 15%. Widely distributed. Metabolized in liver. Primarily excreted in urine. Not removed by hemodialysis. Half-life: *PO:* 2.5 hrs; *IV:* 2–2.5 hrs (half-life increased with impaired renal function).

USES/*UNLABELED*

Short-term treatment of active duodenal ulcer. Prevention of duodenal ulcer recurrence. Treatment of active benign gastric ulcer, pathologic GI hypersecretory conditions, acute gastroesophageal reflux disease (GERD) including erosive esophagitis. Maintenance of healed erosive esophagitis. **Bismuth citrate:** Treatment of duodenal ulcers associated with *H. Pylori. Prophylaxis of aspiration pneumonia.*

PRECAUTIONS

CONTRAINDICATIONS: None significant. **CAUTIONS:** Impaired renal/hepatic function, elderly. ▷**LIFESPAN CONSIDERATIONS:** **Pregnancy/Lactation:** Unknown if drug crosses placenta or is distributed in breast milk. **Pregnancy Category B. Children:** No age-related precautions noted. **Elderly:** Confusion more likely in those with liver or renal impairment.

INTERACTIONS

DRUG: Antacids may decrease absorption (do not give within 1 hr). May decrease absorption of **ketoconazole** (give at least 2 hrs after). **HERBAL:** None known. **FOOD:** None known. **LAB VALUES:** Interferes with skin tests using allergen extracts. May increase liver function tests, creatinine, gamma-glutamyl transpeptidase.

AVAILABILITY (Rx)

TABLETS: 75 mg **(OTC),** 150 mg, 300 mg. **TABLETS (effervescent):** 150 mg. **CAPSULES:** 150 mg, 300 mg. **SYRUP:** 15 mg/ml. **GRANULES (effervescent):** 150 mg. **INJECTION:** 25 mg/ml, 0.5 mg/ml, 100 ml infusion.

Bismuth citrate: TABLETS: 400 mg.

ADMINISTRATION/HANDLING

PO:

• Give without regard to meals. Best given after meals or at bedtime. • Do not administer within 1 hr of magnesium-or aluminum-containing antacids (decreases absorption by 33%).

IM:

• May be given undiluted. • Give deep IM into large muscle mass.

IV 🍴

Storage:

• IV solutions appear clear, colorless to yellow (slight darkening does not affect potency). • IV infusion (piggyback) is stable for 48 hrs at room temperature (discard if discolored or precipitate forms).

Reconstitution:

• For IV push, dilute each 50 mg with 20 ml 0.9% NaCl, D_5W, $D_5W/0.45\%$ NaCl, $D_{10}W$, lactated Ringer's, or 5% $NaHCO_3$. • For intermittent IV infusion (piggyback), dilute each 50 mg with 50 ml 0.9% NaCl, D_5W, $D_5W/0.45\%$ NaCl, $D_{10}W$, lactated Ringer's, or 5% $NaHCO_3$. • For IV infusion, dilute with 250–1,000 ml 0.9% NaCl, D_5W, $D_5W/0.45\%$ NaCl, $D_{10}W$, lactated Ringer's, or 5% $NaHCO_3$.

Rate of administration:

• Administer IV push over minimum of 5 min (prevents arrhythmias, hypotension). • Infuse IV piggyback over 15–20 min. • Infuse IV infusion over 24 hrs.

IV INCOMPATIBILITIES ⊘

Amphotericin B complex (Abelcet, Ambisome, Amphotec).

IV COMPATIBILITIES

Diltiazem (Cardizem), dobutamine (Dobutrex), dopamine (Intropin), heparin, lorazepam (Ativan), midazolam (Versed), nitroglycerin, norepinephrine (Levophed), propofol (Diprivan).

INDICATIONS/ROUTES/DOSAGE

Duodenal, gastric ulcers:

IV: **Adults, elderly:** 50 mg q6–8h. **Children:** 2–4 mg/kg/day.

PO: **Adults, elderly:** *(Treatment):* 150 mg 2/times day or 200 mg at bedtime. **Children:** *(Treatment):* 2–4 mg/kg 2 times/day. **Maximum:** *(Treatment):* 300 mg/day. *(Prophylaxis):* 150 mg/day.

GERD:

PO: **Adults, elderly:** 150 mg 2 times/day or 300 mg at bedtime. **Children:** 4–10 mg/kg/day. **Maximum:** 300 mg/day.

Erosive esophagitis:

PO: **Adults, elderly:** 150 mg 4 times/day. **Children:** 4–10 mg/kg/day. **Maximum:** 600 mg/day.

Hypersecretory conditions:

PO: **Adults, elderly:** 150 mg 2 times/day up to 6 g/day.

Dosage in renal impairment (creatinine clearance <50 ml/min):

PO: 150 mg q24h.

IM/IV: 50 mg q18–24h.

SIDE EFFECTS

OCCASIONAL (2%): Diarrhea. ***RARE*** (1%): Constipation, headache (may be severe).

ADVERSE REACTIONS/TOXIC EFFECTS

Reversible hepatitis, blood dyscrasias occur rarely.

NURSING IMPLICATIONS

BASELINE ASSESSMENT:

Do not confuse medication with Xanax (alprazolam).

INTERVENTION/EVALUATION:

Monitor serum SGOT (AST), SGPT (ALT) levels. Assess mental status in elderly.

PATIENT/FAMILY TEACHING:

Smoking decreases effectiveness of medication. Do not take medicine within 1 hr of magnesium- or aluminum-containing antacids. Transient burning/itching may occur with IV administration. Report headache. Avoid alcohol, aspirin.

---

remifentanil hydrochloride

(Ultiva)

See Classification section under: Opioid analgesics

R

---

repaglinide

reh-**pah**-glih-nide
(Prandin)

▶CLASSIFICATION

PHARMACOTHERAPEUTIC: Antihyperglycemic. ***CLINICAL:*** Antidiabetic (see p. 40C)

ACTION/*THERAPEUTIC EFFECT*

Stimulates release of insulin from beta cells of the pancreas by depolarizing beta cells, leading to an opening of calcium channels. Resulting calcium influx induces insulin secretion, *lowering glucose concentration.*

PHARMACOKINETICS

Rapidly and completely absorbed from GI tract. Protein binding: 98%. Metabolized in liver to inactive metabolites. Excreted primarily in feces with a lesser amount in urine. Unknown if removed by hemodialysis. Half-life: 1 hr.

USES

Adjunct to diet and exercise to lower blood glucose in pts with type 2 diabetes mellitus. Used as monotherapy or in combination with metformin (Glucophage).

PRECAUTIONS

CONTRAINDICATIONS: Diabetic ketoacidosis, type 1 diabetes mellitus. ***CAUTIONS:*** Hepatic/renal function impairment.

▷*LIFESPAN CONSIDERATIONS:*
Pregnancy/Lactation: Unknown if distributed in breast milk. **Pregnancy Category C. Children:** Safety and efficacy not established. **Elderly:** No age-related precautions noted, but hypoglycemia more difficult to recognize.

INTERACTIONS

DRUG: Antifungal agents (**ketoconazole, miconazole**), antibacterial agents (**erythromycin**) may reduce repaglinide metabolism. **Rifampin, barbiturates, carbamazepine** increase repaglinide metabolism. **NSAIDs, salicylates, sulfonamides, chloramphenicol, warfarin, probenecid, MAOIs, beta-blockers** may increase effect. **Diuretics, corticosteroids, phe-**nothiazines, thyroid medication, estrogens, oral contraceptives, phenytoin, nicotinic acid, sympathomimetics, calcium channel blockers, isoniazid** may produce hyperglycemia. ***HERBAL:*** None known. ***FOOD:*** Food decreases repaglinide plasma concentration. ***LAB VALUES:*** None significant.

AVAILABILITY (Rx)

TABLETS: 0.5 mg, 1 mg, 2 mg.

ADMINISTRATION/HANDLING

PO:

• Ideally, give within 15 min of a meal but may be given immediately before a meal to as long as 30 min before a meal.

INDICATIONS/ROUTES/DOSAGE

Diabetes mellitus:

PO: **Adults, elderly:** 0.5–4 mg 2–4 times/day. **Maximum:** 16 mg/day.

SIDE EFFECTS

FREQUENT (6–10%): Upper respiratory infection, headache, rhinitis, bronchitis, back pain. ***OCCASIONAL*** (3–5%): Diarrhea, dyspepsia, sinusitis, nausea, arthralgia, urinary tract infection. ***RARE*** (2%): Constipation, vomiting, paresthesia, allergy.

ADVERSE REACTIONS/TOXIC EFFECTS

Hypoglycemia occurs in 16% of pts. Chest pain occurs rarely.

NURSING IMPLICATIONS

BASELINE ASSESSMENT:

Check fasting blood glucose and glycosylated Hgb (HbA$_1$C) periodically to determine minimum effective dose. Discuss lifestyle to determine extent of learning, emotional needs. Assure follow-up instruction if pt/family do not thoroughly understand diabetes management or glucose-testing technique. At least 1 wk should elapse to assess response to drug before new dose adjustment is made.

INTERVENTION/EVALUATION:

Monitor blood glucose and food intake. Assess for hypoglycemia (cool wet skin, tremors, dizziness, anxiety, headache, tachycardia, numbness in mouth, hunger, diplopia) or hyperglycemia (polyuria, polyphagia, polydipsia, nausea, vomiting, dim vision, fatigue, deep rapid breathing). Be alert to conditions that alter glucose requirements: fever, increased activity or stress, surgical procedures.

PATIENT/FAMILY TEACHING:

Diabetes mellitus requires lifelong control. Prescribed diet and exercise is principal part of treatment; do not skip or delay meals. Continue to adhere to dietary instructions, a regular exercise program, and regular testing of urine or blood glucose. When taking combination drug therapy with a sulfonylurea or insulin, have a source of glucose available to treat symptoms of low blood sugar.

ACTION/*THERAPEUTIC EFFECT*

High concentration of neutralizing and protective antibodies specific for respiratory syncytial virus (RSV).

USES

Prevents serious lower respiratory tract infections caused by RSV in children <24 mos with bronchopulmonary dysplasia or history of premature birth.

AVAILABILITY (Rx)

INJECTION: 2,500 mcg RSV immune globulin.

INDICATIONS/ROUTES/DOSAGE

RSV:

IV INFUSION: **Children (<24 mo):** 750 mg/kg (15 ml/kg). Initially, 1.5 ml/kg/hr for first 15 min; increase to 3 ml/kg/hr for next 15 min, then 6 ml/kg/hr for remainder of infusion. Administer moly for total of 5 doses beginning in September or October.

SIDE EFFECTS

OCCASIONAL (2–6%): Fever, vomiting, wheezing. *RARE* (<1%): Diarrhea, rash, tachycardia, hypertension, hypoxia, injection site inflammation.

R

---

respiratory syncytial immune globulin

(Respigam)

▶CLASSIFICATION

PHARMACOTHERAPEUTIC:
Immune serum. ***CLINICAL:*** Respiratory agent

---

reteplase, recombinant

rhet-eh-place
(Retavase)
Do not confuse with Restasis.

▶CLASSIFICATION

PHARMACOTHERAPEUTIC:
Tissue plasminogen activator.
CLINICAL: Thrombolytic (see p. 30C)

ACTION/*THERAPEUTIC EFFECT*

Activates fibrinolytic system by directly cleaving plasminogen to generate plasmin, an enzyme that degrades the fibrin of the thrombus, *exerting thrombolytic action.*

PHARMACOKINETICS

Rapidly cleared from plasma. Eliminated primarily by the liver and kidney. Half-life: 13–16 min.

USES

Management of acute myocardial infarction (AMI) for improvement of ventricular function following AMI, reduction of incidence of CHF and reduction of mortality associated with AMI.

PRECAUTIONS

CONTRAINDICATIONS: Active internal bleeding, history of CVA, recent intracranial or intraspinal surgery or trauma, intracranial neoplasm, arteriovenous malformation or aneurysm, bleeding diathesis or severe uncontrolled hypertension (increases risk of bleeding). ***CAUTIONS:*** Recent major surgery (coronary artery bypass graft, OB delivery, organ biopsy), cerebrovascular disease, recent GI or GU bleeding, hypertension, mitral stenosis with atrial fibrillation, acute pericarditis, bacterial endocarditis, hepatic/renal impairment, diabetic retinopathy, ophthalmic hemorrhaging, septic thrombophlebitis, occluded AV cannula at an infected site, advanced age, those receiving oral anticoagulants.

▷***LIFESPAN CONSIDERATIONS:***
Pregnancy/Lactation: Unknown if distributed in breast milk. **Pregnancy Category C. Children:** Safety and efficacy not established. **Elderly:** More susceptible to bleeding; caution advised.

INTERACTIONS

DRUG: Heparin, warfarin plate-let aggregation antagonists (e.g., aspirin, dipyridamole, abciximab) increases risk of bleeding. ***HERBAL:*** Ginkgo biloba may increase risk of bleeding. ***FOOD:*** None significant. ***LAB VALUES:*** Plasminogen and fibrinogen levels may decrease.

AVAILABILITY (Rx)

POWDER FOR INJECTION: 10.8 units (18.8 mg).

ADMINISTRATION/HANDLING

IV ▦

Storage:

• Use within 4 hrs of reconstitution.
• Discard any unused portion.

Reconstitution:

• Reconstitute only with Sterile Water for Injection immediately before use. • Reconstituted solution contains 1 unit/ml. • Slight foaming may occur; let stand for a few mins to allow bubbles to dissipate.

Rate of administration:

• Give through an IV line in which no other medications are being administered simultaneously. • Give as a 10 unit plus 10 unit double bolus, with each IV bolus administered over 2 min period. • Give the second bolus 30 min after the first bolus injection. • Do not add other medications to the bolus injection solution. • Do not give second bolus if serious bleeding occurs after first IV bolus is given.

IV INCOMPATIBILITY ⊘

Do not mix with any other medications.

INDICATIONS/ROUTES/DOSAGE

Acute MI:

IV BOLUS: Adults, elderly: 10

units over 2 min, then repeat 10 units 30 min after initiation of first bolus injection.

SIDE EFFECTS

FREQUENT: Bleeding at superficial sites (venous injection sites, catheter insertion sites, venous cutdowns, arterial punctures, sites of recent surgical procedures).

ADVERSE REACTIONS/TOXIC EFFECTS

Bleeding at internal sites (intracranial, retroperitoneal, GI, GU, or respiratory) occurs occasionally. Lysis or coronary thrombi may produce atrial or ventricular dysrhythmias, stroke.

NURSING IMPLICATIONS

BASELINE ASSESSMENT:

Obtain baseline B/P, apical pulse. Evaluate 12 lead EKG, CPK, CPK-MB, electrolytes. Assess hematocrit, platelet count, thrombin (TT), activated thromboplastin (APTT), prothrombin time (PT), plasminogen and fibrinogen level before therapy is instituted. Type and hold blood.

INTERVENTION/EVALUATION:

Carefully monitor all needle puncture sites, catheter insertion sites for bleeding. Continuous cardiac monitoring for arrhythmias, B/P, pulse, respiration is essential until pt is stable. Check peripheral pulses, lung sounds. Monitor for chest pain relief; notify physician of continuation or recurrence of chest pain (note location, type, intensity). Avoid any trauma that may increase risk of bleeding (injections, shaving).

Rh₀(D) immune globulin IV (human)

(WinRho SD)

▶CLASSIFICATION

CLINICAL: Immune serum

ACTION/THERAPEUTIC EFFECT

Gamma globulin (IgG) fraction containing antibodies to Rh₀(D) antigen-negative individuals. *Increases platelets in idiopathic thrombocytopenic purpura (ITP).* Exact mechanism unknown.

USES

Pregnancy/other obstetric conditions: Suppresses Rh isoimmunization in nonsensitized Rh₀(D) antigen-negative women, reduces hemolytic disease in Rh₀(D)-positive fetus in present and future pregnancies. **Transfusion:** Suppresses isoimmunization transfusion with Rh₀(D) antigen-positive RBCs or blood components containing Rh₀(D)-positive RBCs. Treatment of nonsplenectomized Rh₀(D) antigen-positive children with chronic or acute ITP, adults with chronic ITP, or children and adults with ITP secondary to HIV infection in clinical conditions to prevent excessive hemorrhage.

PRECAUTIONS

CONTRAINDICATIONS: Hypersensitivity to immune globulin, IgA deficiency. **CAUTIONS:** Thrombocytopenia, bleeding disorders. Hgb <8 g/dl.

INTERACTIONS

DRUG: May interfere with immune response to **live virus vaccines.** **HERBAL:** None significant. **FOOD:** None significant. **LAB VALUES:** None significant.

R

AVAILABILITY (Rx)

INJECTION: 600 IU (120 mcg), 1,500 IU (300 mcg).

ADMINISTRATION/HANDLING

IV 🚱

Storage:

• Refrigerate vials (do not freeze).
• Once reconstituted, stable for 12 hrs at room temperature.

Reconstitution:

• Reconstitute 120 mcg and 300 mcg with 2.5 ml NaCl (8.5 ml for 1,000 mcg vial). • Gently swirl; do not shake.

Rate of administration:

• Infuse over 3–5 min.

IM:

• Reconstitute 120 mcg and 300 mcg with 2.5 ml NaCl (8.5 ml for 1,000 mcg vial). • Administer into deltoid muscle of upper arm or anterolateral aspect of upper thigh.

INDICATIONS/ROUTES/DOSAGE

Pregnancy:

IV/IM: Adults: 1,500 IU (300 mcg) at 28 wks gestation. Give at 12 wk intervals if administered early in pregnancy, 600 IU (120 mcg) as soon as possible after delivery of confirmed Rh$_o$(D) antigen-positive baby, and within 72 hrs of delivery.

Other obstetric conditions:

IV/IM: Adults: 600 IU (120 mcg) immediately after abortion, amniocentesis, or other manipulations late in pregnancy (after 34 wks gestation) associated with increased risk of Rh isoimmunization. Give within 72 hrs after the event. Administer 1,500 IU (300 mcg) immediately after amniocentesis before 34 wks gestation or after chorionic villus sampling. Repeat q12wks during the pregnancy. In case of threatened abortion, give as soon as possible.

Transfusion:

Note: Within 72 hrs after exposure of incompatible blood transfusion or massive fetal hemorrhage.

IV: Adults: 3,000 IU (600 mcg) q8h until total dose given.

IM: Adults: 6,000 IU (1,200 mcg) q12h until total dose given.

ITP:

IV: Adults, children: Initially, 250 IU (50 mcg)/kg. If hemoglobin <10 g/dl, give 125–200 IU (25–40 mcg)/kg. Additional doses give 125–300 IU (25–60 mcg)/kg.

SIDE EFFECTS

OCCASIONAL (1–7%): *Rh isoimmunization suppression:* Discomfort, slight swelling at injection site, slight elevation of temperature. *ITP:* Headache, chills, fever.

ADVERSE REACTIONS/TOXIC EFFECTS

None significant.

Rh$_o$(D) immune globulin IGIM

(RhoGAM, BayRho-D Full Dose)

▶CLASSIFICATION

PHARMACOTHERAPEUTIC: Immune globulin. **CLINICAL:** Hemolytic disease prophylactic

ACTION/*THERAPEUTIC EFFECT*

Suppresses the immune response of Rh$_o$(D)-negative pts to Rh$_o$(D)-positive red blood cells, *neutralizing micro-organisms and their toxins,* participating in antibody-dependent cytolytic reactions.

USES/*UNLABELED*

For prevention of Rh hemolytic disease of the newborn or in pts who have undergone spontaneous or induced abortion. Also used to prevent isoimmunization in Rh$_o$(D)-negative individuals who have been transfused with Rh$_o$(D)-positive red blood cells. *Treatment of immune thrombocytopenia purpura in Rh$_o$(D) antigen-positive pts.*

PRECAUTIONS

CONTRAINDICATIONS: History of allergic response to gamma globulin or anti-immunoglobulin A (IgA) antibodies, allergic response to thimerosal, pts with isolated immunoglobulin A (IgA) deficiency, those who have severe thrombocytopenia and any coagulation disorder. **CAUTIONS:** Prior systemic allergic reactions following administration of human immunoglobulin preparations. Pre-existing renal dysfunction, diabetes.

INTERACTIONS

DRUG: Live virus vaccines may potentiate virus replication, increase vaccine side effects, decrease pt's antibody response to vaccine. **HERBAL:** None significant. **FOOD:** None significant. **LAB VALUES:** None significant.

AVAILABILITY (Rx)

(Rho-Gam): **SOLUTION FOR INJECTION:** 5% ± 1% gamma globulin. *(BayRho-D Full Dose):* **SOLUTION FOR INJECTION:** 15–18% protein.

ADMINISTRATION/HANDLING
IM:
Storage:
• Store at room temperature. Dis-

card if particulate matter or discoloration is present.

Administration:
• Remove syringe from package by lifting syringe by barrel, not by plunger. Twist plunger rod clockwise until threads are seated. Push the plunger rod forward a few millimeters to break any friction seal between rubber stopper and the glass syringe barrel. Expel air bubbles and proceed with injection. • Do not inject IV. Do not inject the neonate. Inject preferably in anterolateral aspect of upper thigh or deltoid muscle of upper arm. Generally, avoid the gluteal region (risk of injury to sciatic nerve). If gluteal region is used, avoid the central region; use only upper, outer quadrant. • Inject entire contents of vial or syringe IM. • If transfusing Rh$_o$(D)-positive red cells to an Rh$_o$(D)-negative pt, the volume of Rh-positive whole blood is multiplied by the Hct of the donor unit giving the volume of RBCs transfused. The RBC volume is divided by 15 ml, providing the number of vials or syringes to be given. The total volume can be given in divided doses at different sites at one time, or total dose may be divided and injected at intervals within 72 hrs of fetomaternal hemorrhage or transfusion.

IV INCOMPATIBILITIES ⊘
Do not mix with any other medications.

INDICATIONS/ROUTES/DOSAGE
Postpartum prophylaxis:
IM: Adults: Administer 1 vial or syringe (300 mcg) preferably within 72 hrs of delivery or miscarriage.

R

Antenatal prophylaxis:

IM: **Adults:** Administer 1 vial or syringe (300 mcg) preferably at approximately 28 wks of gestation. Follow with another dose preferably within 72 hrs following delivery if the infant is Rh-positive.

Transfusion:

IM: **Adults:** Administer within 72 hrs after exposure of incompatible blood transfusion.

SIDE EFFECTS

OCCASIONAL (1–7%): Discomfort, slight swelling at injection site, slight elevation of temperature.

ADVERSE REACTIONS/TOXIC EFFECTS

Anaphylactic reactions occur rarely but incidence increased when given large IM doses or in pts receiving repeated injections of immune globulin. Epinephrine should be readily available.

NURSING IMPLICATIONS

BASELINE ASSESSMENT:

Inquire about history of exposure to hemolytic condition. Have epinephrine readily available.

PATIENT/FAMILY TEACHING:

Explain rationale for therapy. Local pain or muscle tenderness may occur at IM injection site.

ribavirin

rye-bah-**vi**-rin
(Rebetol, Virazole)
Do not confuse with riboflavin.

FIXED-COMBINATION(S)

With interferon, alfa 2b **(Rebetron)**

▶CLASSIFICATION

PHARMACOTHERAPEUTIC: Synthetic nucleoside. *CLINICAL:* Antiviral (see p. 59C)

ACTION/THERAPEUTIC EFFECT

Appears to be virustatic through disruption of RNA and DNA synthesis, *interfering with viral replication, protein synthesis.*

USES/UNLABELED

Severe lower respiratory tract infections due to respiratory syncytial viruses in select infants, children. *Treatment of influenza A or B.*

PRECAUTIONS

CONTRAINDICATIONS: Potential for pregnancy. *CAUTIONS:* Use care in assisted ventilation because of mechanical problems associated with precipitate and "rainout" when fluid accumulates in tubing.

INTERACTIONS

DRUG: May have antagonistic effect with **zidovudine**. *HERBAL:* None known. *FOOD:* None known. *LAB VALUES:* None significant.

AVAILABILITY (Rx)

POWDER FOR RECONSTITUTION (Aerosol): 6 g/100 ml. *CAPSULES.*

ADMINISTRATION/HANDLING

Inhalation:

Note: May be given via nasal or oral inhalation.

• Solution appears clear and colorless, is stable for 24 hrs at room temperature. Discard solution for nebulization after 24 hrs. • Discard if discolored or cloudy. • Add 50–100 ml Sterile Water for Injection or inhalation to 6 g vial. • Transfer to a flask, serving as reservoir for aerosol generator. • Further dilute to final volume of 300 ml, giving a solution concentration of 20 mg/ml. • Use only aerosol generator available from manufacturer of drug. • Do not give concomitantly with other drug solutions for nebulization. • Discard reservoir solution when fluid levels are low and at least q24h. • Controversy over safety in ventilator-dependent pts; only experienced personnel should administer.

INDICATIONS/ROUTES/DOSAGE

Severe lower respiratory tract infection caused by RSV:

INHALATION: Children, infants: Use with Viratek small particle aerosol generator at a concentration of 20 mg/ml (6 g reconstituted with 300 ml sterile water) 12–18 hrs/day for 3 days or up to 7 days.

SIDE EFFECTS

OCCASIONAL: Rash, conjunctivitis, reticulocytosis. ***RARE:*** Hypotension, digitalis toxicity.

ADVERSE REACTIONS/TOXIC EFFECTS

Cardiac arrest, apnea and ventilator dependence, bacterial pneumonia, pneumonia, pneumothorax occur rarely. If therapy exceeds 7 days, anemia may occur.

NURSING IMPLICATIONS

BASELINE ASSESSMENT:
Obtain respiratory tract secretions before giving first dose or at least during first 24 hrs of therapy. Assess respiratory status for baseline.

INTERVENTION/EVALUATION:
Monitor I&O, fluid balance carefully. Check hematology reports for anemia due to reticulocytosis when therapy exceeds 7 days. For ventilator-assisted pts watch for "rainout" in tubing and empty frequently; be alert to impaired ventilation and gas exchange due to drug precipitate. Assess skin for rash. Monitor B/P, respirations; assess lung sounds.

PATIENT/FAMILY TEACHING:
Report immediately any difficulty breathing, or itching/swelling/redness of eyes.

rifabutin

rye-fah-**byew**-tin
(Mycobutin)
Do not confuse with rifampin.

▶CLASSIFICATION

PHARMACOTHERAPEUTIC: Antitubercular. ***CLINICAL:*** Antibacterial (antimycobacterial)

ACTION/*THERAPEUTIC EFFECT*

Inhibits DNA-dependent RNA polymerase, an enzyme in susceptible strains of *E. coli* and *Bacillus subtilis, preventing M avium complex (MAC) disease.*

PHARMACOKINETICS

Readily absorbed from GI tract (high-fat meals slow absorption). Protein binding: 85%. Widely distributed. Crosses blood-brain barrier. Extensive intracellular tissue uptake. Metabolized in liver to active metabolite. Excreted in urine;

R

eliminated in feces. Unknown if removed by hemodialysis. Half-life: 16–69 hrs.

USES

Prevention of disseminated *Mycobacterium avium* complex (MAC) disease in those with advanced HIV infection.

PRECAUTIONS

CONTRAINDICATIONS: Hypersensitivity to other rifamycins (e.g., rifampin). Active tuberculosis. ***CAUTIONS:*** Safety in children not established.

▷***LIFESPAN CONSIDERATIONS:*** **Pregnancy/Lactation:** Unknown if drug crosses placenta or is excreted in breast milk. **Pregnancy Category B. Children/Elderly:** No age-related precautions noted.

INTERACTIONS

DRUG: May decrease effects of **oral contraceptives.** May decrease concentration of **zidovudine** (does not affect inhibition of HIV by zidovudine). ***HERBAL:*** None known. ***FOOD:*** None known. ***LAB VALUES:*** May increase SGOT (AST), SGPT (ALT), alkaline phosphatase. May cause anemia, neutropenia, leukopenia, thrombocytopenia.

AVAILABILITY (Rx)

CAPSULES: 150 mg.

ADMINISTRATION/HANDLING
PO:

• Give without regard to food. Give with food GI irritation occurs.
• May mix with applesauce if pt is unable to swallow capsules whole.

INDICATIONS/ROUTES/DOSAGE
MAC:

PO: Adults, elderly, adolescents:

300 mg/day as single dose or in two divided doses.

SIDE EFFECTS

FREQUENT (30%): Red-orange/red-brown discoloration of urine, feces, saliva, skin, sputum, sweat, or tears. ***OCCASIONAL*** (3–11%): Rash, nausea, abdominal pain, diarrhea, dyspepsia (heartburn, indigestion, epigastric pain), belching headache, altered taste. ***RARE*** (≤2%): Anorexia, flatulence, fever, myalgia, vomiting, insomnia.

ADVERSE REACTIONS/TOXIC EFFECTS

Hepatitis, thrombocytopenia occur rarely.

NURSING IMPLICATIONS

BASELINE ASSESSMENT:

Chest x-ray, sputum or blood cultures, biopsy of suspicious node must be done to rule out active tuberculosis (given in active tuberculosis may cause resistance to both rifabutin and rifampin). Obtain baseline CBC, hepatic function tests.

INTERVENTION/EVALUATION:

Monitor lab values. Avoid IM injections, rectal temperatures, other trauma that may induce bleeding. Check temperature and notify physician of flulike syndrome, rash, or GI intolerance.

PATIENT/FAMILY TEACHING:

Urine, feces, saliva, sputum, perspiration, tears, skin may be discolored brown-orange. Soft contact lenses may be permanently discolored. Rifabutin may decrease efficacy of oral contraceptives; nonhormonal methods should be considered. Avoid crowds, those with infection. Notify physician immediately of signs and symptoms of MAC and tuberculosis: night sweats, fatigue, fever, weight loss, abdominal pain. Report any yellowing of skin or eyes.

rifampin

rif-**am**-pin
(Rifadin, Rimactane, Rofact✤)
Do not confuse with rifabutin, Rifamate, rifapentine, Ritalin.

FIXED-COMBINATION(S)

With isoniazid, an antitubercular **(Rifamate);** with isoniazid and pyrazinamide, antituberculars **(Rifater)**

▶CLASSIFICATION
CLINICAL: Antitubercular

ACTION/*THERAPEUTIC EFFECT*

Interferes with bacterial RNA synthesis by binding to DNA-dependent RNA polymerase, preventing attachment of the enzyme to DNA, thereby blocking RNA transcription. *Bactericidal activity occurs in susceptible microorganisms.*

PHARMACOKINETICS

Well absorbed from GI tract (food delays absorption). Protein binding: 80%. Widely distributed. Metabolized in liver to active metabolite. Primarily eliminated via biliary system. Not removed by hemodialysis. Half-life: 3–5 hrs.

USES/*UNLABELED*

In conjunction with at least one other antitubercular agent for initial treatment and retreatment of clinical tuberculosis. Eliminates *Neisseria* meningococci from the nasopharynx of asymptomatic carriers in situations with high risk of meningococcal meningitis (prophylaxis, not cure). Recommended by WHO as adjunctive therapy with dapsone for leprosy. *Prophylaxis of H. Influenza type b infection, treatment of atypical mycobacterial infection, serious infections caused by Staphylococcus species.*

PRECAUTIONS

CONTRAINDICATIONS: Hypersensitivity to rifampin or any rifamycins, intermittent therapy. *CAUTIONS:* Hepatic dysfunction, active/treated alcoholism. Dosage not established in children <5 yrs of age.
▷*LIFESPAN CONSIDERATIONS:*
Pregnancy/Lactation: Crosses placenta; is distributed in breast milk. **Pregnancy Category C. Children/Elderly:** No age-related precautions noted.

INTERACTIONS

DRUG: **Alcohol, hepatotoxic medications** may increase risk of hepatotoxicity. May increase clearance of **aminophylline, theophylline.** May decrease effects of **oral anticoagulants, oral hypoglycemics, chloramphenicol, digoxin, disopyramide, mexiletine, quinidine, tocainide, fluconazole, methadone, phenytoin, verapamil.** *HERBAL:* None known. *FOOD:* None known. *LAB VALUES:* May increase SGOT (AST), SGPT (ALT), alkaline phosphatase, bilirubin, BUN, uric acid.

AVAILABILITY (Rx)

CAPSULES: 150 mg, 300 mg. *POWDER FOR INJECTION:* 600 mg.

R

ADMINISTRATION/HANDLING

PO:

• Preferably give 1 hr before or 2 hrs after meals with 8 oz water (may give with food to decrease GI upset; will delay absorption). • For those unable to swallow capsules, contents may be mixed with applesauce, jelly. • Administer at least 1 hr before antacids, esp. those containing aluminum.

IV 💊

Storage:

• Reconstituted vial is stable for 24 hrs. • Use diluted solution within 4 hrs.

Reconstitution:

• Reconstitute 600 mg vial with 10 ml Sterile Water for Injection to provide concentration of 60 mg/ml. • Withdraw desired dose and further dilute with 500 ml D_5W.

Rate of administration:

• For IV infusion only. Avoid IM, SubQ administration. • Avoid extravasation (local irritation, inflammation). • Infuse over 3 hrs (may dilute with 100 ml D_5W and infuse over 30 min).

IV INCOMPATIBILITY ⊘

Diltiazem (Cardizem).

INDICATIONS/ROUTES/DOSAGE

Tuberculosis:

IV/PO: Adults, elderly: 10 mg/kg/day. **Maximum:** 600 mg/day. **Children:** 10–20 mg/kg/day in divided doses q12–24h.

Meningococcal prophylaxis:

IV/PO: Adults, elderly: 600 mg q12h for 2 days. **Children:** 20 mg/kg/day in divided doses q12–24h. **Maximum:** 600 mg/dose. **Infants <1 mo:** 10 mg/kg/day in divided doses q12h for 2 days.

Staphylococcal infections:

IV/PO: Adults, elderly: 600 mg once daily. **Children:** 15 mg/kg/day in divided doses q12h.

SIDE EFFECTS

EXPECTED: Red-orange/red-brown discoloration of urine, feces, saliva, skin, sputum, sweat, or tears. ***OCCASIONAL*** (2–5%): Hypersensitivity reaction (pruritus, flushing, rash). ***RARE*** (1–2%): Diarrhea, dyspepsia, nausea, fungal overgrowth (sore mouth/tongue).

ADVERSE REACTIONS/TOXIC EFFECTS

Hepatotoxicity (risk increased with isoniazid combination), hepatitis, blood dyscrasias, Stevens-Johnson syndrome, antibiotic-associated colitis occur rarely.

NURSING IMPLICATIONS

BASELINE ASSESSMENT:

Question for hypersensitivity to rifampin, rifamycins. Assure collection of diagnostic specimens. Evaluate initial hepatic function and CBC results.

INTERVENTION/EVALUATION:

Assess IV site at least hrly during infusion; restart at another site at the first sign of irritation/inflammation. Monitor hepatic function tests and assess for hepatitis: jaundice, anorexia, nausea, vomiting, fatigue, weakness (hold rifampin and inform physician at once). Report hypersensitivity reactions promptly: any type skin eruption, pruritus, flu-like syndrome with high dosage. Monitor frequency, consistency of stools esp. with potential for antibiotic-associated colitis.

Monitor CBC results for blood dyscrasias and be alert for infection (fever, sore throat), bleeding/bruising, or unusual tiredness/weakness.

PATIENT/FAMILY TEACHING:

Preferably take on empty stomach with 8 oz water 1 hr before or 2 hrs after meal (with food if GI upset). Avoid alcohol during treatment. Do not take *any* other medications without consulting physician, including antacids; must take rifampin at least 1 hr before antacid. Urine, feces, sputum, sweat, tears may become red-orange; soft contact lenses may be permanently stained. Notify physician of *any* new symptom, immediately for yellow eyes/skin, fatigue, weakness, nausea/vomiting, sore throat, fever, flu, unusual bruising/bleeding. If taking oral contraceptives check with physician (reliability may be affected).

rifapentine

rif-ah-**pen**-teen
(Priftin)

▶CLASSIFICATION
CLINICAL: Antitubercular

ACTION/*THERAPEUTIC EFFECT*

Inhibits DNA-dependent RNA polymerase in *M. tuberculosis.* Interferes with bacterial RNA synthesis, preventing attachment of enzyme to DNA, thereby blocking RNA transcription. *Bactericidal activity.*

USES

Treatment of pulmonary tuberculosis in combination with at least one other antituberculosis medication.

INTERACTIONS

DRUG: None significant. ***HERBAL:*** None known. ***FOOD:*** None known. ***LAB VALUES:*** None significant.

AVAILABILITY (Rx)
TABLETS: 150 mg.

INDICATIONS/ROUTES/DOSAGE

Note: Use only with another antituberculosis agent.

Tuberculosis:

PO: Adults, elderly: Intensive phase: 600 mg 2 times/wk for 2 mos (interval no less than 3 days). ***Continuation phase:*** 600 mg weekly for 4 mos.

SIDE EFFECTS

RARE (<4%): Red-orange/red-brown discoloration of urine, feces, saliva, skin, sputum, sweat, or tears, arthralgia, pain, nausea, vomiting, headache, dyspepsia (heartburn, indigestion, epigastric pain), hypertension, dizziness, diarrhea.

ADVERSE REACTIONS/TOXIC EFFECTS

Hyperuricemia, neutropenia, proteinuria, hematuria occur rarely.

NURSING IMPLICATIONS

BASELINE ASSESSMENT:
Evaluate initial hepatic function and CBC results.

INTERVENTION/EVALUATION:
Monitor frequency, consistency of stools. Assess for nausea, vomiting, GI upset, diarrhea.

R

PATIENT/FAMILY TEACHING:

Urine, feces, sputum, sweat, tears may become red-orange; soft contact lenses may be permanently stained. If taking oral contraceptives check with physician (reliability may be affected).

rimantadine hydrochloride

rye-**man**-tah-deen
(Flumadine)
Do not confuse with flunisolide, flutamide, ranitidine.

▶CLASSIFICATION
CLINICAL: Antiviral

ACTION/*THERAPEUTIC EFFECT*

Appears to exert inhibitory effect early in viral replication cycle. May inhibit uncoating of virus, *preventing replication of influenza A virus.*

PHARMACOKINETICS

Readily absorbed from GI tract. Protein binding: 40%. Metabolized in liver. Primarily excreted in urine. Not removed by hemodialysis. Half-life: 20–65 hrs (half-life increased in severe liver and/or renal impairment).

USES

Adults: Prophylaxis and treatment of illness due to influenza A virus. ***Children:*** Prophylaxis against influenza A virus.

PRECAUTIONS

CONTRAINDICATIONS: Hypersensitivity to amantadine, rimantadine. ***CAUTIONS:*** Pts with renal, liver impairment; history of seizures (increased incidence of seizures).

▷*LIFESPAN CONSIDERATIONS:*
Pregnancy/Lactation: Avoid use in nursing mothers. Potentially carcinogenic. Unknown if drug crosses placenta or is excreted in breast milk. **Pregnancy Category C. Children:** No age-related precautions noted in those >1 yr of age. **Elderly:** More likely to experience CNS and GI side effects.

INTERACTIONS

DRUG:* Acetaminophen, aspirin** may decrease concentrations. **Cimetidine** may increase concentrations. ***HERBAL: None known. ***FOOD:*** None known. ***LAB VALUES:*** None significant.

AVAILABILITY (Rx)

TABLETS: 100 mg. ***SYRUP:*** 50 mg/5 ml.

ADMINISTRATION/HANDLING
PO:

• Give without regard to food.

INDICATIONS/ROUTES/DOSAGE
Prophylaxis against influenza A virus:

***PO:* Adults, elderly, children >10 yrs:** 100 mg 2 times/day. **Severe hepatic/renal impairment, elderly nursing home pts:** 100 mg/day. **Children <10 yrs:** 5 mg/kg once daily. **Maximum:** 150 mg.

Treatment of influenza virus A:

***PO:* Adults, elderly:** 100 mg 2 times/day for 7 days. **Severe hepatic/renal impairment, elderly nursing home pts:** 100 mg/day for 7 days.

SIDE EFFECTS

OCCASIONAL (2–3%): Insomnia, nausea, nervousness, impaired concentration, dizziness. **RARE** (<2%): Vomiting, anorexia, dry mouth, abdominal pain, asthenia (loss of strength, energy), fatigue.

ADVERSE REACTIONS/TOXIC EFFECTS

None significant.

NURSING IMPLICATIONS

INTERVENTION/EVALUATION:

Assess for nervousness and evaluate sleep pattern for insomnia. Provide assistance if dizziness occurs.

PATIENT/FAMILY TEACHING:

Avoid contact with those who are at high risk for influenza A (rimantadine-resistant virus may be shed during therapy). Do not drive or perform tasks that require alert response if dizziness or decreased concentration occurs. Do not take aspirin, acetaminophen, or compounds containing these drugs.

risedronate sodium

rize-droe-nate
(Actonel)

▶CLASSIFICATION

PHARMACOTHERAPEUTIC: Biphosphonate. **CLINICAL:** Calcium regulator

ACTION/THERAPEUTIC EFFECT

Binds to bone hydroxyapatite and inhibits osteoclasts. *Reduces bone turnover (number of sites at which bone is remodeled) and bone resorption.*

USES

Treatment of Paget's disease of bone (osteitis deformans). Treatment/prophylaxis for postmenopausal, glucocorticoid-induced osteoporosis.

PRECAUTIONS

CONTRAINDICATIONS: Hypersensitivity to other biphosphonates (etidronate, tiludronate, risedronate, alendronate), renal impairment when serum creatinine clearance 5mg/dl, hypocalcemia. **CAUTIONS:** GI diseases (duodenitis, dysphagia, esophagitis, gastritis, ulcers (drug may exacerbate these conditions), severe renal impairment.

INTERACTIONS

DRUG: Antacids with **calcium, magnesium, aluminum, vitamin D** may decrease absorption. **HERBAL:** None known. **FOOD:** None known. **LAB VALUES:** None significant.

AVAILABILITY (Rx)

TABLETS: 5 mg, 30 mg.

INDICATIONS/ROUTES/DOSAGE

Note: Must take with 6–8 oz water 30 min before first food or drink of the day. Avoid lying down for at least 30 min after taking.

Paget's disease:

PO: Adults, elderly: 30 mg/day for 2 mos. Retreatment may occur after 2 mo post-treatment observation period.

Osteoporosis:

PO: Adults, elderly: 5 mg/day.

R

SIDE EFFECTS

FREQUENT (30%): Arthralgia. ***OCCASIONAL*** (8–12%): Rash, flu-like symptoms, peripheral edema. ***RARE*** (3–5%): Bone pain, sinusitis, asthenia, (loss of strength, energy), dry eye, tinnitus.

ADVERSE REACTIONS/TOXIC EFFECTS

Hypocalcemia, hypophosphatemia, significant GI disturbances result from overdosage.

NURSING IMPLICATIONS

BASELINE ASSESSMENT:

Hypocalcemia, vitamin D deficiency must be corrected before therapy. Obtain lab baselines, esp. electrolytes, renal function.

INTERVENTION/EVALUATION:

Check electrolytes (esp. calcium and alkaline phosphatase serum levels). Check I&O, BUN, creatinine in pts with impaired renal function.

PATIENT/FAMILY TEACHING:

Instruct pt that expected benefits occur only when medication is taken with full glass (6–8 oz) of plain water, first thing in the morning and at least 30 min before first food, beverage, or medication of the day. Any other beverage (mineral water, orange juice, coffee) significantly reduces absorption of medication. Do not lie down for at least 30 min after taking medication (potentiates delivery to stomach, reduces risk of esophageal irritation). Consider weight-bearing exercises, modify behavioral factors (e.g., cigarette smoking, alcohol consumption).

risperidone

ris-**pear**-ih-doan
(Risperdal)
Do not confuse with reserpine.

▶CLASSIFICATION

PHARMACOTHERAPEUTIC: Benzisoxazole derivative. ***CLINICAL:*** Antipsychotic (see p. 56C)

ACTION/*THERAPEUTIC EFFECT*

Action may be due to dopamine and serotonin receptor antagonism. *Suppresses behavioral response in psychosis.*

PHARMACOKINETICS

Well absorbed from GI tract (unaffected by food). Protein binding: 90%. Extensively metabolized in liver to active metabolite. Primarily excreted in urine. Half-life: 3–20 hrs; metabolite: 21–30 hrs (half-life increased in elderly).

USES

Management of manifestations of psychotic disorders.

PRECAUTIONS

CONTRAINDICATIONS: Cardiac pts, those with cerebrovascular disease, dehydration, hypovolemia, use of antihypertensives. ***CAUTIONS:*** History of seizures. May mask signs of drug overdose, intestinal obstruction.

▷***LIFESPAN CONSIDERATIONS:*** **Pregnancy/Lactation:** Unknown if drug crosses placenta or is excreted in breast milk. Recommend against breast feeding. **Pregnancy Category C. Children:** Safety and efficacy not established. **Elderly:** More susceptible to postural hypotension. Age-related renal or liver impairment may require dosage adjustment.

INTERACTIONS

DRUG: May decrease effects of **levodopa, dopamine agonists. Carbamazepine** may decrease concentration. **Clozapine** may increase concentration. **Alcohol, CNS depressants** may increase CNS depression. **Paroxetine** can increase concentration, risk of extrapyramidal symptoms. ***HERBAL:*** None known. ***FOOD:*** None known. ***LAB VALUES:*** May increase creatine phosphatase, uric acid, triglycerides, SGOT (AST), SGPT (ALT), prolactin. May decrease potassium, sodium, protein, glucose. May cause EKG changes.

AVAILABILITY (Rx)

TABLETS: 0.25 mg, 0.5 mg, 1 mg, 2 mg, 3 mg, 4 mg. ***ORAL SOLUTION:*** 1 mg/ml.

ADMINISTRATION/HANDLING
PO:
• Give without regard to food.

INDICATIONS/ROUTES/DOSAGE
Antipsychotic:

PO: Adults: Initially, 1 mg 2 times/day for 1 day; then, 2 mg 2 times/day for 1 day; then, 3 mg 2 times/day for 1 day. Further adjustments of 1 mg 2 times/day made at at least 1 wk intervals. Maximum effect in range of 4–6 mg/day. **Elderly, debilitated, pts with severe liver/renal impairment, risk of hypotension:** Initially, 0.5 mg 2 times/day for 1 day; then, 1 mg 2 times/day for 1 day; then, 1.5 mg 2 times/day for 1 day. Further adjustments made at at least 1 wk intervals.

SIDE EFFECTS

FREQUENT (13–26%): Agitation, anxiety, insomnia, headache, constipation. ***OCCASIONAL*** (4–10%): Dyspepsia, rhinitis, drowsiness, dizziness, nausea, vomiting, rash, abdominal pain, dry skin, tachycardia. ***RARE*** (2–3%): Visual disturbances, fever, back pain, pharyngitis, cough, arthralgia, angina, aggressive reaction.

ADVERSE REACTIONS/TOXIC EFFECTS

Neuroleptic malignant syndrome (NMS): hyperpyrexia, muscle rigidity, change in mental status, irregular pulse or B/P, tachycardia, diaphoresis, cardiac dysrhythmias, rhabdomyolysis, acute renal failure. Tardive dyskinesia (protrusion of tongue, puffing of cheeks, chewing/puckering of the mouth).

NURSING IMPLICATIONS

BASELINE ASSESSMENT:

Renal and liver function tests should be done before therapy. Assess behavior, appearance, emotional status, response to environment, speech pattern, thought content.

INTERVENTION/EVALUATION:

Monitor for fine tongue movement (may be first sign of tardive dyskinesia, which may be irreversible). Supervise suicidal risk pt closely during early therapy (as depression lessens, energy level improves, increasing suicide potential). Assess for therapeutic response (greater interest in surroundings, improved self-care, increased ability to concentrate, relaxed facial expression). Monitor for potential neuroleptic malignant syndrome (NMS):

R

fever, muscle rigidity, irregular B/P or pulse, altered mental status.

PATIENT/FAMILY TEACHING:

Do not drive or perform tasks requiring alert response until assured that drug does not cause impairment.

ritodrine hydrochloride

rih-toe-dreen
(Yutopar)
Do not confuse with ranitidine.

▶**CLASSIFICATION**

PHARMACOTHERAPEUTIC: Uterine active agent. *CLINICAL:* Uterine relaxant

ACTION/*THERAPEUTIC EFFECT*

Beta$_2$-adrenergic stimulant that relaxes uterine smooth muscle, altering cellular calcium balance affecting smooth muscle contractility, *suppressing uterine contractions.*

USES

Prolongs gestation by inhibiting uterine contractions in preterm labor.

PRECAUTIONS

CONTRAINDICATIONS: Before 20th week of pregnancy, maternal cardiac arrhythmias, uncontrolled hypertension, bronchial asthma treated with betamimetics or steroids, hypovolemia. When continuation of pregnancy is hazardous to mother or fetus: eclampsia, severe pre-eclampsia, antepartum hemorrhage, intrauterine fetal death, pulmonary hypertension, pheochromocytoma, hyperthyroidism,

cardiac disease, chorioamnionitis, uncontrolled diabetes mellitus. With injection, sulfite sensitivity (often with aspirin sensitivity). *CAUTIONS:* Migraine headache, diabetes mellitus, concomitant use of potassium-depleting diuretics.

INTERACTIONS

DRUG: **Beta-adrenergic blockers** antagonize effects. **Glucocorticoids** enhance fetal lung maturity; may increase risk of pulmonary edema in mother. *HERBAL:* None known. *FOOD:* None known. *LAB VALUES:* May increase SGOT (AST), SGPT (ALT), FFA, blood glucose, serum insulin. May decrease potassium.

AVAILABILITY (Rx)

INJECTION: 10 mg/ml, 15 mg/ml.

ADMINISTRATION/HANDLING
IV 🝙

Storage:
• Stable for 48 hrs at room temperature after dilution. Do not use if discolored or if precipitate forms.

Reconstitution:
• Dilute 15 ml concentrate (150 mg) in 500 ml of D_5W to provide concentration of 0.3 mg/ml. Due to potential for pulmonary edema, NaCl-containing solutions are used only when dextrose is medically undesirable (e.g., diabetes mellitus).

Rate of administration:
• Place pt in left lateral position to prevent hypotension. • Begin with 0.05 mg/min (10 gtt/min), gradually increase by 0.05 mg/min (10 gtt/min) q10min until desired effect is achieved or maternal heart rate reaches 130 beats per min.

IV INCOMPATIBILITY ⊘

Do not mix with any other medications.

INDICATIONS/ROUTES/DOSAGE

Usual parenteral dosage:

IV INFUSION: **Adults:** Initially, 0.05 mg/min (10 ml/hr); gradually increase by 0.05 mg/min (10 ml/hr) q10min until desired result reached. **Range:** 0.15–0.35 mg/min (30–70 ml/hr). Continue for 12 hrs after uterine contractions cease.

SIDE EFFECTS

FREQUENT: Increased maternal and fetal heart rates, widening maternal pulse pressure (80–100%); palpitations (33%); nausea, vomiting, headache, erythema (10–15%). ***OCCASIONAL*** (3–10%): Tremors, jitteriness, chest pain/tightness, constipation, diarrhea, bloating, sweating, chills, weakness. *Neonate:* Hypo/hyperglycemia, ileus, hypocalcemia, hypotension. ***RARE:*** Impaired liver function.

ADVERSE REACTIONS/TOXIC EFFECTS

Ketoacidosis occurs infrequently. Pulmonary edema (may be fatal, esp. with preexisting cardiopulmonary disease or concomitant use of corticosteroids), anaphylactic shock, hepatitis occur rarely.

NURSING IMPLICATIONS

BASELINE ASSESSMENT:

Assess baseline vitals, glucose and potassium levels, EKG, fetal heart rate. Check lungs, determine hydration status. Determine frequency, duration, and strength of contractions.

INTERVENTION/EVALUATION:

Take temperature at start and conclusion of IV infusion. Monitor vitals, fetal heart rate q15min until stable, then hrly until infusion is complete. Check uterine contractions frequently throughout the infusion. Assess lungs for rales; pay particular attention to evidence of impending pulmonary edema (persistent tachycardia, fluid retention [I&O], increased respiratory rate/shortness of breath). Monitor potassium and glucose levels.

PATIENT/FAMILY TEACHING:

Keep pt, family informed of therapeutic response during infusion. Explain importance of left lateral position during IV infusion.

ritonavir

rih-**tone**-ah-vir
(Norvir)
Do not confuse with Retrovir.

▶CLASSIFICATION

PHARMACOTHERAPEUTIC: Protease inhibitor. ***CLINICAL:*** Antiviral (see pp. 59C, 96C)

ACTION/*THERAPEUTIC EFFECT*

Inhibits HIV-1 and HIV-2 proteases, rendering the enzymes incapable of processing the polypeptide precursor that leads to production of immature HIV particles, *slowing HIV replication, reducing progression of HIV infection.*

PHARMACOKINETICS

Slowly absorbed following PO administration (extent of absorption increased with food). Protein binding: 98–99%. Extensively metabolized by liver to active metabolite.

Primarily eliminated in feces. Unknown if removed by hemodialysis. Half-life: 2.7–5 hrs.

USES

Used in combination with nucleoside analogues or as monotherapy for treatment of HIV infection.

PRECAUTIONS

CONTRAINDICATIONS: Hypersensitivity to drug; amiodarone, astemizole, bepridil, bupropion, cisapride, clozapine, encainide, flecainide, meperidine, piroxicam, propafenone, propoxyphene, quinidine, rifabutin, and terfenadine increase risk of arrhythmias, hematologic abnormalities, seizures. Alprazolam, clorazepate, diazepam, estrazolam, flurazepam, midazolam, triazolam, and zolpidem may produce extreme sedation and respiratory depression. ***CAUTIONS:*** Impaired hepatic function. ▷***LIFESPAN CONSIDERATIONS:*** **Pregnancy/Lactation:** Breast feeding not recommended (possibility of HIV transmission). **Pregnancy Category B. Children:** No age-related precautions noted in those >2 yrs of age. **Elderly:** Information not available.

INTERACTIONS

DRUG: May produce disulfiramlike reaction if taken with **disulfiram** or drugs causing disulfiramlike reaction (e.g., **metronidazole). Enzyme inducers (e.g., nevirapine, phenobarbital, carbamazepine, dexamethasone, phenytoin, rifampin, rifabutin)** may increase metabolism, decrease efficacy. May decrease effectiveness of **theophylline, oral contraceptives.** May increase concentration of **desipramine, fluoxetine, other antidepressants. *HERBAL:* St. John's wort** may decrease concentration, effect. ***FOOD:*** None known. ***LAB VALUES:*** May alter SGPT (ALT), SGOT (AST), creatinine clearance, GGT, CPK, uric acid, triglycerides.

AVAILABILITY (Rx)

SOFT GELATIN CAPSULES: 100 mg. ***ORAL SOLUTION:*** 80 mg/ml.

ADMINISTRATION/HANDLING
PO:

• Store capsules, solution in refrigerator. • Protect from light. • Refrigeration of oral solution is recommended but not necessary if used within 30 days and stored below 77°F. • Give without regard to meals (preferably give with food). • May improve taste of oral solution by mixing with chocolate milk, Ensure, or Advera within 1 hr of dosing.

INDICATIONS/ROUTES/DOSAGE
HIV infection:

PO: Adults: 600 mg 2 times/day. If nausea becomes apparent upon initiation of 600 mg twice daily, give 300 mg twice daily for 1 day, 400 mg twice daily for 2 days, 500 mg twice daily for 1 day, then 600 mg twice daily thereafter.

Children <12 yrs: Initially, 250 mg/m^2/dose 2 times/day. Increase by 50 mg/m^2/dose up to 400 mg/m^2/dose. **Maximum:** 600 mg/dose 2 times/day.

SIDE EFFECTS

FREQUENT: GI disturbances (nausea, diarrhea, vomiting, anorexia, abdominal pain), neurologic disturbances (taste perversion, circumoral and peripheral paresthesias, esp. around lips, hands, or feet), headache, dizziness, fatigue, weakness. ***OCCASIONAL:*** Allergic reaction, flu syndrome, hypotension.

ADVERSE REACTIONS/TOXIC EFFECTS

None significant.

NURSING IMPLICATIONS

BASELINE ASSESSMENT:

Pts beginning combination therapy with ritonavir and nucleosides may promote GI tolerance by beginning ritonavir alone and subsequently adding nucleosides before completing 2 wks of ritonavir monotherapy. Obtain baseline laboratory testing, esp. liver function tests, triglycerides before beginning ritonavir therapy and at periodic intervals during therapy. Offer emotional support.

INTERVENTION/EVALUATION:

Closely monitor for evidence of GI disturbances or neurologic abnormalities (particularly paresthesias). Monitor clinical chemistry tests for marked laboratory abnormalities.

PATIENT/FAMILY TEACHING:

Continue therapy for full length of treatment. Doses should be evenly spaced. Ritonavir is not a cure for HIV infection, nor does it reduce risk of transmission to others. Pts may continue to acquire illnesses associated with advanced HIV infection. If possible, take ritonavir with food. Taste of solution may be mixed with chocolate, Ensure, or Advera.

rituximab

rye-**tucks**-ih-mab
(Rituxan)

▶**CLASSIFICATION**

PHARMACOTHERAPEUTIC: Monoclonal antibody. ***CLINICAL:*** Antineoplastic (see p. 73C)

ACTION/*THERAPEUTIC EFFECT*

Binds to CD20, the antigen found on surface of B lymphocytes and B-cell non-Hodgkin's lymphomas, *producing cytotoxicity, reducing tumor size.*

PHARMACOKINETICS

Rapidly depletes B-cells. Half-life: 59.8 hrs after first infusion and 174 hrs after fourth infusion.

USES

Treatment of relapsed or refractory low-grade or follicular B-cell non-Hodgkins' lymphoma.

PRECAUTIONS

CONTRAINDICATIONS: Hypersensitivity to murine proteins. ***CAUTIONS:*** Those with history of cardiac disease.

▷***LIFESPAN CONSIDERATIONS:*** **Pregnancy/Lactation:** Has potential to cause fetal B-cell depletion. Unknown if distributed in breast milk. Those with childbearing potential should use contraceptive methods during treatment and up to 12 mos following therapy. **Pregnancy Category C. Children:** Safety and efficacy not established. **Elderly:** No age-related precautions noted.

INTERACTIONS

DRUG: None significant. ***HERBAL:*** None known. ***FOOD:*** None known. ***LAB VALUES:*** None significant.

AVAILABILITY (Rx)

INJECTION: 10 mg/ml.

R

♣ - Canadian trade name   ✳ - see also www.wbsaunders.com/SIMON/SaundersNDH

ADMINISTRATION/HANDLING

IV 🖾

Storage:

Note: Do not give by IV push or bolus.

• Refrigerate vials. • Diluted solution is stable for 24 hrs if refrigerated and at room temperature for an additional 12 hrs.

Reconstitution:

• Dilute with 0.9% NaCl or D_5W to provide a final concentration of 1–4 mg/ml into infusion bag.

Rate of administration:

• Infuse at rate of 50 mg/hr. May increase infusion rate in 50 mg/hr increments q30min to maximum 400 mg/hr. • Subsequent infusion can be given at 100 mg/hr and increased by 100 mg/hr increments q30min to maximum 400 mg/hr.

IV INCOMPATIBILITY ⊘

Do not mix with any other medications.

INDICATIONS/ROUTES/DOSAGE

Note: Pretreatment with acetaminophen and diphenhydramine before each infusion may prevent infusion-related effects.

Non-Hodgkins' lymphoma:

IV INFUSION: **Adults:** 375 mg/m^2 given once weekly for 4–8 wks. May be retreated with second 4 wk course.

SIDE EFFECTS

FREQUENT: Fever (49%), chills (32%), headache (14%), asthenia (16%), angioedema (13%), hypotension (10%), nausea (18%), rash/pruritus (10%). *OCCASIONAL* (<10%): Myalgia, dizziness, abdominal pain, throat irritation, vomiting, neutropenia, rhinitis, bronchospasm, urticaria.

ADVERSE REACTIONS/TOXIC EFFECTS

Hypersensitivity reaction produces hypotension, bronchospasm, angioedema. Cardiac arrhythmias may occur, particularly in those with history of preexisting cardiac conditions.

NURSING IMPLICATIONS

BASELINE ASSESSMENT:

Pretreatment with acetaminophen and diphenhydramine before each infusion may prevent infusion-related effects. CBC, platelet count should be obtained at regular interval during therapy.

INTERVENTION/EVALUATION:

Monitor for an infusion-related symptoms complex consisting mainly of fever, chills, rigors that generally occurs 30 min to 2 hrs of beginning first infusion. Slowing drip rate or slowing infusion resolves symptoms.

rivastigmine tartrate

rye-vah-**stig**-meen
(Exelon)

▶CLASSIFICATION

PHARMACOTHERAPEUTIC: Cholinesterase inhibitor. *CLINICAL:* Anti-Alzheimer's dementia agent

ACTION/*THERAPEUTIC EFFECT*

Increases the concentration of acetylcholine through reversible inhibition of its hydrolysis by cholinesterase, *enhancing cholinergic function.*

PHARMACOKINETICS

Rapidly and completely absorbed. Protein binding: 60%. Widely distributed throughout the body. Rapidly and extensively metabolized. Primarily excreted in urine. Half-life: 1.5 hrs.

USES

Treatment of mild to moderate dementia of the Alzheimer's type.

PRECAUTIONS

CONTRAINDICATIONS: None significant. ***CAUTIONS:*** Severe renal or liver impairment, those with sick-sinus syndrome, supraventricular cardiac conditions, asthma, COPD.

▷***LIFESPAN CONSIDERATIONS:*** **Pregnancy/Lactation:** Unknown if distributed in breast milk. **Pregnancy Category B. Children:** Not indicated in children. **Elderly:** No age-related precautions.

INTERACTIONS

DRUG: May interfere with **anticholinergic medications.** May have additive effect with **bethanecol. HERBAL:** None known. ***FOOD:*** None known. ***LAB VALUES:*** None significant.

AVAILABILITY (Rx)

CAPSULES: 1.5 mg, 3 mg, 4.5 mg, 6 mg. ***ORAL SOLUTION:*** 2 mg/ml.

ADMINISTRATION/HANDLING

Note: Oral solution and capsules may be interchanged at equal doses.

PO:

• Give with food in divided doses morning and evening.

Oral solution:

• Using oral syringe (provided by manufacturer), withdraw prescribed amount rivastigmine from container. • May be swallowed directly from syringe or mixed in small glass of water, cold fruit juice, or soda (use within 4 hrs of mixing).

INDICATIONS/ROUTES/DOSAGE

Alzheimer's disease:

PO: Adults, elderly: Initially, 1.5 mg twice daily. May increase after minimum of 2 wks to 3 mg twice daily. Subsequent increases to 4.5 mg and 6 mg twice daily may be made after a minimum of 2 wks at the previous dose. **Maximum:** 6 mg twice daily.

SIDE EFFECTS

FREQUENT (17–47%): Nausea, vomiting, dizziness, diarrhea, headache, anorexia. ***OCCASIONAL*** (6–13%): Abdominal pain, insomnia, dyspepsia (heartburn, indigestion, epigastric pain), confusion, urinary tract infection, depression. ***RARE*** (3–5%): Anxiety, somnolence, constipation, malaise, hallucinations, tremor, flatulence, rhinitis, hypertension, flulike symptoms, weight decrease, syncope.

ADVERSE REACTIONS/TOXIC EFFECTS

Overdosage can produce cholinergic crisis characterized by severe nausea, vomiting, salivation, sweating, bradycardia, hypotension, respiratory depression, convulsions.

R

NURSING IMPLICATIONS

BASELINE ASSESSMENT:

Obtain baseline vital signs. Obtain history of peptic ulcer, urinary obstruction, asthma, COPD. Assess cognitive, behavioral, and functional deficits.

INTERVENTION/EVALUATION:

Monitor for cholinergic reaction: GI discomfort/cramping, feeling of facial warmth, excessive salivation and sweating, lacrimation, pallor, urinary urgency, dizziness. Assess eyes for pupillary contraction. Monitor for nausea, diarrhea, headache, insomnia.

PATIENT/FAMILY TEACHING:

Report nausea, vomiting, diarrhea, sweating, increased salivary secretions, severe abdominal pain, dizziness.

rizatriptan benzoate

rise-ah-**trip**-tan
(Maxalt, Maxalt-MLT)

▶CLASSIFICATION

PHARMACOTHERAPEUTIC:
Serotonin receptor agonist. ***CLINICAL:*** Antimigraine (see p. 53C)

ACTION/*THERAPEUTIC EFFECT*

Binds selectively to vascular receptors producing a vasoconstrictive effect on cranial blood vessels, *producing relief of migraine headache.*

PHARMACOKINETICS

Well absorbed following PO administration. Protein binding: 14%. Crosses blood-brain barrier. Metabolized by the liver to inactive metabolite. Eliminated primarily in urine with lesser amount excreted in feces. Half-life: 2–3 hrs.

USES

Treatment of acute migraine attack with or without aura.

PRECAUTIONS

CONTRAINDICATIONS: Coronary artery disease, uncontrolled hypertension, ischemic heart disease (angina pectoris, history of MI, silent ischemia), Prinzmetal's angina, concurrent use (or within 24 hrs) of ergotamine-containing preparations, concurrent (or within 2 wks) of MAO therapy, hemiplegic or basilar migraine, within 24 hrs of another serotonin receptor agonist. ***CAUTIONS:*** Mild-to-moderate renal/hepatic impairment, pt profile suggesting cardiovascular risks.
▷***LIFESPAN CONSIDERATIONS:***
Pregnancy/Lactation: Unknown if distributed in breast milk. **Pregnancy Category C. Children:** Safety and efficacy not established. **Elderly:** No age-related precautions noted.

INTERACTIONS

DRUG: **Ergotamine-containing drugs** may produce vasospastic reaction. **MAO inhibitors, propranolol** may dramatically increase plasma concentration of rizatriptan. Combined use of **fluoxetine, fluvoxamine, paroxetine, sertraline** may produce weakness, hyperreflexia, incoordination. ***HERBAL:*** None known. ***FOOD:*** Food delays peak drug concentrations by 1 hr. ***LAB VALUES:*** None significant.

AVAILABILITY (Rx)

TABLETS: 5 mg, 10 mg. ***ORAL DISINTEGRATING TABLETS:*** 5 mg, 10 mg.

ADMINISTRATION/HANDLING
PO:

• The oral disintegrating tablet is packaged in an individual aluminum pouch. • Open packet with dry hands and place tablet onto tongue to be dissolved and swal-

---

𝒫 - see color pill atlas

lowed with saliva. Administration with water is not necessary.

INDICATIONS/ROUTES/DOSAGE

Migraine:

PO: **Adults >18 yrs:** 5–10 mg. Separate doses by at least 2 hrs. **Maximum:** 30 mg/24 hrs.

SIDE EFFECTS

FREQUENT (7–9%): Dizziness, somnolence, tingling in extremities, fatigue. *OCCASIONAL* (3–6%): Nausea, paresthesia, sensation of chest pressure, dry mouth. *RARE* (2%): Headache, neck/throat/jaw pressure, photosensitivity.

ADVERSE REACTIONS/TOXIC EFFECTS

Cardiac events (ischemia, coronary artery vasospasm, MI), noncardiac vasospasm-related reactions (hemorrhage, stroke) occur rarely but particularly in those with hypertension, obesity, smokers, diabetes, strong family history of coronary artery disease, male >40 yrs, postmenopausal women.

NURSING IMPLICATIONS

BASELINE ASSESSMENT:

Question regarding history of peripheral vascular disease, renal/hepatic impairment. Question pt regarding onset, location, and duration of migraine and possible precipitating symptoms.

INTERVENTION/EVALUATION:

Monitor for evidence of dizziness. Assess for relief of migraine headache and potential for photophobia, phonophobia (sound sensitivity, nausea, vomiting).

PATIENT/FAMILY TEACHING:

Take a single dose as soon as symptoms of an actual migraine attack appear. Medication is intended to relieve migraine, not to prevent or reduce number of attacks. Avoid tasks that require alertness, motor skills until response to drug is established. If heart throbbing, pain/tightness in chest or throat, or pain or weakness of extremities occurs, contact physician immediately. Do not remove the blister from the orally disintegrating tablet until just prior to dosing. Use protective measures (e.g., sunscreen, protective clothing) against exposure to UV/sunlight.

rocuronium bromide

(Zemuron)

See Classification section under: Neuromuscular blockers (p. 103C)

rofecoxib

row-feh-**cox**-ib
(Vioxx)
Do not confuse with Zyvox.

▶CLASSIFICATION

PHARMACOTHERAPEUTIC: Nonsteroidal anti-inflammatory. *CLINICAL:* Antiarthritic, analgesic, antidysmenorrheal (see p. 107C)

ACTION/THERAPEUTIC EFFECT

Produces analgesic and anti-inflammatory effect by inhibiting prostaglandin synthesis, *reducing inflammatory response and inten-*

sity of pain stimulus reaching sensory nerve endings.

PHARMACOKINETICS

Rapid, complete absorption from GI tract. Protein binding: 87%. Primarily metabolized in liver. Primarily eliminated in urine with a lesser amount excreted in feces. Not removed by hemodialysis. Half-life: 17 hrs.

USES

Relief of signs and symptoms of osteoarthritis. Management of acute pain in adults. Treatment of primary dysmenorrhea.

PRECAUTIONS

CONTRAINDICATIONS: History of hypersensitivity to aspirin, NSAIDs, sulfonamides. *CAUTIONS:* Impaired renal/hepatic function, history of GI tract disease, predisposition to fluid retention.
▷*LIFESPAN CONSIDERATIONS:* **Pregnancy/Lactation:** Unknown if drug is distributed in breast milk. Avoid use during third trimester (may adversely affect fetal cardiovascular system: premature closure of ductus arteriosus). **Pregnancy Category C. Children:** Safety and efficacy not established. **Elderly:** GI bleeding or ulceration more likely to cause serious adverse effects. Age-related renal impairment may increase risk of liver or renal toxicity; decreased dosage recommended.

INTERACTIONS

DRUG: May increase effects of **anticoagulants. Aspirin** may increase risk of GI side effects, bleeding. *HERBAL:* May decrease effects of **feverfew. Ginkgo biloba** may increase risk of bleeding. *FOOD:* None known. *LAB VALUES:*

May prolong bleeding time. May increase alkaline phosphatase, LDH, liver function tests. May decrease sodium, hemoglobin, hematocrit.

AVAILABILITY (Rx)

TABLETS: 12.5 mg, 25 mg, 50 mg. *SUSPENSION:* 12.5 mg/5 ml, 25 mg/5 ml.

ADMINISTRATION/HANDLING

PO:
* Give without regard to meals.

INDICATIONS/ROUTES/DOSAGE

Osteoarthritis:
PO: Adults: Initially, 12.5 mg/day. May increase dose to 25 mg/day. **Maximum:** 25 mg/day.

Acute pain, dysmenorrhea:
PO: Adults: Initially, 50 mg/day.

SIDE EFFECTS

FREQUENT (5–6%): Nausea (with or without vomiting), diarrhea, abdominal distress. *OCCASIONAL* (3%): Dyspepsia (heartburn, indigestion, epigastric pain). *RARE* (<2%): Constipation, flatulence.

ADVERSE REACTIONS/TOXIC EFFECTS

None significant.

NURSING IMPLICATIONS

BASELINE ASSESSMENT:

Assess onset, type location, duration of pain, inflammation. Inspect appearance of affected joints for immobility, deformities, skin condition.

INTERVENTION/EVALUATION:

Monitor for evidence of nausea, dyspepsia. Monitor pattern of daily bowel activity and stool consistency. Evaluate for therapeutic response: relief of pain, stiffness, swelling, increase in joint mobility, reduced joint tenderness, improved grip strength. Monitor blood pressure.

PATIENT/FAMILY TEACHING:

Avoid aspirin, alcohol during therapy (increase risk of GI bleeding). If GI upset occurs, take with food, milk.

ropinirole hydrochloride

roh-**pin**-ih-role
(Requip)

▶**CLASSIFICATION**

PHARMACOTHERAPEUTIC:
Dopamine agonist. *CLINICAL:*
Antiparkinson

ACTION/*THERAPEUTIC EFFECT*

Stimulates dopamine receptors in the striatum, *relieving signs/symptoms of Parkinson's disease.*

PHARMACOKINETICS

Rapidly absorbed after PO administration. Protein binding: 40%. Extensively distributed throughout the body. Extensively metabolized. Steady-state concentrations achieved within 2 days. Eliminated in urine. Unknown if removed by hemodialysis. Half-life: 6 hrs.

USES

Treatment of signs and symptoms of idiopathic Parkinson's disease.

PRECAUTIONS

CONTRAINDICATIONS: None significant. *CAUTIONS:* History of orthostatic hypotension, syncope, hallucinations, esp. in elderly, CNS depressants.

▷*LIFESPAN CONSIDERATIONS:*
Pregnancy/Lactation: Distributed in breast milk. Drug activity possible in nursing infant. **Pregnancy Category C. Children:** Safety and efficacy not established. **Elderly:** No age-related precautions noted, but hallucinations appear to occur more.

INTERACTIONS

DRUG: Additive side effects with **CNS depressants.** Increases **levodopa** concentration. **Estrogens** reduce ropinirole clearance. **Ciprofloxacin** increases ropinirole concentration. **Cimetidine, diltiazem, enoxacin, erythromycin, fluvoxamine, mexiletine, norfloxacin, tacrine** alters ropinirole's concentration. **Phenothiazines, butyrophenones, thioxanthenes, metaclopramide** diminishes effectiveness of ropinirole. *HERBAL:* None known. *FOOD:* Time to maximum plasma levels is increased by 2.5 hrs when taken with food (extent of absorption not affected). **Food** may decrease the occurrence of nausea. *LAB VALUES:* May increase alkaline phosphatase.

AVAILABILITY (Rx)

TABLETS: 0.25 mg, 0.5 mg, 1 mg, 2 mg, 5 mg.

ADMINISTRATION/HANDLING

PO:

• Ascending-dose schedule should increase very gradually at weekly intervals: **Week 1:** 0.25 mg 3 times/day to total daily dose 0.75 mg. **Week 2:** 0.5 mg 3 times/day to total daily dose 1.5 mg. **Week 3:** 0.75 mg 3 times/day to total daily dose 2.25 mg. **Week 4:** 1 mg 3 times/day to total daily dose 3 mg.
• Discontinue medication gradually at 7 day intervals. Decrease frequency from 3 times/day to 2

R

times/day for 4 days. For the remaining 3 days, decrease frequency to once daily prior to complete withdrawal.

INDICATIONS/ROUTES/DOSAGE

Parkinson's disease:

PO: **Adults, elderly:** Initially, 0.25 mg 3 times/day. Do not increase dose more frequently than q7days. After week 4, daily dosage may be increased, if needed, by 1.5–3 mg/day per week to total daily dose of 24 mg/day.

SIDE EFFECTS

FREQUENT (40–60%): Nausea, dizziness, excessive drowsiness. *OCCASIONAL* (5–12%): Syncope, vomiting, fatigue, viral infection, dyspepsia, increased sweating, weakness, orthostatic hypotension, abdominal discomfort, pharyngitis, abnormal vision, dry mouth, hypertension, hallucinations, confusion. *RARE* (≤4%): Anorexia, peripheral edema, memory loss, rhinitis, sinusitis, palpitations, impotence.

ADVERSE REACTIONS/TOXIC EFFECTS

None significant.

NURSING IMPLICATIONS

INTERVENTION/EVALUATION:

Instruct pt to rise from lying to sitting or sitting to standing position slowly to prevent risk of postural hypotension. Assess for clinical improvement. Assist with ambulation if dizziness occurs. Assess for clinical reversal of symptoms (improvement of tremor of head/hands at rest, masklike facial expression, shuffling gait, muscular rigidity).

PATIENT/FAMILY TEACHING:

Drowsiness, dizziness may be an initial response to drug. Postural hypotension may occur more frequently during initial therapy. Avoid tasks that require alertness, motor skills until response to drug is established. If nausea occurs, take medication with food. Inform pt that hallucinations may occur, more so in the elderly than in younger pts with Parkinson's disease.

rosiglitazone maleate

rose-ih-**glit**-ah-zone
(Avandia)

►CLASSIFICATION

CLINICAL: Antidiabetic (see p. 40C)

ACTION/*THERAPEUTIC EFFECT*

Improves target cell response to insulin without increasing pancreatic insulin secretion. Decreases hepatic glucose output, increases insulin-dependent glucose utilization in skeletal muscle, *lowering blood glucose concentration.*

PHARMACOKINETICS

Rapidly absorbed. Protein binding: >99%. Metabolized in liver. Excreted primarily in urine with a lesser amount in feces. Not removed by hemodialysis. Half-life: 3–4 hrs.

USES

Adjunct to diet and exercise to lower blood glucose in those with Type 2 noninsulin-dependent diabetes mellitus (NIDDM). Used as monotherapy or in combination with metformin or insulin to improve glycemic control.

PRECAUTIONS

CONTRAINDICATIONS: Diabetic ketoacidosis, Type 1 diabetes mellitus, active liver disease, or increased serum transaminase levels (ALT [SGPT] >2.5 times the normal serum level). ***CAUTIONS:*** Hepatic function impairment, congestive heart failure, edematous pts.

▷***LIFESPAN CONSIDERATIONS:***
Pregnancy/Lactation: Unknown if drug crosses placenta or is distributed in breast milk. Not recommended in pregnant or nursing women. **Pregnancy Category C. Children:** Safety and efficacy not established. **Elderly:** No age-related precautions noted in the elderly.

INTERACTIONS

DRUG: None significant. ***HERBAL:*** None known. ***FOOD:*** None significant. ***LAB VALUES:*** May decrease hemoglobin, hematocrit, bilirubin, AST (SGOT), alkaline phosphatase. Less than 1% experience ALT (SGPT) values ≤3 times normal level.

AVAILABILITY (RX)

TABLETS: 2 mg, 4 mg, 8 mg.

ADMINISTRATION/HANDLING

PO:
• Give without regard to meals.

INDICATIONS/ROUTES/DOSAGE

Diabetes mellitus, combination therapy:

***PO:>* Adults, elderly:** Initially, 4 mg as a single daily dose or in divided doses twice daily. May in-

crease to 8 mg/day after 12 wks of therapy if fasting glucose is not adequately controlled.

MONOTHERAPY: Initially, 4 mg as single daily dose or in divided doses twice daily. May increase to 8 mg/day after 12 wks of therapy.

SIDE EFFECTS

FREQUENT (9%): Upper respiratory tract infection. ***OCCASIONAL*** (2–4%): Headache, edema, back pain, fatigue, sinusitis, diarrhea.

ADVERSE REACTIONS/TOXIC EFFECTS

None significant.

NURSING IMPLICATIONS

BASELINE ASSESSMENT:

Obtain liver enzyme levels prior to initiation of therapy and periodically thereafter. Assure follow-up instruction if pt/family do not thoroughly understand diabetes management or glucose-testing technique.

INTERVENTION/EVALUATION:

Monitor blood glucose, hemoglobin, liver function tests, esp. SGOT, SGPT. Assess for hypoglycemia (cool wet skin, tremors, dizziness, anxiety, headache, tachycardia, numbness in mouth, hunger, diplopia) or hyperglycemia (polyuria, polyphagia, polydipsia, nausea, vomiting, dim vision, fatigue, deep rapid breathing). Be alert to conditions that alter glucose requirements: fever, increased activity or stress, surgical procedures.

PATIENT/FAMILY TEACHING:

Diabetes mellitus requires lifelong control. Prescribed diet and exercise are principal part of

R

treatment; do not skip or delay meals. Wear medical alert identification. Continue to adhere to dietary instructions, a regular exercise program, and regular testing of urine or blood glucose. When taking combination drug therapy with a sulfonylurea or insulin, have a source of glucose available to treat symptoms of low blood sugar.

salmeterol

sal-**met**-er-all
(<u>Serevent</u>, Serevent Diskus)
Do not confuse with Serentil.

FIXED-COMBINATION(S)

With fluticasone, a corticosteroid **(Advair)**

►CLASSIFICATION

PHARMACOTHERAPEUTIC: Sympathomimetic (adrenergic agonist). *CLINICAL:* Bronchodilator (see p. 63C)

ACTION/*THERAPEUTIC EFFECT*

Stimulates beta$_2$-adrenergic receptors in the lungs resulting in relaxation of bronchial smooth muscle; *relieving bronchospasm, reducing airway resistance.*

PHARMACOKINETICS

Onset	Peak	Duration
Inhalation		
10–20 min	3 hrs	12 hrs

Primarily acts in lung; low systemic absorption. Protein binding: 95%. Metabolized by hydroxylation. Primarily eliminated in feces. Half-life: 5.5 hrs.

USES

Maintenance of asthma, prevention of exercise-induced bronchospasm, bronchospasm in pts with reversible obstructive airway disease. Long-term maintenance treatment of bronchospasm associated with COPD, including emphysema and chronic bronchitis.

PRECAUTIONS

CONTRAINDICATIONS: History of hypersensitivity to sympathomimetics. *CAUTIONS:* Not for acute symptoms. May cause paradoxical bronchospasm. Pts with cardiovascular disorders (e.g., coronary insufficiency, arrhythmias, hypertension), seizure disorder, thyrotoxicosis.

▷*LIFESPAN CONSIDERATIONS:* **Pregnancy/Lactation:** Unknown if excreted in breast milk. **Pregnancy Category C. Children:** No age-related precautions in those >4 yrs of age. **Elderly:** Lower doses may be needed due to increased sympathetic sensitivity (may be more susceptible to tachycardia or tremors).

INTERACTIONS

DRUG: May decrease effects of **beta-adrenergic blockers. HERBAL:** Ma Huang (Ephedra) may increase CNS stimulation. *FOOD:* None known. *LAB VALUES:* May decrease serum potassium levels.

AVAILABILITY (Rx)

AEROSOL: 21 mcg/actuation. *AEROSOL POWDER:* 50 mcg.

ADMINISTRATION/HANDLING
Inhalation:

• Shake container well, exhale completely through mouth; place mouthpiece into mouth and close lips, holding inhaler upright. • Inhale deeply through mouth while fully depressing the top of canister. Hold breath as long as possible before exhaling slowly. • Wait 2 min before inhaling second dose (allows for deeper bronchial penetration). • Rinse mouth with water immediately after inhalation (prevents mouth/throat dryness).

INDICATIONS/ROUTES/DOSAGE
Maintenance of bronchodilation, prevention of asthma symptoms:
INHALATION: **Adults, elderly, children >12 yrs:** 2 inhalations 2 times/day, morning and evening about 12 hrs apart. **Children 4–12 yrs:** 1 inhalation 2 times/day.

Prevention of exercise-induced bronchospasm:
INHALATION: **Adults, elderly, children >12 yrs:** 2 inhalations at least 30–60 min before exercise.

Long-term maintenance treatment of COPD-induced bronchospasm:
INHALATION: **Adults:** 2 inhalations q12h.

SIDE EFFECTS
FREQUENT (28%): Headache. *OCCASIONAL* (≤3–7%): Cough, tremor, dizziness, vertigo, throat dryness/irritation, pharyngitis. *RARE* (<3%): Palpitations, tachycardia, shakiness, nausea, heartburn, GI distress, diarrhea.

ADVERSE REACTIONS/TOXIC EFFECTS
May prolong QT interval (may lead to ventricular arrhythmias). May cause hypokalemia, hyperglycemia.

NURSING IMPLICATIONS

INTERVENTION/EVALUATION:
Monitor rate, depth, rhythm, tape of respiration; quality and rate of pulse, B/P. Assess lungs for wheezing, rales, rhonchi. Periodically evaluate potassium levels.

PATIENT/FAMILY TEACHING:
Not for relief of acute episodes. Keep canister at room temperature (cold decreases effects). Do not stop medication or exceed recommended dosage. Notify physician promptly of chest pain, dizziness, or failure to respond to medication. Wait at least one full min before second inhalation. Administer dose 30 to 60 min before exercise when used to prevent exercise-induced bronchospasm. Avoid excessive use of caffeine derivatives: coffee, tea, colas, chocolate.

salsalate

sal-sah-late
(Disalcid, Mono-Gesic)

▶CLASSIFICATION

PHARMACOTHERAPEUTIC: Nonsteroidal anti-inflammatory. *CLINICAL:* Analgesic, anti-inflammatory

S

ACTION/*THERAPEUTIC EFFECT*
Produces analgesic, anti-inflammatory effect by inhibiting prostaglandin synthesis, reducing inflammatory response and intensity of pain stimulus reaching sensory nerve endings.

USES

Symptomatic treatment of acute and/or chronic rheumatoid arthritis and osteoarthritis, related inflammatory conditions.

PRECAUTIONS

CONTRAINDICATIONS: Chickenpox/flu in children/teenagers. ***CAUTIONS:*** None significant.

INTERACTIONS

DRUG: **Alcohol, NSAIDs** may increase risk of GI effects (e.g., ulceration). **Urinary alkalinizers, antacids** increase excretion. **Anticoagulants, heparin, thrombolytics** increase risk of bleeding. Large dose may increase effect of **insulin, oral hypoglycemics. Valproic acid, platelet aggregation inhibitors** may increase risk of bleeding. May increase toxicity of **methotrexate, zidovudine. Ototoxic medications, vancomycin** may increase ototoxicity. May decrease effect of **probenecid, sulfinpyrazone.** ***HERBAL:*** **Ginkgo biloba** may increase risk of bleeding. ***FOOD:*** None known. ***LAB VALUES:*** May alter SGOT (AST), SGPT (ALT), alkaline phosphatase, uric acid; prolong prothrombin time, bleeding time. May decrease cholesterol, potassium, T_3, T_4.

AVAILABILITY (Rx)

CAPSULES: 500 mg. ***TABLETS:*** 500 mg, 750 mg.

INDICATIONS/ROUTES/DOSAGE

Rheumatoid arthritis, osteoarthritis:

PO: Adults, elderly: Initially: 3 g/day in 2–3 divided doses. **Maintenance:** 2–4 g/day.

SIDE EFFECTS

OCCASIONAL: Nausea, dyspepsia (heartburn, indigestion, epigastric pain).

ADVERSE REACTIONS/TOXIC EFFECTS

Tinnitus may be first sign that blood salicylic acid concentration is reaching/exceeding upper therapeutic range. May also produce vertigo, headache, confusion, drowsiness, sweating, hyperventilation, vomiting, diarrhea. Severe overdosage may result in electrolyte imbalance, hyperthermia, dehydration, blood pH imbalance. Low incidence of GI bleeding, peptic ulcer.

NURSING IMPLICATIONS

BASELINE ASSESSMENT:

Do not give to children/teenagers who have flu/chickenpox (increases risk of Reye's syndrome). Assess type, location, duration of pain, inflammation. Inspect appearance of affected joints for immobility, deformities, and skin condition.

INTERVENTION/EVALUATION:

Assess for evidence of nausea, dyspepsia. Evaluate for therapeutic response: relief of pain/stiffness/swelling, increase in joint mobility, reduced joint tenderness, improved grip strength.

PATIENT/FAMILY TEACHING:

Do not crush/chew capsules or film-coated tablets. Avoid antacids (decreases drug effectiveness). Report ringing in ears, persistent GI pain. Avoid alcohol.

---

saquinavir

sah-**quin**-ah-vir
(Fortovase, Invirase)
Do not confuse with Sinequan.

▶CLASSIFICATION
PHARMACOTHERAPEUTIC:
Protease inhibitor. **CLINICAL:**
Antiretroviral (see pp. 59C, 96C)

ACTION/*THERAPEUTIC EFFECT*

Inhibits HIV protease, rendering
the enzyme incapable of processing the polyprotein precursor to
generate functional proteins in
HIV-infected cells, *slowing HIV
replication, reducing progression
of HIV infection.*

PHARMACOKINETICS

Poorly absorbed following oral
administration (high-caloric/high-
fat meal increases absorption).
Protein binding: 99%. Metabolized
in liver to inactive metabolite. Primarily eliminated in feces. Unknown if removed by hemodialysis.

USES

Used in combination with nucleoside analogues for treatment of
advanced HIV infection in selected pts.

PRECAUTIONS

CONTRAINDICATIONS: Clinically significant hypersensitivity to
drug. **CAUTIONS:** Impaired hepatic function.

▷**LIFESPAN CONSIDERATIONS:**
Pregnancy/Lactation: Breast
feeding not recommended (possibility of HIV transmission). **Pregnancy Category B. Children:**
Safety and efficacy not established. **Elderly:** Information not
available.

INTERACTIONS

DRUG: Ketoconazole increases
saquinavir concentration. **Rifampin, phenobarbital, phenytoin,
dexamethasone, carbamazepine**
may reduce saquinavir plasma
concentration. May increase **calcium channel blockers, clindamycin, dapsone, quinidine,
triazolam** plasma concentrations.
HERBAL: St. John's wort, garlic
may decrease concentrations, effect. **FOOD: Grapefruit juice** may
increase saquinavir concentrations. **LAB VALUES:** May elevate
serum transaminase, lower glucose level, alter CPK.

AVAILABILITY (Rx)

**CAPSULES, SOFT GELATIN CAP-
SULES:** 200 mg.

ADMINISTRATION/HANDLING
PO:

• Give within 2 hrs after a full meal
(if taken without food in stomach,
may result in no antiviral activity).

INDICATIONS/ROUTES/DOSAGE

Note: Complete prescribing information for saquinavir should be
consulted before concurrent therapy with zidovudine (AZT), zalcitabine (ddC).

HIV infection (combination
therapy):

PO: Adults, elderly: *Fortovase:*
1,200 mg 3 times/day. **Saquinavir:**
Three 200 mg capsules given 3
times daily within 2 hrs after a full
meal. Do not give <600 mg/day
(does not produce antiviral activity). *Recommended daily doses of*

S

---

ddC or AZT: ddC 0.75 mg 3 times daily; AZT 200 mg 3 times daily.

SIDE EFFECTS

OCCASIONAL: Diarrhea, abdominal discomfort or pain, nausea, photosensitivity, buccal mucosa ulceration. ***RARE:*** Confusion, ataxia, weakness, headache, rash.

ADVERSE REACTIONS/TOXIC EFFECTS

None significant.

NURSING IMPLICATIONS

BASELINE ASSESSMENT:

Obtain baseline laboratory testing, esp. liver function tests, before beginning saquinavir therapy and at periodic intervals during therapy. Offer emotional support. Obtain medication history.

INTERVENTION/EVALUATION:

Closely monitor for evidence of GI discomfort. Monitor stool frequency and consistency (watery, loose, soft). Inspect mouth for signs of mucosal ulceration. Monitor clinical chemistry tests for marked laboratory abnormalities. If serious or severe toxicities occur, interrupt therapy, contact physician.

PATIENT/FAMILY TEACHING:

Continue therapy for full length of treatment. Doses should be evenly spaced. Saquinavir is not a cure for HIV infection, nor does it reduce risk of transmission to others. Pts may continue to acquire illnesses associated with advanced HIV infection. Take within 2 hrs after a full meal. Avoid coadministration with grapefruit products.

---

sargramostim (granulocyte macrophage colony stimulating factor; GM-CSF)

sar-gra-**moh**-stim
(Leukine, Prokine)
Do not confuse with Leukeran.

▶CLASSIFICATION

PHARMACOTHERAPEUTIC: Colony-stimulating factor. ***CLINICAL:*** Hematopoietic, antineutropenic

ACTION/*THERAPEUTIC EFFECT*

Stimulates proliferation/differentiation of hematopoietic cells to activate mature granulocytes and macrophages, *assisting bone marrow in making new WBCs.* Chemotactic, antifungal, and antiparasite activities increase. Increases cytotoxicity of monocytes to certain neoplastic cells; *activates neutrophils to inhibit tumor cell growth.*

PHARMACOKINETICS

Detected in serum within 5 min after SubQ administration. Half-life: *IV:* 1 hr; *SubQ:* 3 hrs.

USES/*UNLABELED*

Accelerates myeloid recovery in pt with non-Hodgkin's lymphoma, acute lymphoblastic leukemia, and Hodgkin's disease undergoing autologous bone marrow transplantation. Used in pts with allogenic or autologous bone marrow transplantation where engraftment is delayed or has failed. Shortens time of neutrophil recovery following induction chemo-

---

therapy in pts with AML. Mobilizes autologous peripheral blood progenitor cells (PBPC) following induction of chemotherapy in pt >55 yrs with acute myelogenous leukemia; used in myeloid reconstitution after allogenic bone marrow transplantation. *Treatment of AIDS-related neutropenia; chronic, severe neutropenia, drug-induced neutropenia; myelodysplastic syndrome.*

PRECAUTIONS

CONTRAINDICATIONS: Excessive leukemic myeloid blasts in bone marrowith peripheral blood (>10%), known hypersensitivity to GM-CSF, yeast-derived products, any component of drug, 24 hrs before/after chemotherapy, 12 hrs before/after radiation therapy. ***CAUTIONS:*** Preexisting cardiac disease, hypoxia, preexisting fluid retention, pulmonary infiltrates, CHF, impaired renal/hepatic function.

▷***LIFESPAN CONSIDERATIONS:*** **Pregnancy/Lactation:** Unknown if drug crosses placenta or is distributed in breast milk. **Pregnancy Category C. Children:** Safety and efficacy not established. **Elderly:** No age-related precautions noted.

INTERACTIONS

DRUG: **Lithium, steroids** may increase effect. ***HERBAL:*** None known. ***FOOD:*** None known. ***LAB VALUES:*** May decrease albumin. May increase bilirubin, creatinine, liver enzymes.

AVAILABILITY (Rx)

POWDER FOR INJECTION: 250 mcg, 500 mcg. ***LIQUID FOR INJECTION:*** 500 mcg/ml.

ADMINISTRATION/HANDLING
IV 📺

Storage:
• Refrigerate powder, reconstituted solution, diluted solution for injection. Do not shake. Do not use past expiration date. • Reconstituted solutions are clear, colorless. • Use within 6 hrs; discard unused portions. Use 1 dose/vial; do not reenter vial.

Reconstitution:
• To 250 mcg/500 mcg vial, add 1 ml Sterile Water for Injection (preservative free). • Direct Sterile Water for Injection to side of vial, gently swirl contents to avoid foaming; do not shake/vigorously agitate. • After reconstitution, further dilute with 0.9% NaCl. If final concentration <10 mcg/ml, add 1 mg albumin/ml 0.9% NaCl to provide a final albumin concentration of 0.1%. **Note:** Albumin is added before addition of sargramostim (prevents drug adsorption to components of drug delivery system).

Rate of administration:
• Give each single dose over 2, 4, or 24 hrs as directed by physician.

IV INCOMPATIBILITIES ⊘
Amphotericin B complex (Abelcet, Ambisome, Amphotec), cefoperazone (Cefobid), chlorpromazine (Thorazine).

IV COMPATIBILITIES
Calcium gluconate, dopamine (Intropin), heparin, magnesium, potassium chloride.

INDICATIONS/ROUTES/DOSAGE
Usual parenteral dosage:

IV INFUSION: **Adults, elderly:** 250 mcg/m²/day for 21 days (as a 2 hr infusion). Begin 2–4 hrs after autologous bone marrow infusion and not less than 24 hrs after last dose of chemotherapy or not less than 12 hrs after last radiation treatment. Discontinue if blast cells appear or underlying disease progresses.

Bone marrow transplantation failure/engraftment delay:

IV INFUSION: **Adults, elderly:** 250 mcg/m^2/day for 14 days. Infuse over 2 hrs. May repeat after 7 days of therapy if engraftment not occurred with 500 mcg/m^2/day for 14 days.

Mobilization or post PBPC transplant:

IV/SUBQ: **Adults:** 250 mcg/m^2/day.

Allogeneic transplantation:

IV INFUSION: **Adults:** 250 mcg/m^2/day for 21 days starting 2–4 hrs after bone marrow infusion and not less than 24 hrs after last chemotherapy dose or 12 hrs after last radiation dose.

Aplastic anemia:

IV/SUBQ: **Adults, elderly:** 15–480 mcg/m^2/day.

Cancer chemotherapy recovery:

IV/SUBQ: 3–15 mcg/kg/day for 10 days.

SIDE EFFECTS

FREQUENT: GI disturbances, (nausea, diarrhea, vomiting, stomatitis, anorexia, abdominal pain), arthralgia/myalgia, headache, malaise, rash, pruritus. ***OCCASIONAL:*** Peripheral edema, weight gain, dyspnea, asthenia (loss of strength), fever, leukocytosis, capillary leak syndrome (e.g., fluid retention, irritation at local injection site, peripheral edema). ***RARE:*** Rapid/irregular heartbeat, thrombophlebitis.

ADVERSE REACTIONS/TOXIC EFFECTS

Pleural/pericardial effusion occurs rarely following infusion.

NURSING IMPLICATIONS

BASELINE ASSESSMENT:

Monitor for supraventricular arrhythmias during administration (particularly in those with history of cardiac arrhythmias). Assess closely for dyspnea during and immediately following infusion (particularly in those with history of lung disease). If dyspnea occurs during infusion, cut infusion rate by half. If dyspnea continues, stop infusion immediately. If neutrophil count exceeds 20,000 cells/mm^3 or platelet count exceeds 500,000/mm^3, stop infusion or reduce dose by half, based on clinical condition of pt. Blood counts return to normal or baseline 3–7 days after discontinuation of therapy.

INTERVENTION/EVALUATION:

Monitor urinalysis reports, alkaline phosphatase, serum creatinine, bilirubin, SGOT (AST), SGPT (ALT) levels, CBC diligently. Assess for peripheral edema, particularly behind medial malleolus (usually first area showing peripheral edema), skin turgor, mucous membranes for hydration status. Assess muscle strength. Monitor daily bowel activity, stool consistency (watery, loose, soft, semisolid, solid).

saw palmetto

Also known as American dwarf palm tree, cabbage palm, sabal, zu-zhong

►CLASSIFICATION
HERBAL

ACTION/*EFFECT*

Appears to inhibit 5 alpha-reductase and prevent conversion of testosterone to dihydrotestosterone (DHT), *reducing prostate growth*. Also has anti-androgenic, antiproliferative, and anti-inflammatory properties.

USES

Symptoms of benign prostate hyperplasia (BPH). Also used as a mild diuretic, sedative, anti-inflammatory agent, and antiseptic.

PRECAUTIONS

CONTRAINDICATIONS: Pregnancy, lactation due to antiandrogenic and estrogenic activity. ***CAUTIONS:*** None significant.
▷***LIFESPAN CONSIDERATIONS:*** **Pregnancy/Lactation:** Contraindicated. **Children:** Safety and efficacy not established. **Elderly:** No age-related precautions noted.

INTERACTIONS

DRUG: May interfere with **oral contraceptives** and **hormone therapy.** ***HERBAL:*** None significant. ***FOOD:*** None significant. ***LAB VALUES:*** None significant.

AVAILABILITY (OTC)

CAPSULES: 80 mg, 160 mg, 500 mg. ***BERRIES. FLUID EXTRACT. TEA.***

INDICATIONS/ROUTES/DOSAGE
BPH:

PO: Adults, elderly: 160 mg 2 times/day or 320 mg once/day.

SIDE EFFECTS

Mild anorexia, dizziness, nausea, vomiting, constipation, diarrhea, headache, impotence, hypersensitivity reactions, back pain.

ADVERSE REACTIONS/TOXIC EFFECTS

None significant.

NURSING IMPLICATIONS

BASELINE ASSESSMENT:

Determine use of oral contraceptives, hormone replacement therapy (may interfere). Assess pt's urinary patterns.

INTERVENTION/EVALUATION:

Assess for hypersensitivity reactions. Monitor symptoms of BHP (e.g., frequent/painful urination, hesitancy, urgency). Watch for decreased nocturia, improved urinary flow, decreased residual urine volume.

PATIENT/FAMILY TEACHING:

Should be taken with food. Obtain a prostate-specific antigen (PSA) before using.

scopolamine

sko-**poll**-ah-meen
(Trans-Derm Scop)

▶CLASSIFICATION
PHARMACOTHERAPEUTIC: Anticholinergic. ***CLINICAL:*** Antinausea, antiemetic

ACTION/*THERAPEUTIC EFFECT*

Reduces excitability of labyrinthine receptors, depressing conduction in vestibular cerebellar pathway, *preventing nausea/vomiting induced by motion*.

USES
Prevention of motion sickness.

S

PRECAUTIONS

CONTRAINDICATIONS: Narrow-angle glaucoma, sensitivity to belladonna alkaloids. **CAUTIONS:** Liver, renal impairment, pyloric, urinary bladder neck or intestinal obstruction.

INTERACTIONS

DRUG: CNS depressants may increase CNS depression. **Antihistamines, tricyclic-antidepressants** may increase anticholinergic effects. **HERBAL:** None significant. **FOOD:** None significant. **LAB VALUES:** May interfere with gastric secretion test.

AVAILABILITY (Rx)

TRANSDERMAL SYSTEM: 1.5 mg.

INDICATIONS/ROUTES/DOSAGE

Prevention of motion sickness:

PO: Adults: 1–2 tablets an hr before travel provide effect for several hrs.

TRANSDERMAL: Adults: 1 system q72h.

SIDE EFFECTS

FREQUENT (>15%): Dry mouth, drowsiness, blurred vision. **RARE** (1–5%): Dizziness, restlessness, hallucinations, confusion, difficulty urinating, rash.

ADVERSE REACTION/TOXIC EFFECTS

None significant.

NURSING IMPLICATIONS

BASELINE ASSESSMENT:

Assess for use of other CNS depressants, drugs with anticholinergic action, history of narrow-angle glaucoma.

INTERVENTION/EVALUATION:

Monitor liver, renal function.

BASELINE ASSESSMENT:

Caution driving/operating machinery (may cause drowsiness, disorientation, confusion). Proper administration of patch. Use only 1 patch at a time; do not cut. Wash hands after administration.

secobarbital sodium

(Seconal)

See Classification section under: Sedative-Hypnotics

selegiline hydrochloride

sell-**eh**-geh-leen
(Eldepryl, Novo-Selegiline ♣)
Do not confuse with enalapril, Stelazine.

▶CLASSIFICATION

CLINICAL: Antiparkinson

ACTION/THERAPEUTIC EFFECT

Irreversibly inhibits monoamine oxidase type B activity. Increases dopaminergic action, *assisting in reduction in tremor, akinesia (absence of sense of movement), posture and equilibrium disorders, rigidity of parkinsonism.*

PHARMACOKINETICS

Rapidly absorbed from GI tract. Crosses blood-brain barrier. Metabolized in liver to active metabolites. Primarily excreted in urine. Half-life: 16–69 hrs.

USES

Adjunctive to levodopa/carbidopa in treatment of Parkinson's disease.

PRECAUTIONS

CONTRAINDICATIONS: None significant. **CAUTIONS:** History of peptic ulcer disease, dementia, psychosis, tardive dyskinesia, profound tremor, cardiac dysrhythmias.
▷**LIFESPAN CONSIDERATIONS:** **Pregnancy/Lactation:** Unknown if drug crosses placenta or is distributed in breast milk. **Pregnancy Category C. Children:** Safety and efficacy not established. **Elderly:** No age-related precautions noted.

INTERACTIONS

DRUG: Fluoxetine may cause mania, serotonin syndrome (mental changes, restlessness, diaphoresis, diarrhea, fever). **Meperidine** may cause a potentially fatal reaction (e.g., excitation, sweating, rigidity, hypertension or hypotension, coma, and death). **HERBAL:** None known. **FOOD: Tyramine-rich foods** may produce hypertensive reactions. **LAB VALUES:** None significant.

AVAILABILITY (Rx)

CAPSULES: 5 mg. **TABLETS:** 5 mg.

ADMINISTRATION/HANDLING

PO:
• Give without meals.

INDICATIONS/ROUTES/DOSAGE

Note: Therapy should begin with lowest dosage, then be increased in gradual increments over 3–4 wks.

Parkinsonism:

PO: Adults: 10 mg/day in divided doses (5 mg at breakfast and lunch). **Elderly:** Initially, 5 mg in morning. May increase up to 10 mg/day.

SIDE EFFECTS

FREQUENT (4–10%): Nausea, dizziness, lightheadedness, faintness, abdominal discomfort. **OCCASIONAL** (2–3%): Confusion, hallucinations, dry mouth, vivid dreams, dyskinesia (impairment of voluntary movement). **RARE** (1%): Headache, generalized aches, anxiety, diarrhea, insomnia.

ADVERSE REACTIONS/TOXIC EFFECTS

Overdosage may vary from CNS depression (sedation, apnea, cardiovascular collapse, death) to severe paradoxical reaction (hallucinations, tremor, seizures). Impaired motor coordination (loss of balance, blepharospasm [blinking], facial grimace, feeling of heavy leg/stiff neck, involuntary movements), hallucinations, confusion, depression, nightmares, delusions, overstimulation, sleep disturbance, anger occurs in some pts.

NURSING IMPLICATIONS   S

INTERVENTION/EVALUATION:

Be alert to neurologic effects (headache, lethargy, mental confusion, agitation). Monitor for evidence of dyskinesia (difficulty with movement). Assess for clinical reversal of symptoms (improvement of tremor of head/hands at rest, masklike facial expression, shuffling gait, muscular rigidity).

PATIENT/FAMILY TEACHING:

Tolerance to feeling of light-headedness develops during therapy. To reduce hypotensive effect, rise slowly from lying to sitting position and permit legs to dangle momentarily before standing. Avoid tasks that require alertness, motor skills until response to drug is established. Dry mouth, drowsiness, dizziness may be an expected response of drug. Avoid alcoholic beverages during therapy. Coffee/tea may help reduce drowsiness.

senna

sen-ah
(Senokot, Senolax)

FIXED-COMBINATION(S)

With docusate, a stool softener (**Gentlax-S, Senokap DSS, Senokot-S**)

▶CLASSIFICATION

PHARMACOTHERAPEUTIC:
GI stimulant. *CLINICAL:* Laxative (see p. 101C)

ACTION/THERAPEUTIC EFFECT

Increases peristalsis by direct effect on intestinal smooth musculature (stimulates intramural nerve plexi). Builds fluid and ion accumulation in colon, *promoting laxative effect.*

PHARMACOKINETICS

	Onset	Peak	Duration
PO	6–12 hrs	—	—
Rectal	0.5–2 hrs	—	—

Minimal absorption after oral administration. Hydrolyzed to active form by enzymes of colonic flora.

Absorbed drug metabolized in liver; eliminated in feces via biliary system.

USES

Facilitates defecation in those with diminished colonic motor response, for evacuation of colon for rectal, bowel examination, elective colon surgery.

PRECAUTIONS

CONTRAINDICATIONS: Abdominal pain, nausea, vomiting, appendicitis, intestinal obstruction. *CAUTIONS:* None significant.

▷*LIFESPAN CONSIDERATIONS:*
Pregnancy/Lactation: Unknown if distributed in breast milk. **Pregnancy Category C. Children:** Safety and efficacy not established in those <6 yrs of age. **Elderly:** No age-related precautions noted; monitor signs of dehydration/electrolyte loss.

INTERACTIONS

DRUG: May decrease transit time of concurrently administered **oral medication**, decreasing absorption. *HERBAL:* None known. *FOOD:* None known. *LAB VALUES:* May increase glucose, may decrease potassium.

AVAILABILITY (OTC)

TABLETS: 187 mg, 217 mg, 374 mg, 600 mg. *GRANULES:* 326 mg/tsp. *SUPPOSITORY:* 652 mg. *SYRUP:* 218 mg/5 ml. *LIQUID:* 33.3 mg/ml.

ADMINISTRATION/HANDLING
PO:

• Give on an empty stomach (faster results). • Offer at least 6–8 glasses of water/day (aids stool softening). • Avoid giving within 1 hr of other oral medication (decreases drug absorption).

Rectal:
• If suppository is too soft, chill for 30 min in refrigerator or run cold water over foil wrapper. • Moisten suppository with cold water before inserting well up into rectum.

INDICATIONS/ROUTES/DOSAGE
Laxative:
*PO: **Adults, elderly:*** 2 tablets (or 1 tsp granules) at bedtime. **Maximum:** 4 tablets (2 tsp) 2 times/day. **Children:** 1 tablet ($^1/_2$ tsp granules) at bedtime.
*PO: **Adults, elderly:** (Syrup):* 10–15 ml at bedtime. **Children 5–15 yrs:** 5–10 ml at bedtime. **Children 1–5 yrs:** 2.5–5 ml at bedtime. **Children 1 mo–1 yr:** 1.25–2.5 ml at bedtime.
*RECTAL: **Adults, elderly:*** 1 suppository at bedtime, may repeat in 2 hrs. **Children:** $^1/_2$ suppository at bedtime.

SIDE EFFECTS
FREQUENT: Pink-red, red-violet, red-brown, or yellow-brown discoloration of urine. ***OCCASIONAL:*** Some degree of abdominal discomfort, nausea, mild cramps, griping, faintness.

ADVERSE REACTIONS/TOXIC EFFECTS
Long-term use may result in laxative dependence, chronic constipation, loss of normal bowel function. Chronic use/overdosage may result in electrolyte disturbances (hypokalemia, hypocalcemia, metabolic acidosis/alkalosis), persistent diarrhea, malabsorption, weight loss. Electrolyte disturbance may produce vomiting, muscle weakness.

NURSING IMPLICATIONS

INTERVENTION/EVALUATION:
Encourage adequate fluid intake. Assess bowel sounds for peristalsis. Monitor stool frequency, consistency (watery, loose, soft, semisolid, solid). Assess for abdominal disturbances. Monitor serum electrolytes in those exposed to prolonged, frequent, or excessive use of medication.

PATIENT/FAMILY TEACHING:
Urine may turn pink-red, red-violet, red-brown, or yellow-brown (only temporary and not harmful). Institute measures to promote defecation (increase fluid intake, exercise, high-fiber diet). Laxative effect generally occurs in 6–12 hrs, but may take 24 hrs. Suppository produces evacuation in 30 min to 2 hrs. Do not take other oral medication within 1 hr of taking this medicine (decreased effectiveness).

sertraline hydrochloride &

sir-trah-leen
(Zoloft)
Do not confuse with Serentil.

▶CLASSIFICATION
PHARMACOTHERAPEUTIC:
Serotonin reuptake inhibitor. ***CLINICAL:*** Antidepressant, antipanic, obsessive-compulsive adjunct (see p. 36C)

ACTION/*THERAPEUTIC EFFECT*
Blocks reuptake of the neurotransmitter serotonin at CNS neuronal presynaptic membranes, increas-

ing availability at postsynaptic receptor sites, *producing antidepressant effect, reducing obsessive compulsive behavior, decreasing anxiety.*

PHARMACOKINETICS

Incompletely, slowly absorbed from GI tract (food increases absorption). Protein binding: 98%. Widely distributed. Undergoes extensive first-pass metabolism in liver to active compound. Excreted in urine, eliminated in feces. Not removed by hemodialysis. Half-life: 26 hrs.

USES

Treatment of major depressive disorders, panic disorder, obsessive compulsive disorder (OCD). Post traumatic stress disorder.

PRECAUTIONS

CONTRAINDICATIONS: During or within 14 days of MAO inhibitor antidepressant therapy. **CAUTIONS:** Severe hepatic/renal impairment.

▷**LIFESPAN CONSIDERATIONS:** **Pregnancy/Lactation:** Unknown if drug crosses placenta or is distributed in breast milk. **Pregnancy Category C. Children:** No age-related precautions in those >6 yrs of age. **Elderly:** No age-related precautions noted, but lower initial doses recommended.

INTERACTIONS

DRUG: May increase concentration, toxicity of **highly protein-bound medications (e.g., digoxin, warfarin). MAO inhibitors** may cause serotonin syndrome (mental changes, restlessness, diaphoresis, shivering, diarrhea, fever), confusion, agitation, hyperpyretic convulsions. **HERBAL:** St. **John's wort** may increase risk of

adverse effects. **FOOD:** None known. **LAB VALUES:** May increase SGOT (AST), SGPT (ALT), total cholesterol, triglycerides. May decrease uric acid.

AVAILABILITY (Rx)

TABLETS: 50 mg, 100 mg. **ORAL CONCENTRATE:** 20 mg/ml.

ADMINISTRATION/HANDLING
PO:

• Give with food or milk if GI distress occurs.

INDICATIONS/ROUTES/DOSAGE
Antidepressant, OCD:

PO: Adults, children 13–17 yrs: Initially, 50 mg/day with morning or evening meal. May increase by 50 mg/day at 7 day intervals. **Elderly, children 6–12 yrs:** Initially, 25 mg/day. May increase by 25–50 mg/day at 7 day intervals.

Panic disorder, post-traumatic stress disorder:

PO: Adults, elderly: Initially, 25 mg/day. May increase by 50 mg/day at 7 day intervals. **Range:** 50–200 mg/day. **Maximum:** 200 mg/day.

SIDE EFFECTS

FREQUENT (12–26%): Headache, nausea, diarrhea, insomnia, drowsiness, dizziness, fatigue, rash, dry mouth. **OCCASIONAL** (4–6%): Anxiety, nervousness, agitation, tremor, dyspepsia, excessive sweating, vomiting, constipation, abnormal ejaculation, change in vision, change in taste. **RARE** (<3%): Flatulence, urinary frequency, paresthesia, hot flashes, chills.

ADVERSE REACTIONS/TOXIC EFFECTS

None significant.

NURSING IMPLICATIONS

BASELINE ASSESSMENT:

For those on long-term therapy, liver/renal function tests, blood counts should be performed periodically.

INTERVENTION/EVALUATION:

Supervise suicidal risk pt closely during early therapy (as depression lessens, energy level improves, increasing suicide potential). Assess appearance, behavior, speech pattern, level of interest, mood. Monitor pattern of daily bowel activity, stool consistency. Assist with ambulation if dizziness occurs.

PATIENT/FAMILY TEACHING:

Dry mouth may be relieved by sugarless gum, sips of tepid water. Report headache, fatigue, tremor, sexual dysfunction. Avoid tasks that require alertness, motor skills until response to drug is established. Take with food if nausea occurs. Inform physician if pregnancy occurs. Avoid alcohol. Do not take OTC medications without consulting physician.

sevelamer hydrochloride

seh-**vell**-ah-mur
(Renagel)
Do not confuse with Reglan, Regonol.

▶**CLASSIFICATION**

PHARMACOTHERAPEUTIC: Polymeric phosphate binder. **CLINICAL:** Antihyperphosphatemia

ACTION/*THERAPEUTIC EFFECT*

Binds/removes dietary phosphorus in GI tract and eliminates phosphorus through normal digestive process. *Decreases incidence of hypercalcemic episodes in pts receiving calcium acetate treatment.*

PHARMACOKINETICS

Not absorbed systemically. Unknown if removed by hemodialysis.

USES

Reduction of serum phosphorous in pts with end-stage renal disease (ESRD).

PRECAUTIONS

CONTRAINDICATIONS: Bowel obstruction, hypophosphatemia. **CAUTIONS:** Dysphagia, severe GI tract motility disorders, major GI tract surgery, swallowing disorders.

▷**LIFESPAN CONSIDERATIONS:** **Pregnancy/Lactation:** Not distributed in breast milk **Pregnancy Category C. Children:** Safety and efficacy not established. **Elderly:** No age-related precautions noted.

INTERACTIONS

DRUG: None significant. **HERBAL:** None known. **FOOD:** None known. **LAB VALUES:** None significant.

AVAILABILITY (Rx)

CAPSULES: 403 mg. **TABLETS:** 400 mg, 800 mg.

ADMINISTRATION/HANDLING

PO:

• Give with meals. • Do not take capsule apart prior to administration (contents expand in water). • Space other medication by ≥1 hr before or 3 hrs after sevelamer.

S

INDICATIONS/ROUTES/DOSAGE
Hyperphosphatemia:

PO: Adults, elderly: 2–4 capsules with each meal depending on severity of hyperphosphatemia.

SIDE EFFECTS

FREQUENT (11–20%): Infection, pain, hypotension, diarrhea, dyspepsia, nausea, vomiting. **OCCASIONAL** (1–10%): Headache, constipation, hypertension, thrombosis, increased coughing.

ADVERSE REACTIONS/TOXIC EFFECTS

None significant.

NURSING IMPLICATIONS

BASELINE ASSESSMENT:
Obtain baseline serum phosphorus level; assess for any bowel obstruction.

INTERVENTION/EVALUATION:
Serum phosphorus, bicarbonate, chloride, calcium levels.

PATIENT/FAMILY TEACHING:
Take with meals, swallow whole.

sibutramine

sigh-**bew**-trah-meen
(Meridia)

►CLASSIFICATION
PHARMACOTHERAPEUTIC: CNS stimulant. **CLINICAL:** Anorexiant

ACTION/THERAPEUTIC EFFECT
Inhibits reuptake of serotonin (enhancing satiety) and norepinephrine (raises metabolic rate) centrally, inducing, maintaining weight loss.

USES
Management of obesity, including weight loss and maintenance of weight loss, when used in conjunction with a reduced-calorie diet.

PRECAUTIONS
CONTRAINDICATIONS: Anorexia nervosa, uncontrolled hypertension, use of MAOIs. **CAUTIONS:** CHF, cardiac arrhythmias, CAD, history of stroke, liver or renal impairment.

INTERACTIONS
DRUG: Appetite suppressants (avoid), **MAOIs** (contraindicated). **HERBAL:** None significant. **FOOD:** None significant. **LAB VALUES:** May increase liver function tests, HDL. May decrease uric acid.

AVAILABILITY (Rx)
CAPSULES: 5 mg, 10 mg, 15 mg.

INDICATIONS/ROUTES/DOSAGE
Weight loss:

PO: Adults: Initially, 10 mg/day. May increase up to 15 mg/day. **Maximum:** 20 mg/day.

SIDE EFFECTS
FREQUENT (10–30%): Headache, dry mouth, anorexia, constipation, insomnia, rhinitis, pharyngitis. **OCCASIONAL** (5–9%): Back pain, flu syndrome, dizziness, nausea, asthenia (loss of strength, energy), arthralgia, nervousness, dyspepsia, sinusitis, abdominal pain, anxiety, dysmenorrhea. **RARE** (2–4%): Depression, rash, cough, sweating, tachycardia, migraine, increased B/P, paresthesia, altered taste.

NURSING IMPLICATIONS

BASELINE ASSESSMENT:

Assess use of MAOIs, other medical problems, esp. anorexia nervosa, uncontrolled hypertension.

INTERVENTION/EVALUATION:

Monitor for allergic reaction (e.g., rash, hives).

PATIENT/FAMILY TEACHING:

Do not increase dose if effect diminishes. Notify physician of allergic reactions. Use caution in driving/operating machinery until effect of drug is known (may cause dizziness, drowsiness, impaired judgment).

sildenafil citrate

sill-**den**-ah-fill
(<u>Viagra</u>)
Do not confuse with Vaniqa.

▶**CLASSIFICATION**

CLINICAL: Erectile dysfunction adjunct

ACTION/*THERAPEUTIC EFFECT*

Inhibits type V cyclic GMP, a specific phosphodiesterase, the predominant isoenzyme in human corpus cavernosum in the penis. *Relaxes smooth muscle, increases blood flow, facilitating an erection.*

USES/*UNLABELED*

Treatment of male erectile dysfunction. *Treatment of sexual dysfunction from SSRI (antidepressants), diabetic gastroparesis.*

PRECAUTIONS

CONTRAINDICATIONS: Those concurrently using sodium nitroprusside or organic nitrates in any form. **CAUTIONS:** Renal or hepatic function impairment, anatomic deformation of the penis, those that may be predisposed to priapism (sickle cell anemia, multiple myeloma, leukemia).

INTERACTIONS

DRUG: Cimetidine, erythromycin, itraconazole, ketoconazole may increase sildenafil plasma concentration. Potentiates hypotensive effects of **nitrates. HERBAL:** None known. **FOOD:** Rate of absorption is reduced and time to maximum effectiveness is delayed by 1 hr when taken with a high-fat meal. **LAB VALUES:** None significant.

AVAILABILITY (Rx)

TABLETS: 25 mg, 50 mg, 100 mg.

ADMINISTRATION/HANDLING

PO:

• May take approx. 1 hr before sexual activity but may be taken anywhere from 4 hrs to 30 min before sexual activity.

INDICATIONS/ROUTES/DOSAGE

Erectile dysfunction:

PO: Adults: 50 mg ($\frac{1}{2}$–4 hrs prior to sexual activity). **Range:** 25–100 mg.

SIDE EFFECTS

OCCASIONAL (10–16%): Headache, flushing. (3–7%): Dyspepsia (heartburn, indigestion, epigastric pain), nasal congestion, urinary tract infection, abnormal vision, diarrhea. **RARE** (2%): Dizziness, rash.

S

ADVERSE REACTIONS/TOXIC EFFECTS

None significant.

NURSING IMPLICATIONS

BASELINE ASSESSMENT:

Assess cardiovascular status before initiating treatment for erectile dysfunction.

PATIENT/FAMILY TEACHING:

Sildenafil has no effect in the absence of sexual stimulation.

silver sulfadiazine

sul-fah-**dye**-ah-zeen
(Flamazine ♣, Flint SSD, Silvadene)

▶CLASSIFICATION

PHARMACOTHERAPEUTIC:
Anti-infective. ***CLINICAL:*** Burn preparation

ACTION/*THERAPEUTIC EFFECT*

Acts upon cell wall and cell membrane to *produce bactericidal effect.* Silver is released slowly in concentrations selectively toxic to bacteria.

USES/*UNLABELED*

Prevention, treatment of infection in second-and third-degree burns, protection against conversion from partial-to full-thickness wounds (infection causes extended tissue destruction). *Treatment of minor bacterial skin infection, dermal ulcer.*

PRECAUTIONS

CONTRAINDICATIONS: None significant. ***CAUTIONS:*** Impaired renal/hepatic function, G-6-PD deficiency, premature neonates, infants <2 mos.

INTERACTIONS

DRUG:* Collagenase, papain, sutilains** may be inactivated. ***HERBAL: None known. ***FOOD:*** None known. ***LAB VALUES:*** None significant.

AVAILABILITY (Rx)

CREAM: 10 mg per gm.

ADMINISTRATION/HANDLING

Topical:

• Apply to cleansed, debrided burns using sterile glove. • Keep burn areas covered with silver sulfadiazine cream at all times; reapply to areas where removed by pt activity. • Dressings may be ordered on individual basis.

INDICATIONS/ROUTES/DOSAGE

Usual topical dosage:

***TOPICAL:* Adults, elderly:** Apply 1–2 times/day.

SIDE EFFECTS

Side effects characteristic of all sulfonamides may occur when systemically absorbed, e.g., extensive burn areas (over 20% of body surface): anorexia, nausea, vomiting, headache, diarrhea, dizziness, photosensitivity, joint pain. ***FREQUENT:*** Burning feeling at treatment site. ***OCCASIONAL:*** Brown-gray skin discoloration, rash, itching. ***RARE:*** Increased sensitivity of skin to sunlight.

ADVERSE REACTIONS/TOXIC EFFECTS

If significant systemic absorption occurs, less often but serious are hemolytic anemia, hypoglycemia, diuresis, peripheral neuropathy,

Stevens-Johnson syndrome, agranulocytosis, disseminated lupus erythematosus, anaphylaxis, hepatitis, toxic nephrosis. Fungal superinfections may occur. Interstitial nephritis occurs rarely.

NURSING IMPLICATIONS

BASELINE ASSESSMENT:
Determine initial CBC, renal/hepatic function test results.

INTERVENTION/EVALUATION:
Evaluate fluid balance, renal function: Check I&O, renal function tests and report changes promptly. Monitor vital signs. Check serum sulfonamide concentrations carefully. Assess burns, surrounding areas for pain, burning, itching, rash (antihistamines may provide relief, silver sulfadiazine therapy should continue unless reactions severe). Check CBC results.

PATIENT/FAMILY TEACHING:
Therapy must be continued until healing is satisfactory or the site is ready for grafting.

simethicone

sye-**meth**-ih-cone
(Alka-Seltzer Gas Relief, Gas-X, Genasym, Maalox AntiGas, Mylanta Gas, Ovol♣, Phazyme)

FIXED-COMBINATION(S)
With aluminum and magnesium hydroxide, antacids **(Digel, Gelusil, Maalox Plus, Mylanta);** with loperamide, an antidiarrheal **(Imodium Advanced);** with magaldrate, an antacid **(Riopan)**

▶CLASSIFICATION
CLINICAL: Antiflatulent

ACTION/*THERAPEUTIC EFFECT*
Changes surface tension of gas bubbles allowing for easier elimination of gas. *Disperses, prevents formation of gas pockets in GI tract.*

PHARMACOKINETICS
Does not appear to be absorbed from GI tract. Excreted unchanged in feces.

USES/*UNLABELED*
Treatment of flatulence, gastric bloating, postop gas pain or when gas retention may be problem (i.e., peptic ulcer, spastic colon, air swallowing). *Adjunct to gastroscopy, bowel radiography.*

PRECAUTIONS
CONTRAINDICATIONS: None significant. ***CAUTIONS:*** None significant.
▷***LIFESPAN CONSIDERATIONS:***
Pregnancy/Lactation: Unknown if drug crosses placenta or is distributed in breast milk. **Pregnancy Category C. Children/Elderly:** None known.

INTERACTIONS
DRUG: None significant. ***HERBAL:*** None known. ***FOOD:*** None known. ***LAB VALUES:*** None significant.

AVAILABILITY (OTC)
SOFTGEL: 125 mg, 166 mg. ***SUSPENSION:*** 40 mg/0.6 ml. ***TABLETS (chewable):*** 80 mg, 125 mg, 150 mg, 166 mg.

ADMINISTRATION/HANDLING
PO:
• Give after meals and at bedtime as needed. Chewable tablets are to be chewed thoroughly before

S

swallowing. Enteric-coated tablets are swallowed whole; do not crush. • Shake suspension well before using.

INDICATIONS/ROUTES/DOSAGE

Antiflatulent:

PO: Adults, elderly, children >12 yrs: 40–125 mg after meals and at betime. **Maximum:** 500 mg/day. **Children 2–12 yrs:** 40 mg 4 times/day. **Children <2 yrs:** 20 mg 4 times/day.

SIDE EFFECTS

None significant.

ADVERSE REACTIONS/TOXIC EFFECTS

None significant.

NURSING IMPLICATIONS

INTERVENTION/EVALUATION:
Evaluate for therapeutic response: relief of flatulence, abdominal bloating.

simvastatin

sim-vah-**stay**-tin
(Zocor)
Do not confuse with Cozaar.

▶CLASSIFICATION

PHARMACOTHERAPEUTIC: HMG-CoA reductase inhibitor. *CLINICAL:* Antihyperlipidemic (see p. 50C)

ACTION/THERAPEUTIC EFFECT

Interferes with cholesterol biosynthesis by inhibiting the conversion of the enzyme HMG-CoA to mevalonate. *Decreases LDL, cholesterol, VLDL, plasma triglycerides, slight increase in HDL concentration.*

PHARMACOKINETICS

Well absorbed from GI tract. Protein binding: 95%. Undergoes extensive first-pass metabolism. Hydrolyzed to active metabolite. Primarily eliminated in feces. Unknown if removed by hemodialysis.

USES

Adjunct to diet therapy to decrease elevated total and LDL cholesterol concentrations in those with primary hypercholesterolemia (types IIa and IIb), lowers triglyceride levels, increases HDL. Reduces deaths, prevents heart attacks in pts with heart disease, high cholesterol. Decreases risk of mortality by decreasing coronary death, risk of nonfatal myocardial infarction, need for myocardial revascularization procedures. Decreases risk for stroke/TIA.

PRECAUTIONS

CONTRAINDICATIONS: Pregnancy, active liver disease or unexplained, persistent elevations of liver function tests, <18 yrs. *CAUTIONS:* History of liver disease, substantial alcohol consumption. Withholding/discontinuing simvastatin may be necessary when pt is at risk for renal failure secondary to rhabdomyolysis. Severe metabolic, endocrine, or electrolyte disorders. ▷*LIFESPAN CONSIDERATIONS:* **Pregnancy/Lactation:** Contraindicated in pregnancy (suppression of cholesterol biosynthesis may cause fetal toxicity) and lactation. Risk of serious adverse reactions in nursing infants. **Pregnancy Category X. Children:** Safety and efficacy not established. **Elderly:** No age-related precautions noted.

INTERACTIONS

DRUG: Increased risk of rhabdomyolysis, acute renal failure with **cyclosporine, erythromycin, gemfibrozil, niacin, other immunosuppressants. Erythromycin, itraconazole, ketoconazole** may increase concentration, cause muscle pain, inflammation or weakness. ***HERBAL:*** None known. ***FOOD:*** None known. ***LAB VALUES:*** May increase creatinine kinase, serum transaminase concentrations.

AVAILABILITY (Rx)

TABLETS: 5 mg, 10 mg, 20 mg, 40 mg, 80 mg.

ADMINISTRATION/HANDLING

PO:

• Give without regard to meals. • Administer in evening.

INDICATIONS/ROUTES/DOSAGE

Note: Before initiating therapy, pt should be on standard cholesterol-lowering diet for minimum of 3–6 mos. Continue diet throughout simvastatin therapy.

Hyperlipidemia/decreased mortality:

PO: Adults: Initially, 10–20 mg/day in evening. Dosage adjustment at 4 wk intervals. **Elderly:** Initially, 10 mg/day. May increase by 5–10 mg/day q4wks. **Range:** 5–80 mg/day. **Maximum:** 80 mg/day.

SIDE EFFECTS

Generally well tolerated. Side effects usually mild and transient. ***OCCASIONAL*** (2–3%): Headache, abdominal pain/cramps, constipation, upper respiratory infection. ***RARE*** (<2%): Diarrhea, flatulence, asthenia (loss of strength and energy), nausea/vomiting.

ADVERSE REACTIONS/TOXIC EFFECTS

Potential for lens opacities. Hypersensitivity reaction, hepatitis occurs rarely.

NURSING IMPLICATIONS

BASELINE ASSESSMENT:

Question for possibility of pregnancy before initiating therapy (Pregnancy Category X). Question history of hypersensitivity to simvastatin. Assess baseline lab results: cholesterol, triglycerides, liver function tests.

INTERVENTION/EVALUATION:

Monitor cholesterol and triglyceride lab results for therapeutic response. Monitor liver function tests. Determine pattern of bowel activity. Check for headache.

PATIENT/FAMILY TEACHING:

Use appropriate contraceptive measures (Pregnancy Category X). Periodic lab tests are essential part of therapy.

sirolimus

sigh-row-**lie**-mus
(Rapamune)

▶CLASSIFICATION

CLINICAL: Immunosuppressant

ACTION/*THERAPEUTIC EFFECT*

Inhibits T-lymphocyte proliferation induced by stimulation of cell surface receptors, mitogens, alloanti-

S

gens, lymphokines. Prevents activation of enzyme TOR, a key regulatory kinase in cell cycle progression. *Inhibits T and B cell proliferation (essential components of immune response).*

USES

Prophylaxis of organ rejection in pts after renal transplants in combination with cyclosporine and corticosteroids.

PRECAUTIONS

CONTRAINDICATIONS: Hypersensitivity to sirolimus, current malignancy. ***CAUTIONS:*** Chickenpox, herpes zoster, impaired liver function, infection.

INTERACTIONS

DRUG: **Cyclosporine, diltiazem, ketoconazole** may increase concentration, toxicity. **Rifampin** may decrease concentration effect. ***HERBAL:*** None significant. ***FOOD:*** **Grapefruit juice** may decrease metabolism. ***LAB VALUES:*** May decrease Hct, Hgb, platelets. May increase serum creatinine, cholesterol, triglycerides.

AVAILABILITY (Rx)

ORAL SOLUTION: 1 mg/ml. ***TABLETS:*** 1 mg.

INDICATIONS/ROUTES/DOSAGE

Prophylaxis of organ rejection:
PO: **Adults: Loading dose:** 6 mg. **Maintenance:** 2 mg/day. **Children ≥13 yrs <40 kg:** 3 mg/m^2 loading dose; then, 1 mg/m^2/day.

SIDE EFFECTS

OCCASIONAL: Hypercholesterolemia, hyperlipidemia, hypertension, rash. **(High dose 5 mg/day):** Anemia, arthralgia, diarrhea, hypokalemia, thrombocytopenia.

ADVERSE REACTIONS/TOXIC EFFECTS

None significant.

NURSING IMPLICATIONS

BASELINE ASSESSMENT:

Assess if pregnant, breast-feeding, using medications, esp. cyclosporine, diltiazem, ketoconazole, rifampin. Determine if pt has chickenpox, herpes zoster, malignancy, infection.

INTERVENTION/EVALUATION:

Monitor liver function.

PATIENT/FAMILY TEACHING:

Avoid those with colds or other infections. Do not drink grapefruit juice or eat grapefruit. Close monitoring by physician is important.

---

sodium bicarbonate

►CLASSIFICATION

PHARMACOTHERAPEUTIC: Alkalinizing agent. ***CLINICAL:*** Antacid

ACTION/*THERAPEUTIC EFFECT*

Increases plasma bicarbonate, buffers excess hydrogen ion concentration, *increases pH, reverses acidosis.* **Urinary alkalizer:** Increases excretion of free bicarbonate in urine, *increases urinary pH.* **Antacid:** Neutralizes existing quantities of stomach acid, *increases pH of stomach contents.*

PHARMACOKINETICS

After administration, sodium bicarbonate dissociates to sodium and bicarbonate ions. Forms/ex-

---

cretes CO_2 (with increased hydrogen ions combines to form carbonic acid, then dissociates to CO_2, which is excreted by lungs). Plasma concentration regulated by kidney (ability to excrete/make bicarbonate).

USES

Corrects metabolic acidosis occurring in severe renal disease and for advanced cardiac life support during cardiopulmonary resuscitation. Used in treatment of drug intoxicants and hyperacidity, associated stomach upset. Treatment of symptoms of peptic ulcer disease; reduces uric acid crystallization (prophylactic).

PRECAUTIONS

CONTRAINDICATIONS: Metabolic/respiratory alkalosis, hypocalcemia, excessive chloride loss due to vomiting/diarrhea/GI suction. ***CAUTIONS:*** CHF, edematous states, renal insufficiency, those on corticosteroid therapy.
▷***LIFESPAN CONSIDERATIONS:*** **Pregnancy/Lactation:** May produce hypernatremia, increase tendon reflexes in neonate/fetus whose mother is a chronic, high-dose user. May be distributed in breast milk. **Pregnancy Category C. Children:** No age-related precautions noted. Do not use as antacid in those <6 yrs of age. **Elderly:** Age-related renal impairment may require caution.

INTERACTIONS

DRUG: May decrease excretion **of quinidine, ketoconazole, tetracyclines. Calcium-containing products** may result in milk-alkali syndrome. May increase excretion of **salicylates, lithium.** May decrease effect of **methenamine.**

HERBAL: None known. ***FOOD:*** **Milk, milk products** may result in milk-alkali syndrome. ***LAB VALUES:*** May increase serum, urinary pH.

AVAILABILITY (OTC)

TABLETS: 325 mg, 520 mg, 650 mg. ***INJECTION (Rx):*** 0.5 mEq/ml (4.2%), 0.6 mEq/ml (5%), 0.9 mEq/ml (7.5%), 1 mEq/ml (8.4%).

ADMINISTRATION/HANDLING

PO:
• *Chewable tablets:* Thoroughly chew tablets before swallowing (follow with glass of water or milk).

IV 🏧

Storage:
• Store at room temperature.

Reconstitution:
• May give undiluted.

Rate of administration:
• For IV push, give up to 1 mEq/kg over 1–3 min for cardiac arrest. • For IV infusion, do not exceed rate of infusion of 50 mEq/hr. For children <2 yrs, premature infants, neonates, administer by slow infusion, up to 8 mEq/daily.

IV INCOMPATIBILITIES ⊘

Amiodarone (Cordarone), amphotericin B complex (Abelcet, Ambisome, Amphotec), ciprofoxacin (Cipro), diltiazem (Cardizem), idarubicin (Idamycin), midazolam (Versed), nalbuphine (Nubain), ondansetron (Zofran), verapamil (Isoptin), vinorelbine (Navelbine).

IV COMPATIBILITIES

Acyclovir (Zovirax), astreonam (Azactam), cefepime (Maxipime), ceftriaxone (Rocephin), heparin, insulin, milrinone (Primacor), potassium chloride, propofol (Diprivan), vancomycin (Vancocin).

INDICATIONS/ROUTES/DOSAGE

Note: May give by IV push, IV infusion, or orally. Dose individualized (based on severity of acidosis, laboratory values, pt age, weight, clinical conditions). Do not fully correct bicarbonate deficit during first 24 hrs (may cause metabolic alkalosis).

Cardiac arrest:

IV: **Adults, elderly:** Initially, 1 mEq/kg (as 7.5–8.4% solution). May repeat with 0.5 mEq/kg q10min during continued arrest. Postresuscitation phase based on arterial blood pH, $PaCO_2$ base deficit. **Children, infants:** Initially, 1 mEq/kg.

Metabolic acidosis (less severe):

IV INFUSION: **Adults, elderly, older children:** 2–5 mEq/kg over 4–8 hrs. May repeat based on laboratory values.

Acidosis (associated with chronic renal failure):

Note: Give when plasma bicarbonate <15 mEq/L.

PO: **Adults, elderly:** Initially, 20–36 mEq/day in divided doses.

Renal tubular acidosis (prevents renal failure, osteomalacia):

PO: **Adults, elderly:** 4–6 g/day in divided doses or 0.5–10 mEq/kg/day in divided doses (higher doses for proximal renal tubular acidosis).

Alkalinization of urine:

PO: **Adults, elderly:** Initially, 4 g, then 1–2 g q4h. **Maximum:** 16 g/day. **Children:** 84–840 mg/kg/day in divided doses.

Antacid:

PO: **Adults, elderly:** 300 mg to 2 g 1–4 times/day.

SIDE EFFECTS

FREQUENT: Abdominal distention, flatulence, belching.

ADVERSE REACTIONS/TOXIC EFFECTS

Excessive/chronic use may produce metabolic alkalosis (irritability, twitching, numbness/tingling of extremities, cyanosis, slow/with shallow respiration, headache, thirst, nausea). Fluid overload results in headache, weakness, blurred vision, behavioral changes, incoordination, muscle twitching, rise in B/P, decrease in pulse rate, rapid respirations, wheezing, coughing, distended neck veins. Extravasation may occur at IV site, resulting in necrosis, ulceration.

NURSING IMPLICATIONS

BASELINE ASSESSMENT:

Do not give other oral medication within 1–2 hrs of antacid administration.

INTERVENTION/EVALUATION:

Monitor blood and urine pH, CO_2 level, serum electrolytes, plasma bicarbonate, and $PaCO_2$ levels. Watch for signs of metabolic alkalosis, fluid overload. Assess for clinical improvement of metabolic acidosis (relief from hyperventilation, weakness, disorientation). Assess pattern of daily bowel activity, stool consistency. Monitor serum phosphate, calcium, uric acid levels. Assess for relief of gastric distress.

PATIENT/FAMILY TEACHING:

Chewable tablets: Chew tablets thoroughly before swallowing (may be followed by water or milk). Tablets may discolor stool. Maintain adequate fluid intake.

sodium chloride

(Ocean Mist, Salinex, Sodium chloride✤)

▶CLASSIFICATION

CLINICAL: Electrolyte, ophthalmic adjunct, bronchodilator

ACTION/ *THERAPEUTIC EFFECT*

Sodium (a major cation of extracellular fluid) primarily *controls water distribution, fluid/electrolyte balance, osmotic pressure of body fluids.* Associated with chloride and bicarbonate, *maintains acid-base balance.*

PHARMACOKINETICS

Well absorbed from GI tract. Widely distributed. Primarily excreted in urine.

USES

Parenteral: Source of hydration; prevent/treats sodium and chloride deficiencies (hypertonic for severe deficiencies). Prevents muscle cramps/heat prostration occurring with excessive perspiration. **Hypotonic:** Hydrating solution, used to assess renal function status and manage hyperosmolar diabetes. Diluent for reconstitution. **Nasal:** Restores moisture, relieves dry and inflamed nasal membranes. **Ophthalmic:** Therapy in reduction of corneal edema, diagnostic aid in ophthalmoscopic exam.

PRECAUTIONS

CONTRAINDICATIONS: Hypernatremia, fluid retention. **CAUTIONS:** CHF, circulatory insufficiency, kidney dysfunction, hypoproteinemia.

Do not use NaCl preserved with benzyl alcohol in neonates.

▷*LIFESPAN CONSIDERATIONS:*
Pregnancy/Lactation: Pregnancy Category C. Children/Elderly: No age-related precautions noted.

INTERACTIONS

DRUG: Hypertonic saline and oxytocics may cause uterine hypertonus, possible uterine ruptures or lacerations. **HERBAL:** None known. **FOOD:** None known. **LAB VALUES:** None significant.

AVAILABILITY (OTC)

TABLETS: 650 mg, 1 g, 2.25 g. **TABLETS (slow-release):** 600 mg. **NASAL SOLUTION:** 0.4%, 0.6%, 0.75%. **OPHTHALMIC SOLUTION:** 2%, 5%. **OPHTHALMIC OINTMENT:** 5%. **INJECTION (concentrate) (Rx):** 14.6%, 23.4%. **INJECTION (infusion) (Rx):** 0.45%, 0.9%, 3%, 5%. **IRRIGATION (Rx):** 0.45%, 0.9%.

ADMINISTRATION/HANDLING

PO:

• Do not crush or break enteric-coated or extended-release tablets.

Nasal:

• Instruct pt to begin inhaling slowly just before releasing medication into nose. • Inhale slowly, then release air gently through mouth. • Continue technique for 20–30 sec.

Ophthalmic:

• Place finger on lower eyelid and pull out until pocket is formed between eye and lower lid. Hold dropper above pocket and place prescribed number of drops (or apply thin strip of ointment) in pocket. Instruct pt to close eyes

S

✤ - Canadian trade name   ✳ - see also www.wbsaunders.com/SIMON/SaundersNDH

gently so medication will not be squeezed out of sac. • When lower lid is released, have pt keep eye open without blinking for at least 30 sec for solution; for ointment have pt close eye and roll eyeball around to distribute medication. • When using drops, apply gentle finger pressure to lacrimal sac (bridge of the nose, inside corner of the eye) for 1–2 min after administration of solution (reduces systemic absorption).

IV 📋

• Hypertonic solutions (3% or 5%) is administered via large vein; avoid infiltration; do not exceed 100 ml/hr. • Vials containing 2.5–4 mEq/ml (concentrated NaCl) must be diluted with D_5W or $D_{10}W$ before administration.

INDICATIONS/ROUTES/DOSAGE

Usual parenteral dosage:

Note: Dosage based on age, weight, clinical condition, fluid, electrolyte, acid-base status.

IV INFUSION: **Adults, elderly:** (0.9 or 0.45%): 1–2 L/day. (3 or 5%): 100 ml over 1 hr; assess serum electrolyte concentration before additional fluid is given.

Usual oral dosage:

PO: **Adults, elderly:** 1–2 g 3 times/day.

Usual nasal dosage:

INTRANASAL: **Adults, elderly:** Take as needed.

Usual ophthalmic dosage:

OPHTHALMIC: **Adults, elderly:** *(solution):* 1–2 drops q3–4h. *(ointment):* Once/day or as directed.

SIDE EFFECTS

FREQUENT: Facial flushing. *OCCASIONAL:* Fever, irritation/phlebitis/extravasation at injection site.

Ophthalmic: Temporary burning/irritation.

ADVERSE REACTIONS/TOXIC EFFECTS

Too-rapid administration may produce peripheral edema, CHF, pulmonary edema. Excessive dosage produces hypokalemia, hypervolemia, hypernatremia.

NURSING IMPLICATIONS

BASELINE ASSESSMENT:
Assess fluid balance (I&O, edema).

INTERVENTION/EVALUATION:
Monitor fluid balance (e.g., I&O, daily weight, edema, lung sounds), IV site for extravasation. Monitor serum electrolytes, acid-base balance, B/P. Hypernatremia associated with edema, weight gain, elevated B/P; hyponatremia associated with muscle cramps, nausea, vomiting, dry mucous membranes.

PATIENT/FAMILY TEACHING:
Temporary burning, irritation may occur upon instillation of eye medication. Discontinue eye medication if severe pain, headache, rapid change in vision (side and straight ahead), sudden appearance of floating spots, acute redness of eyes, pain on exposure to light, or double vision occurs and contact physician.

sodium ferric gluconate complex

(Ferrlecit)

▶CLASSIFICATION

PHARMACOTHERAPEUTIC: Trace element. ***CLINICAL:*** Hematinic

ACTION/*THERAPEUTIC EFFECT*

Repletes total body content of iron. Iron is necessary for normal hemoglobin synthesis to maintain O_2 transport, *for metabolism and synthesis of DNA.*

USES

Treatment of iron deficiency anemia in pts undergoing chronic hemodialysis who are receiving supplemental erythropoietin therapy.

PRECAUTIONS

CONTRAINDICATIONS: All anemias not associated with iron deficiency. ***CAUTIONS:*** Pts with iron overload.
▷***LIFESPAN CONSIDERATIONS:***
Pregnancy/Lactation: Unknown if distributed in breast milk. **Pregnancy Category B. Children:** Safety and efficacy not established. **Elderly:** No age-related precautions noted; lower initial doses recommended.

INTERACTIONS

DRUG: None significant. ***HERBAL:*** None known. ***FOOD:*** None known. ***LAB VALUES:*** None significant.

AVAILABILITY (Rx)

AMPULES: 12.5 mg/ml elemental iron.

ADMINISTRATION/HANDLING
IV 💊
Storage:
• Store at room temperature. • Use immediately after dilution.

Reconstitution:
• Must be diluted. • Test dose: dilute 25 mg (2 ml) with 50 ml 0.9% NaCl. • Recommended dose: dilute 125 mg (10 ml) with 100 ml 0.9% NaCl.

Rate of administration:
• Infuse test dose and recommended dose over 1 hr.

IV INCOMPATIBILITY ⊘
Do not mix with any other medications.

INDICATIONS/ROUTES/DOSAGE

Note: Initially, a 25 mg test dose is diluted in 50 ml 0.9% NaCl and given over 60 min. May give IV undiluted without test dose.

IV INFUSION: Adults, elderly: 125 mg in 100 ml 0.9% NaCl infused over 1 hr. Minimum cumulative dose 1 g elemental iron given over 8 sessions at sequential dialysis treatment. (May be given during dialysis session itself.)

SIDE EFFECTS

FREQUENT (>3%): Flushing, hypotension, hypersensitivity reaction. ***OCCASIONAL*** (1–3%): Injection site reaction, headache, abdominal pain, chills, flulike syndrome, dizziness, leg cramps, dyspnea, nausea, vomiting, diarrhea, myalgia, pruritus, edema.

ADVERSE REACTIONS/TOXIC EFFECTS

Rarely, potentially fatal hypersensitivity reaction characterized by cardiovascular collapse, cardiac arrest, dyspnea, bronchospasm, angioedema, urticaria. Hypotension associated with flushing, lightheadedness, fatigue, weakness, or severe pain in chest, back, or groin with rapid administration of iron.

S

NURSING IMPLICATIONS

BASELINE ASSESSMENT:
Do not give concurrently with oral iron form (excessive iron may produce excessive iron storage [hemosiderosis]). Be alert to those with rheumatoid arthritis or iron deficiency anemia (acute exacerbation of joint pain and swelling may occur).

INTERVENTION/EVALUATION:
Monitor serum ferritin levels.

PATIENT/FAMILY TEACHING:
Stools frequently become black with iron therapy; this is harmless unless accompanied by red streaking, sticky consistency of stool, abdominal pain or cramping, which should be reported to physician.

sodium polystyrene sulfonate

(Kayexalate, SPS)

►**CLASSIFICATION**

PHARMACOTHERAPEUTIC: Cation exchange resin. *CLINICAL:* Antihyperkalemic

ACTION/*THERAPEUTIC EFFECT*
Resin either passes through intestine or is retained in colon; *releases sodium ions in exchange for primarily potassium ions.* Occurs from 2–12 hrs after PO administration, longer after rectal administration.

USES
Treatment of hyperkalemia.

PRECAUTIONS

CONTRAINDICATIONS: None significant. *CAUTIONS:* Those who cannot tolerate increase in sodium (CHF, severe hypertension, marked edema).

▷*LIFESPAN CONSIDERATIONS:*
Pregnancy/Lactation: Unknown if drug crosses placenta or is distributed in breast milk. **Pregnancy Category N/A. Children:** No age-related precautions noted. **Elderly:** May be at increased risk of fecal impaction.

INTERACTIONS

DRUG: **Cation-donating antacids, laxatives (e.g., magnesium hydroxide)** may decrease effect, cause systemic alkalosis (pts with renal impairment). *HERBAL:* None known. *FOOD:* None known. *LAB VALUES:* May decrease magnesium, calcium.

AVAILABILITY (Rx)
SUSPENSION: 15 g/60 ml. *POWDER.*

ADMINISTRATION/HANDLING
PO:
• Give with 20–100 ml sorbitol (facilitates passage of resin through intestinal tract, prevents constipation, aids in potassium removal, increases palatability). • Do not mix with foods, liquids containing potassium.

Rectal:
• After initial cleansing enema, insert large rubber tube into rectum well into sigmoid colon, tape in place. • Introduce suspension (with 100 ml sorbitol) via gravity. • Flush with 50–100 ml fluid and clamp. • Retain for several hrs if possible. • Irrigate colon with nonsodium-containing solution to remove resin.

⏀ - see color pill atlas   underscored - top 100 prescribed drug

INDICATIONS/ROUTES/DOSAGE

Hyperkalemia:

PO: **Adults, elderly:** 60 ml (15 g) 1–4 times/day.

RECTAL: **Adults, elderly:** 30–50 g as needed q6h.

Usual pediatric dosage:

PO/RECTAL: Based on 1 g resin binding approx. 1 mEq potassium: 1 g/kg q6h.

SIDE EFFECTS

High dosage: Anorexia, nausea, vomiting, constipation. *High dosage in elderly:* Fecal impaction (severe stomach pain with nausea/vomiting). *OCCASIONAL:* Diarrhea, sodium retention (decreased urination, peripheral edema, increased weight).

ADVERSE REACTIONS/TOXIC EFFECTS

Serious potassium deficiency may occur. Early signs of hypokalemia: irritable confusion, delayed thought processes, often associated with lengthened QT interval and widening, flattening, or conversion of T wave and prominent U waves. Hypocalcemia (abdominal/muscle cramps) occurs occasionally. Arrhythmias, severe muscle weakness may be noted.

NURSING IMPLICATIONS

BASELINE ASSESSMENT:

Does not rapidly correct severe hyperkalemia (may take hrs to days). Consider other measures in medical emergency (IV calcium, IV sodium bicarbonate, glucose, insulin, dialysis).

INTERVENTION/EVALUATION:

Frequent potassium levels within each 24 hrs should be main-tained, monitored. Assess pt's clinical condition, EKG (valuable in determining when treatment should be discontinued). In addition to checking serum potassium, monitor magnesium, calcium levels. Monitor daily bowel activity, stool consistency (fecal impaction may occur in those on high doses, particularly in elderly).

somatrem

soe-ma-trem
(Protropin)
Do not confuse with Proloprim, Protamine, Protopam, somatropin.

▶CLASSIFICATION

PHARMACOTHERAPEUTIC: Polypeptide hormone. *CLINICAL:* Growth stimulator

ACTION/THERAPEUTIC EFFECT

Stimulates linear growth. Increases number, size of muscle cells, increases red cell mass. Affects carbohydrate metabolism (antagonizes action of insulin), fats (increases mobilization of fats), and proteins (increases cellular protein synthesis).

USES

Long-term treatment of children who have growth failure due to endogenous growth hormone deficiency.

PRECAUTIONS

CONTRAINDICATIONS: None significant. *CAUTIONS:* Diabetes mellitus, untreated hypothyroidism, malignancy.

S

INTERACTIONS

DRUG: **Corticosteroids** may inhibit growth response. ***HERBAL:*** None significant. ***FOOD:*** None significant. ***LAB VALUES:*** May increase alkaline phosphatase, serum inorganic phosphorus, parathyroid hormone.

AVAILABILITY (Rx)

POWDER FOR INJECTION: 5 mg, 10 mg.

INDICATIONS/ROUTES/DOSAGE

Usual parenteral dosage:

IM/SᴜʙQ: Up to 0.1 mg/kg (0.26 IU/kg) 3 times/wk.

SIDE EFFECTS

FREQUENT: 30% of pts develop persistent antibodies to growth hormone (generally does not cause failure to respond to somatrem). ***OCCASIONAL:*** Headache, muscle pain, weakness, mild hyperglycemia, allergic reaction (rash, itching), pain/swelling at injection site, pain in hip/knee.

NURSING IMPLICATIONS

BASELINE ASSESSMENT:

Thyroid function, blood glucose levels.

INTERVENTION/EVALUATION:

Monitor bone age, calcium, parathyroid, phosphorus, renal function, glucose, growth rate, thyroid function, decreased wasting in AIDS.

PATEINT/FAMILY TEACHING:

Correct procedure to reconstitute for IM/SubQ administration. Safe handling and disposal of needles. Need for regular follow-up with physician.

---

somatropin

soe-mah-**troe**-pin
(Humatrope, Norditropin, Nutropin, Nutropin AQ, Nutropin Depot, Saizen)
Do not confuse with somatrem, sumatriptan.

▶CLASSIFICATION

PHARMACOTHERAPEUTIC: Polypeptide hormone. ***CLINICAL:*** Growth stimulator

ACTION/THERAPEUTIC EFFECT

Stimulates linear growth. Increases number, size of muscle cells, increases red cell mass. Affects carbohydrate metabolism (antagonizes action of insulin), fats (increases mobilization of fats), and proteins (increases cellular protein synthesis).

USES

Long-term treatment of children who have growth failure due to endogenous growth hormone deficiency or associated with chronic renal insufficiency (Nutropin only). Long-term therapy in adults with growth hormone deficiency. Long-term treatment of short stature associated with Turner's syndrome, treatment of AIDS-wasting syndrome.

PRECAUTIONS

CONTRAINDICATIONS: None significant. ***CAUTIONS:*** Diabetes mellitus, untreated hypothyroidism, malignancy.

INTERACTIONS

DRUG: **Corticosteroids** may inhibit growth response. ***HERBAL:*** None significant. ***FOOD:*** None

---

significant. ***LAB VALUES:*** May increase alkaline phosphatase, serum inorganic phosphorus, parathyroid hormone.

INDICATIONS/ROUTES/DOSAGE
Growth hormone deficiency:

IM/SubQ: (Humatrope): Up to 0.06 mg/kg 3 times/wk.

SubQ: (Nutropin): 0.3 mg/kg/wk.

SubQ: (Nutropin Depot): 1.5 mg/kg/mo or 0.75 mg/kg 2 times/mo.

SubQ: Adults: 0.04 mg/kg/wk in 6–7 injections/wk. **Maximum:** 0.08 mg/kg/wk.

Chronic renal insufficiency:

SubQ: (Nutropin): 0.35 mg/kg/wk.

Turner's syndrome:

SubQ: 0.375 mg/kg/wk divided into 3–7 equal doses/wk.

AIDS-wasting syndrome:

SubQ: 4–6 mg at bedtime.

SIDE EFFECTS

FREQUENT: Development of persistent antibodies to growth hormone (generally does not cause failure to respond to somatropin); hypercalciuria during first 2–3 mos of therapy. ***OCCASIONAL:*** Headache, muscle pain, weakness, mild hyperglycemia, allergic reaction (rash, itching), pain/swelling at injection site, pain in hip/knee.

NURSING IMPLICATIONS

BASELINE ASSESSMENT:

Thyroid function, blood glucose levels.

INTERVENTION/EVALUATION:

Monitor bone age, calcium, parathyroid, phosphorus, renal function, glucose, growth rate,

thyroid function, decreased wasting in AIDS.

PATIENT/FAMILY TEACHING:

Correct procedure to reconstitute for IM/SubQ administration. Safe handling and disposal of needles. Need for regular follow-up with physician.

sotalol hydrochloride

sew-tah-lol
(Betapace, Sotacor ♣)
Do not confuse with Stadol.

▶CLASSIFICATION

PHARMACOTHERAPEUTIC: Beta-adrenergic blocking agent. ***CLINICAL:*** Antiarrhythmic (see pp. 14C, 61C)

ACTION/*THERAPEUTIC EFFECT*

Prolongs action potential and effective refractory period, QT interval. Decreases heart rate, AV nodal conduction; increases AV nodal refractoriness, *producing antiarrhythmic activity.*

PHARMACOKINETICS

Well absorbed from GI tract. Protein binding: None. Widely distributed. Primarily excreted unchanged in urine. Removed by hemodialysis. Half-life: 12 hrs (half-life increased in elderly, pts with impaired renal function).

USES/*UNLABELED*

Treatment of documented, life-threatening ventricular arrhythmias. *Treatment of chronic angina pectoris, hypertension, hypertrophic cardiomyopathy, myocardial infarction, pheochromocytoma, tremors, anxiety, thyrotoxicosis, mitral*

S

valve prolapse syndrome. Maintenance of normal heart rhythm in chronic or recurring atrial fibrillation or flutter.

PRECAUTIONS

CONTRAINDICATIONS: Bronchial asthma, uncontrolled cardiac failure, sinus bradycardia, second-and third-degree heart block, cardiogenic shock, long QT syndrome (unless functioning pacemaker present). **CAUTIONS:** Pts with history of ventricular tachycardia, ventricular fibrillation, cardiomegaly, CHF, diabetes mellitus, excessive prolongation of QT interval, hypokalemia, and hypomagnesium. Severe, prolonged diarrhea. Pts with sick-sinus syndrome; pts at risk of developing thyrotoxicosis. Avoid abrupt withdrawal.

▷**LIFESPAN CONSIDERATIONS:**
Pregnancy/Lactation: Crosses placenta; excreted in breast milk. **Pregnancy Category B** (Category D if used in second or third trimester). **Children:** Safety and efficacy not established. **Elderly:** Age-related peripheral vascular disease may increase susceptibility to decreased peripheral circulation.

INTERACTIONS

DRUG: Antiarrhythmics, phenothiazine, tricyclic antidepressants may increase prolonged QT interval. May increase proarrhythmia with **digoxin. Calcium channel blockers** may increase effect on AV conduction, B/P. May mask signs of hypoglycemia, prolong effect of **insulin, oral hypoglycemics.** May inhibit effects of **sympathomimetics.** May potentiate rebound hypertension noted after discontinuing **clonidine. HERBAL:** None known. **FOOD:**

None known. **LAB VALUES:** May increase glucose, alkaline phosphatase, LDH, SGOT (AST), SGPT (ALT), lipoproteins, triglycerides.

AVAILABILITY (Rx)

TABLETS: 80 mg, 120 mg, 160 mg, 240 mg

ADMINISTRATION/HANDLING
PO:
• Give without regard to food.

INDICATIONS/ROUTES/DOSAGE
Antiarrhythmic:

PO: Adults, elderly: Initially, 80 mg 2 times/day. May increase gradually at 2–3 day intervals. **Range:** 240–320 mg/day. **Note:** Some pts may require 480–640 mg/day. Dosing more than 2 times/day usually not necessary due to long half-life.

Dosage in renal impairment:

Creatinine Clearance	Dosage Interval
30–60 ml/min	24 hrs
10–30 ml/min	36–48 hrs
<10 ml/min	Individualized

SIDE EFFECTS

FREQUENT: Decreased sexual ability, drowsiness, difficulty sleeping, unusual tiredness/weakness. **OCCASIONAL:** Depression, cold hands/feet, diarrhea, constipation, anxiety, nasal congestion, nausea, vomiting. **RARE:** Altered taste, dry eyes, itching, numbness of fingers, toes, scalp.

ADVERSE REACTIONS/TOXIC EFFECTS

Bradycardia, CHF, hypotension, bronchospasm, hypoglycemia, prolonged QT interval, torsade de pointes, ventricular tachycardia, premature ventricular complexes.

NURSING IMPLICATIONS

BASELINE ASSESSMENT:

Pt must be on continuous cardiac monitoring upon initiation of therapy. Do not administer without consulting physician if pulse is below 60 beats/min.

INTERVENTION/EVALUATION:

Diligently monitor arrhythmias. Assess B/P for hypotension, pulse for bradycardia. Assess for CHF: dyspnea, peripheral edema, jugular vein distention, increased weight, rales in lungs, decreased urine output.

sparfloxacin

spar-**flocks**-ah-sin
(Zagam)
Do not confuse with Zyban.

▶**CLASSIFICATION**

PHARMACOTHERAPEUTIC:
Fluoroquinolone. *CLINICAL:* Antibiotic (see p. 22C)

ACTION/THERAPEUTIC EFFECT

Inhibits the DNA enzyme, gyrase, in susceptible microorganisms, interfering with bacterial DNA replication and repair, *producing bactericidal activity.*

PHARMACOKINETICS

Well absorbed following PO administration. Protein binding: 45%. Widely distributed. Metabolized in the liver. Excreted primarily in the urine with a lesser amount eliminated in the feces. Half-life: 16–30 hrs.

USES

Treatment of community-acquired pneumonia, acute bacterial exacerbation of chronic bronchitis.

PRECAUTIONS

CONTRAINDICATIONS: History of hypersensitivity to fluoroquinolone antibiotics, cinoxacin, nalidixic acid. *CAUTIONS:* Impaired renal/hepatic function.

▷*LIFESPAN CONSIDERATIONS:*
Pregnancy/Lactation: Distributed in breast milk. May cause adverse effects in nursing infant. **Pregnancy Category C. Children:** Safety and efficacy not established. **Elderly:** Age-related renal impairment may require dosage adjustment.

INTERACTIONS

DRUG: **Erythromycin, phenothiazines, tricyclic antidepressants** may cause torsades de pointes. **Antacids, iron preparations, sucralfate** may decrease sparfloxacin serum levels (give sparfloxacin at least 4 hrs after any of these medications). *HERBAL:* None known. *FOOD:* None known. *LAB VALUES:* May increase SGOT (AST), SGOT (ALT), alkaline phosphatase, WBC count.

AVAILABILITY (Rx)

TABLETS: 200 mg.

ADMINISTRATION/HANDLING

PO:

• Give without regard to meals. • Do not crush or break film-coated tablets.

INDICATIONS/ROUTES/DOSAGE

Bronchitis, pneumonia:

PO: **Adults ≥18 yrs, elderly:** Initially, two 200 mg tablets as a loading dose on first day. Then one 200 mg tablet q24h for a total of 10 days.

S

Dosage in renal impairment (creatinine clearance <50 ml/min):

PO: **Adults ≥18 yrs, elderly:** Initially, two 200 mg tablets as a loading dose on first day. Then one 200 mg tablet q48h for a total of 9 days.

SIDE EFFECTS

FREQUENT (4–8%): Photosensitivity, diarrhea, nausea, headache. ***RARE*** (1–2%): Dyspepsia, dizziness, insomnia, abdominal pain, change in taste.

ADVERSE REACTIONS/TOXIC EFFECTS

Superinfection (particularly enterococcal or fungal overgrowth of nonsusceptible organisms) due to altered bacterial balance may occur (genital-anal pruritus, ulceration or changes in oral mucosa, moderate to severe diarrhea, new or increased fever). Hypersensitivity reactions have occurred in those receiving fluoroquinolone therapy.

NURSING IMPLICATIONS

BASELINE ASSESSMENT:

Question for hypersensitivity to sparfloxacin or other fluoroquinolones.

INTERVENTION/EVALUATION:

Be alert for superinfection (e.g., genital/anal pruritus, ulceration or changes in oral mucosa, moderate to severe diarrhea, new or increased fever). Provide symptomatic relief for nausea. Evaluate change in taste sensation.

PATIENT/FAMILY TEACHING:

Do not take antacids 2 hrs before or after taking medication (reduces/destroys effectiveness). Avoid excessive sunlight/artificial ultraviolet light (reaction may occur up to several wks after stopping therapy). Continue medication for full length of treatment. Sugarless gum, hard candy may relieve bad taste.

spironolactone

spear-own-oh-**lak**-tone
(Aldactone, Novospiroton✦)

FIXED-COMBINATION(S)

With hydrochlorothiazide, a thiazide diuretic **(Aldactazide, Spironazide)**

▶CLASSIFICATION

PHARMACOTHERAPEUTIC: Aldosterone antagonist. ***CLINICAL:*** Potassium-sparing diuretic, antihypertensive, antihypokalemic (see p. 84C)

ACTION/*THERAPEUTIC EFFECT*

Competitively inhibits action of aldosterone. Interferes with sodium reabsorption in distal tubule, *increasing potassium retention while promoting sodium and water excretion.*

PHARMACOKINETICS

Onset	Peak	Duration
PO		
24–48 hrs	48–72 hrs	48–72 hrs

Well absorbed from GI tract (increased with food). Protein binding: 91–98%. Metabolized in liver to active metabolite. Primarily excreted in urine. Unknown if removed by hemodialysis. Half-life: 0–24 hrs.

USES/*UNLABELED*

Treatment of excessive aldosterone production, essential hypertension, edema due to CHF, CHF, cirrhosis of liver/nephrotic syndrome. Adjunct to potassium-losing diuretics or to potentiate action of other diuretics. Diagnosis of hyperaldosteronism. *Treatment of polycystic ovary syndrome, female hirsutism.*

PRECAUTIONS

CONTRAINDICATIONS: Acute renal insufficiency/impairment, anuria, BUN/creatinine over twice normal values levels, hyperkalemia. ***CAUTIONS:*** Hepatic/renal impairment.

▷***LIFESPAN CONSIDERATIONS:***
Pregnancy/Lactation: Active metabolite excreted in breast milk; nursing not advised. **Pregnancy Category D. Children:** No age-related precautions noted. **Elderly:** May be more susceptible to develop hyperkalemia. Age-related renal impairment may require cautious use.

INTERACTIONS

DRUG: May decrease effect of **anticoagulants, heparin. NSAIDs** may decrease antihypertensive effect. **ACE inhibitors (e.g., captopril), potassium-containing medications, potassium supplements** may increase potassium. May decrease **lithium** clearance, increase toxicity. May increase **digoxin** half-life. ***HERBAL:*** None known. ***FOOD:*** None known. ***LAB VALUES:*** May increase BUN, calcium excretion, creatinine, glucose, magnesium, potassium, uric acid. May decrease sodium.

AVAILABILITY (Rx)

TABLETS: 25 mg, 50 mg, 100 mg.

ADMINISTRATION/HANDLING
PO:

• Oral suspension containing crushed tablets in cherry syrup is stable for up to 30 days if refrigerated. • Drug absorption enhanced if taken with food. • Scored tablets may be crushed. • Do not crush or break film-coated tablets.

INDICATIONS/ROUTES/DOSAGE
Diuretic, hypertension:

PO: **Adults, elderly:** 25–200 mg/day in 1–2 divided doses. **Children:** 1.5–3.3 mg/kg/day in divided doses q6–12h. **Neonates (*Diuretic):*** 1–3 mg/kg/day q12–24h.

CHF:

PO: **Adults, elderly:** 25 mg/day

Diagnosis of primary aldosteronism:

PO: **Adults, elderly:** 100–400 mg/day in 1–2 divided doses. **Children:** 100–400 mg/m^2/day in 1–2 divided doses.

SIDE EFFECTS

FREQUENT: Hyperkalemia for those on potassium supplements or those with renal insufficiency; dehydration, hyponatremia, lethargy. ***OCCASIONAL:*** Nausea, vomiting, anorexia, cramping, diarrhea, headache, ataxia, drowsiness, confusion, fever. ***Male:*** Gynecomastia, impotence, decreased libido. ***Female:*** Menstrual irregularities/amenorrhea, postmenopausal bleeding, breast tenderness. ***RARE:*** Rash, urticaria, hirsutism.

ADVERSE REACTIONS/TOXIC EFFECTS

Severe hyperkalemia may produce arrhythmias, bradycardia, tented T waves, widening QRS, ST depression. These can proceed to cardiac standstill or ventricular fibrillation. Cirrhosis pts at risk for hepatic decompensation if dehydration/hyponatremia occurs. Those with primary aldosteronism may experience rapid weight loss, severe fatigue during high-dose therapy.

NURSING IMPLICATIONS

BASELINE ASSESSMENT:

Weigh pt; initiate strict I&O. Evaluate hydration status by assessing mucous membranes, skin turgor. Obtain baseline electrolytes, renal/hepatic functions, urinalysis. Assess for edema; note location and extent. Check baseline vital signs, note pulse rate/regularity.

INTERVENTION/EVALUATION:

Monitor electrolyte values, esp. for increased potassium. Monitor B/P levels. Monitor for hyponatremia: mental confusion, thirst, cold/clammy skin, drowsiness, dry mouth. Monitor for hyperkalemia: colic, diarrhea, muscle twitching followed by weakness/paralysis, arrhythmias. Obtain daily weight. Note changes in edema, skin turgor.

PATIENT/FAMILY TEACHING:

Expect increase in volume, frequency of urination. Therapeutic effect takes several days to begin and can last for several days when drug is discontinued. This may not apply if pt is on a potassium-losing drug concomitantly (diet and use of supplements should be established by physician). Notify physician for irregular/slow pulse, electrolyte imbalance (signs noted above). Avoid foods high in potassium such as whole grains (cereals), legumes, meat, bananas, apricots, orange juice, potatoes (white, sweet), raisins.

stavudine (d4T)

stay-view-deen
(Zerit)

▶**CLASSIFICATION**

PHARMACOTHERAPEUTIC: Nucleoside reverse transcriptase inhibitor. ***CLINICAL:*** Antiviral (see pp. 59C, 95C)

ACTION/*THERAPEUTIC EFFECT*

Inhibits HIV reverse transcriptase via viral DNA chain termination. Also inhibits RNA- and DNA-dependent DNA polymerase, an enzyme necessary for viral HIV replication, *slowing HIV replication, reducing progression of HIV infection.*

PHARMACOKINETICS

Rapidly, completely absorbed following PO administration. Equally distributed into extravascular spaces. Undergoes minimal metabolism. Excreted in urine. Half-life: 1.5 hrs (half-life increased with impaired renal function).

USES

Treatment of adults with advanced HIV infection who are intolerant or have experienced deterioration with other drug therapy. First-line component in treatment of HIV.

PRECAUTIONS

CONTRAINDICATIONS: None significant. ***CAUTIONS:*** History of peripheral neuropathy.

▷***LIFESPAN CONSIDERATIONS:*** **Pregnancy/Lactation:** Breast feeding not recommended (possibility of HIV transmission). **Pregnancy Category C. Children:** No age-related precautions noted. **Elderly:** Information not available.

INTERACTIONS

DRUG: None significant. **HERBAL:** None known. **FOOD:** None known. **LAB VALUES:** Commonly increases SGOT (AST), SGPT (ALT). May decrease neutrophil count.

AVAILABILITY (Rx)

CAPSULES: 15 mg, 20 mg, 30 mg, 40 mg. **ORAL SOLUTION:** 1 mg/ml.

ADMINISTRATION/HANDLING
PO:

• Give without regard to meals.

INDICATIONS/ROUTES/DOSAGE
HIV infection:

PO: Adults >60 kg: 40 mg twice daily. **Adults <60 kg:** 30 mg twice daily. If peripheral neuropathy or elevated hepatic transaminases present, stop therapy. If symptoms resolve completely, resume treatment using following schedule: **Adults >60 kg:** 20 mg twice daily. **Adults <60 kg:** 15 mg twice daily. **Children >30 kg:** Same as adults; **<30 kg:** 2 mg/kg/day.

Dosage in renal impairment:

Dose and/or frequency is modified based on creatinine clearance, pt weight.

Creatinine Clearance	>60 kg	<60 kg
>50	40 mg q12h	30 mg q12h
26–50	20 mg q12h	15 mg q12h
10–25	20 mg q24h	15 mg q24h

SIDE EFFECTS

FREQUENT: Headache (55%), diarrhea (50%), chills/fever (38%), nausea/vomiting, myalgia (35%), rash (33%), asthenia [loss of strength, energy] (28%), insomnia, abdominal pain (26%), anxiety (22%), arthralgia (18%), back pain (20%), sweating (19%), malaise (17%), depression (14%). **OCCASIONAL:** Anorexia, weight loss, nervousness, dizziness, conjunctivitis, dyspepsia, dyspnea. **RARE:** Constipation, vasodilation, confusion, migraine, urticaria, abnormal vision.

ADVERSE REACTIONS/TOXIC EFFECTS

Peripheral neuropathy, characterized by numbness, tingling, or pain in hands or feet, occurs frequently (15–21%). Ulcerative stomatitis (erythema/ulcers of oral mucosa, glossitis, gingivitis), pneumonia, benign skin neoplasms occur occasionally. Pancreatitis occurs rarely.

NURSING IMPLICATIONS

BASELINE ASSESSMENT:

Obtain baseline laboratory testing, esp. liver function tests, before beginning stavudine therapy and at periodic intervals during therapy. Offer emotional support. Question pt for previous history of peripheral neuropathy.

INTERVENTION/EVALUATION:

Monitor for peripheral neuropathy (characterized by numbness, tingling, or pain in hands or feet). Symptoms resolve promptly if therapy is discontinued (symptoms may worsen temporarily after drug is withdrawn). If symptoms resolve completely, reduced dosage may be resumed. Assess for headache, nausea, skin rash. Monitor skin

S

for evidence of rash, signs of chills/fever. Determine pattern of bowel activity and stool consistency. Assess for muscle or joint aches, dizziness, sleep pattern. Assess eating pattern; monitor for weight loss. Check eyes for signs of conjunctivitis.

PATIENT/FAMILY TEACHING:

Continue therapy for full length of treatment. Doses should be evenly spaced. Do not take any medications, including OTC drugs, without consulting physician. Stavudine is not a cure for HIV infection, nor does it reduce risk of transmission to others. Pt may continue to experience illnesses, including opportunistic infections.

st. john's wort

Also known as amber, demon chaser, goatweed, hardhay, rosin rose, tipton weed.

▶ CLASSIFICATION
HERBAL

ACTION/EFFECT

Inhibits COMT (catechol-O-methyl transferase) and MAO (monoamine oxidase); modulates effects of serotonin by inhibiting serotonin reuptake and 5-HT3 and 5-HT4 antagonism, *producing antidepressant effect.*

USES

Treatment of depression, including secondary effects of depression (fatigue, loss of appetite, anxiety, nervousness, insomnia).

PRECAUTIONS

CONTRAINDICATIONS: Pregnancy, breast-feeding (may cause increased muscle tone of uterus; infants may experience colic, drowsiness, lethargy. *CAUTIONS:* Bipolar disorder, schizophrenia.
▷ *LIFESPAN CONSIDERATIONS:* **Pregnancy/Lactation:** Contraindicated. **Children:** Safety and efficacy not established. Avoid use. **Elderly:** No age-related precautions noted.

INTERACTIONS

DRUG: **Antidepressants** may increase therapeutic effect. **Cyclosporine** may cause organ rejection. **Digoxin** may cause CHF exacerbation. **ACE inhibitors** may cause hypertension. May decrease concentration/effect of **indinavir**. *HERBAL:* **Ginseng, chamomile, goldenseal, kava kava, valerian** may increase therapeutic and adverse effects. *FOOD:* Large doses with **tyramine-containing food** may cause a hypertensive crisis. *LAB VALUES:* May increase INR/PT in pts treated with warfarin.

AVAILABILITY

CAPSULES: 150 mg, 300 mg, *LIQUID EXTRACT. TINCTURE.*

INDICATIONS/ROUTES/DOSAGE
Depression:

PO: **Adults, elderly:** 300 mg 3 times/day is the most common.

SIDE EFFECTS

Abdominal cramps, insomnia, vivid dreams, restlessness, anxiety, agitation, irritability, fatigue, dry mouth, headache, dizziness, photosensitivity, confusion.

ADVERSE REACTIONS/TOXIC EFFECTS

None significant.

NURSING IMPLICATIONS

BASELINE ASSESSMENT:
Assess if pt is pregnant or breast-feeding, has history of psychiatric disease. Determine medication usage (many potential interactions). Assess mental status: mood, memory, anxiety level.

INTERVENTION/EVALUATION:
Monitor changes in depressive state, behavior, and signs of side effects.

PATIENT/FAMILY TEACHING:
Do not abruptly discontinue (may increase adverse effects). Check with physician before taking any medications (many interactions). Avoid foods high in tyramine (e.g., aged cheese, pickled products, beer, and wine). Therapeutic effect may take 4- 6 wks. Avoid the sun or use sun screen or protective clothing (photosensitive).

streptokinase

strep-toe-**kine**-ace
(Kabikinase, Streptase)

▶CLASSIFICATION

PHARMACOTHERAPEUTIC:
Enzyme. ***CLINICAL:*** Thrombolytic (see p. 30C)

ACTION/THERAPEUTIC EFFECT

Activates fibrinolytic system by converting plasminogen to plasmin (enzyme that degrades fibrin clots). Acts indirectly by forming complex with plasminogen, which converts plasminogen to plasmin. Action occurs within thrombus, on its surface, and in circulating blood. *Resultant effect destroys thrombi.*

PHARMACOKINETICS

Rapidly cleared from plasma by antibodies, reticuloendothelial system. Route of elimination unknown. Duration of action continues for several hrs after discontinuing medication. Half-life: 23 min.

USES

Management of acute myocardial infarction (lyses thrombi obstructing coronary arteries, decreases infarct size, improves ventricular function after MI, decreases CHF, mortality associated with MI). Lysis of diagnosed pulmonary emboli, acute/extensive thrombi of deep veins, and acute arterial thrombi/emboli. Clears totally/partially occluded arteriovenous cannulae.

PRECAUTIONS

CONTRAINDICATIONS: Active internal bleeding, recent (within 2 mos) cerebrovascular accident, intracranial/intraspinal surgery, intracranial neoplasm, severe uncontrolled hypertension. ***CAUTIONS:*** Recent (10 days) major surgery/GI bleeding, obstetrical delivery, organ biopsy, trauma (cardiopulmonary resuscitation); uncontrolled arterial hypertension, left heart thrombus, endocarditis, severe hepatic/renal disease, pregnancy, elderly, cerebrovascular disease, diabetic retinopathy, thrombophlebitis, occluded AV cannula at infected site.

▷***LIFESPAN CONSIDERATIONS:***

S

Pregnancy/Lactation: Use only when benefit outweighs potential risk to fetus. Unknown if drug crosses placenta or is distributed in breast milk. **Pregnancy Category C. Children:** Safety and efficacy not established. **Elderly:** May have increased risk of intracranial hemorrhage; caution recommended.

INTERACTIONS

DRUG: **Anticoagulants, heparin** may increase risk of hemorrhage. **Platelet aggregation inhibitors (e.g., aspirin)** may increase risk of bleeding. *HERBAL:* None known. *FOOD:* None known. *LAB VALUES:* Decreases plasminogen and fibrinogen level during infusion, decreasing clotting time (confirms presence of lysis).

AVAILABILITY (Rx)

POWDER FOR INJECTION: 250,000 IU, 600,000 IU, 750,000 IU, 1.5 million IU.

ADMINISTRATION/HANDLING

Note: Must be administered within 12–14 hrs of clot formation (little effect on older, organized clots).

IV 🔟

Storage:

• Store vials at room temperature. • Reconstitute vials immediately before use. Slight flocculation may occur; does not affect safe use of the drug. Discard solution that has large amount of flocculation. • Solution for IV push may be used within 8 hrs of reconstitution. • Discard unused portion.

Reconstitution:

ARTERIOVENOUS CANNULA OCCLUSION:

• Dilute 250,000 IU vial with 2 ml 0.9% NaCl. Add diluent slowly to side of vial, roll and tilt to avoid foaming. Do not shake vial.

USES OTHER THAN CANNULA OCCLUSION:

• Reconstitute vial with 5 ml D$_5$W or 0.9% NaCl (preferred). Add diluent slowly to side of vial, roll and tilt to avoid foaming. Do not shake vial. • May further dilute with 50–500 ml in 45 ml increments of D$_5$W or 0.9% NaCl.

Rate of administration:

ARTERIOVENOUS CANNULA OCCLUSION:

• Give IV push slowly into each occluded limb of cannula. • Clamp for 2 hrs, then aspirate contents, flush with 0.9% NaCl.

IV INJECTION FOR CORONARY ARTERY THROMBI:

• Give 1.5 million IU over 60 min.

CORONARY ARTERY THROMBI:

• Give bolus dose over 25–30 sec usiong coronary catheter. Follow with 2,000 IU/min for 60 min.

DVT, PULMONARY ARTERIAL EMBOLISM ARTERIAL THROMBI:

• Give single dose over 25–30 min. Follow with maintenance dose of 100,00 or more every hr for 24–72 hrs. • Monitor B/P during infusion (hypotension may be severe, occurs in 1–10%). Decrease of infusion rate may be necessary. • If uncontrolled hemorrhage occurs, discontinue infusion immediately (slowing rate of infusion may produce worsening hemorrhage). Do not use dextran to control hemorrhage.

IV INCOMPATIBILITY ⊘

Do not mix with any other medications.

IV COMPATIBILITIES

Dobutamine (Dobutrex), dopamine (Intropin), heparin, lidocaine, nitroglycerin.

INDICATIONS/ROUTES/DOSAGE

Note: Do not use from 5 days to 6 mos of previous streptokinase treatment of streptococcal infection (pharyngitis, rheumatic fever, acute glomerulonephritis secondary to streptococcal infection).

Acute evolving transmural myocardial infarction (give as soon as possible after symptoms occur):

IV INFUSION: **Adults, elderly: (1.5 million units diluted to 45 ml):** 1.5 million IU infused over 60 min.

INTRACORONARY INFUSION: **Adults, elderly: (250,000 units diluted to 125 ml):** Initially, 20,000 IU (10 ml) bolus; then, 2,000 IU/min for 60 min. **Total dose:** 140,000 IU.

Pulmonary embolism, deep vein thrombosis, arterial thrombosis/embolism (give within 7 days after onset):

IV INFUSION: **Adults, elderly: (1.5 million units diluted to 90 ml):** Initially, 250,000 IU infused over 30 min; then, 100,000 IU/hr for 24–72 hrs for arterial thrombosis/embolism, 24–72 hrs for pulmonary embolism, 72 hrs for deep vein thrombosis.

INTRACORONARY INFUSION: **Adults, elderly: (1.5 million units diluted to 45 ml):** Initially, 250,000 IU infused over 30 min; then, 100,000 IU/hr for maintenance.

SIDE EFFECTS

FREQUENT: Fever, superficial bleeding at puncture sites, de-creased B/P. *OCCASIONAL:* Allergic reaction (rash, wheezing), bruising.

ADVERSE REACTIONS/TOXIC EFFECTS

Severe internal hemorrhage may occur. Lysis of coronary thrombi may produce atrial/ventricular arrhythmias.

NURSING IMPLICATIONS

BASELINE ASSESSMENT:

Assess hematocrit, platelet count, thrombin (TT), activated thromboplastin (APTT), prothrombin (PT) time, fibrinogen level, before therapy is instituted. If heparin is component of treatment, discontinue before streptokinase is instituted (TT/APTT should be less than twice normal value before institution of therapy).

INTERVENTION/EVALUATION:

Assess clinical response, vital signs q4h or per protocol. Handle pt carefully and as infrequently as possible to prevent bleeding. Do not obtain B/P in lower extremities (possible deep vein thrombi). Monitor TT, PT, APTT, fibrinogen level q4h after initiation of therapy. Check stool for occult blood. Assess for decrease in B/P, increase in pulse rate, complaint of abdominal/back pain, severe headache (may be evidence of hemorrhage). Question for increase in amount of discharge during menses. Assess area of thromboembolus for color, temperature. Assess peripheral pulses, skin for bruises and petechiae. Check for excessive bleeding from minor cuts, scratches. Assess urine output for hematuria.

S

streptomycin sulfate

(Streptomycin)

See Classification section under: Antibiotics: Aminoglycosides (p. 17C)

streptozocin

strep-toe-**zoe**-sin
(Zanosar)

▶**CLASSIFICATION**

PHARMACOTHERAPEUTIC: Nitrosurea. *CLINICAL:* Antineoplastic (see p. 74C)

ACTION/*THERAPEUTIC EFFECT*

Inhibits DNA synthesis with significantly affecting RNA or protein synthesis by cross-linking strands of DNA, *promoting cell death.* Cell cycle-phase nonspecific.

PHARMACOKINETICS

Rapidly distributed primarily in liver, kidneys, intestine, pancreas. Metabolized in liver. Primarily excreted in urine. Half-life: 35 min; metabolite: 40 min.

USES/*UNLABELED*

Treatment of metastatic islet cell carcinoma of pancreas. *Treatment of carcinoid tumor.*

PRECAUTIONS

CONTRAINDICATIONS: None significant. *EXTREME CAUTION:* Impaired renal function. *CAUTIONS:* Impaired hepatic function.
▷*LIFESPAN CONSIDERATIONS:*
Pregnancy/Lactation: If possible, avoid use during pregnancy, esp.

first trimester. Unknown whether distributed in breast milk. Breast feeding not recommended. **Pregnancy Category C. Children:** Safety and efficacy not established. **Elderly:** Age-related renal impairment may require caution.

INTERACTIONS

DRUG: **Nephrotoxic medications** may increase nephrotoxicity. May decrease effects of **phenytoin. Live virus vaccines** may potentiate virus replication, increase vaccine side effects, decrease pt's antibody response to vaccine. *HERBAL:* None known. *FOOD:* None known. *LAB VALUES:* May increase SGOT (AST), SGPT (ALT), alkaline phosphatase, bilirubin, LDH, BUN, creatinine, urinary protein. May decrease albumin, phosphate concentrations.

AVAILABILITY (Rx)
POWDER FOR INJECTION: 1 g.

ADMINISTRATION/HANDLING

Note: May give by IV injection or infusion. Wear gloves when preparing solution (topical contact may be carcinogenic hazard). If powder or solution comes in contact with skin, wash immediately, thoroughly with soap, water. May be carcinogenic, mutagenic, or teratogenic. Handle with extreme care during preparation/administration.

IV ⚕

Storage:

• Refrigerate unopened vials. • Solution appears clear to pale gold. Discard if color changes to dark brown (indicates decomposition). • Discard solution within 12 hrs after reconstitution.

Reconstitution:

• Reconstitute 1 g vial with 9.5 ml D_5W or 0.9% NaCl to provide concentration of 100 mg/ml. • For IV infusion, further dilute with 10–200 ml D_5W or 0.9% NaCl solution.

Rate of administration:

• For IV push, administer over 10–15 min. • Infuse piggyback over 15 min–6 hrs. • Extravasation may produce severe tissue necrosis. Apply warm compresses to reduce severity of irritation at IV site.

IV INCOMPATIBILITIES ⊘

Allopurinol (Aloprim), aztreonam (Azactam), cefepime (Maxipime), piperacillin/tazobactam (Zosyn).

IV COMPATIBILITIES

Granisetron (Kytril), ondansetron (Zofran).

INDICATIONS/ROUTES/DOSAGE

Note: Dosage individualized based on clinical response, tolerance to adverse effects. When used in combination therapy, consult specific protocols for optimum dosage, sequence of drug administration. Dosage based on body surface area (BSA).

Daily:

IV: **Adults, elderly:** 500 mg/m² of BSA for 5 consecutive days q6wks.

Weekly:

IV: **Adults, elderly:** Initially, 1 g/m² BSA weekly for 2 wks. May increase up to 1.5 g/m² BSA.

SIDE EFFECTS

FREQUENT (>90%): Severe nausea, vomiting (usually begins 1–4 hrs after administration; may persist over 24 hrs). *OCCASIONAL:* A burning sensation originating at IV site and moving up arm (occurs particularly with rapid IV injection), diarrhea, confusion, lethargy, depression, particularly in those

receiving continuous IV infusion over 5 days.

ADVERSE REACTIONS/TOXIC EFFECTS

High incidence of nephrotoxicity manifested by azotemia, anuria, proteinuria, hyperchloremia, hypophosphatemia. Proximal renal tubular acidosis evidenced by glycosuria, acetonuria, aminoaciduria. Mild to moderate bone marrow depression manifested as hematologic toxicity (leukopenia, thrombocytopenia, anemia). Severe myelosuppression, hepatotoxicity occur rarely.

NURSING IMPLICATIONS

BASELINE ASSESSMENT:

Phenothiazine antiemetics is only minimally effective in preventing/reducing nausea, vomiting; droperidol, metoclopramide appear to be more effective. Obtain renal function tests, electrolytes, CBC before and weekly during therapy. Obtain hepatic function tests before therapy.

INTERVENTION/EVALUATION:

Monitor urinalysis, creatinine clearance, BUN, serum creatinine, electrolyte, CBC. (Earliest sign of renal toxicity is mild proteinuria, glycosuria.) Inform physician if urine is positive for proteinuria or if vomiting exceeds 600–800 ml/8 hrs. Monitor for hematologic toxicity (fever, sore throat, signs of local infection, easy bruising, unusual bleeding from any site), symptoms of anemia (excessive tiredness, weakness).

PATIENT/FAMILY TEACHING:

Do not have immunizations without physician's approval (drug

S

lowers body's resistance). Avoid contact with those who have recently received live virus vaccine. Promptly report fever, sore throat, signs of local infection, easy bruising/unusual bleeding from any site. Increase fluid intake (decreases risk of nephrotoxicity).

succinylcholine chloride

(Anectine, Quelicin)

See Classification section under: Neuromuscular blockers (p. 103C)

sucralfate

sue-**kral**-fate
(Carafate, Novo-Sucralate✿, Sulcrate✿)
Do not confuse with Cafergot.

▶**CLASSIFICATION**

CLINICAL: Antiulcer

ACTION/*THERAPEUTIC EFFECT*

Forms adhesive gel that adheres to ulcer site. *Gel protects damaged mucosa from further destruction by absorbing gastric acid, pepsin, bile salts* and reacting with exudation of proteins.

PHARMACOKINETICS

Minimally absorbed from GI tract. Eliminated in feces with small amount excreted in urine. Not removed by hemodialysis.

USES/*UNLABELED*

Short-term treatment (up to 8 wks) of duodenal ulcer. Maintenance therapy of duodenal ulcer after healing of acute ulcers. *Treatment of gastric ulcer, rheumatoid arthritis (relieves GI symptoms associated with NSAIDs), prevents/treatment of stress-related mucosal damage esp. ICU pts, treatment of gastroesophageal reflux.*

PRECAUTIONS

CONTRAINDICATIONS: None significant. *CAUTIONS:* None significant.
▷*LIFESPAN CONSIDERATIONS:*
Pregnancy/Lactation: Unknown if drug crosses placenta or is distributed in breast milk. **Pregnancy Category B. Children:** Safety and efficacy not established. **Elderly:** No age-related precautions noted.

INTERACTIONS

DRUG: **Antacids** may interfere with binding (do not give within half hr). May decrease absorption of **digoxin, phenytoin, quinolones (e.g., ciprofloxacin), theophylline** (do not give within 2–3 hrs of sucralfate). *HERBAL:* None known. *FOOD:* None known. *LAB VALUES:* None significant.

AVAILABILITY (Rx)

TABLETS: 1 g. *ORAL SUSPENSION:* 500 mg/5 ml.

ADMINISTRATION/HANDLING

PO:

• Administer 1 hr before meals and at bedtime. • Tablets may be crushed/dissolved in water. • Avoid antacids 1/2 hr before or after giving sucralfate.

INDICATIONS/ROUTES/DOSAGE

Note: 1 g = 10 ml suspension.

Duodenal ulcers, active:

PO: Adults, elderly: 1 g 4 times/day (before meals and at bedtime) for up to 8 wks.

Duodenal ulcers, maintenance:
PO: Adults, elderly: 1 g 2 times/day.

SIDE EFFECTS
FREQUENT (2%): Constipation.
OCCASIONAL (<2%): Dry mouth, backache, diarrhea, dizziness, drowsiness, nausea, indigestion, skin rash/hives/itching, stomach discomfort.

ADVERSE REACTIONS/TOXIC EFFECTS
None significant.

NURSING IMPLICATIONS

INTERVENTION/EVALUATION:
Monitor stool consistency and frequency.

PATIENT/FAMILY TEACHING:
Take medication on an empty stomach. Antacids may be given as an adjunct but should not be taken for 30 min before or after sucralfate (formation of sucralfate gel is activated by stomach acid). Dry mouth may be relieved by sour hard candy or sips of tepid water.

sufentanil citrate

(Sufenta)

See Classification section under: Opioid analgesics

sulconazole nitrate

(Exelderm)

See Classification section under: Antifungals: topical

sulfacetamide sodium ✳

sul-fah-**see**-tah-mide
(AK-Sulf, Bleph-10, Cetamide✤, Diosulf✤, Isopto Cetamide, Ophthacet, Sodium Sulamyd, Sulfair)

FIXED-COMBINATION(S)

With phenylephrine hydrochloride, a sympathomimetic **(Vasosulf);** with prednisolone, a steroid **(Blephamide, Cetapred, Metimyd, Optimyd, Sulphrin, Vasocidin)**

▶CLASSIFICATION

PHARMACOTHERAPEUTIC: Sulfonamide. **CLINICAL:** Ophthalmic, topical agent

ACTION/*THERAPEUTIC EFFECT*
Interferes with synthesis of folic acid that bacteria require for growth, *preventing further bacterial growth.* Bacteriostatic.

USES/*UNLABELED*
Treatment of corneal ulcers, conjunctivitis and other superficial infections of the eye, prophylaxis after injuries to the eye/removal of foreign bodies, adjunctive therapy for trachoma and inclusion conjunctivitis. **Topical lotion:** Seborrheic dermatitis, seborrheic sicca (dandruff), secondary bacterial skin infections. **Ophthalmic:** *Treatment of bacterial blepharitis, blepharoconjunctivitis, bacterial keratitis, keratoconjunctivitis.*

PRECAUTIONS
CONTRAINDICATIONS: Hypersensitivity to sulfonamides or any component of preparation (some

S

products contain sulfite). **CAUTIONS:** Extremely dry eye. Application of lotion to large infected, denuded, or debrided areas.

INTERACTIONS

DRUG: Silver-containing preparations. **HERBAL:** None known. **FOOD:** None known. **LAB VALUES:** None significant.

AVAILABILITY (Rx)

OPHTHALMIC OINTMENT: 10%.
OPHTHALMIC SOLUTION: 10%, 15%, 30%.

INDICATIONS/ROUTES/DOSAGE

Usual ophthalmic dosage:

OPHTHALMIC: Adults, elderly, children >2 mos: OINTMENT: Apply small amount in lower conjunctival sac 1–4 times/day and at bedtime. **SOLUTION:** 1–3 drops to lower conjunctival sac q2–3h.

SIDE EFFECTS

FREQUENT: Transient ophthalmic burning, stinging. **OCCASIONAL:** Headache. **RARE:** Hypersensitivity: erythema, rash, itching, swelling, photosensitivity.

ADVERSE REACTIONS/TOXIC EFFECTS

Superinfection, drug-induced lupus erythematosus, Stevens-Johnson syndrome occur rarely; nephrotoxicity with high dermatologic concentrations.

NURSING IMPLICATIONS

BASELINE ASSESSMENT:

Question for hypersensitivity to sulfonamides, any ingredients of preparation (e.g., sulfite).

INTERVENTION/EVALUATION:

Withhold medication and notify physician at once of hypersensitivity reaction (redness, itching, urticaria, rash). Assess for fever, joint pain, or sores in mouth—hold drug, inform physician.

PATIENT/FAMILY TEACHING:

May have transient burning, stinging upon ophthalmic application; may cause sensitivity to light; wear sunglasses, avoid bright light. Notify physician of *any* new symptom, esp. swelling, itching, rash, joint pain, fever. For topical skin/scalp treatment, cleanse (shampoo) area before application to ensure direct contact with affected area.

sulfasalazine

sul-fah-**sal**-ah-zeen
(Azulfidine, Azulfidine EN-tabs, Salazopyrin✦, SAS-500✦)
Do not confuse with azathioprine, sulfadiazine, sulfisoxazole.

▶CLASSIFICATION

PHARMACOTHERAPEUTIC: Sulfonamide. **CLINICAL:** Anti-inflammatory

ACTION/THERAPEUTIC EFFECT

Blocks prostaglandin synthesis, *producing anti-inflammatory and antibacterial effect.*

PHARMACOKINETICS

Poorly absorbed from GI tract. Cleaved in colon by intestinal bacterial forming sulfapyridine and mesalamine (5-ASA). Absorbed in colon. Widely distributed. Metabolized in liver. Primarily excreted in urine. Half-life: sulfapyridine: 6–14 hrs; 5-ASA: 0.6–1.4 hrs.

USES/*UNLABELED*

Treatment of ulcerative colitis, inflammatory bowel disease, rheumatoid arthritis. *Treatment of ankylosing spondylitis.*

PRECAUTIONS

CONTRAINDICATIONS: Hypersensitivity to salicylates, sulfonamides, sulfonylureas, thiazide or loop diuretics, carbonic anhydrase inhibitors, sunscreens containing PABA, local anesthetics, pregnancy at term, severe hepatic/renal dysfunction, porphyria, intestinal/urinary tract obstruction, children <2 yrs. ***CAUTIONS:*** Severe allergies, bronchial asthma, impaired hepatic/renal function, G-6-PD deficiency.

▷*LIFESPAN CONSIDERATIONS:* **Pregnancy/Lactation:** May produce infertility, oligospermia in men while on medication. Readily crosses placenta; if given near term, may produce jaundice, hemolytic anemia, kernicterus. Excreted in breast milk. Do not nurse premature infant or those with hyperbilirubinemia or G-6-PD deficiency. **Pregnancy Category B** (Category D if given near term). **Children/Elderly:** No age-related precautions noted in those >2 yrs of age.

INTERACTIONS

DRUG: May increase effects of **oral anticoagulants, anticonvulsants, oral hypoglycemics, methotrexate. Hemolytics** may increase toxicity. **Hepatotoxic medications** may increase hepatotoxicity. ***HERBAL:*** None known. ***FOOD:*** None known. ***LAB VALUES:*** None significant.

AVAILABILITY (Rx)

TABLETS: 500 mg. ***ORAL SUSPENSION:*** 250 mg/5 ml.

ADMINISTRATION/HANDLING
PO:
• Space doses evenly (intervals not to exceed 8 hrs). • Administer after meals if possible (prolong intestinal passage). • Swallow enteric-coated tablets whole; do not chew. • Give with 8 oz water; encourage several glasses of water between meals.

INDICATIONS/ROUTES/DOSAGE
Ulcerative colitis:

PO: **Adults, elderly:** *(Treatment):* 1 g 3–4 times/day in divided doses q4–6h. **Maximum:** 6 g/day. *(Maintenance):* 2 g/day in divided doses q6–12h. **Children:** *(Treatment):* 40–75 mg/kg/day in divided doses q4–6h. **Maximum:** 6 g/day. *(Maintenance):* 30–50 mg/kg/day in divided doses q4–8h. **Maximum:** 2 g/day.

Rheumatoid arthritis:

PO: **Adults, elderly:** Initially, 0.5–1 g/day for 1 wk. Increase by 0.5 g/wk, up to 3 g/day.

Juvenile rheumatoid arthritis:

PO: **Children:** Initially, 10 mg/kg/day. May increase by 10 mg/kg/day at weekly intervals. **Range:** 30–50 mg/kg/day. **Maximum:** 2 g/day.

SIDE EFFECTS

FREQUENT (33%): Anorexia, nausea, vomiting, headache, oligospermia (generally reversed by withdrawal of drug). ***OCCASIONAL*** (3%): Hypersensitivity reaction: rash, urticaria, pruritus, fever, anemia. ***RARE*** (<1%): Tinnitus, hypoglycemia, diuresis, photosensitivity.

ADVERSE REACTIONS/TOXIC EFFECTS

Anaphylaxis, Stevens-Johnson syndrome, hematologic toxicity (leukopenia, agranulocytosis); hepatotoxicity, nephrotoxicity occur rarely.

NURSING IMPLICATIONS

BASELINE ASSESSMENT:

Question for hypersensitivity to medications (see Contraindications). Check initial urinalysis, CBC, hepatic and renal function tests.

INTERVENTION/EVALUATION:

Check I&O, urinalysis, renal function tests; assure adequate hydration (minimum output 1,500 ml/24 hr) to prevent nephrotoxicity. Assess skin for rash (discontinue drug/notify physician at first sign). Check pattern of bowel activity, stool consistency (dosage may need to be increased if diarrhea continues/recurs). Monitor CBC closely; assess for/report immediately hematologic effects: bleeding, bruising, fever, sore throat, pallor, weakness, purpura, jaundice.

PATIENT/FAMILY TEACHING:

May cause orange-yellow discoloration of urine, skin. Space doses evenly around the clock. Take after food with 8 oz water; drink several glasses of water between meals. Continue for full length of treatment; may be necessary to take drug even after symptoms relieved. Follow-up, lab tests are essential. In event of dental/other surgery inform dentist/surgeon of sulfasalazine therapy. Avoid exposure to sun/ultraviolet light until photosensitivity determined (may last for months after last dose).

sulindac

suel-**in**-dak
(Apo-Sulin✹, Clinoril, Novo Sundac✹)
Do not confuse with Clozaril.

▶CLASSIFICATION

PHARMACOTHERAPEUTIC: Nonsteroidal anti-inflammatory. **CLINICAL:** Anti-inflammatory, antigout (see p. 107C)

ACTION/THERAPEUTIC EFFECT

Produces analgesic and anti-inflammatory effect by inhibiting prostaglandin synthesis, *reducing inflammatory response and intensity of pain stimulus reaching sensory nerve endings.*

PHARMACOKINETICS

Onset	Peak	Duration
PO (antirheumatic)		
7 days	2–3wks	—

Well absorbed from GI tract. Metabolized in liver to active metabolite. Primarily excreted in urine. Not removed by hemodialysis. Half-life: 7.8 hrs; metabolite: 16.4 hrs.

USES

Treatment of pain of rheumatoid arthritis, osteoarthritis, ankylosing spondylitis, acute painful shoulder, bursitis/tendinitis, acute gouty arthritis.

PRECAUTIONS

CONTRAINDICATIONS: Active peptic ulcer, GI ulceration, chronic inflammation of GI tract, GI bleeding disorders, history of hypersensitivity to aspirin/NSAIDs. **CAU-**

TIONS: Impaired renal/hepatic function, history of GI tract disease, predisposition to fluid retention.

▷*LIFESPAN CONSIDERATIONS:*
Pregnancy/Lactation: Unknown if drug is excreted in breast milk. Avoid use during third trimester (may adversely affect fetal cardiovascular system: premature closure of ductus arteriosus). **Pregnancy Category B** (Category D if used in third trimester or near delivery). **Children:** Safety and efficacy not established. **Elderly:** GI bleeding or ulceration more likely to cause serious adverse effects. Age-related renal impairment may increase risk of liver or renal toxicity; lower dosage recommended.

INTERACTIONS

DRUG: May increase effects of **oral anticoagulants, heparin, thrombolytics.** May decrease effect of **antihypertensives, diuretics. Salicylates, aspirin** may increase risk of GI side effects, bleeding. **Bone marrow depressants** may increase risk of hematologic reactions. May increase concentration, toxicity of **lithium.** May increase **methotrexate** toxicity. **Probenecid** may increase concentration. **Antacids** may decrease concentration. **HERBAL: Ginkgo biloba** may increase risk of bleeding. May reduce effects of **feverfew. FOOD:** None known. **LAB VALUES:** May increase alkaline phosphatase, liver function tests.

AVAILABILITY (Rx)
TABLETS: 150 mg, 200 mg.

ADMINISTRATION/HANDLING
PO:
• Give with food, milk, or antacids if GI distress occurs.

INDICATIONS/ROUTES/DOSAGE
Rheumatoid arthritis, osteoarthritis, ankylosing spondylitis:

PO: Adults, elderly: Initially, 150 mg 2 times/day, up to 400 mg/day.

Acute painful shoulder, gouty arthritis, bursitis, tendinitis:

PO: Adults, elderly: 200 mg 2 times/day.

SIDE EFFECTS

FREQUENT (3–9%): Diarrhea/constipation, indigestion, nausea, maculopapular rash, dermatitis, dizziness, headache. **OCCASIONAL** (1–3%): Anorexia, GI cramps, flatulence.

ADVERSE REACTIONS/TOXIC EFFECTS

GI bleeding, peptic ulcer occur infrequently. Nephrotoxicity (glomerular nephritis, interstitial nephritis, and nephrotic syndrome) may occur in those with preexisting impaired renal function. Acute hypersensitivity reaction (fever, chills, joint pain) occurs rarely.

NURSING IMPLICATIONS

BASELINE ASSESSMENT:

Assess onset, type, location, and duration of pain, fever, or inflammation. Inspect appearance of affected joints for immobility, deformities, and skin condition.

INTERVENTION/EVALUATION:

Assist with ambulation if dizziness occurs. Monitor pattern of daily bowel activity, stool consistency. Assess for evidence of rash. Evaluate for therapeutic response: relief of pain, stiffness, swelling, increase in joint mobility, reduced joint tenderness, improved grip strength.

S

PATIENT/FAMILY TEACHING:
Therapeutic antiarthritic effect noted 1–3 wks after therapy begins. Avoid aspirin, alcohol during therapy (increases risk of GI bleeding). If GI upset occurs, take with food, milk.

sumatriptan succinate injection

sue-mah-**trip**-tan
(Imitrex)
Do not confuse with somatropin.

►**CLASSIFICATION**

PHARMACOTHERAPEUTIC:
Serotonin receptor agonist. **CLINICAL:** Antimigraine (see pp. 53C, 54C)

ACTION/THERAPEUTIC EFFECT

Binds selectively to vascular receptors producing a vasoconstrictive effect on cranial blood vessels, *producing relief of migraine headache.* Efficiency of relief unaffected by aura, duration of attack, concurrent use of other antimigraine medications (e.g., beta-blockers).

PHARMACOKINETICS

	Onset	Peak	Duration
SubQ	<10 min	<2 hrs	—
PO	1–1.5 hrs	2–4 hrs	—

Rapidly absorbed after SubQ administration. Widely distributed, protein binding (10–21%). Undergoes first-pass hepatic metabolism; excreted in urine. Half-life: 2 hrs.

USES

Acute treatment of migraine headache with or without aura; treatment of cluster headaches.

PRECAUTIONS

CONTRAINDICATIONS: IV use, those with ischemic heart disease (angina pectoris, history of myocardial infarction), silent ischemia, Prinzmetal's angina, uncontrolled hypertension, concurrent ergotamine-containing preparations, hemiplegic or basilar migraine. **CAUTIONS:** Hepatic, renal impairment. Pt profile suggesting cardiovascular risks.
▷**LIFESPAN CONSIDERATIONS:**
Pregnancy/Lactation: Unknown if distributed in breast milk. **Pregnancy Category C. Children:** Safety and efficacy not established. **Elderly:** No age-related precautions noted.

INTERACTIONS

DRUG: Ergotamine-containing drugs may produce vasospastic reaction. **Monoamine oxidase inhibitors** may increase concentration, half-life. **HERBAL:** None known. **FOOD:** None known. **LAB VALUES:** None significant.

AVAILABILITY (Rx)

TABLETS: 25 mg, 50 mg. **INJECTION:** 12 mg/ml. **NASAL SPRAY:** 5 mg, 20 mg.

ADMINISTRATION/HANDLING
PO:

• Swallow tablets whole. • Take with full glass of water.

Nasal:

• Unit contains only one spray—do not test before use. • Gently blow nose to clear nasal passages. • With head upright, close one nostril with index finger. Breathe out gently through mouth. • Insert nozzle into open nostril about ½ inch. Do not press blue plunger yet. • Close mouth and while taking a breath through nose, release spray dosage by firmly pressing the blue plunger. • Remove nozzle from nose and gently breathe in through nose and out through mouth for 10–20 sec. Do not breathe in deeply.

SubQ:

• Follow pt instructions provided by manufacturer using auto-injection device.

INDICATIONS/ROUTES/DOSAGE

Vascular headache:

SUBQ: **Adults, elderly:** 6 mg. **Maximum:** No more than two 6 mg injections within a 24 hr period separated by at least 1 hr between injections.

PO: **Adults, elderly:** 50 mg. **Maximum single dose:** 100 mg. May repeat no sooner than 2 hrs. **Maximum:** 200 mg/24 hrs.

NASAL: **Adults, elderly:** 5–20 mg; may repeat in 2 hrs. **Maximum:** 40 mg/24 hrs.

SIDE EFFECTS

FREQUENT: Oral (5–10%): Tingling, nasal discomfort. *SubQ* (>10%): Injection site reactions, tingling, warm, hot sensation, dizziness, vertigo. *Nasal* (>10%): Bad, unusual taste, nausea, vomiting. *OCCASIONAL: Oral* (1–5%): Flushing, weakness, visual disturbances. *SubQ* (2–10%): Burning sensation, numbness, chest discomfort, drowsiness, weakness. *Nasal* (1–5%): Discomfort of nasal cavity/throat, dizziness. *RARE: Oral* (<1%): Agitation, eye irritation, dysuria. *SubQ* (<2%): Anxiety, fatigue, sweating, muscle cramps, muscle pain. *Nasal* (<1%): Burning sensation.

ADVERSE REACTIONS/TOXIC EFFECTS

Excessive dosage may produce tremor, redness of extremities, reduced respirations, cyanosis, convulsions, paralysis. Serious arrhythmias occur rarely, but particularly in those with hypertension, obesity, smokers, diabetics, and those with strong family history of coronary artery disease.

NURSING IMPLICATIONS

BASELINE ASSESSMENT:

Question pt regarding history of peripheral vascular disease, renal/hepatic impairment, or possibility of pregnancy. Question pt regarding onset, location, and duration of migraine and possible precipitating symptoms.

INTERVENTION/EVALUATION:

Evaluate for relief of migraine headache and resulting photophobia, phonophobia (sound sensitivity), nausea and vomiting.

PATIENT/FAMILY TEACHING:

Teach pt proper loading of autoinjector, injection technique, and discarding of syringe. Do not use >2 injections during any 24 hr period and allow at least 1 hr between injections. If experience wheezing, heart throbbing, skin rash, swelling of eyelids/face/lips, pain/tightness in chest or throat, contact physician immediately.

S

---

tacrine hydrochloride

tay-crin
(Cognex)

▶CLASSIFICATION

PHARMACOTHERAPEUTIC:
Cholinesterase inhibitor. ***CLINI-CAL:*** Antidementia

ACTION/*THERAPEUTIC EFFECT*

Elevates acetylcholine concentrations in cerebral cortex by slowing degeneration of acetylcholine released by still intact cholinergic neurons (Alzheimer's disease involves degeneration of cholinergic neuronal pathways). *Resultant effect slows Alzheimer's disease process.*

USES

Symptomatic treatment of pts with Alzheimer's disease.

PRECAUTIONS

CONTRAINDICATIONS: Known hypersensitivity to cholinergics; current treatment with other cholinesterase inhibitors; severe, active liver disease; active, untreated gastric/duodenal ulcers; mechanical obstruction of intestine/urinary tract; pregnancy, nursing, or childbearing potential. ***CAUTIONS:*** Known liver dysfunction, asthma, COPD, seizure disorders, bradycardia, hyperthyroidism, cardiac arrhythmias, history of gastric/intestinal ulcers, alcohol abuse.

INTERACTIONS

DRUG: May increase **theophylline** concentration; **cimetidine** may increase tacrine concentrations; may interfere with **anticholinergics;** may increase adverse effects of **NSAIDs. *HERBAL:*** None known. ***FOOD:*** None known. ***LAB VALUES:*** Increases SGOT (AST), SGPT (ALT); alters hematocrit, hemoglobin, electrolytes.

AVAILABILITY (Rx)

CAPSULES: 10 mg, 20 mg, 30 mg, 40 mg.

ADMINISTRATION/HANDLING

PO:

• Give without regard to food.

INDICATIONS/ROUTES/DOSAGE

Alzheimer's disease:

***PO:* Adults, elderly:** Initially, 10 mg 4 times/day for 6 wks; then 20 mg 4 times/day for 6 wks; then 30 mg 4 times/day for 12 wks; then to maximum of 40 mg 4 times/day if needed.

Note: If medication is stopped for >14 days, must retitrate as noted above.

SIDE EFFECTS

FREQUENT (11–28%): Headache, nausea, vomiting, diarrhea, dizziness. ***OCCASIONAL*** (4–9%): Fatigue, chest pain, dyspepsia, anorexia, abdominal pain, flatulence, constipation, confusion, agitation, rash, depression, ataxia (muscular incoordination), insomnia, rhinitis, myalgia. ***RARE*** (<3%): Weight loss, anxiety, cough, facial flushing, urinary frequency, back pain, tremor.

ADVERSE REACTIONS/TOXIC EFFECTS

Overdose can cause cholinergic crises (increased salivation, lacrimation, urination, defecation, bradycardia, hypotension, increased muscle weakness). Treatment aimed at general supportive measures, use of anticholinergics (e.g., atropine).

NURSING IMPLICATIONS

BASELINE ASSESSMENT:

Assess cognitive, behavioral, and functional deficits of pt. Assess liver function.

INTERVENTION/EVALUATION:

Monitor cognitive, behavioral, and functional status of pt. Monitor SGOT (AST), SGPT (ALT). EKG evaluation, periodic rhythm strips in pts with underlying arrhythmias. Monitor for symptoms of ulcer, GI bleeding.

PATIENT/FAMILY TEACHING:

Take at regular intervals, between meals (may take with meals if GI upset occurs). Do not reduce or stop medication; do not increase dosage without physician direction. Do not smoke (reduces plasma concentration of tacrine). Inform family of local chapter of Alzheimer's Disease Association (provides a guide to services for these pts).

tacrolimus

tack-row-**lee**-mus
(Prograf, Protopic)

▶CLASSIFICATION

PHARMACOTHERAPEUTIC:
Immunologic agent. ***CLINICAL:***
Immunosuppressant

ACTION/*THERAPEUTIC EFFECT*

Binds to intracellular protein, forming a complex, inhibiting phosphatase activity. This effect results in inhibition of T-lymphocyte activation, suppressing immunologically mediated inflammatory response, assisting in prevention of liver transplant rejection.

PHARMACOKINETICS

Variably absorbed following oral administration (food reduces absorption). Protein binding: 75–97%. Extensively metabolized in the liver. Excreted in urine. Not removed by hemodialysis. Half-life: 11.7 hrs.

USES/*UNLABELED*

Prophylaxis of organ rejection in pts receiving allogeneic liver transplants, kidney transplants. Should be used concurrently with adrenal corticosteroids. ***Topical:*** Atopic dermatitis. *Bone marrow, cardiac, pancreas, pancreatic island cell, and small bowel transplantation. Treatment of autoimmune disease, severe recalcitrant psoriasis.*

PRECAUTIONS

CONTRAINDICATIONS: Hypersensitivity to tacrolimus, hypersensitivity to HCO-60 polyoxyl 60 hydrogenated castor oil (used in vehicle for injection), cyclosporine (increased risk of ototoxicity). ***CAUTIONS:*** Immunosuppressed pts, renal/hepatic function impairment.

▷***LIFESPAN CONSIDERATIONS:***
Pregnancy/Lactation: Crosses placenta. Neonatal hyperkalemia, renal dysfunction noted in neonates. Excreted in breast milk. Avoid nursing. **Pregnancy Category C. Children:** May require higher doses (decreased bioavailability, increased clearance). May make post-transplant lymphoproliferative disorder more common (esp. those <3 yrs of age). **Elderly:** Age-related renal impairment may require dosage adjustment.

T

INTERACTIONS

DRUG: **Aminoglycosides, amphotericin B, cisplatin** increase risk of renal dysfunction. **Cyclosporine** increases risk of nephrotoxicity. **Antifungals, bromocriptine, calcium channel blockers, cimetidine, clarithromycin, cyclosporine, danazol, diltiazem, erythromycin, methylprednisolone, metoclopramide** increase tacrolimus blood levels. **Carbamazepine, phenobarbital, phenytoin, rifamycins** decrease tacrolimus blood levels. Other immunosuppressants may increase risk of infection or development of lymphomas. **Live virus vaccines** may potentiate virus replication, increase vaccine side effects, decrease pt's antibody response to vaccine. **HERBAL: Echinacea** may decrease effects. **FOOD:** None known. **LAB VALUES:** May increase creatinine, BUN, WBCs, glucose. May decrease thrombocytes, RBCs, magnesium. Alters potassium level.

AVAILABILITY (Rx)

CAPSULES: 1 mg, 5 mg. **INJECTION:** 5 mg/ml. **OINTMENT:** 0.03%, 0.1%.

ADMINISTRATION/HANDLING

IV 🏥

Storage:

• Store diluted infusion solution in glass or polyethylene containers and discard after 24 hrs. • Do not store in a PVC container (decreased stability, potential for extraction).

Reconstitution:

• Dilute with an appropriate amount (between 250–1,000 ml, depending on desired dose) 0.9% NaCl or D_5W to provide a concentration between 0.004 and 0.02 mg/ml.

Rate of administration:

• Give as continuous IV infusion. • Continuously monitor pt for anaphylaxis for at least 30 min following start of infusion. • Stop infusion immediately at first sign of hypersensitivity reaction.

IV INCOMPATIBILITY ⊘

Do not mix with any other medications.

IV COMPATIBILITIES

Calcium gluconate, diphenhydramine (Benadryl), dobutamine (Dobutrex), dopamine (Intropin), furosemide (Lasix), heparin, lorazepam (Ativan), multivitamins, nitroglycerin, potassium chloride.

INDICATIONS/ROUTES/DOSAGE

Note: In pts unable to take capsules, initiate therapy with IV infusion. Give oral dose 8–12 hrs after discontinuing IV infusion. Titrate dosing based on clinical assessments of rejection and tolerability. In pts with hepatic/renal function impairment, give lowest IV and oral dosing range (delay dosing up to 48 hrs or longer in pts with postop oliguria).

Liver transplantation:

IV INFUSION: Adults, elderly: 0.05–0.1 mg/kg/day with initial dose given no sooner than 6 hrs after transplant. Give adult pts doses at lower end of dosing range. Give in combination with adrenal corticosteroids. Transfer to oral therapy when oral tolerance is apparent (usually occurs within 2–3 days).

PO: Adults: 0.15–0.3 mg/kg/day given in 2 divided daily doses q12h. Give initial dose no sooner than 6 hrs after transplant. Give in combination with adrenal corticosteroids.

Pediatric dosage (without preexisting renal or hepatic dysfunction):

IV INFUSION: 0.05–1.5 mg/kg/day.

PO: 0.3 mg/kg/day.

Atopic dermatitis:

TOPICAL: **Adults, elderly, children ≥2 yrs:** 0.03% ointment to affected area 2 times/day. Continue for 1 wk after symptoms have cleared.

SIDE EFFECTS

FREQUENT (>30%): Headache, tremor, insomnia, paresthesia, diarrhea, nausea, constipation, vomiting, abdominal pain, hypertension. *OCCASIONAL* (10–29%): Rash, pruritus, anorexia, asthenia, peripheral edema.

ADVERSE REACTIONS/TOXIC EFFECTS

Nephrotoxicity, pleural effusion occur frequently. Overt nephrotoxicity characterized by increasing serum creatinine, decrease in urine output. Thrombocytopenia, leukocytosis, anemia, atelectasis occur occasionally. Neurotoxicity, including tremor, headache, mental status changes, occur commonly. Sepsis, infection occur occasionally. Significant anemia, thrombocytopenia, leukocytosis may occur.

NURSING IMPLICATIONS

BASELINE ASSESSMENT:

Assess medical history, esp. renal function, drug history, esp. other immunosuppressants. Have aqueous solution of epinephrine 1:1,000 available at bedside as well as O_2 before beginning IV infusion. Assess pt continuously for first 30 min following start of infusion and at frequent intervals thereafter.

INTERVENTION/EVALUATION:

Closely monitor pts with impaired renal function. Monitor lab values, esp. serum creatinine, serum potassium levels. CBC with differential, hepatic function tests. Monitor I&O closely. CBC should be performed weekly during first mo of therapy, twice moly during second and third mos of treatment, then moly throughout the first yr. Report any major change in assessment of pt. Routinely watch for any change from normal.

PATIENT/FAMILY TEACHING:

Contact physician if unusual bleeding or bruising, sore throat, mouth sores, abdominal pain, or fever occurs.

tamoxifen citrate

tam-**ox**-ih-fen
(Apo-Tamox✢, Nolvadex, Nolvaldex-D✢, Novo-Tamoxifen✢, Tamofen✢, Tamone✢)

▶**CLASSIFICATION**

PHARMACOTHERAPEUTIC: Nonsteroidal antiestrogen. *CLINICAL:* Antineoplastic (see p. 74C)

ACTION/*THERAPEUTIC EFFECT*

Competes with estradiol for binding to estrogen in tissues containing high concentration of receptors (e.g., breasts, uterus, vagina).

Reduces DNA synthesis, estrogen response.

PHARMACOKINETICS

Well absorbed from GI tract. Metabolized in liver. Primarily eliminated in feces via biliary system. Half-life: 7 days.

USES

Treatment of metastatic breast carcinoma in women/men. Effective in delaying recurrence following total mastectomy and axillary dissection or segmental mastectomy, axillary dissection and breast irradiation in women with axillary node-negative breast carcinoma. Prevention of breast cancer in high-risk women.

PRECAUTIONS

CONTRAINDICATIONS: None significant. ***CAUTIONS:*** Leukopenia, thrombocytopenia, increased risk of uterine cancer.
▷***LIFESPAN CONSIDERATIONS:***
Pregnancy/Lactation: If possible, avoid use during pregnancy, esp. first trimester. May cause fetal harm. Unknown if distributed in breast milk. Breast feeding not recommended. **Pregnancy Category D. Children:** Not prescribed in this pt population. **Elderly:** No age-related precautions noted.

INTERACTIONS

DRUG: Estrogens may decrease effect. ***HERBAL:*** None known. ***FOOD:*** None known. ***LAB VALUES:*** May increase calcium, cholesterol, triglycerides.

AVAILABILITY (Rx)

TABLETS: 10 mg, 20 mg.

ADMINISTRATION/HANDLING

PO:
• Give without regard to food.

INDICATIONS/ROUTES/DOSAGE

Breast cancer:
***PO:* Adults, elderly:** 20–40 mg/day. Give doses >20 mg/day in divided doses.

Prevention of breast cancer:
***PO:* Adults, elderly:** 20 mg/day.

SIDE EFFECTS

FREQUENT: Women (>10%): Hot flashes, nausea, vomiting. ***OCCASIONAL: Women*** (1–9%): Changes in menstrual period, genital itching, vaginal discharge, endometrial hyperplasia/polyps. ***Males:*** Impotence, decreased sexual interest. ***Men/Women:*** Headache, nausea, vomiting, rash, bone pain, confusion, weakness, sleepiness.

ADVERSE REACTIONS/TOXIC EFFECTS

Retinopathy, corneal opacity, decreased visual acuity noted in those receiving extremely high doses (240–320 mg/day) for >17 mos.

NURSING IMPLICATIONS

BASELINE ASSESSMENT:

An estrogen receptor assay should be done before therapy is begun. CBC, platelet count, serum calcium levels should be checked before and periodically during therapy.

INTERVENTION/EVALUATION:

Be alert to increased bone pain and assure adequate pain relief. Monitor I&O, weight; check for edema, esp. of dependent areas. Assess for hypercalcemia (increased urine volume, excessive thirst, nausea, vomiting, constipation, hypotonicity of muscles, deep bone or flank pain, renal stones).

PATIENT/FAMILY TEACHING:

Report vaginal bleeding/discharge/itching, leg cramps, weight gain, shortness of breath, weakness. May initially experience increase in bone, tumor pain (appears to indicate good tumor response). Contact physician if nausea/vomiting continues at home. Nonhormone contraceptives are recommended during treatment.

tamsulosin hydrochloride

tam-sul-**owe**-sin
(Flomax)
Do not confuse with Fosamax, Volmax.

▶CLASSIFICATION

PHARMACOTHERAPEUTIC: Alpha$_1$-adrenergic blocker. *CLINICAL:* Benign prostatic hyperplasia agent

ACTION/*THERAPEUTIC EFFECT*

An alpha$_1$ antagonist, targets receptors around bladder neck and prostate capsule, *resulting in relaxation of smooth muscle, improvement in urinary flow, symptoms of prostate hyperplasia.*

PHARMACOKINETICS

Well absorbed following PO administration. Protein binding: 94–99%. Widely distributed. Protein binding 94–99%. Metabolized

in liver. Primarily excreted in urine. Unknown if removed by hemodialysis. Half-life: 9–13 hrs.

USES

Treatment of signs and symptoms of benign prostatic hyperplasia.

PRECAUTIONS

CONTRAINDICATIONS: History of sensitivity to tamsulosin. *CAUTIONS:* Renal/hepatic function impairment.
▷*LIFESPAN CONSIDERATIONS:* **Pregnancy/Lactation:** Not indicated for use in women. **Children:** Not indicated in this pt population. **Elderly:** No age-related precautions noted.

INTERACTIONS

DRUG: Other **alpha-blocking agents (prazosin, terazosin, doxazosin)** may have additive effect. May alter effects of **warfarin.** *HERBAL:* None known. *FOOD:* None known. *LAB VALUES:* None significant.

AVAILABILITY (Rx)

CAPSULES: 0.4 mg.

ADMINISTRATION/HANDLING

PO:

• Give at the same time each day, 1–2 hrs following the same meal. • Do not crush or open capsule unless directed by physician.

INDICATIONS/ROUTES/DOSAGE

Benign prostatic hypertrophy:

PO: Adults: 0.4 mg once daily, approximately 30 min after same meal each day. Dosage may be increased to 0.8 mg once daily.

SIDE EFFECTS

FREQUENT: (7–9%): Dizziness, drowsiness. *OCCASIONAL* (3–5%):

Headache, anxiety, insomnia, postural hypotension. **RARE** (<2%): Nasal congestion, pharyngitis, rhinitis, nausea, vertigo, impotence.

ADVERSE REACTIONS/TOXIC EFFECTS

First-dose syncope (hypotension with sudden LOC) may occur 30–90 min after giving initial dose. May be preceded by tachycardia (120–160 beats/min).

NURSING IMPLICATIONS

BASELINE ASSESSMENT:

Question for sensitivity to tamsulosin, use of other alpha-blocking agents, warfarin.

INTERVENTION/EVALUATION:

Assist with ambulation if dizziness occurs. Monitor renal function lab values.

PATIENT/FAMILY TEACHING:

Take at the same time each day, 30 min after a meal. Use caution when getting up from sitting or lying position. Avoid tasks that require alertness, motor skills until response to drug is established. Do not chew, crush, or open capsule.

tazarotene

tay-zah-**row**-teen
(Tazorac)

▶CLASSIFICATION

PHARMACOTHERAPEUTIC: Retinoid. **CLINICAL:** Antipsoriasis, antiacne

ACTION/THERAPEUTIC EFFECT

Modulates differentiation and proliferation of epithelial tissue; binds selectively to retinoic acid receptors. *Restores normal differentiation of the epidermis and reduction in epidermal inflammation.*

USES

Treatment of stable plaque psoriasis in pts with at least 20% body surface area involvement. Treatment of mild to moderate facial acne.

AVAILABILITY (Rx)

GEL: 0.05%, 0.1%.

INDICATIONS/ROUTES/DOSAGE
Psoriasis:

TOPICAL: Adults: Thin film applied once daily in the evening; only cover the lesions, and area should be dry before application.

Acne:

TOPICAL: Adults: Thin film applied to affected areas once daily in the evening, after face is gently cleansed and dried.

SIDE EFFECTS

FREQUENT (10–30%): *Acne:* Desquamation, burning or stinging, dry skin, itching, erythema. *Psoriasis:* Itching, burning or stinging, erythema, worsening of psoriasis, irritation, skin pain. **OCCASIONAL** (1–9%): *Acne:* Irritation, skin pain, fissuring, localized edema, skin discoloration. *Psoriasis:* Rash, desquamation, contact dermatitis, skin inflammation, fissuring, bleeding, dry skin.

NURSING IMPLICATIONS

BASELINE ASSESSMENT:

Assess for sensitivity to tazarotene. Determine if pt is taking medications that may increase sensitivity (e.g., ...holones.

...N/EVALUATION:

...nprovement of pso-..., any burning or ...medication.

...AMILY TEACHING:

...continue if skin irritation, pruritus, skin redness is excessive; contact physician. For external use only. Avoid contact with eyes, eyelids, mouth. Photosensitization may occur; use sunscreen, protective clothing.

telmisartan

tell-mih-**sar**-tan
(Micardis)

FIXED-COMBINATION(S)

With hydrochlorothiazide, a diuretic **(Micardis HCT)**

▶ **CLASSIFICATION**

PHARMACOTHERAPEUTIC: Angiotensin II receptor antagonist. **CLINICAL:** Antihypertensive (see p. 7C)

ACTION/THERAPEUTIC EFFECT

Potent vasodilator. An angiotensin II receptor (type AT_1) antagonist; blocks vasoconstrictor and aldosterone-secreting effects of angiotensin II, inhibiting the binding of angiotensin II to the AT_1 receptors, *producing vasodilation, decreased peripheral resistance, decrease in B/P.*

PHARMACOKINETICS

Rapidly and completely absorbed following oral administration. Protein binding: >99%. Undergoes hepatic metabolism to inactive metabolite. Excreted in feces. Unknown if removed by hemodialysis. Half-life: 24 hrs.

USES/UNLABELED

Treatment of hypertension alone or in combination with other antihypertensives. *Treatment of heart failure.*

PRECAUTIONS

CONTRAINDICATIONS: None significant. **CAUTIONS:** Biliary obstructive disorders, hepatic insufficiency.

▷**LIFESPAN CONSIDERATIONS:**
Pregnancy/Lactation: May cause fetal harm. Unknown if excreted in breast milk. **Category C (first trimester), Category D (second and third trimesters). Children:** Safety and efficacy not established. **Elderly:** No age-related precautions noted.

INTERACTIONS

DRUG: Increases **digoxin** plasma concentration. Slightly decreases **warfarin** plasma concentration. **HERBAL:** None known. **FOOD:** None known. **LAB VALUES:** May increase in serum creatinine. May decrease hemoglobin, hematocrit.

AVAILABILITY (Rx)

TABLETS: 40 mg, 80 mg.

ADMINISTRATION/HANDLING
PO:

• Give without regard to meals.

INDICATIONS/ROUTES/DOSAGE

Note: May be given concurrently with other antihypertensives. If B/P is not controlled by telmisartan alone, a diuretic may be added.

T

Hypertension:
PO: Adults, elderly: 40 mg once daily. **Dose range:** 20–80 mg.

SIDE EFFECTS

OCCASIONAL (3–7%): Upper respiratory tract infection, sinusitis, back/leg pain, diarrhea. ***RARE*** (1%): Dizziness, headache, fatigue, nausea, heartburn, myalgia, cough, peripheral edema.

ADVERSE REACTIONS/TOXIC EFFECTS

Overdosage may manifest as hypotension and tachycardia; bradycardia occurs less often.

NURSING IMPLICATIONS

BASELINE ASSESSMENT:

Obtain B/P and apical pulse immediately before each dose, in addition to regular monitoring (be alert to fluctuations). If excessive reduction in B/P occurs, place pt in supine position, feet slightly elevated. Assess medication history (esp. diuretic). Question for history of hepatic/renal impairment, renal artery stenosis. Obtain BUN, serum creatinine, hemoglobin, and vital signs, particularly B/P, pulse rate.

INTERVENTION/EVALUATION:

Maintain hydration (offer fluids frequently). Assess for evidence of upper respiratory infection. Assist with ambulation if dizziness occurs. Monitor all blood serum levels. Assess B/P for hypertension/hypotension.

PATIENT/FAMILY TEACHING:

Inform female pt regarding consequences of second-and third-trimester exposure to telmisartan. Report pregnancy to physician as soon as possible. Avoid task. alertness, motor skill dizziness effect). Report infection (sore throat, fever) lifelong control. Caution aga ercising during hot weather (dehydration, hypotension).

temazepam

tem-**az**-eh-pam
(Restoril)
Do not confuse with Vistaril, Zestril.

▶CLASSIFICATION

PHARMACOTHERAPEUTIC:
Benzodiazepine **(Schedule IV).**
CLINICAL: Sedative-hypnotic
(see p. 123C)

ACTION/*THERAPEUTIC EFFECT*

Enhances action of inhibitory neurotransmitter gamma-amino-butyric acid (GABA), *producing hypnotic effect due to CNS depression.*

PHARMACOKINETICS

Well absorbed from GI tract. Protein binding: 96%. Widely distributed. Crosses blood-brain barrier. Metabolized in liver. Primarily excreted in urine. Not removed by hemodialysis. Half-life: 8–15 hrs.

USES

Short-term treatment of insomnia (up to 5 wks). Reduces sleep-induction time, number of nocturnal awakenings; increases length of sleep.

PRECAUTIONS

CONTRAINDICATIONS: Acute narrow-angle glaucoma, acute alcohol intoxication. ***CAUTIONS:*** Impaired renal/hepatic function.

▷***LIFESPAN CONSIDERATIONS:***
Pregnancy/Lactation: Crosses placenta; may be distributed in breast milk. Chronic ingestion during pregnancy may produce withdrawal symptoms, CNS depression in neonates. **Pregnancy Category X. Children:** Not recommended in those <18 yrs of age. **Elderly:** Use small initial doses with gradual dosage increases to avoid ataxia or excessive sedation.

INTERACTIONS

DRUG: **Alcohol, CNS depressants** may increase CNS depressant effect. ***HERBAL:*** **Kava kava, valerian** may increase CNS effects. ***FOOD:*** None known. ***LAB VALUES:*** None significant.

AVAILABILITY (Rx)

CAPSULES: 7.5 mg, 15 mg, 30 mg.

ADMINISTRATION/HANDLING

PO:
• Give without regard to meals. • Capsules may be emptied and mixed with food.

INDICATIONS/ROUTES/DOSAGE

Hypnotic:
***PO:* Adults >18 yrs:** 15–30 mg at bedtime. **Elderly/debilitated:** 7.5–15 mg at bedtime.

SIDE EFFECTS

FREQUENT: Drowsiness, sedation, rebound insomnia (may occur for 1–2 nights after drug is discontinued), dizziness, confusion, euphoria. ***OCCASIONAL:*** Weakness, anorexia, diarrhea. ***RARE:*** Paradoxical CNS excitement, restlessness (particularly noted in elderly/debilitated).

ADVERSE REACTIONS/TOXIC EFFECTS

Abrupt or too-rapid withdrawal may result in pronounced restlessness, irritability, insomnia, hand tremors, abdominal/muscle cramps, sweating, vomiting, seizures. Overdosage results in somnolence, confusion, diminished reflexes, coma.

NURSING IMPLICATIONS

BASELINE ASSESSMENT:

Question for possibility of pregnancy before initiating therapy (Pregnancy Category X). Assess B/P, pulse, respirations immediately before administration. Raise bed rails. Provide environment conducive to sleep (back rub, quiet environment, low lighting).

INTERVENTION/EVALUATION:

Assess sleep pattern of pt. Assess elderly/debilitated for paradoxical reaction, particularly during early therapy. Evaluate for therapeutic response: decrease in number of nocturnal awakenings, increase in length of sleep.

PATIENT/FAMILY TEACHING:

Smoking reduces drug effectiveness. Rebound insomnia may occur when drug is discontinued after short-term therapy. Avoid alcohol and other CNS depressants. Inform physician if you are or are planning to become pregnant.

T

temozolomide

teh-moe-**zoll**-oh-mide
(Temodar)

▶CLASSIFICATION

PHARMACOTHERAPEUTIC: Imidazotetrazine derivative. **CLINICAL:** Antineoplastic (see p. 74C)

ACTION/*THERAPEUTIC EFFECT*

Pro-drug, converted to highly active cytotoxic metabolite. Cytotoxic effect associated with methylation of DNA. *Inhibits DNA replication, causing cell death.*

PHARMACOKINETICS

Rapidly, completely absorbed following oral administration. Protein binding: 15%. Peak plasma concentration occurs in 1 hr. Weakly bound to plasma proteins. Penetrates across blood-brain barrier. Primarily eliminated in urine and, to a much lesser extent, in feces.

USES

Treatment of refractory anaplastic astrocytoma in adults whose disease has relapsed after initial therapy with other agents.

PRECAUTIONS

CONTRAINDICATIONS: Hypersensitivity to dacarbazine. **CAUTIONS:** Severe renal impairment, severe hepatic impairment.
▷*LIFESPAN CONSIDERATIONS:*
Pregnancy/Lactation: May cause fetal harm. May produce malformation of external organs, soft tissue, skeleton. If possible, avoid use during pregnancy. Unknown if drug is excreted in breast milk. **Pregnancy Category D. Children:** Safety and efficacy not established. **Elderly:** In those >70 yrs, may experience a higher risk of developing grade 4 neutropenia and grade 4 thrombocytopenia.

INTERACTIONS

DRUG: Valproic acid decreases temozolomide clearance. **Live virus vaccines** may potentiate virus replication, increase vaccine side effects, decrease pt's antibody response to vaccine. **HERBAL:** None known. **FOOD:** Food decreases drug rate, absorption. **LAB VALUES:** May decrease hemoglobin, WBCs, platelets, neutrophils.

AVAILABILITY (Rx)

CAPSULES: 5 mg, 20 mg, 100 mg, 250 mg.

ADMINISTRATION/HANDLING

• Food reduces rate, extent of absorption, increases risk of nausea, vomiting. • For best results, administration should occur at bedtime. • Do not open capsules; if capsules are accidentally opened or damaged, avoid inhalation or contact with skin or mucous membranes.

INDICATIONS/ROUTES/DOSAGE

Anaplastic astrocytoma:

PO: Adults: Initially, 150 mg/m^2 daily for 5 consecutive days of a 28 day treatment cycle. If myelosuppression is not severe on day 22, dose may increase to 200 mg/m^2 and be repeated at 4 wk intervals.

SIDE EFFECTS

FREQUENT (33–53%): Nausea, vomiting, headache, fatigue, constipation. **OCCASIONAL** (10–16%): Diarrhea, asthenia (loss of strength, energy), fever, dizziness, peripheral edema, incoordination, insomnia. **RARE** (5–9%): Paresthesia, drowsiness, anorexia, urinary in-

---

continence, anxiety, pharyngitis, cough.

ADVERSE REACTIONS/TOXIC EFFECTS

Myelosuppression is characterized by neutropenia and thrombocytopenia with elderly and women showing the higher incidence of developing severe myelosuppression. Usually occurs within the first few cycles; is not cumulative. Nadir occurs approximately 26–28 days, with recovery 14 days of nadir.

NURSING IMPLICATIONS

BASELINE ASSESSMENT:

Prior to dosing, absolute neutrophil count (ANC) must be ≥1,500 and platelet count ≥100,000. Potential for nausea, vomiting readily controlled with antiemetic therapy.

INTERVENTION/EVALUATION:

Obtain a CBC on day 22 (21 days after the first dose) or within 48 hrs of that day and weekly until ANC is ≥1500 and platelet count ≥100,000. Monitor for hematologic toxicity (fever, sore throat, signs of local infection, easy bruising, or unusual bleeding from any site), symptoms of anemia (excessive tiredness, weakness).

PATIENT/FAMILY TEACHING:

To reduce nausea and vomiting, take temozolomide on an empty stomach. Do not open capsules. Promptly report fever, sore throat, signs of local infection, easy bruising, or unusual bleeding from any site. Avoid crowds, those with infection. Do not have immunizations without physician's approval.

tenecteplase

ten-**eck**-teh-place
(TNKase)

▶CLASSIFICATION

PHARMACOTHERAPEUTIC:
Tissue plasminogen activator.
CLINICAL: Thrombolytic (see p. 30C)

ACTION/THERAPEUTIC EFFECT

A tissue plasminogen activator (tPA) produced by recombinant DNA that binds to fibrin and converts plasminogen to plasmin, an enzyme that *degrades fibrin clots, fibrinogen, other plasma proteins.*

PHARMACOKINETICS

Extensively distributed to tissues. Completely eliminated by hepatic metabolism. Half-life: 11–20 min.

USES

Reduction of mortality associated with acute myocardial infarction (AMI).

PRECAUTIONS

CONTRAINDICATIONS: Active internal bleeding, history of CVA, intracranial/intraspinal surgery/trauma within 2 mos, intracranial neoplasm, arteriovenous malformation, aneurysm, known bleeding diathesis, severe uncontrolled hypertension. **CAUTIONS:** Patients previously received tenecteplase, severe liver impairment.

▷**LIFESPAN CONSIDERATIONS:**
Pregnancy/Lactation: Unknown if distributed in breast milk. **Pregnancy Category C. Children:** Safety and efficacy not established. **Elderly:** May have in-

T

creased intracranial hemorrhage, stroke, major bleeding; caution advised.

INTERACTIONS

DRUG: **Anticoagulants (e.g., heparin, warfarin), aspirin, dipyridamole, GP IIb/IIIa inhibitors** increase risk of bleeding. ***HERBAL:*** **Ginkgo biloba** may increase risk of bleeding. ***FOOD:*** None known. ***LAB VALUES:*** Decreases plasminogen and fibrinogen level during infusion, decreasing clotting time (confirms presence of lysis). Decreases hemoglobin and hematocrit.

AVAILABILITY (Rx)

POWDER FOR INJECTION: 50 mg.

ADMINISTRATION/HANDLING
IV 🖤

Storage:

• Store at room temperature. • If possible, use immediately but may refrigerate up to 8 hrs after reconstitution. • Appears as colorless to pale yellow solution. Do not use if discolored or contains particulates. • Discard after 8 hrs.

Reconstitution:

• Add 10 ml Sterile Water for Injection without preservative to vial to provide concentration of 5 mg/ml. Gently swirl until dissolved. Do not shake. • If foaming occurs, vial should be left undisturbed for several minutes.

Rate of administration:

• Administer as IV push over 5 sec.

IV INCOMPATIBILITY ⊘

Do not mix with any other medications.

INDICATIONS/ROUTES/DOSAGE

Note: Give as a single IV bolus over 5 sec. Precipitate may occur when given in an IV line containing dextrose. Flush with saline prior to and after administration.

Acute myocardial infarction:

IV: Adults: Dosage is based on the weight of the pt. Treatment to be initiated as soon as possible after onset of AMI symptoms.

Weight (kg)	(mg)	(ml)
<60	30	6
≥60 to <70	35	7
≥70 to <80	40	8
≥80 to <90	45	9
≥90	50	10

SIDE EFFECTS

FREQUENT: Bleeding (major: 4.7%; minor 21.8%).

ADVERSE REACTIONS/TOXIC EFFECTS

Bleeding at internal sites (intracranial, retroperitoneal, GI, GU, or respiratory) may occur. Lysis or coronary thrombi may produce atrial or ventricular dysrhythmias, stroke.

NURSING IMPLICATIONS

BASELINE ASSESSMENT:

Obtain baseline B/P, apical pulse. Record weight. Evaluate 12 lead EKG, CPK, CPK-MB, electrolytes. Assess hematocrit, platelet count, thrombin (TT), activated thromboplastin (APTT), prothrombin time (PT), fibrinogen level, before therapy is instituted. Type and hold blood.

INTERVENTION/EVALUATION:

Continuous cardiac monitoring for arrhythmias, B/P, pulse and respirations q15min until stable, then hrly. Check peripheral pulses, heart and lung sounds. Monitor chest pain relief and notify physician of continuation or recurrence (note location, type, and intensity). Assess for bleeding: overt blood, blood in any body substance. Monitor PTT per protocol. Maintain B/P; avoid any trauma that might increase risk of bleeding (injections, shaving, etc.). Assess neurologic status.

teniposide

ten-**ih**-poe-side
(Vumon)

▶**CLASSIFICATION**

PHARMACOTHERAPEUTIC: Podophyllotoxin derivative. ***CLINICAL:*** Antineoplastic (see p. 74C)

ACTION/THERAPEUTIC EFFECT

Induces single- and double-stranded breaks in DNA, inhibiting or altering DNA synthesis, *preventing cells from entering mitosis.* Phase specific acting in late S and early G_2 phases of cell cycle.

PHARMACOKINETICS

Protein binding: >99%. Does not efficiently cross blood-brain barrier. Metabolized extensively in liver. Primarily excreted in urine. Unknown if removed by hemodialysis. Half-life: 5 hrs.

USES

In combination with other antineoplastic agents, induction therapy in pts with refractory childhood acute lymphoblastic leukemia.

PRECAUTIONS

CONTRAINDICATIONS: Hypersensitivity to etoposide, teniposide, or Cremophor EL (polyoxyethylated castor oil); platelet count <50,000 mm^3; absolute neutrophil count <500/mm^3. ***CAUTIONS:*** Pts with brain tumors/neuroblastoma (increased risk of anaphylaxis), retreating pts with hypersensitivity reaction to teniposide, Down syndrome, decreased liver function.

▷***LIFESPAN CONSIDERATIONS:*** **Pregnancy/Lactation:** If possible, avoid use during pregnancy, esp. during first trimester. May cause fetal harm. Breast feeding not recommended. Unknown whether excreted in breast milk. **Pregnancy Category D. Children:** Down syndrome pts may be more sensitive to effects. **Elderly:** No information available.

INTERACTIONS

DRUG: May increase intracellular accumulation of **methotrexate.** May increase severity of peripheral neuropathy with **vincristine. Bone marrow depressants** may increase bone marrow depression. **Live virus vaccines** may potentiate virus replication, increase vaccine side effects, decrease pt's antibody response to vaccine. ***HERBAL:*** None known. ***FOOD:*** None known. ***LAB VALUES:*** None significant.

AVAILABILITY (Rx)

INJECTION: 50 mg.

ADMINISTRATION/HANDLING

Note: Administer by slow IV infusion. Wear gloves when preparing solution. If powder or solution comes in contact with skin, wash

T

---

immediately and thoroughly with soap, water.

IV 💊

Storage:

• Refrigerate unopened ampules. • Protect from light. • Reconstituted solutions stable for 24 hrs at room temperature. • Discard if precipitation occurs. • Use 1 mg/ml solution within 4 hrs of preparation (reduces potential for precipitation). • Do not refrigerate reconstituted solution.

Reconstitution:

• Dilute with D_5W or 0.9% NaCl to provide a final concentration of 0.1, 0.2, 0.4, or 1 mg/ml. • Avoid contact of undiluted teniposide with plastic (may cause softening/cracking and possible drug leakage).

Rate of administrations:

• Prepare/administer in non-DEHP-containing LVP containers such as glass or polyolefin plastic bags/containers. Avoid use of PVC containers. • Give by IV infusion only over at least 30–60 min (decreases hypotension). • Avoid contact with other drugs/fluids. • Monitor for anaphylactic reaction during infusion (chills, fever, dyspnea, sweating, lacrimation, sneezing, throat/back/chest pain).

IV INCOMPATIBILITY ⊘

Idarubicin (Idamycin).

IV COMPATIBILITIES

Allopurinol (Aloprim), calcium gluconate, dexmethasone (Decadron), ondansetron (Zofran), potassium chloride.

INDICATIONS/ROUTES/DOSAGE

Dosage individualized based on clinical response, tolerance to adverse effects. When used in com-

bination therapy, consult specific protocols for optimum dosage, sequence of drug administration.

SIDE EFFECTS

FREQUENT (>30%): Mucositis, nausea, vomiting, diarrhea, anemia. **OCCASIONAL** (3–5%): Alopecia, rash. **RARE** (<3%): Liver dysfunction, fever, renal dysfunction, peripheral neurotoxicity.

ADVERSE REACTIONS/TOXIC EFFECTS

Bone marrow depression manifested as hematologic toxicity (principally leukopenia, neutropenia, thrombocytopenia) with increased risk of infection or bleeding. Hypersensitivity reaction, including anaphylaxis (chills, fever, tachycardia, bronchospasm, dyspnea, facial flushing).

NURSING IMPLICATIONS

BASELINE ASSESSMENT:

Assess hematology (platelet count, hemoglobin, WBC, differential), renal and hepatic function tests before and frequently during therapy.

INTERVENTION/EVALUATION:

Have antihistamines, corticosteroids, epinephrine, IV fluids, and other supportive measures readily available for first dose (possible life-threatening anaphylaxis as evidenced by chills, fever, tachycardia, bronchospasm, dyspnea, hyper/hypotension, facial flushing). Monitor for myelosuppression: unusual bleeding or bruising; anemia (excessive tiredness, weakness). Pretreat with antiemetics for nausea, vomiting but be alert to hypotension and CNS depression that may occur with these drug combinations (be-

cause of benzyl alcohol in teniposide, esp. with high doses).

PATIENT/FAMILY TEACHING:

Avoid crowds, those with infection. Do not have immunizations
without physician's approval.
Promptly report fever, signs of
infection, easy bruising, unusual
bleeding from any site, difficulty
breathing. Avoid pregnancy.
Alopecia is reversible, but new
hair growth may have different
color or texture.

tenofovir disoproxil fumarate

ten-**oh**-fah-vir
(Viread)

▶CLASSIFICATION

PHARMACOTHERAPEUTIC:
Nucleotide analog. **CLINICAL:**
Antiviral (see pp. 59C, 95C)

ACTION/*THERAPEUTIC EFFECT*

Inhibits HIV-1 protease, rendering
the enzymes incapable of processing the polypeptide precursor
to generate functional proteins in
HIV-infected cells, *slowing HIV
replication, reducing viral load.*

USES

Used in combination with nucleoside analogues or as monotherapy
for treatment of HIV infection.

PRECAUTIONS

CONTRAINDICATIONS: None
significant. **CAUTIONS:** Impaired
hepatic or renal function.

INTERACTIONS

DRUG: None significant. **HERBAL:**
None significant. **FOOD:** Food in-
creases bioavailability. **LAB VAL-
UES:** May elevate serum transami-
nase. May alter SGPT (ALT),
SGOT (AST), creatinine clearance,
GGT, CPK, uric acid, triglycerides.

AVAILABILITY (Rx)

TABLETS: 300 mg.

ADMINISTRATION/HANDLING

PO:

• Give with food.

INDICATIONS/ROUTES/DOSAGE

HIV infection:

PO: Adults, elderly: 300 mg once
daily.

SIDE EFFECTS

OCCASIONAL: GI disturbances
(nausea, diarrhea, vomiting, flatulence).

ADVERSE REACTIONS/TOXIC
EFFECTS

Lactic acidosis, hepatomegaly
with steatosis (excess fat in liver)
occur rarely; may be severe.

NURSING IMPLICATIONS

BASELINE ASSESSMENT:

Obtain baseline laboratory testing, esp. liver function tests,
triglycerides before beginning
tenofovir therapy and at periodic
intervals during therapy. Offer
emotional support.

INTERVENTION/EVALUATION:

Closely monitor for evidence of
GI discomfort. Monitor stool frequency and consistency (watery,
loose, soft). Monitor clinical
chemistry tests for marked laboratory abnormalities.

T

PATIENT/FAMILY TEACHING:

Continue therapy for full length of treatment. Doses should be evenly spaced. Tenofovir is not a cure for HIV infection, nor does it reduce risk of transmission to others. Pts may continue to acquire illnesses associated with advanced HIV infection. Take tenofovir with food.

terazosin hydrochloride 🖊

tear-**aye**-zoe-sin
(Apo-Terazosin✦, <u>Hytrin</u>)

▶CLASSIFICATION

PHARMACOTHERAPEUTIC:
Alpha-adrenergic blocker. **CLINICAL:** Antihypertensive, benign prostatic hyperplasia agent (see p. 52C)

ACTION/THERAPEUTIC EFFECT

Blocks alpha-adrenergic receptors. **Hypertension:** Produces vasodilation, decreases peripheral resistance, *resulting in decreased B/P.* **Benign prostatic hypertrophy:** Targets receptors around bladder neck and prostate, *resulting in relaxation of smooth muscle, improvement in urinary flow.*

PHARMACOKINETICS

	Onset	Peak	Duration
PO	15 min	1–2 hrs	12–24 hrs

Rapidly, completely absorption from GI tract. Protein binding: 90–94%. Metabolized in liver to active metabolite. Primarily eliminated in feces via biliary system; excreted in urine. Not removed by hemodialysis. Half-life: 12 hrs.

USES

Treatment of mild to moderate hypertension. Used alone or in combination with other antihypertensives. Treatment of benign prostatic hypertrophy.

PRECAUTIONS

CONTRAINDICATIONS: None significant. **CAUTIONS:** Chronic renal failure, impaired hepatic function.

▷**LIFESPAN CONSIDERATIONS:**
Pregnancy/Lactation: Unknown if drug crosses placenta or is distributed in breast milk. **Pregnancy Category C. Children:** Safety and efficacy not established. **Elderly:** No age-related precautions noted but may be more sensitive to hypotensive effects.

INTERACTIONS

DRUG: Estrogen, NSAIDs, sympathomimetics may decrease effect. **Hypotension-producing medications** may increase antihypertensive effect. **HERBAL:** None known. **FOOD:** None known. **LAB VALUES:** May decrease albumin, total protein, hemoglobin, hematocrit, WBC.

AVAILABILITY (Rx)

CAPSULES: 1 mg, 2 mg, 5 mg, 10 mg.

ADMINISTRATION/HANDLING
PO:

• Give without regard to food. • Tablets may be crushed. • Administer first dose at bedtime (minimizes risk of fainting due to "first-dose syncope").

INDICATIONS/ROUTES/DOSAGE

Note: If medication is discontinued for several days, retitrate initially using 1 mg dose at bedtime.

Hypertension:

PO: Adults, elderly: Initially, 1 mg at bedtime. Slowly increase dose to desired levels. **Range:** 1–5 mg/day as single or 2 divided doses. **Maximum:** 20 mg.

Benign prostatic hypertrophy:

PO: Adults, elderly: Initially, 1 mg at bedtime. May increase up to 10 mg/day. **Maximum:** 20 mg/day.

SIDE EFFECTS

FREQUENT (5–9%): Dizziness, headache, unusual tiredness. ***RARE*** (<2%): Peripheral edema, orthostatic hypotension, back/joint pain, blurred vision, nausea, vomiting, nasal congestion, drowsiness.

ADVERSE REACTIONS/TOXIC EFFECTS

"First-dose syncope" (hypotension with sudden LOC) generally occurs 30–90 min after giving initial dose of ≥2 mg, a too-rapid increase in dose, or addition of another hypotensive agent to therapy. May be preceded by tachycardia (120–160 beats/min).

NURSING IMPLICATIONS

BASELINE ASSESSMENT:

Give first dose at bedtime. If initial dose is given during daytime, pt must remain recumbent for 3–4 hrs. Assess B/P, pulse immediately before each dose, and q15–30min until stabilized (be alert to B/P fluctuations).

INTERVENTION/EVALUATION:

Monitor pulse diligently ("first-dose syncope" may be preceded by tachycardia). Assist with ambulation if dizziness occurs. Assess for peripheral edema of hands, feet (usually, first area of low extremity swelling is behind medial malleolus in ambulatory, sacral area in bedridden).

PATIENT/FAMILY TEACHING:

Noncola carbonated beverage, unsalted crackers, dry toast may relieve nausea. Nasal congestion may occur. Full therapeutic effect may not occur for 3–4 wks. Use caution driving, performing tasks requiring mental alertness. Use caution rising from sitting position. Report dizziness, palpitations.

terbinafine hydrochloride

tur-**bin**-ah-feen
(Lamisil, Lamisil Derma Gel)
Do not confuse with Lamictal, terbutaline.

▶CLASSIFICATION

CLINICAL: Antifungal (see p. 43C)

ACTION/*THERAPEUTIC EFFECT*

Fungicidal. Inhibits the enzyme, squalene epoxidase, interfering with biosynthesis in fungi, *resulting in fungal cell death.*

USES

Systemic: Treatment of onychomycosis (fungal disease of nails due to dermatophytes). ***Topical:*** Treatment of *Tinea cruris* (jock itch), *T. pedis* (athlete's foot), *T. corporis* (ringworm). ***Derma Gel:*** Treatment of *T. corporis, T. pedis,* and *T. versicolor.*

PRECAUTIONS

CONTRAINDICATIONS: Oral: Preexisting liver disease or renal impairment (creatinine clearance ≤50 ml/min). Safety in children <12 yrs not established. ***CAUTIONS:*** None significant.

INTERACTIONS

DRUG:* Alcohol, other hepatotoxic medications** may increase risk of hepatotoxicity. **Liver enzyme inhibitors** may decrease clearance (e.g., **cimetidine**). **Liver enzyme inducers** may increase clearance (e.g., **rifampin**). ***HERBAL: None known. ***FOOD:*** None known. ***LAB VALUES:*** May increase SGPT (ALT), SGOT (AST).

AVAILABILITY (Rx)

TABLETS: 250 mg. ***CREAM:*** 1%. ***TOPICAL SOLUTION:*** 1%.

INDICATIONS/ROUTES/DOSAGE

Note: Topical therapy used for minimum 1 wk, not to exceed 4 wks.

T. pedis:

***TOPICAL:* Adults, elderly, adolescents:** Apply 2 times/day until signs/symptoms significantly improved.

T. cruris, T. corporis:

***TOPICAL:* Adults, elderly, adolescents:** Apply 1–2 times/day until signs/symptoms significantly improved.

Onychomycosis:

***PO:* Adults, elderly, adolescents:** 250 mg/day for 6 wks (fingernails), 12 wks (toenails).

SIDE EFFECTS

FREQUENT (13%): ***Oral:*** Headache. ***OCCASIONAL*** (3–6%): ***Oral:*** Diarrhea, rash, dyspepsia, pruritus, taste disturbance, nausea. ***RARE: Oral:*** Abdominal pain, flatulence, urticaria, visual disturbance. ***Topical:*** Irritation, burning, itching, dryness.

ADVERSE REACTIONS/TOXIC EFFECTS

Hepatobiliary dysfunction (including cholestatic hepatitis), serious skin reactions, severe neutropenia occur rarely. Ocular lens and retina changes have been noted.

NURSING IMPLICATIONS

BASELINE ASSESSMENT:

Liver function tests should be obtained in pts receiving treatment for >6 wks.

INTERVENTION/EVALUATION:

Check for therapeutic response. Discontinue medication, notify physician if local reaction occurs (irritation, redness, swelling, itching, oozing, blistering, burning). Monitor liver function tests in pts receiving treatment for >6 wks.

PATIENT/FAMILY TEACHING:

Keep areas clean and dry; wear light clothing to promote ventilation. Separate personal items. Avoid topical cream contact with eyes, nose, mouth, or other mucous membranes. Rub well into affected, surrounding area. Do not cover with occlusive dressing. Notify physician if skin irritation, diarrhea occurs.

terbutaline sulfate

tur-**byew**-ta-leen
(Brethine, Bricanyl)
Do not confuse with Brethaire, terbinafine, tolbutamide.

►CLASSIFICATION

PHARMACOTHERAPEUTIC:
Sympathomimetic (adrenergic
agonist). *CLINICAL:* Bronchodilator, premature labor inhibitor
(see p. 63C)

ACTION/*THERAPEUTIC EFFECT*

Bronchospasm: Stimulates beta₂-
adrenergic receptors, *relaxes bronchial smooth muscle, relieves bronchospasm, reduces airway resistance.*
Labor: Relaxes uterine muscle, inhibiting uterine contractions.

USES

Symptomatic relief of reversible
bronchospasm due to bronchial
asthma, bronchitis, emphysema.
Delays premature labor in pregnancies between 20 and 34 wks.

PRECAUTIONS

CONTRAINDICATIONS: History
of hypersensitivity to sympathomimetics. *CAUTIONS:* Impaired
cardiac function, diabetes mellitus,
hypertension, hyperthyroidism,
history of seizures.

INTERACTIONS

DRUG: **Tricyclic antidepressants**
may increase cardiovascular effects. **MAO inhibitors** may increase risk of hypertensive crises.
May decrease effects of **beta-
blockers. Digoxin, sympathomimetics** may increase risk of arrhythmias. *HERBAL:* None known.
FOOD: None known. *LAB VALUES:*
May decrease serum potassium
levels.

AVAILABILITY (Rx)

TABLETS: 2.5 mg, 5 mg. *INJEC-
TION:* 1 mg/ml.

ADMINISTRATION/HANDLING

PO:

• Give without regard to food
(give with food if GI upset occurs).
• Tablets may be crushed.

SubQ:

• Do not use if solution appears
discolored. • Inject SubQ into lateral deltoid region.

INDICATIONS/ROUTES/DOSAGE

Bronchospasm:

*PO: Adults, elderly, children >15
yrs:* Initially, 2.5 mg 3–4 times/day.
Maintenance: 2.5–5 mg 3 times/
day q6h while awake. **Maximum:**
15 mg/day. **Children 12–15 yrs:**
2.5 mg 3 times/day. **Maximum:**
7.5 mg/day. **Children <12 yrs:** Initially, 0.05 mg/kg/dose q8h. May
increase up to 0.15 mg/kg/dose.
Maximum: 5 mg.

SuBQ: Adults: Initially, 0.25 mg.
Repeat in 15–30 min if substantial
improvement does not occur.
Maximum: No more than 0.5 mg/
4 hrs. **Children <12 yrs:** 0.005–
0.01 mg/kg/dose to a maximum of
0.4 mg/dose q15–20min for 2
doses.

SIDE EFFECTS

FREQUENT (23–38%): Tremor,
shakiness, nervousness. *OCCA-
SIONAL* (10–11%): Drowsiness,
headache, nausea, heartburn,
dizziness. *RARE* (1–3%): Flushing,
weakness, drying or irritation of
oropharynx noted with inhalation
therapy.

ADVERSE REACTIONS/TOXIC
EFFECTS

Too frequent or excessive use
may lead to loss of bronchodilating effectiveness and/or severe,
paradoxical bronchoconstriction.

T

Excessive sympathomimetic stimulation may cause palpitations, extrasystoles, tachycardia, chest pain, slight increase in B/P followed by a substantial decrease, chills, sweating, and blanching of skin.

NURSING IMPLICATIONS

BASELINE ASSESSMENT:

Bronchospasm: Offer emotional support (high incidence of anxiety due to difficulty in breathing and sympathomimetic response to drug).

INTERVENTION/EVALUATION:

Bronchospasm: Monitor rate, depth, rhythm, type of respiration; quality and rate of pulse. Assess lung sounds for rhonchi, wheezing, rales. Monitor arterial blood gases. Observe lips, fingernails for blue or dusky color in light-skinned pts; gray in dark-skinned pts. Observe for clavicular retractions, hand tremor. Evaluate for clinical improvement (quieter, slower respirations, relaxed facial expression, cessation of clavicular retractions).

PATIENT/FAMILY TEACHING:

Bronchospasm: Increase fluid intake (decreases lung secretion viscosity). Do not take >2 inhalations at any one time (excessive use may produce paradoxical bronchoconstriction or a decreased bronchodilating effect). Rinsing mouth with water immediately after inhalation may prevent mouth/throat dryness. Avoid excessive use of caffeine derivatives (chocolate, coffee, tea, cola, cocoa).

terconazole

ter-**con**-ah-zole
(Terazol)
Do not confuse with
tioconazole.

▶CLASSIFICATION
CLINICAL: Antifungal

ACTION/THERAPEUTIC EFFECT
Disrupts fungal cell membrane permeability, *producing antifungal activity.*

USES
Treatment of vulvovaginal candidiasis (moniliasis).

AVAILABILITY [Rx]
VAGINAL TABLETS: 80 mg. *VAGINAL CREAM:* 0.4%, 0.8%.

INDICATIONS/ROUTES/DOSAGE
Vulvovaginal candidiasis:

INTRAVAGINAL: **Adults, elderly:** *TABLET:* 1 suppository vaginally at bedtime for 3 days. *CREAM (0.4%):* 1 applicatorful at bedtime for 7 days; 0.8% for 3 days.

SIDE EFFECTS
FREQUENT (>10%): Headache, vulvovaginal burning. *OCCASIONAL* (1–10%): Dysmenorrhea, pain in female genitalia, abdominal pain, fever, itching. *RARE* (<1%): Chills.

testolactone

tes-toe-**lack**-tone
(Teslac)
Do not confuse with
testosterone.

►CLASSIFICATION

PHARMACOTHERAPEUTIC:
Androgen. ***CLINICAL:*** Antineoplastic

ACTION

Inhibits steroid aromatase activity, an enzyme that reduces estrone synthesis (estrone is major source of estrogen in postmenopausal women).

USES

Adjunctive therapy in treatment of advanced disseminated breast carcinoma in postmenopausal women when hormonal therapy is indicated, and in premenopausal women where ovarian function has been terminated.

PRECAUTIONS

CONTRAINDICATIONS: Breast cancer in men. ***CAUTIONS:*** Renal, liver, cardiac disease.

INTERACTIONS

DRUG: May increase effects of **oral anticoagulants. *HERBAL:*** None known. ***FOOD:*** None known. ***LAB VALUES:*** May increase calcium, creatinine, 17-ketosteroids. May decrease estradiol.

AVAILABILITY (Rx)

TABLETS: 50 mg.

INDICATIONS/ROUTES/DOSAGE

Breast carcinoma:

PO: Adults, elderly: 250 mg 4 times/day.

SIDE EFFECTS

RARE: Maculopapular erythema, increase in B/P, alopecia, nail growth disturbances, paresthesia, aches, edema of extremities, glossitis, anorexia, hot flashes, nausea, vomiting, diarrhea.

ADVERSE REACTIONS/TOXIC EFFECTS

None significant.

NURSING IMPLICATIONS

INTERVENTION/EVALUATION:

Monitor plasma calcium levels (hypercalcemia is evidence of active remission of bone metastasis). Assess for signs of hypercalcemia (decreased muscle tone, bone/flank pain, thirst, excessive urination). Assess skin for maculopapular erythema.

PATIENT/FAMILY TEACHING:

Therapeutic effects usually noted in 6–12 wks. Therapy should continue for at least 3 mos. If alopecia occurs, it is reversible, but new hair growth may have different color or texture.

testosterone

tess-**toss**-ter-own
(Andronaq, Delatestryl♣, Histerone)

testosterone cypionate
(Depotest, Depo-Testosterone)

testosterone enanthate
(Delatest)

testosterone propionate
(Testex)

T

testosterone transdermal

(Androderm, Testoderm, Testoderm TTS)
Do not confuse with testolactone.

FIXED-COMBINATION(S)

Testosterone cypionate with estradiol cypionate, an estrogen **(dep-Androgyn, De-Comberol, Duratestrin);** testosterone enanthate with estradiol cypionate **(Deladumone)**

▶CLASSIFICATION

PHARMACOTHERAPEUTIC: Androgen. *CLINICAL:* Sex hormone

ACTION/*THERAPEUTIC EFFECT*

Stimulates spermatogenesis, development of male secondary sex characteristics, sexual maturation at puberty. Stimulates production of RBCs. *Initiates male puberty, corrects hormonal deficiency, suppresses tumor growth in breast cancer.*

PHARMACOKINETICS

Well absorbed after IM administration. Protein binding: 98%. Metabolized in liver (undergoes first-pass metabolism). Primarily excreted in urine. Unknown if removed by hemodialysis. Half-life: 10–20 min.

USES

Replacement therapy in treatment of delayed male puberty. Treatment of hypogonadism, breast cancer in women who have been postmenopausal 1–5 yrs.

PRECAUTIONS

CONTRAINDICATIONS: Serious cardiac, renal, or hepatic dysfunction. Do not use for men with carcinomas of the breast or prostate. *EXTREME CAUTION:* In children because of bone maturation effects. *CAUTIONS:* Epilepsy, migraine, or other conditions aggravated by fluid retention; metastatic breast cancer or immobility increases risk of hypercalcemia.

▷*LIFESPAN CONSIDERATIONS:* **Pregnancy/Lactation:** Contraindicated during lactation. **Pregnancy Category X. Children:** Safety and efficacy not established; use with caution. **Elderly:** May increase risk of hyperplasia or stimulate growth of occult prostate carcinoma.

INTERACTIONS

DRUG: May increase effect of **oral anticoagulants. Hepatotoxic medications** may increase hepatotoxicity. *HERBAL:* None known. *FOOD:* None known. *LAB VALUES:* May increase SGOT (AST), alkaline phosphatase, bilirubin, calcium, potassium, sodium, hemoglobin, hematocrit, LDL. May decrease HDL.

AVAILABILITY (Rx)

INJECTION: Aqueous suspension: 50 mg/ml, 100 mg/ml. *Cypionate:* 100 mg/ml, 200 mg/ml. *Enanthate:* 200 mg/ml. *Propionate:* 100 mg/ml. *PELLETS FOR SUBQ IMPLANTATION:* 75 mg. *TRANSDERMAL GEL:* (25 mg (2.5 g gel/pack), 50 mg (5 g gel/pack). *TRANSDERMAL SYSTEM:* 2.5 mg/day, 4 mg/day, 5 mg/day, 6 mg/day.

ADMINISTRATION/HANDLING
IM:

• Give deep in gluteal muscle. • Do *not* give IV. • Warming and shaking redissolves crystals that may form in long-acting preparations. • Wet needle of syringe may cause solution to become cloudy; this does not affect potency.

Transdermal:

Testoderm:

• Apply to clean, dry scrotal skin that has been dry-shaved (optimal skin contact). Testoderm TTS may be applied to arm, back, or upper buttock.

Androderm:

• Apply to clean, dry area on skin on back, abdomen, upper arms, or thighs. • Do not apply to bony prominences (e.g., shoulder) or oily, damaged, irritated skin. Do not apply to scrotum. • Rotate application site with 7 day interval to same site.

INDICATIONS/ROUTES/DOSAGE

Male hypogonadism:

IM: Adults, elderly: (Aqueous/propionate): 10–25 mg 2–3 times/wk. ***(Cypionate/enanthate):*** 50–400 mg q2–4wks. ***(Transdermal system):*** Initially, 5–6 mg/day. ***(Pellets):*** 150–450 mg q3mos. ***(Transdermal gel):*** Initially, 5 g. May increase to 10 g. **Children: *(Cypionate/enanthate):*** *Initial pubertal growth:* 40–50 mg/m²/dose qmo. *Terminal growth phase:* 100 mg/m²/dose qmo. ***Maintenance virilizing dose:*** 100 mg/m²/dose 2 times/mo.

Delayed puberty:

IM: 40–50 mg/m²/dose qmo for 6 mos.

Breast carcinoma:

IM: Adults: (Aqueous): 50–100 mg 3 times/wk. ***(Cypionate/enanthate):*** 200–400 mg q2–4wks. ***(Propionate):*** 50–100 mg 3 times/wk.

SIDE EFFECTS

FREQUENT: Gynecomastia, acne, amenorrhea or other menstrual irregularities. ***Females:*** hirsutism, deepening of voice, clitoral enlargement (may not be reversible when drug discontinued). ***OCCASIONAL:*** Edema, nausea, insomnia, oligospermia, priapism, male pattern of baldness, bladder irritability, hypercalcemia in immobilized pts or those with breast cancer, hypercholesterolemia, inflammation and pain at IM injection site. ***Transdermal:*** Itching, erythema, skin irritation. ***RARE:*** Polycythemia with high dosage, hypersensitivity.

ADVERSE REACTIONS/TOXIC EFFECTS

Peliosis hepatitis (liver, spleen replaced with blood-filled cysts), hepatic neoplasms and hepatocellular carcinoma have been associated with prolonged high-dosage, anaphylactoid reactions.

NURSING IMPLICATIONS

BASELINE ASSESSMENT:

Establish baseline weight, B/P, hemoglobin, and hematocrit. Check liver function test results, electrolytes, and cholesterol if ordered. Wrist x-rays may be ordered to determine bone maturation in children.

INTERVENTION/EVALUATION:

Weigh daily and report weekly gain of >5 lbs; evaluate for edema. Monitor I&O. Check B/P at least 2 times/day. Assess electrolytes, cholesterol, hemoglobin, and hematocrit (periodically for high dosage), liver function test results. With breast cancer or immobility, check for hypercalcemia (lethargy, muscle weakness, confusion, irritability). Assure adequate intake of protein, calories. Assess for virilization. Monitor sleep patterns. Check injection site for redness, swelling, or pain.

PATIENT/FAMILY TEACHING:

Regular visits to physician and monitoring tests are necessary. Do not take any other medications without consulting physician. Teach diet high in protein, calories. Food may be tolerated better in small, frequent feedings. Weigh daily, report 5 lbs/gain/wk. Notify physician if nausea, vomiting, acne, or ankle swelling occurs. *Females:* Promptly report menstrual irregularities, hoarseness, deepening of voice. *Males:* Report frequent erections, difficulty urinating, gynecomastia.

tetracaine

(Pontocaine)

See Classification section under: Anesthetics: local (p. 4C)

tetracycline hydrochloride

tet-rah-**sigh**-klin
(Achromycin, Actisite, Apo-Tetra✚, Novotetra✚, Panmycin, Robitet, Sumycin, Topicycline)

▶CLASSIFICATION

PHARMACOTHERAPEUTIC: Tetracycline. ***CLINICAL:*** Antibiotic

ACTION/*THERAPEUTIC EFFECT*

Inhibits protein synthesis by binding to ribosomes, *preventing bacterial cell growth.* Bacteriostatic.

PHARMACOKINETICS

Readily absorbed from GI tract. Protein binding: 30–60%. Widely distributed. Excreted in urine; eliminated in feces via biliary system. Not removed by hemodialysis. Half-life: 6–11 hrs (half-life increased with impaired renal function).

USES

Treatment of inflammatory acne vulgaris, Lyme disease, mycoplasma disease, Legionella, Rocky Mountain spotted fever, Chlamydial infection in pts with gonorrhea.

PRECAUTIONS

CONTRAINDICATIONS: Hypersensitivity to tetracyclines, sulfite, children ≤age 8 yrs. ***CAUTIONS:*** Sun/ultraviolet light exposure (severe photosensitivity reaction).

▷***LIFESPAN CONSIDERATIONS:*** **Pregnancy/Lactation:** Readily crosses placenta, is distributed in breast milk. Avoid use in women during last half of pregnancy. May produce permanent teeth discoloration/enamel hypoplasia, inhibit fetal skeletal growth in children ≤8 yrs. **Pregnancy Category D. Children:** Not recommended in those ≤8 yrs of age; may cause permanent staining of teeth, enamel hypoplasia, decreased linear skeletal growth rate. **Elderly:** No age-related precautions noted.

INTERACTIONS

DRUG: **Cholestyramine, colestipol** may decrease absorption. May decrease effect of **oral contraceptives. Carbamazepine, phenytoin** may decrease concentrations. ***HERBAL:*** **St. John's wort** may increase risk of photosensitivity. ***FOOD:*** **Dairy products** inhibit absorption. ***LAB VALUES:*** May increase BUN, SGOT

(AST), SGPT (ALT), alkaline phosphatase, amylase, bilirubin concentrations.

AVAILABILITY (Rx)

CAPSULES: 250 mg, 500 mg. *TABLETS:* 250 mg, 500 mg. *TOPICAL SOLUTION. TOPICAL OINTMENT:* 3%.

ADMINISTRATION/HANDLING

PO:
• Give capsules, tablets with full glass of water 1 hr before or 2 hrs after meals, milk.

Topical:
• Cleanse area gently before application. • Apply only to affected area.

INDICATIONS/ROUTES/DOSAGE

Note: Space doses evenly around the clock.

Usual dosage:

PO: **Adults, elderly:** 1–3 g/day in 2–4 divided doses. **Children >8 yrs:** 25–50 mg/kg/day in 2–4 divided doses.

Dosage in renal impairment:

Creatinine Clearance	Dosage Interval
50–80 ml/min	q8–12h
10–50 ml/min	q12–24h
<10 ml/min	q24h

Usual topical dosage:

TOPICAL: **Adults, elderly:** Apply 2 times/day in morning, evening.

SIDE EFFECTS

FREQUENT: Dizziness, lightheadedness, diarrhea, nausea, vomiting, stomach cramps, increased sensitivity of skin to sunlight. *Topical:* Dry scaly skin, stinging, burning feeling. *OCCASIONAL:* Pigmentation of skin, mucus membranes, itching in rectal/genital area, sore mouth/tongue. *Topical:* Pain, redness, swelling, other skin irritation.

ADVERSE REACTIONS/TOXIC EFFECTS

Superinfection (esp. fungal), anaphylaxis, increased intracranial pressure, bulging fontanelles occur rarely in infants.

NURSING IMPLICATIONS

BASELINE ASSESSMENT:
Question for history of allergies, esp. tetracyclines, sulfite.

INTERVENTION/EVALUATION:
Assess skin for rash. Determine pattern of bowel activity and stool consistency. Monitor food intake, tolerance. Be alert for superinfection: diarrhea, ulceration, or changes of oral mucosa, anal/genital pruritus. Monitor B/P and LOC because of potential for increased intracranial pressure.

PATIENT/FAMILY TEACHING:
Continue antibiotic for full length of treatment. Space doses evenly. Take oral doses on empty stomach (1 hr before or 2 hrs after food/beverages). Drink full glass of water with capsules and avoid bedtime doses. Notify physician in event of diarrhea, rash, other new symptom. Protect skin from sun exposure. Consult physician before taking any other medication. *Topical:* Skin may turn yellow with Topicycline application (washing removes solution); fabrics may be stained by heavy application. Do not apply to deep/open wounds.

T

tetrahydrozyline hydrochloride

tet-rah-high-**droz**-ah-leen
(Tyzine, Visine)
Do not confuse with Visken.

FIXED-COMBINATION(S)

With benzalkonium chloride, a wetting agent, and edetate disodium, a chelating agent **(Murine Plus, Visine A.C.)**

▶CLASSIFICATION

PHARMACOTHERAPEUTIC: Vasoconstrictor. **CLINICAL:** Ophthalmic decongestant

ACTION/THERAPEUTIC EFFECT

Stimulates alpha-adrenergic receptors in sympathetic nervous system. **Ophthalmic:** Constricts arterioles, *reduces redness, irritation.* **Intranasal:** Constricts arterioles, *reduces congestion.*

USES

Ophthalmic: Relief of itching, minor irritation and to control hyperemia in pts with superficial corneal vascularity. Combination solutions relieve discomfort due to minor eye irritations and symptoms related to dry eyes. **Intranasal:** Relief of nasal congestion of rhinitis, the common cold, sinusitis, hay fever, or other allergies; reduces swelling and improves visualization for surgery or diagnostic procedures; opens obstructed eustachian ostia in pts with ear inflammation.

PRECAUTIONS

CONTRAINDICATIONS: Children <2 yrs of age (the 0.1% nasal solution is contraindicated in children <6 yrs of age); angle closure glaucoma or other serious eye diseases. **CAUTIONS:** Cardiac disease, hyperthyroidism, hypertension, diabetes mellitus, cerebral arteriosclerosis, bronchial asthma, MAO inhibitors.

INTERACTIONS

DRUG: Maprotiline, tricyclic antidepressants may increase pressor effects. **MAO inhibitors** may cause severe hypertensive reaction. **HERBAL: Ma Huang (Ephedra)** may increase CNS stimulation. **FOOD:** None known. **LAB VALUES:** None significant.

AVAILABILITY (OTC)

NASAL SOLUTION: 0.05%, 0.1%.
OPHTHALMIC SOLUTION: 0.05%.

ADMINISTRATION/HANDLING

Ophthalmic:

• Instruct pt to tilt head backward and look up. • Place finger on lower eyelid and pull out until a pocket is formed between eye and lower lid. Hold dropper above pocket and place correct number of drops into pocket. Close eye gently. • Apply gentle finger pressure to lacrimal sac (bridge of the nose, inside corner of the eye) for 1–2 min. • Remove excess solution around eye with tissue.

Intranasal:

• Drops should be administered with pt in lateral, head-low position or reclining with head tilted back as far as possible. • Pt should maintain same position for 5 min, then drops applied to other nostril. • Dropper containers should be used by only one person; tips of dispensers or droppers should be rinsed well with hot water after use.

INDICATIONS/ROUTES/DOSAGE

Usual nasal dosage:

Adults, elderly, children >6 yrs: 2–4 drops (0.1% solution) to each nostril q4–6h (no sooner than q3h). **Children, 2–6 yrs:** 2–3 drops (0.05% solution) to each nostril q4–6h (no sooner than q3h).

Usual ophthalmic dosage:

Adults, elderly, children: 1–2 drops (0.05%) 2–4 times/day.

SIDE EFFECTS

OCCASIONAL: Intranasal: Transient burning, stinging, sneezing, dryness of mucosa. ***Ophthalmic:*** Irritation, blurred vision, mydriasis. Systemic sympathomimetic effects may occur with either route: headache, hypertension, weakness, sweating, palpitations, tremors. Prolonged use may result in rebound congestion.

ADVERSE REACTIONS/TOXIC EFFECTS

Overdosage may result in CNS depression with drowsiness, decreased body temperature, bradycardia, hypotension, coma, apnea.

NURSING IMPLICATIONS

PATIENT/FAMILY TEACHING:

Overuse of vasoconstrictors may produce rebound congestion, hyperemia. Avoid excessive dosage, prolonged or too frequent use. ***Ophthalmic:*** Remove contact lenses before administration. Do not use with wetting agents for contact lenses. Discontinue and consult physician immediately if ocular pain or visual changes occur, if condition worsens or continues >72 hrs. ***Intranasal:*** Discontinue and consult physician if rebound congestion occurs.

thalidomide

thah-**lid**-owe-mide
(Thalomid)

▶CLASSIFICATION

PHARMACOTHERAPEUTIC: Immunomodulator. ***CLINICAL:*** Immunosuppressive

ACTION/*THERAPEUTIC EFFECT*

Exact mechanism unknown. Has sedative, anti-inflammatory, and immunosuppressive activity. Action may be due to selective inhibition of the production of tumor necrosis factor alpha.

USES/*UNLABELED*

Treatment of leprosy. *Wasting syndrome of HIV or cancer, recurrent aphthous ulcers in HIV pts, multiple myeloma, Crohn's disease.*

PRECAUTIONS

CONTRAINDICATIONS: Sensitivity to thalidomide, neutropenia, peripheral neuropathy; pregnancy. ***CAUTIONS:*** History of seizures.

INTERACTIONS

DRUG: Alcohol, CNS depressants may increase sedative effects. Medication associated with peripheral neuropath (e.g., **INH, lithium, metronmidazole, phenytoin**). Medications decreasing effectiveness of oral contraceptives (e.g., **carbamazepine, protease inhibitors, refampin**). ***HERBAL:*** None significant. ***FOOD:*** None signifcant. ***LAB VALUES:*** None significant.

AVAILABILITY (Rx)

CAPSULES: 50 mg.

INDICATIONS/ROUTES/DOSAGE

AIDS-related muscle wasting:
PO: Adults: 100–200 mg daily.

T

SIDE EFFECTS

FREQUENT: Drowsiness, dizziness, mood changes, constipation, xerostimia, peripheral neuropathy. **OCCASIONAL:** Increased appetite, weight gain, headache, loss of libido, edema of face and limbs, nausea, hair loss, dry skin, skin rash, hypothyroidism.

ADVERSE REACTIONS/TOXIC EFFECTS

Neutropenia, peripheral neuropathy.

NURSING IMPLICATIONS

BASELINE ASSESSMENT:
Assess for hypersensitivity to thalidomide, if pregnant (contraindicated). Determine use of other medications (many interactions).

INTERVENTION/EVALUATION:
Monitor WBC, peripheral neuropathy, nerve conduction studies, HIV viral load.

PATIENT/FAMILY TEACHING:
Avoid use of alcoholic beverages, other drugs causing drowsiness. Pregnancy test within 24 hrs prior to starting thalidomide, then q2–4wks in women of childbearing age. Discontinue and call physician if symptoms of peripheral neuropathy occur.

thiamine hydrochloride (vitamin B₁)

thigh-ah-min
(Betalin, Betaxin ♣)

▶CLASSIFICATION

PHARMACOTHERAPEUTIC: Water-soluble vitamin. **CLINICAL:** Vitamin B complex (see p. 127C)

ACTION/THERAPEUTIC EFFECT

Combines with adenosine triphosphate (ATP) in liver, kidney, leukocytes to form thiamine diphosphate, *necessary for carbohydrate metabolism.*

PHARMACOKINETICS

Readily absorbed from GI tract primarily in duodenum, after IM administration. Widely distributed. Metabolized in liver. Primarily excreted in urine.

USES

Prevention/treatment of thiamine deficiency (e.g., beriberi, alcoholic with altered sensorium).

PRECAUTIONS

CONTRAINDICATIONS: None significant. **CAUTIONS:** None significant.
▷**LIFESPAN CONSIDERATIONS:**
Pregnancy/Lactation: Crosses placenta; unknown if excreted in breast milk. **Pregnancy Category A** (Category C if used in doses above RDA). **Children/Elderly:** No age-related precautions noted.

INTERACTIONS

DRUG: None significant. **HERBAL:** None known. **FOOD:** None known. **LAB VALUES:** None significant.

AVAILABILITY (OTC)

TABLETS: 5 mg, 10 mg, 25 mg, 50 mg, 100 mg, 250 mg, 500 mg. **INJECTION (Rx):** 100 mg/ml.

ADMINISTRATION/HANDLING

Note: IM/IV administration used only in acutely ill or those unresponsive to PO route (GI malabsorption syndrome). IM route preferred to IV use. Give by IV push, or add to most IV solutions and give as infusion.

IV COMPATIBILITIES

Famotidine (Pepcid), multivitamins.

INDICATIONS/ROUTES/DOSAGE

Dietary supplement:

PO: **Adults, elderly:** 1–2 mg/day. **Children:** 0.5–1 mg/day. **Infants:** 0.3–0.5 mg/day.

Thiamine deficiency:

PO: **Adults, elderly:** 5–30 mg/ day, in single or 3 divided doses, for 1 mo. **Children:** 10–50 mg/day in 3 divided doses.

Critically ill/malabsorption syndrome:

IM/IV: **Adults, elderly:** 5–100 mg, 3 times/day. **Children:** 10–25 mg/ day.

Metabolic disorders:

PO: **Adults, elderly, children:** 10–20 mg/day; up to 4 g in divided doses/day.

SIDE EFFECTS

FREQUENT: Pain, induration, tenderness at IM injection site.

ADVERSE REACTIONS/TOXIC EFFECTS

Rare, severe hypersensitivity reaction with IV administration may result in feeling of warmth, pruritus, urticaria, weakness, sweating, nausea, restlessness, tightness of throat, angioedema (swelling of face/lips), cyanosis, pulmonary edema, GI tract bleeding, cardiovascular collapse.

NURSING IMPLICATIONS

INTERVENTION/EVALUATION:

Monitor lab values for erythrocyte activity, EKG readings. Assess for clinical improvement (improved sense of well-being, weight gain). Observe for reversal of deficiency symptoms (**neurologic:** peripheral neuropathy, hyporeflexia, nystagmus, ophthalmoplegia, ataxia, muscle weakness; **cardiac:** venous hypertension, bounding arterial pulse, tachycardia, edema; **mental:** confused state).

PATIENT/FAMILY TEACHING:

Discomfort may occur with IM injection. Foods rich in thiamine include pork, organ meats, whole grain and enriched cereals, legumes, nuts, seeds, yeast, wheat germ, rice bran.

thioguanine

thigh-oh-**guan**-een
(Thioguanine)

See Classification section under: Antineoplastics (p. 74C)

thiopental sodium

(Pentothal)

See Classification section under: Anesthetics: general (p. 3C)

T

thioridazine

thigh-oh-**rid**-ah-zeen
(Apo-Thioridazine✿, Mellaril)
Do not confuse with Mebaral,
thiothixene, Thorazine.

▶CLASSIFICATION

PHARMACOTHERAPEUTIC:
Phenothiazine. ***CLINICAL:*** Antipsychotic, sedative, antidyskinetic (see p. 56C)

ACTION/*THERAPEUTIC EFFECT*

Blocks dopamine at postsynaptic receptor sites, *suppressing
behavioral response in psychosis, reducing locomotor activity,
aggressiveness, suppressing conditioned responses.* Possesses
strong anticholinergic, sedative
effects.

USES

Treatment of refractory schizophrenic pts.

PRECAUTIONS

CONTRAINDICATIONS: Severe
CNS depression, comatose states,
severe cardiovascular disease,
bone marrow depression, subcortical brain damage. ***CAUTIONS:*** Impaired respiratory/hepatic/renal/
cardiac function, alcohol withdrawal, history of seizures, urinary
retention, glaucoma, prostatic
hypertrophy, hypocalcemia (increases susceptibility to dystonias).
May prolong QT interval.

INTERACTIONS

***DRUG:* Alcohol, CNS depres-
sants** may increase CNS, respiratory depression, hypotensive
effects. **Tricyclic antidepres-

sants, MAO inhibitors** may increase sedative, anticholinergic
effects. **Antithyroid agents** may
increase risk of agranulocytosis.
Extrapyramidal symptoms (EPS)
may increase with **EPS-producing medications. Hypotensives**
may increase hypotension. May
decrease **levodopa** effects. **Lithium** may decrease absorption,
produce adverse neurologic
effects. ***HERBAL:*** None known.
FOOD: None known. ***LAB VAL-
UES:*** May cause EKG changes.
Therapeutic blood serum level:
0.2–2.6 mcg/ml; toxic blood
serum level: N/E.

INDICATIONS/ROUTES/DOSAGE
Psychosis:

***PO:* Adults, elderly, children >12
yrs:** Initially, 25–100 mg 3 times/
day. Gradually increase. **Maximum:** 800 mg/day. **Children 2–12
yrs:** Initially, 0.5 mg/kg/day in 2–3
divided doses. **Maximum:** 3 mg/
kg/day.

SIDE EFFECTS

Generally well tolerated with only
mild and transient effects. ***OCCA-
SIONAL:*** Drowsiness during early
therapy, dry mouth, blurred vision,
lethargy, constipation or diarrhea,
nasal congestion, peripheral edema, urinary retention. ***RARE:*** Ocular changes, skin pigmentation
(those on high doses for prolonged periods).

ADVERSE REACTIONS/TOXIC
EFFECTS

Prolongation of QT interval may
produce torsade de pointes (a
form of ventricular tachycardia)
and sudden death.

NURSING IMPLICATIONS

BASELINE ASSESSMENT:

Avoid skin contact with solution (contact dermatitis). Assess behavior, appearance, emotional status, response to environment, speech pattern, thought content.

INTERVENTION/EVALUATION:

Monitor B/P for hypotension. Assess for extrapyramidal symptoms. Monitor WBC, differential count for blood dyscrasias. Monitor for fine tongue movement (may be early sign of tardive dyskinesia). Supervise suicidal risk pt closely during early therapy (as depression lessens, energy level improves, but suicide potential increases). Assess for therapeutic response (interest in surroundings, improvement in self-care, increased ability to concentrate, relaxed facial expression). Therapeutic blood serum level: 0.2–2.6 mcg/ml; toxic blood serum level: N/E.

PATIENT/FAMILY TEACHING:

Full therapeutic effect may take up to 6 wks. Urine may darken. Do not abruptly withdraw from long-term drug therapy. Report visual disturbances. Sugarless gum, sips of tepid water may relieve dry mouth. Drowsiness generally subsides during continued therapy. Avoid tasks that require alertness, motor skills until response to drug is established.

thiotepa

thigh-oh-**teh**-pah
(Thioplex, Thiotepa)

▶CLASSIFICATION

PHARMACOTHERAPEUTIC:
Alkylating agent. ***CLINICAL:***
Antineoplastic (see p. 74C)

ACTION/*THERAPEUTIC EFFECT*

Binds with many intracellular structures. Cross-links strands of DNA, RNA, disrupting protein synthesis, *producing malignant cell death.* Cell cycle-phase nonspecific.

USES/*UNLABELED*

Treatment of superficial papillary carcinoma of urinary bladder, adenocarcinoma of breast and ovary, Hodgkin's disease, lymphosarcoma. Intracavitary injection to control pleural, pericardial, or peritoneal effusions due to metastatic tumors. *Treatment of lung carcinoma.*

PRECAUTIONS

CONTRAINDICATIONS: Existing hepatic, renal, bone marrow damage unless drug administered in low doses, concurrent use with alkylating agents or radiation therapy until pt recovers from myelosuppression. ***CAUTIONS:*** None significant.

INTERACTIONS

DRUG: May decrease effect of **antigout** medications. **Bone marrow depressants** may increase bone marrow depression. **Live virus vaccines** may potentiate virus replication, increase vaccine side effects, decrease pt's antibody response to vaccine. ***HERBAL:*** None known. ***FOOD:*** None known. ***LAB VALUES:*** May increase uric acid.

AVAILABILITY (Rx)

POWDER FOR INJECTION: 15 mg.

ADMINISTRATION/HANDLING

Note: May be carcinogenic, mutagenic, or teratogenic. Handle with extreme care during preparation/administration.

IV 💊

Note: Give by IV, intrapleural, intraperitoneal, intrapericardial, or intratumor injection; intravesical instillation.

Storage:

• Refrigerate unopened vials. • Reconstituted solution appears clear to slightly opaque; is stable for 5 days if refrigerated. Discard if solution appears grossly opaque or precipitate forms.

Reconstitution:

• Reconstitute 15 mg vial with 1.5 ml Sterile Water for Injection to provide concentration of 10 mg/ml. Shake solution gently; let stand to clear.

Rate of administration:

• For IV push, administer each 60 mg or fraction thereof over 1 min. • For intracavitary use, IV infusion, perfusion therapy, further dilute with D_5W, 0.9% NaCl.

IV INCOMPATIBILITIES ⊘

Do not mix with any other medications.

IV COMPATIBILITIES

Allopurinol (Aloprim), calcium gluconate, dexamethasone (Decadron), diphenhydramine (Benadryl), granisetron (Kytril), magnesium, ondansetron (Zofran), potassium chloride.

INDICATIONS/ROUTES/DOSAGE

Note: Dosage individualized based on clinical response, tolerance to adverse effects. When used in combination therapy, consult specific protocols for optimum dosage, sequence of drug administration.

Initial treatment:

IV: Adults, elderly: 0.3–0.4 mg/kg q1–4wks. Maintenance dose adjusted weekly on basis of blood counts. **Children:** 25–65 mg/m^2 as a single dose q3–4wks.

INTRACAVITARY: Adults, elderly: 0.6–0.8 mg/kg q1–4wks.

SIDE EFFECTS

OCCASIONAL: Pain at injection site, headache, dizziness, hives, rash, nausea, vomiting, anorexia, stomatitis. **RARE:** Alopecia, cystitis, hematuria following intravesical dosing.

ADVERSE REACTIONS/TOXIC EFFECTS

Hematologic toxicity manifested as leukopenia, anemia, thrombocytopenia, pancytopenia due to bone marrow depression. Although WBC falls to lowest point at 10–14 days after initial therapy, bone marrow effects not evident for 30 days. Stomatitis, ulceration of intestinal mucosa may be noted.

NURSING IMPLICATIONS

BASELINE ASSESSMENT:

Interrupt therapy if WBC falls below 3,000/mm^3, platelet count below 150,000/mm^3, WBC or platelet count declines rapidly. Obtain hematologic status at least weekly during therapy and for 3 wks after therapy discontinued.

INTERVENTION/EVALUATION:

Monitor uric acid serum levels, hematology tests. Assess for stomatitis (burning/erythema of oral mucosa at inner margin of lips, sore throat, difficulty swallowing, oral ulceration). Monitor for hematologic toxicity: infection (fever, sore throat, signs of local infection), easy bruising, unusual bleeding from any site, symptoms of anemia (excessive tiredness, weakness). Assess skin for rash, hives.

PATIENT/FAMILY TEACHING:

Maintain fastidious oral hygiene. Do not have immunizations without physician's approval (drug lowers body's resistance). Avoid crowds, those with infection. Promptly report fever, sore throat, signs of local infection, easy bruising, unusual bleeding from any site.

thiothixene

thigh-oh-**thicks**-een
(Navane)
Do not confuse with thioridazine.

▶CLASSIFICATION

CLINICAL: Antipsychotic (see p. 56C)

ACTION/THERAPEUTIC EFFECT

Blocks postsynaptic dopamine receptor sites in brain. Has alpha-adrenergic blocking effects; depresses release of hypothalamic, hypophyseal hormones. *Suppresses behavioral response in psychosis.*

PHARMACOKINETICS

	Onset	Peak	Duration
IM	—	1–6 hrs	—

Well absorbed from GI tract, after IM administration. Widely distrib-uted. Metabolized in liver. Primarily excreted in urine. Unknown if removed by hemodialysis. Half-life: 34 hrs.

USES

Symptomatic management of psychotic disorders.

PRECAUTIONS

CONTRAINDICATIONS: Comatose states, circulatory collapse, CNS depression, blood dyscrasias. **EXTREME CAUTION:** History of seizures. **CAUTIONS:** Severe cardiovascular disorders, alcoholic withdrawal, pt exposure to extreme heat, glaucoma, prostatic hypertrophy.

▷**LIFESPAN CONSIDERATIONS:**
Pregnancy/Lactation: Crosses placenta; distributed in breast milk. **Pregnancy Category C. Children:** May develop neuromuscular or extrapyramidal symptoms, esp. dystonias. **Elderly:** More prone to orthostatic hypotension, anticholinergic effects (e.g., dry mouth), sedation or extrapyramidal symptoms.

INTERACTIONS

DRUG: Alcohol, CNS depressants may increase CNS, respiratory depression, increase hypotension. **Extrapyramidal symptom (EPS)–producing medications** may increase risk of EPS. May inhibit effects of **levodopa.** May increase cardiac effects with **quinidine. HERBAL:** None known. **FOOD:** None known. **LAB VALUES:** May decrease uric acid.

AVAILABILITY (Rx)

CAPSULES: 1 mg, 2 mg, 5 mg, 10 mg, 20 mg. **ORAL CONCENTRATE:** 5 mg/ml.

T

ADMINISTRATION/HANDLING
PO:
• Give without regard to meals. • Avoid skin contact with oral solution (contact dermatitis).

INDICATIONS/ROUTES/DOSAGE
Pschosis:
PO: Adults, elderly, children >12 yrs: Initially, 2 mg 3 times/day. **Maximum:** 60 mg/day.

SIDE EFFECTS
Hypotension, dizziness, fainting occur frequently after first injection, occasionally after subsequent injections, rarely with oral dosage. *FREQUENT:* Transient drowsiness, dry mouth, constipation, blurred vision, nasal congestion. *OCCASIONAL:* Diarrhea, peripheral edema, urinary retention, nausea. *RARE:* Ocular changes, skin pigmentation (those on high dosage for prolonged periods).

ADVERSE REACTIONS/TOXIC EFFECTS
Frequently noted extrapyramidal symptom is akathisia (motor restlessness, anxiety). Occurring less frequently is akinesia (rigidity, tremor, salivation, masklike facial expression, reduced voluntary movements). Infrequently noted are dystonias: torticollis (neck muscle spasm), opisthotonos (rigidity of back muscles), and oculogyric crisis (rolling back of eyes). Tardive dyskinesia (protrusion of tongue, puffing of cheeks, chewing/puckering of mouth) occurs rarely but may be irreversible. Risk is greater in female geriatric pts. Grand mal seizures may occur in epileptic pts (risk higher with IM administration).

NURSING IMPLICATIONS

BASELINE ASSESSMENT:
Assess behavior, appearance, emotional status, response to environment, speech pattern, thought content.

INTERVENTION/EVALUATION:
Supervise suicidal risk pt closely during early therapy (as depression lessens, energy level improves, increasing suicide potential). Monitor B/P for hypotension. Assess for peripheral edema. Assess stools; prevent constipation. Monitor for EPS, tardive dyskinesia (see Adverse Reactions/Toxic Effects) and potentially fatal, rare neuroleptic malignant syndrome: fever, irregular pulse or B/P, muscle rigidity, altered mental status. Assess for therapeutic response (interest in surroundings, improvement in self-care, increased ability to concentrate, relaxed facial expression).

PATIENT/FAMILY TEACHING:
Full therapeutic effect may take up to 6 wks. Report visual disturbances. Sugarless gum, sips of tepid water may relieve dry mouth. Drowsiness generally subsides during continued therapy. Avoid tasks that require alertness, motor skills until response to drug is established. Avoid alcohol and other CNS depressants.

thyroid

(Armour Thyroid, S-P-T, Thyrar)

See Classification section under: Thyroid (p. 126C)

tiagabine

tie-**ag**-ah-bean
(Gabitril)

►CLASSIFICATION

CLINICAL: Anticonvulsant (see p. 33C)

ACTION/*THERAPEUTIC EFFECT*

Blocks reuptake of gamma aminobutyric acid (GABA) in the presynaptic neurons, the major inhibitory neurotransmitter in the CNS, increasing GABA levels at postsynaptic neurons, *inhibiting seizures.*

USES

Adjunctive therapy for treatment of partial seizures.

PRECAUTIONS

CONTRAINDICATIONS: None significant. **CAUTIONS:** Hepatic function impairment.

INTERACTIONS

DRUG: May alter **valproate** effect. **Carbamazepine, phenytoin, phenobarbital** may increase tiagabine clearance. **HERBAL:** None known. **FOOD:** None known. **LAB VALUES:** None significant.

AVAILABILITY (Rx)

TABLETS: 2 mg, 4 mg, 12 mg, 16 mg, 20 mg.

INDICATIONS/ROUTES/DOSAGE

Partial seizures:

PO: Adults: Initially, 4 mg once daily. May increase by 4–8 mg/day at weekly intervals. **Maximum:** 56 mg/day. **Children (12–18 yrs):** Initially, 4 mg once daily, may increase by 4 mg at week 2 and by 4–8 mg/week thereafter. **Maximum:** 32 mg/day.

SIDE EFFECTS

FREQUENT (20–34%): Dizziness, asthenia (loss of strength, energy), somnolence, nervousness, confusion, headache, infection, tremor. **OCCASIONAL:** Nausea, diarrhea, stomach pain, trouble concentrating, weakness.

ADVERSE REACTIONS/TOXIC EFFECTS

Overdosage characterized by agitation, confusion, hostility, weakness. Full recovery occurs within 24 hrs.

NURSING IMPLICATIONS

BASELINE ASSESSMENT:

Review history of seizure disorder (intensity, frequency, duration, LOC). Observe frequently for recurrence of seizure activity. Initiate seizure precautions.

INTERVENTION/EVALUATION:

For those on long-term therapy, liver/renal function tests, blood counts should be performed periodically. Assist with ambulation if dizziness occurs. Assess for clinical improvement (decrease in intensity/frequency of seizures).

PATIENT/FAMILY TEACHING:

If dizziness occurs, change positions slowly from recumbent to sitting position before standing. Avoid tasks that require alertness, motor skills until response to drug is established. Avoid alcohol.

T

---

ticarcillin disodium

(Ticar)

**See Classification section
under: Antibiotics:
penicillins**

ticarcillin disodium/
clavulanate potassium

tie-car-**sill**-in/klah-view-**lan**-ate
(Timentin)

▶CLASSIFICATION

PHARMACOTHERAPEUTIC:
Penicillin. ***CLINICAL:*** Antibiotic
(see p. 27C)

ACTION/*THERAPEUTIC EFFECT*

Ticarcillin: Binds to bacterial cell
wall inhibiting bacterial cell wall
synthesis, *causing cell lysis, death.*
Clavulanate: Inhibits bacterial
beta-lactamase *protecting ticarcillin from enzymatic degradation.*
Bactericidal.

PHARMACOKINETICS

Widely distributed. Protein binding: 45–65%. Minimal metabolism
in liver. Primarily excreted unchanged in urine. Removed by hemodialysis. Half-life: 1–1.2 hrs
(half-life increased with impaired
renal function).

USES

Treatment of septicemia, skin/skin
structure, bone and joint, lower
respiratory, urinary tract infections, endometritis.

PRECAUTIONS

CONTRAINDICATIONS: Hypersensitivity to any penicillin. ***CAU-
TIONS:*** History of allergies, esp.
cephalosporins.

▷*LIFESPAN CONSIDERATIONS:*
Pregnancy/Lactation: Readily
crosses placenta, appears in cord
blood, amniotic fluid. Distributed
in breast milk in low concentrations. May lead to allergic sensitization, diarrhea, candidiasis, skin
rash in infant. **Pregnancy Category B. Children:** Safety and efficacy not established in those <3
mos of age. **Elderly:** Age-related
renal impairment may require
dosage adjustment.

INTERACTIONS

DRUG: **Anticoagulants, heparin,
thrombolytics, NSAIDs** may increase risk of hemorrhage with
high doses of ticarcillin. **Probenecid**
may increase concentration, risk of
toxicity. ***HERBAL:*** None known.
FOOD: None known. ***LAB VALUES:***
May cause positive Coombs' test.
May increase SGOT (AST), SGPT
(ALT), alkaline phosphatase, bilirubin, creatinine, LDH, bleeding time.
May decrease potassium, sodium,
uric acid.

AVAILABILITY (Rx)

POWDER FOR INJECTION: 3.1 g.
SOLUTION FOR INFUSION: 3.1
g/100 ml.

ADMINISTRATION/HANDLING
IV

Storage:

• Solution appears colorless to
pale yellow (if solution darkens, indicates loss of potency). • IV infusion (piggyback) is stable for 24
hrs at room temperature, 3 days if
refrigerated. • Discard if precipitate forms.

Reconstitution:

• Available in ready to use containers. • For IV infusion (piggyback), reconstitute each 3.1 g vial with 13 ml Sterile Water for Injection or 0.9% NaCl to provide concentration of 200 mg ticarcillin and 6.7 mg clavulanic acid per ml. • Shake vial to assist reconstitution. • Further dilute with 50–100 ml D_5W or 0.9% NaCl.

Rate of administration:

• Infuse over 30 min. • Because of potential for hypersensitivity/anaphylaxis, start initial dose at few drops/min, increase slowly to ordered rate; stay with pt first 10–15 min, then check q10min.

IV INCOMPATIBILITIES $\oslash$

Amphotericin B complex (Abelcet, Ambisome, Amphotec), vancomycin (Vancocin).

IV COMPATIBILITIES

Diltiazem (Cardizem), heparin, insulin, propofol (Diprivan).

INDICATIONS/ROUTES/DOSAGE

Systemic infections:

IV: Adults, elderly: 3.1 g (3 g ticarcillin) q4–6h. **Maximum:** 18–24 g/day. **Children >3 mo:** 200–300 mg (as ticarcillin) q4–6h.

UTI:

IV: Adults, elderly: 3.1 g q6–8h.

Dosage in renal impairment:

Creatinine Clearance	Dosage Interval
10–30 ml/min	q8h
<10 ml/min	q12h

SIDE EFFECTS

FREQUENT: Phlebitis, thrombophlebitis with IV dose, rash, urticaria, pruritus, taste/smell disturbances. ***OCCASIONAL:*** Nausea, diarrhea, vomiting. ***RARE:*** Headache, fatigue, hallucinations, bruising/bleeding.

ADVERSE REACTIONS/TOXIC EFFECTS

Overdosage may produce seizures, neurologic reactions. Superinfections, potentially fatal antibiotic-associated colitis may result from bacterial imbalance. Severe hypersensitivity reactions, including anaphylaxis, occur rarely.

NURSING IMPLICATIONS

BASELINE ASSESSMENT:

Question for history of allergies, esp. penicillins, cephalosporins.

INTERVENTION/EVALUATION:

Hold medication and promptly report rash (hypersensitivity) or diarrhea (with fever, abdominal pain, mucus and blood in stool may indicate antibiotic-associated colitis). Assess food tolerance. Provide mouth care, sugarless gum or hard candy to offset taste, smell effects. Evaluate IV site for phlebitis (heat, pain, red streaking over vein). Monitor I&O, urinalysis, renal function tests. Assess for bleeding: overt bleeding, bruising or tissue swelling; check hematology reports. Monitor electrolytes, particularly potassium. Be alert for superinfection: increased fever, onset of sore throat, diarrhea, vomiting, ulceration or other oral changes, anal/genital pruritus.

PATIENT/FAMILY TEACHING:

Continue antibiotic for full length of treatment. Space doses evenly. Notify physician in event of rash, diarrhea, bleeding, bruising, or other new symptom.

ticlopidine hydrochloride

tie-**clow**-pih-deen
(Apo-Ticlopidine ✦, Ticlid)

►CLASSIFICATION

PHARMACOTHERAPEUTIC:
Aggregation inhibitor. *CLINICAL:* Antiplatelet (see p. 30C)

ACTION/*THERAPEUTIC EFFECT*

Inhibits release of platelet granule constituents, platelet-platelet interactions, and adhesion to endothelium and atheromatous plaque, *preventing platelet aggregation.*

USES/*UNLABELED*

To reduce risk of stroke in those who have experienced strokelike warnings or those with history of thrombotic stroke. *Treatment of intermittent claudication, subarachnoid hemorrhage, sickle cell disease.*

PRECAUTIONS

CONTRAINDICATIONS: Hematopoietic disorders (neutropenia, thrombocytopenia), presence of hemostatic disorder, active pathologic bleeding (bleeding peptic ulcer, intracranial bleeding), severe liver impairment. *CAUTIONS:* Those at risk of increased bleeding from trauma, surgery, pathologic conditions.

INTERACTIONS

DRUG: May increase risk of bleeding with **oral anticoagulants, heparin, thrombolytics, aspirin. HERBAL:** None known. *FOOD:* None known. *LAB VALUES:* May increase alkaline phosphatase, bilirubin, liver function tests, cholesterol, triglycerides. May prolong bleeding time. May decrease neutrophil, platelet count.

AVAILABILITY (Rx)

TABLETS: 250 mg.

ADMINISTRATION/HANDLING

PO:
• Give with food or just after meals (bioavailability increased, GI discomfort decreased).

INDICATIONS/ROUTES/DOSAGE

Prevention of stroke:
PO: **Adults, elderly:** 250 mg 2 times/day.

SIDE EFFECTS

FREQUENT (5–13%): Diarrhea, nausea, dyspepsia (heartburn, indigestion, GI discomfort, bloating). *RARE* (1–2%): Vomiting, flatulence, pruritus, dizziness.

ADVERSE REACTIONS/TOXIC EFFECTS

Neutropenia occurs in approx. 2% of pts. Thrombotic thrombocytopenia purpura (TTD), agranulocytosis, hepatitis, cholestatic jaundice, tinnitus occur rarely.

NURSING IMPLICATIONS

BASELINE ASSESSMENT:

Drug should be discontinued 10–14 days before surgery if antiplatelet effect is not desired.

INTERVENTION/EVALUATION:

Monitor bowel activity, stool consistency. Assist with ambulation if dizziness occurs. Monitor heart sounds by auscultation. Assess B/P for hypotension. Assess skin for flushing, rash.

PATIENT/FAMILY TEACHING:
If nausea occurs, cola, unsalted crackers, or dry toast may relieve effect. Therapeutic response may not be achieved before 2–3 mos of continuous therapy. Report any unusual bleeding/bruising.

tiludronate

tie-**lew**-dro-nate
(Skelid)

►CLASSIFICATION
PHARMACOTHERAPEUTIC: Bone resorption inhibitor. **CLINICAL:** Calcium regulator

ACTION/*THERAPEUTIC EFFECT*
Inhibits functioning osteoclasts through disruption of cytoskeletal ring structure and inhibition of osteoclastic proton pump, *inhibiting bone resorption.*

USES
Treatment of Paget's disease of bone (osteitis deformans).

PRECAUTIONS
CONTRAINDICATIONS: GI disease (e.g., dysphagia, gastric ulcer), impaired renal function. **CAUTIONS:** Hyperparathyroidism, hypocalcemia, vitamin D deficiency.

INTERACTIONS
DRUG: Aluminum- or magnesium-containing antacids, **calcium, salicylates** may interfere with tiludronate absorption. **HERBAL:** None known. **FOOD:** None known. **LAB VALUES:** None significant

AVAILABILITY (Rx)
TABLETS: 200 mg.

INDICATIONS/ROUTES/DOSAGE
Paget's disease:

PO: Adults: 400 mg once daily for 3 mos. Must take with 6–8 oz plain water. Do not take within 2 hrs of food intake. Avoid taking aspirin, calcium supplements, mineral supplements, and antacids within 2 hrs of taking tiludronate.

SIDE EFFECTS
FREQUENT (6–9%): Nausea, diarrhea, generalized body pain, back pain, headache. **OCCASIONAL:** Rash, dyspepsia, vomiting, rhinitis, sinusitis, dizziness.

NURSING IMPLICATIONS

BASELINE ASSESSMENT:
Assess if pt is pregnant, using medications (esp. aluminum, magnesium, calcium, salicylates). Determine baseline renal function. Assess for GI disease.

INTERVENTION/EVALUATION:
Monitor alkaline phosphatase to assess effectiveness of medication.

PATIENT/FAMILY TEACHING:
Take with 6–8 oz water. Check with physician if calcium and vitamin D supplements are necessary.

timolol maleate

tim-oh-lol
(Apo-Timol ♣, Betimol, Blocadren, Timoptic, Timoptic XE)
Do not confuse with atenolol, Viroptic.

FIXED-COMBINATION(S)

With hydrochlorothiazide, a diuretic **(Timolide)**; with dorzolamide, a carbonic anhydrase inhibitor **(Cosopt)**

▶CLASSIFICATION

PHARMACOTHERAPEUTIC:
Beta-adrenergic blocker. ***CLINICAL:*** Antihypertensive, antimigraine, antiglaucoma (see pp. 46C, 61C)

ACTION/*THERAPEUTIC EFFECT*

Blocks beta$_1$-adrenergic receptors, *slowing sinus heart rate, decreasing cardiac output, decreasing B/P.* Blocks beta$_2$-adrenergic receptors, *increasing airway resistance.* Decreases myocardial ischemia severity by decreasing O_2 requirements. *Reduces intraocular pressure (IOP).*

PHARMACOKINETICS

Onset	Peak	Duration
Eye drops		
30 min	1–2 hrs	12–24 hrs

Well absorbed from GI tract. Protein binding: <10%. Minimal absorption following ophthalmic administration. Metabolized in liver. Primarily excreted in urine. Not removed by hemodialysis. Half-life: 4 hrs. **Ophthalmic:** Systemic absorption may occur.

USES/*UNLABELED*

Management of mild to moderate hypertension. Used alone or in combination with diuretics, esp. thiazide type. Reduces cardiovascular mortality in those with definite/suspected acute MI. Prophylaxis of migraine headache. **Ophthalmic:** Reduces IOP in management of open-angle glaucoma, aphakic glaucoma, ocular hypertension, secondary glaucoma. *Systemic:* Treatment of chronic angina pectoris, cardiac arrhythmias, hypertrophic cardiomyopathy, pheochromocytoma, tremors, anxiety, thyrotoxicosis, migraines. **Ophthalmic:** *With miotics decreases IOP in acute/chronic angle closure glaucoma, treatment of secondary glaucoma, malignant glaucoma, angle closure glaucoma during/after iridectomy.*

PRECAUTIONS

CONTRAINDICATIONS: Bronchial asthma, COPD, uncontrolled cardiac failure, sinus bradycardia, heart block greater than first degree, cardiogenic shock, CHF unless secondary to tachyarrhythmias, those on MAO inhibitors. Precautions also apply to oral and ophthalmic administration (due to systemic absorption of ophthalmic). ***CAUTIONS:*** Inadequate cardiac function, impaired renal/hepatic function, hyperthyroidism.
▷***LIFESPAN CONSIDERATIONS:***
Pregnancy/Lactation: Distributed in breast milk; not for use in nursing women because of potential for serious adverse effect on nursing infant. Avoid use during first trimester. May produce bradycardia, apnea, hypoglycemia, hypothermia during delivery, small birth weight infants. **Pregnancy Category C** (Category D if used in second or third trimester). **Children:** Safety and efficacy not established. **Elderly:** Age-related peripheral vascular disease increases susceptibility to decreased peripheral circulation.

INTERACTIONS

DRUG: **Diuretics, other hypotensives** may increase hypotensive effect. **Sympathomimetics, xanthines** may mutually inhibit effects.

May mask symptoms of hypoglycemia, prolong hypoglycemic effect of **insulin, oral hypoglycemics. NSAIDs** may decrease antihypertensive effect. **HERBAL:** None known. **FOOD:** None known. **LAB VALUES:** May increase ANA titer, SGOT (AST), SGPT (ALT), alkaline phosphatase, LDH, bilirubin, BUN, creatinine, potassium, uric acid, lipoproteins, triglycerides.

AVAILABILITY (Rx)

TABLETS: 5 mg, 10 mg, 20 mg. **OPHTHALMIC SOLUTION:** 0.25%, 0.5%. **OPHTHALMIC GEL:** 0.25%, 0.5%.

ADMINISTRATION/HANDLING

PO:
• Give without regard to meals. • Tablets may be crushed.

Ophthalmic:
Note: When using gel, invert container, shake once prior to each use.

• Place finger on lower eyelid and pull out until pocket is formed between eye and lower lid. • Hold dropper above pocket and place prescribed number of drops or amount of prescribed gel into pocket. Instruct pt to close eyes gently so medication will not be squeezed out of sac. • Apply gentle finger pressure to the lacrimal sac at inner canthus for 1 min following installation (lessens risk of systemic absorption).

INDICATIONS/ROUTES/DOSAGE

Hypertension:
PO: Adults, elderly: Initially, 10 mg 2 times/day, alone or in combination with other therapy. Gradually increase at intervals of not less than 1 wk. **Maintenance:** 20–60 mg/day in 2 divided doses.

Myocardial infarction:
PO: Adults, elderly: 10 mg 2 times/day, beginning within 1–4 wks after infarction.

Migraine prophylaxis:
PO: Adults, elderly: Initially, 10 mg 2 times/day. **Range:** 10–30 mg/day.

Glaucoma:
OPHTHALMIC: Adults, elderly, children: 1 drop of 0.25% solution in affected eye(s) 2 times/day. May be increased to 1 drop of 0.5% solution in affected eye(s) 2 times/day. When IOP is controlled, dosage may be reduced to 1 drop 1 time/day. If pt is transferred to timolol from another antiglaucoma agent, administer concurrently for 1 day. Discontinue other agent on following day. *Timoptic XE:* **Adults, elderly:** 1 drop/day.

SIDE EFFECTS

FREQUENT: Decreased sexual ability, drowsiness, difficulty sleeping, unusual tiredness/weakness. **Ophthalmic:** Eye irritation, visual disturbances. **OCCASIONAL:** Depression, cold hands/feet, diarrhea, constipation, anxiety, nasal congestion, nausea, vomiting. **RARE:** Altered taste, dry eyes, itching, numbness of fingers, toes, scalp.

ADVERSE REACTIONS/TOXIC EFFECTS

Oral form may produce profound bradycardia, hypotension, bronchospasm. Abrupt withdrawal may result in sweating, palpitations, headache, tremulousness. May precipitate CHF, myocardial infarction in those with cardiac disease, thyroid storm in those with thyrotoxicosis, peripheral ischemia in those with existing peripheral vascular disease. Hypo-

T

glycemia may occur in previously controlled diabetics. Ophthalmic overdosage may produce brady-cardia, hypotension, broncho-spasm, acute cardiac failure.

NURSING IMPLICATIONS

BASELINE ASSESSMENT:

Assess B/P, apical pulse immediately before drug is administered (if pulse is 60/min or below, or systolic B/P is below 90 mm Hg, withhold medication, contact physician).

INTERVENTION/EVALUATION:

Assess pulse for strength/weakness, irregular rate, bradycardia. Monitor EKG for cardiac arrhythmias, particularly PVCs. Monitor stool frequency and consistency. Monitor I&O (increase in weight, decrease in urine output may indicate CHF). Assess for nausea, diaphoresis, headache, fatigue. **Ophthalmic:** Monitor B/P and pulse regularly.

PATIENT/FAMILY TEACHING:

Do not abruptly discontinue medication. Compliance with therapy regimen is essential to control glaucoma, hypertension, angina, arrhythmias. Avoid tasks that require alertness, motor skills until response to drug is established. Report shortness of breath, excessive fatigue, prolonged dizziness/headache. Do not use nasal decongestants, OTC cold preparations (stimulants) without physician approval. Restrict salt, alcohol intake. **Ophthalmic:** Teach pt how to instill drops correctly, how to take pulse. Transient stinging, discomfort may occur upon instillation.

tinzaparin sodium

tin-zah-**pare**-inn
(Innohep)

►CLASSIFICATION

PHARMACOTHERAPEUTIC: Low molecular weight heparin. **CLINICAL:** Anticoagulant (see p. 29C)

ACTION/THERAPEUTIC EFFECT

Produces anticoagulation by inhibition of factor Xa. Tinzaparin causes less inactivation of thrombin, inhibition of platelets, and bleeding than standard heparin. Does not significantly influence bleeding time, prothrombin time (PT), activated partial thromboplastin time (APTT).

PHARMACOKINETICS

Well absorbed following SubQ administration. Primarily eliminated in urine. Half-life: 3–4 hrs.

USES

Treatment of acute symptomatic deep vein thrombosis (DVT) with or without pulmonary embolism, when given in conjunction with warfarin.

PRECAUTIONS

CONTRAINDICATIONS: Active major bleeding, concurrent heparin therapy, thrombocytopenia associated with positive in vitro test for antiplatelet antibody, hypersensitivity to heparin or pork products. **CAUTIONS:** Conditions with increased risk of hemorrhage, history of heparin-induced thrombocytopenia, impaired renal function, elderly, uncontrolled arterial hypertension, history of recent GI ulceration and hemorrhage.

▷*LIFESPAN CONSIDERATIONS:*
Pregnancy/Lactation: Use with caution, particularly during last trimester, immediate postpartum period (increased risk of maternal hemorrhage). Unknown if distributed in breast milk. **Pregnancy Category B. Children:** Safety and efficacy not established. **Elderly:** May be more susceptible to bleeding.

INTERACTIONS

DRUG: **Anticoagulants, platelet inhibitors** may increase bleeding (use with care). *HERBAL:* None known. *FOOD:* **Ginkgo biloba** may increase risk of bleeding. *LAB VALUES:* Reversible increases in SGOT (AST), SGPT (ALT), alkaline phosphatase, lactic dehydrogenase (LDH).

AVAILABILITY (Rx)

INJECTION: 20,000 IU/ml.

ADMINISTRATION/HANDLING

Note: Do not mix with other injections or infusions. Do not give IM.

SubQ:

• Parenteral form appears clear and colorless to pale yellow. • Store at room temperature. • Instruct pt to lie down before administering by deep SubQ injection. • Introduce entire length of needle ($1/2$ inch) into skin fold held between thumb and forefinger, holding skin fold during injection. • Inject between left and right anterolateral and left and right posterolateral abdominal wall.

INDICATIONS/ROUTES/DOSAGE

Deep vein thrombosis (DVT):
SubQ: Adults, elderly: 175 IU/kg

given once daily. Continue at least 6 days and until pt is sufficiently anticoagulated with warfarin (INR 2 or greater for 2 consecutive days).

SIDE EFFECTS

FREQUENT (16%): Injection site reaction (inflammation, oozing, nodules, skin necrosis). *RARE* (<2%): Nausea, asthenia (unusual tiredness or weakness), constipation, epistaxis (nosebleed).

ADVERSE REACTIONS/TOXIC EFFECTS

Accidental overdosage may lead to bleeding complications ranging from local ecchymoses to major hemorrhage. *Antidote:* Dose of protamine sulfate (1% solution) should be equal to the dose of tinzaparin injected. One mg protamine sulfate neutralizes 100 IU of tinzaparin. A second dose of 0.5 mg/mg protamine sulfate may be given if APTT tested 2–4 hrs after the first infusion remains prolonged.

NURSING IMPLICATIONS

BASELINE ASSESSMENT:
Assess CBC, including platelet count. Determine initial B/P.

INTERVENTION/EVALUATION:
Periodically monitor CBC, platelet count. Assess for any sign of bleeding: bleeding at surgical site, hematuria, blood in stool, bleeding from gums, petechiae, bruising, bleeding from injection sites.

PATIENT/FAMILY TEACHING:
Usual length of therapy is 7–10 days. Do not take any OTC medication (esp. aspirin) without consulting physician.

T

tioconazole

tie-oh-**con**-ah-zole
(Gynecure♣, Monostat-1,
Trosyd♣, Vagistat)
Do not confuse with
terconazole.

▶CLASSIFICATION

PHARMACOTHERAPEUTIC:
Imidazole derivative. **CLINI-
CAL:** Antifungal

ACTION/*THERAPEUTIC EFFECT*
Inhibits synthesis of ergosterol
(vital component of fungal cell formation), *damaging fungal cell
membrane. Fungistatic.*

USES
Treatment of vulvovaginal candidiasis (moniliasis).

INTERACTIONS
DRUG: None significant. **HERBAL:**
None known. **FOOD:** None known.
LAB VALUES: None significant.

AVAILABILITY (OTC)
VAGINAL OINTMENT: 6.5%.

INDICATIONS/ROUTES/DOSAGE
Vulvovaginal candidiasis:
INTRAVAGINAL: Adults, elderly:
1 applicatorful just before bedtime
as a single dose.

SIDE EFFECTS
FREQUENT (25%): Headache.
OCCASIONAL (1–6%): Burning,
itching. **RARE** (<1%): Irritation,
vaginal pain, dysuria, dryness of
vaginal secretions, vulvar edema/
swelling.

tirofiban

tie-**row**-fih-ban
(Aggrastat)
Do not confuse with Aggrenox.

▶CLASSIFICATION

PHARMACOTHERAPEUTIC:
Glycoprotein (GP) IIb/IIIa inhibitor. **CLINICAL:** Antiplatelet,
antithrombotic (see p. 30C)

ACTION/*THERAPEUTIC EFFECT*
Inhibits binding of the platelet glycoprotein (GP) IIb/IIIa receptor
(the major platelet surface receptor involved in platelet aggregation), *inhibiting platelet aggregation.* Inhibition persists over the
duration of the maintenance infusion and is reversible after infusion
is completed.

PHARMACOKINETICS
Poorly bound to plasma proteins;
unbound fraction in plasma: 35%.
Limited metabolism. Primarily
eliminated in the urine (65%) and,
to a lesser amount, in the feces.
Half-life: 2 hrs. Clearance is significantly decreased in severe renal
impairment (creatinine clearance <
30 ml/min). Removed by hemodialysis.

USES
In combination with heparin, treatment of acute coronary syndrome,
including those to be managed
medically and those undergoing
percutaneous transluminal coronary angioplasty (PTCA) or atherectomy.

PRECAUTIONS
CONTRAINDICATIONS: Active internal bleeding or a history of

bleeding diathesis within previous 30 days, history of thrombocytopenia following prior exposure to tirofiban, stroke, major surgical procedure within previous 30 days, severe hypertension, history of intracranial hemorrhage, intracranial neoplasm, arteriovenous malformation or aneurysm. **CAUTIONS:** Pts with platelets <150,000/mm^3, hemorrhagic retinopathy. Concomitant use of drugs affecting hemostasis (e.g., warfarin), renal function impairment.

▷**LIFESPAN CONSIDERATIONS:** **Pregnancy/Lactation:** Unknown if distributed in breast milk. **Pregnancy Category B. Children:** Safety and efficacy not established. **Elderly:** Increased risk of bleeding; caution advised.

INTERACTIONS

DRUG: Drugs that affect hemostasis (e.g., **aspirin, NSAIDs, heparin, thrombolytics, warfarin). HERBAL:** None known. **FOOD:** None known. **LAB VALUES:** Decreases hemoglobin, hematocrit, platelets.

AVAILABILITY (Rx)

INJECTION PREMIX: 25 mg/500 ml (50 mcg/ml). **VIAL:** 250 mcg/ml.

ADMINISTRATION/HANDLING

IV 🔟

Storage:
• Store at room temperature • Protect from light. • Use only clear solution. • Discard unused solution 24 hrs following start of infusion.

Reconstitution:
Note: Heparin and tirobifan can be administered through the same IV line.

Injection for solution (250 mcg/ml):
• Withdraw and discard 100 ml from a 500 ml bag 0.9% NaCl or D$_5$W and replace this volume with 100 ml of tirobifan (from two 50 ml vials) or withdraw and discard 50 ml from a 250 ml bag and replace with 50 ml of tirobifan (from one 50 ml vial) to achieve a final concentration of 50 mcg/ml. • Mix well before administration.
Injection (50 mcg/ml) premix in 500 ml IntraVia container:
• To open the IntraVia container, tear off the dust cover. • Check for leaks by squeezing the inner bag firmly; if any leak is found or if the solution is not clear, discard the solution. • Do not add other drugs or remove solution directly from the bag with a syringe. Do not use plastic containers in series connections (may result in air embolism by drawing air from the first container if it is empty of solution).

Rate of administration:
• For loading dose, give 0.4 mcg/kg/min for 30 min. • For maintenance infusion, give 0.1 mcg/kg/min.

IV INCOMPATIBILITY 🚫

Do not mix with any other medications.

INDICATIONS/ROUTES/DOSAGE

Inhibition of platelet aggregation:
IV: Adults, elderly: Give at initial rate of 0.4 mcg/kg/min for 30 min and then continue at 0.1 mcg/kg/min through procedure and for 12–24 hrs following procedure.

Severe renal insufficiency (creatinine clearance < 30 ml/min): Half the usual rate of infusion.

SIDE EFFECTS

OCCASIONAL (3–6%): Pelvis

T

---

pain, bradycardia, dizziness, leg pain. **RARE** (1–2%): Edema/swelling, vasovagal reaction, sweating, nausea, fever, headache.

ADVERSE REACTIONS/TOXIC EFFECTS

Overdosage manifested as primarily minor mucocutaneous bleeding and bleeding at the femoral artery access site. Thrombocytopenia occurs rarely.

NURSING IMPLICATIONS

BASELINE ASSESSMENT:

Assess platelet count, hemoglobin, hematocrit, APTT, renal function prior to treatment, within 6 hrs following the loading dose and at least daily thereafter during therapy. If platelet count <90,000/mm³, additional platelet counts should be obtained routinely to avoid thrombocytopenia. If thrombocytopenia occurs, drug therapy and heparin should be discontinued.

INTERVENTION/EVALUATION:

Monitor APTT 6 hrs after the beginning of the heparin infusion. Adjust heparin dosage to maintain APTT at approx. 2 times control. Diligently monitor for potential bleeding, particularly at other arterial and venous puncture sites, IM injection site. If possible, urinary catheters, NG tubes should be avoided. Maintain complete bed rest with head of the bed elevated at 30°.

tizanidine

tih-**zan**-ih-deen
(Zanaflex)

▶CLASSIFICATION

PHARMACOTHERAPEUTIC:
Skeletal muscle relaxant. ***CLINICAL:*** Antispastic

ACTION/*THERAPEUTIC EFFECT*

Increases presynaptic inhibition of spinal motor neurons mediated by alpha₂ adrenergic agonists, reducing facilitation to postsynaptic motor neurons, *reducing muscle spasticity.*

USES

Acute and intermittent management of muscle spasticity (spasms, stiffness, rigidity). *Spasticity associated with multiple sclerosis and spinal cord injury.*

PRECAUTIONS

CONTRAINDICATIONS: None significant. ***CAUTIONS:*** Renal insufficiency, hepatic function impairment, elderly (clearance is decreased 4-fold).

INTERACTIONS

DRUG: Oral contraceptives may reduce tizanidine clearance. May increase serum levels/toxicity of **phenytoin. Alcohol, CNS depressants** may increase CNS depressant effects. **Antihypertensives** may increase tizanidine's hypotensive potential. ***HERBAL:*** None known. ***FOOD:*** None known. ***LAB VALUES:*** May increase ALT (SGPT), AST (SGOT), alkaline phosphatase.

AVAILABILITY (Rx)

TABLETS: 4 mg.

INDICATIONS/ROUTES/DOSAGE

Muscle spasticity:

PO: Adults, elderly: Initially 4 mg, gradually increased in 2–4 mg increments and repeated q6–8h. **Maximum:** 3 doses/day or 36 mg total in 24 hrs.

SIDE EFFECTS

FREQUENT (41–49%): Dry mouth, somnolence, asthenia (loss of strength, weakness). ***OCCASIONAL*** (4–16%): Dizziness, urinary tract infection, constipation. ***RARE*** (3%): Nervousness, amblyopia (dimness of vision), pharyngitis, rhinitis, vomiting, urinary frequency.

ADVERSE REACTIONS/TOXIC EFFECTS

Hypotension with a reduction in either diastolic or systolic B/P and may be associated with bradycardia, orthostatic hypotension, and, rarely, syncope. As dosage increases, risk of hypotension increases and is noted within 1 hr after dosing.

NURSING IMPLICATIONS

BASELINE ASSESSMENT:

Record onset, type, location, and duration of muscular spasm. Check for immobility, stiffness, swelling. Obtain baseline liver function tests, alkaline phosphatase, and total bilirubin.

INTERVENTION/EVALUATION:

Assist with ambulation at all times. For those on long-term therapy, liver/renal function tests should be performed periodically. Evaluate for therapeutic response (decreased intensity of skeletal muscle pain/tenderness, improved mobility, decrease in spasticity). For those at increased risk of orthostatic hypotension, instruct pt to rise slowly from lying to sitting and from sitting to supine position.

PATIENT/FAMILY TEACHING:

Avoid tasks that require alertness, motor skills until response to drug is established. Avoid sudden changes

tobramycin sulfate

tow-bra-**my**-sin
(Nebcin, Tobi, Tobrex)

FIXED-COMBINATION(S)

With dexamethasone, a steroid **(TobraDex)**

▶CLASSIFICATION

PHARMACOTHERAPEUTIC: Aminoglycoside. ***CLINICAL:*** Antibiotic (see p. 18C)

ACTION/*THERAPEUTIC EFFECT*

Irreversibly binds to protein on bacterial ribosome, *interfering in protein synthesis of susceptible microorganisms.*

PHARMACOKINETICS

Rapid, complete absorption after IM administration. Protein binding: <30%. Widely distributed (does not cross blood-brain barrier, low concentrations in CSF). Excreted unchanged in urine. Removed by hemodialysis. Half-life: 2–4 hrs (half-life increased with impaired renal function, neonates; decreased in cystic fibrosis, burn or febrile pts).

USES

Skin/skin structure, bone, joint, respiratory tract infections; postop, burn, intra-abdominal infections, complicated urinary tract infections, septicemia, meningitis. ***Ophthalmic:*** Superficial eye infections: blepharitis, conjunctivitis,

T

keratitis, corneal ulcers. ***Inhalation:*** Bronchopulmonary infections in pts with cystic fibrosis.

PRECAUTIONS

CONTRAINDICATIONS: Hypersensitivity to aminoglycosides (cross-sensitivity). ***CAUTIONS:*** Elderly, neonates due to renal insufficiency/immaturity; neuromuscular disorders (potential for respiratory depression), prior hearing loss, vertigo, renal impairment. Cumulative effects may occur with concurrent ophthalmic and systemic administration.
▷***LIFESPAN CONSIDERATIONS:***
Pregnancy/Lactation: Readily crosses placenta; distributed in breast milk. May cause fetal nephrotoxicity. **Pregnancy Category D.** Ophthalmic form should not be used in nursing mothers and only when specifically indicated in pregnancy. **Pregnancy Category B. Children:** Immature renal function in neonates and premature infants may increase risk of toxicity. **Elderly:** Age-related renal impairment may increase risk of toxicity; dosage adjustment recommended.

INTERACTIONS

DRUG:* Other aminoglycosides, nephrotoxic, ototoxic-producing medications** may increase toxicity. May increase effects of **neuromuscular blocking agents.** ***HERBAL: None known. ***FOOD:*** None known. ***LAB VALUES:*** May increase BUN, SGPT (ALT), SGOT (AST), bilirubin, creatinine, LDH concentrations; may decrease serum calcium, magnesium, potassium, sodium concentrations. Therapeutic blood serum level: Peak: 5–20 mcg/ml; trough: 0.5–2 mcg/ml. Toxic blood serum level: Peak: >20 mcg/ml; trough: >2 mcg/ml.

AVAILABILITY (Rx)

INJECTION: 10 mg/ml, 40 mg/ml. ***POWDER FOR INJECTION:*** 1.2 g. ***OPHTHALMIC SOLUTION:*** 0.3%. ***OPHTHALMIC OINTMENT:*** 3 mg/g. ***INHALATION SOLUTION:*** 300 mg/5 ml.

ADMINISTRATION/HANDLING

Note: Coordinate peak and trough lab draws with administration times.

IM:

• To minimize discomfort, give deep IM slowly. • Less painful if injected into gluteus maximus rather than lateral aspect of thigh.

IV ▥

Storage:
• Store vials at room temperature.
• Solutions may be discolored by light/air (does not affect potency).

Reconstitution:
• Dilute with 50–200 ml D$_5$W, 0.9% NaCl. Amount of diluent for infants, children depends upon individual need.

Rate of administration:
• Infuse over 20–60 min.

Ophthalmic:

• Place finger on lower eyelid and pull out until a pocket is formed between eye and lower lid. • Hold dropper above pocket and place correct number of drops ($1/4$–$1/2$ inch ointment) into pocket. Have pt close eye gently.

• ***Solution:*** Apply digital pressure to lacrimal sac for 1–2 min (minimizes drainage into nose and throat, reducing risk of systemic effects.) ***Ointment:*** Close eye for 1–2 min, rolling eyeball (increases contact area of drug to eye). • Remove excess solution or ointment around eye with tissue.

IV INCOMPATIBILITIES 🚫

Amphotericin B complex (Abelcet, Ambisome, Amphotec), heparin, hetastarch (Hespan), indomethacin (Indocin), propofol (Diprivan), sargramostim (Leukine, Prokine).

IV COMPATIBILITIES

Amiodarone (Cordarone), calcium gluconate, diltiazem (Cardizem), magnesium, midazolam (Versed).

INDICATIONS/ROUTES/DOSAGE

Note: Space parenteral doses evenly around the clock. Dosage based on ideal body weight. Peak, trough level is determined periodically to maintain desired serum concentrations (minimizes risk of toxicity). *Recommended peak level:* 4–10 mcg/ml; *trough level:* 1–2 mcg/ml.

Moderate to severe infections:
IM/IV: **Adults, elderly:** 3 mg/kg/day in divided doses q8h.

Life-threatening infections:
IM/IV: **Adults, elderly:** Up to 5 mg/kg/day in divided doses q6–8h.

Usual dosage for children, infants:
IM/IV: **Children, infants:** 6–7.5 mg/kg/day in 3–4 divided doses.

Dosage in renal impairment:
Dose and/or frequency is modified based on degree of renal impairment, serum concentration of drug. After loading dose of 1–2 mg/kg, maintenance dose/frequency based on serum creatinine/creatinine clearance.

Usual ophthalmic dosage:
OPHTHALMIC OINTMENT: **Adults, elderly:** Thin strip to conjunctiva q8–12h (q3–4h for severe infections).

OPHTHALMIC SOLUTION: **Adults, elderly:** 1–2 drops q4h (2 drops every hr for severe infections).

Usual inhalation dosage:
Adults: 60–80 mg twice daily for 28 days, then off for 28 days.

SIDE EFFECTS

OCCASIONAL: Pain, induration at IM injection site; phlebitis, thrombophlebitis with IV administration; hypersensitivity reaction (rash, fever, urticaria, pruritus). *Ophthalmic:* Tearing, itching, redness, swelling of eyelid. *RARE:* Hypotension, nausea, vomiting.

ADVERSE REACTIONS/TOXIC EFFECTS

Nephrotoxicity (evidenced by increased BUN and serum creatinine, decreased creatinine clearance) may be reversible if drug stopped at first sign of symptoms; irreversible ototoxicity (tinnitus, dizziness, ringing/roaring in ears, reduced hearing) and neurotoxicity (headache, dizziness, lethargy, tremors, visual disturbances) occur occasionally. Risk is greater with higher dosages, prolonged therapy, or if solution is applied directly to mucosa. Superinfections, particularly with fungi, may result from bacterial imbalance via any route of administration; anaphylaxis.

NURSING IMPLICATIONS

BASELINE ASSESSMENT:

Dehydration must be treated before parenteral therapy is begun. Question for history of allergies, esp. to aminoglycosides and sulfite (and parabens for topical/ophthalmic routes). Establish baseline for hearing acuity.

INTERVENTION/EVALUATION:

Monitor I&O (maintain hydration), urinalysis (casts, RBCs, WBCs, decrease in specific gravity). Monitor results of peak/trough blood tests. Therapeutic blood serum level: Peak: 5–20 mcg/ml; trough: 0.5–2 mcg/ml. Toxic blood serum level: Peak: >20 mcg/ml; trough: >2 mcg/ml. Be alert to ototoxic and·neurotoxic symptoms (see Adverse Reactions/Toxic Effects). Evaluate IV site for phlebitis (heat, pain, red streaking over vein). Assess for rash. Be alert for superinfection particularly genital/anal pruritus, changes of oral mucosa, diarrhea. When treating pts with neuromuscular disorders, assess respiratory response carefully. (***Ophthalmic:*** assess for redness, swelling, itching, tearing).

PATIENT/FAMILY TEACHING:

Continue antibiotic for full length of treatment. Space doses evenly. Discomfort may occur with IM injection. Notify physician in event of any hearing, visual, balance, urinary problems even after therapy is completed. ***Ophthalmic:*** Blurred vision/tearing may occur briefly after application. Contact physician if tearing, redness, or irritation continues.

tocainide hydrochloride

toe-**kay**-nied
(Tonocard)

►CLASSIFICATION

PHARMACOTHERAPEUTIC: Amide-type local anesthetic. ***CLINICAL:*** Antiarrhythmic (see p. 12C)

ACTION/*THERAPEUTIC EFFECT*

Shortens action potential duration, decreases effective refractory period, automaticity in His-Purkinje system of myocardium by blocking sodium transport across myocardial cell membranes, *suppressing ventricular arrhythmias.*

USES

Suppression, prevention of ventricular arrhythmias including frequent unifocal/multifocal coupled premature ventricular contractions and paroxysmal ventricular tachycardia.

PRECAUTIONS

CONTRAINDICATIONS: Hypersensitivity to local anesthetics, second-or third-degree AV block. ***CAUTIONS:*** CHF, elderly, severe respiratory depression, bradycardia, incomplete heart block.

INTERACTIONS

DRUG: Other **antiarrhythmics** may increase risk of adverse cardiac effects. **Beta-adrenergic blockers** may increase pulmonary wedge pressure, decrease cardiac index. ***HERBAL:*** None known. ***FOOD:*** None known. ***LAB VALUES:*** None significant. Therapeutic blood serum level: 4–10 mcg/ml; toxic blood serum level: N/E.

AVAILABILITY (Rx)

TABLETS: 400 mg, 600 mg.

INDICATIONS/ROUTES/DOSAGE

Note: When giving tocainide in those receiving IV lidocaine, give single 600 mg dose 6 hrs before cessation of lidocaine and repeat in 6 hrs. Then give standard tocainide maintenance doses.

Ventricular arrhythmias:

*PO: **Adults, elderly:*** Initially, 400 mg q8h. **Maintenance:** 1.2–1.8 g/day in divided doses q8h. **Maximum:** 2,400 mg/day.

SIDE EFFECTS

Generally well tolerated. *FREQUENT* (3–10%): Minor, transient lightheadedness, dizziness, nausea, paresthesia, rash, tremor. *OCCASIONAL* (1–3%): Clammy skin, night sweats, joint pain. *RARE* (<1%): Restlessness, nervousness, disorientation, mood changes, ataxia (muscular incoordination), visual disturbances.

ADVERSE REACTIONS/TOXIC EFFECTS

High dosage may produce bradycardia/tachycardia, hypotension, palpitations, increased ventricular arrhythmias, PVCs, chest pain, exacerbation of CHF.

NURSING IMPLICATIONS

BASELINE ASSESSMENT:

Assess pulse for strength/weakness, irregular rate. Monitor EKG for cardiac changes, particularly shortening of QT interval. Notify physician of any significant interval changes.

INTERVENTION/EVALUATION:

Monitor fluid and electrolyte serum levels. Assess hand movement for sign of tremor (usually first clinical sign that maximum dose is being reached). Assess sleeping pt for night sweats. Question for tingling/numbness in hands/feet. Assess skin for rash, clamminess. Observe for CNS disturbances (restlessness, disorientation, mood changes, incoordination). Assess for evidence of CHF: dyspnea (particularly on exertion or lying down), night cough, peripheral edema, distended neck veins. Monitor I&O (increase in weight, decrease in urine output may indicate CHF). Monitor for therapeutic serum level (3–10 mcg/ml). Therapeutic blood serum level: 4–10 mcg/ml; toxic blood serum level: N/E.

PATIENT/FAMILY TEACHING:

Avoid tasks that require alertness, motor skills until response to drug is established. Side effects generally disappear with continued therapy. Unsalted crackers, dry toast may relieve nausea.

tolazamide

(Tolinase, Tolamide)
See Classification section under: Antidiabetic agents (p. 39C)

tolazoline hydrochloride

toe-**laze**-oh-lean
(Priscoline)
Do not confuse with tolazamide.

▶CLASSIFICATION
PHARMACOTHERAPEUTIC: Peripheral vasodilator. *CLINICAL:* Antihypertensive

ACTION/THERAPEUTIC EFFECT

Directly relaxes vascular smooth muscle, *causes vasodilation, decreases peripheral resistance.* Has moderate alpha-adrenergic blocking activity.

PHARMACOKINETICS

Rapidly, completely absorbed. Concentrated primarily in liver, kidney. Excreted unchanged in urine. Half-life: 3–10 hrs.

USES

Treatment of persistent pulmonary vasoconstriction and hypertension of newborn (persistent fetal circulation). Improves oxygenation.

PRECAUTIONS

CONTRAINDICATIONS: None significant. **CAUTIONS:** Known/suspected mitral stenosis.

▷**LIFESPAN CONSIDERATIONS:** **Newborns:** No age-related precautions noted.

INTERACTIONS

DRUG: Antagonizes vasoconstriction caused by **dopamine.** Decreases effects of **metaraminol, ephedrine, phenylephrine. HERBAL:** None known. **FOOD:** None known. **LAB VALUES:** None significant.

AVAILABILITY (Rx)

INJECTION: 25 mg/ml.

ADMINISTRATION/HANDLING
IV 🎍

Storage:

• Store at room temperature.

Reconstitution:

• May give undiluted as IV push through Y-tube or three-way stopcock of running IV infusion. • May further dilute with 0.9% or 0.45% NaCl, D_5W, 6% dextran in dextrose or NaCl, fructose in water or NaCl, invert sugar in water or NaCl, Ionosol, lactated Ringer's, protein hydrolysate 5%, Ringer's injection, sodium lactate 1/6 molar and given as intermittent IV infusion (piggyback). • Amount of dilutent based on total dose, pediatric fluid needs.

Rate of administration:

• Give loading dose over 10 min. • Give maintenance infusion at 1–2 mg/kg/hr. • Monitor B/P diligently for systemic hypotension. If hypotension occurs, place in supine position with feet elevated, give IV fluids. • Do not administer epinephrine. • Tolazoline may cause "epinephrine reversal" (further B/P decrease followed by rebound hypertension).

IV INCOMPATIBILITY ⊘

Indomethacin (Indocin).

IV COMPATIBILITIES

Ampicillin (Polycillin), calcium gluconate, dobutamine (Dobutrex), dopamine (Intropin), furosemide (Lasix), gentamicin (Garamycin).

INDICATIONS/ROUTES/DOSAGE
Persistent fetal circulation:

IV: Newborn: Initially, 1–2 mg/kg via scalp vein or upper extremity vein over 10 min; then, IV infusion of 1–2 mg/kg/hr.

SIDE EFFECTS

OCCASIONAL: Nausea, diarrhea, vomiting, increased pilomotor activity (goose bumps), peripheral vasodilation (flushing), tachycardia. **RARE:** Mydriasis.

ADVERSE REACTIONS/TOXIC EFFECTS

GI hemorrhage, hypochloremic alkalosis, cardiac arrhythmias, hypotension, oliguria, hepatitis, thrombocytopenia, leukopenia may occur.

BASELINE ASSESSMENT:
Obtain B/P immediately before each dose, in addition to regular monitoring (be alert to fluctuations). If excessive reduction in B/P occurs, place pt in supine position with feet elevated, give IV fluids.

INTERVENTION/EVALUATION:
Monitor vital signs, O_2ation, acid-base balance, fluid and electrolytes.

tolbutamide

(Orinase, Oramide)
See Classification section under: Antidiabetic agents (p. 39C)

tolcapone

toll-cah-pone
(Tasmar)

▶CLASSIFICATION
PHARMACOTHERAPEUTIC:
Antidyskinetic. **CLINICAL:** Antiparkinson agent

ACTION/THERAPEUTIC EFFECT
Inhibits the enzyme COMT, sustaining plasma levels and thereby increasing the duration of action of levodopa, resulting in greater effect, *relieving signs and symptoms of Parkinson's disease.*

PHARMACOKINETICS
Rapidly absorbed following PO administration. Protein binding: 99%. Metabolized in liver. Eliminated primarily in urine (60%) and to a lesser amount (40%) in feces. Unknown if removed by hemodialysis. Half-life: 2–3 hrs.

USES
Adjunctive therapy to levodopa and carbidopa for treatment of signs and symptoms of idiopathic Parkinson's disease.

PRECAUTIONS
CONTRAINDICATIONS: None significant. **CAUTIONS:** Severe renal impairment, severe liver impairment, those with history of hallucinations, baseline hypotension, history of orthostatic hypotension.

▷**LIFESPAN CONSIDERATIONS:**
Pregnancy/Lactation: Unknown if distributed in breast milk. **Pregnancy Category C. Children:** Not used in children. **Elderly:** May have increased risk of hallucinations.

INTERACTIONS
DRUG: Increases levodopa duration of action. **HERBAL:** None known. **FOOD:** Food given 1 hr before or 2 hrs after tolcapone administration decreases bioavailability by 10–20%. **LAB VALUES:** May increase AST (SGOT), ALT (SGPT).

AVAILABILITY (Rx)
TABLETS: 100 mg, 200 mg.

ADMINISTRATION/HANDLING
PO:
• Give without regard to food.

INDICATIONS/ROUTES/DOSAGE
Note: May combine tolcapone with both the immediate and sustained-release form of levodopa/carbidopa.

T

Parkinson's disease:

PO: Adults, elderly: Initially, 100–200 mg 3 times/day. **Maximum:** 600 mg/day. For those with moderate to severe cirrhosis of liver, do not increase to 200 mg 3 times/day.

SIDE EFFECTS

Note: Frequency of occurrence increases with dosage amount. Following is based on 200 mg dose.

FREQUENT: Nausea (35%), (16–25%): Insomnia, somnolence, anorexia, diarrhea, muscle cramps, orthostatic hypotension, excessive dreaming. **OCCASIONAL** (4–11%): Headache, vomiting, confusion, hallucinations, constipation, increased sweating, urine discoloration (bright yellow), dry eyes, abdominal pain, dizziness, flatulence. **RARE** (2–3%): Dyspepsia, neck pain, hypotension, fatigue, chest discomfort.

ADVERSE REACTIONS/TOXIC EFFECTS

Upper respiratory infection, urinary tract infection occur occasionally (5–7%). Too-rapid withdrawal from therapy may produce withdrawal emergent hyperpyrexia characterized by elevated temperature, muscular rigidity, altered consciousness. An increase in dyskinesia (impaired voluntary movement) or dystonia (impaired muscular tone) occur frequently.

NURSING IMPLICATIONS

BASELINE ASSESSMENT:

Serum transaminase levels should be monitored q2wks for the first yr, q4wks for the next 6 mos, and q8wks thereafter. Treatment should be discontinued if ALT (SGPT) exceeds the upper limit of normal or clinical signs of onset of hepatic failure occur. If hallucination occurs may be eliminated if levodopa dosage is reduced. Hallucinations generally are accompanied by confusion and, to a lesser extent, insomnia.

INTERVENTION/EVALUATION:

Instruct pt to rise from lying to sitting or sitting to standing position slowly to prevent risk of postural hypotension. Assist with ambulation if dizziness occurs. Assess for clinical reversal of symptoms (improvement of tremor of head/hands at rest, masklike facial expression, shuffling gait, muscular rigidity).

PATIENT/FAMILY TEACHING:

If nausea occurs, take medication with food. Drowsiness, dizziness, nausea may be an initial response of drug but diminishes or disappears with continued treatment. Postural hypotension may occur more frequently during initial therapy. Avoid tasks that require alertness, motor skills until response to drug is established. Hallucinations may occur, more so in the elderly than in younger pts with Parkinson's disease and typically within the first 2 wks of therapy. Inform physician if possibility of pregnancy occurs. Urine will change color to a bright yellow.

tolmetin sodium

toll-meh-tin
(Tolectin)

▶CLASSIFICATION

PHARMACOTHERAPEUTIC: Nonsteroidal anti-inflammatory. **CLINICAL:** Antiarthritic (see p. 107C)

ACTION/*THERAPEUTIC EFFECT*

Produces analgesic and anti-inflammatory effect by inhibiting prostaglandin synthesis, *reducing inflammatory response and intensity of pain stimulus reaching sensory nerve endings.*

USES/*UNLABELED*

Relief of pain, disability associated with rheumatoid arthritis, juvenile rheumatoid arthritis, osteoarthritis. *Treatment of ankylosing spondylitis, psoriatic arthritis.*

PRECAUTIONS

CONTRAINDICATIONS: History of hypersensitivity to aspirin or other NSAIDs, those severely incapacitated, bedridden, wheelchair bound. **CAUTIONS:** Impaired renal function, impaired cardiac function, coagulation disorders, history of upper GI disease.

INTERACTIONS

DRUG: May increase effects of **oral anticoagulants, heparin, thrombolytics.** May decrease effect of **antihypertensives, diuretics. Salicylates, aspirin** may increase risk of GI side effects, bleeding. **Bone marrow depressants** may increase risk of hematologic reactions. May increase concentration, toxicity of **lithium.** May increase **methotrexate** toxicity. **Probenecid** may increase concentration. **Antacids** may decrease concentration. **HERBAL:** Ginkgo biloba may increase risk of bleeding. May decrease **feverfew** effect. **FOOD:** None known. **LAB VALUES:** May increase BUN, potassium, liver function tests. May decrease hemoglobin, hematocrit. May prolong bleeding time.

AVAILABILITY (Rx)

TABLETS: 200 mg, 600 mg. **CAPSULES:** 400 mg.

ADMINISTRATION/HANDLING

PO:
• May give with food, milk, or antacids if GI distress occurs.

INDICATIONS/ROUTES/DOSAGE

Rheumatoid arthritis, osteoarthritis:

PO: Adults, elderly: Initially, 400 mg 3 times/day (including 1 dose upon arising, 1 dose at bedtime). Adjust dose at 1–2 wk intervals. **Maintenance:** 600–1,800 mg/day in 3–4 divided doses.

Juvenile rheumatoid arthritis:

PO: Children >2 yrs: Initially, 20 mg/kg/day in 3–4 divided doses. **Maintenance:** 15–30 mg/kg/day in 3–4 divided doses.

SIDE EFFECTS

OCCASIONAL (3–11%): Nausea, vomiting, diarrhea, abdominal cramping, dyspepsia (heartburn, indigestion, epigastric pain), flatulence, dizziness, headache, weight decrease or increase. **RARE** (<3%): Constipation, anorexia, rash, pruritus.

ADVERSE REACTIONS/TOXIC EFFECTS

Peptic ulcer, GI bleeding, gastritis, severe hepatic reaction (cholestasis, jaundice) occur rarely. Nephrotoxicity (dysuria, hematuria, proteinuria, nephrotic syndrome) and severe hypersensitivity reaction (fever, chills, bronchospasm) occur rarely.

T

NURSING IMPLICATIONS

BASELINE ASSESSMENT:

Assess onset, type, location, and duration of pain/inflammation. Inspect appearance of affected joints for immobility, deformities, and skin condition.

INTERVENTION/EVALUATION:
Monitor pattern of daily bowel activity, stool consistency. Assist with ambulation if dizziness occurs. Monitor for evidence of GI distress. Evaluate for therapeutic response (relief of pain, stiffness, swelling; increase in joint mobility, reduced joint tenderness, improved grip strength).

PATIENT/FAMILY TEACHING:
Therapeutic effect noted in 1–3 wks. Avoid tasks that require alertness, motor skills until response to drug is established. If GI upset occurs, take with food, milk. Avoid aspirin, alcohol during therapy (increases risk of GI bleeding). Report headache, GI distress.

tolnaftate

(Tinactin, Aftate)
See Classification section under: Antifungals: topical (p. 43C)

tolterodine tartrate

toll-**tear**-oh-deen
(Detrol)

▶**CLASSIFICATION**
PHARMACOTHERAPEUTIC:
Muscarinic receptor antagonist.
CLINICAL: Antispasmotic

ACTION/THERAPEUTIC EFFECT
Exhibits potent antimuscarinic activity by interceding by way of cholinergic muscarinic receptors, thereby relaxing urinary bladder contraction, *decreasing urinary frequency, urgency.*

PHARMACOKINETICS
Rapidly, well absorbed following oral administration. Protein binding: 96%. Extensive first-pass hepatic metabolism to active metabolite. Primarily excreted in urine. Unknown if removed by hemodialysis. Half-life: 1.9–3.7 hrs.

USES
Treatment of those with an overactive bladder with symptoms of urinary frequency, urgency or urge incontinence.

PRECAUTIONS
CONTRAINDICATIONS: Urinary retention, uncontrolled narrow-angle glaucoma. *CAUTIONS:* Renal function impairment, clinically significant bladder outflow obstruction (risk of urinary retention), GI obstructive disorders, e.g., pyloric stenosis (risk of gastric retention), treated narrow-angle glaucoma.
▷*LIFESPAN CONSIDERATIONS:*
Pregnancy/Lactation: Unknown if distributed in breast milk. Recommended to discontinue during nursing. **Children:** Safety and efficacy not established. **Elderly:** No age-related precautions noted.

INTERACTIONS
DRUG: **Clarithromycin, erythromycin, itraconazole, ketoconazole, miconazole** may increase concentration of tolterodine. **Fluoxetine** may inhibit metabolism of tolterodine. *HERBAL:* None known. *FOOD:* None known. *LAB VALUES:* None significant.

AVAILABILITY (Rx)

TABLETS: 1 mg, 2 mg. **_CAPSULES (extended-release):_** 2 mg, 4 mg.

ADMINISTRATION/HANDLING

PO:
• May give without regard to food.

INDICATIONS/ROUTES/DOSAGE

Overactive bladder:

_PO:_ Adults, elderly: 1–2 mg twice daily. **Severe hepatic impairment:** 1 mg twice daily. **_EXTENDED-RELEASE:_** 2–4 mg once daily.

SIDE EFFECTS

FREQUENT: (40%): Dry mouth. **_OCCASIONAL_** (4–11%): Headache, dizziness, fatigue, constipation, dyspepsia (heartburn, indigestion, epigastric discomfort), upper respiratory infection, urinary tract infection, abnormal vision (including accommodation, dry eyes), nausea, diarrhea. **_RARE_** (3%): Somnolence, chest/back pain, arthralgia, rash, weight gain, dry skin.

ADVERSE REACTIONS/TOXIC EFFECTS

Overdosage can result in severe anticholinergic effects, including GI cramping, feeling of facial warmth, excessive salivation, sweating, lacrimation, pallor, urinary urgency, blurred vision and QT interval prolongation.

NURSING IMPLICATIONS

INTERVENTION/EVALUATION:
Assist with ambulation if dizziness occurs. Question for change in vision.

PATIENT/FAMILY TEACHING:
Sips of tepid water or sour hard candy may relieve dry mouth. Report nausea, constipation, and visual abnormalities.

topiramate

toe-**pie**-rah-mate
(Topamax)

▶CLASSIFICATION

CLINICAL: Anticonvulsant (see p. 33C)

ACTION/THERAPEUTIC EFFECT

Blocks repetitive, sustained firing of neurons by enhancing the ability of gamma aminobutyric acid (GABA) to induce a flux of chloride ions into the neurons, *decreasing seizure frequency.*

PHARMACOKINETICS

Rapidly absorbed following PO administration. Protein binding: 13–17%. Not extensively metabolized. Primarily excreted unchanged in the urine. Removed by hemodialysis. Half-life: 21 hrs.

USES

Adjunctive therapy for the treatment of partial-onset seizures, tonic-clonic seizures, seizures associated with Lennox-Gastant syndrome.

PRECAUTIONS

CONTRAINDICATIONS: None significant. **_CAUTIONS:_** Sensitivity to topiramate, impaired liver/renal function, predisposition to renal calculi.

▷**_LIFESPAN CONSIDERATIONS:_**
Pregnancy/Lactation: Unknown if distributed in breast milk. **Preg-**

T

nancy **Category C. Children:** No age-related precautions noted in those >2 yrs of age. **Elderly:** Age-related renal impairment may require dosage adjustment.

INTERACTIONS

DRUG: **Phenytoin, valproic acid, carbamazepine** may decrease topiramate concentration. **Carbonic anhydrase inhibitors** may increase risk of renal calculi. May decrease effectiveness of **oral contraceptives. Alcohol, CNS depressants** may increase CNS depression. *HERBAL:* None known. *FOOD:* None known. *LAB VALUES:* None significant.

AVAILABILITY (Rx)

TABLETS: 25 mg, 100 mg, 200 mg. *SPRINKLE CAPSULES:* 15 mg, 25 mg.

ADMINISTRATION/HANDLING

PO:

• Do not break tablets (bitter taste). • Give without regard to meals. • Capsules may be swallowed whole or contents sprinkled on a teaspoonful of soft food and swallowed immediately and not chewed.

INDICATIONS/ROUTES/DOSAGE

Partial seizures:

PO: **Adults, elderly, children >17 yrs:** Initially, 25–50 mg for 1 wk. May increase by 25–50 mg/day at weekly intervals. **Maximum:** 1,600 mg/day. **Children 2–16 yrs:** Initially, 1–3 mg/kg/day (**Maximum:** 25 mg). May increase by 1–3 mg/kg/day at weekly intervals. **Maintenance:** 5–9 mg/kg/day in 2 divided doses.

Tonic-clonic seizures:

PO: **Adults, elderly, children:** Individual and titrated.

Note: Reduce dose by 50% if creatinine clearance <70 ml/min.

SIDE EFFECTS

FREQUENT (10–30%): Somnolence, dizziness, ataxia, nervousness, nystagmus (involuntary eye movement), diplopia (double vision), paresthesia, nausea, tremor. *OCCASIONAL* (3–9%): Confusion, breast pain, dysmenorrhea, dyspepsia, depression, asthenia (loss of strength), pharyngitis, weight loss, anorexia, rash, back/abdominal/leg pain, difficulty with coordination, sinusitis, agitation, flulike symptoms. *RARE* (2–3%): Mood disturbances (irritability, depression), dry mouth, aggressive reaction.

ADVERSE REACTIONS/TOXIC EFFECTS

Psychomotor slowing, difficulty with concentration, language problems, esp. word-finding difficulties, and memory disturbances occur occasionally. These events are generally mild to moderate but may be severe enough to require withdrawal from drug therapy.

NURSING IMPLICATIONS

BASELINE ASSESSMENT:

Review history of seizure disorder (intensity, frequency, duration, LOC). Provide safety precautions, quiet, dark environment. Question sensitivity to topiramate, pregnancy, use of other anticonvulsant medication (esp. carbamazepine, valproic acid, phenytoin, carbonic anhydrase inhibitors). Assess renal function. Instruct pt to use alternative/additional means of contraception (topiramate decreases effectiveness of oral contraceptives).

INTERVENTION/EVALUATION:

Observe frequently for recurrence of seizure activity. Assess for clinical improvement (decrease in intensity/frequency of seizures). Monitor renal function tests (BUN, creatinine). Assist with ambulation if dizziness occurs.

PATIENT/FAMILY TEACHING:

Avoid tasks that require alertness, motor skills until response to drug is established (may cause dizziness, drowsiness, impaired thinking). Avoid use of alcohol, other CNS depressants. Do not abruptly discontinue (may precipitate seizures). Strict maintenance of drug therapy is essential for seizure control. Drowsiness usually diminishes with continued therapy. Do not break tablets (bitter taste). Maintain adequate fluid intake (decreases risk of renal stone formation).

topotecan

toe-**poh**-teh-can
(Hycamtin)

▶CLASSIFICATION

PHARMACOTHERAPEUTIC:
DNA topoisomerase inhibitor.
CLINICAL: Antineoplastic (see p. 74C)

ACTION/THERAPEUTIC EFFECT

Interacts with topoisomerase I, an enzyme, which relieves torsional strain in DNA by inducing reversible single-strand breaks. Binds to topoisomerase-DNA complex preventing relegation of these single-strand breaks. Double-strand DNA damage occurring during DNA synthesis *produces cytoxic effect.*

PHARMACOKINETICS

Protein binding: 35%. Following IV administration, hydrolyzed to active form. Excreted in urine. Half-life: 2–3 hrs (half-life increased with impaired renal function).

USES

Treatment of metastatic carcinoma of ovary after failure of initial or recurrent chemotherapy. Treatment of sensitive, relapsed small cell lung cancer.

PRECAUTIONS

CONTRAINDICATIONS: Baseline neutrophil count <1,500 cells/mm^3, pregnancy, breast feeding, severe bone marrow depression. **CAUTIONS:** Mild bone marrow depression, liver or renal impairment.
▷**LIFESPAN CONSIDERATIONS:**
Pregnancy/Lactation: May cause fetal harm. Avoid pregnancy; discontinue nursing. **Pregnancy Category D. Children:** Safety and efficacy not established. **Elderly:** Store vials at room temperature in original cartons. Reconstituted vials diluted for infusion stable at room temperature, ambient lighting for 24 hrs. Age-related renal impairment may require dosage adjustment.

INTERACTIONS

DRUG: Other **myelosuppressants** may increase risk of myelosuppression. Concurrent use of **cisplatin** may increase severity of myelosuppression. **Live virus vaccines** may potentiate virus replication, increase vaccine side effects, decrease antibody response to vaccine. **HERBAL:** None known. **FOOD:** None known. **LAB VALUES:** May decrease neutrophil, leukocyte, thrombocyte, RBC levels. May increase SGOT (AST), SGPT (ALT), bilirubin.

AVAILABILITY (Rx)

POWDER FOR INJECTION: 4 mg (single-dose vial).

ADMINISTRATION/HANDLING
IV
Storage:

• Store vials at room temperature in original cartons. • Reconstituted vials diluted for infusion stable at room temperature, ambient lighting for 24 hrs.

Reconstitution:

• Reconstitute each 4 mg vial with 4 ml Sterile Water for Injection. • Further dilute with 50–100 ml 0.9% NaCl or D_5W.

Rate of administration:

• Administer all doses as IV infusion over 30 min. • Extravasation associated with only mild local reactions (erythema, bruising).

IV INCOMPATIBILITY ⊘

Do not mix with any other medications.

IV COMPATIBILITY

Gemcitabine (Gemzar).

INDICATIONS/ROUTES/DOSAGE

Note: Do not give topotecan if baseline neutrophil count <1,500 cells/mm³ and platelet count <100,000/mm³.

Carcinoma of ovary; small cell lung cancer:

IV INFUSION: Adults, elderly: 1.5 mg/m² over 30 min daily for 5 consecutive days, beginning on day 1 of a 21 day course. Minimum of four courses recommended. If severe neutropenia occurs during treatment, reduce dose by 0.25 mg/m² for subsequent courses or as an alternative, give G-CSF following the subsequent course beginning day 6 of the course (24 hrs after completion of topotecan administration).

Note: No dosage adjustment necessary in pts with mild renal impairment (creatinine clearance 40–60 ml/min).

Moderate renal impairment (creatinine clearance 20–39 ml/min):

IV INFUSION: Adults, elderly: 0.75 mg/m².

SIDE EFFECTS

FREQUENT: Nausea (77%), vomiting (58%), diarrhea, total alopecia (42%), headache (21%), dyspnea (21%). **OCCASIONAL:** Paresthesia (9%), constipation, abdominal pain (3%). **RARE:** Anorexia, malaise, arthralgia, asthenia, myalgia.

ADVERSE REACTIONS/TOXIC EFFECTS

Severe neutropenia (<500 cells/mm³) occurs in 60% of pts (develops at median of 11 days after day 1 of initial therapy). Thrombocytopenia (<25,000/mm³) occurs in 26% of pts and severe anemia (< 8 g/dl) occurs in 40% of pts (develops at median of 15 days after day 1 of initial therapy).

NURSING IMPLICATIONS

BASELINE ASSESSMENT:

Offer emotional support to pt and family. Assess CBC with differential, hemoglobin, and platelet count before each dose. Myelosuppression may precipitate life-threatening hemorrhage, infection, anemia. If platelet count drops, avoid even slightest trauma to body (injection site, assisting movement). Premedicate with antiemetics on day of treatment, starting at least 30 min prior to administration.

INTERVENTION/EVALUATION:

Monitor frequently for CBC with differential during treatment. Assess for bleeding, signs of infection, anemia. Monitor hydration status, I/O, electrolytes (diarrhea, vomiting are common side effects). Monitor CBC with differential, hemoglobin, platelets for evidence of myelosuppression. Assess response to medication; provide interventions, e.g., small, frequent meals/antiemetics for nausea and vomiting. Question for complaints of headache. Assess breathing pattern for evidence of dyspnea.

PATIENT/FAMILY TEACHING:

Explain that alopecia is reversible, but new hair may have different color, texture. Inform pt of possible late diarrhea causing dehydration, electrolyte depletion. Provide antiemetic/antidiarrheal regimen for subsequent use. Notify physician if diarrhea, vomiting continues at home. Do not have immunizations without physician's approval (drug lowers body's resistance). Avoid contact with those who have recently received live virus vaccine.

toremifene citrate

tore-mih-feen
(Fareston)

▶ **CLASSIFICATION**

PHARMACOTHERAPEUTIC: Nonsteroidal antiestrogen. ***CLINICAL:*** Antineoplastic (see p. 74C)

ACTION/*THERAPEUTIC EFFECT*

Interacts with estrogen receptors to serve as an antiestrogen, depleting cytosolic estrogen receptors, resulting in *cytostatic effects on tumor growth.*

PHARMACOKINETICS

Well absorbed following oral administration. Metabolized in the liver. Eliminated in feces. Half-life: approx. 5 days.

USES

Treatment of advanced breast cancer in postmenopausal women with estrogen receptor–positive disease.

PRECAUTIONS

CONTRAINDICATIONS: History of thromboembolic disease. ***CAUTIONS:*** Preexisting endometrial hyperplasia, leukopenia, thrombocytopenia.

▷ ***LIFESPAN CONSIDERATIONS:*** **Pregnancy/Lactation:** Unknown if distributed in breast milk. **Pregnancy Category D. Children:** Safety and efficacy not established. Not prescribed in this pt population. **Elderly:** No age-related precautions noted.

INTERACTIONS

DRUG: **Warfarin** may increase prothrombin time. **Carbamazepine, phenobarbital, phenytoin** may decrease concentration. ***HERBAL:*** None known. ***FOOD:*** None known. ***LAB VALUES:*** May increase alkaline phosphatase, AST (SGOT), bilirubin, calcium.

T

AVAILABILITY [Rx]

TABLETS: 60 mg.

ADMINISTRATION/HANDLING

PO:

• Give without regard to food.

INDICATIONS/ROUTES/DOSAGE

Breast cancer:

PO: Adults: 60 mg daily until disease progression is observed.

SIDE EFFECTS

FREQUENT: Hot flashes (35%), sweating (20%), nausea (14%), vaginal discharge (13%), dizziness, dry eyes (9%). **OCCASIONAL** (2–5%): Edema, vomiting, vaginal bleeding. **RARE:** Nausea, vomiting, fatigue, depression, lethargy, anorexia.

ADVERSE REACTIONS/TOXIC EFFECTS

Cataracts, glaucoma, decreased visual acuity may occur. May produce hypercalcemia.

NURSING IMPLICATIONS

BASELINE ASSESSMENT:

An estrogen receptor assay should be done before therapy is begun. CBC, platelet count, serum calcium levels should be checked before and periodically during therapy.

INTERVENTION/EVALUATION:

Assess for hypercalcemia (increased urine volume, excessive thirst, nausea, vomiting, constipation, hypotonicity of muscles, deep bone or flank pain, renal stones).

PATIENT/FAMILY TEACHING:

Report vaginal bleeding/discharge/itching, leg cramps, weight gain, shortness of breath, weakness. Contact physician if nausea/vomiting continues. Non-hormone contraceptives are recommended during treatment.

torsemide

tore-seh-mide
(Demadex)

►CLASSIFICATION

PHARMACOTHERAPEUTIC: Loop diuretic. **CLINICAL:** Antihypertensive, antiedema (see p. 84C)

ACTION/*THERAPEUTIC EFFECT*

Diuretic: Enhances excretion of sodium, chloride, potassium, water at ascending limb of loop of Henle, *producing diuretic effect.* **Antihypertensive:** Reduces plasma, extracellular fluid volume, *lowering B/P.*

PHARMACOKINETICS

	Onset	Peak	Duration
PO	1 hr	1–2 hrs	6–8 hrs
IV	10 min	1 hr	6–8 hrs

Rapidly, well absorbed from GI tract. Protein binding: 97–99%. Metabolized in liver. Primarily excreted in urine. Not removed by hemodialysis. Half-life: 3.3 hrs.

USES

Treatment of hypertension either alone or in combination with other antihypertensives. Edema associated with CHF, renal disease, hepatic cirrhosis, chronic renal failure.

PRECAUTIONS

CONTRAINDICATIONS: Anuria, hepatic coma, severe electrolyte depletion. **EXTREME CAUTION:**

Hypersensitivity to sulfonamides. **CAUTIONS:** Elderly, cardiac pts, pts with history of ventricular arrhythmias, pts with hepatic cirrhosis, ascites. Renal impairment, systemic lupus erythematosus. Safety in children not known.

▷**LIFESPAN CONSIDERATIONS:**
Pregnancy/Lactation: Unknown if drug is excreted in breast milk. **Pregnancy Category B. Children:** Safety and efficacy not established. **Elderly:** No age-related precautions noted.

INTERACTIONS

DRUG: May increase antihypertensive effect of **other antihypertensives. NSAIDs, probenecid** may decrease effect. May increase risk of **digoxin**-induced arrhythmias (due to hypokalemia). **Amphotericin** may increase risk nephrotoxicity. Effects of **anticoagulants, heparin, thrombolytics** may be decreased, **hypokalemia-causing medications** may increase risk of hypokalemia; may increase risk of **lithium** toxicity. **Nephrotoxic/ototoxic medications** may increase nephrotoxicity/ototoxicity. **HERBAL:** None known. **FOOD:** None known. **LAB VALUES:** May increase uric acid, BUN, creatinine. May decrease calcium, chloride, magnesium, potassium, sodium.

AVAILABILITY (Rx)

TABLETS: 5 mg, 10 mg, 20 mg, 100 mg. **INJECTION:** 10 mg/ml.

ADMINISTRATION/HANDLING

PO:

• Give without regard to food. Give with food to avoid GI upset, preferably with breakfast (prevents nocturia).

IV 🖩

Storage:

• Store at room temperature.

Rate of administration:

Note: Flush IV line with 0.9% NaCl before and after administration.

• May give undiluted as IV push over 2 min. • For continuous IV infusion, dilute with 0.9% or 0.45% NaCl or D_5W and infuse over 24 hrs. • A too-rapid IV rate, high doses may cause ototoxicity; administer IV rate *slowly*.

IV INCOMPATIBILITY ⊘

Do not mix with any other medications.

IV COMPATIBILITY

Milrinone (Primacor).

INDICATIONS/ROUTES/DOSAGE

Hypertension:

PO: Adults, elderly: Initially, 5 mg/day. May increase to 10 mg/day if no response in 4–6 wks. If no response, additional antihypertensive added.

Congestive heart failure:

IV/PO: Adults, elderly: Initially, 10–20 mg/day. May increase by approximately doubling dose until desired diuretic dose attained. (Dose >200 mg not adequately studied.)

Chronic renal failure:

IV/PO: Adults, elderly: Initially, 20 mg/day. May increase by approximately doubling dose until desired diuretic dose attained. (Dose >200 mg not adequately studied.)

Hepatic cirrhosis:

IV/PO: Adults, elderly: Initially, 5 mg/day (with aldosterone antagonist or potassium-sparing diuretic). May increase by approximately doubling dose until desired diuretic dose attained. (Dose >40 mg not adequately studied.)

SIDE EFFECTS

FREQUENT (3–10%): Headache, dizziness, rhinitis. **OCCASIONAL** (1–3%): Asthenia, insomnia, nervousness, diarrhea, constipation, nausea, dyspepsia, edema, EKG changes, sore throat, cough, arthralgia, myalgia. **RARE** (<1%): Syncope, hypotension, arrhythmias.

ADVERSE REACTIONS/TOXIC EFFECTS

Ototoxicity may occur with a too-rapid IV rate or with high doses; must be administered slowly. Overdosage produces acute, profound water loss, volume and electrolyte depletion, dehydration, decreased blood volume, circulatory collapse.

NURSING IMPLICATIONS

BASELINE ASSESSMENT:

Assess baseline. Check electrolyte levels, esp. potassium. Obtain baseline weight; check for edema, rales in lungs.

INTERVENTION/EVALUATION:

Monitor B/P, electrolytes (esp. potassium), I&O, weight. Notify physician of any hearing abnormality. Note extent of diuresis. Assess lungs for rales. Check for signs of edema, particularly of dependent areas. Although less potassium is lost with torsemide than furosemide, assess for signs of hypokalemia (change of muscle strength, tremor, muscle cramps, change in mental status, cardiac arrhythmias).

PATIENT/FAMILY TEACHING:

Take medication in morning to prevent nocturia. Expect increased frequency and volume of urination. Report irregular heartbeats, signs of hypokalemia (see above), muscle weakness, cramps, nausea, or dizziness. Do not take other medications (including OTC drugs) without consulting physician. Eat foods high in potassium such as whole grains (cereals), legumes, meat, bananas, apricots, orange juice, potatoes (white, sweet), raisins.

tramadol hydrochloride &

tray-mah-doal
(Ultram)
Do not confuse with Toradol, Ultane.

FIXED-COMBINATION(S)

With acetaminophen, an analgesic **(Ultracet)**

▶CLASSIFICATION

CLINICAL: Analgesic

ACTION/THERAPEUTIC EFFECT

Binds to μ-opiate receptors and inhibits reuptake of norepinephrine and serotonin. *Reduces intensity of pain stimuli incoming from sensory nerve endings, altering pain perception and emotional response to pain.*

PHARMACOKINETICS

	Onset	Peak	Duration
PO	<1 hr	2–3 hrs	4–6 hrs

Rapidly, almost completely absorbed following PO administration. Protein binding: 20%. Extensively metabolized in liver to active metabolite (reduced in pts with advanced cirrhosis). Primarily excreted in urine. Minimally removed by hemodialysis. Half-life: 6–7 hrs.

USES

Management of moderate to moderately severe pain.

PRECAUTIONS

CONTRAINDICATIONS: Acute intoxication with alcohol, hypnotics, centrally acting analgesics, opioids or psychotropic drugs. *EXTREME CAUTION:* CNS depression, anoxia, advanced liver cirrhosis, epilepsy, respiratory depression, acute alcoholism, shock. *CAUTIONS:* Sensitivity to opioids, increased intracranial pressure, impaired hepatic/renal function, acute abdominal conditions, opioid-dependent pts.

▷*LIFESPAN CONSIDERATIONS:* **Pregnancy/Lactation:** Crosses placenta; distributed in breast milk. **Pregnancy Category C. Children:** Safety and efficacy not established. **Elderly:** Age-related renal impairment may require dosage adjustment.

INTERACTIONS

DRUG: **Alcohol, CNS depressants** may increase CNS effects or respiratory depression, hypotension. **MAO inhibitors** increase tramadol concentration. **Carbamazepine** increases tramadol metabolism, decreases concentration. *HERBAL:* None known. *FOOD:* None known. *LAB VALUES:* May increase creatinine, liver enzymes. May decrease hemoglobin, proteinuria.

AVAILABILITY (Rx)

TABLETS: 50 mg.

ADMINISTRATION/HANDLING

PO:
• Give without regard to meals.

INDICATIONS/ROUTES/DOSAGE

Moderate to moderately severe pain:

PO: **Adults, elderly:** 50–100 mg q4–6h. **Maximum <75 yrs:** 400 mg/day. **Maximum >75 yrs:** 300 mg/day.

Renal function impairment (creatinine clearance <30 ml/min):

Note: Dialysis pts can receive their regular dose on day of dialysis.

PO: **Adults, elderly:** Increase dosing interval to 12 hrs. **Maximum daily dose:** 200 mg.

Hepatic function impairment:

PO: **Adults, elderly:** 50 mg q12h.

SIDE EFFECTS

FREQUENT (15–25%): Dizziness/vertigo, nausea, constipation, headache, somnolence. *OCCASIONAL* (5–10%): Vomiting, pruritus, CNS stimulation (nervousness, anxiety, agitation, tremor, euphoria, mood swings, hallucinations), asthenia, sweating, dyspepsia, dry mouth, diarrhea. *RARE* (<5%): Malaise, vasodilation, anorexia, flatulence, rash, visual disturbance, urinary retention/frequency, menopausal symptoms.

ADVERSE REACTIONS/TOXIC EFFECTS

Overdosage results in respiratory depression, seizures. Prolonged duration of action, cumulative effect may occur in those with impaired hepatic, renal function.

T

♣ - Canadian trade name ✴ - see also www.wbsaunders.com/SIMON/SaundersNDH

NURSING IMPLICATIONS

BASELINE ASSESSMENT:

Assess onset, type, location, and duration of pain. Effect of medication is reduced if full pain recurs before next dose. Assess drug history, esp. carbamazepine, CNS depressant medication, MAO inhibitors. Review past medical history, esp. epilepsy/seizures. Assess renal/liver function lab values.

INTERVENTION/EVALUATION:

Assist with ambulation if dizziness, vertigo occurs. Dry crackers, cola may relieve nausea. Question bowel activity, frequency. Palpate bladder for urinary retention. Monitor pattern of daily bowel activity and stool consistency. Sips of tepid water may relieve dry mouth. Assess for clinical improvement and record onset of relief of pain.

PATIENT/FAMILY TEACHING:

Avoid tasks that require alertness, motor skills until response to drug is established.

trandolapril

tran-**doal**-ah-prill
(Mavik)

FIXED-COMBINATION(S)

With verapamil, a calcium channel blocker **(Tarka)**

▶**CLASSIFICATION**

PHARMACOTHERAPEUTIC:
Angiotensin-converting enzyme (ACE) inhibitor. ***CLINICAL:*** Antihypertensive, CHF agent (see p. 6C)

ACTION/*THERAPEUTIC EFFECT*

Suppresses renin-angiotensin-aldosterone system (prevents conversion of angiotensin I to angiotensin II, a potent vasoconstrictor; may also inhibit angiotensin II at local vascular and renal sites). Decreases plasma angiotensin II, increases plasma renin activity, decreases aldosterone secretion. *Reduces peripheral arterial resistance, pulmonary capillary wedge pressure; improves cardiac output, exercise tolerance.*

PHARMACOKINETICS

Slowly absorbed from GI tract. Protein binding: 80%. Metabolized in liver, GI mucosa to active metabolite. Primarily excreted in urine. Removed by hemodialysis. Half-life: 6–10 hrs.

USES

Treatment of hypertension. Used alone or in combination with other antihypertensives. Treatment of congestive heart failure (CHF).

PRECAUTIONS

CONTRAINDICATIONS: History of angioedema with previous treatment with ACE inhibitors. ***CAUTIONS:*** Renal impairment, those with sodium depletion or on diuretic therapy, dialysis, hypovolemia, coronary or cerebrovascular insufficiency.

▷***LIFESPAN CONSIDERATIONS:***
Pregnancy/Lactation: Crosses placenta; distributed in breast milk. May cause fetal/neonatal mortality/morbidity. **Pregnancy Category C** (first trimester); **Pregnancy Category D** (second and third trimesters). **Children:** Safety and efficacy not established. **Elderly:** No age-related precautions noted.

INTERACTIONS

DRUG:* Alcohol, diuretics, hypotensive agents** may increase effects. **NSAIDs** may decrease effect. **Potassium-sparing diuretics, potassium supplements** may cause hyperkalemia. May increase **lithium** concentration, toxicity. ***HERBAL: None known. ***FOOD:*** None known. ***LAB VALUES:*** May increase potassium, SGOT (AST), SGPT (ALT), alkaline phosphatase, bilirubin, BUN, creatinine. May decrease sodium. May cause positive ANA titer.

AVAILABILITY (Rx)

TABLETS: 1 mg, 2 mg, 4 mg.

ADMINISTRATION/HANDLING

PO:

• Give without regard to meals. • Tablets may be crushed.

INDICATIONS/ROUTES/DOSAGE

Hypertension (without diuretic):

***PO:* Adults, elderly:** Initially, 1 mg once daily in nonblack pts, 2 mg once daily in black pts. Adjust dose at least at 7 day intervals. **Maintenance:** 2–4 mg/day. **Maximum:** 8 mg/day.

CHF:

***PO:* Adults, elderly:** Initially, 0.5–1 mg, titrated to target dose of 4 mg/day.

SIDE EFFECTS

FREQUENT (23–35%): Dizziness, cough. ***OCCASIONAL*** (3–11%): Hypotension, dyspepsia (heartburn, epigastric pain, indigestion), syncope, asthenia (loss of strength), tinnitus. ***RARE*** (<1%): Palpitations, insomnia, drowsiness, nausea, vomiting, constipation, flushed skin.

ADVERSE REACTIONS/TOXIC EFFECTS

Excessive hypotension ("first-dose syncope") may occur in those with CHF, severely salt/volume depleted. Angioedema (swelling of face/lips), hyperkalemia occur rarely. Agranulocytosis, neutropenia may be noted in those with impaired renal function or collagen vascular disease (systemic lupus erythematosus, scleroderma). Nephrotic syndrome may be noted in those with history of renal disease.

NURSING IMPLICATIONS

BASELINE ASSESSMENT:

Obtain B/P immediately before each dose, in addition to regular monitoring (be alert to fluctuations). Renal function tests should be performed before therapy begins. In those with renal impairment, autoimmune disease, or taking drugs that affect leukocytes or immune response, CBC and differential count should be performed before therapy begins and q2wks for 3 mos, then periodically thereafter.

INTERVENTION/EVALUATION:

If excessive reduction in B/P occurs, place pt in supine position with legs elevated. Assist with ambulation if dizziness occurs. Assess for urinary frequency. Auscultate lung sounds for rales, wheezing in those with CHF. Monitor urinalysis for proteinuria. Monitor serum potassium levels in those on concurrent diuretic therapy. Monitor pattern of daily bowel activity and stool consistency.

T

PATIENT/FAMILY TEACHING:
Report any sign of infection (sore throat, fever). Several wks may be needed for full therapeutic effect of B/P reduction. Skipping doses or voluntarily discontinuing drug may produce severe, rebound hypertension. To reduce hypotensive effect, rise slowly from lying to sitting position and permit legs to dangle from bed momentarily before standing. Report facial swelling, difficulty swallowing. Avoid potassium supplements/salt substitutes.

tranylcypromine sulfate

tran-ill-**sip**-roe-meen
(Parnate)

▶CLASSIFICATION

PHARMACOTHERAPEUTIC:
MAO inhibitor. ***CLINICAL:*** Antidepressant (see p. 35C)

ACTION/*THERAPEUTIC EFFECT*

Inhibits MAO enzyme (assists in metabolism of sympathomimetic amines) at CNS storage sites. Levels of epinephrine, norepinephrine, serotonin, dopamine increased at neuron receptor sites, *producing antidepressant effect.*

USES

Symptomatic treatment of severe depression in hospitalized or closely supervised pts who have not responded to other antidepressant therapy, including electroconvulsive therapy.

PRECAUTIONS

CONTRAINDICATIONS: Pts >60 yrs, debilitated/hypertensive pts, cerebrovascular/cardiovascular disease, foods containing tryptophan/tyramine, within 10 days of elective surgery, pheochromocytoma, CHF, history of liver disease, abnormal liver function tests, severe renal impairment, history of severe/recurrent headache. ***CAUTIONS:*** Impaired renal function, history of seizures, parkinsonian syndrome, diabetic pts, hyperthyroidism.

INTERACTIONS

DRUG: **Alcohol, CNS depressants** may increase CNS depressant effects. **Tricyclic antidepressants, fluoxetine, trazodone** may cause serotonin syndrome. May increase effect of **oral hypoglycemics, insulin.** B/P may increase with **buspirone. Caffeine-containing medications** may increase cardiac arrhythmias, hypertension. May precipitate hypertensive crises with **carbamazepine, cyclobenzaprine, maprotiline, other MAO inhibitors. Meperidine, other opioid analgesics** may produce immediate excitation, sweating, rigidity, severe hypertension or hypotension, severe respiratory distress, coma, convulsions, vascular collapse, death. May increase CNS stimulant, vasopressor effects. **Tyramine, foods with pressor amines (e.g., aged cheese)** may cause sudden, severe hypertension. ***HERBAL:*** None known. ***FOOD:*** None known. ***LAB VALUES:*** None significant.

AVAILABILITY (Rx)
TABLETS: 10 mg.

INDICATIONS/ROUTES/DOSAGE
PO: Adults, elderly: 30 mg/day in

---

divided doses. May increase dose by 10 mg/day at intervals of 1–3 wks. **Maximum:** 60 mg/day.

SIDE EFFECTS

FREQUENT: Postural hypotension, restlessness, GI upset, insomnia, dizziness, lethargy, weakness, dry mouth, peripheral edema. ***OCCASIONAL:*** Flushing, increased perspiration, rash, urinary frequency, increased appetite, transient impotence. ***RARE:*** Visual disturbances.

ADVERSE REACTIONS/TOXIC EFFECTS

Hypertensive crisis may be noted by hypertension, occipital headache radiating frontally, neck stiffness/soreness, nausea, vomiting, sweating, fever/chilliness, clammy skin, dilated pupils, palpitations. Tachycardia/bradycardia, constricting chest pain may also be present. Antidote for hypertensive crisis: 5–10 mg phentolamine IV injection.

NURSING IMPLICATIONS

BASELINE ASSESSMENT:

Periodic liver function tests should be performed in those requiring high dosage and/or undergoing prolonged therapy. MAO inhibitor therapy should be discontinued for 7–14 days before elective surgery.

INTERVENTION/EVALUATION:

Assess appearance, behavior, speech pattern, level of interest, mood. Supervise suicidal risk pt closely during early therapy (as depression lessens, energy level improves, increasing suicide potential). Monitor for occipital headache radiating frontally, and/or neck stiffness or soreness

(may be first signal of impending hypertensive crisis). Monitor blood pressure diligently for hypertension. Assess skin temperature for fever. Discontinue medication immediately if palpitations or frequent headaches occur.

PATIENT/FAMILY TEACHING:

Antidepressant relief may be noted during first week of therapy; maximum benefit noted within 3 wks. Report headache, neck stiffness/soreness immediately. To avoid orthostatic hypotension, change from lying to sitting position slowly and dangle legs momentarily before standing. Avoid foods that require bacteria/molds for their preparation/preservation or those that contain tyramine, e.g., cheese, sour cream, beer, wine, pickled herring, liver, figs, raisins, bananas, avocados, soy sauce, yeast extracts, yogurt, papaya, broad beans, meat tenderizers, or excessive amounts of caffeine (coffee, tea, chocolate), or OTC preparations for hay fever, colds, weight reduction.

---

trastuzumab

traz-**two**-zoo-mab
(Herceptin)

▶CLASSIFICATION

PHARMACOTHERAPEUTIC: Monoclonal antibody. ***CLINICAL:*** Antineoplastic (see p. 74C)

ACTION/*THERAPEUTIC EFFECT*

Inhibits proliferation of human tumor cells that overexpress HER-2 (HER-2 protein overexpression is

T

seen in 25–30% of primary breast cancer pts). Mediates antibody-dependent cellular cytotoxicity.

PHARMACOKINETICS

Half-life: 5.8 days (range: 1–32 days).

USES

Treatment of metastatic breast cancer pts whose tumors overexpress HER-2 protein and who have received one or more chemotherapy regimens. May be used with paclitaxel without previous treatment for metastatic disease.

PRECAUTIONS

CONTRAINDICATIONS: Preexisting cardiac disease. ***CAUTIONS:*** Previous cardiotoxic drug or radiation therapy to chest wall, those with known hypersensitivity to trastuzumab.

▷***LIFESPAN CONSIDERATIONS:*** **Pregnancy/Lactation:** Unknown if distributed in breast milk. **Pregnancy Category B. Children:** Safety and efficacy not established. **Elderly:** Age-related cardiac dysfunction may require cautious use.

INTERACTIONS

DRUG: **Cyclophosphamide, doxorubicin** or **epirubicin** may increase risk of developing cardiac dysfunction. ***HERBAL:*** None known. ***FOOD:*** None known. ***LAB VALUES:*** None significant.

AVAILABILITY (Rx)

LYOPHILIZED POWDER: 440 mg.

ADMINISTRATION/HANDLING

IV 🏛

Storage:

• Refrigerate vial. • Reconstituted solution appears colorless to pale yellow. • Solution is stable for 28 days if refrigerated after reconstitution with Bacteriostatic Water for Injection (if using Sterile Water for Injection without preservative, use immediately; discard unused portions). • Stable for 24 hrs in 0.9% NaCl if refrigerated.

Reconstitution:

• Reconstitute with 20 ml Bacteriostatic Water for Injection to yield concentration of 21 mg/ml. • Add calculated dose to 250 ml 0.9% NaCl (do not use D_5W). • Gently mix contents in bag.

Rate of administration:

• Do not give IV push or bolus. • Give loading dose (4 mg/kg) over 90 min. Give maintenance infusion (2 mg/kg) over 30 min.

IV INCOMPATIBILITIES ⊘

Avoid use with D_5W. Do not mix with any other medications.

INDICATIONS/ROUTES/DOSAGE

Note: Do not give as IV bolus or IV push. Do *not* use dextrose solutions.

Breast cancer:

IV INFUSION: **Adults, elderly:** Initially, 4 mg/kg as 90 min infusion, then weekly infusion of 2 mg/kg as 30 min infusion.

SIDE EFFECTS

FREQUENT (>20%): Pain, asthenia, fever, chills, headache, abdominal pain, back pain, infection, nausea, diarrhea, vomiting, cough, dyspnea. ***OCCASIONAL*** (5–15%): Tachycardia, CHF, flulike symptoms, anorexia, edema, bone pain, arthralgia, insomnia, dizziness, paresthesia, depression, rhinitis, pharyngitis, sinusitis. ***RARE*** (<5%): Allergic reaction, anemia, leukopenia, neuropathy, herpes simplex.

ADVERSE REACTIONS/TOXIC EFFECTS

Cardiomyopathy, development of ventricular dysfunction and CHF occur rarely. Pancytopenia may occur.

NURSING IMPLICATIONS

BASELINE ASSESSMENT:

Evaluate left ventricular function. Obtain baseline echocardiogram, EKG, MUGA scan. CBC, platelet count should be obtained at regular interval during therapy.

INTERVENTION/EVALUATION:

Frequently monitor for deteriorating cardiac function. Assess for asthenia (loss of strength, energy). Assist with ambulation if asthenia occurs. Monitor for fever, chills, abdominal pain, back pain. Offer antiemetics if nausea, vomiting occurs. Monitor daily bowel activity, stool consistency.

PATIENT/FAMILY TEACHING:

Do not have immunizations without physician's approval (lowers body's resistance). Avoid contact with those who have recently taken oral polio vaccine. Avoid crowds, those with infection.

travoprost

(Travatan)

See Classification section under: Antiglaucoma agents (p. 45C)

trazodone hydrochloride

tra-zoh-doan
(Desyrel)
Do not confuse with Delsym, Zestril.

►CLASSIFICATION
Antidepressant (see p. 36C)

ACTION/*THERAPEUTIC EFFECT*

Blocks reuptake of serotonin by CNS presynaptic neuronal membranes, increasing availability at postsynaptic neuronal receptor sites. Resulting enhancement of synaptic activity *produces antidepressant effect.*

PHARMACOKINETICS

Well absorbed from GI tract. Protein binding: 85–95%. Metabolized in liver. Primarily excreted in urine. Unknown if removed by hemodialysis. Half-life: 5–9 hrs.

USES/*UNLABELED*

Treatment of depression exhibited as persistent, prominent dysphoria (occurring nearly every day for at least 2 wks) manifested by 4 of 8 symptoms: appetite change, sleep pattern change, increased fatigue, impaired concentration, feelings of guilt or worthlessness, loss of interest in usual activities, psychomotor agitation or retardation, suicidal tendencies. *Treatment of neurogenic pain.*

PRECAUTIONS

CONTRAINDICATIONS: Recovery phase of MI, surgical pts, electroconvulsive therapy. ***CAUTIONS:*** Cardiovascular disease, MAO inhibitor therapy.

T

▷*LIFESPAN CONSIDERATIONS:*
Pregnancy/Lactation: Crosses placenta; minimally distributed in breast milk. **Pregnancy Category C. Children:** Safety and efficacy not established in those <6 yrs of age. **Elderly:** More likely to experience sedative or hypotensive effects; lower dosage recommended.

INTERACTIONS

DRUG: **Alcohol, CNS depressant–producing medications** may increase CNS depression. May increase effects of **antihypertensives.** May increase concentration of **digoxin, phenytoin.** *HERBAL:* **St. John's wort** may increase adverse effects. *FOOD:* None known. *LAB VALUES:* May decrease neutrophil, leukocyte counts.

AVAILABILITY (Rx)

TABLETS: 50 mg, 100 mg, 150 mg, 300 mg.

ADMINISTRATION/HANDLING

PO:

• Give shortly after snack, meal (reduces risk of dizziness, lightheadedness). • Tablets may be crushed.

INDICATIONS/ROUTES/DOSAGE

Antidepressant:

PO: **Adults:** Initially, 150 mg daily in equally divided doses. Increase by 50 mg/day at 3–4 day intervals until therapeutic response is achieved. **Maximum:** 600 mg/day. **Children 6–18 yrs:** Initially, 1.5–2 mg/kg/day in divided doses. May increase gradually to 6 mg/kg/day in 3 divided doses.

Usual elderly dosage:

PO: Initially, 25–50 mg at bedtime. May increase by 25–50 mg q3–7days. **Range:** 75–150 mg/day.

SIDE EFFECTS

FREQUENT (3–9%): Drowsiness, dry mouth, lightheadedness/dizziness, headache, blurred vision, nausea/vomiting. *OCCASIONAL* (1–3%): Nervousness, fatigue, constipation, generalized aches and pains, mild hypotension.

ADVERSE REACTIONS/TOXIC EFFECTS

Priapism (painful, prolonged penile erection), decreased/increased libido, retrograde ejaculation, impotence have been noted rarely. Appears to be less cardiotoxic than other antidepressants, although arrhythmias may occur in pts with preexisting cardiac disease.

NURSING IMPLICATIONS

BASELINE ASSESSMENT:

For those on long-term therapy, liver/renal function tests, blood counts should be performed periodically.

INTERVENTION/EVALUATION:

Supervise suicidal risk pt closely during early therapy (as depression lessens, energy level improves, increasing suicide potential). Assess appearance, behavior, speech pattern, level of interest, mood. Monitor WBC and neutrophil count (drug should be stopped if levels fall below normal). Assist with ambulation if dizziness or lightheadedness occurs.

PATIENT/FAMILY TEACHING:

Immediately discontinue medication and consult physician if priapism occurs. Change positions slowly to avoid hypotensive effect. Tolerance to sedative and anticholinergic effects usually develops during early therapy. Photosensitivity to sun may occur. Dry mouth may be relieved by sugarless gum, sips of tepid water. Report visual disturbances. Do not abruptly discontinue medication. Avoid tasks that require alertness, motor skills until response to drug is established. Avoid alcohol.

tretinoin

tret-ih-noyn
(Avita, Renova, Retin-A, Retin-A Micro, Stieva-A✿, Vesanoid, Vitamin A Acid✿)
Do not confuse with trientine.

FIXED-COMBINATION(S)

With octyl methoxycinnamate and oxybenzone, moisturies, and SPF-12, a sunscreen **(Retin-A Regimen Kit)**

▶CLASSIFICATION

PHARMACOTHERAPEUTIC: Retinoid. **CLINICAL:** Antiacne, transdermal, antineoplastic (see p. 74C)

ACTION/THERAPEUTIC EFFECT

Antiacne: Decreases cohesiveness of follicular epithelial cells. Increases turnover of follicular epithelial cells, *causing expulsion of blackheads.* Bacterial skin counts are not altered. **Transdermal:** Exerts its effects on growth and differentiation of epithelial cells, *alleviating fine wrinkles, hyperpigmentation.* **Antineoplastic:** Induces maturation, decreases proliferation of acute promyelocytic leukemia (APL) cells, *followed by repopulation of bone marrow and* *blood by normal hematopoietic cells.*

PHARMACOKINETICS

Topical: Minimally absorbed. **PO:** Well absorbed following PO administration. Primarily excreted in urine. Half-life: 0.5–2 hrs.

USES/*UNLABELED*

Topical: Treatment of acne vulgaris, esp. grades I–III in which blackheads, papules, pustules predominate. **Transdermal:** Treatment of fine wrinkles, hyperpigmentation. **Antineoplastic:** Induction of remission in pts with acute promyelocytic leukemia (APL). *Treatment of disorders of keratinization, including photo-aged skin, liver spots.*

PRECAUTIONS

CONTRAINDICATIONS: Sensitivity to parabens (used as preservative in gelatin capsule). **EXTREME CAUTION: Topical:** Eczema, sun exposure. **CAUTIONS: Topical:** Those with considerable sun exposure in their occupation or hypersensitivity to sun. **PO:** Elevated cholesterol/triglycerides.

▷*LIFESPAN CONSIDERATIONS:*
Pregnancy/Lactation: Topical: Use during pregnancy only if clearly needed. Unknown if excreted in breast milk; exercise caution in nursing mother. **Pregnancy Category C (Topical). PO:** Teratogenic, embryotoxic effect. **Pregnancy Category D. Children/Elderly:** Safety and efficacy not established.

INTERACTIONS

DRUG: Topical: Keratolytic agents (e.g., sulfur, benzoyl peroxide, salicylic acid), medicated soaps, shampoos, astringents, spice or lime cologne, permanent wave solutions, hair depilatories may increase skin irritation. **Photosensitive medication (thiazides, tetracyclines, fluoroquinolones, phenothiazines, sulfonamides)** augments phototoxicity. *PO:* **Ketoconazole** may increase tretinoin concentration. *HERBAL:* None known. *FOOD:* None known. *LAB VALUES: PO:* Leukocytosis occurs commonly (40%). May elevate liver function tests, cholesterol, triglycerides.

AVAILABILITY [Rx]

CAPSULES: 10 mg. *CREAM:* 0.025%, 0.05%, 0.1%. *CREAM (Avita):* 0.025%. *(Renova):* 0.05%. *GEL:* 0.025%, 0.01%. *(Retin-A Micro):* 0.1%. *LIQUID:* 0.05%.

ADMINISTRATION/HANDLING

PO:

* Do not crush or break capsule.

Topical:

* Thoroughly cleanse area before applying tretinoin. * Lightly cover only the affected area. Liquid may be applied with fingertip, gauze, or cotton, taking care to avoid running onto unaffected skin. * Keep medication away from eyes, mouth, angles of nose, mucous membranes. * Wash hands immediately after application.

INDICATIONS/ROUTES/DOSAGE

Acne:

TOPICAL: **Adults:** Apply once daily at bedtime.

Acute promyelocytic leukemia:

PO: **Adults:** 45 mg/m^2/day given as two evenly divided doses until complete remission is documented. Discontinue therapy 30 days after complete remission or after 90 days of treatment, whichever comes first.

SIDE EFFECTS

Topical: Temporary change in pigmentation, photosensitivity. Local inflammatory reactions (peeling, dry skin, stinging, erythema, pruritus) are to be expected and are reversible with discontinuation of tretinoin. *FREQUENT, PO* (54–87%): Headache, fever, dry skin/oral mucosa, bone pain, nausea, vomiting, rash. *OCCASIONAL, PO* (6–26%): Mucositis, earache or feeling of fullness in ears, flushing, pruritus, increased sweating, visual disturbances, hypo/hypertension, dizziness, anxiety, insomnia, alopecia, skin changes. *RARE* (6%): Change in visual acuity, temporary hearing loss.

ADVERSE REACTIONS/TOXIC EFFECTS

PO: Retinoic acid syndrome (fever, dyspnea, weight gain, abnormal chest auscultatory findings [pulmonary infiltrates, pleural or pericardial effusions], episodic hypotension) occurs commonly (25%) as does leukocytosis (40%). Syndrome generally occurs during first mo of therapy (sometimes occurs following first dose). High-dose steroids (dexamethasone 10 mg IV) at first suspicion of syndrome reduces morbidity, mortality. Pseudo tumor cerebri may be noted, esp. in children (headache, nausea, vomiting, visual disturbances). *Topical:* Possible tumorigenic potential when combined with ultraviolet radiation.

NURSING IMPLICATIONS

BASELINE ASSESSMENT:

PO: Inform women of childbearing potential of risk to fetus if pregnancy occurs. Instruct in need for use of two reliable forms of contraceptives concurrently during therapy and for 1 mo after discontinuation of therapy, even in infertile, premenopausal women. Pregnancy test should be obtained within 1 wk prior to institution of therapy. Obtain initial liver function tests, cholesterol, triglyceride levels.

INTERVENTION/EVALUATION:

PO: Monitor liver function tests, hematologic, coagulation profiles, cholesterol, triglycerides. Monitor signs/symptoms of pseudo tumor cerebri in children.

PATIENT/FAMILY TEACHING:

Topical: Avoid exposure to sunlight or sunbeds; use sunscreens and protective clothing. Affected areas should also be protected from wind, cold. If skin is already sunburned, do not use until fully recovered. Keep tretinoin away from eyes, mouth, angles of nose and mucous membranes. Do not use medicated, drying, or abrasive soaps; wash face no more than 2–3 times/day with bland soap. Avoid use of preparations containing alcohol, menthol, spice, or lime such as shaving lotions, astringents, perfume. Mild redness, peeling are expected; decrease frequency or discontinue medication if excessive reaction occurs. Nonmedicated cosmetics may be used; however, cosmetics must be removed before tretinoin application. Improvement noted during first 24 wks of therapy. **Antiacne:** Therapeutic results noted in 2–3 wks; optimal results in 6 wks.

triamcinolone

try-am-**sin**-oh-lone
(Aristocort, Kenacort)

triamcinolone diacetate

(Amcort, Aristocort Intralesional, Trilone)

triamcinolone acetonide

(Aristocort, Azmacort, Kenalog, Nasacort AQ, Triaderm ♣)

triamcinolone hexacetonide

(Aristospan)
Do not confuse with
Triaminicin, Triaminicol.

FIXED-COMBINATION(S)

Triamcinolone acetonide with nystatin, an antifungal **(Myco-Aricin, Myco II, Myco-Biotic, Mycogen II, Nystolone)**

▶CLASSIFICATION

PHARMACOTHERAPEUTIC:
Adrenocortical steroid. ***CLINI-CAL:*** Anti-inflammatory (see pp. 64C, 79C, 82C)

ACTION/*THERAPEUTIC EFFECT*

Inhibits accumulation of inflammatory cells at inflammation sites, phagocytosis, lysosomal enzyme release and synthesis and/or release of mediators of inflammation. *Prevents/suppresses cell-mediated immune reactions. Decreases/prevents tissue response to inflammatory process.*

USES

Substitution therapy in deficiency states: Acute/chronic adrenal insufficiency, congenital adrenal hyperplasia, adrenal insufficiency secondary to pituitary insufficiency. ***Nonendocrine disorders:*** Arthritis, rheumatic carditis, allergic, collagen, intestinal tract, liver,

T

ocular, renal, and skin diseases, bronchial asthma, cerebral edema, malignancies. Allergic rhinitis. **Inhalation:** Maintenance prophylaxis of asthma.

PRECAUTIONS

CONTRAINDICATIONS: Hypersensitivity to any corticosteroid or tartrazine, systemic fungal infection, peptic ulcers (except life-threatening situations). IM injection, oral inhalation not for children <6 yrs of age. Avoid immunizations, smallpox vaccination. **Topical:** Marked circulation impairment. **CAUTIONS:** History of tuberculosis (may reactivate disease), hypothyroidism, cirrhosis, nonspecific ulcerative colitis, CHF, hypertension, psychosis, renal insufficiency. Prolonged therapy should be discontinued slowly.

INTERACTIONS

DRUG: Amphotericin may increase hypokalemia. May decrease effect of **oral hypoglycemics, insulin, diuretics, potassium supplements.** May increase **digoxin** toxicity (due to hypokalemia). **Hepatic enzyme inducers** may decrease effect. **Live virus vaccines** may potentiate virus replication, increase vaccine side effects, decrease pt's antibody response to vaccine. **HERBAL:** None known. **FOOD:** None known. **LAB VALUES:** May decrease calcium, potassium, thyroxine. May increase cholesterol, lipids, glucose, sodium, amylase.

AVAILABILITY (Rx)

TABLETS: 1 mg, 2 mg, 4 mg, 8 mg. **SYRUP:** 4 mg/5 ml. **AEROSOL (respiratory inhalant), NASAL SPRAY, OINTMENT:** 0.025%, 0.1%, 0.5%. **CREAM:** 0.025%, 0.1%, 0.5%. **LOTION:** 0.025%, 0.1%.

ACETONIDE: INJECTION: 3 mg/ml, 10 mg/ml, 40 mg/ml.

DIACETATE: INJECTION: 25 mg/ml, 40 mg/ml.

HEXACETONE: INJECTION: 5 mg/ml, 20 mg/ml.

ADMINISTRATION/HANDLING
PO:

• Give with food or milk. • Single doses given before 9 AM; multiple doses at evenly spaced intervals.

IM:

• Do *not* give IV. • Give deep IM in gluteus maximus.

Inhalation:

• Shake container well; exhale as completely as possible. • Place mouthpiece fully into mouth, holding inhaler upright, inhale deeply and slowly while pressing the top of the cannister and hold breath as long as possible before exhaling; then exhale slowly. • Wait 1 min between inhalations when multiple inhalations ordered (allows for deeper bronchial penetration). • Rinse mouth with water immediately after inhalation.

Topical:

• Gently cleanse area before application. • Use occlusive dressings only as ordered. • Apply sparingly and rub into area thoroughly.

INDICATIONS/ROUTES/DOSAGE
Usual oral dosage:

PO: Adults, elderly: 4–60 mg/day.

Triamcinolone diacetate:

IM: Adults, elderly: 40 mg/wk.

INTRA-ARTICULAR, INTRALESIONAL: Adults, elderly: 5–40 mg.

Triamcinolone acetonide:

IM: Adults, elderly: Initially, 2.5–60 mg/day.

INTRA-ARTICULAR: Adults, elderly: Initially, 2.5–40 mg up to 100 mg.

Triamcinolone hexacetonide:

INTRA-ARTICULAR: Adults, elderly: 2–20 mg.

Control of bronchial asthma:

INHALATION: Adults, elderly: 2 inhalations 3–4 times/day. **Children 6–12 yrs:** 1–2 inhalations 3–4 times/day. **Maximum:** 12 inhalations/day.

Rhinitis:

INTRANASAL: Adults, children >6 yrs: 2 sprays each nostril daily.

Usual topical dosage:

TOPICAL: Adults, elderly: Sparingly 2–4 times/day. May give 1–2 times/day or intermittent therapy.

SIDE EFFECTS

FREQUENT: Insomnia, heartburn, nervousness, abdominal distention, increased sweating, acne, mood swings, increased appetite, facial flushing, delayed wound healing, increased susceptibility to infection, diarrhea/constipation. **OCCASIONAL:** Headache, edema, change in skin color, frequent urination. **RARE:** Tachycardia, allergic reaction (rash, hives), psychic changes, hallucinations, depression. *Topical:* Allergic contact dermatitis.

ADVERSE REACTIONS/TOXIC EFFECTS

Long-term therapy: Muscle wasting (esp. arms, legs), osteoporosis, spontaneous fractures, amenorrhea, cataracts, glaucoma, peptic ulcer, CHF. **Abrupt withdrawal following long-term therapy:** anorexia, nausea, fever, headache, joint pain, rebound inflammation, fatigue, weakness, lethargy, dizziness, orthostatic hypotension. Anaphylaxis with parenteral administration occurs rarely. Sudden discontinuance may be fatal. Blindness has occurred rarely after intralesional injection around face, head.

NURSING IMPLICATIONS

BASELINE ASSESSMENT:

Question for hypersensitivity to any of the corticosteroids or tartrazine (Kenacort). Obtain baselines for height, weight, B/P, glucose, electrolytes. Check results of initial tests, e.g., TB skin test, x-rays, EKG.

INTERVENTION/EVALUATION:

Monitor I&O, daily weight; assess for edema. Check vitals at least 2 times/day. Be alert to infection: sore throat, fever, or vague symptoms. Monitor electrolytes. Watch for hypocalcemia (muscle twitching, cramps, positive Trousseau's or Chvostek's signs) or hypokalemia (weakness and muscle cramps, numbness/tingling, esp. in lower extremities, nausea and vomiting, irritability, EKG changes). Assess emotional status, ability to sleep. Check lab results for blood coagulability and clinical evidence of thromboembolism. Provide assistance with ambulation.

PATIENT/FAMILY TEACHING:

Take with food or milk. Do not change dose/schedule or stop taking drug, must taper off gradually under medical supervision. Notify physician of fever, sore throat, muscle aches, sudden weight gain/swelling. With dietician give instructions for

T

prescribed diet (usually sodium restricted with high vitamin D, protein, and potassium). Maintain careful personal hygiene, avoid exposure to disease or trauma. Severe stress (serious infection, surgery, or trauma) may require increased dosage. Inform dentist or other physicians of triamcinolone therapy now or within past 12 mos. **Topical:** Apply after shower/bath for best absorption. Do not cover unless physician orders; do not use tight diapers, plastic pants or coverings. Avoid contact with eyes.

triamterene

try-**am**-tur-een
(Dyrenium)
Do not confuse with diazoxide, Maxidex, trimipramine.

FIXED-COMBINATION(S)

With hydrochlorothiazide, a thiazide diuretic **(Dyazide, Maxzide)**

▶CLASSIFICATION

PHARMACOTHERAPEUTIC:
Potassium-sparing diuretic. ***CLINICAL:*** Antiedema (see p. 84C)

ACTION/THERAPEUTIC EFFECT

Competitively inhibits action of aldosterone. Interferes with sodium reabsorption in distal tubule, *increasing potassium retention while promoting sodium and water excretion.*

PHARMACOKINETICS

	Onset	Peak	Duration
PO	2–4 hrs	6–8 hrs	12–16 hrs

Incompletely absorbed from GI tract. Widely distributed. Metabolized in liver. Primarily eliminated in feces via biliary route. Half-life: 5–7 hrs (half-life increased with impaired renal function).

USES/UNLABELED

Treatment of edema associated with CHF, hepatic cirrhosis, nephrotic syndrome, steroid-induced edema, idiopathic edema, edema due to secondary hyperaldosteronism. May be used alone or with other diuretics. *Treatment adjunct for hypertension, prophylaxis/treatment of hypokalemia.*

PRECAUTIONS

CONTRAINDICATIONS: Severe or progressive renal disease, severe hepatic disease, preexisting or drug-induced hyperkalemia. ***CAUTIONS:*** Impaired hepatic or kidney function, history of renal calculi, diabetes mellitus.

▷***LIFESPAN CONSIDERATIONS:***
Pregnancy/Lactation: Crosses placenta; distributed in breast milk. Nursing is not advised. **Pregnancy Category D. Children:** Safety and efficacy not established. **Elderly:** May be at increased risk for developing hyperkalemia.

INTERACTIONS

DRUG: May decrease effect of **anticoagulants, heparin. NSAIDs** may decrease antihypertensive effect. **ACE inhibitors (e.g., captopril), potassium-containing medications, potassium supplements** may increase potassium. May decrease **lithium** clearance, increase toxicity. ***HERBAL:*** None known. ***FOOD:*** None known. ***LAB VALUES:*** May increase BUN, calcium excretion, creatinine, glucose, magnesium, potassium, uric acid. May decrease sodium.

AVAILABILITY (Rx)

CAPSULES: 50 mg, 100 mg.

ADMINISTRATION/HANDLING

PO:

• Give with food if GI disturbances occur. • Do not crush or break capsules.

INDICATIONS/ROUTES/DOSAGE

Edema, hypertension:

PO: Adults, elderly: 25–100 mg/day in 1 or 2 divided doses. **Maximum:** 300 mg/day. **Children:** 2–4 mg/kg/day in 1 or 2 divided doses. **Maximum:** 6 mg/kg/day or 300 mg/day.

SIDE EFFECTS

OCCASIONAL: Tiredness, nausea, diarrhea, abdominal distress, leg aches, headache. **RARE:** Anorexia, weakness, rash, dizziness.

ADVERSE REACTIONS/TOXIC EFFECTS

May produce hyponatremia (drowsiness, dry mouth, increased thirst, lack of energy) or severe hyperkalemia (irritability, anxiety, heaviness of legs, paresthesia, hypotension, bradycardia, tented T waves, widening QRS, ST depression). Agranulocytosis, nephrolithiasis, thrombocytopenia occur rarely.

NURSING IMPLICATIONS

BASELINE ASSESSMENT:

Assess baseline electrolytes, particularly check for low potassium. Assess renal/hepatic functions. Assess edema (note location, extent), skin turgor, mucous membranes for hydration status. Assess muscle strength, mental status. Note skin temperature, moisture. Obtain baseline weight. Initiate strict I&O. Note pulse rate/regularity.

INTERVENTION/EVALUATION:

Monitor B/P, vital signs, electrolytes (particularly potassium), I&O, weight. Note extent of diuresis. Watch for changes from initial assessment (hyperkalemia may result in muscle strength changes, tremor, muscle cramps), change in mental status (orientation, alertness, confusion), cardiac arrhythmias. Monitor potassium level, particularly during initial therapy. Weigh daily. Assess lung sounds for rhonchi, wheezing.

PATIENT/FAMILY TEACHING:

Expect increase in volume and frequency of urination. Therapeutic effect takes several days to begin and can last for several days when drug is discontinued. Avoid prolonged exposure to sunlight. Report severe or persistent weakness, headache, dry mouth, nausea, vomiting, fever, sore throat, unusual bleeding/bruising.

triazolam

try-**aye**-zoe-lam
(Apo-Triazo✚, Halcion)
Do not confuse with Haldol, Healon.

▶CLASSIFICATION

PHARMACOTHERAPEUTIC: Benzodiazepine **(Schedule IV).** **CLINICAL:** Sedative-hypnotic (see p. 123C)

T

ACTION/*THERAPEUTIC EFFECT*

Enhances action of inhibitory neurotransmitter gamma-aminobutyric acid (GABA), *producing hypnotic effect due to CNS depression.*

PHARMACOKINETICS

Well absorbed from GI tract. Protein binding: 89%. Widely distributed (crosses blood-brain barrier). Metabolized in liver (undergoes first-pass liver extraction). Primarily excreted in urine. Not removed by hemodialysis. Half-life: 1.5–5.5 hrs.

USES

Short-term treatment of insomnia (up to 6 wks). Reduces sleep-induction time, number of nocturnal awakenings; increases length of sleep.

PRECAUTIONS

CONTRAINDICATIONS: Acute narrow-angle glaucoma, acute alcohol intoxication. ***CAUTIONS:*** Impaired renal/hepatic function.
▷*LIFESPAN CONSIDERATIONS:*
Pregnancy/Lactation: Crosses placenta; may be distributed in breast milk. Chronic ingestion during pregnancy may produce withdrawal symptoms, CNS depression in neonates. **Pregnancy Category X. Children:** Not recommended in those <18 yrs of age. **Elderly:** Use small initial doses with gradual increases to avoid ataxia or excessive sedation.

INTERACTIONS

DRUG: **Alcohol, CNS depressants** may increase CNS depressant effect. ***HERBAL:*** **Kava kava, valerian** may increase CNS depression. ***FOOD:*** **Grapefruit/grapefruit juice** may alter absorption. ***LAB VALUES:*** None significant.

AVAILABILITY (Rx)

TABLETS: 0.125 mg, 0.25 mg.

ADMINISTRATION/HANDLING

PO:

• Give without regard to meals. • Tablets may be crushed. • Grapefruit juice may alter absorption.

INDICATIONS/ROUTES/DOSAGE

Hypnotic:

PO: **Adults >18 yrs:** 0.125–0.5 mg at bedtime. **Elderly:** 0.0625–0.125 mg at bedtime.

SIDE EFFECTS

FREQUENT: Drowsiness, sedation, headache, dizziness, nervousness, lightheadedness, incoordination, nausea. ***OCCASIONAL:*** Euphoria, tachycardia, abdominal cramps, visual disturbances. ***RARE:*** Paradoxical CNS excitement, restlessness, particularly noted in elderly, debilitated.

ADVERSE REACTIONS/TOXIC EFFECTS

Abrupt or too-rapid withdrawal may result in pronounced restlessness, irritability, insomnia, hand tremors, abdominal/muscle cramps, sweating, vomiting, seizures. Overdosage results in somnolence, confusion, diminished reflexes, coma.

NURSING IMPLICATIONS

BASELINE ASSESSMENT:

Question for possibility of pregnancy before initiating therapy (Pregnancy Category X). Assess B/P, pulse, respirations immediately before administration. Raise bed rails. Provide environment conducive to sleep (backrub, quiet environment, low lighting).

INTERVENTION/EVALUATION:

Assess sleep pattern of pt. Assess elderly/debilitated for paradoxical reaction, particularly during early therapy. Evaluate for therapeutic response to insomnia: decrease in number of nocturnal awakenings, increase in length of sleep.

PATIENT/FAMILY TEACHING:

Smoking reduces drug effectiveness. Rebound insomnia may occur when drug is discontinued after short-term therapy. Avoid alcohol and other CNS depressants. Inform physician if you are or are planning to become pregnant. May experience disturbed sleep for 1–2 nights after discontinuing triazolam. Avoid concomitant grapefruit juice.

trifluoperazine hydrochloride

try-floo-oh-**pear**-ah-zeen
(Apo-Trifluoperazine✦,
Stelazine)
Do not confuse with selegiline,
triflupromazine.

▶**CLASSIFICATION**

PHARMACOTHERAPEUTIC:
Penothiazine derivative. **CLINICAL:** Antipsychotic, antianxiety
(see p. 56C)

ACTION/THERAPEUTIC EFFECT

Blocks dopamine at postsynaptic receptor sites, *suppressing behavioral response in psychosis, reducing locomotor activity/aggressiveness, suppressing conditioned responses.* Has strong extrapyra-midal, antiemetic action; weak anticholinergic, sedative effects.

USES

Management of psychotic disorders, nonpsychotic anxiety.

PRECAUTIONS

CONTRAINDICATIONS: Severe CNS depression, comatose states, severe cardiovascular disease, bone marrow depression, subcortical brain damage. ***CAUTIONS:*** Impaired respiratory/hepatic/renal/cardiac function, alcohol withdrawal, history of seizures, urinary retention, glaucoma, prostatic hypertrophy, hypocalcemia (increases susceptibility to dystonias).

INTERACTIONS

DRUG: **Alcohol, CNS depressants** may increase CNS, respiratory depression, hypotensive effects. **Tricyclic antidepressants, MAO inhibitors** may increase sedative, anticholinergic effects. **Antithyroid agents** may increase risk of agranulocytosis. Extrapyramidal symptoms (EPS) may increase with **EPS-producing medications. Hypotensives** may increase hypotension. May decrease **levodopa** effects. **Lithium** may decrease absorption, produce adverse neurologic effects. ***HERBAL:*** None known. ***FOOD:*** None known. ***LAB VALUES:*** May cause EKG changes.

INDICATIONS/ROUTES/DOSAGE
Psychotic disorders:
PO: Adults, elderly, children >12 yrs: Initially, 2–5 mg 1–2 times/day. **Range:** 15–20 mg/day. **Maximum:** 40 mg/day. **Children 6–12 yrs:** Initially, 1 mg 1–2 times/day. **Maintenance:** Up to 15 mg/day.

SIDE EFFECTS

FREQUENT: Hypotension, dizziness, and fainting occur frequently after first injection, occasionally after subsequent injections, and rarely with oral dosage. **OCCASIONAL:** Drowsiness during early therapy, dry mouth, blurred vision, lethargy, constipation or diarrhea, nasal congestion, peripheral edema, urinary retention. **RARE:** Ocular changes, skin pigmentation (those on high doses for prolonged periods).

ADVERSE REACTIONS/TOXIC EFFECTS

Extrapyramidal symptoms appear dose related (particularly high dosage) and are divided into 3 categories: akathisia (inability to sit still, tapping of feet, urge to move around); parkinsonian symptoms (masklike face, tremors, shuffling gait, hypersalivation); and acute dystonias: torticollis (neck muscle spasm), opisthotonos (rigidity of back muscles), and oculogyric crisis (rolling back of eyes). Dystonic reaction may also produce profuse sweating, pallor. Tardive dyskinesia (protrusion of tongue, puffing of cheeks, chewing/puckering of the mouth) occurs rarely (may be irreversible). Abrupt withdrawal following long-term therapy may precipitate nausea, vomiting, gastritis, dizziness, tremors. Blood dyscrasias, particularly agranulocytosis, mild leukopenia (sore mouth/gums/throat) may occur. May lower seizure threshold.

NURSING IMPLICATIONS

BASELINE ASSESSMENT:

Avoid skin contact with oral concentrate (contact dermatitis). Assess behavior, appearance, emotional status, response to environment, speech pattern, thought content.

INTERVENTION/EVALUATION:

Monitor B/P for hypotension. Assess for extrapyramidal symptoms. Monitor WBC for blood dyscrasias. Monitor for fine tongue movement (may be early sign of tardive dyskinesia). Supervise suicidal risk pt closely during early therapy (as depression lessens, energy level improves, increasing suicide potential). Assess for therapeutic response (interest in surroundings, improvement in self-care, increased ability to concentrate, relaxed facial expression).

PATIENT/FAMILY TEACHING:

Maximum therapeutic response occurs in 2–3 wks. Urine may darken. Do not abruptly withdraw from long-term drug therapy. Report visual disturbances. Sugarless gum, sips of tepid water may relieve dry mouth. Drowsiness generally subsides during continued therapy. Avoid tasks that require alertness, motor skills until response to drug is established. Avoid alcohol.

---

trihexyphenidyl hydrochloride

try-hex-eh-**fen**-ih-dill
(Apo-Trihex ♣, Artane)

▶CLASSIFICATION

PHARMACOTHERAPEUTIC: Anticholinergic. **CLINICAL:** Antiparkinson

ACTION/*THERAPEUTIC EFFECT*

Blocks central cholinergic receptors (aids in balancing cholinergic and dopaminergic activity). *Decreases salivation, relaxes smooth muscle.*

USES

Adjunctive treatment for all forms of Parkinson's disease, including postencephalitic, arteriosclerotic, idiopathic forms. Controls symptoms of drug-induced extrapyramidal symptoms.

PRECAUTIONS

CONTRAINDICATIONS: Angle closure glaucoma, GI obstruction, paralytic ileus, intestinal atony, severe ulcerative colitis, prostatic hypertrophy, myasthenia gravis, megacolon. ***CAUTIONS:*** Treated open-angle glaucoma, autonomic neuropathy, pulmonary disease, esophageal reflux, hiatal hernia, heart disease, hyperthyroidism, hypertension.

INTERACTIONS

DRUG: **Alcohol, CNS depressants** may increase sedative effect. **Amantadine, anticholinergics, MAO inhibitors** may increase anticholinergic effects. **Antacids, antidiarrheals** may decrease absorption, effects. ***HERBAL:*** None known. ***FOOD:*** None known. ***LAB VALUES:*** None significant.

AVAILABILITY (Rx)

TABLETS: 2 mg, 5 mg. ***ELIXIR:*** 2 mg/5 ml.

INDICATIONS/ROUTES/DOSAGE

Parkinsonism:

Note: Do not use sustained-release capsules for initial therapy. Once stabilized, may switch, on mg-for-mg basis, giving a single daily dose after breakfast or 2 divided doses 12 hrs apart.

PO: Adults, elderly: Initially, 1 mg on first day. May increase by 2 mg/day at 3–5 day intervals up to 6–10 mg/day (12–15 mg/day in pts with postencephalitic parkinsonism).

Drug-induced extrapyramidal symptoms:

PO: Adults, elderly: Initially, 1 mg/day. **Range:** 5–15 mg/day in 3–4 divided doses.

SIDE EFFECTS

Note: Elderly (>60 yrs) tend to develop mental confusion, disorientation, agitation, psychotic-like symptoms. ***FREQUENT:*** Drowsiness, dry mouth. ***OCCASIONAL:*** Blurred vision, urinary retention, constipation, dizziness, headache, muscle cramps. ***RARE:*** Skin rash, seizures, depression.

ADVERSE REACTIONS/TOXIC EFFECTS

Hypersensitivity reaction (eczema, pruritus, rash, cardiac disturbances, photosensitivity) may occur. Overdosage may vary from CNS depression (sedation, apnea, cardiovascular collapse, death) to severe paradoxical reaction (hallucinations, tremor, seizures).

NURSING IMPLICATIONS

INTERVENTION/EVALUATION:
Be alert to neurologic effects: headache, lethargy, mental confusion, agitation. Monitor children closely for paradoxical reaction. Assess for clinical reversal of symptoms (improvement of tremor of head/hands at rest, masklike facial expression, shuffling gait, muscular rigidity).

T

PATIENT/FAMILY TEACHING:
Avoid tasks that require alertness, motor skills until response to drug is established. Dry mouth, drowsiness, dizziness may be an expected response of drug. Avoid alcoholic beverages during therapy. Sugarless gum, sips of tepid water may relieve dry mouth. Coffee/tea may help reduce drowsiness.

trimethobenzamide hydrochloride

try-meth-oh-**benz**-ah-mide
(Tigan)

▶CLASSIFICATION

PHARMACOTHERAPEUTIC:
Anticholinergic. **CLINICAL:** Antiemetic

ACTION/THERAPEUTIC EFFECT

Acts at the chemoreceptor trigger zone in CNS (medulla oblongata), *relieving nausea and vomiting.*

PHARMACOKINETICS

	Onset	Peak	Duration
PO	10–40 min	—	3–4 hrs
IM	15–30 minn	—	2–3 hrs

Partially absorbed from GI tract. Distributed primarily to liver. Metabolic fate unknown. Excreted in urine.

USES

Control of nausea and vomiting.

PRECAUTIONS

CONTRAINDICATIONS: Hypersensitivity to benzocaine or similar local anesthetics; parenteral form in children, suppositories in premature infants or neonates. **CAUTIONS:** Elderly, debilitated, dehydration, electrolyte imbalance, high fever.

▷**LIFESPAN CONSIDERATIONS:**
Pregnancy/Lactation: Unknown whether drug crosses placenta or is distributed in breast milk. **Pregnancy Category C.**

INTERACTIONS

DRUG: CNS depression–producing medications may increase CNS depression. **HERBAL:** None known. **FOOD:** None known. **LAB VALUES:** None significant.

AVAILABILITY (Rx)

CAPSULES: 100 mg, 250 mg. **SUPPOSITORIES:** 100 mg, 200 mg. **INJECTION:** 100 mg/ml.

ADMINISTRATION/HANDLING
PO:
• Give without regard to meals. • Do not crush or break capsule form.

IM:
• Give deep IM into large muscle mass, preferably upper outer gluteus maximus.

Rectal:
• If suppository is too soft, chill for 30 min in refrigerator or run cold water over foil wrapper. • Moisten suppository with cold water before inserting well up into rectum.

INDICATIONS/ROUTES/DOSAGE
Note: Do not use IV route (produces severe hypotension).

Nausea, vomiting:

PO: Adults, elderly: 250 mg 3–4 times/day. **Children 30–100 lbs:** 100–200 mg 3–4 times/day.

IM: Adults, elderly: 200 mg 3–4 times/day.

RECTAL: **Adults, elderly:** 200 mg 3–4 times/day. **Children 30–100 lbs:** 100–200 mg 3–4 times/day. **Children <30 lbs:** 100 mg 3–4 times/day. Do not use in premature or newborn infants.

SIDE EFFECTS

Note: Elderly (>60 yrs) tend to develop mental confusion, disorientation, agitation, psychotic-like symptoms.
FREQUENT: Drowsiness. *OCCASIONAL:* Blurred vision, diarrhea, dizziness, headache, muscle cramps. *RARE:* Skin rash, seizures, depression, opisthotonus, Parkinson's syndrome, Reye's syndrome (vomiting, seizures).

ADVERSE REACTIONS/TOXIC EFFECTS

Hypersensitivity reaction manifested as extrapyramidal symptoms (muscle rigidity, allergic skin reactions) occurs rarely. Children may experience dominant paradoxical reaction (restlessness, insomnia, euphoria, nervousness, tremors). Overdosage may vary from CNS depression (sedation, apnea, cardiovascular collapse, death) to severe paradoxical reaction (hallucinations, tremor, seizures).

NURSING IMPLICATIONS

BASELINE ASSESSMENT:

Assess for dehydration if excessive vomiting occurs (poor skin turgor, dry mucous membranes, longitudinal furrows in tongue).

INTERVENTION/EVALUATION:

Check B/P, esp. in elderly (increased risk of hypotension). Assess children closely for paradoxical reaction. Monitor serum electrolytes in those with severe vomiting. Assess skin turgor, mucous membranes to evaluate hydration status. Assess for extrapyramidal symptoms (hypersensitivity). Measure I&O and assess any vomitus.

PATIENT/FAMILY TEACHING:

Report visual disturbances, headache. Dry mouth is expected response to medication. Relief from nausea/vomiting generally occurs within 30 min of drug administration.

trimethoprim

try-**meth**-oh-prim
(Primsol, Proloprim, Trimpex)

FIXED-COMBINATION(S)

With sulfamethoxazole, a sulfonamide **(Bactrim, Septra)**

▶CLASSIFICATION

PHARMACOTHERAPEUTIC: Folate antagonist. *CLINICAL:* Urinary tract agent, antibacterial

ACTION/*THERAPEUTIC EFFECT*

Blocks bacterial biosynthesis of nucleic acids and proteins by interfering with metabolism of folinic acid, *producing antibacterial activity.*

PHARMACOKINETICS

Rapidly, completely absorbed from GI tract. Protein binding: 42–46%. Widely distributed including CSF. Metabolized in liver. Primarily excreted in urine. Moderately removed by hemodialysis. Half-life: 8–10 hrs (half-life increased with impaired renal function, newborns; decreased in children).

T

USES/*UNLABELED*

Treatment of initial acute uncomplicated urinary tract infections (UTIs). *Prophylaxis of bacterial UTI, treatment of pneumonia caused by Pneumocystis carinii.*

PRECAUTIONS

CONTRAINDICATIONS: Infants <2 mos, megaloblastic anemia due to folic acid deficiency. ***CAUTIONS:*** Impaired renal or hepatic function, children who have X chromosome with mental retardation, pts who have possible folic acid deficiency.

▷***LIFESPAN CONSIDERATIONS:*** **Pregnancy/Lactation:** Readily crosses placenta; distributed in breast milk. **Pregnancy Category C. Children:** Safety and efficacy not established. **Elderly:** No age-related precautions noted. May increase incidence of thrombocytopenia.

INTERACTIONS

DRUG: **Folate antagonists (e.g., methotrexate)** may increase risk of myeloblastic anemia. ***HERBAL:*** None known. ***FOOD:*** None known. ***LAB VALUES:*** May increase BUN, SGOT (AST), SGPT (ALT), serum bilirubin, creatinine concentration.

AVAILABILITY (Rx)

TABLETS: 100 mg, 200 mg. ***ORAL SOLUTION:*** 50 mg/5 ml.

ADMINISTRATION/HANDLING
PO:

• Space doses evenly to maintain constant level in urine. • Give without regard to meals (if stomach upset occurs, give with food).

INDICATIONS/ROUTES/DOSAGE
Acute, uncomplicated UTIs:
PO: Adults, elderly: 100 mg q12h or 200 mg once daily for 10 days.

Dosage in renal impairment:

Creatinine Clearance	Dosage
>30 ml/min	No change
15–30 ml/min	50 mg q12h

SIDE EFFECTS

OCCASIONAL: Nausea, vomiting, diarrhea, decreased appetite, stomach cramps, headache. ***RARE:*** Hypersensitivity reaction (rash, itching), methemoglobinemia (blue color on fingernails, lips, or skin, pale skin, sore throat, fever, unusual tiredness).

ADVERSE REACTIONS/TOXIC EFFECTS

Stevens-Johnson syndrome, erythema multiforme, exfoliative dermatitis, anaphylaxis occur rarely. Hematologic toxicity (thrombocytopenia, neutropenia, leukopenia, megaloblastic anemia) .more likely to occur in elderly, debilitated, alcoholics, those with impaired renal function or receiving prolonged high dosage.

NURSING IMPLICATIONS

BASELINE ASSESSMENT:
Assess hematology baseline reports.

INTERVENTION/EVALUATION:
Assess skin for rash. Evaluate food tolerance. Monitor hematology reports, renal, hepatic test results if ordered. Check for developing signs of hematologic toxicity: pallor, fever, sore throat, malaise, bleeding, or bruising.

PATIENT/FAMILY TEACHING:
Space doses evenly. Complete full length of therapy (may be

10–14 days). May take on empty stomach or with food if stomach upset occurs. Avoid sun/ultraviolet light; use sunscreen, wear protective clothing. Immediately report pallor, tiredness, sore throat, bleeding, bruising or discoloration of skin, fever to physician.

trimetrexate glucuronate

try-meh-**trex**-ate
(Neutrexin)
Do not confuse with Neurontin.

▶CLASSIFICATION

PHARMACOTHERAPEUTIC:
Folate antagonist. *CLINICAL:*
Anti-infective

ACTION/*THERAPEUTIC EFFECT*

Inhibits the enzyme dihydrofolate reductase (DHFR), *disrupting purine, DNA, RNA, protein synthesis, with consequent cell death.*

PHARMACOKINETICS

Following IV administration, distributed readily into ascitic fluid. Metabolized in liver. Eliminated in urine. Unknown if removed by hemodialysis. Half-life: 11–20 hrs.

USES/*UNLABELED*

Alternative therapy with concurrent leucovorin administration for treatment of moderate to severe *Pneumocystis carinii pneumonia* (PCP) in immunocompromised pts, including pts with acquired immunodeficiency syndrome (AIDS), who are intolerant of, or are refractory to, trimethoprim-sulfamethoxazole (TMP/SMZ)

therapy or for whom TMP/SMZ is contraindicated. *Treatment of non small cell lung, prostate, and colorectal cancer.*

PRECAUTIONS

CONTRAINDICATIONS: Clinically significant hypersensitivity to trimetrexate, leucovorin, or methotrexate. *CAUTIONS:* Fertility impairment, pts with hematologic, renal, hepatic impairment.
▷*LIFESPAN CONSIDERATIONS:*
Pregnancy/Lactation: May cause fetal harm. Unknown if drug crosses placenta or is distributed in breast milk. **Pregnancy Category D. Children:** Safety and efficacy not established. **Elderly:** Information not available.

INTERACTIONS

DRUG: **Erythromycin, rifampin, rifabutin, ketoconazole, flucnazole, acetaminophen** may alter timetrexate plasma concentration. **Cimetidine** reduces trimetrexate metabolism. **Clotrimazole, ketoconazole, miconazole** may inhibit trimetrexate metabolism. *HERBAL:* None known. *FOOD:* None known. *LAB VALUES:* May increase SGOT (AST), SGPT (ALT), alkaline phosphatase, bilirubin, BUN, serum creatinine. May decrease hemoglobin, hematocrit, leukocytes, platelet counts.

AVAILABILITY (Rx)

POWDER FOR INJECTION: 25 mg.

ADMINISTRATION/HANDLING
IV 🔲

Note: If solution comes in contact with skin or mucosa, wash with soap and water immediately. Use proper cytoxic disposal technique. Do not reconstitute with solution containing either chloride ion or leucovorin, since precipitate occurs instantly.

Storage:

• Store vials for parenteral use at room temperature. • After reconstitution, solution is stable under refrigeration or at room temperature for up to 24 hrs. • Reconstituted solution appears as pale greenish yellow. • Inspect for particulate matter. Discard if cloudiness or precipitate is present. • Do not freeze reconstituted solution. Discard unused portion after 24 hrs.

Reconstitution:

• Reconstitute each 25 mg vial with 2 ml D_5W or Sterile Water for Injection to provide concentration of 12.5 mg/ml. Complete dissolution should occur within 30 sec. • Filter the reconstituted solution prior to further dilution. • Further dilute with D_5W to yield a final concentration of 0.25–2 mg/ml.

Rate of administration:

• Give diluted solution by IV infusion over 60–90 min. • Flush IV line thoroughly with at least 10 ml D_5W before and after administering trimetrexate.

IV INCOMPATIBILITIES ⊘

Foscarnet (Foscavir), indomethacin (Indocin).

INDICATIONS/ROUTES/DOSAGE

Note: Even though trimetrexate and leucovorin are given concurrently, they must be administered separately or precipitate will occur instantly; flush IV line thoroughly with 10 ml D_5W between infusions. Dilute leukovorin according to leukovorin instructions and give over 5–10 min q6h.

PCP:

IV INFUSION: Adults: Trimetrexate: 45 mg/m² once daily over 60–90 min. **Leukovorin:** 20 mg/m² over 5–10 min q6h for total daily dose of 80 mg/m², or orally as 4 doses of 20 mg/m² spaced equally throughout the day. Round up the oral dose to the next higher 25 mg increment. **Recommended course of therapy:** 21 days trimetrexate, 24 days leucovorin.

Note: In event of hematologic, renal, hepatic toxicities, doses of trimetrexate and leukovorin should be modified.

SIDE EFFECTS

OCCASIONAL (2–8%): Fever, rash, pruritus, nausea, vomiting, confusion. **RARE** (<2%): Fatigue.

ADVERSE REACTIONS/TOXIC EFFECTS

Trimetrexate given without concurrent leucovorin may result in serious or fatal hematologic, hepatic, and/or renal complications, including bone marrow suppression, oral and GI mucosal ulceration, and renal and hepatic dysfunction. In event of overdose, stop trimetrexate and give leucovorin 40 mg/m² q6h for 3 days. Anaphylaxis occurs rarely.

NURSING IMPLICATIONS

BASELINE ASSESSMENT:

Leucovorin therapy must extend for 72 hrs past the last dose of trimetrexate. Blood tests should be performed twice weekly during therapy. To allow for full therapeutic effect of trimetrexate to occur, zidovudine treatment should be discontinued during trimetrexate therapy.

INTERVENTION/EVALUATION:

Closely monitor neutrophil count, platelet count, liver function tests (SGOT, SGPT, alkaline phosphatase), renal values (serum creatinine, BUN) for development of serious toxicities. Carefully assess and treat pts with nephrotoxic, myelosuppressive, or hepatotoxic drugs given during trimetrexate therapy.

PATIENT/FAMILY TEACHING:

Use two forms of contraception during therapy. Avoid persons with bacterial infections. Immediately contact physician if fever, chills, cough or hoarseness, lower back or side pain, or painful urination occurs. Report any unusual bleeding or bruising, black tarry stools, blood in urine or stools, pinpoint red spots on skin.

---

triptorelin pamoate

trip-toe-**ree**-linn
(Trelstar Depot)

▶CLASSIFICATION

PHARMACOTHERAPEUTIC: Gonadotropin-releasing hormone analog. **CLINICAL:** Antineoplastic

ACTION/THERAPEUTIC EFFECT

Through a negative feedback mechanism, triptorelin inhibits gonadotropin hormone secretion. Initially, a transient surge in circulating levels of luteinizing hormone (LH), follicle-stimulating hormone (FSH), testosterone, and estradiol occurs. Chronic administration results in decreased LH and FSH, marked reduction in testosterone and estradiol levels. *Suppresses abnormal growth of prostate tissue.*

USES

Treatment of advanced prostate cancer.

PRECAUTIONS

CONTRAINDICATIONS: Hypersensitivity to luteinizing hormone releasing hormone (LHRH) agonists or LHRH. **CAUTIONS:** None significant.

INTERACTIONS

DRUG: Hyperprolactinemic drugs reduce number of pituitary GnRH receptors. **HERBAL:** None known. **FOOD:** None known. **LAB VALUES:** May mislead pituitary-gonadal function test results. Increases transient testosterone levels (usually during first week of treatment, declines thereafter).

AVAILABILITY (Rx)

INJECTION: 3.75 mg.

INDICATIONS/ROUTES/DOSAGE

Prostate cancer:

IM: Adults, elderly: 3.75 mg once monthly.

SIDE EFFECTS

FREQUENT (>5%): Hot flushes, skeletal pain, headache, impotence. **OCCASIONAL** (2–5%): Insomnia, vomiting, leg pain, fatigue. **RARE** (<2%): Dizziness, emotional lability, diarrhea, urinary retention, urinary tract infections, anemia, pruritus.

ADVERSE REACTIONS/TOXIC EFFECTS

Bladder outlet obstruction, bone pain, hematuria, spinal cord compression with weakness or paralysis of lower extremities may occur.

T

NURSING IMPLICATIONS

INTERVENTION/EVALUATION:

Obtain serum testosterone, prostatic acid phosphatase (PAP) levels periodically during therapy. Serum testosterone and PAP levels should increase during first week of therapy. Testosterone level then should decrease to baseline level or less within 2 wks, PAP level within 4 wks. Monitor pt closely for worsening signs and symptoms of prostatic cancer, esp. during first week of therapy (due to transient increase in testosterone).

PATIENT/FAMILY TEACHING:

Hot flushes tend to decrease during continued therapy. A temporary exacerbation of signs/symptoms of disease may occur during first few wks of therapy.

tubocurarine chloride

(Tubarine)

See Classification section under: Neuromuscular blockers (p. 103C)

valacyclovir 🔗

val-ah-**sigh**-klo-veer
(Valtrex)

▶CLASSIFICATION

PHARMACOTHERAPEUTIC: Antiviral. ***CLINICAL:*** Antiherpes virus agent (see p. 59C)

ACTION/*THERAPEUTIC EFFECT*

Converted to acyclovir triphosphate, becoming part of DNA chain, *interfering with DNA synthesis and viral replication of herpes simplex and varicella zoster virus.* Virustatic.

PHARMACOKINETICS

Rapidly absorbed following PO administration. Protein binding: 13–18%. Rapidly converted by hydrolysis to active compound, acyclovir. Widely distributed to tissues/body fluids (including CSF). Primarily eliminated in urine. Removed by hemodialysis. Half-life: 2.5–3.3 hrs (half-life increased with impaired renal function).

USES

Treatment of herpes zoster (shingles) in immunocompetent adults. Episodic treatment of recurrent genital herpes in immunocompetent adults. Prevention of recurrent genital herpes. Treatment of initial genital herpes.

PRECAUTIONS

CONTRAINDICATIONS: Hypersensitivity or intolerance to valacyclovir, acyclovir, or components of formulation. ***CAUTIONS:*** Bone marrow or renal transplantation, advanced HIV infections, renal or hepatic impairment, dehydration, fluid/electrolyte imbalance, concurrent use of nephrotoxic agents, neurologic abnormalities.

▷*LIFESPAN CONSIDERATIONS:*
Pregnancy/Lactation: May cross placenta; may be distributed in breast milk. **Pregnancy Category B. Children:** Safety and efficacy not established. **Elderly:** Age-related renal impairment may require dosage adjustment.

INTERACTIONS

DRUG: **Probenecid, cimetidine**

🔗 - see color pill atlas   underscored - top 100 prescribed drug may increase acyclovir concentration. **HERBAL:** None known. **FOOD:** None known. **LAB VALUES:** None significant.

AVAILABILITY (Rx)

TABLETS: 500 mg.

ADMINISTRATION/HANDLING

PO:

• Give without regard to meals. • Do not crush or break tablets.

INDICATIONS/ROUTES/DOSAGE

Note: Therapy should be initiated at first sign of shingles (most effective within 48 hrs of onset of zoster rash).

Herpes zoster (shingles):

PO: **Adults, elderly:** 1 g 3 times daily for 7 days.

Recurrent genital herpes:

PO: **Adults, elderly:** 500 mg twice daily for 3 days.

Prevention of herpes:

PO: **Adults, elderly:** 500–1,000 mg/day.

Initial treatment of genital herpes:

PO: **Adults, elderly:** 1 g twice daily for 10 days.

Dosage in renal impairment:

Creatinine Clearance	Herpes Zoster	Genital Herpes
≥50	1 g q8h	500 mg q12h
30–49	1 g q12 h	500 mg q12h
10–29	1 g q24h	500 mg q24h
<10	500 mg q24h	500 mg q24h

SIDE EFFECTS

Herpes zoster: FREQUENT (10–17%): Nausea, headache. **OCCASIONAL** (3–7%): Vomiting, diarrhea, constipation (≥50 yrs), asthenia, dizziness (≥50 yrs). **RARE** (1–3%): Abdominal pain, anorexia. **Genital herpes: FREQUENT** (17%): Headache. **OCCASIONAL** (3–8%): Nausea, diarrhea, dizziness. **RARE** (1–3%): Asthenia, abdominal pain.

ADVERSE REACTIONS/TOXIC EFFECTS

None significant.

NURSING IMPLICATIONS

BASELINE ASSESSMENT:

Question history of allergies, particularly to valacyclovir, acyclovir. Tissue cultures for herpes zoster and herpes simplex should be done before giving first dose (therapy may proceed before results are known). Assess medical history, esp. advanced HIV infection, bone marrowith renal transplantation, hepatic/renal function.

INTERVENTION/EVALUATION:

Evaluate cutaneous lesions. Manage herpes zoster with strict isolation. Provide analgesics and comfort measures for herpes zoster; esp. exhausting to elderly. Encourage fluids. Keep pt's fingernails short, hands clean.

PATIENT/FAMILY TEACHING:

Drink adequate fluids. Do not touch lesions with fingers to avoid spreading infection to new site. **Genital herpes:** Continue therapy for full length of treatment. Space doses evenly. Avoid sexual intercourse during duration of lesions to prevent infecting partner. Valacyclovir does not cure herpes. Notify physician if lesions do not improve or recur. Pap smears should be done at least annually due to increased risk of cancer of cervix in women with genital herpes. Initiate treatment at first sign of a recurrent episode of genital herpes or herpes zoster (early treatment, that is, within first 24–48 hrs, is imperative for therapeutic results).

valdecoxib

(Bextra)

See New Drug Supplement.

valerian

Also known as amantilla, all-heal, garden heliotrope, valeriana.

▶CLASSIFICATION

HERBAL

ACTION/EFFECT

Appears to inhibit enzyme system responsible for catabolism of GABA, increasing GABA concentration and decreasing CNS activity, *producing sedative effects*. Also has anxiolytic, antidepressant, anticonvulsant effects.

USES

Used as a sedative for insomnia, sleeping disorders associated with anxiety, restlessness. Also used for depression and attention deficit hyperactivity disorder (ADHD).

PRECAUTIONS

CONTRAINDICATIONS: Insufficient data on pregnancy/lactation (avoid use); liver disease. *CAUTIONS:* None significant.

▷*LIFESPAN CONSIDERATIONS:*
Pregnancy/Lactation: Contrain-

dicated. **Children:** Safety and efficacy not established; avoid use. **Elderly:** No age-related precautions noted.

INTERACTIONS

DRUG: **Alcohol, barbiturates, benzodiazepines** may cause additive effect, increase adverse effects. *HERBAL:* **Chamomile, ginseng, kava kava, melatonin, St. John's wort** may enhance therapeutic effect/adverse effects. *FOOD:* None significant. *LAB VALUES:* None significant.

AVAILABILITY (OTC)

CAPSULES. TABLETS. EXTRACT. TEA. TINCTURE.

INDICATIONS/ROUTES/DOSAGE

Sedation:

PO: **Adults, elderly:** *(extract):* 400–900 mg 1/2–1 hr before bedtime or 1 cup tea taken several times/day.

SIDE EFFECTS

Headache, excitability, insomnia, hangover, cardiac disturbances.

ADVERSE REACTIONS/TOXIC EFFECTS

Trouble walking, hypothermia, increased muscle relaxation.

NURSING IMPLICATIONS

BASELINE ASSESSMENT:

Determine if pt is using other CNS depressants, esp. benzodiazepine. Assess baseline liver function.

INTERVENTION/EVALUATION:

Monitor effectiveness in decreasing insomnia. Assess for hypersensitivity reaction, liver function tests.

PATIENT/FAMILY TEACHING:

Up to 4 wks may be needed for significant relief. Avoid driving/operating machinery. Inform physician if pregnant or breast-feeding. Taper doses slowly; do not discontinue abruptly.

valganciclovir hydrochloride

val-gan-**sye**-klo-vir
(Valcyte)

▶CLASSIFICATION

PHARMACOTHERAPEUTIC: Synthetic nucleoside. **CLINI-CAL:** Antiviral (see p. 59C)

PHARMACOKINETICS

Well absorbed and rapidly converted to ganciclovir by intestinal and hepatic enzymes. Widely distributed. Slowly metabolized intracellularly. Primarily excreted unchanged in urine. Removed by hemodialysis. Half-life: 18 hrs (half-life increased with impaired renal function).

ACTION/*THERAPEUTIC EFFECT*

Converted intracellularly; competes with viral DNA esterases and incorporates directly into growing viral DNA chains, *interfering with DNA synthesis and viral replication.*

USES

Treatment of cytomegalovirus (CMV) retinitis in autoimmunodeficiency syndrome (AIDS).

PRECAUTIONS

CONTRAINDICATIONS: Hypersensitivity to ganciclovir or acyclovir. ***CAUTIONS:*** Extreme caution in children because of long-term carcinogenicity, reproductive toxicity. Renal impairment, pre-existing cytopenias, or history of cytopenic reactions to other drugs; elderly (at greater risk of renal impairment).

▷***LIFESPAN CONSIDERATIONS:*** **Pregnancy/Lactation:** Effective contraception should be used during therapy; valganciclovir should not be used during pregnancy. Nursing should be discontinued. May be resumed no sooner than 72 hrs after the last dose of valganciclovir. **Pregnancy Category C. Children:** Safety and efficacy not established in those <12 yrs. **Elderly:** Age-related renal impairment may require dosage adjustment.

INTERACTIONS

DRUG: **Bone marrow depressants** may increase bone marrow depression. May increase risk of seizures with **imipenem-cilastatin.** May increase hematologic toxicity with **zidovudine. Probenecid** reduces renal clearance of valganciclovir. Concurrent use of amphotericin B or cyclosporine may produce nephrotoxicity. ***HERBAL:*** None significant. ***FOOD:*** Food maximizes drug bioavailability. ***LAB VALUES:*** May decrease WBCs, Hgb, Hct, platelet count, serum creatinine.

AVAILABILITY (Rx)

TABLETS: 450 mg.

ADMINISTRATION/HANDLING

PO:

• Do not break or crush tablets (potential carcinogen). Avoid touching to skin . Wash skin with soap and water if contact occurs. • Give with food.

V

INDICATIONS/ROUTES /DOSAGE

CMV retinitis
(normal renal function):

PO: Adults: Initially, 900 mg (2 450 mg tablets) twice daily for 21 days with food. **Maintenance:** 900 mg once daily with food.

Dosage in renal impairment:

Creatinine Clearance	Induction Dosage	Maintenance Dosage
≥60 ml/min	900 mg twice/day	900 mg once/day
40–59 ml/min	450 mg twice/day	450 mg once/day
25–39 ml/min	450 mg once/day	450 mg q2day
10–24 ml/min	450 mg q2day	450 mg twice weekly

SIDE EFFECTS

FREQUENT (9–16%): Diarrhea, neutropenia, headache. *OCCASIONAL* (3–8%): Nausea, anemia, thrombocytopenia. *RARE* (<3%): Insomnia, paresthesia, vomiting, abdominal pain, pyrexia.

ADVERSE REACTIONS/TOXIC EFFECTS

Hematologic toxicity, mainly neutropenia; anemia, thrombocytopenia may occur. Retinal detachment occurs rarely. Overdose may result in renal toxicity. May decrease sperm production, fertility.

NURSING IMPLICATIONS

BASELINE ASSESSMENT:

Evaluate hematologic, blood chemistry baselines, serum creatinine.

INTERVENTION/EVALUATION:

Monitor I&O and assure adequate hydration (minimum 1,500 ml/24 hrs). Diligently evaluate CBC for decreased WBCs, Hgb, Hct, decreased platelets. Question pt regarding vision, therapeutic improvement, or complications.

PATIENT/FAMILY TEACHING:

Valganciclovir provides suppression, not cure, of CMV retinitis. Frequent blood tests are necessary during therapy because of toxic nature of drug. Ophthalmologic exam every 4–6 wks during treatment is advised. It is essential to report any new symptom promptly. May temporarily or permanently inhibit sperm production in men, suppress fertility in women. Barrier contraception should be used during and for 90 days after therapy because of mutagenic potential.

---

valproic acid

val-**pro**-ick
(Depakene)

valproate sodium

(Depakene syrup)

divalproex sodium

(Depacon, Depakote, Epival✦)

▶CLASSIFICATION

CLINICAL: Anticonvulsant, antimanic, antimigraine (see p. 33C)

ACTION/*THERAPEUTIC EFFECT*

Directly increases concentration of the inhibitory neurotransmitter gamma-aminobutyric acid (GABA), *producing anticonvulsant effect.*

PHARMACOKINETICS

Well absorbed from GI tract. Protein binding: 80–90%. Metabolized in liver. Primarily excreted in urine. Not removed by hemodialysis. Half-life: 6–16 hrs (half-life may be increased with impaired liver function, elderly, children <18 mos).

USES/*UNLABELED*

Prophylaxis of absence seizures (petit mal), myoclonic, tonic-clonic seizure control. Used principally as adjunct with other anticonvulsant agents. Treatment of manic episodes with bipolar disorders, complex partial seizures. Prophylaxis of migraine headaches. *Treatment of myoclonic, simple partial, tonic-clonic seizures.*

PRECAUTIONS

CONTRAINDICATIONS: Hepatic disease. ***CAUTIONS:*** History of hepatic disease, bleeding abnormalities.

▷*LIFESPAN CONSIDERATIONS:* **Pregnancy/Lactation:** Crosses placenta; distributed in breast milk. **Pregnancy Category D. Children:** Increased risk of hepatotoxicity in those <2 yrs of age. **Elderly:** No age-related precautions, but lower doses recommended.

INTERACTIONS

***DRUG:* Alcohol, CNS depressants** may increase CNS depressant effects. May increase risk of bleeding with **anticoagulants, heparin, thrombolytics, platelet aggregation inhibitors.** May increase concentration of **amitriptyline, primidone. Carbamazepine** may decrease concentration. **Hepatotoxic medications** may increase risk of hepatotoxicity. May alter **phenytoin** protein binding, increasing toxicity. Phenytoin may

decrease effect. ***HERBAL:*** None known. ***FOOD:*** None known. ***LAB VALUES:*** May increase SGOT (AST), SGPT (ALT), LDH, bilirubin. Therapeutic blood serum level: 50–100 mcg/ml; toxic blood serum level: >100 mcg/ml.

AVAILABILITY (Rx)

CAPSULES: 250 mg (valproic acid). ***SYRUP:*** 250 mg/5 ml (valproic acid). ***TABLETS (delayed-release):*** 125 mg, 250 mg, 500 mg (divalproex). ***CAPSULES (sprinkle):*** 125 mg (divalproex). ***INJECTION:*** 100 mg/ml.

ADMINISTRATION/HANDLING
PO:

• Give with food if GI distress occurs. • Do not crush, chew, or break enteric-coated tablets. • Do not mix solution with carbonated drinks (may produce local mouth irritation, unpleasant taste).

IV 💊
Storage:

• Store vials at room temperature. • Diluted solutions stable for 24 hrs. • Discard unused portion.

Reconstitution:

• Dilute each single dose with at least 50 ml D_5W, 0.9% NaCl, or lactated Ringer's.

Rate of administration:

• Infuse over 60 min. • Do not exceed 20 mg/min. Too-rapid infusion increases side effects.

IV INCOMPATIBILITY ⊘

Do not mix with any other medications.

INDICATIONS/ROUTES/DOSAGE
Anticonvulsant:

PO: Adults, elderly, children: Initially, 15 mg/kg daily (if dosage exceeds 250 mg daily, give in two or more equally divided doses). Increase at 1 wk intervals by 5–10 mg/kg daily until seizures are controlled or unacceptable effects occur. **Maximum daily dose:** 60 mg/kg.

Manic episodes:

PO: Adults, elderly: Initially, 750 mg/day in divided doses. **Maximum:** 60 mg/kg/day.

Migraines:

PO: Adults: 250 mg 2 times/day. **Maximum:** 1,000 mg/kg/day.

EXTENDED-RELEASE: Initially, 500 mg/day for 7 days. May increase up to 1,000 mg/day.

SIDE EFFECTS

FREQUENT: Epilepsy: Abdominal pain, irregular menses, diarrhea, transient alopecia, indigestion, nausea, vomiting, trembling, weight change. **OCCASIONAL:** Constipation, dizziness, drowsiness, headache, skin rash, unusual excitement, restlessness. **RARE:** Mood changes, double vision, nystagmus, spots before eyes, unusual bleeding/bruising. **Mania: FREQUENT** (19–22%): Nausea, somnolence. **OCCASIONAL** (6–12%): Asthenia, abdominal pain, dyspepsia (heartburn, indigestion, epigastric distress), rash.

ADVERSE REACTIONS/TOXIC EFFECTS

Hepatotoxicity may occur, particularly in the first 6 mos of therapy. May not be preceded by abnormal liver function tests, but may be noted as loss of seizure control, malaise, weakness, lethargy, anorexia, and vomiting. Blood dyscrasias may occur.

NURSING IMPLICATIONS

BASELINE ASSESSMENT:

Anticonvulsant: Review history of seizure disorder (intensity, frequency, duration, LOC). Initiate safety measures, quiet dark environment. CBC, platelet count should be performed before and 2 wks after therapy begins, then 2 wks after maintenance dose is given. **Antimanic:** Assess behavior, appearance, emotional status, response to environment, speech pattern, thought content. **Antimigraine:** Question pt regarding onset, location, and duration of migraine and possible precipitating symptoms.

INTERVENTION/EVALUATION:

Anticonvulsant: Observe frequently for recurrence of seizure activity. Monitor liver function, CBC, platelet count. Assess skin for bruising, petechiae. Monitor for clinical improvement (decrease in intensity or frequency of seizures). **Antimanic:** Assess for therapeutic response (interest in surroundings, increased ability to concentrate, relaxed facial expression). **Antimigraine:** Evaluate for relief of migraine headache and resulting photophobia, phonophobia, nausea, vomiting. Therapeutic blood serum level: 50–100 mcg/ml; toxic blood serum level: >100 mcg/ml.

PATIENT/FAMILY TEACHING:

Do not abruptly withdraw medication following long-term use (may precipitate seizures). Strict maintenance of drug therapy is essential for seizure control. Drowsiness usually disappears during continued therapy. Avoid tasks that require alertness, motor skills until response to drug is established. Avoid alcohol. Carry identification card/bracelet to note anticonvulsant therapy.

valrubicin

val-**rue**-bih-sin
(Valstar)
Do not confuse with valsartan.

▶CLASSIFICATION

PHARMACOTHERAPEUTIC: Anthracycline antibiotic. **CLINICAL:** Antineoplastic (see p. 75C)

ACTION/THERAPEUTIC EFFECT

Following intracellular penetration, inhibits incorporation of nucleosides into nucleic acids. *Causes chromosomal damage, arresting cell cycle in G2 phase, interfering with DNA.*

USES

Intravesical therapy of BCG-refractory carcinoma in situ of urinary bladder in pts for whom cystectomy is unacceptable.

PRECAUTIONS

CONTRAINDICATIONS: Severe irritated bladder, perforated bladder, small bladder capacity, urinary tract infection, sensitivity to valrubicin. **CAUTIONS:** None significant.

AVAILABILITY (Rx)

SOLUTION FOR INTRAVESICAL INSTILLATION: 40 mg/ml.

INDICATIONS/ROUTES/DOSAGE

Note: Not for IM/IV use.

Bladder cancer:

INTRAVESICAL: Adults, elderly: 800 mg once weekly for 6 wks.

SIDE EFFECTS

Local intravesical reaction: FREQUENT (>10%): Local bladder symptoms, urinary frequency, dysuria, urinary urgency, hematuria, bladder pain, cystitis, bladder spasms. **OCCASIONAL** (<10%): Nocturia, local burning, urethral pain, pelvic pain, gross hematuria.

Systemic: FREQUENT (5–15%): Abdominal pain, nausea, urinary tract infection. **OCCASIONAL** (2–5%): Diarrhea, vomiting, urinary retention, microscopic hematuria, asthenia, headache, malaise, back pain, chest pain, dizziness, rash, anemia, fever, vasodilation. **RARE** (1%): Flatus, peripheral edema, increased glucose, pneumonia, myalgia.

NURSING IMPLICATIONS

BASELINE ASSESSMENT:

Assess if pt is sensitive to valrubicin, is pregnant, or is breastfeeding (not recommended). Assess other medications, conditions (see Contraindications).

valsartan

val-**sar**-tan
(Diovan)

FIXED-COMBINATION(S)

With hydrochlorothiazide, a diuretic **(Diovan HCT)**

▶CLASSIFICATION

PHARMACOTHERAPEUTIC: Angiotensin II receptor antagonist. **CLINICAL:** Antihypertensive (see p. 7C)

V

ACTION/*THERAPEUTIC EFFECT*

Potent vasodilator. An angiotensin II receptor (type AT_1) antagonist; blocks vasoconstrictor and aldosterone-secreting effects of angiotensin II, inhibiting the binding of angiotensin II to the AT_1 receptors, *producing vasodilation, decreased peripheral resistance, decrease in B/P.*

PHARMACOKINETICS

Poorly absorbed following PO administration. Food decreases peak plasma concentration. Protein binding: 95%. Metabolized in the liver. Recovered primarily in feces and, to a lesser extent, in urine. Unknown if removed by hemodialysis. Half-life: 6 hrs.

USES

Treatment of hypertension alone or in combination with other antihypertensives. Treatment of heart failure.

PRECAUTIONS

CONTRAINDICATIONS: None significant. *CAUTIONS:* Renal/hepatic function impairment, renal arterial stenosis, severe CHF, dehydration.
▷*LIFESPAN CONSIDERATIONS:*
Pregnancy/Lactation: May cause fetal harm. Unknown if distributed in breast milk. **Pregnancy Category C** (Category D if used in second or third trimester). **Children:** Safety and efficacy not established. **Elderly:** No age-related precautions noted.

INTERACTIONS

DRUG: Diuretics produce additive hypotensive effects. *HERBAL:* None known. *FOOD:* None known. *LAB VALUES:* May increase liver enzymes, bilirubin, creatinine, potassium. May decrease hemoglobin, hematocrit.

AVAILABILITY (Rx)

CAPSULES: 80 mg, 160 mg.

ADMINISTRATION/HANDLING

PO:
• Give without regard to meals.

INDICATIONS/ROUTES/DOSAGE

Note: May be given concurrently with other antihypertensives. If B/P is not controlled by valsartan alone, a diuretic may be added.

Hypertension:

PO: Adults, elderly, mildly impaired renal or hepatic function: 80 mg once daily in pts who are not volume depleted. **Dose range:** 80–320 mg once daily.

SIDE EFFECTS

RARE (1–2%): Insomnia, fatigue, heartburn, abdominal pain, dizziness, headache, diarrhea, nausea, vomiting, arthralgia, edema.

ADVERSE REACTIONS/TOXIC EFFECTS

Overdosage may manifest as hypotension and tachycardia; bradycardia occurs less often. Institute supportive measures. Viral infection, upper respiratory infection (cough, pharyngitis, sinusitis, rhinitis) occur rarely.

NURSING IMPLICATIONS

BASELINE ASSESSMENT:

Obtain B/P and apical pulse immediately before each dose, in addition to regular monitoring (be alert to fluctuations). If excessive reduction in B/P occurs, place pt in supine position, feet slightly elevated. Question possibility of pregnancy (see Pregnancy Category). Assess medication history (esp. diuretic). Question for history of hepatic/renal impairment, renal artery stenosis, history of severe CHF. Obtain BUN, serum creatinine, SGOT (AST), SGPT (ALT), alkaline phosphatase, bilirubin, hemoglobin, hematocrit, and vital signs, particularly B/P, pulse rate.

INTERVENTION/EVALUATION:

Maintain hydration (offer fluids frequently). Assess for evidence of upper respiratory infection. Monitor all blood serum levels. Assess B/P for hypertension/hypotension.

PATIENT/FAMILY TEACHING:

Inform female pt regarding consequences of second- and third-trimester exposure to valsartan. Report pregnancy to physician as soon as possible. Report any sign of infection (sore throat, fever). Do not stop taking medication. Need for lifelong control. Caution against exercising during hot weather (risk of dehydration, hypotension).

vancomycin hydrochloride

van-koe-**my**-sin
(Vancocin, Vancoled)

▶CLASSIFICATION

CLINICAL: Tricyclic glycopeptide antibiotic

ACTION/THERAPEUTIC EFFECT

Inhibits cell wall synthesis by binding to bacterial cell wall, altering cell membrane permeability, inhibiting RNA synthesis, *producing bacterial cell death.* Bactericidal.

PHARMACOKINETICS

PO: Poorly absorbed from GI tract. Primarily eliminated in feces. **Parenteral:** Widely distributed. Protein binding: 55%. Primarily excreted unchanged in urine. Not removed by hemodialysis. Half-life: 4–11 hrs (half-life increased with impaired renal function).

USES/UNLABELED

Systemic: Treatment of respiratory tract, bone, skin/soft tissue infections, endocarditis, peritonitis, septicemia. Given prophylactically to those at risk for bacterial endocarditis (if penicillin contraindicated) when undergoing dental, respiratory, GI, GU, biliary surgery/invasive procedures. **PO:** Treatment of antibiotic colitis, pseudomembranous colitis, antibiotic-associated diarrhea, staphylococcal enterocolitis. *Treatment of brain abscess, staphylococcal/streptococcal meningitis, perioperative infections.*

PRECAUTIONS

CONTRAINDICATIONS: None significant. **CAUTIONS:** Renal dysfunction, preexisting hearing impairment, concurrent therapy with other ototoxic/nephrotoxic medications.

▷**LIFESPAN CONSIDERATIONS:**
Pregnancy/Lactation: Drug crosses placenta; unknown if distributed in breast milk. **Pregnancy Category C. Children:** Close monitoring of serum levels recommended in premature neonates and young infants. **Elderly:** Age-related renal impairment may increase risk of ototoxicity and nephrotoxicity; dosage adjustment recommended.

V

INTERACTIONS

DRUG: Oral: Cholestyramine, colestipol may decrease effect. **Parenteral: Aminoglycosides, amphotericin, aspirin, bumetanide, carmustine, cisplatin, cyclosporine, ethacrynic acid, furosemide, streptozocin** may increase ototoxicity and/or nephrotoxicity. **HERBAL:** None known. **FOOD:** None known. **LAB VALUES:** May increase BUN. Therapeutic blood serum level: Peak: 20–40 mcg/ml; trough: 5–15 mcg/ml. Toxic blood serum level: Peak: >40 mcg/ml; trough: >15 mcg/ml.

AVAILABILITY (Rx)

CAPSULES: 125 mg, 250 mg. **POWDER FOR ORAL SOLUTION:** 1 g, 10 g. **POWDER FOR INJECTION:** 500 mg, 1 g.

ADMINISTRATION/HANDLING

PO:

• Generally not given for systemic infections because of poor absorption from GI tract; however, some pts with colitis may have effective absorption. • Powder for oral solution may be reconstituted, given by mouth or NG tube. • Oral solution is stable for 2 wks if refrigerated. • Do not use powder for oral solution for IV administration.

IV

Note: Give by intermittent IV infusion (piggyback) or continuous IV infusion. Do not give IV push (may result in exaggerated hypotension).

Storage:

• IV infusion (piggyback) is stable for 24 hrs at room temperature, 96 hrs if refrigerated. • Discard if precipitate forms.

Reconstitution:

• For intermittent IV infusion (piggyback), reconstitute each 500 mg vial with 10 ml Sterile Water for Injection (20 ml for 1 g vial) to provide concentration of 50 mg/ml. • Further dilute each 500 mg with at least 100 ml D_5W, 0.9% NaCl, lactated Ringer's.

Rate of administration:

• Infuse each 500 mg over at least 1 hr. • Monitor B/P closely during IV infusion. • ADD-Vantage vials should not be used in neonates, infants, children requiring <500 mg dose.

IV INCOMPATIBILITIES ⊘

Albumin, amphotericin B complex (Abelcet, Ambisome, Amphotec), aztreonam (Azactam), cefazolin (Ancef), cefepime (Maxipime), cefotaxime (Claforan), cefotetan (Cefotan), cefoxitin (Mefoxin), ceftazidime (Fortaz), ceftriaxone (Rocephin), cefuroxime (Zinacef), foscarnet (Foscavir), heparin, idarubicin (Idamycin), nafcillin (Nafcil), piperacillin/tazobactam (Zosyn), ticarcillin/clavulanate (Timentin).

IV COMPATIBILITIES

Amiodarone (Cordarone), calcium gluconate, diltiazem (Cardizem), lorazepam (Ativan), magnesium, midazolam (Versed), multivitamins, propofol (Diprivan).

INDICATIONS/ROUTES/DOSAGE

Usual parenteral dosage:

IV: Adults, elderly: 500 mg q6h or 1 g q12h. **Children >1 mo:** 40 mg/kg/day in divided doses q6–8h. **Maximum:** 2 g/day. **Neonates:** 15 mg/kg initially, then 10 mg/kg q8–12h.

Dosage in renal impairment:

After a loading dose, subsequent

---

dose and/or frequency is modified based on degree of renal impairment, severity of infection, serum concentration of drug.

Staphylococcal enterocolitis, antibiotic-associated pseudomembranous colitis caused by *Clostridium difficile*:

PO: **Adults, elderly:** 0.5–2 g/day in 3–4 divided doses for 7–10 days. **Children:** 40 mg/kg/day in 3–4 divided doses for 7–10 days. **Maximum:** 2 g/day.

SIDE EFFECTS

FREQUENT: PO: Bitter/unpleasant taste, nausea, vomiting, mouth irritation (oral solution). *RARE: Systemic:* Phlebitis, thrombophlebitis, pain at peripheral IV site. Necrosis may occur with extravasation. Dizziness, vertigo, tinnitus, chills, fever, rash. *PO:* Rash.

ADVERSE REACTIONS/TOXIC EFFECTS

Nephrotoxicity (change in amount/frequency of urination, nausea, vomiting, increased thirst, anorexia); ototoxicity (deafness due to damage to auditory branch of eighth cranial nerve); red-neck syndrome (too rapid injection): redness on face/neck/arms/back; chills, fever, fast heartbeat, nausea, vomiting, itching, rash, unpleasant taste.

NURSING IMPLICATIONS

BASELINE ASSESSMENT:

Avoid other ototoxic and nephrotoxic medications if possible. Obtain culture and sensitivity test before giving first dose (therapy may begin before results are known). Peak and trough levels are usually ascertained with fifth dose.

INTERVENTION/EVALUATION:

Monitor renal function tests, I&O. Assess skin for rash. Check hearing acuity, balance. Monitor B/P carefully during infusion. Evaluate IV site for phlebitis (heat, pain, red streaking over vein). Therapeutic blood serum level: Peak: 20–40 mcg/ml; trough: 5–15 mcg/ml. Toxic blood serum level: Peak: >40 mcg/ml; trough: >15 mcg/ml.

PATIENT/FAMILY TEACHING:

Continue therapy for full length of treatment. Doses should be evenly spaced. Notify physician in event of tinnitus, rash, signs and symptoms of nephrotoxicity. Lab tests are important part of total therapy.

varicella vaccine

(Varivax)

See Classification section under: Immunizations

vasopressin

vay-sew-**press**-in
(Pitressin, Pressyn✿)

▶CLASSIFICATION

PHARMACOTHERAPEUTIC: Posterior pituitary hormone. *CLINICAL:* Vasopressor, antidiuretic

ACTION/*THERAPEUTIC EFFECT*

Increases reabsorption of water by the renal tubules *resulting in decreased urinary flow rate,* increased urine osmolality. Urea is also reab-

---

✿ - Canadian trade name   ✳ - see also www.wbsaunders.com/SIMON/SaundersNDH

sorbed by the collecting ducts. Directly stimulates contraction of smooth muscle, *preventing abdominal distention, intestinal paresis.* Causes vasoconstriction with reduced blood flow in coronary, peripheral, cerebral, and pulmonary vessels, but particularly in portal and splanchnic vessels. In large doses, may cause mild uterine contractions.

PHARMACOKINETICS

	Onset	Peak	Duration
IM/SubQ	—	—	2–8 hrs
IV	—	—	0.5–1 hr

Distributed throughout extracellular fluid. Metabolized in liver, kidney. Primarily excreted in urine. Half-life: 10–20 min.

USES/*UNLABELED*

Treatment of adult shock-refractory ventricular fibrillation (Class IIb). Prevents/controls polydipsia, polyuria, dehydration in pts with neurogenic diabetes insipidus. Stimulates peristalsis in the prevention or treatment of postop abdominal distention, intestinal paresis. *Adjunct in treatment of acute, massive hemorrhage.*

PRECAUTIONS

CONTRAINDICATIONS: Chronic nephritis with nitrogen retention. **CAUTIONS:** Migraine, epilepsy, heart failure, asthma, or any condition in which rapid addition of extracellular water may be a risk. Extreme caution in pts with vascular disease, esp. coronary artery disease.

▷**LIFESPAN CONSIDERATIONS:** **Pregnancy/Lactation:** Caution in giving to nursing woman. **Pregnancy Category B. Children/Elderly:** Caution due to risk of water intoxication/hyponatremia.

INTERACTIONS

DRUG: Carbamazepine, chlor- **propamide, clofibrate** may increase effects. **Demeclocycline, lithium, norepinephrine** may decrease effect. **HERBAL:** None known. **FOOD:** None known. **LAB VALUES:** None significant.

AVAILABILITY (Rx)

INJECTION: 20 units/ml.

ADMINISTRATION/HANDLING

SubQ/IM:
• Give with 1–2 glasses of water to reduce side effects.

IV 💊

Storage:
• Store at room temperature.

Reconstitution:
• Dilute with D_5W in water or 0.9% NaCl to concentration of 0.1–1 units/ml.

Rate of administration:
• Give as IV infusion.

IV INCOMPATIBILITIES ⊘

Amphotericin B complex (Abelcet, Ambisome, Amphotec), diazepam (Valium), etomidate (Amidate), furosemide (Lasix), thiopentothal.

IV COMPATIBILITIES

Dobutamine (Dobutrex), dopamine (Intropin), heparin, lorazepam (Ativan), midazolam (Versed), milrinone (Primacor), verapamil (Calan, Isoptin).

INDICATIONS/ROUTES/DOSAGE

Cardiac arrest:
IV: Adults, elderly: 40 units as a one-time dose.

Diabetes insipidus:
Note: May administer intranasally on cotton pledgets, by nasal spray; individualize dosage.

IM/SubQ: Adults, elderly: 5–10 units, 2–4 times/day. **Range:** 5–60 units/day. **Children:** 2.5–10 units, 2–4 times/day.

IV INFUSION: **Adults, children:** 0.5 milliunits/kg/hr. May double dose q30min. **Maximum:** 10 milliunits/kg/hr.

Abdominal distention:

IM: **Adults, elderly:** Initially, 5 units. Subsequent doses of 10 units q3–4h.

GI hemorrhage:

IV INFUSION: **Adults, elderly:** Initially, 0.2–0.4 units/min progressively increased to 0.9 units/min. **Children:** 0.002–0.005 units/kg/min. Titrate as needed. **Maximum:** 0.01 units/kg/min.

SIDE EFFECTS

FREQUENT: Pain at injection site with vasopressin tannate. *OCCASIONAL:* Stomach cramps, nausea, vomiting, diarrhea, dizziness, diaphoresis, paleness, circumoral pallor, trembling, "pounding" in head, eructation, flatulence. *RARE:* Chest pain, confusion. *Allergic reaction:* Rash or hives, pruritus, wheezing or difficulty breathing, swelling of mouth, face, feet, hands. Sterile abscess with vasopressin tannate.

ADVERSE REACTIONS/TOXIC EFFECTS

Anaphylaxis, myocardial infarction, and water intoxication have occurred. Elderly and very young at higher risk for water intoxication.

NURSING IMPLICATIONS

BASELINE ASSESSMENT:

Establish baselines for weight, B/P, pulse, electrolytes, urine specific gravity.

INTERVENTION/EVALUATION:

Monitor I&O closely, restrict in-take as necessary to prevent water intoxication. Weigh daily if indicated. Check B/P and pulse 2 times/day. Monitor electrolytes, urine specific gravity. Evaluate injection site for erythema, pain, abscess. Report side effects to physician for dose reduction. Be alert for early signs of water intoxication (drowsiness, listlessness, headache). Hold medication and report immediately any chest pain/allergic symptoms.

PATIENT/FAMILY TEACHING:

Promptly report headache, chest pain, shortness of breath, or other symptom. Stress importance of I&O.

---

vecuronium bromide

(Norcuron)

See Classification section under: Neuromuscular blockers (p. 103C)

---

venlafaxine

ven-lah-**facks**-een
(Effexor, Effexor XR)

▶CLASSIFICATION

PHARMACOTHERAPEUTIC: Phenethylamine derivative. *CLINICAL:* Antidepressant (see p. 36C)

ACTION/THERAPEUTIC EFFECT

Potentiates CNS neurotransmitter activity. Inhibits reuptake of serotonin, norepinephrine (weakly inhibits dopamine reuptake), *producing antidepressant activity.*

V

PHARMACOKINETICS

Well absorbed from GI tract. Protein binding: 25–30%. Metabolized in liver to active metabolite. Primarily excreted in urine. Not removed by hemodialysis. Half-life: 3–7 hrs; metabolite: 9–13 hrs (half-life increased impaired hepatic or renal disease).

USES

Treatment of depression exhibited as persistent, prominent dysphoria (occurring nearly every day for at least 2 wks) manifested by 4 of 8 symptoms: change in appetite, change in sleep pattern, increased fatigue, impaired concentration, feelings of guilt or worthlessness, loss of interest in usual activities, psychomotor agitation or retardation, or suicidal tendencies. Psychotherapy augments therapeutic result. **Venlafaxine XR:** Treatment of generalized anxiety disorder.

PRECAUTIONS

CONTRAINDICATIONS: Children <18 yrs of age, those currently receiving MAO inhibitors. **CAUTIONS:** Renal, hepatic impairment, history of mania, seizures, those with metabolic or hemodynamic disease, hypertension, history of drug abuse.

▷**LIFESPAN CONSIDERATIONS:**
Pregnancy/Lactation: Unknown if excreted in breast milk. **Pregnancy Category C. Children:** Safety and efficacy not established. **Elderly:** No age-related precautions noted.

INTERACTIONS

DRUG: MAO inhibitors may cause hyperthermia, rigidity, myoclonus, autonomic instability (including rapid fluctuations of vital signs), mental status changes, coma, extreme agitation. May cause neuroleptic malignant syndrome (wait 14 days after discontinuing MAOIs to start or wait 7 days after discontinuing venlafaxine before starting MAOIs). **HERBAL: St. John's wort** may increase sedative-hypnotic effect. **FOOD:** None known. **LAB VALUES:** May increase serum cholesterol, uric acid, alkaline phosphatase, SGOT (AST), SGPT (ALT), bilirubin, BUN. May decrease sodium, phosphate. May alter glucose, potassium.

AVAILABILITY (Rx)

TABLETS: 25 mg, 37.5 mg, 50 mg, 75 mg, 100 mg. **Effexor XR (extended-release):** 37.5 mg, 75 mg, 150 mg.

ADMINISTRATION/HANDLING
PO:

• Give without regard to food. Give with food or milk if GI distress occurs. • Scored tablet may be crushed. • Do not crush extended-release capsules.

INDICATIONS/ROUTES/DOSAGE

Note: Decrease dose by 50% in pts with moderate liver impairment; 25% in mild to moderate renal impairment (50% in pts on dialysis, withholding dose until completion of dialysis). When discontinuing the medication, taper slowly over 2 wks.

Depression:

PO: Adults, elderly: Initially, 75 mg/day in 2–3 divided doses with food. May increase by 75 mg/day no sooner than 4 day intervals. **Maximum:** 375 mg/day in 3 divided doses. **EXTENDED-RELEASE:** 75

mg/day as single dose. May increase by 75 mg/day at intervals of at least 4 days. **Maximum:** 225 mg/day.

Anxiety disorder:

PO: Adults: 37.5–225 mg/day.

SIDE EFFECTS

FREQUENT (>20%): Nausea, somnolence, headache, dry mouth. *OCCASIONAL* (10–20%): Dizziness, insomnia, constipation, sweating, nervousness, asthenia (loss of strength, energy), ejaculatory disturbance, anorexia. *RARE* (<10%): Anxiety, blurred vision, diarrhea, vomiting, tremor, abnormal dreams, impotence.

ADVERSE REACTIONS/TOXIC EFFECTS

Sustained increase in diastolic B/P (10–15 mm Hg) occurs occasionally.

NURSING IMPLICATIONS

BASELINE ASSESSMENT:

Obtain initial weight and B/P. Assess appearance, behavior, speech pattern, level of interest, mood.

INTERVENTION/EVALUATION:

Assess sleep pattern for evidence of insomnia. Check during waking hrs for somnolence or dizziness and anxiety; provide assistance as necessary. Supervise suicidal risk pt closely during early therapy (as depression lessens, energy level improves, increasing suicide potential). Assess appearance, behavior, speech pattern, level of interest, mood for therapeutic response.

PATIENT/FAMILY TEACHING:

Take with food to minimize GI distress. Do not increase, decrease, or suddenly stop medication. Do not drive or perform tasks that require alert response until response to drug is established. Inform physician if breast feeding, pregnant or planning to become pregnant. Avoid alcohol.

verapamil hydrochloride

ver-**ap**-ah-mill
(Apo-Verap✢, Calan, Chronovera✢, Covera-HS, Isoptin, Novoveramil✢, Verelan, Verelan PM)
Do not confuse with Intropin, Virilon, Vivarin, Voltaren.

FIXED-COMBINATION(S)

With trandolapril, an angiotensin inhibitor **(Tarka)**

▶CLASSIFICATION

PHARMACOTHERAPEUTIC: Calcium channel blocker. *CLINICAL:* Antihypertensive, antianginal, antiarrhythmic, hypertropic cardiomyopathy therapy adjunct (see pp. 14C, 66C)

ACTION/*THERAPEUTIC EFFECT*

Inhibits calcium ion entry across cell membranes of cardiac and vascular smooth muscle (dilates coronary arteries, peripheral arteries, arterioles). *Decreases heart rate, myocardial contractility, slows SA and AV conduction. Decreases total peripheral vascular resistance by vasodilation.*

PHARMACOKINETICS

	Onset	Peak	Duration
PO	30 min	1–2 hrs	6–8 hrs
Extended-release			
	30 min	—	—
IV	1–2 min	3–5 min	10–60 min

Well absorbed from GI tract. Protein binding: 90% (Neonates: 60%). Undergoes first-pass metabolism in liver. Metabolized in liver to active metabolite. Primarily excreted in urine. Not removed by hemodialysis. Half-life: *oral:* 2.8–7.4 hrs; *IV:* 2–5 hrs.

USES/*UNLABELED*

Parenteral: Management of supraventricular tachyarrhythmias, temporary control of rapid ventricular rate in atrial flutter/fibrillation. ***PO:*** Management of spastic (Prinzmetal's variant) angina, unstable (crescendo, preinfarction) angina, chronic stable angina (effort-associated angina), hypertension, prevention of recurrent PSVT, and (with digoxin) control of ventricular resting rate in those with atrial flutter and/or fibrillation. *Treatment of hypertrophic cardiomyopathy, vascular headaches.*

PRECAUTIONS

CONTRAINDICATIONS: Sick-sinus syndrome/second-or third-degree AV block (except in presence of pacemaker), cardiogenic shock, severe hypotension (<90 mm Hg, systolic), severe CHF (unless secondary to supraventricular tachycardia). ***CAUTIONS:*** Impaired renal, hepatic function.

▷***LIFESPAN CONSIDERATIONS:*** **Pregnancy/Lactation:** Crosses placenta; is distributed in breast milk. Breast feeding not recommended. **Pregnancy Category C. Children:** No age-related precautions noted. **Elderly:** Age-related renal impairment may require cautious use.

INTERACTIONS

DRUG: **Beta-blockers** may have additive effect. May increase **digoxin** concentration. **Procainamide, quinidine** may increase risk of QT interval prolongation. **Carbamazepine, quinidine, theophylline** may increase concentration, toxicity. **Disopyramide** may increase negative inotropic effect. ***HERBAL:*** None known. ***FOOD:*** **Grapefruit/grapefruit juice** may increase concentrations. ***LAB VALUES:*** PR interval may be increased. Therapeutic blood serum level: 0.08–0.3 mcg/ml; toxic blood serum level: N/E.

AVAILABILITY (Rx)

TABLETS: 40 mg, 80 mg, 120 mg. ***TABLETS (sustained-release):*** 120 mg, 180 mg, 240 mg. ***CAPSULES (sustained-release):*** 120 mg, 180 mg, 240 mg, 360 mg. ***VERELAN PM:*** 100 mg, 200 mg, 300 mg. ***INJECTION:*** 5 mg/2 ml.

ADMINISTRATION/HANDLING
PO:

• Give sustained-release tablets with food. Verelan may be taken without regard to food. • Do not crush or break sustained-released tablets. Do not break capsules. • Verelan may be opened and sprinkled on food. • Grapefruit juice can increase concentration.

IV 🕮

Storage:
• Store vials at room temperature.

Reconstitution:
• May give undiluted.

Rate of administration:

• Administer IV push >2 min for adults, children; give >3 min for elderly. • Continuous EKG monitoring during IV injection is required for children, recommended for adults. • Monitor EKG for rapid ventricular rates, extreme bradycardia, heart block, asystole, prolongation of PR interval. Notify physician of any significant changes. • Monitor B/P q5–10min. • Pt should remain recumbent for at least 1 hr following IV administration.

IV INCOMPATIBILITIES ⊘

Amphotericin B complex (Abelcet, Ambisome, Amphotec), nafcillin (Nafcil), propofol (Diprivan), sodium bicarbonate.

IV COMPATIBILITIES

Amiodarone (Cordarone), calcium gluconate, digoxin (Lanoxin), dopamine (Intropin), heparin, magnesium, milrinone (Primacor), multivitamins, potassium chloride.

INDICATIONS/ROUTES/DOSAGE

Supraventricular tachyarrhythmias:

IV: Adults, elderly: Initially, 5–10 mg, repeat in 30 min with 10 mg dose. **Children 1–15 yrs:** 0.1 mg/kg. May repeat in 30 min. **Maximum second dose:** 10 mg. Not recommended in children <1 yr.

Arrhythmias:

PO: Adults, elderly: 240–480 mg/day in 3–4 divided doses.

Angina:

PO: Adults, elderly: Initially, 80–120 mg 3 times/day (40 mg in elderly, pts with liver dysfunction). Titrate to optimal dose. **Maintenance:** 240–480 mg/day in 3–4 divided doses. *Covera-HS:* 180–480 mg/day at bedtime.

Hypertension:

PO: Adults, elderly: Initially, 40–80 mg 3 times/day. **Maintenance:** Up to 480 mg/day. *Covera-HS:* 180–480 mg/day at bedtime.

EXTENDED-RELEASE TABLETS: 120–240 mg/day up to 480 mg/day in 2 divided doses.

Verelan PM: 100–300 mg/day.

SIDE EFFECTS

FREQUENT (7%): Constipation. **OCCASIONAL** (2–4%): Dizziness, lightheadedness, headache, asthenia (loss of strength, energy), nausea, peripheral edema, hypotension. **RARE** (<1%): Bradycardia, dermatitis/rash.

ADVERSE REACTIONS/TOXIC EFFECTS

Rapid ventricular rate in atrial flutter/fibrillation, marked hypotension, extreme bradycardia, CHF, asystole, and second-and third-degree AV block occur rarely.

NURSING IMPLICATIONS

BASELINE ASSESSMENT:
Concurrent therapy of sublingual nitroglycerin may be used for relief of anginal pain. Record onset, type (sharp, dull, squeezing), radiation, location, intensity, and duration of anginal pain and precipitating factors (exertion, emotional stress). Check B/P for hypotension, pulse for bradycardia immediately before giving medication.

INTERVENTION/EVALUATION:
Assess pulse for strength/weakness, irregular rate. Monitor EKG for cardiac changes, particularly prolongation of PR interval. No-

V

tify physician of any significant interval changes. Assist with ambulation if dizziness occurs. Assess for peripheral edema behind medial malleolus (sacral area in bedridden pts). For those taking oral form, check stool consistency, frequency. Therapeutic blood serum level: 0.08–0.3 mcg/ml; toxic blood serum level: N/E.

PATIENT/FAMILY TEACHING:

Do not abruptly discontinue medication. Compliance with therapy regimen is essential to control anginal pain. To avoid hypotensive effect, rise slowly from lying to sitting position, wait momentarily before standing. Avoid tasks that require alertness, motor skills until response to drug is established. Contact physician/nurse if irregular heartbeat, shortness of breath, pronounced dizziness, nausea, or constipation occurs. Avoid concomitant grapefruit juice.

vidarabine

vy-**dare**-ah-been
(Ara-A, Vira-A)
Do not confuse with cytarabine.

▶CLASSIFICATION
CLINICAL: Antiviral

ACTION/THERAPEUTIC EFFECT

Appears to interfere with viral DNA synthesis, *regenerating corneal epithelium.*

USES

Treatment of keratitis, keratoconjunctivitis caused by herpes simplex virus, types 1 and 2.

PRECAUTIONS

CONTRAINDICATIONS: None significant. **CAUTIONS:** None significant.

INTERACTIONS

DRUG: None significant. **HERBAL:** None known. **FOOD:** None known. **LAB VALUES:** None significant.

AVAILABILITY (Rx)

OPHTHALMIC OINTMENT: 3%.

INDICATIONS/ROUTES/DOSAGE
Usual ophthalmic dosage:

OPHTHALMIC: Adults, elderly: 0.5 inch into lower conjunctival sac 5 times/day at 3 hr intervals. After reepithelialization, treat additional 7 days at dosage of 2 times/day.

SIDE EFFECTS

FREQUENT: Burning, itching, irritation. **OCCASIONAL:** Foreign body sensation, tearing, sensitivity to light, pain, photophobia.

ADVERSE REACTIONS/TOXIC EFFECTS

None significant.

NURSING IMPLICATIONS

INTERVENTION/EVALUATION:

Assess for irritation, itching, burning.

PATIENT/FAMILY TEACHING:

Notify physician if there is no improvement in 7 days or if burning, irritation, pain develops. Do not stop or increase doses. Ointment should be continued for 5–7 days after infection is gone to prevent recurrence of infection. A temporary haze may occur after application to eye; sunglasses will decrease sensitivity to light. Use other eye products, including makeup, only with advice of physician. Refrigerate, avoid freezing; if using another eye ointment, wait at least 10 min between dosing.

vinblastine sulfate

vin-**blass**-teen
(Velban, Velbe✦, Velsar)
Do not confuse with vincristine, vinorelbine.

▶CLASSIFICATION

PHARMACOTHERAPEUTIC:
Vinca alkaloid. ***CLINICAL:*** Antineoplastic (see p. 75C)

ACTION/*THERAPEUTIC EFFECT*

Blocks mitosis by arresting cells in metaphase of cell division, *inhibiting cellular division.* Interferes with amino acid metabolism, synthesis of nucleic acids, protein. Cell cycle-specific for M phase of cell division. Has some immunosuppressive activity.

PHARMACOKINETICS

Does not cross blood-brain barrier. Protein binding: 75%. Metabolized in liver to active metabolite. Primarily eliminated in feces via biliary system. Half-life: 24.8 hrs.

USES/*UNLABELED*

Treatment of disseminated Hodgkin's disease, non-Hodgkin's lymphoma, advanced stage of mycosis fungoides, advanced carcinoma of testis, Kaposi's sarcoma, Letterer-Siwe disease, breast carcinoma, choriocarcinoma. *Treatment of neuroblastoma, carcinoma of bladder, lung, head/neck, renal; germ cell ovarian tumors, chronic myelocytic leukemia.*

PRECAUTIONS

CONTRAINDICATIONS: Severe leukopenia, bacterial infection, significant granulocytopenia unless a result of disease being treated. ***EXTREME CAUTION:*** Debilitated, elderly (high susceptibility to leukopenia).
▷*LIFESPAN CONSIDERATIONS:*
Pregnancy/Lactation: If possible, avoid use during pregnancy, esp. first trimester. Breast feeding not recommended. **Pregnancy Category D. Children/Elderly:** No age-related precautions noted.

INTERACTIONS

DRUG: May decrease effect of **antigout medications. Bone marrow depressants** may increase bone marrow depression. **Live virus vaccines** may potentiate virus replication, increase vaccine side effects, decrease pt's antibody response to vaccine. ***HERBAL:*** None known. ***FOOD:*** None known. ***LAB VALUES:*** May increase uric acid.

AVAILABILITY (Rx)

POWDER FOR INJECTION: 10 mg. ***INJECTION:*** 1 mg/ml.

ADMINISTRATION/HANDLING

Note: May be carcinogenic, mutagenic, or teratogenic. Handle with extreme care during preparation/administration. Give by IV injection. Leakage from IV site into surrounding tissue may produce extreme irritation. Avoid eye contact with solution (severe eye irritation, possible corneal ulceration may result). If eye contact occurs, immediately irrigate eye with water.

V

IV 🍴

Storage:

• Refrigerate unopened vials. • Solutions appear clear, colorless. • Following reconstitution, solution is stable for 30 days if refrigerated. • Discard if precipitate forms, discoloration occurs.

Reconstitution:

• Reconstitute 10 mg vial with 10 ml 0.9% NaCl preserved with phenol or benzyl alcohol to provide concentration of 1 mg/ml.

Rate of administration:

• Inject into tubing of running IV infusion or directly into vein over 1 min. • Do not inject into extremity with impaired or potentially impaired circulation caused by compression or invading neoplasm, phlebitis, varicosity. • Rinse syringe, needle with venous blood before withdrawing needle (minimizes possibility of extravasation). • Extravasation may result in cellulitis, phlebitis. Large amount of extravasation may result in tissue sloughing. If extravasation occurs, give local injection of hyaluronidase and apply warm compresses.

IV INCOMPATIBILITIES ⊘

Cefepime (Maxipime), furosemide (Lasix).

IV COMPATIBILITIES

Allopurinol (Aloprim), granisetron (Kytril), heparin, ondansetron (Zofran).

INDICATIONS/ROUTES/DOSAGE

Note: Dosage individualized based on clinical response, tolerance to adverse effects. When used in combination therapy, consult specific protocols for optimum dosage, sequence of drug administration. Reduce dose if serum bilirubin >3 mg/dl. Repeat dosage at intervals of no less than 7 days and if the WBC count is at least 4,000/mm³.

Induction of remission:

IV: **Adults, elderly:** Initially, 3.7 mg/m² as single dose. Increase dose at weekly intervals of about 1.8 mg/m² until desired response is attained, WBC count falls below 3,000/mm³, or maximum weekly dose of 18.5 mg/m² is reached. **Children:** Initially, 2.5 mg/m² as single dose. Increase dose at weekly intervals of about 1.25 mg/m² until desired response is attained, WBC count falls below 3,000/mm³, or maximum weekly dose of 7.5–12.5 mg/m² is reached.

Maintenance dose:

IV: **Adults, elderly, children:** Use one increment less than dose required to produce leukocyte count of 3,000/mm³. Each subsequent dose given when leukocyte count returns to 4,000/mm³ and at least 7 days has elapsed since previous dose.

SIDE EFFECTS

FREQUENT: Nausea, vomiting, alopecia. ***OCCASIONAL:*** Constipation/diarrhea, rectal bleeding, paresthesia, headache, malaise, weakness, dizziness, pain at tumor site, jawith face pain, mental depression, dry mouth. GI distress, headache, paresthesia occurs 4–6 hrs after administration, persists for 2–10 hrs. ***RARE:*** Dermatitis, stomatitis, phototoxicity, hyperuricemia.

ADVERSE REACTIONS/TOXIC EFFECTS

Hematologic toxicity manifested most commonly as leukopenia, less frequently as anemia. WBC falls to lowest point 4–10 days after initial therapy with recovery within another 7–14 days (high doses may require 21 day recovery period). Thrombocytopenia is usually slight, transient, with rapid recovery within few days. Hepatic insufficiency may increase risk of toxicity. Acute shortness of breath, bronchospasm may occur, particularly when administered concurrently with mitomycin.

NURSING IMPLICATIONS

BASELINE ASSESSMENT:

Nausea, vomiting easily controlled by antiemetics. Discontinue therapy if WBC, thrombocyte counts fall abruptly (unless drug is clearly destroying tumor cells in bone marrow). Obtain CBC weekly or before each dosing.

INTERVENTION/EVALUATION:

If WBC falls below 2,000/mm^3, assess diligently for signs of infection. Assess for stomatitis (burning erythema of oral mucosa at inner margin of lips, sore throat, difficulty swallowing, oral ulceration). Monitor for hematologic toxicity: infection (fever, sore throat, signs of local infection); easy bruising, unusual bleeding from any site; symptoms of anemia (excessive tiredness, weakness). Assess frequency and consistency of stools; avoid constipation.

PATIENT/FAMILY TEACHING:

Immediately report any pain or burning at injection site during administration. Pain at tumor site may occur during or shortly after injection. Do not have immunizations without physician approval (drug lowers body's resistance). Avoid crowds, those with infection. Promptly report fever, sore throat, signs of local infection, easy bruising, unusual bleeding from any site. Alopecia is reversible, but new hair growth may have different color or texture. Contact physician if nausea/vomiting continues at home. Avoid constipation by increasing fluids, bulk in diet, exercise as tolerated.

vincristine sulfate

vin-**cris**-teen
(Oncovin, Vincasar PFS)
Do not confuse with Ancobon, vinblastine.

▶CLASSIFICATION

PHARMACOTHERAPEUTIC: Vinca alkaloid. ***CLINICAL:*** Antineoplastic (see p. 75C).

ACTION/*THERAPEUTIC EFFECT*

Blocks mitosis by arresting cells in metaphase stage, *inhibiting cellular division*. Interferes with amino acid metabolism, nucleic acid synthesis. Cell cycle-specific for M phase of cell division. Has some immunosuppressive effect.

PHARMACOKINETICS

Does not cross blood-brain barrier. Protein binding: 75%. Metabolized in liver. Primarily eliminated in feces via biliary system. Half-life: 10–37 hrs.

USES/*UNLABELED*

Treatment of acute leukemia, disseminated Hodgkin's disease, advanced non-Hodgkin's lymphomas, neuroblastoma, rhabdomyosarcoma, Wilms' tumor. *Treatment of chronic lymphocytic, myelocytic leukemia, carcinoma of breast, lung, ovarian, cervical, colorectal, malignant melanoma, multiple myeloma, germ cell ovarian tumors, mycosis fungoides, idiopathic thrombocytopenia purpura.*

PRECAUTIONS

CONTRAINDICATIONS: Those receiving radiation therapy through ports that include liver. ***EXTREME CAUTION:*** Hepatic impairment.

▷***LIFESPAN CONSIDERATIONS:*** **Pregnancy/Lactation:** If possible, avoid use during pregnancy, esp. first trimester. May cause fetal harm. Breast feeding not recommended. **Pregnancy Category D. Children:** No age-related precautions noted. **Elderly:** More susceptible to neurotoxic effects.

INTERACTIONS

DRUG: May decrease effect of **antigout medications. Live virus vaccines** may potentiate virus replication, increase vaccine side effects, decrease pt's antibody response to vaccine. Asparaginase, neurotoxic medications may increase neurotoxicity. Doxorubicin may increase myelosuppression. ***HERBAL:*** None known. ***FOOD:*** None known. ***LAB VALUES:*** May increase uric acid.

AVAILABILITY (Rx)

INJECTION: 1 mg/ml.

ADMINISTRATION/HANDLING
IV 🎖

Note: May be carcinogenic, mutagenic, or teratogenic. Handle with extreme care during preparation/administration. Give by IV injection. Use extreme caution in calculating, administering vincristine. Overdose may result in serious or fatal outcome.

Storage:
• Refrigerate unopened vials. • Solutions appear clear, colorless. • Discard if precipitate forms or discoloration occurs.

Reconstitution:
• May give undiluted.

Rate of administration:
• Inject dose into tubing of running IV infusion or directly into vein >1 min. • Do not inject into extremity with impaired or potentially impaired circulation caused by compression or invading neoplasm, phlebitis, varicosity. • Extravasation produces stinging, burning, edema at injection site. Terminate immediately, locally inject hyaluronidase and apply heat (disperses drug, minimizes discomfort, cellulitis).

IV INCOMPATIBILITIES ⊘

Cefepime (Maxipime), furosemide (Lasix), idarubicin (Idamycin).

IV COMPATIBILITIES

Allopurinol (Aloprim), granisetron (Kytril), heparin, ondansetron (Zofran).

INDICATIONS/ROUTES/DOSAGE

Note: Dosage individualized based on clinical response, tolerance to adverse effects. When used in combination therapy, consult specific protocols for optimum dosage, sequence of drug administration.

Usual dosage (administer at weekly intervals):
IV: **Adults, elderly:** 0.4–1.4 mg/m². **Maximum:** 2 mg. **Children:** 1–2 mg/m². **Children <10 kg or**

body surface area <1 m2: 0.05 mg/kg.

Hepatic function impairment:

Reduce dose by 50% in those with direct serum bilirubin concentration <3 mg/dl.

SIDE EFFECTS

Peripheral neuropathy occurs in nearly every pt (first clinical sign: depression of Achilles tendon reflex). *FREQUENT:* Peripheral paresthesia, alopecia, constipation or obstipation (upper colon impaction with empty rectum), abdominal cramps, headache, jaw pain, hoarseness, double vision, ptosis (drooping of eyelid), urinary tract disturbances. *OCCASIONAL:* Nausea, vomiting, diarrhea, abdominal distention, stomatitis, fever. *RARE:* Mild leukopenia, mild anemia, thrombocytopenia.

ADVERSE REACTIONS/TOXIC EFFECTS

Acute shortness of breath, bronchospasm may occur (esp. when used in combination with mitomycin). Prolonged or high-dose therapy may produce foot/wrist drop, difficulty walking, slapping gait, ataxia, muscle wasting. Acute uric acid nephropathy may be noted.

NURSING IMPLICATIONS

BASELINE ASSESSMENT:

Monitor serum uric acid levels, renal, hepatic function studies, hematologic status. Assess Achilles tendon reflex. Assess stools for consistency, frequency. Monitor for ptosis, blurred vision. Question pt regarding urinary changes.

PATIENT/FAMILY TEACHING:

Immediately report any pain or burning at injection site during administration. Alopecia is reversible, but new hair growth may have different color/texture. Contact physician if nausea/vomiting continues at home. Teach signs of peripheral neuropathy.

vinorelbine

vin-oh-**rell**-bean
(Navelbine)
Do not confuse with vinblastine.

▶CLASSIFICATION

CLINICAL: Antineoplastic (see p. 75C)

ACTION/*THERAPEUTIC EFFECT*

Interferes with mitotic microtubule assembly, *preventing cellular division.*

PHARMACOKINETICS

Following IV administration, widely distributed. Protein binding: 80–90%. Metabolized in liver. Primarily eliminated via biliary/fecal route. Half-life: 28B43 hrs.

USES/*UNLABELED*

Single agent or in combination with cisplatin for treatment with unresectable, advanced, non small cell lung cancer (NSCLC). *Treatment of breast cancer, cisplatin-resistant ovarian carcinoma, Hodgkin's disease.*

PRECAUTIONS

CONTRAINDICATIONS: Pretreatment granulocyte count <1,000 cells/mm^3. *EXTREME CAUTION:* Immunocompromised pts. *CAUTIONS:*

Existing or recent chickenpox, herpes zoster, infection, leukopenia, impaired pulmonary function, severe hepatic injury or impairment.

▷**LIFESPAN CONSIDERATIONS:**
Pregnancy/Lactation: If possible, avoid use during pregnancy, esp. during first trimester. May cause fetal harm. Breast feeding not recommended. Unknown whether excreted in breast milk. **Pregnancy Category D. Children:** Safety and efficacy not established. **Elderly:** No age-related precautions noted.

INTERACTIONS

DRUG: Significantly increased risk of granulocytopenia when **cisplatin** is used concurrently with vinorelbine. **Mitomycin** may produce acute pulmonary reaction. **Bone marrow depressants** may increase risk of bone marrow depression. **Live virus vaccines** may potentiate virus replication, increase vaccine side effects, decrease pt's antibody response to vaccine. **HERBAL:** None known. **FOOD:** None known. **LAB VALUES:** Decreases granulocytes, leukocytes, thrombocytes, RBCs. May increase total bilirubin, SGOT (AST), liver function tests.

AVAILABILITY (Rx)

INJECTION: 10 mg/ml (1 ml, 5 ml vials).

ADMINISTRATION/HANDLING
IV 💊

Note: Extremely important that IV needle or catheter is correctly positioned before administration. Leaking into surrounding tissue produces extreme irritation, local tissue necrosis, or thrombophlebitis. Wear gloves when preparing solution. If solution comes in contact with skin or mucosa, wash immediately and thoroughly with soap, water.

Storage:

• Refrigerate unopened vials. • Protect from light. • Unopened vials are stable at room temperature for 72 hrs. • Do not administer if particulate matter is noted. • Diluted vinorelbine may be used for up to 24 hrs under normal room light when stored in polypropylene syringes or polyvinyl chloride bags at room temperature.

Reconstitution:

• Must be diluted and administered via a syringe or IV bag. • *Syringe dilution:* Dilute calculated vinorelbine dose with D_5W or 0.9% NaCl to a concentration between 1.5 and 3 mg/ml. • *IV bag dilution:* Dilute calculated vinorelbine dose with D_5W, 0.45% or 0.9% NaCl, 5% dextrose and 0.45% NaCl, Ringer's or lactated Ringer's to a concentration between 0.5 and 2 mg/ml.

Rate of administration:

• Administer diluted vinorelbine over 6–10 min into side port of free-flowing IV closest to IV bag followed by flushing with 75–125 ml of one of the solutions. • If extravasation occurs, stop injection immediately; give remaining portion of the dose into another vein.

IV INCOMPATIBILITIES ⊘

Acyclovir (Zovirax), allopurinol (Aloprim), amphotericin B (Fungizone), amphotericin B complex (Abelcet, Ambisome, Amphotec), ampicillin (Omnipen), cefazolin (Ancef), cefoperazone (Cefobid), cefotetan (Cefotan), ceftriaxone (Rocephin), cefuroxime (Zinacef), fluorouracil, furosemide (Lasix), ganciclovir (Cytovene), methylprednisolone (Solu-Medrol), sodium bicarbonate.

IV COMPATIBILITIES

Calcium gluconate, filgrastim (Neupogen), granisetron (Kytril), ondansetron (Zofran).

INDICATIONS/ROUTES/DOSAGE

Note: Granulocyte count should be ≥1,000 cells/mm^3 before vinorelbine administration. Dosage adjustments should be based on granulocyte count obtained on day of treatment, as follows:

Granulocytes (cells/mm^3) on Days of Treatment	Dose (mg/m^2)
≥1,500	30
1,000–1,499	15
<1,000	Do not administer.

Non small cell lung cancer:

IV INJECTION: **Adults, elderly:** 30 mg/m^2, given over 6–10 min, administered weekly.

SIDE EFFECTS

FREQUENT: Asthenia (35%), mild or moderate nausea (34%), constipation (29%), injection site reaction manifested as erythema, pain, vein discoloration (28%), fatigue (27%), peripheral neuropathy manifested as paresthesia, hypresthesia (25%), diarrhea (17%), alopecia (12%). ***OCCASIONAL:*** Phlebitis (10%), dyspnea (7%), loss of deep tendon reflexes (5%). ***RARE:*** Chest pain, jaw pain, myalgia, arthralgia, rash.

ADVERSE REACTIONS/TOXIC EFFECTS

Bone marrow depression is manifested mainly as granulocytopenia (may be severe); other hematologic toxicity (neutropenia, thrombocytopenia, leukopenia, anemia) increases risk of infection, bleeding. Acute shortness of breath, severe bronchospasm occurs infrequently, particularly when there is preexisting pulmonary dysfunction.

NURSING IMPLICATIONS

BASELINE ASSESSMENT:

Review medication history. Assess hematology (CBC, platelet count, hemoglobin, differential) values before giving each dose. Granulocyte count should be ≥1,000 cells/mm^3 before vinorelbine administration. Granulocyte nadirs occur between 7 and 10 days after dosing. Do not give hematologic growth factors within 24 hrs before administration of chemotherapy or no earlier than 24 hrs after cytotoxic chemotherapy. Advise women of childbearing potential to avoid pregnancy during drug therapy.

INTERVENTION/EVALUATION:

Diligently monitor injection site for swelling, redness, pain at injection site. Frequently monitor for myelosuppression both during and after therapy: infection (fever, sore throat, signs of local infection); unusual bleeding or bruising; anemia (excessive tiredness, weakness). Monitor pts developing severe granulocytopenia for evidence of infection or fever. Crackers, dry toast, sips of cola may help relieve nausea. Assess bowel activity and frequency. Check injection site for reaction. Question for tingling, burning, numbness of hands/feet (peripheral neuropathy). Pt complaint of "walking on glass" is sign of hyperesthesia.

PATIENT/FAMILY TEACHING:

Notify nurse immediately if redness, swelling, pain occur at in-

V

jection site. Avoid crowds, those with infection. Do not have immunizations without physician's approval. Promptly report fever, signs of infection, easy bruising, unusual bleeding from any site, difficulty breathing. Avoid pregnancy. Alopecia is reversible, but new hair growth may have different color or texture.

vitamin A

(Aquasol A)
Do not confuse with Anusol.

▶CLASSIFICATION

PHARMACOTHERAPEUTIC:
Fat-soluble vitamin. **CLINICAL:**
Nutritional supplement (see p. 127C)

ACTION/*THERAPEUTIC EFFECT*

May be a cofactor in biochemical reactions. *Essential for normal function of retina. Necessary for visual adaptation to darkness, bone growth, testicular and ovarian function, embryonic development, preserves integrity of epithelial cells.*

PHARMACOKINETICS

Absorption dependent on bile salts, pancreatic lipase, dietary fat. Transported in blood to liver, stored in parenchymal liver cells, then transported in plasma as retinol, as needed. Metabolized in liver. Excreted in bile and to a lesser amount in urine.

USES

Treatment of vitamin A deficiency (biliary tract or pancreatic disease, sprue, colitis, hepatic cirrhosis, celiac disease, regional enteri-

tis, extreme dietary inadequacy, partial gastrectomy, cystic fibrosis).

PRECAUTIONS

CONTRAINDICATIONS: Hypervitaminosis A, oral use in malabsorption syndrome. **CAUTIONS:**
Renal impairment.

▷**LIFESPAN CONSIDERATIONS:**
Pregnancy/Lactation: Crosses placenta; distributed in breast milk. **Pregnancy Category A** (Category X if doses above RDA). **Children/Elderly:** Caution with higher doses.

INTERACTIONS

DRUG: Cholestyramine, colestipol, mineral oil may decrease absorption. **Isotretinoin** may increase toxicity. **HERBAL:** None known. **FOOD:** None known. **LAB VALUES:** May increase BUN, calcium, cholesterol, triglycerides. May decrease erythrocyte, leukocyte counts.

AVAILABILITY (OTC)

CAPSULES: 8,000 units, 10,000 units, 25,000 units, 50,000 units. **TABLETS:** 5,000 units, 10,000 units, 15,000 units. **INJECTION:** 50,000 units/2 ml.

ADMINISTRATION/HANDLING

Note: IM administration used only in acutely ill or those unresponsive to oral route (GI malabsorption syndrome).

PO:

• Do not crush or break capsule form. • Give without regard to food.

IM:

• For IM injection in adults, if dosage is 1 ml (50,000 IU), may give in deltoid muscle; if dosage is

>1 ml, give in gluteus maximus muscle. The anterolateral thigh is site of choice for infants and children <7 mos.

INDICATIONS/ROUTES/DOSAGE
Severe deficiency with xerophthalmia:

IM: **Adults, elderly, children >8 yrs:** 50,000–100,000 units/day for 3 days, then 50,000 units/day for 14 days. **Children 1–8 yrs:** 5,000–15,000 units/day for 10 days.

PO: **Adults, elderly, children >8 yrs:** 500,000 units/day for 3 days, then 50,000 units/day for 14 days, then 10,000–20,000 units/day for 2 mo. **Children 1–8 yrs:** 5,000 units/kg/day for 5 days or until recovery occurs.

Malabsorption syndrome:

PO: **Adults, elderly, children >8 yrs:** 50,000 units/day.

Dietary supplement:

PO: **Adults, elderly:** 4,000–5,000 units/day. **Children 7–10 yrs:** 3,300–3,500 units/day. **Children 4–6 yrs:** 2,500 units/day. **Children 6 mos–3 yrs:** 1,500–2,000 units/day. **Neonates to 6 mos:** 1,500 units/day.

SIDE EFFECTS
None significant.

ADVERSE REACTIONS/TOXIC EFFECTS
Chronic overdosage produces malaise, nausea, vomiting, drying/cracking of skin/lips, inflammation of tongue/gums, irritability, loss of hair, night sweats. Bulging fontanelles in infants noted.

NURSING IMPLICATIONS

INTERVENTION/EVALUATION:
Closely supervise for overdosage symptoms during prolonged daily administration over 25,000 IU. Monitor for therapeutic serum vitamin A levels (80–300 IU/ml).

PATIENT/FAMILY TEACHING:
Foods rich in vitamin A include cod, halibut, tuna, shark (naturally occurring vitamin A found only in animal sources). Avoid taking mineral oil, cholestyramine (Questran) while taking vitamin A.

vitamin D calcifediol

(Calderol)

calcitriol

(Calcijex, Rocaltrol)

dihydrotachysterol

(DHT, Hytakerol)

ergocalciferol

(Calciferol, Deltalin, Drisdol)

paricalcitol

(Zemplar)

▶ CLASSIFICATION

PHARMACOTHERAPEUTIC: Fat-soluble vitamin. ***CLINICAL:*** Nutritional supplement (see p. 128C)

ACTION/*THERAPEUTIC EFFECT*
Essential for absorption and utilization of calcium and phosphate, normal calcification of bone, regulation of serum calcium concentration (with parathyroid, calcitonin).

PHARMACOKINETICS
Readily absorbed from small intestine. Concentrated primarily in liver, fat depots. Activated in liver,

V

kidney. Eliminated via biliary system; excreted in urine. Half-life: calcifediol: 10–22 days; calcitriol: 3–6 hrs; ergocalciferol: 19–48 hrs.

USES

Prevention and treatment of vitamin D deficiency (may lead to rickets and osteomalacia), chronic hypocalcemia, hypophosphatemia, rickets, and osteodystrophy associated with chronic renal failure, familial hypophosphatemia or hypoparathyroidism. **Paricalcitol:** Prevention/treatment of secondary hypoparathyroidism associated with chronic renal failure.

PRECAUTIONS

CONTRAINDICATIONS: Hypercalcemia, vitamin D toxicity, malabsorption syndrome, hypervitaminosis D, decreased renal function, abnormal sensitivity to vitamin D effects (those with idiopathic hypercalcemia). **CAUTIONS:** Those with kidney stones, coronary disease, renal function impairment, arteriosclerosis, hypoparathyroidism, those with tartrazine sensitivity.

▷**LIFESPAN CONSIDERATIONS:**
Pregnancy/Lactation: Unknown if drug crosses placenta; is distributed in breast milk. **Pregnancy Category A** (Category D if used in doses above RDA). **Children:** May be more sensitive to effects. **Elderly:** No age-related precautions noted.

INTERACTIONS

DRUG: Aluminum-containing antacid (long-term use) may increase aluminum concentration, aluminum bone toxicity. **Magnesium-containing antacids** may increase magnesium concentration. **Calcium-containing preparations, thiazide diuretics** may increase

risk of hypercalcemia. **HERBAL:** None known. **FOOD:** None known. **LAB VALUES:** May increase calcium, cholesterol, phosphate, magnesium. May decrease alkaline phosphatase.

AVAILABILITY (Rx)

Calcifediol: CAPSULES: 20 mcg, 50 mcg.

Calcitriol: CAPSULES: 0.25 mcg, 0.5 mcg. **ORAL SOLUTION:** 1 mcg/ml. **INJECTION:** 1 mcg/ml, 2 mcg/ml.

Dihydrotachysterol: TABLETS: 0.125 mg, 0.2 mg, 0.4 mg. **CAPSULES:** 0.125 mg. **ORAL SOLUTION:** 0.2 mg/ml.

Ergocalciferol: LIQUID (OTC): 8,000 units/ml. **CAPSULES:** 50,000 units. **INJECTION:** 500,000 units/ml.

Paricalcitol: INJECTION: 5 mcg/ml.

ADMINISTRATION/HANDLING
PO:

• Give without regard to food. • Swallow whole; do not crush/chew.

INDICATIONS/ROUTES/DOSAGE
Note: 1 mcg = 40 units.

Dietary supplement:

PO: Adults, elderly, children: 10 mcg (400 units)/day. **Neonates:** 10–20 mcg (400–800 units)/day.

Renal failure:

PO: Adults, elderly: 0.5 mcg/day. **Children:** 0.1–1 mcg/day.

Hypoparathyroidism:

PO: Adults, elderly: 625 mcg–5 mg/day (with calcium supplements). **Children:** 1.25–5 mg/day (with calcium supplements).

Vitamin D–dependent rickets:

PO: Adults, elderly: 250 mcg–1.5 mg/day. **Children:** 75–125 mcg/day. **Maximum:** 1,500 mcg/day.

Nutritional rickets/osteomalacia:

PO: Adults, elderly, children: 25–125 mcg/day for 8–12 wks. **Adults, elderly (malabsorption):** 250–7,500 mcg/day. **Children (malabsorption):** 250–625 mcg/day.

Vitamin D–resistant rickets:

PO: Adults, elderly: 250–1,500 mcg/day (with phosphate supplements). **Children:** Initially 1,000–2,000 mcg/day (with phosphate supplements). May increase at 3–4 mo intervals in 250–600 mcg increments.

SIDE EFFECTS

None significant.

ADVERSE REACTIONS/TOXIC EFFECTS

Early signs of overdosage manifested as weakness, headache, somnolence, nausea, vomiting, dry mouth, constipation, muscle and bone pain, metallic taste sensation. Later signs of overdosage evidenced by polyuria, polydipsia, anorexia, weight loss, nocturia, photophobia, rhinorrhea, pruritus, disorientation, hallucinations, hyperthermia, hypertension, cardiac arrhythmias.

NURSING IMPLICATIONS

BASELINE ASSESSMENT:

Therapy should begin at lowest possible dose.

INTERVENTION/EVALUATION:

Monitor serum calcium and urinary calcium levels, serum phosphate, magnesium, creatinine, alkaline phosphatases and BUN determinations (therapeutic serum calcium level: 9–10 mg/dl). Estimate daily dietary calcium intake. Encourage adequate fluid intake.

PATIENT/FAMILY TEACHING:

Foods rich in vitamin D include vegetable oils, vegetable shortening, margarine, leafy vegetables, milk, eggs, meats. Do not take mineral oil while on vitamin D therapy. If on chronic renal dialysis, do not take magnesium-containing antacids during vitamin D therapy. Drink plenty of liquids.

vitamin E

(Aquasol E)
Do not confuse with Anusol.

▶CLASSIFICATION

PHARMACOTHERAPEUTIC: Fat-soluble vitamin. ***CLINICAL:*** Nutritional supplement (see p. 128C)

ACTION/*THERAPEUTIC EFFECT*

Essential nutritional element. An antioxidant, *protects cells from oxidation, preserves red blood cell wall integrity, protecting them against hemolysis.* May act as cofactor in enzyme systems.

PHARMACOKINETICS

Variably absorbed from GI tract (requires bile salts, dietary fat, normal pancreatic function). Primarily concentrated in adipose tissue. Metabolized in liver. Primarily eliminated via biliary system.

USES/*UNLABELED*

Treatment of vitamin E deficiency. *Decreases severity of tardive dyskinesia.*

PRECAUTIONS

CONTRAINDICATIONS: None significant. ***CAUTIONS:*** None significant.

V

▷**LIFESPAN CONSIDERATIONS:**
Pregnancy/Lactation: Unknown if drug crosses placenta or is distributed in breast milk. **Pregnancy Category A** (Category C if used in doses above RDA). **Children/Elderly:** No age-related precautions noted in normal dosages.

INTERACTIONS

DRUG: May impair hematologic response in pts with iron deficiency anemia. **Iron** (large doses) may increase vitamin E requirements. **Cholestyramine, colestipol, mineral oil** may decrease absorption. **HERBAL:** None known. **FOOD:** None known. **LAB VALUES:** None significant.

AVAILABILITY (OTC)

CAPSULES: 100 units, 200 units, 400 units, 600 units, 800 units, 1,000 units. **TABLETS:** 100 units, 200 units, 400 units, 500 units, 800 units. **ORAL DROPS:** 15 units/0.3 ml.

ADMINISTRATION/HANDLING
PO:
• Do not crush or break tablets/capsules. • Give without regard to food.

INDICATIONS/ROUTES/DOSAGE
Vitamin E deficiency:
PO: Adults, elderly: 60–75 units/day. **Children:** 1 unit/kg/day.

SIDE EFFECTS
None significant.

ADVERSE REACTIONS/TOXIC EFFECTS

Chronic overdosage produces fatigue, weakness, nausea, headache, blurred vision, flatulence, diarrhea.

NURSING IMPLICATIONS

PATIENT/FAMILY TEACHING:

Foods rich in vitamin E include vegetable oils, vegetable shortening, margarine, leafy vegetables, milk, eggs, meats.

vitamin K

phytonadione
(vitamin K₁)

fy-toe-na-**dye**-own
(AquaMEPHYTON, Konakion, Mephyton)
Do not confuse with melphalan, mephenytoin.

▶CLASSIFICATION

PHARMACOTHERAPEUTIC: Fat-soluble vitamin. **CLINICAL:** Nutritional supplement, antidote (drug-induced hypoprothrombinemia), antihemorrhagic

ACTION/*THERAPEUTIC EFFECT*

Necessary for hepatic formation of coagulation factors II, VII, IX, and X, *essential for normal clotting of blood.*

PHARMACOKINETICS

Readily absorbed from GI tract (duodenum), after IM, SubQ administration. Metabolized in liver. Excreted in urine, eliminated via biliary system. **Parenteral:** Controls hemorrhage within 3–6 hrs, normal prothrombin time in 12–14 hrs. **PO:** Effect in 6–10 hrs.

USES

Prevention, treatment of hemorrhagic states in neonates; antidote for hemorrhage induced by oral anticoagulants, hypoprothrombinemic states due to vitamin K deficiency. Will not counteract anticoagulation effect of heparin.

PRECAUTIONS

CONTRAINDICATIONS: Last few wks of pregnancy, neonates. **CAUTIONS:** Those with asthma, impaired hepatic function.
▷**LIFESPAN CONSIDERATIONS:** **Pregnancy/Lactation:** Crosses placenta; distributed in breast milk. **Pregnancy Category C. Children/Elderly:** No age-related precautions noted.

INTERACTIONS

DRUG: Broad-spectrum antibiotics, high-dose salicylates may increase vitamin K requirements. May decrease effect of **oral anticoagulants. Cholestyramine, colestipol, mineral oil, sucralfate** may decrease absorption. **HERBAL:** None known. **FOOD:** None known. **LAB VALUES:** None significant.

AVAILABILITY (Rx)

TABLETS: 5 mg. **INJECTION:** 2 mg/ml, 10 mg/ml.

ADMINISTRATION/HANDLING
PO:
• Scored tablets may be crushed.

SUBQ/IM:
• Inject into anterolateral aspect of thigh/deltoid region.

IV 🕎
Note: Restrict to emergency use only.

Storage:
• Store at room temperature.

Reconstitution:
• May dilute with preservative-free NaCl or D_5W immediately before use. Do not use other diluents. Discard unused portions.

Rate of administration:
• Administer slow IV at rate of 1 mg/min. • Monitor continuously for hypersensitivity, anaphylactic reaction during and immediately following IV administration.

IV INCOMPATIBILITY ⊘

No known incompatibility noted via Y-site administration.

IV COMPATIBILITIES

Heparin, potassium chloride.

INDICATIONS/ROUTES/DOSAGE
Note: IV route for emergency use only.
Oral anticoagulant overdose:
IV/SUBQ/PO: Adults, elderly: 2.5–10 mg/dose. May repeat in 6–8 hrs if given IV/SubQ or 12–48 hrs if given orally. **Children:** 0.5–5 mg depending on need for further anticoagulation, severity of bleeding.

Vitamin K deficiency:
IV/IM/SUBQ: Adults, elderly: 10 mg. **Children:** 1–2 mg/dose.
PO: Adults, elderly: 2.5–25 mg/24 hrs. **Children:** 2.5–5 mg/24 hrs.

Hemorrhagic disease in newborn:
IM/SUBQ: (Treatment): 1–2 mg/dose/day. **(Prophylaxis):** 0.5–1 mg within 1 hr of birth. May repeat in 6–8 hrs if necessary.

SIDE EFFECTS
Note: PO or SubQ administration less likely to produce side effects than IM or IV route.

OCCASIONAL: Pain, soreness, swelling at IM injection site; re-

V

peated injections: pruritic erythema; flushed face, unusual taste.

ADVERSE REACTIONS/TOXIC EFFECTS

May produce hyperbilirubinemia in newborn (esp. premature infants). Rarely, severe reaction occurs immediately following IV administration (cramp-like pain, chest pain, dyspnea, facial flushing, dizziness, rapid/weak pulse, rash, profuse sweating, hypotension; may progress to shock, cardiac arrest).

NURSING IMPLICATIONS

INTERVENTION/EVALUATION:

Monitor prothrombin time routinely in those taking anticoagulants. Assess skin for bruises, petechiae. Assess gums for gingival bleeding, erythema. Monitor urine output for hematuria. Assess hematocrit, platelet count, urine/stool culture for occult blood. Assess for decrease in B/P, increase in pulse rate, complaint of abdominal or back pain, severe headache (may be evidence of hemorrhage). Question for increase in amount of discharge during menses. Assess peripheral pulses, skin for bruises, petechiae. Check for excessive bleeding from minor cuts, scratches. Assess urine output for hematuria.

PATIENT/FAMILY TEACHING:

Discomfort may occur with parenteral administration. **Adults:** Use electric razor, soft toothbrush to prevent bleeding. Report any sign of red or dark urine, black or red stool, coffee-ground vomitus, red-speckled mucus from cough. Do not use any OTC medication without physician approval (may interfere with platelet aggrega-

tion). Foods rich in vitamin K_1 include leafy green vegetables, meat, cow's milk, vegetable oil, egg yolks, tomatoes.

warfarin sodium

war-fair-in
(<u>Coumadin</u>, Warfilone ♣)
Do not confuse with Kemadrin.

▶CLASSIFICATION

PHARMACOTHERAPEUTIC: Coumarin derivative. ***CLINICAL:*** Anticoagulant (see p. 29C)

ACTION/*THERAPEUTIC EFFECT*

Interferes with hepatic synthesis of vitamin K–dependent clotting factors, resulting in depletion of coagulation factors II, VII, IX, X. *Prevents further extension of formed existing clot; prevents new clot formation or secondary thromboembolic complications.*

PHARMACOKINETICS

	Onset	Peak	Duration
PO	—	1.5–3 days	2–5 days

Well absorbed from GI tract. Metabolized in liver. Primarily excreted in urine. Not removed by hemodialysis. Half-life: 1.5–2.5 days.

USES/*UNLABELED*

Prophylaxis, treatment of venous thrombosis, pulmonary embolism. Treatment of thromboembolism associated with chronic atrial fibrillation. Adjunct in treatment of coronary occlusion. Prophylaxis/treatment of thromboembolic complications associated with cardiac valve replacement. Reduces risk of death, recurrent MI, stroke, embolization after myocardial infarction. *Prophylaxis vs. recurrence cerebral embolism, myocardial reinfarction, treatment adjunct in transient ischemic attacks.*

PRECAUTIONS

CONTRAINDICATIONS: Bleeding abnormalities, hemophilia, thrombocytopenia, brain/spinal cord surgery, spinal anesthesia, eye surgery; bleeding from GI, respiratory, or GU tract; threatened abortion, aneurysm, ascorbic acid deficiency, acute nephritis, cerebrovascular hemorrhage, eclampsia, pre-eclampsia, blood dyscrasias, hypertension, severe hepatic disease, pericardial effusion, bacterial endocarditis, visceral carcinoma, following spinal puncture, IUD insertion, or any potential for bleeding abnormalities. **CAUTIONS:** Factors increasing risk of hemorrhage, active tuberculosis, severe diabetes, GI tract ulcer disease, during menstruation, postpartum period. Long-term use may increase bone fractures.
▷**LIFESPAN CONSIDERATIONS:**
Pregnancy/Lactation: Contraindicated in pregnancy (fetal/neonatal hemorrhage, intrauterine death). Crosses placenta; is distributed in breast milk. **Pregnancy Category D. Children:** More susceptible to effects. **Elderly:** Increased risk of hemorrhage; lower dosage recommended.

INTERACTIONS

DRUG: Increased effect with: **Acetaminophen (regular use), allopurinol, amiodarone, anabolic steroids, androgens, aspirin, cefamandole, cefoperazone, chloral hydrate, chloramphenicol, cimetidine, clofibrate, danazol, dextrothyroxine, diflunisal, disulfiram, erythromycin, fenoprofen, gemfibrozil, indomethacin, methimazole, metronidazole, oral hypoglycemics, phenytoin, plicamycin, PTU, quinidine, salicylates, sulfinpyrazone, sulfonamides, sulindac.** Decreased effect with: **Barbiturates, carbamazepine, cholestyramine, colestipol, estramustine, estrogens, griseofulvin, primidone, rifampin, vitamin K. HERBAL: Feverfew, garlic, ginkgo biloba, ginseng** may increase risk of bleeding. **FOOD:** None known. **LAB VALUES:** None significant.

AVAILABILITY (Rx)

TABLETS: 1 mg, 2 mg, 2.5 mg, 3 mg, 5 mg, 6 mg, 7.5 mg, 10 mg.
INJECTION: 5 mg vials.

ADMINISTRATION/HANDLING

PO:

• Scored tablets may be crushed.
• Give without regard to food. If GI upset occurs, give with food.

INDICATIONS/ROUTES/DOSAGE

Note: Dosage highly individualized, based on prothrombin time (PT), INR.

PO/IV: Adults: Initially, 10–15 mg, then adjust dose. **Maintenance:** 2–10 mg/day based on prothrombin determinations.

Usual elderly dosage:

PO/IV: Adults: 2–5 mg/day (maintenance).

SIDE EFFECTS

OCCASIONAL: GI distress (nausea, anorexia, abdominal cramps, diarrhea). **RARE:** Hypersensitivity reaction (dermatitis, urticaria, esp. in those sensitive to aspirin).

ADVERSE REACTIONS/TOXIC EFFECTS

Bleeding complications ranging from local ecchymoses to major

W

hemorrhage. Drug should be discontinued immediately and vitamin K (phytonadione) administered. *Mild hemorrhage:* 2.5–10 mg PO/IM/IV. *Severe hemorrhage:* 10–15 mg IV and repeated q4h, as necessary. Hepatotoxicity, blood dyscrasias, necrosis, vasculitis, local thrombosis occur rarely.

NURSING IMPLICATIONS

BASELINE ASSESSMENT:

Cross-check dose with co-worker. Determine INR before administration and daily after therapy initiation. When stabilized, follow with INR determination q4–6wks.

INTERVENTION/EVALUATION:

Monitor INR reports diligently. Assess hematocrit, platelet count, urine/stool culture for occult blood, SGOT (AST), SGPT (ALT), regardless of route of administration. Be alert to complaints of abdominal back pain, severe headache (may be signs of hemorrhage). Decrease in B/P, increase in pulse rate may also be sign of hemorrhage. Question for increase in amount of discharge during menses. Assess area of thromboembolus for color, temperature. Assess peripheral pulses, skin for bruises, petechiae. Check for excessive bleeding from minor cuts, scratches. Assess gums for erythema, gingival bleeding. Assess urine output for hematuria.

PATIENT/FAMILY TEACHING:

Take medication exactly as prescribed. Do not take or discontinue any other medication except on advice of physician. Avoid alcohol, salicylates, or drastic dietary changes. Do not change from one brand to another. Consult with physician before surgery or dental work. Urine may become red-orange. Notify physician if bleeding, bruising, red or brown urine, black stools occur. Use electric razor, soft toothbrush to prevent bleeding. Report any sign of red or dark urine, black or red stool, coffee-ground vomitus, red-speckled mucus from cough. Do not use any OTC medication without physician approval (may interfere with platelet aggregation).

yohimbe

Also known as johimbi, aphrodien, corynine

▶CLASSIFICATION
HERBAL

ACTION/*EFFECT*

Produces genital blood vessel dilation, nerve impulse transmission to genital area, *improving sexual vigor.* Increases penile blood flow, central sympathetic excitation impulses to genital tissues, *affecting impotence.*

USES

Aphrodisiac, impotence, exhaustion, angina, diabetic neuropathy, postural hypotension.

PRECAUTIONS

CONTRAINDICATIONS: Pregnancy/lactation (may have uterine relaxant effect, cause fetal toxicity), angina, heart disease, benign prostatic hypertrophy, depression, renal/liver disease. ***CAUTIONS:***

Anxiety, diabetes mellitus, hypertension, post-traumatic stress disorder, schizophrenia.
▷*LIFESPAN CONSIDERATIONS:*
Pregnancy/Lactation: Contraindicated; avoid use. **Children:** Safety and efficacy not established; avoid use. **Elderly:** Age-related renal/liver impairment may require discontinuing.

INTERACTIONS

DRUG: May interfere with drugs for diabetes, **antihypertensives.** May antagonize effect of **clonidine.** Additive effects with **MAOIs, sympathomimetics, tricyclic antidepressants.** *HERBAL:* **Ginkgo, St. John's wort** can have additive therapeutic/adverse effects. **Ephedra** may increase risk of hypertensive crises. *FOOD:* Tyramine-containing foods (e.g., aged cheese, chianti wine), caffeine-containing products, coffee, tea, chocolate may increase risk of hypertensive crises. *LAB VALUES:* None significant.

AVAILABILITY (OTC)

TABLETS: 5 mg. *LIQUID:* 5 mg/5 ml.

INDICATIONS/ROUTES /DOSAGE

Impotence:

PO: **Adults, elderly:** 15–30 mg/day in divided doses.

SIDE EFFECTS

Excitement, tremors, insomnia, anxiety, hypertension, tachycardia, dizziness, headache, irritability, salivation, dilated pupils, nausea, vomiting, hypersensitivity reaction.

ADVERSE REACTIONS/TOXIC EFFECTS

Paralysis, severe hypotension, irregular heartbeats, cardiac failure. Overdose can be fatal.

NURSING IMPLICATIONS

BASELINE ASSESSMENT:

Assess if pt is pregnant/breastfeeding (contraindicated). Determine other medical conditions, including angina, heart disease, benign prostatic hypertrophy. Assess baseline renal/liver function, medications (see Interactions).

INTERVENTION/EVALUATION:

Monitor renal/liver functions, blood pressure. Assess for hypersensitivity reaction.

PATIENT/FAMILY TEACHING:

Avoid use of other medications without checking with physician. Do not take OTC medications. Inform physician if pregnant/breast-feeding.

---

zafirlukast

zay-**fur**-leu-cast
(Accolate)
Do not confuse with Accupril, Aclovate.

▶CLASSIFICATION

PHARMACOTHERAPEUTIC: Leukotriene receptor antagonist. *CLINICAL:* Anti-asthma (see p. 64C)

ACTION/*THERAPEUTIC EFFECT*

Binds to leukotriene receptors. Inhibits bronchoconstriction due to sulfur dioxide, cold air, specific antigens (grass, cat dander, ragweed) *reducing airway edema,*

Y
Z

---

smooth muscle constriction, altered cellular activity associated with inflammatory process.

PHARMACOKINETICS

Rapidly absorbed following PO administration (food reduces absorption). Protein binding: 99%. Extensively metabolized in liver. Primarily excreted in feces. Unknown if removed by hemodialysis. Half-life: 10 hrs.

USES

Prophylaxis, chronic treatment of bronchial asthma.

PRECAUTIONS

CONTRAINDICATIONS: None significant. ***CAUTIONS:*** Impaired hepatic function.

▷***LIFESPAN CONSIDERATIONS:*** **Pregnancy/Lactation:** Distributed in breast milk. Do not administer to breast-feeding women. **Pregnancy Category B. Children:** Safety and efficacy not established in those <12 yrs of age. **Elderly:** No age-related precautions noted.

INTERACTIONS

DRUG: **Aspirin** increases concentration. Coadministration of **warfarin** increases prothrombin time (PT). **Erythromycin, theophylline** decreases concentration. ***HERBAL:*** None known. ***FOOD:*** None known. ***LAB VALUES:*** May increase SGPT (ALT).

AVAILABILITY (Rx)

TABLETS: 10 mg, 20 mg.

ADMINISTRATION/HANDLING

PO:

• Give 1 hr before or 2 hrs after meals. • Do not crush or break tablets.

INDICATIONS/ROUTES/DOSAGE

Bronchial asthma:

PO: **Adults, elderly, children >12 yrs:** 20 mg twice daily. **Children 5–12 yrs:** 10 mg twice daily.

SIDE EFFECTS

FREQUENT (13%): Headache. ***OCCASIONAL*** (3%): Nausea, diarrhea. ***RARE*** (<3%): Generalized pain, asthenia, myalgia, fever, dyspepsia, vomiting, dizziness.

ADVERSE REACTIONS/TOXIC EFFECTS

Coadministration of inhaled corticosteroids increases risk of upper respiratory infection.

NURSING IMPLICATIONS

BASELINE ASSESSMENT:

Obtain medication history. Assess liver function lab values.

INTERVENTION/EVALUATION:

Monitor rate, depth, rhythm, type of respiration; quality and rate of pulse. Assess lung sounds for rhonchi, wheezing, rales. Observe lips, fingernails for blue or dusky color in light-skinned pts; gray in dark-skinned pts. Monitor liver function tests.

PATIENT/FAMILY TEACHING:

Increase fluid intake (decreases lung secretion viscosity). Take as prescribed, even during symptom-free periods. Do not use for acute asthma episodes. Do not alter/stop other asthma medications. Nursing mothers should not breast-feed. Report nausea, jaundice, abdominal pain, flulike symptoms, or worsening of asthma.

---

zalcitabine

zal-**site**-ah-bean
(Hivid)

▶CLASSIFICATION

PHARMACOTHERAPEUTIC:
Nucleoside reverse transcriptase
inhibitor. ***CLINICAL:*** Antiretroviral (see pp. 59C, 95C)

ACTION/*THERAPEUTIC EFFECT*

Intracellularly converted to active
metabolite. Inhibits viral DNA synthesis, *preventing replication of
human immunodeficiency virus
(HIV-1).*

PHARMACOKINETICS

Readily absorbed from GI tract
(food decreases absorption). Proteing binding: <4%. Undergoes
phosphorylation intracellularly to
the active metabolite. Primarily
excreted in urine. Unknown if removed by hemodialysis. Half-life:
1–3 hrs; metabolite: 2.6–10 hrs
(half-life increased with impaired
renal function).

USES

Management of adult pts with advanced HIV disease who are either intolerant to zidovudine or
have disease progression while
receiving zidovudine.

PRECAUTIONS

CONTRAINDICATIONS: Pts with
moderate/severe peripheral neuropathy, children <13 yrs (safety
not known). ***EXTREME CAUTION:***
Those with low CD4 cell counts
(risk of peripheral neuropathy is
greater), preexisting neuropathy.
CAUTIONS: Pts with history of
pancreatitis or increased amylase,
history of ethanol abuse. History

of CHF, baseline cardiomyopathy,
decreased renal function, liver disease.

▷***LIFESPAN CONSIDERATIONS:***
Pregnancy/Lactation: Unknown
if drug crosses placenta or is distributed in breast milk. Avoid
breast feeding in HIV-positive
women. **Pregnancy Category C.**
Children: No age-related precautions in those <6 mos of age;
dosage not established. **Elderly:**
Age-related renal impairment
may require dosage adjustment.

INTERACTIONS

DRUG: Medications associated
with peripheral neuropathy may
increase risk (**e.g., cisplatin,
disulfiram, phenytoin, vincristine).** Medications causing pancreatitis may increase risk (e.g.,
IV pentamidine). ***HERBAL:*** None
known. ***FOOD:*** None known. ***LAB
VALUES:*** May increase SGOT
(AST), SGPT (ALT), alkaline phosphatase, amylase, lipase, triglyceride, bilirubin concentrations.
May decrease phosphates, magnesium, calcium. May alter sodium, glucose levels.

AVAILABILITY (Rx)

TABLETS: 0.375 mg, 0.75 mg.

ADMINISTRATION/HANDLING

PO:

• Best taken on empty stomach
(food decreases absorption). •
May take with food to decrease GI
distress. • Space doses evenly
around the clock.

INDICATIONS/ROUTES/DOSAGE

HIV infection:

PO: **Adults:** 0.75 mg q8h (may be
given with zidovudine). **Children
<13 yrs:** 0.01 mg/kg q8h. **Range:**
0.005–0.01 mg/kg q8h.

Z

Dosage in renal impairment:

Based on creatinine clearance.

Creatinine Clearance	Dose
10–40 ml/min	0.75 mg q12h
<10 ml/min	0.75 mg q24h

SIDE EFFECTS

FREQUENT (11–28%): Peripheral neuropathy, fever, fatigue, headache, rash. **OCCASIONAL** (5–10%): Diarrhea, abdominal pain, oral ulcers, cough, pruritus, myalgia, weight loss, nausea, vomiting. **RARE** (1–4%): Fatigue, nasal discharge, dysphagia, depression, night sweats, confusion.

ADVERSE REACTIONS/TOXIC EFFECTS

Peripheral neuropathy occurs commonly (17–31%), characterized by numbness, tingling, burning, and pain of lower extremities. May be followed by sharp shooting pain and progress to severe continuous burning pain that may be irreversible if the drug is not discontinued in time. Pancreatitis, leukopenia, neutropenia, eosinophilia, thrombocytopenia occur rarely.

NURSING IMPLICATIONS

BASELINE ASSESSMENT:

Offer emotional support to pt and family. Monitor CBC, triglycerides, and serum amylase levels before and during therapy.

INTERVENTION/EVALUATION:

Stop medication and notify physician immediately if signs and symptoms of peripheral neuropathy develop: numbness, tingling, burning, or shooting pains of extremities, loss of vibratory sense or ankle reflex. Although rare, be alert to impending potentially fatal pancreatitis: increasing serum amylase, rising triglycerides, nausea, vomiting, abdominal pain (withhold medication and notify physician). Assess for therapeutic response: weight gain, increased energy, decreased fatigue. Assess CBC for evidence of blood dyscrasias.

PATIENT/FAMILY TEACHING:

Not a cure for HIV; may continue to contract illnesses associated with advanced HIV infection. Does not preclude the need to continue practices to prevent transmission of HIV. Report promptly any signs and symptoms of peripheral neuropathy or pancreatitis (see Adverse Reactions/Toxic Effects). Women of childbearing age should use contraception.

zaleplon

zale-eh-plon
(Sonata)

▶CLASSIFICATION

PHARMACOTHERAPEUTIC:
Nonbenzodiazepine. **CLINICAL:**
Hypnotic (see p. 124C)

ACTION/THERAPEUTIC EFFECT

Enhances action of inhibitory neurotransmitter gamma-aminobutyric acid (GABA), *producing hypnotic effect.*

USES

Short-term treatment of insomnia (7–10 days). Decreases sleep onset time (no effect on number of nocturnal awakenings, total sleep time).

PRECAUTIONS

CONTRAINDICATIONS: Severe hepatic impairment. ***CAUTIONS:*** Mild-to-moderate hepatic function in those experiencing signs/symptoms of depression, those hypersensitive to aspirin (allergic-type reaction).

INTERACTIONS

DRUG: Alcohol, CNS depressants may increase CNS depressant effect. **Rifampin** reduces zaleplon concentration. **Cimetidine** increases zaleplon effect. ***HERBAL:*** None known. ***FOOD: High-fat/heavy meal*** delays sleep onset time by approx. 2 hrs. ***LAB VALUES:*** None significant.

AVAILABILITY (Rx)

CAPSULES: 5 mg, 10 mg.

ADMINISTRATION/HANDLING
PO:

• Giving drug with or immediately after a high-fat meal results in slower absorption. • Capsules may be emptied and mixed with food.

INDICATIONS/ROUTES/DOSAGE
Hypnotic:

PO: Adults >18 yrs: 10 mg immediately before bedtime or after going to bed. **Elderly/debilitated, hepatic function impaired, those taking concurrent cimetidine:** 5 mg at bedtime.

SIDE EFFECTS

EXPECTED: Drowsiness, sedation, mild rebound insomnia on first night after drug is discontinued. ***FREQUENT*** (7–28%): Nausea, headache, myalgia, dizziness. ***OCCASIONAL*** (3–5%): Abdominal pain, asthenia (loss of strength/energy), dyspepsia, eye pain, pares-thesia. ***RARE*** (2%): Tremors, amnesia, hyperacusis (acute sense of hearing), fever, dysmenorrhea.

ADVERSE REACTIONS/TOXIC EFFECTS

May produce abnormal thinking/behavior changes. Taking medication while ambulating may result in memory impairment, hallucination, impaired coordination, dizziness, lightheadedness. Overdosage results in somnolence, confusion, diminished reflexes, coma.

NURSING IMPLICATIONS

BASELINE ASSESSMENT:
Raise bed rails. Provide environment conducive to sleep (back rub, quiet environment, low lighting).

INTERVENTION/EVALUATION:
Assess sleep pattern.

PATIENT/FAMILY TEACHING:
Do not exceed prescribed dosage. Do not take with or immediately after a high-fat/heavy meal. Rebound insomnia may occur when drug is discontinued after short-term therapy. Avoid alcohol and other CNS depressants.

zanamivir

zah-**nam**-ih-vur
(Relenza)

►CLASSIFICATION

PHARMACOTHERAPEUTIC: Antiviral. ***CLINICAL:*** Anti-influenza (see p. 59C)

Z

ACTION/*THERAPEUTIC EFFECT*

Appears to inhibit the influenza virus enzyme, neuraminidase, essential for viral replication, and *prevents viral release from infected cells.*

PHARMACOKINETICS

Systemically absorbed. Protein binding: <10%. Excreted unchanged in urine. Unabsorbed drug excreted in feces. Half-life: 2.5–5 hrs.

USES

Treatment of uncomplicated acute illness due to influenza virus in adults and adolescents >12 yrs who have been symptomatic for <2 days. Prevention of influenza A and B.

PRECAUTIONS

CONTRAINDICATIONS: None significant. ***CAUTIONS:*** COPD, asthma.
▷*LIFESPAN CONSIDERATIONS:*
Pregnancy/Lactation: Unknown if crosses placenta or distributed in breast milk. **Pregnancy Category B. Children:** Safety and efficacy not established in those <12 yrs of age. **Elderly:** No age-related precautions noted.

INTERACTIONS

DRUG: None significant. ***HERBAL:*** None known. ***FOOD:*** None known. ***LAB VALUES:*** May increase liver enzymes, CPK.

AVAILABILITY (Rx)

BLISTERS OF POWDER FOR INHALATION: 5 mg.

ADMINISTRATION/HANDLING
Inhalation:

• Using the Diskhaler device provided, exhale completely; then, holding mouthpiece 1 inch away from lips, inhale and hold breath as long as possible before exhaling. • Rinse mouth with water immediately after inhalation (prevents mouth/throat dryness). • Store at room temperature.

INDICATIONS/ROUTES/DOSAGE
Treatment of influenza virus:

***INHALATION:* Adults, elderly, children ≥7 yrs:** 2 inhalations (one 5 mg blister per inhalation for a total dose of 10 mg) twice daily (approx. 12 hrs apart) for 5 days.

Prevention of influenza virus:

***INHALATION:* Adults, elderly:** 1 inhalation given once daily for at least 7 days.

SIDE EFFECTS

OCCASIONAL (2–3%): Diarrhea, sinusitis, nausea, bronchitis, cough, dizziness, headache. ***RARE*** (<1.5%): Malaise, fatigue, fever, abdominal pain, myalgia, arthralgia, urticaria.

ADVERSE REACTIONS/TOXIC EFFECTS

May produce neutropenia. Bronchospasm may occur in those with history of COPD, bronchial asthma.

NURSING IMPLICATIONS

BASELINE ASSESSMENT:

Those requiring an inhaled bronchodilator at the same time as zanamivir should use the bronchodilator before zanamivir administration.

INTERVENTION/EVALUATION:

Provide assistance if dizziness occurs. Monitor bowel activity and stool consistency.

PATIENT/FAMILY TEACHING:

Avoid contact with those who are at high risk for influenza. Continue treatment for the full 5 day course. Doses should be evenly spaced. In pts with respiratory disease, an inhaled bronchodilator should be readily available.

zidovudine

zye-**dough**-view-deen
(Apo-Zidovudine✤, AZT, Novo-AZT✤, Retrovir)
Do not confuse with
Combivent, ritonavir.

FIXED-COMBINATION(S)

With lamivudine, an antiviral **(Combivir)**; with abacavir and lamivudine, antivirals **(Trizivir)**

▶CLASSIFICATION

PHARMACOTHERAPEUTIC: Nucleoside reverse transcriptase inhibitor. *CLINICAL:* Antiretroviral (see pp. 59C, 95C)

ACTION/*THERAPEUTIC EFFECT*

Interferes with viral RNA-dependent DNA polymerase, an enzyme necessary for viral HIV replication, *slowing HIV replication, reducing progression of HIV infection.*

PHARMACOKINETICS

Rapidly, completely absorbed from GI tract. Protein binding: 25–38%. Undergoes first-pass metabolism in liver. Widely distributed. Crosses blood-brain barrier, CSF. Primarily excreted in urine. Minimal removal by hemodialysis. Half-life: 0.8–1.2 hrs (half-life increased with impaired renal function).

USES/*UNLABELED*

IV: Management of select adult pts with symptomatic HIV infection (AIDS, advanced HIV disease). *PO:* Management of pts with HIV infection having evidence of impaired immunity. HIV-infected children (>3 mos) who have HIV-related symptoms or asymptomatic with abnormal lab values showing significant HIV-related immunosuppression. Prevents maternal-fetal HIV transmission. *Prophylaxis in occupational exposure at risk of acquiring HIV.*

PRECAUTIONS

CONTRAINDICATIONS: Life-threatening allergies to zidovudine or components of preparation. *CAUTIONS:* Bone marrow compromise, renal and hepatic dysfunction, decreased hepatic blood flow.

▷*LIFESPAN CONSIDERATIONS:* **Pregnancy/Lactation:** Unknown if drug crosses placenta or is distributed in breast milk. Unknown if fetal harm or effects on fertility can occur. **Pregnancy Category C. Children:** No age-related precautions noted. **Elderly:** Information not available.

INTERACTIONS

DRUG: **Bone marrow depressants, ganciclovir** may increase myelosuppression. **Clarithromycin** may decrease concentrations. **Probenecid** may increase concentrations, risk of toxicity. *HERBAL:* None known. *FOOD:* None known. *LAB VALUES:* May increase mean corpuscular volume.

Z

CAPSULES: 100 mg. *TABLETS:* 300 mg. *SYRUP:* 50 mg/5 ml. *INJECTION:* 10 mg/ml.

ADMINISTRATION/HANDLING
PO:

• Keep capsules in cool, dry place. Protect from light. • Food, milk do not affect GI absorption. • Space doses evenly around the clock.

IV 💊

Storage:

• After dilution, IV solution is stable for 24 hrs at room temperature; 48 hrs if refrigerated. • Use within 8 hrs if stored at room temperature; 24 hrs if refrigerated. • Do not use if particulate matter is present or discoloration occurs.

Reconstitution:

• Must dilute before administration. • Remove calculated dose from vial and add to D_5W to provide a concentration no greater than 4 mg/ml.

Rate of administration:

• Infuse over 1 hr.

IV INCOMPATIBILITY ⊘

Do not mix with any other medications.

IV COMPATIBILITIES

Lorazepam (Ativan), pentamidine (Pentam IV), potassium chloride, co-trimethoxazole (Bactrim, Septra), trimetrexate (Neutrexin).

INDICATIONS/ROUTES/DOSAGE
HIV:

IV: Adults, elderly, children >12 yrs: 1–2 mg/kg/dose q4h. **Children ≤12 yrs:** 120 mg/m²/dose q6h. **Neonates:** 1.5 mg/kg/dose q6h.

PO: Adults, elderly, children >12 yrs: 200 mg q8h or 300 mg q12h. **Children ≤12 yrs:** 160 mg/m²/dose q8h. **Range:** 90–180 mg/m²/dose q6–8h. **Neonates:** 2 mg/kg/dose q6h.

SIDE EFFECTS

COMMON (42–46%): Nausea, headache. *FREQUENT* (16–20%): GI pain, asthenia (loss of strength, energy), rash, fever. *OCCASIONAL* (8–12%): Diarrhea, anorexia, malaise, myalgia, somnolence. *RARE* (5–6%): Dizziness, paresthesia, vomiting, insomnia, dyspnea, altered taste.

ADVERSE REACTIONS/TOXIC EFFECTS

Anemia (occurring most commonly after 4–6 wks of therapy) and granulocytopenia, particularly significant in those with pretherapy low baselines, occur rarely. Nausea, vomiting, neurotoxicity (ataxia, fatigue, lethargy, nystagmus), seizures.

NURSING IMPLICATIONS

BASELINE ASSESSMENT:

Avoid drugs that are nephrotoxic, cytotoxic, or myelosuppressive—may increase risk of toxicity. Obtain specimens for viral diagnostic tests before starting therapy (therapy may begin before results are obtained). Check hematology reports for accurate baseline.

INTERVENTION/EVALUATION:

Monitor hematology reports for anemia and granulocytopenia; check for bleeding. Assess for headache, dizziness. Determine pattern of bowel activity. Evaluate skin for acne or rash. Be alert to development of opportunistic infections, e.g., fever, chills, cough, myalgia. Monitor I&O, renal and liver function tests. Check for insomnia.

PATIENT/FAMILY TEACHING:

Continue therapy for full length of treatment. Doses should be evenly spaced around the clock. Zidovudine does not cure AIDS or HIV disease, acts to reduce symptomatology and slowith arrest progress of disease. Do not take any medications without physician approval; even acetaminophen/aspirin may have serious consequence. Bleeding from gums, nose, or rectum may occur and should be reported to physician immediately. Blood counts are essential because of bleeding potential. Dental work should be done before therapy or after blood counts return to normal (often wks after therapy has stopped).

---

zileuton

zye-**lew**-ton
(Zyflo)

▶CLASSIFICATION

PHARMACOTHERAPEUTIC:
Leukotriene inhibitor. ***CLINI-CAL:*** Anti-asthma (see p. 64C)

ACTION/*THERAPEUTIC EFFECT*

Inhibits the enzyme responsible for producing inflammatory response. Prevents formation of leukotrienes (leukotrienes induce bronchoconstriction response, enhances vascular permeability, stimulates mucus secretion). *Prevents airway edema, smooth muscle contraction, and the inflamma-tory process, relieving signs and symptoms of bronchial asthma.*

PHARMACOKINETICS

	Onset	Peak	Duration
PO	—	2 hrs	—

Rapidly, completely absorbed following PO administration. Protein binding: 93%. Metabolized in the liver. Eliminated in feces. Not removed by dialysis. Half-life: 2.5 hrs.

USES

Prophylaxis and chronic treatment of asthma. Not for use in reversal of bronchospasm in acute asthma attacks, status asthmaticus, exercise-induced bronchospasm.

PRECAUTIONS

CONTRAINDICATIONS: Active liver disease, impaired liver function. ***CAUTIONS:*** History of hypersensitivity to zileuton, alcoholism.
▷***LIFESPAN CONSIDERATIONS:***
Pregnancy/Lactation: Unknown if distributed in breast milk. **Pregnancy Category C. Children:** Safety and efficacy not established in those <12 yrs of age. **Elderly:** No age-related precautions noted.

INTERACTIONS

DRUG: May increase concentration/toxicity of **cyclosporine, calcium channel blockers (i.e., nifedipine), theophylline.** Increases PT in those receiving **warfarin.** May increase effects of **beta-blockers (e.g., propranolol).** ***HERBAL:*** None known. ***FOOD:*** None known. ***LAB VALUES:*** May increase liver transaminase, SGOT (ALT).

AVAILABILITY (Rx)
TABLETS: 600 mg.

ADMINISTRATION/HANDLING
PO:
• Give without regard to food.

INDICATIONS/ROUTES/DOSAGE
Bronchial asthma:
PO: **Adults, elderly, children ≥12 yrs:** One 600 mg tablet 4 times/day. **Total daily dosage:** 2,400 mg.

SIDE EFFECTS

FREQUENT (25%): Headache. **OCCASIONAL** (3–8%): Dyspepsia, nausea, abdominal pain, asthenia (loss of strength), myalgia. **RARE** (1%): Conjunctivitis, constipation, dizziness, flatulence, insomnia.

ADVERSE REACTIONS/TOXIC EFFECTS

Liver dysfunction occurs rarely and may be manifested as right upper quadrant pain, nausea, fatigue, lethargy, pruritus, jaundice or flulike symptoms.

NURSING IMPLICATIONS

BASELINE ASSESSMENT:
Obtain baseline hepatic transaminase level, ALT (SGOT) before therapy begins. Monitor transaminase levels routinely thereafter. Monitor ALT (SGOT) moly for the first 3 mos and q2–3mos for the remainder of the first yr and periodically thereafter during long-term therapy.

INTERVENTION/EVALUATION:
Monitor rate, depth, rhythm, type of respirations, quality and rate of pulse. Assess lung sounds for rhonchi, wheezing, rales. Observe lips, fingernails for blue or dusky color in light-skinned pts, gray in dark-skinned pts. Monitor liver function test results.

PATIENT/FAMILY TEACHING:
Increase fluid intake (decreases lung secretion viscosity). Take as prescribed, even during symptom-free periods as well as during worsening asthma. Do not alter/stop other asthma medications. Drug is not for the treatment of acute asthma attacks.

ziprasidone

zip-**rah**-zih-doan
(Geodon)

▶CLASSIFICATION

PHARMACOTHERAPEUTIC: Piperazine derivative. **CLINICAL:** Antipsychotic (see p. 56C)

ACTION/*THERAPEUTIC EFFECT*

Antagonizes dopamine, serotonin, histamine, and alpha$_1$-adrenergic receptors; inhibits reuptake of serotonin and norepinephrine, *diminishing schizophrenic, antidepressant symptomology.*

PHARMACOKINETICS

Extensively metabolized in liver. Food increases bioavailability. Protein binding: 99%. Half-life: 7 hrs. Not removed by hemodialysis.

USES

Treatment of schizoprenia.

PRECAUTIONS

CONTRAINDICATIONS: Conditions associated with a risk of prolonging the QT interval. **CAUTIONS:**

Pts with bradycardia, hypokalemia, hypomagnesemia may be at greater risk for torsades de pointes.

▷*LIFESPAN CONSIDERATIONS:* **Pregnancy/Lactation:** Unknown if drug crosses placenta or is distributed in breast milk. **Pregnancy Category C**. **Children:** Safety and efficacy not established. **Elderly:** No age-related precautions noted.

INTERACTIONS

DRUG: **Carbamazepine** may decrease concentration. **Ketoconazole** may increase concentration. **Alcohol, CNS depressants** may increase CNS depression. *HERBAL:* None significant. *FOOD:* Food enhances bioavailability. *LAB VALUES:* May produce prolongation of QT interval.

AVAILABILITY (Rx)

CAPSULES: 20 mg, 40 mg, 80 mg.

ADMINISTRATION/HANDLING

PO:

• Give with food (increases bioavailability).

INDICATIONS/ROUTES/DOSAGE

Schizophrenia:

PO: **Adults, elderly:** Initially, 20 mg twice daily with food. Titrate at intervals of no less than 2 days. **Maximum:** 80 mg twice daily.

SIDE EFFECTS

FREQUENT (16–30%): Headache, somnolence, dizziness. *OCCASIONAL:* Rash, orthostatic hypotension, weight gain, restlessness, constipation, dyspepsia (heartburn, gastric upset).

ADVERSE REACTIONS/TOXIC EFFECTS

Prolongation of QT interval as seen in EKG may produce torsades de pointes (a form of ventricular tachycardia). Pts with bradycardia, hypokalemia, hypomagnesemia are at increased risk.

NURSING IMPLICATIONS

BASELINE ASSESSMENT:

Assess pt's behavior, appearance, emotional status, response to environment, speech pattern, thought content. An EKG should be administered to assess for QT prolongation before medication is instituted. Blood chemistry for magnesium, potassium should be obtained before therapy begins and routinely thereafter.

INTERVENTION/EVALUATION:

Assess for therapeutic response (greater interest in surroundings, improved self-care, increased ability to concentrate, relaxed facial expression). Monitor weight.

PATIENT/FAMILY TEACHING:

Do not drive or perform tasks requiring alert response until assured that drug does not cause impairment.

zoledronic acid

zole-eh-**dron**-ick
(Zometa)

▶**CLASSIFICATION**

PHARMACOTHERAPEUTIC: Biphosphonate. *CLINICAL:* Calcium regulator, bone resorption inhibitor

Z

ACTION/*THERAPEUTIC EFFECT*

Inhibits resorption of mineralized bone and cartilage; inhibits increased osteoclastic activity and skeletal calcium release induced by stimulatory factors released by tumors. *Increases urinary calcium and phosphorus excretion and decreases serum calcium and phosphorus levels.*

USES/*UNLABELED*

Treatment of hypercalcemia of malignancy (albumin-corrected serum calcium of >12 mg/dl).

PRECAUTIONS

CONTRAINDICATIONS: Hypersensitivity to other biphosphonates (etidronate, pamidronate, tiludronate, risedronate, alendronate). ***CAUTIONS:*** History of aspirin-sensitive asthma, renal impairment, hypoparathyroidism, risk of hypocalcemia.

INTERACTIONS

DRUG: **Calcium-containing medications, vitamin D** may antagonize effects in treatment of hypercalcemia. ***HERBAL:*** None significant. ***FOOD:*** None significant. ***LAB VALUES:*** May decrease calcium, phosphate, magnesium levels.

AVAILABILITY (Rx)

INJECTION: 4 mg/vial of lyophilized powder.

ADMINISTRATION/HANDLING

Note: Pt should be adequately rehydrated before administration of zoledronic acid.

IV 🔟

Storage:

• Store at room temperature. • If not used immediately, reconstituted solution should be refrigerated; time from reconstitution to end of administration should not exceed 24 hrs.

Reconstitution:

• Reconstitute 4 mg vial with 5 ml Sterile Water for Injection. Allow drug to dissolve before withdrawing. • Further dilute with 100 ml 0.9% NaCl or D_5W.

Rate of administration:

• Adequate hydration is essential in conjunction with zoledronic acid • Administer as an IV infusion over not less than 15 min (increases risk of deterioration in renal function).

IV INCOMPATIBILITY 🚫

Do not mix with any other medications.

INDICATIONS/ROUTES/DOSAGE

Note: Pt should be adequately rehydrated before administration.

Hypercalcemia:

IV INFUSION: **Adults, elderly:** 4 mg given as an IV infusion over no less than 15 min. Retreatment may be considered, but wait at least 7 days to allow for full response to initial dose.

SIDE EFFECTS

FREQUENT (26–44%): Fever, nausea, vomiting, constipation. ***OCCASIONAL*** (10–15%): Hypotension, anxiety, insomnia, flulike syndrome (fever, chills, bone pain, joint pain, muscle aches), nausea, vomiting, constipation. ***RARE:*** Conjunctivitis,

ADVERSE REACTIONS/TOXIC EFFECTS

Renal toxicity may occur if IV infusion is administered in less than 15 min.

NURSING IMPLICATIONS

BASELINE ASSESSMENT:

Establish baseline electrolytes.

INTERVENTION/EVALUATION:

Assess vertebral bone mass (document stabilization/improvement). Monitor serum calcium, phosphate, magnesium, serum creatinine. Assess for fever. Monitor food intake and stool frequency. Check I&O, BUN, creatinine in pts with impaired renal function.

zolmitriptan

zoll-mih-**trip**-tan
(Zomig)

▶CLASSIFICATION

PHARMACOTHERAPEUTIC:
Serotonin receptor agonist.
CLINICAL: Antimigraine (see p. 54C)

ACTION/THERAPEUTIC EFFECT

Binds selectively to vascular receptors producing a vasoconstrictive effect on cranial blood vessels, *producing relief of migraine headache.*

PHARMACOKINETICS

Rapidly but incompletely absorbed following PO administration. Protein binding: 15%. Undergoes first-pass metabolism in the liver to active metabolite. Eliminated primarily in the urine (60%) with lesser amount excreted in the feces (30%). Half-life: 3 hrs.

USES

Treatment of acute migraine attack with or without aura.

PRECAUTIONS

CONTRAINDICATIONS: Coronary artery disease, uncontrolled hypertension, ischemic heart disease (angina pectoris, history of MI, silent ischemia), Prinzmetal's angina, concurrent use (or within 24 hrs) of ergotamine-containing preparations, concurrent (or within 2 wks) of MAO therapy, hemiplegic or basilar migraine, within 24 hrs of another serotonin receptor agonist, Wolff-Parkinson-White syndrome, arrhythmias associated with cardiac conduction pathways disorders. **CAUTIONS:** Mild-to-moderate renal/hepatic impairment, pt profile suggesting cardiovascular risks, controlled hypertension, history of CVA.

▷**LIFESPAN CONSIDERATIONS:**
Pregnancy/Lactation: Unknown if distributed in breast milk. **Pregnancy Category C. Children:** Safety and efficacy not established in those <12 yrs of age. **Elderly:** No age-related precautions noted.

INTERACTIONS

DRUG: Ergotamine-containing drugs may produce vasospastic reaction. **MAO inhibitors** may dramatically increase plasma concentration of zolmitriptan. Combined use of **fluoxetine, fluvoxamine, paroxetine, sertraline** may produce weakness, hyperreflexia, incoordination. **Oral contraceptives** reduce zolmitriptan's clearance, volume of distribution. **HERBAL:** None known. **FOOD:** None known. **LAB VALUES:** None significant.

AVAILABILITY (Rx)

TABLETS: 2.5 mg, 5 mg. **ORAL DISINTEGRATING TABLETS:** 2.5 mg, 5 mg.

Z

ADMINISTRATION/HANDLING
PO:
• Give without regard to food.

INDICATIONS/ROUTES/DOSAGE
Migraine:
PO: **Adults >18 yrs, elderly, children:** Initially, 2.5 mg or less. If headache returns, may repeat dose in 2 hrs. **Maximum:** 10 mg/24 hrs.

SIDE EFFECTS
FREQUENT (6–8%): Dizziness, tingling, neck/throat/jaw pressure, somnolence. ***OCCASIONAL*** (3–5%): Sensation of warm/hot, weakness, chest pressure. ***RARE*** (1–2%): Sweating, myalgia, paresthesia.

ADVERSE REACTIONS/TOXIC EFFECTS
Cardiac events (ischemia, coronary artery vasospasm, MI), noncardiac vasospasm-related reactions (hemorrhage, stroke) occur rarely but particularly in those with hypertension, obesity, smokers, diabetes, strong family history of coronary artery disease, male > 40 yrs, postmenopausal women.

NURSING IMPLICATIONS

BASELINE ASSESSMENT:
Question regarding history of peripheral vascular disease or coronary artery disease, renal/hepatic impairment, use of MAO inhibitors. Question pt regarding onset, location, and duration of migraine and possible precipitating symptoms.

INTERVENTION/EVALUATION:
Monitor for evidence of dizziness. Monitor B/P, esp. in those with liver impairment. Assess for relief of migraine headache and migraine potential for photophobia, phonophobia (sound sensitivity, light sensitivity, nausea, vomiting).

PATIENT/FAMILY TEACHING:
Take a single dose as soon as symptoms of an actual migraine attack appear. Medication is intended to relieve migraine, not to prevent or reduce number of attacks. Lie down in quiet dark room for additional benefit after taking medication. Avoid tasks that require alertness, motor skills until response to drug is established. If heart throbbing, pain/tightness in chest or throat, or pain or weakness of extremities occurs, contact physician immediately.

zolpidem tartrate

zole-pih-dem
(<u>Ambien</u>)
Do not confuse with Amen.

▶CLASSIFICATION

PHARMACOTHERAPEUTIC:
Nonbenzodiazepine. ***CLINICAL:***
Sedative-hypnotic **(Schedule IV)**
(see p. 124C)

ACTION/*THERAPEUTIC EFFECT*
Enhances action of inhibitory neurotransmitter gamma-aminobutyric acid (GABA), *producing hypnotic effect due to CNS depression.* Interacts with GABA receptor, inducing sleep with fewer nightly awakenings, improvement of sleep quality.

PHARMACOKINETICS

Rapidly absorbed from GI tract. Protein binding: 92%. Metabolized in liver; excreted in urine. Not removed by hemodialysis. Half-life: 1.4–4.5 hrs (half-life increased with impaired liver function).

USES

Short-term treatment of insomnia. Reduces sleep-induction time, number of nocturnal awakenings; increases length of sleep, improvement of sleep quality.

PRECAUTIONS

CONTRAINDICATIONS: None significant. **CAUTIONS:** Impaired hepatic function.
▷**LIFESPAN CONSIDERATIONS:** **Pregnancy/Lactation:** Unknown if drug crosses placenta or is distributed in breast milk. **Pregnancy Category B. Children:** Safety and efficacy not established. **Elderly:** More likely to experience falls or confusion; decreased initial doses recommended. Age-related renal impairment may require dosage adjustment.

INTERACTIONS

DRUG: Potentiated effects when used with other **CNS depressants. HERBAL:** None known. **FOOD:** None known. **LAB VALUES:** None significant.

AVAILABILITY (Rx)

TABLETS: 5 mg, 10 mg.

ADMINISTRATION/HANDLING

PO:

• For faster sleep onset, do not give with or immediately after a meal.

INDICATIONS/ROUTES/DOSAGE

Hypnotic:

PO: Adults: 10 mg at bedtime. **Elderly, debilitated:** 5 mg at bedtime.

SIDE EFFECTS

OCCASIONAL (7%): Headache. **RARE** (<2%): Dizziness, nausea, diarrhea, muscle pain.

ADVERSE REACTIONS/TOXIC EFFECTS

Overdosage may produce severe ataxia (clumsiness, unsteadiness), slow heartbeat, diplopia, altered vision, severe drowsiness, nausea, vomiting, difficulty breathing, unconsciousness. Abrupt withdrawal of drug after long-term use may produce weakness, facial flushing, sweating, vomiting, tremor. Tolerance/dependence may occur with prolonged use of high doses.

NURSING IMPLICATIONS

BASELINE ASSESSMENT:

Assess B/P, pulse, respirations. Raise bed rails, provide call light. Provide environment conducive to sleep (back rub, quiet environment, low lighting).

INTERVENTION/EVALUATION:

Assess sleep pattern of pt. Evaluate for therapeutic response to insomnia: decrease in number of nocturnal awakenings, increase in length of sleep.

PATIENT/FAMILY TEACHING:

Do not abruptly withdraw medication following long-term use. Avoid alcohol, tasks that require alertness, motor skills until response to drug is established. Tolerance/dependence may

Z

---

occur with prolonged use of high doses.

zonisamide

zoe-**niss**-ah-mide
(Zonegran)

▶CLASSIFICATION

PHARMACOTHERAPEUTIC:
Succinimide. ***CLINICAL:*** Anti-convulsant (see p. 33C)

ACTION/*THERAPEUTIC EFFECT*

Mechanism of action is unknown. May produce anticonvulsant effects through action at sodium and calcium channels *stabilizing neuronal membranes and suppressing neuronal hypersynchronization.*

PHARMACOKINETICS

Well absorbed following PO administration. Extensively bound to erythrocytes. Protein binding: 40%. Primarily excreted in urine. Half-life: 63 hrs (plasma), 105 hrs (RBCs).

USES

Adjunctive therapy in the treatment of partial seizures in adults with epilepsy.

PRECAUTIONS

CONTRAINDICATIONS: Allergy to sulfonamides. ***CAUTIONS:*** Renal function impairment.

▷*LIFESPAN CONSIDERATIONS:*
Pregnancy/Lactation: Unknown if distributed in breast milk. **Pregnancy Category C. Children:** Safety and efficacy not established in those <16 yrs of age. **Elderly:** No age-related precautions

noted but lower dosages recommended.

INTERACTIONS

DRUG:* Carbamazepine, phenobarbital, phenytoin, valproic acid** may increase metabolism, decrease effect. ***HERBAL: None known. ***FOOD:*** None known. ***LAB VALUES:*** May increase serum creatinine, BUN.

AVAILABILITY (Rx)

CAPSULES: 100 mg.

ADMINISTRATION/HANDLING

PO:

• May take with or without food. • Swallow capsules whole. • Do not give to pts allergic to sulfonamides.

INDICATIONS/ROUTES/DOSAGE

Partial seizures:

***PO:* Adults, children >16 yrs:** Initially, 100 mg/day for 2 wks. May increase by 100 mg/day at intervals of at least 2 wks. **Maximum:** 400 mg/day.

SIDE EFFECTS

FREQUENT (9–17%): Somnolence, dizziness, anorexia, headache, agitation, irritability, nausea. ***OCCASIONAL*** (5–8%): Fatigue, ataxia, confusion, depression, memory/concentration impairment, insomnia, abdominal pain, double vision, diarrhea, speech difficulty. ***RARE*** (3–4%): Paresthesia, nystagmus (involuntary movement of eyeball), anxiety, rash, dyspepsia (heartburn, indigestion, epigastric distress), weight loss.

ADVERSE REACTIONS/TOXIC EFFECTS

Overdosage characterized by bradycardia, hypotension, respiratory depression, comatose state.

Leukopenia, anemia, thrombocytopenia occur rarely.

NURSING IMPLICATIONS

BASELINE ASSESSMENT:

Anticonvulsant: Review history of seizure disorder (intensity, frequency, duration, LOC). Initiate seizure precautions. Liver function tests, CBC, platelet count should be performed before therapy begins and periodically during therapy.

INTERVENTION/EVALUATION:

Observe frequently for recurrence of seizure activity. Assess for clinical improvement (decrease in intensity/frequency of seizures). Assist with ambulation if dizziness occurs.

PATIENT/FAMILY TEACHING:

Strict maintenance of drug therapy is essential for seizure control. Avoid tasks that require alertness, motor skills until response to drug is established. Avoid alcohol.

Z

Appendixes

A
P
P
E
N
D
I
X

1189

(POISON) ANTIDOTE CHART

Poison/Drug	Indications	Antidote	Dosage
acetaminophen	Treatment of acetaminophen overdose to protect against hepatotoxicity.	N-acetylcysteine (Mucomyst)	Dilute to 5% solution with carbonated beverage, fruit juice, or water and administer orally. **Loading:** 140 mg/kg for one dose. **Maintenance:** 70 mg/kg for 17 doses, starting 4 hrs after loading dose and given every 4 hrs.
atropine, anticholinergic agents, antihistamines, plants containing anticholinergic agents	Reverse toxic effects on the central nervous system (CNS) caused by drugs and plants capable of producing anticholinergic poisoning in clinical or toxic dosages (including tricyclic antidepressants).	physostigmine (Antilirium)	**Children:** 0.02 mg/kg IM or slow IV injection (0.5 mg/min). May repeat at 5–10 min intervals until therapeutic response or maximum dose of 2 mg is attained. **Adults:** Slow IV push (1 mg/min): 0.5–2 mg; may repeat if life-threatening signs, including arrhythmias, convulsions, coma, occur.
benzodiazepines	Complete or partial reversal of sedative effects of benzodiazepines when general anesthesia has been induced and/or maintained with benzodiazepines, when sedation has been produced with benzodiazepines for diagnostic and therapeutic procedures, management of benzodiazepine overdosage.	flumazenil (Romazicon)	**IV: Adults, elderly:** Initially, 0.2 mg (2 ml) over 30 seconds; may repeat after 30 seconds with 0.3 mg (3 ml) over 30 seconds if desired level of consciousness not achieved. Further doses of 0.5 mg (5 ml) over 30 seconds may be administered at 60-second intervals. **Maximum:** 3 mg (30 ml) total dose. **Note:** If resedation occurs, repeat dose at 20-min intervals. **Maximum:** 1 mg (given as 0.5 mg/min) at any one time, 3 mg in any 1 hr.

Poison/Drug	Indications	Antidote	Dosage
cyanide, nitroprusside	Begin treatment at first sign of toxicity if exposure is known or strongly suspected.	amyl nitrite, sodium nitrite, sodium thiosulfate (Cyanide Antidote Kit)	First, crush amyl nitrite pearls in gauze and allow patient to inhale for 15 seconds, then remove for 15 seconds. Use a fresh pearl every 3 min. Continue until injection of 10 ml of 3% (300 mg) sodium nitrite in adults. Inject over 2–5 min. Pediatric dose based on hemoglobin level; if normal hemoglobin assumed, then 0.15–0.33 ml/kg sodium nitrite up to 10 ml may be used. After sodium nitrite immediately inject 50 ml of 25% sodium thiosulfate (12.5 g), slow IV, over 10 min. Use 7 g/m^2 maximum of 12.5 g, in children.
digoxin	Treatment of potentially life-threatening digoxin intoxication.	digoxin-immune Fab (Digibind)	Dose in number of vials = steady-state digoxin level in mg/ml × patient weight in kg divided by 100. 4–6 vials adequate to treat 90–95% of patients with chronic digoxin toxicity. If ingested amount is unknown, give 10–20 vials (400–800 mg). Administer IV over 30 min through a 0.22 micron filter. A bolus injection can be given if cardiac arrest is imminent.
ethylene glycol	Ethylene glycol blood levels >20 mg/dl. Blood levels not readily available and suspected ingestion of toxic amounts. Any symptomatic patient with a history of ethylene glycol ingestion.	fomepizole (Antizol)	**Loading:** 15 mg/kg IV over 30 min followed by 10 mg/kg every 12 hrs for 4 doses, then 15 mg/kg every 12 hrs until ethylene glycol levels are below 20 mg/dl.
hydrofluoric acid (HF), fluoride salts	Calcium gluconate 2.5% gel for dermal exposure to HF <20%	calcium gluconate	Massage 2.5% gel into exposed area for 15 min, repeating as

(continued)

Poison/Drug	Indications	Antidote	Dosage
hydrofluoric acid (HF), fluoride salts *(continued)*	concentration. SC injections of calcium gluconate for dermal exposures of HF in >20% concentration or failure to respond to calcium gluconate gel. IV calcium gluconate 10% for serious systemic toxicity following dermal exposure, or ingestion of fluoride salts.		necessary for pain. Infiltrate each cm² of exposed area with 0.5 ml 10% calcium gluconate SC, using a 30-gauge needle. Give 0.1–0.2 ml/kg IV 10% calcium gluconate slowly up to 10 ml. Repeat dose if necessary.
iron	Acute iron intoxication. Chronic iron overload	deferoxamine (Desferal)	**Acute iron intoxication:** *IM:* 1 g, then 0.5 g q4h × 2 doses, then 0.5 g q4–12h. May give IV infusion 10–15 mg/kg/hr Do not exceed 6 g in 24 hrs. **Chronic iron overload:** *IM:* 0.5–1 g daily. *SubQ:* 1–2 g/day (20–40 mg/kg/day) over 8–24 hrs. **Children:** Maximum of 6 g/24 hrs or 2 g/dose.
miscellaneous medications	Treatment of drug overdose	ipecac	**Children (<1 yr):** 5–10 ml, then ½–1 glass water. **Children (>1 yr to 12 yrs):** 15 ml followed by 1–2 glasses water. **Adults:** 15–30 ml followed by 3–4 glasses water. **Note:** Repeat dose (15 ml) once in those older than 1 yr if vomiting does not occur within 20–30 min. Perform gastric lavage if vomiting does not occur within 30–45 min after second dose.
miscellaneous medication poisoning	Treatment of drug poisoning	charcoal, activated	**Adults:** 25–100 g (or 1 g/kg or approximately 10 times the amount of poison ingested) as a suspension (4–8 oz water). Multiple doses may be used in severe poisoning to prevent

Poison/Drug	Indications	Antidote	Dosage
miscellaneous medication poisoning *(continued)*			desorption from the charcoal; also increases GI clearance and rate of elimination of drugs that undergo an enteral recirculation pattern.
opiates, alpha2 agonists (e.g., clonidine)	1. Opiate overdose 2. Coma or respiratory depression of unknown origin.	naloxone (Narcan) nalmefene (Revex)	**Naloxone: Adults:** Give 0.4–2 mg IV bolus. Doses may be repeated every 2–5 min up to 10 mg if no response. **Children:** 0.01 mg/kg. May repeat with 0.1 mg/kg. **Note:** AAP recommends initial dose of 0.1 mg/kg for infants and children up to 5 yrs and weighing <20 kg. **Children >5 yrs or >20 kg:** Recommended initial dose 2 mg. **Nalmefene:** 0.5–1 mg IV every 2 min as needed to a total of 2 mg.
organophosphate insecticides	Synergistic adjunct to atropine therapy. Reverses nicotinic effects such as profound muscle weakness, respiratory depression, and muscle twitching. Organophosphate poisoning. Anticholinesterase drug overdose.	pralidoxim (2-PAM) (Protopam)	**Children:** *IV:* 25–50 mg/kg up to 1 g in 250 ml NaCl over 30 min. **Adults:** *IV:* 1–2 g in 100 ml NaCl over 15–30 min. If pulmonary edema present, may give as a 5% solution slow IV push over not less than 5 min. Dosage may be repeated in 1 hr followed by every 8 hrs if indicated.

CALCULATION OF DOSES

Frequently, dosages ordered do not correspond exactly to what is available and must therefore be calculated.

Ratio/proportions: Most important in setting up this calculation is that the units of measure are the same on both sides of the equation.

Problem: Pt A is to receive 65 mg of a medication only available in an 80 mg/2 ml vial. What volume (ml) needs to be administered to the pt?

STEP 1: Set up ratio.

$$\frac{80}{2\ ml} = \frac{65}{x(ml)}$$

STEP 2: Cross multiply.

$$(80\ mg)(x\ ml) = (65\ mg)(2\ ml)$$
$$80\ x = 130$$

STEP 3: Divide each side of equation by number with x.

$$\frac{80\ x}{80} = \frac{130}{80}$$

STEP 4: Volume to be administered for correct dose.

$$x = 130/80 \text{ or } 1.625\ ml$$

Calculations in micrograms/kilogram per minute: Frequently, medications given by IV infusion are ordered as micrograms/kilogram per minute.

Problem: 63-year-old pt (weight 165 lbs) is to receive Medication A at a rate of 8 micrograms/kilogram per minute (mcg/kg/min). Given a solution containing Medication A in a concentration of 500 mg/250 ml, at what rate (ml/hr) would you infuse this medication?

STEP 1: Convert to same units. In this problem, the dose is expressed in mcg/kg; therefore convert pt weight to kg (1 kg = 2.2 lbs) and drug concentration to mcg (1 mg = 1,000 mcg).

$$165\ lbs \times \frac{1\ kg}{2.2\ lbs} = \frac{165\ kg}{2.2} = 75\ kg$$

$$\frac{500\ mg}{250\ ml} \text{ or } \frac{2\ mg}{ml} \times \frac{1,000\ mcg}{1\ mg} = \frac{2,000\ mcg}{1\ ml} \text{ or } \frac{1\ ml}{2,000\ mcg}$$

STEP 2: Number of micrograms per minute (ml/min).

$$\frac{8 \text{ mcg}}{\text{kg}} \times 75 \text{ kg(pt wt)} = \frac{600 \text{ mcg}}{1 \text{ min}} \text{ or } \frac{1 \text{ min}}{600 \text{ mcg}}$$

STEP 3: Number of milliliters per minute (ml/min).

$$\frac{600 \text{ mcg}}{1 \text{ min}} \times \frac{1 \text{ ml}}{2,000 \text{ mcg}} = \frac{600(\text{ml})}{2,000(\text{min})} = \frac{0.3 \text{ ml}}{\text{min}}$$

STEP 4: Number of milliliters per hour (ml/hr).

$$\frac{0.3 \text{ ml}}{\text{min}} \times \frac{60 \text{ min}}{1 \text{hr}} = \frac{18 \text{ ml}}{\text{hr}}$$

STEP 5: If the number of drops per minute (gtts/min) were desired, and if the IV set delivered 60 drops per milliliter (gtts/ml) (varies with IV set, information provided by manufacturer), then:

$$\frac{0.3 \text{ ml}}{\text{min}} \times \frac{60 \text{ drops}}{\text{ml}} = \frac{18 \text{ drops}}{\text{min}}$$

CONTROLLED DRUGS (UNITED STATES)

Schedule I: Medications having no legal medical use. These substances may be used for research purposes with proper registration (e.g., heroin, LSD).

Schedule II: Medications having a legitimate medical use but are characterized by a very high abuse potential and/or potential for severe physical and psychic dependency. Emergency telephone orders for limited quantities of these drugs are authorized, but the prescriber must provide a written, signed prescription order (e.g., morphine, amphetamines).

Schedule III: Medications having significant abuse potential (less than Schedule II). Telephone orders are permitted (e.g., opiates in combination with other substances such as acetaminophen).

Schedule IV: Medications having a low abuse potential. Telephone orders are permitted (e.g., benzodiazepines, propoxyphene).

Schedule V: Medications having the lowest abuse potential of the controlled substances. Some Schedule V products may be available without a prescription (e.g., certain cough preparations containing limited amounts of an opiate).

DRUGS OF ABUSE

Name (Brand)	Class	Signs and Symptoms	Treatment
Acid (see LSD) Adam (see MDMA) Amphetamine (Adderall, Dexedrine)	Stimulant	Tachycardia, hypertension, diaphoresis, agitation, headache, seizures, dehydration, hypokalemia, lactic acidosis. Severe overdose: hyperthermia, dysrhythmia, shock, rhabdomyolysis, liver necrosis, acute renal failure.	Control agitation, reverse hyperthermia, support hemodynamic function. **Antidote:** No specific antidote.
Angel dust (see phencyclidine) Apache (see fentanyl) Barbiturates (Nembutal, Seconal)	Depressant	Hypotension, hypothermia, apnea, nystagmus, ataxia, hyporeflexia, somnolence, stupor, coma.	Airway management, decontamination, supportive care. **Antidote:** No specific antidote.
Barbs (see barbiturates) Benzodiazepines (Xanax, Valium, Librium, Halcion)	Depressant	Respiratory depression, hypothermia, hypotension, nystagmus, miosis, diplopia, bradycardia, nausea, vomiting, impaired speech and coordination, amnesia, ataxia, somnolence, confusion, depressed deep tendon reflexes.	**Antidote:** Flumazenil (Romazicon) is a specific antidote.
Black tar (see heroin) Horse (see heroin) Boomers (see LSD) Buttons (see mescaline) Cactus (see mescaline) Candy (see benzodiazepines) China girl (see fentanyl) China white (see heroin) Cocaine	Stimulant	Hypertension, tachycardia, mild hyperthermia, mydriasis, pallor, diaphoresis, psychosis, paranoid delusions, mania, agitation, seizures.	Control agitation, seizures, hyperthermia, support hemodynamic function. **Antidote:** No specific antidote.

(continued)

Name (Brand)	Class	Signs and Symptoms	Treatment
Codeine	Opioid	Miosis, respiratory depression, decreased mental status, hypotension, cardiac dysrhythmia, hypoxia, bronchoconstriction, constipation, decreased intestinal motility, ileus, lethargy, coma.	Airway management, hemodynamic support. **Antidote:** Naloxone, nalmefene.
Coke (see cocaine)			
Crank (see amphetamine)			
Crank (see heroin)			
Crystal (see amphetamine)			
Crystal meth (see methamphetamine)			
Cubes (see LSD)			
Downers (see benzodiapepines)			
Ecstasy (see MDMA)			
Fentanyl (Sublimaze)	Opioid	Miosis, respiratory depression, decreased mental status, hypotension, cardiac dysrhythmia, hypoxia, bronchoconstriction, constipation, decreased intestinal motility, ileus, lethargy, coma.	Airway management, hemodynamic support. **Antidote:** Naloxone, nalmefene.
Flunitrazepam (Rohypnol)	Depressant	Drowsiness, slurred speech, impaired judgment and motor skills, hypothermia, hypotension, bradycardia, diplopia, blurred vision, nystagmus, respiratory depression, nausea, constipation, depression, lethargy, headache, ataxia, coma, amnesia, incoordination, tremors, vertigo.	Supportive care, airway control. **Antidote:** Flumazenil (Romazicon)
Forget me pill (see flunitrazepam)			
Goodfellas (see fentanyl)			
Grass (see marijuana)			
Hashish (see marijuana)			
Heroin	Opioid	Miosis, coma, apnea, pulmonary edema, bradycardia, hypotension, pinpoint pupils, CNS depression, seizures.	Airway management. **Antidote:** Naloxone, nalmefene.
Ice (see amphetamine)			

Name (Brand)	Class	Signs and Symptoms	Treatment
LSD	Hallucinogen	Diaphoresis, mydriasis, dizziness, twitching, flushing, hyperreflexia, hypertension, psychosis, behavioral changes, emotional lability, euphoria or dysphoria, paranoia, vomiting, diarrhea, anorexia, restlessness, incoordination, tremors, ataxia.	Airway management, control activity associated with hallucinations, psychosis, panic reaction. **Antidote:** No specific antidote.
Ludes (see methaqualone)			
Magic mushroom (see psilocybin)			
Marijuana	Cannabinoid	Increasd appetite, reduced motility, constipation, urinary retention, seizures, euphoria, somnolence, heightened awareness, relaxation, altered time perception, short-term memory loss, poor concentration, mood alterations, disorientation, decreased strength, ataxia, slurred speech, respiratory depression, coma.	Airway management, supportive care. **Antidote:** No specific antidote.
MDMA (Methylenedioxymethamphetamine)	Stimulant	Euphoria, intimacy, closeness to others, loss of appetite, tachycardia, jaw tension, bruxism, sweating.	**Antidote:** No specific antidote.
Mescaline	Hallucinogen	Diaphoresis, mydriasis, dizziness, twitching, flushing, hyperreflexia, hypertension, psychosis, behavioral changes, emotional instability, euphoria or dysphoria, paranoia, vomiting, diarrhea, anorexia, restlessness, incoordination, tremors, ataxia.	Airway management, control activity associated with hallucinations, psychosis, panic reaction. **Antidote:** No specific antidote.
Meth (see methamphetamine)			
Methamphetamine (Desoxyn)	Stimulant	Hypertension, hyperthermia, hyperpyrexia, agitation, hyperactivity, fasciculation, seizures, coma, tachycardia, dysrhythmias, pale skin, diaphoresis, restlessness, talkativeness, insomnia, headache, coma, delusions, paranoia, aggressive behavior, visual, tactile, or auditory hallucinations.	Airway control, hyperthermia, seizures, dysrhythmias. **Antidote:** No specific antidote.

(continued)

Name (Brand)	Class	Signs and Symptoms	Treatment
Methaqualone (Quaalude)	Depressant	Slurred speech, impaired judgment and motor skills, hypothermia, hypotension, bradycardia, diplopia, blurred vision, nystagmus, mydriasis, respiratory depression, depression, lethargy, headache, ataxia, coma, amnesia, incoordination, hypertonicity, myoclonus, tremors, vertigo.	Airway management, supportive care. **Antidote:** No specific antidote.
Methylphenidate (Ritalin)	Stimulant	Agitation, hypertension, tachycardia, hyperthermia, mydriasis, dry mouth, nausea, vomiting, anorexia, abdominal pain, agitation, hyperactivity, insomnia, euphoria, dizziness, paranoid ideation, social withdrawal, delirium, hallucinations, psychosis, tremors, seizures.	Control agitation, hyperthermia, seizures, support hemodynamic function. **Antidote:** No specific antidote.
Miss Emma (see morphine)			
Mister blue (see morphine)			
Morphine (MS-Contin, Roxanol)	Opioid	Miosis, respiratory depression, decreased mental status, hypotension, cardiac dysrhythmia, hypoxia, bronchoconstriction, constipation, decreased intestinal motility, ileus, lethargy, coma.	Airway management, hemodynamic support. **Antidote:** Naloxone, nalmefene.
Oxy (see oxycodone)			
Oxycodone (Oxycontin)	Opioid	Miosis, respiratory depression, decreased mental status, hypotension, cardiac dysrhythmia, hypoxia, bronchoconstriciton, constipation, decreased intestinal motility, ileus, lethargy, coma.	Airway management, hemodynamic support. **Antidote:** Naloxone, nalmefene.
Oxycotton (see oxycodone)			
Peace pill (see phencyclidine)			
Phencyclidine (PCP)	Hallucinogen	Nystagmus, hypertension, tachycardia, agitation, hallucinations, violent behavior, impaired judgment, delusions, psychosis.	Support blood pressure, manage airway, control agitation. **Antidote:** No specific antidote.
Phennies (see barbiturates)			

Name (Brand)	Class	Signs and Symptoms	Treatment
Pot (see marijuana)			
Propoxyphene (Darvon)	Depressant	Respiratory depression, seizures, cardiac toxicity, miosis, dysrhythmias, nausea, vomiting, anorexia, abdominal pain, constipation, drowsiness, coma, confusion, hallucinations.	Maintain airway, seizures, cardiac toxicity. **Antidote:** Naloxone.
Psilocybin	Hallucinogen	Diaphoresis, mydriasis, dizziness, twitching, flushing, hyperreflexia, hypertension, psychosis, behavioral changes, emotional lability, euphoria or dysphoria, paranoia, vomiting, diarrhea, anorexia, restlessness, incoordination, tremors, ataxia.	Manage airway, control activity associated with hallucinations, psychosis, panic reaction. **Antidote:** No specific antidote.
Purple passion (see psilocybin)			
Quay (see methaqualone)			
Reefer (see marijuana)			
Rock (see cocaine)			
Rocket fuel (see phencyclidine)			
Roofies (see flunitrazepam)			
Rope (see flunitrazepam)			
Rophies (see flunitrazepam)			
Schoolboy (see codeine)			
Snow (see cocaine)			
Speed (see amphetamine)			
STP (see MDMA)			
Tranks (see benzodiazepines)			
Uppers (see amphetamine)			
White girl (see cocaine)			
Yellow jackets (see barbiturates)			
Yellow sunshine (see LSD)			

FDA PREGNANCY CATEGORIES

Note: Medications should be used during pregnancy only if clearly needed.

A: Adequate and well-controlled studies have failed to show a risk to the fetus in the first trimester of pregnancy (also, no evidence of risk has been seen in later trimesters).

B: Animal reproduction studies have failed to show a risk to the fetus, and there are no adequate/well-controlled studies in pregnant women.

C: Animal reproduction studies have shown an adverse effect on the fetus, and there are no adequate/well-controlled studies in humans. However, the benefits may warrant use of the drug in pregnant women despite potential risks.

D: There is positive evidence of human fetal risk based on data from investigational or marketing experience or from studies in humans, but the potential benefits may warrant use of the drug despite potential risks (e.g., use in life-threatening situations in which other medications cannot be used or are ineffective).

X: Animal or human studies have shown fetal abnormalities, and/or there is evidence of human fetal risk based on adverse reaction data from investigational or marketing experience where the risks in using the medication clearly outweigh potential benefits.

HERBAL THERAPIES/INTERACTIONS

The use of herbal therapies is on the increase in the United States. In 1990, an estimated 1 in 3 Americans used at least one form of alternative medicine (of which herbal therapy is part). By 1997, over $12 billion was spent in the United States for vitamins and minerals, herbals, sports supplements or specialty supplements (e.g., glucosamine).

Because of the rise in the use of herbal therapy in the United States, the following is presented to provide some basic information on some of the more popular herbs. Please note this is not an all-inclusive list, which is beyond the scope of this handbook.

Name	Purported Benefit	Interactions	Precautions
Aloe	**Topical:** Promotes burn/wound healing, treatment of cold sores. **Oral:** Laxative, cathartic.	**Topical:** None **Oral:** May increase risk of side effects with cardiac glycosides, antiarrhythmics, diuretics.	**Topical:** None **Oral:** Abdominal pain, diarrhea, reduced potassium levels.
Bilberry	**Topical:** Mild inflammation of mouth/throat. **Oral:** Acute diarrhea, increased visual acuity, angina, atherosclerosis.	May require adjustment of antidiabetic drugs (reduces glucose effect).	May decrease glucose, triglycerides.
Black cohosh*	Manage symptoms of menopause, hypercholesterolemia, peripheral arterial disease, anti-inflammatory and sedative effects.	May further reduce lipids and/or blood pressure when combined with prescription medications.	Side effects: nausea, dizziness, visual changes, migraine.
Capsicum	**Topical:** Pain of shingles; postherpetic, trigeminal, diabetic neuralgias; HIV- associated peripheral neuropathy.	None	Burning, urticaria, irritation to eyes, mucus membranes.
Cat's claw	**Oral:** Diverticulitis, ulcers, hemorrhoids, colitis, gastritis.	Antihypertensives may increase effect.	Diarrhea, hypotension (get up slowly to avoid dizziness).
Catnip	**Topical:** Arthritis, hemorrhoids. **Oral:** Insomnia, migraine, cold, flu, hives, indigestion, cramping, flatulence.	May be additive with other CNS depressants.	Headache, malaise, vomiting (large doses).
Chamomile*	Antispasmodic, sedative, anti-inflammatory, astringent, antibacterial	May increase bleeding with anticoagulants. May increase sedative effect	Anaphylactic reaction if allergic; avoid use if allergic to chrysanthemums, ragweed, and/or asters; delays

*See full herb entry in the A to Z section.   *(continued)*

Name	Purported Benefit	Interactions	Precautions
Chamomile* *(continued)*		with benzodi-azepines.	absorption of medications.
Chastberry	**Oral:** Control of menstrual irregularities, painful menstruation.	May interfere with oral contraceptives, hormone replacement therapy, dopamine antagonists (e.g., antipsychotics).	GI disturbances, rash, itching, headache, increased menstrual flow.
Co-Enzyme Q-10	**Oral:** CHF, angina, diabetes, hypertension; reduces symptoms of chronic fatigue; stimulates immune system in those with AIDS.	May decrease effect of warfarin. Statins may decrease effect.	Reduced appetite, gastritis, nausea, diarrhea.
Cranberry	**Oral:** Prevention, treatment of urinary tract infections; urinary deodorizer.	May increase absorption of vitamin B_{12} in those taking proton pump inhibitors (e.g., Prevacid).	Large doses may cause diarrhea.
DHEA*	Slows aging, boosts energy, controls weight.	None	Side effects: May increase risk of breast/prostate cancer. Women may develop acne, hair growth on face/body.
Dong quai*	Uterine stimulant, antiinflammatory, vasodilator, CNS stimulant, immunosuppressant, analgesic, antipyretic.	May increase effects of warfarin.	Diarrhea, photosensitivity, skin cancer; avoid in pregnancy/lactation; essential oil may contain the carcinogen safrole.
Echinacea*	Prevents/treats colds, flu, bacterial and fungal infections. An immune system stimulator. Aid to wound healing.	May interfere with immunosuppressive therapy.	Not to be used with weakened immune system (e.g., HIV/AIDS, tuberculosis, multiple sclerosis). Habitual or continued use may cause immune system suppression (should only be taken for 2–3 mos or alternating schedule of q2–3wks).
Evening primrose oil	**Oral:** PMS, symptoms of menopause (e.g., hot flashes), psoriasis, rheumatoid arthritis.	Antipsychotics may increase risk of seizures.	Indigestion, nausea, headache. Large doses may cause diarrhea, abdominal pain.
Feverfew*	Relieves migraine. Treatment of fever, headache, menstrual irregularities.	May increase bleeding time with aspirin, dipyridamole, warfarin.	Side effects: headache, mouth ulcers. Should be avoided in pregnancy (stimulates menstruation), nursing mother, infants <2 yrs of age.

*See full herb entry in the A to Z section.

Name	Purported Benefit	Interactions	Precautions
Fish oils	**Oral:** Hypertension, hyperlipidemia, coronary artery disease, rheumatoid arthritis, psoriasis.	May increase risk of bleeding with antiplatelets, anticoagulants. Additive effect with antihypertensives.	Belching, heartburn, nosebleeds. Large doses may cause nausea, diarrhea.
Garlic*	Reduces cholesterol, LDL, triglycerides, increases HDL, lowers B/P, inhibits platelet aggregation. May also possess antibacterial, antiviral, antithrombotic activity.	May increase bleeding time with aspirin, dipyridamole, warfarin.	Side effects: taste, offensive odor. Large doses may cause heartburn, flatulence, other GI distress.
Ginger*	Relieves nausea, effective treatment for motion sickness, anti-inflammatory for arthritis, nausea/voming associated with pregnancy. Possesses ability to lower platelet aggregation; antithrombotic properties.	None	Avoid during pregnancy when bleeding is a concern. Large overdose could potentially depress the CNS, cause cardiac arrhythmias.
Ginko*	Boosts mental prowess by improving memory. Sharpens concentration, pt may think more clearly. Overcomes sexual dysfunction occurring with SSRI antidepressants. May be able to slow progress of Alzheimer's, improve intermittent claudication.	May increase bleeding time with aspirin, dipyridamole, warfarin.	Avoid in pt taking blood thinners or those hypersensitive to poison ivy, cashews, mangos. Side effects: GI disturbances, headache, dizziness, vertigo.
Ginseng*	Boosts energy, sexual stamina; decreases stress, effects of aging.	May affect platelet adhesiveness/blood coagulation. Use caution with anticoagulants. May increase hypoglycemia with insulin.	Avoid in pts receiving anticoagulants, medications that increase B/P. Side effects: breast tenderness, nervousness, headache, increased B/P, abnormal vaginal bleeding.
Glucosamine and chondroitin*	Osteoarthritis	No known interactions but monitor anticoagulant effects.	None known.
Goldenseal	**Topical:** Eczema, itching, acne. **Oral:** UTI, hemorrhoids, gastritis, colitis, mucosal inflammation.	May interfere with antacids, sucralfate, H$_2$ antagonists, proton pump inhibitors.	Constipation, hallucinations. Large doses may cause nausea, vomiting, diarrhea, CNS stimulation, respiratory failure.

*See full herb entry in the A to Z section.   (continued)

Name	Purported Benefit	Interactions	Precautions
Goldenrod	**Oral:** Diuretic, anti-inflammatory, antispasmodic. Prevents urinary tract inflammation, urinary calculi, kidney stones.	May interfere with diuretics.	Allergic reactions.
Grape seed extract	Improves circulation, decreases tissue injury, hemorrhoids. Used as antioxidant to treat hypoxia from atherosclerosis, inflammation.	None	None reported.
Green tea	**Oral:** Improves cognition function, treats nausea, vomiting, headache, weight loss.	May increase risk of bleeding with antiplatelets.	GI upset, constipation.
Hawthorn	Cardiovascular conditions (e.g., atherosclerosis), GI conditions (diarrhea, indigestion, abdominal pain), sleep disorders.	Cardiovascular drugs, digoxin may potentiate or interfere; additive effect with CNS depressants.	Nausea, GI complaints, headache, dizziness, insomnia, agitation.
Kava kava*	Reduces stress, muscle relaxant, relieves anxiety, induces sleep and counters fatigue.	Increases CNS depression with alcohol, sedatives.	Side effects: GI disturbances, temporary discoloration of skin, hair, nails. Do not use in pregnancy, lactation, endogenous depression. Large doses may cause muscle weakness. Chronic use may cause scaly skin resembling psoriasis (reversible). Causes pupil dilation affecting vision (avoid driving, operating heavy machinery). Store in cool, dry place (excess heat/light will alter contents).
Licorice	**Oral:** Inflammation of upper respiratory tract, mucus membranes, ulcers, expectorant.	May decrease effect of antihypertensives. Thiazides may increase potassium loss.	Large doses may cause pseudoaldosteronism (hypertension, headache, lethargy, edema).
Ma huang* (Ephedra)	Controls weight, boosts energy. Treatment of colds, allergies, appetite suppressant.	Increases toxicity with beta blockers, MAOIs, caffeine, theophylline, decongestants, St. John's wort.	Linked to high B/P, headache, seizures. Can cause confusion, insomnia, dizziness, sweating, fever, nausea, vomiting.

*See full herb entry in the A to Z section.

Name	Purported Benefit	Interactions	Precautions
Melatonin*	Aids sleep, prevents jet lag.	Decreases effects of antidepressants.	Side effects: headache, confusion, fatigue. Does not lengthen total sleep time.
Milk thistle	Hepatoprotective, antioxidant, liver disorders, including poisoning (e.g., mushroom), cirrhosis, hepatitis.	None	Mild allergic reactions, laxative effect.
Omega 6 fatty acid	**Oral:** Coronary artery disease, decreases total cholesterol LDL, increases HDL.	None	Increases triglycerides.
SAMe	**Oral:** Depression, heart disease, osteoarthritis, Alzheimer's, Parkinson's; slows aging process.	May increase adverse effects with antidepressants.	Nausea, vomiting, diarrhea, flatulence; headache.
St. John's wort*	Relieves mild to moderate depression, heals wounds.	May cause "serotonin syndrome" (confusion, agitation, chills, fever, sweating, diarrhea, nausea, muscle spasms or twitching), hyperreflexia, tremor with antidepressants, yohimbe.	Side effects: dizziness, dry mouth, increased sensitivity to sunlight. Report symptoms of "serotonin syndrome."
Saw palmetto*	Eases symptoms of large prostate (frequency, dysuria, nocturia).	None	Side effects: upset stomach, headache, erectile dysfunction. Does not reduce size of enlarged prostate. Obtain baseline PSA levels before initiating. Large doses can cause diarrhea.
Shark cartilage	**Oral:** Cancer, arthritis, psoriasis, wound healing.	None	Nausea, vomiting, constipation, dyspepsia, bad taste in mouth.
Soy	Menopausal symptoms; prevents osteoporosis and cardiovascular disease in postmenopausal women; hypertension, hyperlipidemia.	May decrease effects of estrogen replacement therapy.	Constipation, bloating, nausea, allergic reaction.
Valerian*	Aids sleep, relieves restlessness and nervousness. Does not decrease night awakenings.	None	Side effects: heart palpitations, upset stomach, headache, excitability, uneasiness. May cause increased morning drowsiness.

*See full herb entry in the A to Z section.

(continued)

Name	Purported Benefit	Interactions	Precautions
Yohimbe*	Male aphrodisiac. Used to treat impotence, erectile dysfunction, orthostatic hypotension.	Decreases effects of antidepressants, antihypertensives, St. John's wort.	Large doses linked to weakness, paralysis.

*See full herb entry in the A to Z section.

NORMAL LABORATORY VALUES

HEMATOLOGY/COAGULATION

Test	Specimen	Normal Range
Activated partial thromboplastin time (APTT)	Whole blood	25–35 secs
Erythrocyte count (RBC count)	Whole blood	M: 4.3–5.7 million cells/mm^3 F: 3.8–5.1 million cells/mm^3
Hematocrit (HCT, Hct)	Whole blood	M: 39–49% F: 35–45%
Hemoglobin (Hb, Hgb)	Whole blood	M: 13.5–17.5 g/dl F: 12.0–16.0 g/dl
Leucocyte count (WBC count)	Whole blood	4.5–11.0 thousand cells/mm^3
Leucocyte differential count	Whole blood	
Basophils		0–0.75%
Eosinophils		1–3%
Lymphocytes		23–33%
Monocytes		3–7%
Neutrophils-bands		3–5%
Neutrophils-segmented		54–62%
Mean corpuscular hemoglobin (MCH)	Whole blood	26–34 pg/cell
Mean corpuscular hemoglobin concentration (MCHC)	Whole blood	31–37% Hb/cell
Mean corpuscular volume (MCV)	Whole blood	80–100 fL
Partial thromboplastin time (PTT)	Whole blood	60–85 secs
Platelet count (thrombocyte count)	Whole blood	150–450 thousand/mm^3
Prothrombin time (PT)	Whole blood	11–13.5 secs
RBC count (see Erythrocyte count)		

SERUM/URINE VALUES

Test	Specimen	Normal Range
Alanine aminotransferase (ALT, SGPT)	Serum	0–55 units/L
Albumin	Serum	3.5–5 g/dl
Alkaline phosphatase	Serum	M: 53–128 units/L F: 42–98 units/L
Anion gap	Plasma or serum	5–14 mEq/L
Aspartate aminotransferase (AST, SGOT)	Serum	0–50 units/L
Bilirubin (conjugated direct)	Serum	0–0.4 mg/dl
Bilirubin (total)	Serum	0.2–1.2 mg/dl
Calcium (total)	Serum	8.4–10.2 mg/dl
Carbon dioxide (CO_2) total	Plasma or serum	20–34 mEq/L

Test	Specimen	Normal Range
Chloride	Plasma or serum	96–112 mEq/L
Cholesterol (total)	Plasma or serum	<200 mg/dl
C-Reactive protein	Serum	68–8200 ng/ml
Creatine kinase (CK)	Serum	M: 38–174 units/L
		F: 26–140 units/L
Creatine kinase isoenzymes	Serum	Fraction of total: <0.04–0.06
Creatinine	Plasma or serum	M: 0.7–1.3 mg/dl
		F: 0.6–1.1 mg/dl
Creatinine clearance	Plasma or serum and urine	M: 90–139 ml/min/1.73m2
		F: 80–125 ml/min/1.73m2
Free thyroxine index (FTI)	Serum	1.1–4.8
Glucose	Serum	Adults: 70–105 mg/dl
		>60 yrs: 80–115 mg/dl
Hemoglobin A_{1c}	Whole blood	5.6–7.5% of total Hgb
Homovanillic acid (HVA)	Urine, 24 hr	1.4–8.8 mg/day
17–Hydroxycorticosteroids (17–OHCS)	Urine, 24 hr	M: 3–10 mg/day
		F: 2–8 mg/day
Iron	Serum	M: 65–175 mcg/dl
		F: 50–170 mcg/dl
Iron binding capacity, total (TIBC)	Serum	250–450 mcg/dl
Lactate dehydrogenase (LDH)	Serum	0–250 units/L
Magnesium	Serum	1.3–2.3 mg/dl
Oxygen (PO_2)	Whole blood, arterial	83–100 mm Hg
Oxygen saturation	Whole blood, arterial	95–98%
pH	Whole blood, arterial	7.35–7.45
Phosphorus, inorganic	Serum	2.7–4.5 mg/dl
Potassium	Serum	3.5–5.1 mEq/L
Protein (total)	Serum	6–8.5 g/dl
Sodium	Plasma or serum	136–146 mEq/L
Specific gravity	Urine	1.002–1.030
Thyrotropin (hTSH)	Plasma or serum	2–10 mcgU/ml
Thyroxine (T_4) total	Serum	5–12 mcg/dl
Triglycerides (TG)	Serum, after 12 hr fast	20–190 mg/dl
Triiodothyronine resin uptake test (T_3RU)	Serum	22–37%
Urea nitrogen	Plasma or serum	7–25 mg/dl
Urea nitrogen/creatinine ratio	Serum	12/1–20/1
Uric acid	Serum	M: 3.5–7.2 mg/dl
		F: 2.6–6 mg/dl
Vanillylmandelic acid (VMA)	Urine, 24 hr	2–7 mg/day

SIGNS AND SYMPTOMS
OF ELECTROLYTE IMBALANCE

HYPOGLYCEMIA (excessive insulin):

Tremulousness, cold/clammy skin, mental confusion, rapid/shallow respirations, unusual fatigue, hunger, drowsiness, anxiety, headache, muscular incoordination, paresthesia of tongue/mouth/lips, hallucination, increased pulse/blood pressure, tachycardia, seizures, coma.

HYPERGLYCEMIA (insufficient insulin):

Hot/flushed/dry skin, fruity breath odor, excessive urination (polyuria), excessive thirst (polydipsia), acute fatigue, air hunger, deep/labored respirations, mental changes, restlessness, nausea, polyphagia (excessive appetite).

HYPOKALEMIA (potassium level <3.5 mEq/L):

Weakness/paresthesia of extremities, muscle cramps, nausea, vomiting, diarrhea, hypoactive bowel sounds, absent bowel sounds (paralytic ileus), abdominal distention, weak/irregular pulse, postural hypotension, difficulty breathing, disorientation, irritability.

HYPERKALEMIA (potassium level >5.0 mEq/L):

Diarrhea, muscle weakness, heaviness of legs, paresthesia of tongue/hands/feet, slow/irregular pulse, decreased blood pressure, abdominal cramps, oliguria/anuria, respiratory difficulty, cardiac abnormalities.

HYPONATREMIA (sodium level <130 mEq/l):

Abdominal cramping, nausea, vomiting, diarrhea, cold/clammy skin, poor skin turgor, tremulousness, muscle weakness, leg cramps, increased pulse rate, irritability, apprehension, hypotension, headache.

HYPERNATREMIA (sodium level >150 MeQ/L):

Hot/flushed/dry skin, dry mucous membranes, fever, extreme thirst, dry/rough/red tongue, edema, restlessness, postural hypotension, oliguria.

HYPOCALCEMIA (calcium level <8.4 mg/dl):

Circumoral/peripheral numbness and tingling, muscle twitching; Chevostek's sign (facial muscle spasm; test by tapping of facial nerve anterior to earlobe, just below zygomatic arch), muscle cramping, Trousseau's sign (carpopedal spasm), seizures, arrhythmias.

HYPERCALCEMIA (calcium level >10.2 mg/dl):

Muscle hypotonicity, incoordination, anorexia, constipation, confusion, impaired memory, slurred speech, lethargy, acute psychotic behavior, deep bone pain, flank pain.

TECHNIQUES OF MEDICATION ADMINISTRATION

OPHTHALMIC:

Eye Drops:

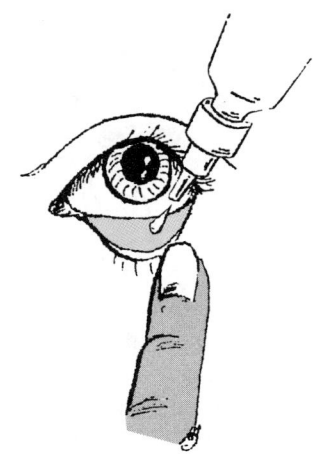

1. Wash hands.
2. Instruct patient to lie down or tilt head backward and look up.
3. Gently pull lower eyelid down until a pocket (pouch) is formed between eye and lower lid (conjunctival sac).
4. Hold dropper above pocket. Without touching tip of eye dropper to eyelid or conjunctival sac, place prescribed number of drops into the center pocket *(placing drops directly onto eye may cause a sudden squeezing of eyelid, with subsequent loss of solution)*. Continue to hold the eyelid for a moment after the drops are applied *(allows medication to distribute along entire conjunctival sac)*.
5. Instruct patient to close eyes gently so medication will not be squeezed out of sac.
6. Apply gentle finger pressure to the lacrimal sac at the inner canthus (bridge of the nose, inside corner of the eye) for 1-2 min *(promotes absorption, minimizes drainage into nose and throat, lessens risk of systemic absorption)*.
7. Remove excess solution around eye with a tissue.
8. Wash hands immediately to remove medication on hands. Never rinse eye dropper.

Eye Ointment:

1. Wash hands.
2. Instruct patient to lie down or tilt head backward and look up.
3. Gently pull lower eyelid down until a pocket (pouch) is formed between eye and lower lid (conjunctival sac).

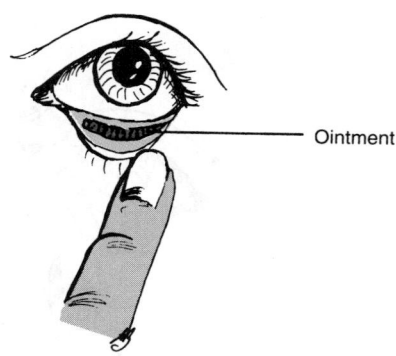

Ointment

4. Hold applicator tube above pocket. Without touching the applicator tip to eyelid or conjunctival sac, place prescribed amount of ointment (1/4–1/2 inch) into the center pocket (*placing ointment directly onto eye may cause discomfort*).
5. Instruct patient to close eye for 1–2 min, rolling eyeball in all directions (*increases contact area of drug to eye*).
6. Inform patient of temporary blurring of vision. If possible, apply ointment just before bedtime.
7. Wash hands immediately to remove medication on hands. Never rinse tube applicator.

OTIC:

1. Ear drops should be at body temperature (wrap hand around bottle to warm contents). *Body temperature instillation prevents startling of patient.*
2. Instruct patient to lie down with head turned so affected ear is upright (*allows medication to drip into ear*).
3. Instill prescribed number of drops toward the canal wall, not directly on eardrum.
4. To promote correct placement of ear drops, pull the auricle down and posterior in children (A) and pull the auricle up and posterior in adults (B).

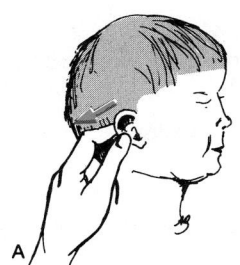
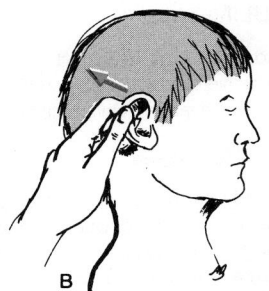

NASAL:

Nose Drops and Sprays:

1. Instruct patient to blow nose to clear nasal passages as much as possible.
2. Tilt head slightly forward if instilling nasal spray, slightly backward if instilling nasal drops.
3. Insert spray tip into 1 nostril, pointing toward inflamed nasal passages, away from nasal septum.
4. Spray or drop medication into 1 nostril while holding other nostril closed and concurrently inspire through nose to permit medication as high into nasal passages as possible.
5. Discard unused nasal solution after 3 mos.

INHALATION:

Aerosol (Multidose Inhalers):

1. Shake container well before each use.
2. Exhale slowly and as completely as possible through the mouth.
3. Place mouthpiece fully into mouth, holding inhaler upright, and close lips fully around mouthpiece.
4. Inhale deeply and slowly through the mouth while depressing the top of the canister with the middle finger.
5. Hold breath as long as possible before exhaling slowly and gently.
6. When two puffs are prescribed, wait 2 min and shake container again before inhaling a second puff *(allows for deeper bronchial penetration)*.
7. Rinse mouth with water immediately after inhalation *(prevents mouth and throat dryness)*.

SUBLINGUAL:

1. Administer while seated.
2. Dissolve sublingual tablet under tongue (do not chew or swallow tablet).
3. Do not swallow saliva until tablet is dissolved.

TOPICAL:

1. Gently cleanse area prior to application.
2. Use occlusive dressings only as ordered.
3. Without touching applicator tip to skin, apply sparingly; gently rub into area thoroughly unless ordered otherwise.
4. When using aerosol, spray area for 3 secs from 15 cm distance; avoid inhalation.

TRANSDERMAL:

1. Apply transdermal patch to clean, dry, hairless skin on upper arm or body (not below knee or elbow).
2. Rotate sites *(prevents skin irritation)*.
3. Do not trim patch to adjust dose.

RECTAL:

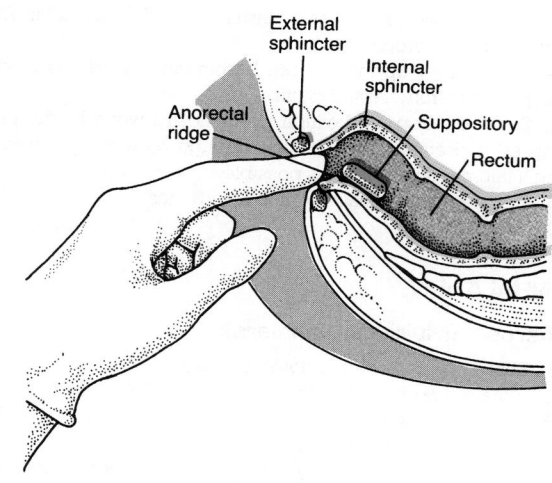

1. Instruct patient to lie in left lateral Sims' position.
2. Moisten suppository with cold water or water-soluble lubricant.
3. Instruct patient to slowly exhale *(relaxes anal sphincter)* while inserting suppository well up into rectum.
4. Inform patient as to length of time (20-30 min) before desire for defecation occurs or <60 min for systemic absorption to occur, depending on purpose for suppository.

SubQ:

1. Use 25–27 gauge, ½–⅝ inch needle; 1–3 ml. Angle of insertion depends on body size: 90° if patient is obese. If patient is very thin, gather the skin at the area of needle insertion and administer also at a 90° angle. A 45° angle may be used in a patient with average weight.
2. Cleanse area to be injected with circular motion.
3. Avoid areas of bony prominence, major nerves, blood vessels.
4. Aspirate syringe before injecting *(to avoid intra-arterial administration)*, except insulin, heparin.
5. Inject slowly; remove needle quickly.

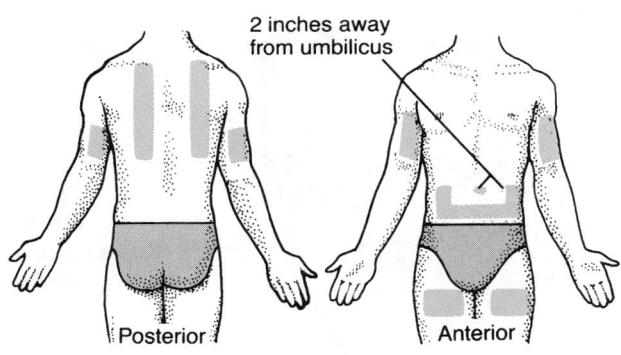

SubQ injection sites

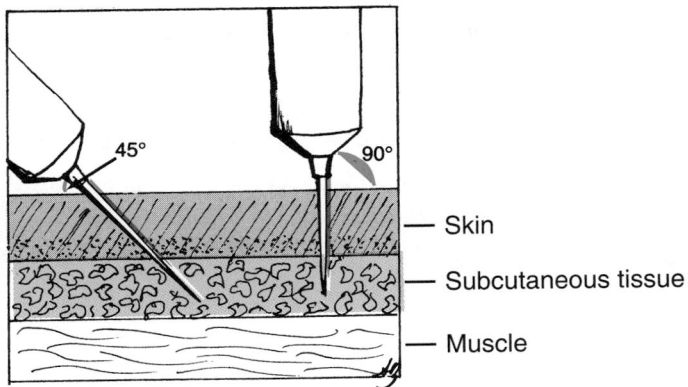

IM:

Injection Sites:

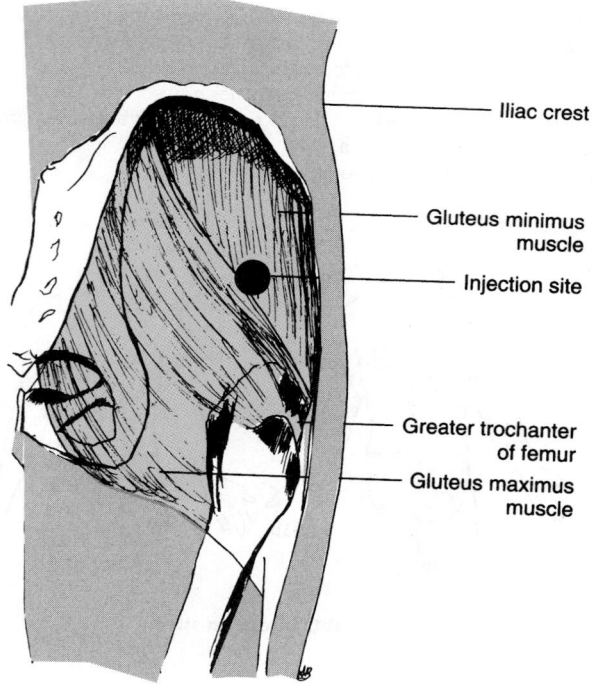

- Iliac crest
- Gluteus minimus muscle
- Injection site
- Greater trochanter of femur
- Gluteus maximus muscle

Dorsogluteal (upper outer quadrant)

1. Use this site if volume to be injected is 1–3 ml. Use 18–23 gauge, 1.25–3 inch needle. Needle should be long enough to reach the middle of the muscle.
2. Do not use this site in children <2 yrs old or in those who are emaciated. Patient should be in prone position.
3. Using 90° angle, flatten the skin area using the middle and index finger and inject between them.

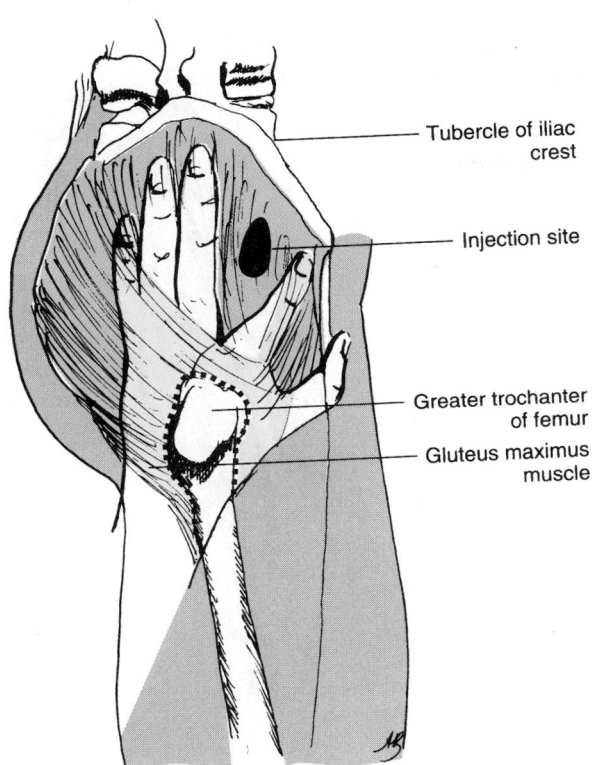

Tubercle of iliac crest

Injection site

Greater trochanter of femur

Gluteus maximus muscle

Ventrogluteal

1. Use this site if volume to be injected is 1–5 ml. Use 20–23 gauge, 1.25–2.5 inch needle. Needle should be long enough to reach the middle of the muscle.
2. Preferred site for adults, children >7 mos. Patient should be in supine lateral position.
3. Using 90° angle, flatten the skin area using the middle and index finger and inject between them.

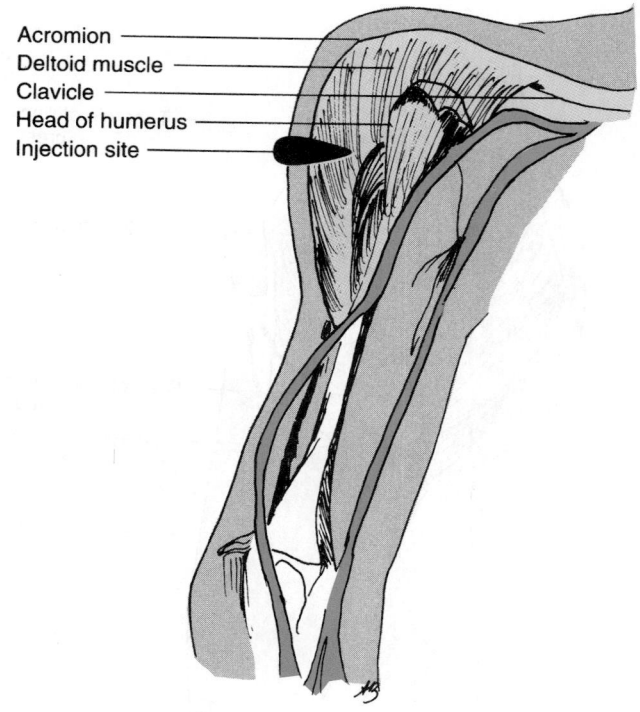

Acromion
Deltoid muscle
Clavicle
Head of humerus
Injection site

Deltoid

1. Use this site if volume to be injected is 0.5–1 ml. Use 23–25 gauge, $1/8$–$1/2$ inch needle. Needle should be long enough to reach the middle of the muscle.
2. Patient may be in prone, sitting, supine, or standing position.
3. Using 90° angle or angled slightly toward acromion, flatten the skin area using the thumb and index finger and inject between them.

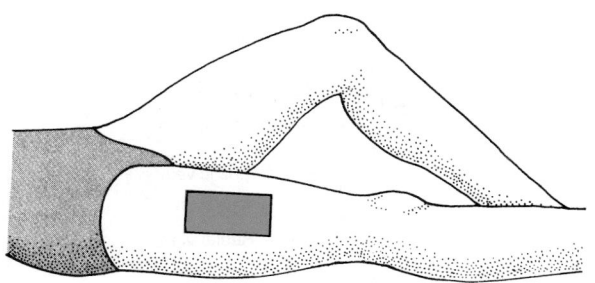

Anterolateral thigh

1. Anterolateral thigh is site of choice for infants and children <7 mos. Use 22–25 gauge, ⅝–1 in needle.
2. Patient may be in supine or sitting position. Using 90° angle, flatten the skin area using the thumb and index finger and inject between them.

Z-TRACK TECHNIQUE:

1. Draw up medication with one needle, and use new needle for injection *(minimizes skin staining)*.
2. Administer deep IM in upper outer quadrant of buttock only (dorsogluteal site).
3. Displace the skin lateral to the injection site before inserting the needle.
4. Withdraw the needle before releasing the skin.

IV:

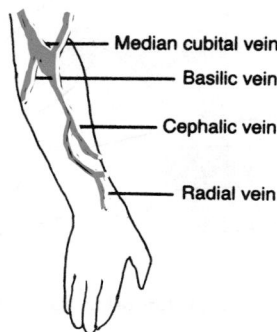

Median cubital vein
Basilic vein
Cephalic vein
Radial vein

1. Medication may be given as direct IV, intermittent (piggyback), or continuous infusion.
2. Ensure that medication is compatible with solution being infused (see IV compatibility chart in this drug handbook).
3. Do not use if precipitate is present or discoloration occurs.
4. Check IV site frequently for correct infusion rate, evidence of infiltration, extravasation.

Intravenous medications are administered by the following:

1. Continuous infusing solution.
2. Piggyback (intermittent infusion).
3. Volume control setup (medication contained in a chamber between the IV solution bag and the patient).
4. Bolus dose (a single dose of medication given through an infusion line or heparin lock). Sometimes this is referred to as an IV push.

Adding medication to a newly prescribed IV bag:

1. Remove the plastic cover from the IV bag.
2. Cleanse rubber port with an alcohol swab.
3. Insert the needle into the center of the rubber port.
4. Inject the medication.
5. Withdraw the syringe from the port.
6. Gently rotate the container to mix the solution.
7. Label the IV including the date, time, medication, and dosage. It should be placed so it is easily read when hanging.
8. Spike the IV tubing and prime the tubing.

Hanging an IV piggyback (IVPB):

1. When using the piggyback method, lower the primary bag at least 6 inches below the piggyback bag.
2. Set the pump as a secondary infusion when entering the rate of infusion and volume to be infused.
3. Most piggyback medications contain 50–100 cc and usually infuse in 20–60 minutes, although larger-volume bags will take longer.

Administering IV medications through a volume control setup (Buretrol):

1. Insert the spike of the volume control set (Buretrol, Soluset, Pediatrol) into the primary solution container.
2. Open the upper clamp on the volume control set and allow sufficient fluid into volume control chamber.
3. Fill the volume control device with 30 cc of fluid by opening the clamp between the primary solution and the volume control device.

Administering an IV bolus dose:

1. If an existing IV is infusing, stop the infusion by pinching the tubing above the port.
2. Insert the needle into the port and aspirate to observe for a blood return.
3. If the IV is infusing properly with no signs of infiltration or inflammation, it should be patent.
4. Blood indicates that the intravenous line is in the vein.
5. Inject the medication at the prescribed rate.
6. Remove the needle and regulate the IV as prescribed.

Hanging an IV Piggyback (PB)

1. When admixture of the medication is ordered, prepare the solution if the pharmacist plans to do so.
2. Set the secondary set to flow into the primary set at the rate of the main solution once the set flows.
3. Most medications come ready to hang as PB ... and should infuse in 30–60 minutes. All other solutions should be ... as appropriate.

Administering IV Medications through a Volume Control Using a Buretrol

1. Prepare medication in the volume control chamber the same as for the ...
2. Open the clamp on the ... chamber and permit the solution to administer to flow into the volume control chamber.
3. Fill the volume control chamber level to the ...

Administering an IV Bolus Dose

1. Prepare the medication in the syringe.
2. Select the injection port that is closest to the patient.
3. Inject the medication slowly ...
4. Rinse the administration ...
5. Inject the medication at the prescribed rate.

New Drug Supplement

anakinra

bosentan

desloratadine

dexmethylphenidate

dimethyl sulfoxide (DMSO)

drotrecogin alfa

ertapenem

fondaparinux sodium

frovatriptan

pimecrolimus

ursodiol (ursodeoxycholic acid)

valdecoxib

anakinra

ana-**kin**-rah
(Kineret)

▶CLASSIFICATION
PHARMACOTHERAPEUTIC:
Interleukin-1 receptor antagonist. ***CLINICAL:*** Anti-inflammatory. Immunomodulator

ACTION/*THERAPEUTIC EFFECT*
Blocks the binding of interleukin-1 (IL-1), a protein which is a major mediator of joint pathology that is present in excess in pts with rheumatoid arthritis, *inhibiting inflammatory response.*

USES/*UNLABELED*
Treatment of signs and symptoms of moderate to severe rheumatoid arthritis.

AVAILABILITY (Rx)
INJECTION: 100 mg/ml syringe.

INDICATIONS/ROUTES/DOSAGE
Rheumatoid arthritis:

SUBQ: **Adults >18 yrs, elderly:** 100 mg/day, given at same time each day.

SIDE EFFECTS
OCCASIONAL: Injection site reactions (redness, inflammation, ecchymosis). ***RARE:*** Headache, abdominal pain, flu-like symptoms.

bosentan

baws-en-tan
(Tracleer)

▶CLASSIFICATION
PHARMACOTHERAPEUTIC:
Amino acid peptide. ***CLINICAL:***
Vasodilator, neurohormonal blocker

ACTION/*THERAPEUTIC EFFECT*
Blocks the peptide endothelin, a potent vasoconstrictor, elevated in pts with pulmonary arterial hypertension, *acting as a vasodilator and neurohormonal blocker, improving overall left ventricular performance.*

USES/*UNLABELED*
Treatment of pulmonary arterial hypertension in pts with CHF, to improve exercise ability, decrease clinical worsening.

AVAILABILITY (Rx)
TABLETS: 62.5 mg, 125 mg.

INDICATIONS/ROUTES /DOSAGE
Pulmonary hypertension:

PO: **Adults, elderly:** 62.5 mg

twice daily. May be titrated up to 125 mg twice daily.

SIDE EFFECTS

OCCASIONAL: Headache, dizziness, blurred vision, flushing, hypotension, elevated liver enzymes. Effects can last up to 6 hrs.

desloratadine

des-low-**rah**-tah-deen
(Clarinex)

►CLASSIFICATION

PHARMACOTHERAPEUTIC: H₁ antagonist. ***CLINICAL:*** Non-sedating antihistamine

ACTION/THERAPEUTIC EFFECT

Exhibits selective peripheral histamine H_1 receptor blocking action. Competes with histamine at receptor site, *preventing allergic response mediated by histamine (rhinitis, urticaria)*. 2.5 to 4 times greater potency than its parent compound, loratadine.

USES

Relief of symptoms of rhinitis (sneezing, rhinorrhea, itching/tearing of eyes, stuffiness) and chronic idiopathic urticaria (hives).

AVAILABILITY (Rx)

TABLETS: 5 mg.

INDICATIONS/ROUTES /DOSAGE

Allergic rhinitis, hives:

PO: **Adults, elderly, children >12 yrs:** 5 mg once daily.

SIDE EFFECTS

FREQUENT (12%): Headache. ***OCCASIONAL*** (3%): Dry mouth, somnolence. ***RARE*** (3%): Fatigue, dizziness, diarrhea, nausea.

dexmethylphenidate

dex-meth-ill-**phen**-ih-date
(Focalin)

►CLASSIFICATION

PHARMACOTHERAPEUTIC: Piperidine derivative. ***CLINICAL:*** CNS stimulant

ACTION/THERAPEUTIC EFFECT

Blocks reuptake of norepinephrine and serotonin and increases release into synapse. *Decreases motor restlessness, enhances ability to pay attention.*

USES

Treatment of attention deficit/hyperactivity disorder (ADHD) in children.

AVAILABILITY (Rx)

TABLETS: 2.5 mg, 5 mg, 10 mg.

INDICATIONS/ROUTES /DOSAGE

Attention deficit/hyperactivity disorder (ADHD):

PO: **Adolescents, children 6–17 yrs:** Initially, 2.5 mg twice daily (5 mg/day). May increase in increments of 2.5–5 mg/day at weekly intervals to a maximum dose of 10 mg twice daily (20 mg/day).

SIDE EFFECTS

RARE (1%): Abdominal pain, fever, anorexia, nausea, twitching, insomnia, tachycardia.

dimethyl sulfoxide (DMSO)

die-**meth**-el sul-**fox**-eyd
(Rimso-50)

►CLASSIFICATION

PHARMACOTHERAPEUTIC: Interstitial cystitis agent. *CLINICAL:* Anti-inflammatory

ACTION

Produces anti-inflammatory, membrane penetration, antifungal activity, cryoprotective effects for living cells and tissue.

USES/*UNLABELED*

Treatment of interstitial cystitis. *Topical treatment of extravasation injury, musculoskeletal injuries, collagen diseases.*

AVAILABILITY (Rx)

SOLUTION: 50% aqueous solution in 50 ml bottle.

INDICATIONS/ROUTES /DOSAGE

Interstitial cystitis:

INSTILLATION: Instill 50 ml directly into bladder by catheter and allow to remain for 15 min. Repeat every 2 wks until therapeutic relief is obtained.

Extravasation:

TOPICAL: **Adults, elderly:** Apply to affected area of extravasation every 4 hrs for 10 days.

SIDE EFFECTS

RARE: Hypersensitivity reaction with topical application.

drotrecogin alfa

dro-trae-**coe**-gin alfa
(Xigris)

►CLASSIFICATION

PHARMACOTHERAPEUTIC: Activated protein C. *CLINICAL:* Antisepsis

ACTION/*THERAPEUTIC EFFECT*

Activates coagulation system, provides protection against thrombosis, *decreasing fibrin/clot formation. Enhances action of tissue plasminogen, producing fibrinolysis. Exhibits profibrinolytic, antirhrombotic, anti-iflammatory activities.*

USES

Treatment of severe sepsis or septic shock with evidence of organ dysfunction.

AVAILABILITY (Rx)

IV. INFUSION: 5 mg, 20 mg vials.

INDICATIONS/ROUTES/DOSAGE

Severe sepsis:

IV INFUSION: **Adults, elderly:** 24 mcg/kg/hr given at a constant rate for 4 days.

SIDE EFFECTS

RARE: Bleeding (intrathoracic, retroperitoneal, genitourinary, gastrointestinal, intra-abdominal).

ertapenem

er-tah-**pen**-em
(Ivanz)

►CLASSIFICATION

PHARMACOTHERAPEUTIC: Carbapenem. *CLINICAL:* Antibiotic

ACTION/*THERAPEUTIC EFFECT*

Inhibits cell wall synthesis, *producing bacterial cell death.*

USES

Treatment of intra-abdominal, skin and skin structure infections, community-acquired pneumonia, complicated urinary tract infection, acute pelvic infection.

AVAILABILITY (Rx)
LYOPHILIZED POWDER: 1 g vial.

ADMINISTRATION
• Dilute each 1 g vial in 50 ml 0.9 NaCl and infuse over 30 min.

INDICATIONS/ROUTES /DOSAGE
Infection:
IM: Adults, elderly: 1 g once daily for up to 7 days.
IV: Adults, elderly: 1 g once daily for up to 14 days.
IM/IV: Adults, elderly with creatinine clearance <30 ml/min: 500 mg daily.

SIDE EFFECTS

OCCASIONAL: Diarrhea, nausea, headache, vaginitis, phlebitis/thrombophlebitis, vomiting.

fondaparinux sodium

fond-dah-**pear**-in-ux
(Arixtra)

▶CLASSIFICATION
PHARMACOTHERAPEUTIC: Factor Xa inhibitor, pentasaccharide. **CLINICAL:** Antithrombotic

ACTION/*THERAPEUTIC EFFECT*
Binds exclusively to antithrombin III, increasing antifactor Xa of antithrombin, resulting in *reduction in thrombin and thrombus development without inhibiting thrombin itself. No effect on APTT, PT, bleeding time.*

USES
Prevention of venous thromboembolism.in orthopedic surgery pts.

AVAILABILITY (Rx)
INJECTION: 2.5 mg/0.5 ml.

INDICATIONS/ROUTES /DOSAGE
Prevention of venous thromboembolism:
SubQ: Adults, elderly: 2.5 mg once daily for 5–9 days postop.

SIDE EFFECTS
RARE: Minor bleeding.

frovatriptan

fro-vah-**trip**-tan
(Frova)

▶CLASSIFICATION
PHARMACOTHERAPEUTIC: Serotonin receptor agonist. **CLINICAL:** Antimigraine (see p. 53C)

ACTION/*THERAPEUTIC EFFECT*
Binds selectively to vascular receptors (serotonin), exhibiting a vasoconstrictive effect on cranial blood vessels, *producing relief of migraine headache.*

USES
In adults, treatment of acute migraine attack with or without aura.

AVAILABILITY (Rx)
TABLETS: 2.5 mg.

INDICATIONS/ROUTES /DOSAGE
Migraine:
PO: Adults: 2.5 mg at onset of migraine. May repeat in 2 hrs. **Maximum:** 7.5 mg/day.

SIDE EFFECTS
OCCASIONAL (8%): Fatigue, headache, flushing, paresthesia.

pimecrolimus

pim-eh-**crow**-leh-mus
(Elidel)

▶CLASSIFICATION
CLINICAL: Anti-inflammatory

ACTION/*THERAPEUTIC EFFECT*
Inhibits release of cytokine, an enzyme that produces an inflammatory reaction (i.e., redness itching), *inducing anti-inflammatory activity.* (May also inhibit T-lymphocyte activation.)

USES
Treatment of atopic dermatitis (eczema).

AVAILABILITY (Rx)
TOPICAL: 1% cream.

INDICATIONS/ROUTES /DOSAGE
Atopic dermatitis (eczema):
TOPICAL: Adults, elderly, adolescents, children 2–17 yrs: Apply to affected area twice daily for up to 3 wks (up to 6 wks in adolescents, children 2–17 yrs).

SIDE EFFECTS
RARE: Application site burning.

ursodiol
(ursodeoxycholic acid)

er-**sew**-dee-ol
(Actigall)

▶CLASSIFICATION
CLINICAL: Gallstone-solubilizing agent

ACTION/*THERAPEUTIC EFFECT*
Suppresses hepatic synthesis, secretion of cholesterol, inhibiting intestinal absorption of cholesterol. *Changes bile in pts with gallstones from cholesterol precipitating (capable of forming crystals) to cholesterol solubilizing (capable of being dissolved).*

USES/*UNLABELED*
Dissolution of radiolucent, noncalcified gallstones when cholecystectomy is an unacceptable method of treatment. Treatment of biliary cirrhosis. Prevention of gallstones. *Treatment of biliary atresia, sclerosing cholangitis, alcoholic cirrhosis, chronic hepatitis; prophylaxis of liver transplant rejection, gallstone formation.*

AVAILABILITY (Rx)
CAPSULES: 300 mg

INDICATIONS/ROUTES /DOSAGE
Usual dosage:
PO: Adults, elderly: 8–10 mg/kg/day in 2–3 divided doses. Treatment may require mos of therapy.

Prevention of gallstones:
PO: Adults, elderly: 300 mg 2 times/day.

SIDE EFFECTS
FREQUENT: Abdominal pain/discomfort (50%), nausea (32%), vomiting (20%), diarrhea (19%). **OCCASIONAL** (3–6%): Fever, anorexia. **RARE** (<2%): Indigestion, loose stool, fatigue, headache.

valdecoxib

val-deh-**cox**-ib
(Bextra)

✣ - Canadian trade name   ✳ - see also www.wbsaunders.com/SIMON/SaundersNDH

▶CLASSIFICATION

PHARMACOTHERAPEUTIC: NSAID. ***CLINICAL:*** Anti-inflammatory, analgesic (see p. 107C)

ACTION/*THERAPEUTIC EFFECT*

Produces analgesic and anti-inflammatory effect by inhibiting prostaglandin synthesis, *reducing inflammatory response and intensity of pain stimulus reaching sensory nerve endings.*

USES/*UNLABELED*

Treatment of arthritis, osteoarthritis, and primary dysmenorrhea.

AVAILABILITY (Rx)

TABLETS: 10 mg, 20 mg.

INDICATIONS/ROUTES /DOSAGE

Osteoarthritis, rheumatoid arthritis:

PO: **Adults, elderly:** 10 mg/day with or without food.

Primary dysmenorrhea:

PO: **Adults, elderly:** 20 mg twice daily.

SIDE EFFECTS

RARE (>2%): Dyspepsia (heartburn, epigastric pain, indigestion), nausea, diarrhea, headache, dizziness, sinusitis, peripheral edema.

GENERAL INDEX

Generic names appear in lower case boldface type. U.S. and Canadian trade names are in regular type. Classifications are in lower case italics. The bold page number is the page number of the main drug entry.

---

bold - generic name   regular type - trade name

---

italics - classification name   **bold page #** - main drug entry

bold - generic name

regular type - trade name

---

bold - generic name   regular type - trade name

italics - classification name   **bold page #** - main drug entry

---

italics - classification name   **bold page #** - main drug entry

italics - classification name   **bold page #** - main drug entry

---

Generic names appear first followed by brand names in parentheses.

Antimigraine agents

Anti-Parkinson agents

Antipsychotic agents

Antipyretic agents

Antiretroviral agents

Lisinopril (Prinivil, Zestril), 668
Losartan (Cozaar), 683
Metoprolol (Lopressor), 736
Milrinone (Primacor), 748
Moexipril (Univasc), 760
Nitroglycerin, 815
Nitroprusside (Nipride), 818
Quinapril (Accupril), 954
Ramipril (Altace), 963

Constipation
Bisacodyl (Dulcolax), 126
Cascara sagrada, 179
Docusate (Colace), 370
Lactulose (Kristalose), 638
Methylcellulose (Citrucel), 723
Milk of magnesia (MOM), 689
Psyllium (Metamucil), 946
Senna (Senokot), 1006

Corticosteroids, inhalant
Beclomethasone (Beclovent, Vanceril), 109
Budesonide (Pulmicort), 142
Flunisolide (AeroBid), 470
Fluticasone (Flovent), 484
Triamcinolone (Azmacort), 1121

Corticosteroids, intranasal
Beclomethasone (Beconase, Vancenase), 109
Budesonide (Rhinocort), 142
Flunisolide (Nasalide), 470
Fluticasone (Flonase), 484
Triamcinolone (Nasacort), 1121

Corticosteroids, systemic
Beclomethasone (Beclovent, Vanceril), 109
Betamethasone (Celestone), 118
Budesonide (Pulmicort, Rhinocort), 142
Cortisone (Cortone), 280
Dexamethasone (Decadron), 324
Fludrocortisone (Florinef), 466
Flunisolide (Aerobid, Nasalide), 470
Fluocinolone (Synalar), 472
Fluocinonide (Lidex), 472
Fluticasone (Flovent), 484

Hydrocortisone (Solu Cortef), 554
Methylprednisolone (Solu Medrol), 728
Prednisolone (Prelone), 916
Prednisone (Deltasone), 918
Triamcinolone (Kenalog), 1121

Crohn's disease
Cyclosporine (Neoral), 293
Hydrocortisone (Cortenema), 554
Infliximab (Remicade), 588
Mesalamine (Asacol, Pentasa), 709
Olsalazine (Dipentum), 835
Sulfasalazine (Azulfidine), 1040

Deep vein thrombosis (DVT)
Dalteparin (Fragmin), 304
Danaparoid (Organan), 305
Enoxaparin (Lovenox), 397
Heparin, 543
Tinzaparin (InnoHep), 1088
Warfarin (Coumadin), 1168

Depression
Amitriptyline (Elavil, Endep), 52
Bupropion (Wellbutrin), 146
Citalopram (Celexa), 248
Clomipramine (Anafranil), 259
Desipramine (Norpramin), 320
Doxepin (Sinequan), 381
Fluoxetine (Prozac), 475
Imipramine (Tofranil), 579
Maprotiline (Ludiomil), 694
Mirtazapine (Remeron), 753
Nefazodone (Serzone), 794
Nortriptyline (Aventyl, Pamelor), 825
Paroxetine (Paxil), 860
Phenelzine (Nardil), 880
Sertraline (Zoloft), 1007
Tranylcypromine (Parnate), 1114
Trazodone (Desyrel), 1117
Venlafaxine (Effexor), 1149

Diabetes mellitus
Acarbose (Precose), 4
Chlorpropamide (Diabinese), 233
Glimepiride (Amaryl), 523
Glipizide (Glucotrol), 524
Glyburide (Micronase), 529
Insulin, 590

Metformin (Glucophage), 714
Miglitol (Glyset), 747
Pioglitazone (Actos), 897
Repaglinide (Prandin), 967
Rosiglitazone (Avandia), 994
Tolazamide (Tolinase), 1097
Tolbutamide (Orinase), 1099

Diarrhea

Bismuth subsalicylate (Pepto-Bismol), 127
Diphenoxylate and atropine (Lomotil), 358
Kaolin-pectin (Kaopectate), 626
Loperamide (Imodium), 675
Octreotide (Sandostatin), 828

Diuretics, loop

Bumetanide (Bumex), 144
Ethacrynic acid (Edecrin), 429
Furosemide (Lasix), 499
Torsemide (Demadex), 1108

Diuretics, potassium sparing

Amiloride (Midamor), 44
Spironolactone (Aldactone), 1028
Triamterene (Dyrenium), 1124

Diuretics, thiazide

Hydrochlorothiazide (HydroDiuril), 550

Duodenal/gastric ulcer

Bismuth subsalicylate (Pepto-Bismol), 127
Cimetidine (Tagamet), 241
Esomeprazole (Nexium), 419
Famotidine (Pepcid), 442
Lansoprazole (Prevacid), 644
Misoprostol (Cytotec), 754
Nizatidine (Axid), 819
Omeprazole (Prilosec), 836
Pantoprazole (Protonix), 858
Rabeprazole (Aciphex), 961
Ranitidine (Zantac), 965
Sucralfate (Carafate), 1038

Edema

Amiloride (Midamor), 44
Bumetanide (Bumex), 144

Chlorthalidone (Hygroton), 233
Ethacrynic acid (Edecrin), 429
Furosemide (Lasix), 499
Hydrochlorothiazide (HydroDiuril), 550
Indapamide (Lozol), 583
Metolazone (Zaroxolyn), 734
Spironolactone (Aldactone), 1028
Torsemide (Demadex), 1108
Triamterine (Dyrenium), 1124

Epilepsy

Acetazolamide (Diamox), 9
Carbamazepine (Tegretol), 167
Clonazepam (Klonopin), 260
Clorazepate (Tranxene), 265
Diazepam (Valium), 334
Gabapentin (Neurontin), 502
Lamotrigine (Lamictal), 642
Levetiracetam (Keppra), 655
Lorazepam (Ativan), 681
Fosphenytoin (Cerebyx), 497
Oxcarbazepine (Trileptal), 846
Phenobarbital, 881
Phenytoin (Dilantin), 889
Primidone (Mysoline), 920
Tiagabine (Gabitril), 1081
Topiramate (Topamax), 1103
Valproic acid (Depakene, Depakote), 1140
Zonisamide (Zonegran), 1186

Esophageal reflux, esophagitis

Cimetidine (Tagamet), 241
Esomeprazole (Nexium), 419
Famotidine (Pepcid), 442
Lansoprazole (Prevacid), 644
Nizatidine (Axid), 819
Omeprazole (Prilosec), 836
Pantoprazole (Protonix), 858
Rabeprazole (Aciphex), 961
Ranitidine (Zantac), 965

Fluoroquinolones

Ciprofloxacin (Cipro), 243
Enoxacin (Penetrex), 397
Gatifloxacin (Tequin), 509
Levofloxacin (Levaquin), 656
Lomefloxacin (Maxaquin), 672
Moxifloxacin (Avelox), 767

Prochlorperazine (Compazine), 928

Promethazine (Phenergan), 932

Trimethobenzamide (Tigan), 1130

Non-nucleoside reverse transcriptase inhibitors (NNRTI)

Delavirdine (Rescriptor), 316

Efavirenz (Sustiva), 392

Nevirapine (Viramune), 802

Nonsteroidal anti-inflammatory drugs (NSAIDs)

Diclofenac (Cataflam, Voltaren), 338

Etolodac (Lodine), 433

Flurbiprofen (Ansaid), 481

Ibuprofen (Advil, Motrin), 567

Indomethacin (Indocin), 586

Ketorolac (Toradol), 653

Naproxen (Anaprox, Naprosyn), 788

Piroxicam (Feldene), 900

Sulindac (Clinoril), 1042

Nucleoside analog reverse transcriptase inhibitors (NRTI)

Abacavir (Ziagen), 1

Didanosine (Videx), 342

Lamivudine (Epivir), 640

Stavudine (Zerit), 1030

Zalcitabine (Hivid), 1173

Zidovudine (Retrovir), 1177

Obsessive compulsive disorder

Citalopram (Celexa), 248

Clomipramine (Anafranil), 259

Fluoxetine (Prozac), 475

Fluvoxamine (Luvox), 488

Sertraline (Zoloft), 1007

Venlafaxine (Effexor), 1149

Osteoporosis

Alendronate (Fosamax), 24

Calcitonin (Miacalcin), 155

Calcium salts, 157

Dihydrotachysterol, 1163

Estradiol (Estrace), 422

Conjugated estrogens (Premarin), 276

Estropipate (Ogen), 426

Etidronate (Didronel), 432

Pamidronate (Aredia), 856

Raloxifene (Evista), 962

Risedronate (Actonel), 981

Tiludronate (Skelid), 1085

Vitamin D, 1163

Paget's disease

Alendronate (Fosamax), 24

Calcitonin (Miacalcin), 155

Etidronate (Didronel), 432

Pamidronate (Aredia), 856

Risedronate (Actonel), 981

Tiludronate (Skelid), 1085

Pain, mild to moderate

Acetaminophen (Tylenol), 7

Aspirin, 83

Celecoxib (Celebrex), 216

Codeine, 271

Diclofenac (Cataflam, Voltaren), 338

Diflunisal (Dolobid), 346

Etodolac (Lodine), 433

Fenoprofen (Nalfon), 448

Flurbiprofen (Ansaid), 481

Ibuprofen (Advil, Motrin), 567

Ketorolac (Toradol), 633

Naproxen (Anaprox, Naprosyn), 788

Propoxyphene (Darvon), 938

Salsalate (Disalcid), 997

Tramadol (Ultram), 1110

Pain, moderate to severe

Alendronate (Fosamax), 24

Butorphanol (Stadol), 151

Etidronate (Didronel), 432

Fentanyl (Sublimaze), 450

Hydromorphone (Dilaudid), 557

Meperidine (Demerol), 704

Methadone (Dolophine), 717

Morphine (MS Contin), 764

Nalbuphine (Nubain), 780

Oxycodone (OxyFast, Roxicodone), 849

Risedronate (Actonel), 981

Tiludronate (Skelid), 1085

Panic attack disorder
Alprazolam (Xanax), 31
Paroxetine (Paxil), 860
Sertraline (Zoloft), 1007

Parkinsonism
Amantadine (Symmetrel), 38
Bromocriptine (Parlodel), 140
Carbidopa/levodopa (Sinemet), 169
Diphenhydramine (Benadryl), 356
Entacapone (Comtan), 399
Pergolide (Permax), 877
Pramipexole (Mirapex), 911
Ropinirole (ReQuip), 993
Selegline (Eldepryl), 1004
Tolcapone (Tasmar), 1099

Penicillins
Amoxicillin (Polymox), 56
Amoxicillin/clavulanic acid
    (Augmentin), 58
Ampicillin (Polycillin), 63
Ampicillin/sulbactam (Unasyn), 65
Cloxacillin (Tegopen), 268
Dicloxacillin (Pathocil), 340
Nafcillin (Unipen), 778
Penicillin G (Pfizerpen), 867
Penicillin V (Pen Vee K, V Cillin K),
    870
Piperacillin/tazobactam (Zosyn),
    898
Ticarcillin/clavulanate (Timentin),
    1082

Peptic ulcer
Bismuth subsalicylate
    (Pepto-Bismol), 127
Cimetidine (Tagamet), 241
Esomeprazole (Nexium), 419
Famotidine (Pepcid), 442
Lansoprazole (Prevacid), 644
Misoprostol (Cytotec), 754
Nizatidine (Axid), 819
Omeprazole (Prilosec), 836
Pantoprazole (Protonix), 858
Rabeprazole (Aciphex), 961
Ranitidine (Zantac), 965
Sucralfate (Carafate), 1038

Pneumonia
Amoxicillin/clavulanate
    (Augmentin), 58
Ampicillin (Polycillin), 63
Azithromycin (Zithromax), 98
Cefaclor (Ceclor), 181
Cefpodoxime (Vantin), 202
Ceftriaxone (Rocephin), 211
Cefuroxime (Kefurox, Zinacef),
    213
Clarithromycin (Biaxin), 253
Co-trimoxazole (Bactrim, Septra),
    283
Dirithromycin (Dynabac), 360
Erythromycin, 415
Gentamicin (Garamycin), 516
Loracarbef (Lorabid), 678
Piperacillin/tazobactam (Zosyn),
    898
Tobramycin (Nebcin), 1093
Vancomycin (Vancocin), 1145

**Pneumonia, *pneumocystis
    carinii***
Atovaquone (Mepron), 90
Clindamycin (Cleocin), 256
Co-trimoxazole (Bactrim, Septra),
    283
Eflornithine (Vaniqa), 393
Pentamidine (Pentam), 871
Trimethoprim (Proloprim), 1131
Trimetrexate (Neutrexin), 1133

Prostatic hyperplasia, benign
Doxazosin (Cardura), 380
Finasteride (Proscar), 458
Leuprolide (Lupron), 651
Prazosin (Minipress), 915
Tamsulosin (Flomax), 1051
Terazosin (Hytrin), 1062

Protease inhibitors
Amprenavir (Agenerase), 67
Indinavir (Crixivan), 584
Lopinavir/ritonavir (Kaletra), 677
Nelfinavir (Viracept), 796
Ritonavir (Norvir), 985
Saquinavir (Fortovase, Invirase),
    999
Tenofovir (Viread), 1061

Levalbuterol (Xopenex), 653
Metaproterenol (Alupent), 713
Norepinephrine (Levophed), 821
Phenylephrine (Neo-Synephrine), 886
Pseudoephedrine (Sudafed), 945
Terbutaline (Brethine), 1064

Thrombosis
Dalteparin (Fragmin), 304
Danaparoid (Orgaran), 305
Enoxaparin (Lovenox), 397
Heparin, 543
Tinzaparin (InnoHep), 1088
Warfarin (Coumadin), 1168

Thyroid
Levothyroxine (Levoxyl, Synthroid), 660
Liothyronine (Cytomel), 666
Thyroid, 1080

Transient ischemic attack
Aspirin, 83
Clopidogrel (Plavix), 264
Ticlopidine (Ticlid), 1084
Warfarin (Coumadin), 1168

Tremor
Atenolol (Tenormin), 86
Chlordiazepoxide (Librium), 227
Diazepam (Valium), 334
Metoprolol (Lopressor), 736
Nadolol (Corgard), 775
Propranolol (Inderal), 940

Tuberculosis
Ethambutol (Myambutol), 430
Isoniazid (INH), 616
Pyrazinamide, 948
Rifabutin (Mycobutin), 975
Rifampin (Rifadin), 977
Rifapentine (Priftin), 979
Streptomycin, 1036

Uric-acid lowering agents
Allopurinol (Zyloprim), 26
Colchicine, 272

Probenecid (Benemid), 922

Urticaria
Cetirizine (Zyrtec), 219
Cimetidine (Tagamet), 241
Clemastine (Tavist), 254
Cyproheptadine (Periactin), 295
Diphenhydramine (Benadryl), 356
Hydroxyzine (Atarax, Vistaril), 563
Loratadine (Claritin), 680
Ranitidine (Zantac), 961

Vertigo
Dimenhydrinate (Dramamine), 354
Diphenhydramine (Benadryl), 356
Meclizine (Antivert), 696
Scopolamine (Trans-Derm Scop), 1003

Vomiting
Chlorpromazine (Thorazine), 231
Dexamethasone (Decadron), 324
Dimenhydrinate (Dramamine), 354
Dolasetron (Anzemet), 372
Dronabinol (Marinol), 388
Droperidol (Inapsine), 389
Granisetron (Kytril), 536
Hydroxyzine (Vistaril), 563
Lorazepam (Ativan), 681
Meclizine (Antivert), 696
Metoclopramide (Reglan), 732
Ondansetron (Zofran), 838
Prochlorperazine (Compazine), 928
Promethazine (Phenergan), 932
Trimethobenzamide (Tigan), 1130

Zollinger-Ellison syndrome
Aluminum salts, 37
Cimetidine (Tagamet), 241
Famotidine (Pepcid), 442
Lansoprazole (Prevacid), 644
Omeprazole (Prilosec), 836
Rabeprazole (Aciphex), 961
Ranitidine (Zantac), 965

SAUNDERS NURSING DRUG HANDBOOK CD-ROM

Welcome to the **Saunders Nursing Drug Handbook CD-ROM**. This software presents over 30 of the most commonly used drugs in a database that resembles the **Saunders Electronic Nursing Drug Cards**. You can view the drug information on screen and print out drug cards in black and white or full color. These portable drug cards can fit in any size pocket! Just one more way to help you keep up with the faster pace of life.

Saunders

An Imprint of Elsevier Science

System Requirements

WINDOWS

Windows 95 or later, 32 Mb RAM, 8 Mb free disk space

CD-ROM drive

SVGA (600 × 800) video minimum 1024 × 768 recommended

MacOS

MacOS 7.55 or later, PowerPC, 24 Mb free RAM recommended, 8 Mb free disk space

CD-ROM drive

600 × 800 or higher video resolution

Software Support

For technical support, call 1 800 692-9010

Monday–Friday. 9 A.M.–5 P.M. central time.

Fax 1 314 579-3316

E-mail: technical.support@harcourt.com

This program has been produced for Windows 95 and later and Mac OS 7.55 or later, single users only.

Brief instructions

This CD will work only when placed into tray-loaded CD-ROM drives. If your computer is set to autorun, just load the CD into the drive. The CD will do the rest!

WINDOWS

* If autorun has been disabled and you have Acrobat Reader 4 installed, open My Computer or use Windows Explorer to access the CD drive. Double-click splash.pdf to start the CD.
* If you do not have Acrobat Reader 4, either open My Computer or use Windows Explorer to navigate as follows on the CD drive: Open the folder Acrors405. Then open the subfolder titled Reader. Double-click on the file Acrord32. When Acrobat Reader opens, use the File menu to open the file splash.pdf on the CD-ROM drive. Then follow the on-screen instructions.

MacOS

* Click on the CD icon located on your desktop. Double-click on "Click Here to Start".

PRODUCT LICENSE AGREEMENT AND WARRANTY
INDIVIDUAL USER

This product is protected by United States Copyright law. Please read the following agreement carefully. It is assumed that by breaking the seal on this software package you have read, understood, and agreed to the product license agreement stated below.

1. Product License. Saunders, Inc. grants the original purchaser the nonexclusive right to use this software and the information contained in it for personal use only. The license for the individual version grants the right for one person to use this software on one computer.

This license does not represent a sale and this software may not be rented or leased.

Use of this product at more than one location by more than one user is specifically prohibited, as is downloading or transmitting this software electronically from one computer to another.

The copyrighted contents of this software may not be reproduced without the accompanying copyright notices. Republication or resale of these contents is specifically prohibited.

2. Limited Warranty. Saunders, Inc. warrantees to the original purchaser that this software is free of defects in materials and of faulty workmanship under normal use for 90 days from the date of purchase. If this physical media is believed to be defective during that period, please notify Saunders, Inc. at the address and/or number below. If Saunders, Inc. determines that there has been a defect in the physical disc/disk or faulty workmanship, the software will be replaced without charge. Return of the disc/disk without authorization by Saunders, Inc. may delay or nullify replacement.

Otherwise, Saunders, Inc. and its licensors disclaim all other warranties, express or implied, including but not limited to any implied warranty of merchantability or fitness for a particular purpose.

Saunders, Inc. and its licensors specifically disclaim any warrant, guarantee, or representation as to the correctness, accuracy, reliability, or timeliness of the contents of the disc/disk or to its use. You as the user assume the entire risk and no information or help provided by Saunders, Inc., its employees, its licensors, agents, distributors, or others associated with the development, production, manufacturing, and distribution shall be considered to create any warranty or liability on behalf of Saunders, Inc.

The only liability and remedy available under this limited warranty are limited solely to replacement of the defective disk/disc and shall not include or extend to any claim for or right to recover any other damages. If any competent jurisdiction determines that the above warranty disclaimer is invalid in any way, then the purchaser and Saunders, Inc. agree that the maximum amount of damage of any kind recoverable shall not exceed the purchase price of the software, as determined by a bill of sale or any other proof of purchase price that must be provided by the purchaser. The remedies available to you against the publisher under the agreement are exclusive.

DRUG COMPATIBILITY IN SAME SYRINGE

Atropine sulfate

C = Compatible
I = Incompatible
Blank = Undocumented

C	Benadryl (diphenhydramine)											
C	C	Compazine (prochlorperazine)										
C	C	C	Demerol (meperidine)									
C	C	C	I	Morphine								
C	C	C			Nubain (nalbuphine)							
C	C	C	C	C	C	Phenergan (promethazine)						
C	C	C		C	C		C	Reglan (metoclopramide)				
C	C	C	C	C	C	C	C		Robinul (glycopyrrolate)			
C	C	C	C	C	C	C			C	Stadol (butorphanol)		
C	C	C	C	C		C		I	C		Talwin (pentazocine)	
C	C	C	C	C			C	I	C	C	C	Thorazine (chlorpromazine)
C	C	I	C	C	C	C	C	C	C		C	Versed (midazolam)
C	C	C	C	C	C	C	C	C	C	C	C	C	Vistaril (hydroxyzine)

Note: Diazepam, barbiturates are incompatible with many medications; consult specialized references.

TABLE OF COMMONLY USED EQUIVALENT VALUES

METRIC WEIGHT/VOLUME

1 kg = 1,000 Gm
1 Gm = 1,000 mg
1 mg = 1,000 mcg
1 mcg = 0.001 mg
1 Liter = 1,000 ml

WEIGHTS

1 oz = 30 Gm
1 Gm = 15 Grains
1 Grain = 60 mg
0.6 mg = 1/100 Grain
0.4 mg = 1/150 Grain
0.3 mg = 1/200 Grain
1 Kg = 2.2 lbs

VOLUME

1 quart = 960 ml
4 fl oz = 120 ml
1 fl oz = 30 ml
1 tsp = 5 ml (approximately)
1 tbs = 15 ml (approximately)
2 tbs = 30 ml (approximately)